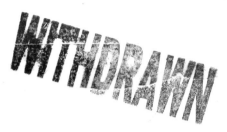
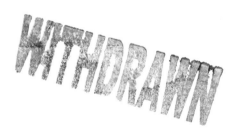
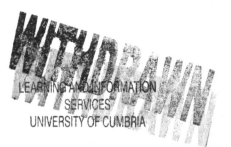

ASSESSMENT OF CHILDHOOD DISORDERS

Assessment of Childhood Disorders

FOURTH EDITION

Edited by
Eric J. Mash
Russell A. Barkley

THE GUILFORD PRESS
New York   London

Library of Congress Cataloging-in-Publication Data

Assessment of childhood disorders / edited by Eric J. Mash, Russell A. Barkley.—4th ed.
  p. ; cm.
  Includes bibliographical references and index.
  ISBN-10: 1-59385-493-5   ISBN-13: 978-1-59385-493-5 (hardcover: alk. paper)
  1. Child psychopathology—Diagnosis.   2. Adolescent psychopathology—
Diagnosis.   3. Psychodiagnostics.   I. Mash, Eric J.   II. Barkley, Russell A., 1949–
  [DNLM: 1. Child Behavior Disorders—diagnosis.   2. Adolescent.   3. Developmental
Disabilities—diagnosis.   4. Mental Disorders—diagnosis. WS 350.6 A845 2007]
  RJ503.5.B43 2007
  618.92′89075—dc22

                                                                    2007006529

In memory of Ronald F. Barkley (1949–2006)

About the Editors

Eric J. Mash, PhD, is Professor of Psychology in the Department of Psychology and Program in Clinical Psychology at the University of Calgary. He is a fellow of the American and Canadian Psychological Associations; has served as an editor, editorial board member, and editorial consultant for many scientific and professional journals; and has written or edited numerous books and journal articles related to children's mental health, child and adolescent psychopathology, child and adolescent psychotherapy, and child and family assessment. Dr. Mash's research has focused on family relationships across a variety of child and family disorders, including attention-deficit/hyperactivity disorder (ADHD), conduct problems, internalizing disorders, and maltreatment. He is a recipient of the Leadership Education in Neurodevelopmental Disabilities Distinguished Alumnus Award from the Oregon Health & Science University.

Russell A. Barkley, PhD, is Research Professor of Psychiatry at the State University of New York Upstate Medical University at Syracuse and Clinical Professor of Psychiatry at the Medical University of South Carolina. He is a Diplomate in three specialties: Clinical Psychology (ABPP), Clinical Child and Adolescent Psychology, and Clinical Neuropsychology (ABCN, ABPP). Dr. Barkley is a clinical scientist, educator, and practitioner who has authored, coauthored, or coedited 20 books and clinical manuals and published more than 200 scientific articles and book chapters related to the nature, assessment, and treatment of ADHD and related disorders. He is the editor of the bimonthly clinical newsletter *The ADHD Report*. Dr. Barkley has presented more than 600 invited addresses internationally and appeared on many nationally televised programs on behalf of children and adults with ADHD. He has received several awards from the American Psychological Association for his contributions to research on ADHD, to clinical practice, and to the dissemination of science.

Contributors

Russell A. Barkley, PhD, Department of Psychiatry, State University of New York Upstate Medical University at Syracuse, Syracuse, New York; Department of Psychiatry, Medical University of South Carolina, Charleston, South Carolina

Andria Botzet, MA, Department of Psychiatry, University of Minnesota, Minneapolis, Minnesota

Bruce F. Chorpita, PhD, Department of Psychology, University of Hawai'i at Manoa, Honolulu, Hawaii

Jill S. Compton, PhD, Department of Psychiatry and Behavioral Sciences, Duke University School of Medicine, Durham, North Carolina

Claire V. Crooks, PhD, Centre for Addiction and Mental Health and University of Western Ontario Centre for Research and Education on Violence Against Women and Children, London, Ontario, Canada

Tamara Fahnhorst, MPH, Department of Psychiatry, University of Minnesota, Minneapolis, Minnesota

Kenneth E. Fletcher, PhD, Department of Psychiatry, University of Massachusetts Medical School, Worcester, Massachusetts

Paul J. Frick, PhD, Department of Psychology, University of New Orleans, New Orleans, Louisiana

David B. Goldston, PhD, Department of Psychiatry and Behavioral Sciences, Duke University School of Medicine, Durham, North Carolina

Beth L. Goodlin-Jones, PhD, MIND Institute, Department of Psychiatry and Behavioral Sciences, University of California, Davis, California

Benjamin L. Handen, PhD, Departments of Psychiatry and Pediatrics, University of Pittsburgh School of Medicine, and Western Psychiatric Institute and Clinic, Pittsburgh, Pennsylvania

Sara J. Hines, PhD, Department of Special Education, University of Maryland, College Park, Maryland

John Hunsley, PhD, School of Psychology, University of Ottawa, Ottawa, Ontario, Canada

Sharon F. Lambert, PhD, Department of Psychology, George Washington University, Washington, DC

Eric J. Mash, PhD, Department of Psychology, University of Calgary, Calgary, Alberta, Canada

Jon M. McClellan, MD, Division of Child and Adolescent Psychiatry, Department of Psychiatry and Behavioral Sciences, University of Washington, Seattle, Washington

Michael G. McDonell, PhD, Division of Child and Adolescent Psychiatry, Department of Psychiatry and Behavioral Sciences, University of Washington, Seattle, Washington

Robert J. McMahon, PhD, Department of Psychology, University of Washington, Seattle, Washington

Sally Ozonoff, PhD, MIND Institute, Department of Psychiatry and Behavioral Sciences, University of California, Davis, California

Carol B. Peterson, PhD, Department of Psychiatry, University of Minnesota, Minneapolis, Minnesota

Karen D. Rudolph, PhD, Department of Psychology, University of Illinois at Urbana–Champaign, Champaign, Illinois

Cheri J. Shapiro, PhD, Department of Psychology, University of South Carolina, Columbia, South Carolina

Rebecca L. Shiner, PhD, Department of Psychology, Colgate University, Hamilton, New York

Bradley H. Smith, PhD, Department of Psychology, University of South Carolina, Columbia, South Carolina

Marjorie Solomon, PhD, MIND Institute, Department of Psychiatry and Behavioral Sciences, University of California, Davis, California

Michael A. Southam-Gerow, PhD, Department of Psychology, Virginia Commonwealth University, Richmond, Virginia

Deborah L. Speece, PhD, Department of Special Education, University of Maryland, College Park, Maryland

Eric Stice, PhD, Department of Psychology, University of Texas at Austin, Austin, Texas; Oregon Research Institute, Eugene, Oregon

Ken C. Winters, PhD, Department of Psychiatry, University of Minnesota, Minneapolis, Minnesota

David A. Wolfe, PhD, Centre for Prevention Science, Centre for Addiction and Mental Health, London, Ontario, Canada; Departments of Psychology and Psychiatry, University of Toronto, Toronto, Ontario, Canada

Vicky Veitch Wolfe, PhD, Child and Adolescent Mental Health Care Program, London Health Sciences, London, Ontario, Canada

Eric Youngstrom, PhD, Department of Psychology, University of North Carolina, Chapel Hill, North Carolina

Preface

Welcome! True to prior editions, this volume focuses on contemporary perspectives on the assessment of childhood psychological disorders. Yet our focus in this edition has also changed somewhat from that of earlier editions. Where previously we sought relatively comprehensive reviews of assessment methods and issues related to various childhood disorders, in this volume we now also focus on "best practices" or state-of-the-art approaches to the evaluation of those disorders. This additional emphasis was necessitated by several developments in the field of assessment, not the least of which is the voluminous extant literature on assessment approaches for each disorder, and for assessment more generally, and the tremendous expansion in the variety of evaluative methods. Our shifting emphasis was also driven by the obvious recognition that evaluators are under increasing pressures to limit the time spent conducting clinical evaluations, requiring that they utilize the best and most cost-effective methods now available while still attending to the clinical issues raised in the evaluation of children generally, and for each disorder more specifically. Yet overall our goal remains the same as in earlier editions: to invite major thought leaders to prepare chapters that reflect the cutting-edge empirically based methods and clinical issues related to evaluating the disorder(s) in which they specialize. We believe that goal has been achieved admirably by the current array of authors participating in this volume. We hope you will agree.

We acknowledge our considerable gratitude to these authors for taking substantial time from their work to update their chapters or prepare entirely new ones. We also wish to thank Seymour Weingarten and Bob Matloff of The Guilford Press for once again permitting us this opportunity to showcase contemporary approaches to assessment. We are further indebted to those working in the production department at Guilford for polishing these chapters to a higher gloss and more consumer-friendly organization and comprehension, particularly Laura Specht Patchkofsky for her matchless production editing skills in shepherding a volume of this complexity to completion and Jacquelyn Coggin for her skillful copy editing. We are also both continually indebted to our wives, Heather Mash and Pat Barkley, for creating a welcoming and supportive home and family life in which our professional activities can flourish. Both have done so for more than three decades—a miraculous feat in contemporary times and with outspoken, overworked, and professionally preoccupied men such as ourselves. There is no way to repay such a debt but we acknowledge it with infinite gratitude here. Finally, to our readers we express our sincerest appreciation for your interest in this volume. We trust you will find it to be a useful and informative guide to the best approaches to the evaluation of children and adolescents with psychological disorders.

Contents

PART I

Introduction

CHAPTER 1

Assessment of Child and Family Disturbance
A Developmental–Systems Approach

Eric J. Mash
John Hunsley

From the time of their conception, children in our society are assessed, evaluated, and labeled with respect to their physical status, behavior, language, cognition, learning, social competence, mood, and personality. These assessments are guided by the implicit assumptions about children's development and behavior held by significant others, and rooted in societal and cultural norms. Parents, other family members, teachers, peers, community members, and health care professionals all participate in this ongoing process, as do the children themselves. For most children, these evaluations occur during everyday social transactions and, to a lesser extent, during periodic formal evaluations best characterized as "routine" (e.g., regular medical checkups, school reports). As a result of these assessments, some children are identified as *deviating* from a normal course of development with regard to their behavior, physical condition, mental development, or conformity to social norms and expectations (Kagan, 1983; Mash & Dozois, 2003). When a negative valence is assigned to these deviations, a child is likely to be informally labeled as belonging to a group of children who display similar characteristics (e.g., "diffi-

cult," "shy," "slow," "overactive"). It is these children and their families who may then come to the attention of society's professional assessors, who utilize special strategies to build upon the informal assessments that led to the referral (e.g., Kamphaus & Campbell, 2006; Kamphaus & Frick, 2005; Mash & Terdal, 1997b; Reynolds & Kamphaus, 2003a, 2003b; Sattler, 1998, 2001; Sattler & Hoge, 2006).

About one in five children and adolescents in the United States suffer from some type of mental health problem during the course of a year (U.S. Department of Health and Human Services, 1999), and about 50% of all mental disorders in adults have an onset prior to age 14 (Kessler, Bergland, Demler, Jin, & Walters, 2005). Although there is much agreement concerning the need for systematic assessments of children and adolescents who display or are at risk for later problems, there has been and continues to be considerable disagreement and debate regarding how childhood disorders should be defined; what child characteristics, adaptations, and contexts should be assessed; by whom and in what situations children should be assessed; what methods should be used;

3

and how assessment information should be integrated, interpreted, and utilized (Jensen, Hoagwood, & Zitner, 2006; Mash & Hunsley, 2005a). Despite these disagreements, there is a general consensus regarding the need for the development of assessment strategies not as an endpoint, but as a prerequisite for planning, implementing, and evaluating effective and efficient services for children (Achenbach & Rescorla, 2006a; Mash & Hunsley, 2005a). Clearly, the value of any clinical assessment procedure ultimately depends on whether it helps the children and families who are being assessed. Such an evidence-based utilitarian approach to the assessment of children and families is a major theme underlying this volume, one that transcends many of the conceptual and methodological differences and preferences that emerge in the current discussion.

This volume examines current approaches to the *developmental–systems assessment* (DSA) of child and adolescent disorders. As described in this chapter, DSA has evolved from the concepts and methods of developmental psychopathology (Cicchetti, 2006), child and family behavioral assessment (Mash & Hunsley, 2004; Mash & Terdal, 1997a; Ollendick & Hersen, 1993), and evidence-based assessment (Hunsley & Mash, 2007; Mash & Hunsley, 2005b), and continues to embrace many of the following fundamental ideas and methods associated with each of these approaches: the use of developmentally sensitive assessments; a focus on the interplay of the child's physical status, affect, behavior, and cognition; the important role of context in assessment, including the child's family (i.e., parent–child interactions, sibling interactions) and larger social systems (i.e., peer relations, influence of teachers, cultural factors); the view of assessment as an ongoing process used to inform decision making; the use of empirically justifiable and feasible assessment methods, multimethod assessment strategies, and multiple informants; an emphasis on assessment information that leads to the design of effective interventions; and the ongoing evaluation of treatment progress and outcomes as an integral part of the assessment process. Our overall purpose in this introductory chapter is to elaborate on these themes, to highlight current principles and practices of DSA with disturbed children and families, and to discuss a number of key issues and concerns surrounding their development and use.

RECENT DEVELOPMENTS

As stated in the introductory chapter to the first edition of this book: "Recognizing the likelihood of ongoing and future changes in assessment strategies related to new empirical findings, emergent ideas, practical concerns, and shifts in the broader sociocultural milieu in which assessments are carried out, this chapter—indeed, this book—should be viewed as a working framework for understanding current approaches to the assessment of children" (Mash & Terdal, 1981, p. 4). This statement is as true today as it was then. As reflected throughout this volume, while retaining certain core elements, DSA has shown dramatic advances since the first edition of this book.

Some of the more notable developments are as follows:

1. An increased emphasis on incorporating developmental considerations into the design, conduct, and interpretation of assessments (Achenbach & Rescorla, 2006a; Peterson, Burbach, & Chaney, 1989; Yule, 1993); the implementation of treatments (Holmbeck, Greenley, & Franks, 2003; Kendall, Lerner, & Craighead, 1984; Luby, 2006); and the conceptualization of child and family psychopathology (e.g., Cicchetti & Cohen, 2006a, 2006b, 2006c; Mash & Barkley, 2003).

2. A heightened interest in issues related to diagnosis and classification. This interest has been accompanied by efforts to integrate DSA and current diagnostic practices in ways that are both sensitive to categorical and dimensional approaches to classification and informed by the limitations associated with current classification systems (Jensen, Hoagwood, et al., 2006; Mash & Terdal, 1997b; Pickles & Angold, 2003).

3. A heightened awareness of the need to assess multiple disorders or symptoms from different disorders in light of the high rates of co-occurrence (comorbidity) for most childhood problems (Kazdin, 2005).

4. A growing recognition of the importance of assessing adaptive functioning, impairment, and, more generally, how children and families are functioning in their daily lives as distinct from symptoms and disorders (Jensen, Hoagwood, et al., 2006; Kazdin, 2005). Such recognition has also led to attention regarding

the extent to which current assessment methods adequately capture important aspects of everyday functioning and quality of life (Bastiaansen, Koot, & Ferdinand, 2005; Kazdin, 2006).

5. A view of DSA as an ongoing decision-making process (Adelman & Taylor, 1988; Carter, Marakovitz, & Sparrow, 2006; Evans & Meyer, 1985) generating interest in the judgmental heuristics that influence this complex information-processing task (Evans, 1985; Kanfer, 1985; Tabachnik & Alloy, 1988), and efforts to develop both clinically and empirically derived decision-making guidelines for specific clinical problems and populations (Frazier & Youngstrom, 2006; Nezu & Nezu, 1993; Sanders & Lawton, 1993).

6. Growing attention to prevention-oriented and socially relevant assessments for high-risk populations (Ialongo et al., 2006; Tuma, Loeber, & Lochman, 2006). Attention emanating from current social concerns has focused on a wide range of groups and issues, including single-parent and stepfamilies, unemployment, children in day care, immigrant families, poverty, accidental injuries, child abductions, sexual abuse, family violence, delinquency, teen violence, adolescent substance abuse, adolescent suicide, and exposure to extreme stressors such as war, torture, and terrorist attacks.

7. An increasing emphasis on understanding the interrelated influences of child and family genetics (Rende & Waldman, 2006), neurobiology (Gunnar & Vazquez, 2006), cognition (Dodge & Pettit, 2003), affect (Dix, 1991; Gottman & Levenson, 1986), and behavior, as assessed within the context of ongoing social interactions (e.g., Bradbury & Fincham, 1987; Gottman, Katz, & Hooven, 1996; Lorber & Slep, 2005).

8. The extension and assimilation of DSA concepts and practices into child health care settings within the general frameworks of developmental pediatrics (Parker, Zucker, & Augustyn, 2005), behavioral pediatrics (Gross & Drabman, 1990), and pediatric psychology (Roberts, 2005).

9. A growing recognition of the need for empirically driven theoretical models as the basis for organizing and implementing assessment strategies with children and families (Mash & Barkley, 2003; McFall, 1986).

10. Increasing technological advances, particularly use of the Internet and computers during both the data-gathering and decision-making phases of assessment (Ancill, Carr, & Rogers, 1985; Whalen et al., 2006). Suggested Internet/computer applications have included gathering interview, self-monitoring, test, and observational data; organizing, synthesizing, and analyzing assessment data, and supporting decision making; monitoring treatment progress and outcomes; and using daily diaries. Technological advances have led to a heightened interest in the utility and feasibility of using actuarial models in clinical decision making (Achenbach, 1985; Frazier & Youngstrom, 2006; Mash, 1985).

11. Conceptual and methodological convergence on an ecologically oriented systems model (Bronfenbrenner, 1986; Hartup, 1986) as the appropriate framework for organizing and understanding assessment information derived from disturbed children and families (Evans, 1985; Wasik, 1984). This has led to a heightened interest in the assessment of whole-family variables (Forman & Hagan, 1984; Mash & Johnston, 1996b; Rodick, Henggeler, & Hanson, 1986) and the relationships among family systems, and between family systems and the broader sociocultural milieu (Cowan & Cowan, 2006; Dunst & Trivette, 1985, 1986; Parke, MacDonald, Beital, & Bhavnagri, 1988).

12. Increased recognition of the growing cultural diversity in North American society (Quintana et al., 2006; Serafica & Vargas, 2006) and the need to consider such diversity, broadly defined, in the assessment and treatment of disturbed children and families (Achenbach & Rescorla, 2006b; Forehand & Kotchick, 1996; Tharp, 1991).

13. Further attention to accountability in assessment and to the development of brief, feasible, and cost-effective assessment strategies (Hayes, 1996; Hayes, Follette, Dawes, & Grady, 1995). Such attention has been fueled by the growing concern for reducing costs within a rapidly changing health care delivery system (Mash & Hunsley, 1993; Strosahl, 1994).

14. Increased emphasis on the treatment evaluation functions of DSA in light of the current emphasis on evidence-based treatment practices (Barrett & Ollendick, 2004; Biglan, Mrazek, Carnine, & Flay, 2003; Buysse & Wesley, 2006; Hibbs & Jensen, 2005; Kazdin & Weisz, 2003; Mash & Barkley, 2006;

Sackett, Straus, Richardson, Rosenberg, & Haynes, 2000). This emphasis has led to heightened attention to the development of meaningful and practical measures for monitoring progress and assessing outcomes in clinical practice (Burlingame, Wells, Lambert, & Cox, 2004; Lambert et al., 2003; Nelson-Gray, 1996; Ogles, Lambert, & Masters, 1996).

It is apparent from this brief overview of developments over the past quarter of a century that current DSA approaches to child and family assessment are complex and varied. These approaches are best conceptualized within an assessment framework that examines the child's development and functioning in the context of the maturational stage of the biological and especially neurological systems, social systems, decisional processes, and practical considerations in which clinical assessments of disturbed children and families are typically conducted.

DEFINING DSA

We use the term "developmental–systems assessment" to describe a range of deliberate assessment strategies for understanding both disturbed and nondisturbed children and their social systems, including families and peer groups. These strategies employ a flexible and ongoing process of hypothesis testing regarding the nature of the problem, its causes, and likely outcome in the absence of intervention, and the anticipated effects of various treatments. It is our view that the generation of better hypotheses to test at the idiographic level can best proceed from an understanding of the general theories and principles of psychological assessment (e.g., Cronbach, 1990; Nunnally & Bernstein, 1994; Urbina, 2004); information concerning normal and abnormal child, and family development (e.g., Cicchetti & Cohen, 2006a, 2006b, 2006c; Mussen, 1983); and knowledge about groups of children and families with similar types of problems, including knowledge about prevalence, core symptoms, developmental features and course, associated characteristics, etiologies, and system parameters (Cicchetti & Cohen, 2006c; Mash & Barkley, 2003). This general view of DSA is reflected throughout the chapters in this volume.

DSA OF CHILD AND FAMILY DISTURBANCE: A PROTOTYPE-BASED VIEW

Rather than attempting to define DSA in terms of its necessary or essential features, we believe that a prototype-based view (e.g., Cantor, Smith, French, & Mezzich, 1980) best depicts the current state of the field. Within such a framework, the general category DSA is based on sets of imperfectly correlated features referred to as "prototypes" (Rosch, 1978). Assessment cases having the largest number of general category features are considered to be the most typical examples of DSA. The prototypical view also recognizes that within the more general category of DSA, there can exist a hierarchically but imperfectly nested set of subcategories, such as "DSA with young children" or "DSA with adolescents." DSA may take many different forms depending on the specific parameters associated with different child and family problems. For example, the prototype for DSA with a 4-year-old child with an oppositional disorder is quite different than that for an adolescent with depression. This view is consistent with the relativistic, contextually based, and idiographic nature of DSA strategies, and with the organization of this volume around categories of commonly occurring childhood disorders.

In the points that follow, we use the prototype-based view to present some of the more commonly occurring conceptual, strategic, and procedural characteristics of DSA (Mash & Terdal, 1997a):

1. DSA is based on conceptualizations of personality and abnormal behavior that emphasize the child's thoughts, feelings, and behaviors as they occur in specific situations, as well as the child's more general personality traits and dispositions (e.g., temperament, psychopathy) (Mischel, 2004; Mischel, Shoda, & Mendoza-Denton, 2002).
2. DSA is predominantly idiographic and individualized. Although comparison to norms is important, a greater relative emphasis is given to understanding the individual child and family than to nomothetic comparisons that describe individual children primarily in relation to group norms.
3. DSA emphasizes the important role of situational influences on behavior. It is recognized that the patterning and organization of an individual's behavior across situations is highly

idiographic (Mischel, 1973); therefore, it is important to describe the child's behaviors, cognitions, and affects as they occur in specific situations. The pragmatic outcomes of an emphasis on situational specificity in DSA have been a greater sensitivity to the measurement of situational dimensions and a corresponding increase in the range of environments sampled; for example, information about home, school, and neighborhood environments has been added to samples of the child's and parent's behavior obtained under highly controlled and standardized testing conditions in the clinic.

4. DSA emphasizes both the consistency and variability of child and family behaviors, cognitions, and affects over time. Because situationally related changes appear to be the norm rather than the exception throughout childhood and adolescence, the predominant DSA view has emphasized the need to consider change, not just stability, particularly during transitional periods of development. That being said, it is important to recognize that consistency can be assessed in relation to many levels of behavior and, depending on the specificity of the behavior under consideration, different results may obtain. If a child's behavior is described in terms of a highly idiographic response topography (e.g., whining), then we may find little consistency over time. In contrast, definitions based on broader response classes that encompass a wide range and pattern of behaviors (e.g., aggression) both within and across age levels may evidence more temporal consistency. Furthermore, if we look at response functions rather than at specific topographies, we may find that phenotypically different responses reflect a dynamic stability in which certain patterns of adjustment are repeated over time. As stated by Garber (1984), "Although there is little evidence of homotypic continuity—symptomatic isomorphism from early childhood—there is some evidence that children may show consistency in their general adaptive or maladaptive pattern of organizing their experiences and interacting with their environment" (p. 34). This organizational–developmental viewpoint has been supported by findings from longitudinal studies of development, which have suggested that patterns expressed in early relationships often repeat themselves over time (Kaye, 1984; Sroufe & Fleeson, 1986). The type of child and family characteristic being assessed also has implications for the question of temporal stability. For example, some characteristics may show stability over time (e.g., achievement motivation, dependence and passivity in females, serious aggressive behavior, and intellectual mastery), whereas others may not (Garber, 1984).

5. DSA is systems-oriented. It is directed at describing and understanding characteristics of the child and family, the contexts in which such characteristics are expressed, and the structural organizations and functional relationships that exist among situations, behaviors, thoughts, and emotions.

6. DSA emphasizes contemporaneous controlling variables relative to historical ones. However, when information about more temporally remote events (e.g., age of onset) facilitates an understanding of current influences, such information is sought and used in assessment. For example, knowing that a mother was physically or sexually abused as a child may help us understand her current attitudes and behavior toward her own child (Crooks & Wolfe, Chapter 14, and Wolfe, Chapter 15, this volume). Similarly, knowledge of early attachment patterns may assist us in understanding a child's current pattern of relational disturbance (Kobak, Cassidy, Lyons-Ruth, & Ziv, 2006).

7. DSA is more often concerned with behaviors, cognitions, and affects as direct samples of the domains of interest rather than as signs of some underlying or remote causes. For example, assessments focusing on a child's cognitive deficiencies, distortions, or misattributions target these characteristics as functional components of the problem to be modified rather than as symptoms of some other problem.

8. DSA focuses on obtaining assessment information that is directly relevant to treatment. Relevance for treatment usually refers to the usefulness of information in identifying treatment goals, selecting targets for intervention, designing and implementing interventions, and evaluating the outcomes of therapy (Carr, 1994; Mace, 1994).

9. DSA recognizes the importance of using multiple informants, including the child, parents, teachers, and peers, as a way to obtain information from different perspectives and settings. Because the data obtained from one source rarely correlate highly with those obtained from other sources, the assessor must be cautious to avoid considering any single source of information as the "gold standard," unless such a position is warranted based on research evidence.

10. DSA relies on a multimethod assessment strategy to capture the diverse aspects of most clinical problems. This approach emphasizes the importance of using a variety of assessment methods, including interviews, questionnaires, and observations (Kamphaus, Petoskey, & Rowe, 2000). However, the inherent value of one method over another is not assumed, but should be based on the purposes and needs associated with specific assessments (McFall, 1986), available resources, the utility of the information obtained, and what method is deemed most useful in a specific setting (Silverman & Ollendick, 2005).

11. DSA is an ongoing self-evaluative process. Instead of conducting assessments on one or two occasions prior to treatment, the need for further assessment is dictated by the effectiveness of the methods in facilitating desired treatment outcomes and the extent to which treatment goals are being met.

12. DSA is empirically anchored. The assessment strategies—in particular, the decision regarding which variables to assess—should be guided by knowledge concerning the characteristics of the child and family being assessed, and the research literature on specific childhood disorders. In the case of assessments that are theoretically driven, theories should be closely tied to empirical evidence. Similarly, decisions regarding the methods used in assessment are also based on their empirically established psychometric properties and their feasibility in relation to specific assessment purposes (Hunsley & Mash, in press).

COMMON ASSESSMENT PURPOSES

Inherent in the view of DSA as an ongoing problem-solving strategy is the recognition that assessments of children and families are always carried out in relation to one or more purposes. Along with the assessor's working assumptions and conceptualizations about normal and abnormal child and family behavior, these purposes determine which individuals, behaviors, and settings are evaluated; the choice of assessment methods; the way findings are interpreted; the specification of assessment and treatment goals; and how the attainment of these goals is evaluated. Questions surrounding the assessment of child and family disturbances can be considered only within the context of the intended assessment purpose(s). Therefore,

decisions regarding the appropriateness or usefulness of particular assessment methods and procedures are always made in relation to the needs of the situation. For example, discussions concerning the relative merits of information obtained via self-report versus direct observation have little meaning outside of a specific set of assessment contexts and purposes.

Many writers have outlined common purposes for which child and family assessments are conducted (e.g., Achenbach & Rescorla, 2006a; Mash & Terdal, 1997a). Broadly conceived, these include (1) diagnosis, or assessment activities focusing on formulating a diagnosis and identifying the nature of the problem; (2) prognosis, or generating predictions concerning future behavior under specified conditions; (3) case conceptualization and treatment planning, or the gathering of information that augments diagnostic information to yield a full clinical case conceptualization to assist in the development and implementation of effective interventions; (4) treatment monitoring and treatment outcome evaluation, or assessments that monitor progress during the course of treatment and evaluate the overall effect of treatment on symptoms, diagnosis, and general functioning, and the treatment's efficiency, acceptability, and satisfaction to consumers. Because these purposes are addressed in relation to each of the specific disorders in the chapters that follow, we comment on them only briefly here.

Diagnosis

The four purposes of assessment we mentioned earlier often occur in phases for individual cases. Initial diagnostic assessments are concerned with questions relating to general screening and administrative decision making (e.g., Can the child be appropriately served by a particular agency or educational program?); whether or not there is a problem (e.g., Does the child's behavior deviate from an appropriate behavioral or social norm?), and the nature and extent of the problem (e.g., What is the child doing or not doing that results in a distressed family or school situation, or impairment in the child's functioning?); and whether the presentation of the problem conforms to one or more categories of a diagnostic classification.

The term "diagnosis" has acquired several meanings (Achenbach, 1985). One of these, *taxonomic diagnosis*, views diagnosis and classification as equivalent, and focuses on the formal assignment of cases to specific categories drawn from either a system of disorder classification such as the *Diagnostic and Statistical Manual of Mental Disorders* (DSM-IV-TR; American Psychiatric Association [APA], 2000) or empirically derived taxometric categories, prototypes, or typologies (Achenbach, 1993). A second and much broader meaning of the term "diagnosis," *problem-solving analysis* or *diagnostic formulation*, considers diagnosis to be an analytic information-gathering process directed at an understanding of the nature of a problem, its possible causes, treatment options, and outcomes. This broader meaning of "diagnosis" is the definition that is most consistent with the concepts and practices of DSA, although DSA also recognizes the utility of taxonomic diagnosis as an organizational framework for applying existing knowledge about a class of cases to a diagnostic formulation for a new case (Achenbach & Rescorla, 2006a; Kazdin, 1983; Mash & Terdal, 1997a; Powers, 1984).

The diagnostic phase within DSA is conducted with the expectation that, with further case formulation, assessment will lead directly to recommendations for subsequent clinical services. Questions often asked during the diagnostic phase of DSA include (1) What is the child doing, thinking, or feeling that causes distress, brings them into conflict with the environment, or impairs functioning? and (2) What are the potential controlling variables for these problems? DSA diagnoses are often highly individualized and based on direct empirical support. The methods employed during the early diagnostic phases of DSA tend to be global and extensive—they have been described as having broad bandwidth but low fidelity—and the use of interviews, global self-report instruments, observational narratives, and simple behavioral code systems is common.

Prognosis

Every child and family assessment carries with it some projection regarding short- and long-term outcomes for the child under varying conditions. Knowledge concerning risk and protective factors, and the likely outcomes for certain behaviors during later periods of development, is required for making judgments about deviance. Because many childhood problems are not intrinsically pathological and are exhibited to some extent by most children, decisions regarding whether or not to treat the problem often depend on prognostic implications. Implicit in any decision about whether to initiate intervention is a projection that things will remain the same, improve, or deteriorate in the absence of treatment, or that outcomes will vary as a function of differing treatments. With children, treatments are often directed at enhancing developmental processes, not just removing symptoms or restoring a previous level of functioning. Information concerning developmental processes (e.g., emotion regulation) may also provide the basis for anticipatory interventions in high-risk situations in which the prognosis is known to be poor. A host of decisions is related to children's mental health and the legal system for which information concerning prognosis is required, for example, assessments of suicide risk (Goldston & Compton, Chapter 7, this volume) or a parent's ability to provide an adequate caregiving environment for their child (Crooks & Wolfe, Chapter 14, this volume).

Questions concerning prognosis are often considered in relation to longitudinal information, as derived, for example, from studies of risk or resilience in high-risk children (Luthar, 2006). For example, children with greater resources (e.g., intellectual ability, stable and supportive families) are generally more competent and show more adaptive patterns of dealing with stress (Masten, Burt, & Coatsworth, 2006). Although such findings can provide a basis for general predictions, their direct applicability to decision making for individual children and their families is not always clear. Studies of individual at-risk children who do well may provide suggestions as to the types of interventions that might be appropriate in high-risk situations.

Longitudinal studies of long-term outcomes for children with different types of disorders also provide information concerning prognosis. For example, the most persistent and pernicious types of conduct disorder are associated with a family history of antisocial behavior, early neuropsychological deficits, comorbid attention-deficit/hyperactivity disorder (ADHD), early onset and variety of antisocial and aggressive symptoms, callous-unemotional traits (deficient guilt, remorse, empathy, etc.), and poor family functioning (Dishion & Patterson, 2006; Moffitt, 2006).

Questions concerning prognosis are frequently raised early in the assessment process. However, such questions are also important following treatment to assess the likelihood that treatment gains will be maintained, especially when long-term maintenance for certain problems is known be poor (e.g., aggression). The systematic assessment of maintenance of treatment effects in the child and family areas has received limited attention to date.

For many children, early problems that can have a severe and lasting negative impact need to be taken very seriously (e.g., Kendall, Hudson, Choudhury, Webb, & Pimentel, 2005). However, the identification of early problems also needs to be viewed with some caution, because the malleability of child behavior also means that for some children these problems may be reduced or even eliminated with treatment or other changes in children's environment.

Case Conceptualization and Treatment Planning

The case conceptualization and treatment planning phase of DSA focuses on obtaining information that is directly relevant to devising effective treatment strategies (Eells, 2007). This gathering of information builds on the previously obtained diagnostic information, and includes further specification and assessment of potential controlling variables (e.g., cognitive distortions or misattributions, patterns of social rewards and punishments), determination of the child's and family's resources for change (e.g., strengths, self-regulatory skills), assessment of potential social and physical resources that can be used in carrying out treatment, assessment of motivation for treatment and readiness for change in both the child and significant others, indication of potential reinforcers, specification of realistic treatment objectives, and recommendations for types of treatments that are likely to be most acceptable and, based on the evidence, most effective for treating specific types of childhood problems. Since parental adherence to treatment recommendations following assessments may be low, it is also important to assess factors that contribute to nonadherence, for example, discontinuity in care, long wait times, or a lack of readiness for change (Geffken, Keeley, Kellison, Storch, & Rodrigue, 2006).

The assessment procedures that characterize this phase are more problem-focused than those in the diagnostic phase, and specific types of problem checklists (e.g., fear survey schedules, measures of hyperactivity–impulsivity, depression inventories, impairment surveys), observational assessments (e.g., command–compliance analogues), and specific behavior codes (e.g., on-task behavior, self-stimulation, aggression) are more likely to be used in this phase than in earlier stages of assessment.

Treatment Monitoring and Treatment Outcome Evaluation

The treatment monitoring and treatment outcome evaluation phase of DSA involves the use of procedures designed to determine whether treatment objectives are being met, whether changes that have occurred can be attributed to specific interventions, whether the changes are long-lasting and generalizable across behaviors and situations, whether the treatment is economically viable, and whether treatments and treatment outcomes are acceptable to the clients.

Assessments for determining whether treatment goals are being met require the measurement of targeted objectives over time. Such measurement indicates the presence or absence of change, which in many cases may be sufficient. However, to determine whether changes are a function of the treatments introduced for individual children and families, it is necessary to observe in a controlled fashion, for example, by using a single-case research design (Freeman & Mash, in press). Although such designs can be extremely useful from a research standpoint, a key question concerns their feasibility in clinical practice and their adequacy in representing the often complex system parameters and relationships that characterize treatment goals in current, evidence-based treatment practices with children and families (Mash & Barkley, 2006).

Evaluations relative to the acceptability of treatments and relevance of treatment changes have been discussed under the rubrics of social validity (Foster & Mash, 1999; Kazdin, 1977; Wolf, 1978), treatment acceptability (Kazdin, 1981, 1984), consumer satisfaction (Kiesler, 1983; LeBow, 1982; McMahon & Forehand, 1983), and clinical significance (Atkins, Bedics, McGlinchey, & Beauchaine, 2005; Kendall, 1999). Such issues are especially pertinent to interventions for children, which must be gauged against ongoing or projected developmental changes. Measurement issues surrounding long-term follow-up are also highly relevant to DSA (Mash & Terdal, 1980). The methods used during the evaluation phase of assessment tend to be highly focused, brief, and specific in comparison to those in earlier assessment phases. The need for reliable, valid, and cost-efficient measures of treatment outcome is becoming increasingly important in the current health care context in which services for children and families are being provided (Daleiden, Chorpita, Donkervoet, Arensdorf, & Brogan, 2006).

The purposes described thus far relate to clinical decision making for individual children, which is characteristically the focus of DSA. There is also a need to recognize that broader societal and institutional purposes often underlie assessment practices with children and families, including classification for administrative record keeping, program development and evaluation, policy planning, quality assurance, and the advancement of scientific knowledge. The types of assessments required to meet these purposes may differ substantially from those required for the clinical assessment of individual children and families.

CHILDREN'S FUNCTIONING AND ITS DETERMINANTS

Childhood Disorders versus Individual Symptoms or Behaviors

The chapters in this volume are organized around the assessment of specific childhood disorders. This organization reflects our view that children and families present themselves for assessment showing characteristic patterns, clusters, or constellations of problems rather than individual symptoms or behaviors (Mash & Dozois, 2003). Both clinical and empirical evidence indicate that broad patterns of child disturbance labeled *externalizing* (e.g., aggression, rule-breaking behavior) and *internalizing* (e.g., anxious–depressed, withdrawn–depressed, somatic complaints) are relatively stable over time and across raters (Achenbach & Rescorla, 2001). For this reason, we believe that assessment best follows an empirically based understanding of characteristic *patterns* of behavior, adjustment, and maladjustment (Kazdin & Kagan, 1994). As a first step in the assessment process, all clinicians engage formally or informally in the identification of behaviors, cognitions, and emotions that cluster together (Barlow, 1986).

We concur with Kanfer's (1979) view that "different problem areas require development of separate methods and conceptualizations that take into account the particular parameters of that area" (p. 39), and that assessment of certain domains may be impeded until conceptual models or data are available to identify the symptoms and associated features that need to be assessed. Empirically derived conceptual models to guide assessments of child and family disorders in both clinical and research contexts are emerging at a rapid rate (see Mash & Barkley, 2003; Mash & Hunsley, 2005a). One of the best-articulated, theory-driven, empirically based models for assessment is represented by Patterson's (1982) work with children and families exhibiting antisocial problems. Through the use of multiple methodologies and statistical methods such as structural equation modeling, a number of important constructs and their relationships have been implicated in the development of children's antisocial behavior (Dishion & Patterson, 2006; Patterson, 1986; Patterson & Bank, 1986). This work suggests the importance of assessing several molar and microvariables when working with antisocial children and their families (e.g., whether the child is rejected or perceived as antisocial by others; the likelihood of the child's unprovoked negative behavior toward parents and siblings, and its duration; the extent to which parents monitor their children and spend time with them; the parents' inept discipline, as reflected in their use of explosive forms of punishment, negative actions and reactions, and inconsistent/erratic behavior; and deviant peer influences). Building on this database, recent models of antisocial behavior have incorporated additional variables (e.g., social-cognitive and emotional processes) that serve to guide assessments of children and adolescents with conduct problems (Dodge & Pettit, 2003). Each chapter in this volume provides one or more conceptual models and an empirical base for the specific disorder under discussion, and the assessment strategies that are presented follow from this framework.

In specifying constellations of problems or "syndromes" as a basis for one's assessment strategies, it is important to recognize that syndromes can be viewed in a number of different ways (Achenbach & Edelbrock, 1978, p. 1294):

1. The syndrome may be viewed as representing a personality or character type that endures beyond the immediate precipitating events requiring professional attention.
2. The syndrome may be viewed as reflecting dimensions or traits, so that children are best described individually in terms of their scores on all syndromes rather than by categorization according to their resemblance to a particular syndrome.
3. The syndrome may be viewed as a reaction type, whose form is as much a function of specific precipitating stresses as of individual characteristics.
4. The syndrome may be viewed as a collection of behaviors that happen to be statistically associated because the environmental contingencies supporting them are statistically associated.

These different views are all consistent with the assumptions underlying DSA, and they are not necessarily independent of one another. It may be that reaction types that become well established early in development eventually emerge as enduring, but not necessarily irreversible, character types. For example, research has suggested that preferential orientations toward others, self, and the object world when confronted with interactive stress may be exhibited by infants as young as 6 months of age (Tronick & Gianino, 1986).

The concept of syndromes in DSA with children and families is also represented by the concepts of *response class* and *response covariation* (e.g., Kazdin, 1982, 1983; Voeltz & Evans, 1982; Wahler, 1975). These notions imply that certain behaviors tend to co-occur, or to be correlated with one another, and/or that certain behaviors tend to covary, such that changes in one are associated with changes in the other. Research into response covariation has suggested indirect paths of clinical intervention—for example, when decreases in a child's noncompliant behavior lead to a reduction in bedwetting (Nordquist, 1971) or stuttering (Wahler, Sperling, Thomas, Teeter, & Luper, 1970). The existence of such response classes has important implications, in that assessment of these relationships may suggest maximally effective courses of intervention.

Although an extensive discussion of the many issues surrounding the concepts of response class and response covariation is beyond the scope of this chapter, several important questions need to be addressed before these concepts can have widespread applicability in the DSA of children and families.

1. First, there is currently little information as to how to identify response classes. Potential response classes have been derived via serendipitous discovery, from clinically described syndromes, from conceptual models or theories about child and family disorders, from statistical methods for grouping data, and through systematic functional analysis. In light of the potentially enormous number of topographically dissimilar responses that could be related, guidelines are needed for limiting the number and range of responses to be assessed.
2. Response class representations are miniature systems, and guidelines are needed for mapping out the structural organizations and functional relationships that describe a particular response class, as well as its relationships to other systems. In this context, discussions and findings relative to the comorbidity of childhood disorders (i.e., the tendency for children to meet diagnostic criteria for multiple disorders) are relevant to understanding relationships among different response classes (e.g., Caron & Rutter, 1991; Youngstrom, Findling, & Calabrese, 2003).
3. Although the focus in DSA has been on "response" classes, we are more often talking about constellations of responses, cognitions, emotions, and physiological reactions. The more varied and complex response classes become, the more they seem to approximate descriptions of clinical disorders as presented in current diagnostic systems.
4. Are response classes to be defined idiographically for each child who is assessed, or can we expect them to have some generality across children?
5. The relationship between response classes and situations has received little attention (Wahler & Graves, 1983). Can we expect response classes to be situation-specific, as some research has suggested (Patterson & Bechtel, 1977), or will some response clusters show generality across situations?
6. Most discussions of response classes have focused on the individual. However, it would be equally feasible to identify response clusters

for more complex social units—for example, parent–child dyads, siblings, couples, or the family.

Although these issues are in need of further investigation, research on response covariation has sensitized assessors to the fact that consideration of only a narrow range of symptoms and behaviors fails to represent adequately the more general network of behaviors, of which this behavior may be a part, or the fact that this network of behaviors may be functionally embedded in larger social systems.

As presented in this volume, the DSA view of child and family disorders focuses on common patterns of behavior and behavior–context disturbances. Rather than emphasizing the use of assessment methods per se, these methods are considered primarily in relation to the specific problems and contexts in which they are to be used. For example, although there are general principles associated with the development and use of particular assessment methods, the nature of an interview with the parent of a depressed child should be different than an interview with the parent of a child with autism. It is believed that an understanding of the specific parameters associated with childhood depression (Rudolph & Lambert, Chapter 5, this volume) or with an autistic disorder (Ozonoff, Goodlin-Jones, & Solomon, Chapter 10, this volume), in concert with knowledge about the general principles of interviewing (e.g., Sattler, 1998), will serve to generate more specialized and ultimately more useful assessments for children experiencing these types of problems.

Impairment in Functioning versus Symptoms and Disorders

In addition to assessing the characteristic patterns of behavior associated with specific childhood disorders, it has become increasingly apparent that assessment of the degree of impairment in children's functioning is essential to defining and understanding their problematic behavior (Jensen, Hoagwood, et al., 2006; Kazdin, 2005). Symptoms and specific impairments are not necessarily highly correlated. Many children who show considerable impairment may not meet the symptom criteria for having a problem and, as a result, may not receive the intervention they clearly need (Angold, Costello, Farmer, Burns, & Erkanli, 1999; Gordon et al., 2006). Similarly, symptom

reduction during treatment does not necessarily correlate with overall improvement in functioning. Thus, the assessment of functional impairment, in addition to symptoms and disorders, is important in determining the impact of the disorder, identifying treatment goals and service needs, and monitoring outcomes. A number of scales designed to assess a child's impairment in functioning may be used for these purposes (Winters, Collett, & Myers, 2005).

Classification and Diagnosis

One of the more controversial areas in the assessment and treatment of disturbed children and families has been the use of diagnostic labels based on global classification systems. Although diagnostic criteria for children have become increasingly differentiated and specific, many concerns remain regarding classification and diagnosis. Over the decades, the same labels have been used to describe different sets of clinical phenomena (Zachary, Levin, Hargreaves, & Greene, 1981), and different labels have been used to describe the same clinical disorder (e.g., hyperactivity, hyperkinesis, attention deficit disorder, ADHD) (Barkley, 2006). Systems for the classification of childhood disorders have received extensive discussion that has increased since the appearance of DSM-III, which included an increased number of child categories (APA, 1980).

There is some agreement regarding the general neglect of meaningful taxonomic frameworks for describing children and families, and the need for classification systems to guide theory, research, and practice. For example, Achenbach and Edelbrock (1978) stated that "the study of psychopathology in children has long lacked a coherent taxonomic framework within which training, treatment, epidemiology, and research could be integrated" (p. 1275). Despite their increased use, all classification systems that have emerged thus far have met with criticism. For example, as Nathan (1986) stated, "For the most part, when more effective treatments have been developed or more light has been shed on etiology, it has not been by virtue of one or another classification scheme that this has come about" (p. 201).

Although DSA acknowledges the need for a classification system of child and family disorders, including widely accepted systems such as DSM-IV-TR (APA, 2000), there continues to be dissatisfaction with the currently available approaches (Doucette, 2002; Kupfer, First, & Regier, 2002; Watson & Clark, 2006). These dissatisfactions with existing classification systems have centered around their lack of fit with many real-world patients, who often present with clusters of symptoms that cross multiple diagnostic categories; empirical inadequacies; their primarily descriptive and relatively atheoretical nature; the complexity of using the system in clinical practice; the subjective–impressionistic criteria used to derive individual categories; the failure to provide empirically derived operational criteria for assignment to categories; the heterogeneity that exists within diagnostic categories; the static nature of the categories when applied to the developing child; the use of diagnostic criteria that are not adjusted for the child's age or sex; the lack of demonstrated relevance for treatment; the potentially undesirable consequences of labeling; a lack of sensitivity to contextual influences, including the role of ethnicity and culture; and a general insensitivity of diagnostic criteria to the relational difficulties that characterize children and families (Beach, Wamboldt, Kaslow, Heyman, & Reiss, 2006; LeBow & Gordon, 2006).

An alternative to current classification schemes has yet to emerge despite these criticisms and the long-standing recognition of the need for alternatives (Adams, Doster, & Calhoun, 1977; Adelman, 1995; Hayes & Follette, 1992; Jensen, Knapp, & Mrazek, 2006). The seeming lack of progress in this area likely reflects the many challenges in developing a viable alternative that would address the aforementioned dissatisfactions, as well as the increasing priority given to the development of evidence-based treatment practices. It is not clear that the development of global classification systems for childhood disorders will do much to facilitate effective intervention at the level of the individual child (cf. Pelham, Fabiano, & Massetti, 2005), although such systems might potentially improve communication, combine data from diverse sources, epidemiological studies, and comparison treatments, and increase understanding of causes (Kessler, 1971).

Efforts to classify childhood disorders have followed several traditions. The first involved the development of clinically derived classification categories based mostly on subjective consensus, as characterized by the systems developed by the Group for the Advancement of Psychiatry (1974), the World Health Organization (1992), the Zero to Three/National Center for Clinical Infant Programs (1994) and Diagnostic Classification of Mental Health and Developmental Disorders of Infancy and Early Childhood (DC:0–3R) Revision Task Force (2005), and the American Psychiatric Association (1980, 1987, 1994, 2000). Although it is beyond the scope of this chapter to review these systems in detail (see Achenbach, 1985; DelCarmen-Wiggins & Carter, 2004), commonly occurring categories are exemplified by those provided in DSM-IV-TR (APA, 2000). These disorders of infancy, childhood, and adolescence include ADHD; disruptive behavior disorders such as oppositional defiant disorder and conduct disorder; feeding and eating disorders such as pica, rumination disorder, and feeding disorders of infancy and childhood; tic disorders such as Tourette's disorder and chronic motor or vocal tic disorder; elimination disorders such as enuresis and encopresis; separation anxiety disorder; selective mutism; reactive attachment disorder, and stereotyped movement disorder. Also included in DSM-IV-TR are developmental and learning disorders such as mental retardation; learning disorders in reading, mathematics, and written expression; developmental coordination disorder; communication disorders such as expressive language disorders, mixed receptive–expressive disorders, language disorder, phonological disorder, and stuttering; and pervasive developmental disorders, including autistic disorder, Rett's disorder, childhood disintegrative disorder, and Asperger's disorder. In addition, many other diagnostic categories for anxiety, mood, and substance use disorders, and relational disturbances used for adult diagnoses are also used for children, with minor modifications in symptom criteria or duration. DSM-IV-TR criteria for assignment to specific categories are presented throughout the chapters of this volume. Generally these criteria include the presence of a specified number of symptoms; a minimum time period during which the specified symptoms must be present; developmental inappropriateness of those symptoms; age or age-of-onset criteria; exclusionary criteria, if the problem is secondary to other disorders; and impairment in functioning.

In recognizing that a simple enumeration of symptoms may not be sufficient for treatment planning or predicting individual outcomes, DSM-IV-TR also provides a multiaxial classification scheme that includes clinical disorders and other conditions that may be a focus of clinical attention (Axis I); personality disorders and mental retardation (Axis II); general medical conditions (Axis III); psychosocial and environmental problems (Axis IV); and global assessment of functioning (Axis V). However, only the first three axes constitute an official diagnostic evaluation, and the amount of differentiation for Axes I and II is disproportionately large when compared with that for Axes IV and V. In addition, although clearly important, Axes IV and V presently have limited or undetermined reliability or validity (Goldman & Skodol, 1992; Van Goor-Lambo, 1987).

Efforts to increase the accuracy and reliability of psychiatric diagnoses have resulted in the development of a number of semistructured and structured interview protocols for obtaining information to assist in making a diagnosis. Many of these are described in the chapters that follow. There has been an increase in the use of these procedures for the identification of groups of children in assessment and treatment outcome studies, and to a lesser extent clinically. In this context, accurate DSM-IV-TR diagnoses offer some direction regarding the range of behaviors/symptoms, settings, and associated features that might then be assessed clinically in a more intensive idiographic fashion (Powers, 1984). It is likely that until assessors are willing, able, and provided with the incentives to invest the time and resources needed to develop and promote a more empirically based classification alternative to DSM-IV-TR and its successor DSM-V (anticipated to appear in 2011) (Kupfer et al., 2002), administrative requirements, the need to communicate with other professionals, and the need for a taxonomy to direct and organize research and clinical activities will all contribute to the use of DSM diagnoses as an important component of DSA with children and families. At present, there is simply no readily available alternative (First, 2005).

A second major approach to the classification of childhood disorders is an empirical one, involving the use of multivariate statistical methods such as factor and cluster analyses (Achenbach, 1993; Achenbach & Rescorla, 2001; McDermott & Weiss, 1995; Reynolds & Kamphaus, 2004). This approach assumes that there are a number of independent dimensions of behavior (i.e., traits), and that all children possess these sets of behavior to varying degrees. In contrast to classification approaches that use clinically derived categories of childhood disorder, the dimensional approach focuses on empirically derived categories of behavioral covariation. Although empirically derived classifications are more objective and potentially more reliable, they also possess associated problems. No classification system can be better than the items that comprise it, and, as noted by Achenbach (1985), "subjective judgment is involved in selecting the samples and attributes to be analyzed, the analytic methods, and the mathematical criteria" (p. 90). Other concerns that need to be addressed include (1) possible interactions between the methods of data collection (e.g., ratings, direct observations, questionnaires), the informants (e.g., parents vs. teachers), or characteristics of the sample (e.g., ethnicity), and the dimensions that emerge, and (2) the lack of sensitivity of global trait dimensions to situational influences (e.g., duration of the disorder, setting in which behavior is rated, when the ratings are made).

Multivariate studies are consistent in identifying two broad dimensions of child behavior labeled "externalizing" and "internalizing." More specific syndromes that have been verified via confirmatory factor analysis include aggressive behavior and rule-breaking behavior (externalizing dimension), anxious–depressed, withdrawn–depressed, somatic complaints (internalizing dimension), and attention problems, thought problems, and social problems (Achenbach & Rescorla, 2001).

Much of the recent impetus for the development of multivariate classification approaches in child and family assessment comes from the extensive work of Achenbach and his colleagues with the Child Behavior Checklist and profile (Achenbach, 1991) and the Achenbach System of Empirically Based Assessment (ASEBA; Achenbach & Rescorla, 2000, 2001). It is not possible here to do justice to the scope and magnitude of this work and the research it has generated (for a detailed discussion of this approach, see Achenbach, 1985, 1993; Achenbach & Rescorla, 2001). Briefly, Achenbach describes a number of advantages associated with utilizing a taxometric integration of prototypical syndromes, in which an individual child may be classified on the basis of the similarity of his or her profile of syndrome scores with the centroid of each previously derived profile type. Beginning with the rationale that child syndromes consist of imperfectly correlated features, the argument is made that a prototype-based view of classification is preferable to one that employs the assignment of individuals to categories based on the presence of a small number of essential or cardinal features. Although it has been recognized that the conceptual derivation of prototypes for syndromes is possible (e.g., Horowitz, Post, French, Wallis, & Siegelman, 1981; Horowitz, Wright, Lowenstein, & Parad, 1981), operational definitions of prototypical syndromes are ideally generated via multivariate statistical analyses. It is argued that the use of quantitative indices, standardized assessment data, and computerized data processing permit the integration of large and complex datasets, reduce the likelihood that information-processing biases influence clinical judgments, and enable the clinician to focus on other, not easily standardized aspects of assessment and treatment.

As reflected throughout this volume, the use of multivariate assessment procedures in the DSA of children and families has increased considerably (e.g., Reynolds & Kamphaus, 2002, 2004) and is a reflection of the increasing availability and relative ease of use of these procedures, the accumulation of evidence for their validity in relation to a variety of assessment purposes, and a growing interest in child and parent perceptions as mediators of behavior and behavior change. Many of the criticisms of the multivariate approach from a DSA perspective have been based on dissatisfaction with the often global and ambiguous content being assessed, the fact that information is heavily based on subjective reports, and the general lack of sensitivity to situational influences. However, these criticisms are not inherent to the approach per se, because it is quite possible to derive "syndromes" that are based on other theories, have different contents, employ other methods, and sample a broader range of settings than is currently the case. Conceivably, syndromes of reaction types specific to particular situations (e.g., profiles of reaction types to stressful family events, social confrontation, medical procedures, or academic tasks) may also be derived.

More serious criticisms of the multivariate strategy within a DSA framework is its nomothetic emphasis on comparisons between an individual child and some group norm, and the limited relevance of this approach in the design of treatment strategies for individual children

(Peterson, 1968). Despite these criticisms, current DSA has integrated standardized multivariate assessments into clinical practice in formulating treatment goals—for example, in cases where the parent's perceptions indicate that the child is deviant, but observations of the child's behavior suggest otherwise (e.g., Mash, Johnston, & Kovitz, 1983)—and as one outcome measure for assessing the impact of treatment on parent and teacher perceptions of the child's behavior.

A third approach to classification follows from a developmental perspective on child psychopathology. Although this perspective is often adopted in clinical practice, it has not had a significant impact on formalized diagnostic practices with children. For example, many of the DSM-IV-TR categories for children are simple extensions of those used to categorize adults, with minor changes to adjust for developmental level, and the focus of the multivariate approaches has been on the categorization of individual behaviors and traits rather than on the patterns of adaptation that characterize different periods of development. The classification system for children from birth to 3 years has a strong developmental emphasis but has not, as yet, been systematically evaluated in research or clinical practice (DC:0–3R Revision Task Force, 2005; Lieberman, Barnard, & Wieder, 2004).

In an insightful developmental perspective on classification, Garber (1984) outlined many of the complexities and challenges that underlie this approach. Central to this view is the need to assess children's levels of functioning within different developmental domains (e.g., emotional, cognitive, social, physical) and their patterns of coping in relation to major developmental tasks (e.g., regulation of biological functions, attachment, dependence, autonomy, self-control, conformity to rules). Children are diagnosed in relation to their successes or failures in negotiating normative developmental expectations and demands, and it is believed that diagnostic models should emphasize adaptations and organizations of behavior at various developmental levels, rather than static traits, signs, or symptoms.

A developmental perspective is quite consistent with the emphasis in DSA on describing children's reactions in relation to situational demands, but it presents some formidable challenges in practice, not the least of which are mapping out and defining "normative" developmental sequences and creating a relevant taxonomy of developmental tasks. Longitudinal studies in child development and developmental psychopathology provide a rich database from which to assess and classify developmental adaptations during the first few years of life, and more recently, during middle childhood and adolescence. This database increases the promise of a developmentally anchored classification system, although this promise is still a long way from being realized. Nevertheless, a developmental perspective on classification, and developmental models more generally, are an integral part of DSA with children and families.

The classification systems we have discussed thus far, especially DSM-IV-TR and the multivariate approaches, have tended to focus exclusively on the child. They are derived from models that generally view disorders as residing in the child rather than in the ongoing and reciprocal interactions between the child and her or his larger social system. However, individual symptomatic and diagnostic variables are limited in characterizing children's mental health outcomes in the absence of information about the child's larger social context, including peer and family relationships; home, school, and neighborhood environments; and cultural and societal factors (Achenbach & Rescorla, 2006b; Hoagwood, Jensen, Petti, & Burns, 1996). Classification models for describing larger social systems, such as the parent–child dyad (Egeland & Sroufe, 1981), sibling relationships (Ellis & DeKeseredy, 1994), the marital relationship (Weiss & Margolin, 1986), and the family (Mash & Johnston, 1996a; Mink, Meyers, & Nihara, 1984; Mink, Nihira, & Meyers, 1983), are available but rarely used in clinical settings. It is believed that these types of classification approaches have the potential to incorporate DSA emphasis on contextual influences into our diagnostic practices. Similarly, there continues to be an enormous need in assessments with children and families for the development of taxonomies that describe situations (Mischel, 1977; Schlundt & McFall, 1987). Most assessment procedures continue to focus on individuals, and the degree of measurement sophistication achieved in describing the situations in which children and families function is still quite primitive, often reflecting global topographical features of the setting, such as home versus school. Elaborated classification schemes that reflect the differentiation

that occurs within settings are needed, and previous work on the ecological assessment of environments should provide some direction in this regard (e.g., Vincent & Trickett, 1983). For example, the Classroom Environment Scale (Moos & Trickett, 2002) examines classroom environments in terms of relationship (e.g., involvement, affiliation, teacher support), personal growth (e.g., task orientation, competition), and system maintenance and change (e.g., order and organization, rule clarity, teacher control, innovation).

On a final note, some efforts have been made to integrate categorical and dimensional approaches in DSA through the development of DSM-oriented scales based on items from multivariate scales judged by expert mental health professionals to be consistent with DSM-IV-TR diagnostic categories (Achenbach & Rescorla, 2001). In addition, there have been discussions regarding possible ways to incorporate multivariate approaches into future revisions of the DSM (First, 2006). The view at this time seems to be that this may likely occur with respect to Axis II personality disorder categories (see Shiner, Chapter 17, this volume), but not Axis I clinical disorder categories (Watson & Clark, 2006). Finally, another alternative may be to give up the notion of one all-encompassing diagnostic system in favor of the idea that different systems of classification may be needed for different purposes, for example, in relation to meeting clinical versus research needs, or for different clinical assessment purposes (e.g., diagnosis vs. case formulation).

Outcomes of Labeling Children

Much has been written about both positive and negative aspects of assigning diagnostic labels to children. On the positive side, it is argued that labels help to summarize and order observations; facilitate communication among professionals with different backgrounds; guide treatment strategies in a global fashion; put clinicians in touch with a preexisting, relevant body of more detailed research and clinical data; and facilitate etiological, epidemiological, and treatment outcome studies (Rains, Kitsuse, Duster, & Friedson, 1975). On the negative side are criticisms regarding how effective current diagnostic labels are in achieving any of the aforementioned purposes, and concerns about the negative effects of assigning labels to children (Hinshaw, 2006). Possible negative effects include how others perceive and react to the children (Bromfield, Weisz, & Messer, 1986), and how the labels influence children's perceptions of themselves and their behavior (Guskin, Bartel, & MacMillan, 1975).

The most important outcomes associated with the labeling of disturbed children may not be the ones associated with labeling or diagnosis by professionals. Rather, the informal labeling processes surrounding child and family behavior, and the interpretations of formal labels by parents, teachers, peers, and children themselves are likely to have the greatest impact (e.g., Coie & Pennington, 1976; Compas, Friedland-Bandes, Bastien, & Adelman, 1981; Dollinger, Thelen, & Walsh, 1980). Further study and assessment of the general beliefs and everyday cognitions of parents and teachers, how parents and teachers use labels to organize their experiences with both normal and disturbed children, and how such labeling influences their responses to and feelings about children are likely to increase our understanding of child and family disturbances (Sigel, McGillicuddy-DeLisi, & Goodnow, 1992). Several lines of research that appear promising in this regard include studies that have examined labeling and attribution processes in parents of disturbed and nondisturbed children (Bugental & Johnston, 2000), and those that have looked at "parents as problem solvers" in common, but demanding, childrearing situations (e.g., crying, noncompliance, refusal, trips to the supermarket) (Holden, 1985a, 1985b). Labeling is a prepotent human response, and there is a need to find methods to assess the usual ways in which those interacting with the children organize child behaviors. In identifying the types of labels used, the conditions under which they are used, and the effects associated with their use, it is likely that we will need to consider the unique characteristics of the interactants, as well as those universal processes that characterize humans as information processors (Kanfer, 1985).

Etiological Assumptions Regarding Childhood Disorders

Several important points concern the relationship between DSA and etiological assumptions about childhood disorders:

1. The first point concerns multiple causality. Given that the child is embedded in a complex and changing system, it is likely that many potentially relevant controlling variables contribute to the problem and need to be assessed, including physical and social-environmental events, and intraorganismic variables of both a neurobiological and a cognitive nature.

2. No a priori assumptions are made regarding the primacy of controlling variables that contribute to child and family disorders. This view rejects particular sets of controlling variables as being more important than others (e.g., physical vs. social causes) either contemporaneously or historically, and is intended to counteract the popular belief in many child assessment and treatment settings that the identification of malfunctioning physical systems through medical examination, neuropsychological testing, or historical information somehow provides a more fundamental explanation for the child's problems. Such an analysis is both incomplete and inaccurate, because it gives greater weight to physical causes in explaining child behavior and ignores potential psychosocial and environmental influences of equal or greater importance.

3. Although no assumptions are made in DSA regarding the primacy of etiological influences, primacy may be given to certain variables when they are suggested by data, or because of their methodological or practical feasibility. Variables that are observable, easily measured, and readily modified may become the focus for assessment when such an approach facilitates remediation of the problem.

4. It is assumed that there is an ongoing and reciprocal interaction among relevant controlling variables, so that attempts to identify *original* causes in assessment are not likely to be fruitful. Putative causes that occur earlier in development (e.g., birth injury or social deprivation) are important, but they are not assumed to be more significant contributors to the child and family's difficulties than contemporaneous physical and social processes.

5. The processes by which relevant controlling variables for most deviant child and family behaviors exert their influence are assumed to be similar and often continuous with those for nondeviant behavior. Principles related to basic biological and social processes are equally applicable in understanding both deviant and nondeviant behavior.

6. Although controlling variables that are contemporaneous and situationally present are frequently emphasized as important influences in DSA, there is also the need to consider both extrasituational and temporally more remote events. For example, stressors such as marital discord have a direct impact on a mother's immediate reaction to her child's behavior (Davies & Cummings, 2006). Passman and Mulhern (1977) have shown that a mother's punitiveness toward her child increases with the amount of external stress to which she is exposed, and Wahler (1980) has reported an inverse relationship between contacts with people outside the family and child behavior problems. Children's behaviors *in situ* represent only one contributor to parental reactions (e.g., Mash & Johnston, 1983), which may be influenced by not only external factors of the types just mentioned (Dunst & Trivette, 1986) but also the general rules, strategies, and propositions that parents apply in interacting with their children (Dix & Ruble, 1989; Geller & Johnston, 1995; Lytton, 1979). These influences may explain why treatment-related changes in children's behavior do not necessarily lead to changes in parental perceptions or reactions to their children.

DIMENSIONS OF DSA

One of the most salient characteristics of developing children is the active interplay that takes place between each child and her or his biological makeup, physical and social environments, and the cultural milieu into which the child is born. Guided by genetic endowment and maturation, relentlessly striving to understand the surrounding physical realities and social expectations, the child is nurtured, shaped, and socialized. No passive partners in this dialogue, children in turn shape their social world, and set their own expectations and demands (Bell & Harper, 1977; Emery, Binkoff, Houts, & Carr, 1983). This developmental engagement is characterized by conflict and equilibrium in the physical, cognitive, emotional, and social domains, and almost always by quantitative and qualitative movement and change. Any assessment of children and families must begin with recognition of the ebb and flow of this developmental dialogue, because it has critical implications for the manner in which child behaviors

are conceptualized, measured, classified, diagnosed, modified, and evaluated. The recognition that child and family behaviors are embedded within normative developmental sequences guided by organizational principles, and that they occur within a nested hierarchical context of interacting micro- and macrosocial influences (Bronfenbrenner, 1986; Cicchetti, 2006), necessitates a view of DSA that reflects both the uniqueness and the multidimensionality of children. This view leads to a number of important generalizations regarding assessment:

1. Developing children represent a unique population that requires special assessment considerations of a conceptual, methodological, and practical nature.

2. The assessment of childhood disorders necessarily involves normative judgments as to what constitutes (a) developmental deviation, (b) performance variation in relation to an appropriate reference group, (c) developmentally appropriate adaptation to a range of situational demands, and (d) unexpected deviation from a projected course of individual development. Of necessity, judgments usually include comparisons of a child with both group and self-referent norms.

3. Assessment of children and their families invariably involves multiple targets, including somatic and physiological states, behaviors, cognitions, and affects.

4. Given the large number and variety of factors at the individual and systems levels implicated for most child and family disorders, decision rules are needed for the selection of meaningful targets for assessment and intervention (Evans, 1985; Mash, 1985). When one considers the potentially infinite number of variables and their interactions that *could* be assessed in disturbed family systems, it is clear that evidence-based decision rules are needed to determine what factors *should* and *should not* be assessed, and by what methods.

5. The situations in which children function are varied and include family, day care, school, formal and informal peer groups, and other neighborhood and community settings. Embedded within each of these global settings are numerous subsettings. In light of this, multisituational analysis is the rule in DSA, and one of the tasks of assessment is to determine which aspects of the child's functioning are unique to

specific contexts, and which occur across situations.

6. The pervasiveness of developmental change and situational variation in children suggests the need to assess patterns of behavior over time, as well as more global situational consistencies, in the family, neighborhood, community, and culture.

Special Considerations in Assessing Children

Although the assessment of children has much in common with the assessment of adults, numerous conditions and constraints are associated with assessing children are not ordinarily encountered when assessing adults, including many unique ethical and legal concerns (e.g., Koocher & Rey-Casserly, 2003; McGivern & Marquart, 2000; Melton, Ehrenreich, & Lyons, 2001; Rae, Brunnquell, & Sullivan, 2003). The uniqueness of child assessment follows from generalizations about children as a group, characteristics of children and their contexts during different periods of development that may interact with the types of assessments being conducted, and common features of situations in which children ordinarily function and in which they are assessed.

Rapid and Uneven Developmental Change

With respect to generalizations about children as a group, a noteworthy characteristic is their rapid and uneven developmental change (Evans & Nelson, 1977). Such change has implications for judgments concerning child deviance and the selection of appropriate methods of assessment. Studies have described both the age trends for many child behaviors and ways in which the social significance and meaning of a problem may vary with the age of the child (e.g., Achenbach & Edelbrock, 1981; Achenbach, Howell, Quay, & Conners, 1991). Many behaviors that are common at an earlier age are considered inappropriate in an older child (e.g., noncompliance, tantrums). Some childhood problems, for example, some types of antisocial behavior, suggest a pattern of "arrested socialization" (Patterson, 1982).

Developmental deviation has been defined empirically in relation to a variation from observed behavioral norms for children of a similar age and gender (Achenbach & Edelbrock, 1981); theoretically, either in terms of a deviation from some expected behavioral pattern characteristic of particular stages of cognitive or psychosexual development (Santostefano, 1978); or in terms of the child's failure to reorganize his or her behavior over time in relation to age-appropriate developmental adaptations (Greenspan & Porges, 1984).

Cross-sectional and longitudinal data describing age trends for a range of normal and problem child behaviors are beginning to accumulate (Bongers, Koot, van der Ende, & Verhulst, 2003). Prior data based exclusively on global parent reports are being buttressed by direct observations of ongoing social interactions. Information concerning proportions of children at different ages exhibiting various problems is also being reinforced with more specific information about children's success or failure in making age-related adaptations, such as the formation of a secure attachment, the development of purposeful communication, and the regulation of emotions. Much of this research conducted in the area of developmental psychopathology is just beginning to find its way into clinical assessments with children and families (Cicchetti & Cohen, 2006c). Making normative judgments in the context of adaptations over time is quite compatible with the assumptions of DSA, because an organizational approach requires careful specification of situational demands (e.g., developmental tasks).

Normative information describing *qualitative* changes across age is needed. Although qualitative change is difficult to assess, it would appear that many childhood problems, such as fears (Southam-Gerow & Chorpita, Chapter 8, this volume), ADHD (Smith, Barkley, & Shapiro, Chapter 2, this volume), and conduct disorder (McMahon & Frick, Chapter 3, this volume), change both qualitatively and quantitatively with age. Judgments regarding deviance and normality need to be made in relation to both types of change.

Rapid and uneven developmental change also carries implications for the stability or instability of assessment information over time. Behavior at one age may not be predictive of behavior at a later time; this is especially true for assessments with very young children. For example, in examining aggressive behavior in males, Olweus (1979) reported that the degree of stability tended to decrease linearly as the interval between the two times of measurement increased, and that stability in aggressive behavior could be broadly described as a positive linear function of the interval covered and the subject's age at the time of the initial measurement.

Plasticity and Modifiability

A second characteristic of children as a group that has implications for assessment and treatment relates to the plasticity and modifiability of infants and young children in relation to environmental influences. Experience can shape both behavior and neural structure and function (Cicchetti & Curtis, 2006). Because children's behavior is under the strong and immediate social control of parents, teachers, and other children, the need for assessment of these environmental influences is usually greater than that in assessments with adults. Yet this process is also reciprocal, in that genetically guided and managed neural structures and functions can influence what is experienced and even determine the very process of learning itself. For instance, the extent to which young children perceive particular stimuli or events as threatening, thus warranting fear or even a flight response, can vary in part due to genetic variation of this trait within the population. However, the extent to which the child has been previously exposed to highly fearful and traumatic events may also sensitize the child to fear reactions in similar future exposures, beyond what his or her genetic endowment may have affected. Hence, modifiability is an interactive and potentially reciprocal process.

Age and Gender

A third characteristic of developing children is their diversity, both within and across ages. There is a need to integrate developmental principles into assessment and treatment (Edelbrock, 1984; Yule, 1993). Developmental characteristics such as a child's age and gender have implications for not only judgments about deviance but also choice of the most appropriate assessment methods. One obvious developmental consideration relates to the constraints placed on the use of child self-report measures as a function of age-related language and cognitive abilities. The nature of children's reaction to being observed and their understanding of assessment purposes also vary with age. Assessments of young children may be affected by the children's wariness of strangers, whereas adolescents may also be wary of assessment by adults, but for quite different reasons.

A child's gender also plays an important role in judgments of deviance, with concomitant implications for the interpretations of assessment information. Norms used to make judgments about child behavior and the overt behavioral reactions of parents and teachers vary as a function of whether a child is male or female. Studies have also revealed differences in the rates and expression of childhood disorders for boys and girls (see Bell, Foster, & Mash, 2005). The dimensions that emerge from multivariate studies of child behavior problems differ for boys and girls after the age of 3 (Achenbach, 1993), and recent work suggests that the same disorder (e.g., depression, conduct disorder) may manifest itself in different ways depending on the sex of the child (Bell et al., 2005).

Common Features of Assessment Situations

Several common features in the types of situations in which children are typically evaluated have implications for assessment (Evans & Nelson, 1977; Mash & Terdal, 1997b). Childhood distress is typically framed in terms of its impact on others. Children are referred by adults, which means that children who are not experiencing subjective distress may not understand the reasons they are being assessed (Reid, Patterson, Baldwin, & Dishion, 1988; Yeh & Weisz, 2001). Adult referral suggests the need to consider factors that have been shown to influence the referral process, including the type and severity of problem, parent and teacher characteristics, social class, and culture.

There is a strong relationship between learning difficulties and behavior problems in childhood, and child assessments are often carried out in the context of cognitive/intellectual evaluations (Reynolds & Kamphaus, 2003a; Sattler & Hoge, 2006) or response to intervention procedures (Speece & Hines, Chapter 13, this volume). The co-occurrence of learning and behavior problems in children reflects the more general observation that problem child behaviors rarely occur in isolation. This means that child assessment is typically multidisciplinary, involving a range of professionals, including educators, psychologists, speech pathologists, and a variety of health personnel.

It is common for children referred for assessment to undergo repeated evaluations. This is especially the case for children with chronic disabilities or conditions, for whom repeated evaluation and planning are often mandated by legislative requirements. Children who display less severe or acute problems also undergo repeated evaluations, reflecting both the fragmentation that is characteristic of mental health delivery systems for children and families, and, more positively, the need to re-evaluate children following behavioral or educational treatment programs. Repeated evaluations necessitate that assessment methods for children be robust across ages and relatively insensitive to the effects of practice.

Normative Comparisons

We have commented a number of times on both the benefits and limitations of normative comparisons. Normative information provides a way to establish an individual child's position on some dimension relative to the performance of other members of a suitable reference group. To make valid normative comparisons, valid norms are needed that reflect the distribution of scores in the populations of interest (Achenbach, 2001). Once this condition is met, it is important to examine issues related to the utility of normative comparisons generally and to the kinds of normative information that are likely to be most useful. Hartmann, Roper, and Bradford (1979) outlined a number of potential uses for normative comparisons in assessment:

1. Normative comparisons are frequently useful in identifying deficient or excessive performance, as would be the case when a child engages in excessively high rates of aggressive behavior. Normative information about rates of aggression in comparable situations by comparable children, depending on social judgments and reactions to the behavior, may serve to identify the child as having a problem.

2. When complaints about children reflect parental expectations that differ markedly from existing norms, as is the case in some abusive family situations (Mash et al., 1983), the focus and type of intervention may differ markedly from that used in the absence of such normative information.

3. When norms suggest that childhood problems are common or transient at particular ages (e.g., early reactions to separation, certain fears, bedwetting), such information may be used to guide decisions regarding the need for intervention. This is not to argue that nor-

mative difficulties are not a real concern for the child and family, or that educative or coping strategies would not be helpful in dealing with these problems. Normative disruptive behavior should not be considered "normal" without careful consideration of the context in which it occurs and its relationship to other responses and other individuals. Most normative behaviors, especially those derived from multivariate studies, are typically presented in terms of their frequency of occurrence for the general population. For example, Edelbrock (1984) noted that "arguing" was reported as a problem by more than half of the parents of nonreferred children, and "the fact that it is such a common complaint about normal children suggests that it should not receive high priority as a target for clinical treatment" (p. 29). However, it is possible that the "functions" of arguing in a group of children referred for treatment are qualitatively different than those in a non-referred population, so that in one group arguing functions as a cue for further escalation of coercive behavior, whereas in another group it may not (Patterson, 1982). Under these circumstances, frequent reports of arguing in non-clinic samples would not provide a sound basis for giving this response a low priority in treatment for clinic-referred children. Nevertheless, in many instances, knowledge that a problem is common and transient suggests that extensive clinical intervention is not required (Achenbach, 2001).

4. When there are norms for skilled versus inept performances, such information may be used to establish both intermediate treatment targets and long-term treatment goals, and to assess whether or not these goals have been met.

5. Norms may be useful for grouping children into relatively homogeneous treatment groups that subsequently could produce greater precision with respect to the most effective types of treatment for children with particular difficulties.

6. Normative information for specific assessment measures may enhance the comparability of findings obtained through different data sources. For example, parent report and direct observation measures may yield equivalent information when the scores on each reflect a similar degree of deviation, as in the case of a child rated one standard deviation above the mean on two different methods use to assess children's aggressive behavior.

7. Normative information may be useful in evaluating the clinical significance or social validity of treatment outcome, for example, to determine whether the treated child's behavior is comparable to that of nonproblem children following treatment. Researchers have noted improvement in the behavior of children with ADHD and conduct disorder with treatment, but a significant number of these children continue to function outside the normative range (Barkley & Guevremont, 1992; Kazdin & Esveldt-Dawson, 1987).

Although these described uses of norms refer primarily to behavior, normative information regarding situational factors may also help to identify some high-risk situations for the development of particular problems. For example, normative information regarding the quality of the child's school environment (e.g., high expectations, good group management, effective feedback and praise, setting of good models of behavior by teachers, pleasant working conditions, and giving students positions of trust and responsibility) may serve as a basis for the detection of early problems when such conditions are deficient, with a subsequent focus on prevention (Rutter, 1979). Similarly, norms regarding the presence or absence of certain family background variables for particular childhood disorders—for example, those related to parental antisocial personality disorder (Frick et al., 1992) or child abuse (Crooks & Wolfe, Chapter 14, this volume)—may also serve to identify high-risk situations. In general, norms for contextual factors have received far less attention than those for individual child behaviors.

Selection of Treatment Goals

The identification of behaviors that are targeted for change has been a hallmark of DSA with children and families. However, many reports begin with a designation of the problem to be treated, with little information about the decisional processes utilized in this selection. A number of important points concerning the selection of target behaviors for treatment as one outcome of the assessment process have been made (Mash & Terdal, 1997a):

1. Models of therapy and assessment that focus on a single target behavior as being synonymous with the goals of treatment provide incomplete representations of both the assessment and change process.

2. An appropriate representation of the problem space for DSA is provided by a systems framework that encompasses a wide range of potentially important responses, individuals, and contexts that might be contributing to the problem.

3. Such systems representations of the child's and family's problems require decision rules for determining how best to conceptualize the system of interest and what aspects of the system should be modified to bring about the most widespread, meaningful, and lasting changes.

4. In practice, decision rules that are often employed in assessment reflect the theoretical preferences and subjective judgments of practicing clinicians (e.g., Nurcombe, Drell, Leonard, & McDermott, 2002). Such clinical decision making is subject to a variety of information-processing errors, many of which stem from the basic limitations (e.g., limited attention and memory) of human information processors to deal with complex datasets under conditions that often involve time pressures and high levels of uncertainty (Achenbach, 1985; Cantor, 1982).

5. An actuarial approach to the selection of treatment goals, and the ways these goals might be most effectively achieved, offers promise as an adjunct to clinical decision making (Achenbach, 1985; Cattell, 1983). The ready availability of computers may facilitate such an approach (Farrell, 1991).

6. If treatment goals are conceptualized in a systems framework, then the derivation of empirically based decision rules for intervention requires that structural and functional interrelationships between different aspects of the system be documented and described. The identification of constellations of target behaviors and response covariations becomes important (Kazdin, 1982, 1985; Voeltz & Evans, 1982).

7. Target behavior selection is conceptualized as a dynamic and ongoing process in which information derived from assessment and the impact of various interventions may be utilized in reformulating treatment goals. Such an approach is consistent with the DSA emphasis on the important relationship between assessment and treatment. Not only does assessment information lead to treatment recommendations but also treatment outcomes are used to determine the need for additional as-

sessment and reformulation of the problem as necessary (Weisz, Chu, & Polo, 2004).

These points emphasize that specification of target behaviors for the individual child, *by itself*, is not likely to provide a complete representation of the family's difficulties or the range of desired treatment goals. Nevertheless, information concerning the types of child behaviors that are often the focus of intervention can be useful within the context of a broader decision-making framework (Mash & Terdal, 1997a). Such information reflects both conceptual and empirical guidelines that commonly underlie target behavior selection.

Some of the more commonly mentioned *conceptual* guidelines for selecting and prioritizing behaviors for treatment include the following:

1. The behavior is considered to be physically dangerous to the child and/or to others in the child's environment.
2. The behavior should provide an entry point into the natural reinforcement community of the child.
3. The behaviors selected should be positive, to avoid a problem focus in treatment.
4. Behaviors viewed as essentials for development should be given high priority. For example, language, cognitive development and school performance, motor skills, rule-governed behavior, problem-solving skills, and peer relationships are common treatment targets. Implicit in this emphasis is the notion that many of these behaviors are embedded in normal developmental sequences, such that the failure to take corrective action early results in cumulative deficits, with the child falling even further behind.
5. Behaviors viewed as essential early elements for more complex response chains have also received priority. Classes of general imitative behavior, compliance, and cognitive styles have been viewed as requisite behaviors that enable a range of other responses.
6. Behaviors that maximize the flexibility of the child in adapting to new, changing environments are viewed as important treatment targets. The emphasis on teaching children general coping skills and self-regulatory strategies is consistent with this notion.
7. Behaviors that dramatically change the existing contingency system for the child (e.g., parent management training), such that

maladaptive environmental reactions to the child are altered, are viewed as likely to contribute to long-term benefit.

Some of the more commonly cited *empirical* criteria for selecting particular child behaviors for treatment include the following:

1. The behaviors are consistent with some developmental or local norms for performance.
2. The behaviors have been shown, as a result of careful task analysis, to be critical components for successful performance; teaching classroom survival skills such as on-task behavior, attending, or peer discussion about class work is an example of this approach.
3. The behaviors are subjectively rated as positive by recognized community standards.
4. The behaviors effectively discriminate between "skilled" and "nonskilled" performers.
5. The behavior's natural history is known to have a poor long-term prognosis.

Multisituational Analysis

Information about the context in which the child's behavior, cognitions, and affects occur is an essential ingredient for any DSA concerned with the assessment of relevant controlling variables to be utilized in the design of effective treatments. Contextual information is crucial, because children function in many different settings. The criterion for what constitutes "competent" performance is likely to vary with the parameters of the situation, suggesting the need for situation-specific measures of behavior (e.g., Dodge, McClaskey, & Feldman, 1985) and ecological assessments (Willems, 1973, 1974). Despite the acknowledged importance of assessing situations in DSA with children and families, it continues to be an area of relative neglect. Greater within-situation differentiation, which recognizes both differences and potential functional similarities in dissimilar environments, will be needed if the potential of situational analysis for the development of effective interventions is to be realized.

One type of molecular situational analysis has examined children's differential responses to varying social stimuli, for example, parents' use of different types of commands or language constructions to direct their children's behavior (Forehand, 1977). Other studies have attempted to identify different types of home, classroom, or institutional situations or task structures that predict particular child responses. For example, home situations in which the mother is occupied; time constraints, such as dinnertime, bedtime, getting dressed, going to school; or situations involving social evaluation, such as visits to others' homes, going to the store, or visits to restaurants increase the likelihood of problem behavior in both normal and disturbed children (DuPaul & Barkley, 1992).

Other studies have examined classroom activity structures that predict different types of child social and academic behavior; examples include instructional arrangements (Greenwood, Delquadri, Stanley, Terry, & Hall, 1985), group versus individual activities (Patterson & Bechtel, 1977), quiet versus noisy conditions (Whalen, Henker, Collins, Finck, & Dotemoto, 1979), self-paced versus other-paced activities (Whalen et al., 1979), room size, seating arrangements, groupings of children based on different levels of ability, and formal versus informal task requirements (Jacob, O'Leary, & Rosenblad, 1978). Similar variables have been examined in institutional and day care environments. In addition, general environmental conditions related to space, noise, and temperature are variables of potential importance. For example, systematic variations in the rates of desirable and undesirable child behavior in the home associated with temporal and climatic variables, such as time of day, day of the week, precipitation, and temperature, have been reported (Russell & Bernal, 1977).

It is likely that situational variation will moderate not only behaviors but also cognitions and affects in family members. For example, in examining cognitions relating to perceptions of equity within the marital relationship, such perceptions may differ depending on the context that is being assessed (sex, finances, etc.). As mentioned previously, there is a need to develop a taxonomy of situations to guide both research and applied work in child and family DSA. In attempting to build such situational taxonomies, the following remarks by Mischel (1977) are of importance:

Depending on one's purpose many different classifications are possible and useful. To seek any single "basic" taxonomy of situations may be as futile as searching for a final or ultimate taxonomy of traits; we can label situations in as many different ways as we can label people. It is important to avoid emerging simply with a trait psychology of situations, in which events and settings, rather than people, are merely given different labels. The task of naming situations cannot substitute for the job of analyzing how conditions and environments interact with people in them. (pp. 337–338)

Expanded Temporal and Contextual Base

DSA assessment focuses on both contemporaneous behavior and controlling, as well as more distal, conditions. Current influences include those that are proximal to the behavior in time and to the situation in which the child's behavior is assessed. For example, an assessment of parent–child interaction may examine controlling variables in terms of the parents' responses to the child in that situation (e.g., cues and consequences). In such an assessment, developmental–historical information may not be given a particularly important role, and the parents' response could be viewed as a direct reaction to the child's immediate behavior in the situation rather than the result of the cumulative effects of many prior experiences with the child, or the parents' belief systems. However, numerous findings indicate that parents' responses are based on more than the immediate behaviors of their children. For example, parents of aggressive children may respond harshly, even when their children are behaving appropriately (Patterson, Reid, & Dishion, 1992). Thus, assessing developmental and historical factors, in addition to parent and child behaviors in the immediate situation, is important to understanding the parent–child interaction.

Similarly, broader contextual factors, such as parental personality, family climate, peer relations, marital relationships, family support, and community conditions, have been shown to be potent sources of influence for child behavior—indeed, as or more important than the reactions of significant others to the child's behavior at the time of its occurrence (Mash & Dozois, 2003). Given the multitude of situationally and temporally remote distal events that have been shown to be important determinants of child and family behavior and of treatment outcomes, a relative emphasis on the assessment of proximal information within a broader developmental, temporal, and social context is essential.

METHODS OF ASSESSMENT

DSA methods are much the same as those used in assessments with children and families more generally. They include unstructured and structured interviews, checklists and questionnaires, self-monitoring procedures, analogue assessments, psychophysiological recordings, and direct observation. The uniqueness of the methods used in DSA is based on the assumptions underlying the approach as we have described them, how the methods are used, and how the results are interpreted and integrated into treatment.

The chapters in this volume provide comprehensive reviews of the methods used to assess a wide spectrum of childhood disorders and problems. In the discussion that follows, we highlight prevalent concerns and issues associated with the use of particular methods. We emphasize again that the major underlying theme of this volume is that methods are best used in relation to specific purposes for children displaying specific types of problems. Nevertheless, because part of the assessment task initially is to identify the problem category that best describes the individual child and his or her family, some methods (e.g., screening instruments, diagnostic interviews, general behavioral checklists) are not problem-specific. In addition, a number of assessment methods have applicability across different problems, which is important because so many children referred for assessment are known to display multiple problems and disorders.

Selection of Methods

When we consider the literature on clinical assessment of children and families, along with writings in child development, abnormal child psychology, developmental psychopathology, education, and child psychotherapy, there is clearly no shortage of available instruments with which to assess children and families (Kazdin, 2005). Numerous checklists and coding systems have been developed to assess child behavior, parent–child interaction, and family interaction. In other areas, such as social support or family stress, the number of available measures is also large. What is lacking at this time seems to be an agreed-upon set of decisional criteria and rules concerning which of the available measures are best suited for particular purposes, and when and how these measures are to be used (Hunsley & Mash, 2007; Mash & Terdal, 1997a).

In practice, the most frequently used decision criteria often equate the quantity and quality of assessment information. This rather crude heuristic assumes that the best assessments sample as many domains as possible, using the widest variety of methods. Traditional test batteries, in which children receive a standardized evaluation that includes an interview with the parent and/or child, an IQ test, a projective personality test, and a test for organicity or perceptual dysfunction, illustrate this approach. Long-standing criticisms of these procedures as being insufficient for diagnosis and treatment have come from clinicians across a range of theoretical orientations (e.g., Santostefano, 1978).

Although there is much empirical support for the notion that different methods of assessment may, and often do, yield different kinds of information, the view that use of multiple methods result in a truer or more useful description of the child and family has not been adequately tested. In some instances, the accumulation of greater amounts of information in the clinical context may actually serve to reduce accuracy, while increasing judgmental confidence (Nisbett, Zukier, & Lemley, 1981). With large amounts of information, the influence of relevant diagnostic data may be diluted by the presence of an increased number of nondiagnostic features. It is important that attention be given to the incremental validity associated with use of multiple methods to avoid redundancy and the perpetuation of potentially unnecessary and costly procedures. "Incremental validity" refers to the extent to which additional information contributes to the prediction of a variable beyond what is possible with other sources of data (Hunsley & Mash, 2007). For example, does obtaining additional assessment information improve the efficiency and outcome of treatment (Hayes & Nelson, 1987, 1989; Hunsley & Meyer, 2003; Johnston & Murray, 2003)?

The many purposes for which assessments with children and families are carried out indicate that referred children need not be assessed in all possible ways (Mash & Hunsley, 2005b). What factors contribute to decision making regarding the selection of methods? Although it is not possible to discuss all factors in detail, the choice of assessment methods for a particular case is based on considerations such as the purpose(s) of the assessment (e.g., screening vs.

treatment evaluation), the nature of the problem (e.g., overt vs. covert, chronic vs. acute), the characteristics of the child (e.g., age, sex, cognitive and language skills) and of the family (e.g., social class, education, single parent vs. intact marriage), the assessment setting (e.g., clinic, home, classroom), characteristics of the assessor (e.g., conceptual preferences, level of training, available time and resources), and characteristics of the method (e.g., standardization, reliability, validity, clinical utility, complexity, sensitivity to treatment change, amount of technical resources or training required for use, feasibility in clinical practice). These and other considerations in selecting particular methods to assess specific childhood disorders are discussed in each of the chapters of this volume.

Interviews with Parents and Others

Regardless of therapeutic orientation, and despite numerous criticisms concerning reliability and validity, the clinical interview continues to be the most universal assessment procedure (Sattler, 1998). However, the interviewer's behaviors and expectations, the kinds of information obtained in the interview, the meaning given to that information, and the degree of standardization vary across therapeutic orientations and purposes (Sattler & Mash, 1998). As an information-gathering procedure, clinical interviews are used flexibly on repeated occasions and are frequently integrated with other types of assessment information, such as observations of family interaction to assess, for example, family problem-solving skills, readiness for change, adherence to treatment, and nonverbal patterns of communication.

Given that a DSA conceptualization of child and family disorders requires an understanding of reciprocal social relationships, and that children are usually referred by adults, it is almost always necessary to obtain descriptions from adults about the nature of the children's difficulties, social circumstances, physical status, and general development. Most typically a child's parent(s), usually the mother and to a lesser extent the father, are the primary informants. However, although less frequently called upon, other adults (e.g., teachers, other family members, friends) and other children (e.g., siblings and peers) may also provide useful and potentially important assessment information (Bierman & McCauley, 1987).

Interviews with parent(s) provide information about the child, the parent, the parent–

child relationship, and family relationships and characteristics more generally. The relative focus in each of these areas varies with the nature of the presenting problem and the purpose(s) for which the interview is conducted. Research has identified relationships between parental characteristics and children's functioning in both family and school settings (e.g., Forehand, Long, Brody, & Fauber, 1986), and between parental affects, such as depression, and child behavior, suggesting that information gathering in the interview needs to include a focus on the child, the parent(s), sibling relationships, and the marriage or couple relationship, as well as relationships between these various family subsystems.

Common purposes of interviews with parents include the following (Haynes & Jensen, 1979): (1) gathering information about parental concerns, expectations, and goals; (2) assessing parental perceptions and feelings about the child's problems, concerns, and goals; (3) identifying possible factors that may elicit or maintain problem behaviors; (4) obtaining historical information about the child's development, problem and nonproblem behaviors, and prior treatment efforts; (5) identifying potentially reinforcing events for both child and parent; (6) educating the parent with respect to the nature of the childhood problem (e.g., ADHD, autism), its prevalence, its prognosis, and its possible etiologies; (7) providing the parent with an adequate rationale for assessment and proposed interventions; (8) assessing the parent's affective state, motivation for changing the situation, readiness for change, and resources for taking an active role in helping to mediate behavior change; (9) obtaining informed consent; (10) providing data for the assessment of treatment outcomes, and (11) communicating with the parent about procedures and setting realistic goals for assessment and intervention.

The many interview purposes described mean that the degree of structure, content, and style of parental interviews will vary greatly for children with different problems and needs, and a lack of uniformity may be the rule rather than the exception. Several general points related to interviews with parents require discussion.

Generality and Flexibility

The first point involves the level of generality and flexibility of the interview. Typically, interviews with parents have been used to determine treatment eligibility (e.g., screening) or as methods of gaining information that facilitate the design of effective treatments (e.g., case formulation). These purposes necessarily define the interview as being general in nature and require the interviewer to adapt to the various concerns raised by parents. The degree of structure and standardization in these types of interviews with parents is usually low, but it can be increased for other interview purposes—for example, when interview information is to be used as an outcome measure, or when the interview is used to make a formal diagnosis. Alternatively, if pretreatment questionnaires include life-history information or ratings of behavior, then initial interviews can be structured around the information obtained from these questionnaires.

A number of guidelines and standardized formats have long been available for interviews with parents (e.g., Kanfer & Grimm, 1977; Wahler & Cormier, 1970). These formats are useful, although many are also quite general and make no a priori assumptions regarding the specific interview content that is likely to be most meaningful. Consistent with the theme of this book, we believe that problem-specific interview formats are needed. For instance, interviews with parents of children with anxiety should focus on anxiety-related symptoms (e.g., Silverman & Ollendick, 2005), and those with parents of children with autism should systematically obtain information about commonly identified problems, situations, and controlling variables associated with autism (Ozonoff, Goodlin-Jones, & Solomon, 2005). Rather than assuming that interviewers have the specific information needed to guide interview content and process, we believe that interview schedules that include disorder- and context-specific information lead to more systematic, standardized, efficient, and useful interviews possessing greater reliability and validity. Such problem-specific interview schedules are described in the chapters of this volume, and others are presented in the comprehensive volume on interviewing by Sattler (1998).

Reliability and Validity

It should be emphasized that questions concerning reliability and validity are meaningful only in relation to the interview purpose. For example, if the purpose of the interview is to gain information about a mother's perception of her child as a possible controlling variable for her reactions to her child, then a lack of correspondence between maternal report and that of other informants is of less concern than it would be if the mother's report is used to assess rates of child behavior over time to assess the impact of treatment.

With respect to reliability, primary concerns relate to issues such as (1) whether information obtained on one occasion is comparable to information obtained on other occasions from the same parent (e.g., stability); (2) whether information obtained from the parent is comparable to information obtained from another informant—for example, mother versus father (i.e., interobserver agreement; Edelbrock, Costello, Dulcan, Conover, & Kalas, 1986); (3) whether the information reported by the parent is consistent with other parental information in the same interview (i.e., internal consistency); and (4) whether the information obtained by one interviewer is comparable to that obtained by another with the same parent, or with data from a self-report measure completed by the parent (i.e., method error).

The first reliability concern is especially relevant in interviews that require parents to report retrospectively on their children's developmental–social history, one of the more common elements of most child assessments (Yarrow, Campbell, & Burton, 1970). It is well established that retrospective reports are likely to be unreliable and frequently distorted in the direction of socially desirable responses and dominant cultural themes (Evans & Nelson, 1977). It has also long been known that the degree of reliability is related to the nature of the events that parents are reporting (e.g., pleasant vs. unpleasant) and the level of specificity of behavior described (Lapouse & Monk, 1958).

Although parental reports may conform to the demand characteristics of the interview situation, such characteristics might not always predict socially desirable responses. For example, there may be a parental bias toward reporting more negative child behaviors and greater parental distress during an initial interview, when eligibility for treatment is being assessed, whereas posttreatment interviews may be associated with an implicit demand to report improvements in child behavior and reductions in parental distress. This latter point is especially important when interview information is to be used as a measure of treatment outcome. Parents of problem children may also be realistic about their children's behavior, in contrast to parents of nonproblem children, who may describe their children in an overly positive fashion. Interinformant agreement between parents or between teachers and parents is difficult to evaluate, because disagreement may reflect true differences in the situation in which each informant observes the child. In general, mothers have been found to be more reliable informants than fathers and usually provide descriptions of their children's behavior that are much more differentiated and situation-specific (McGillicuddy-DeLisi, 1985).

Interviews with other significant adults or with the child's friends, peers, or siblings may be potentially useful but have received little attention in assessment, in part because of ethical concerns associated with obtaining such information. For example, interviews with peers may further stigmatize the child as having a problem, with subsequent changes in how others interact with the child (Martin, 2006). At the same time, data suggest that peer evaluations may be particularly sensitive in identifying children with problems (Bierman & Welsh, 1997; Cowen, Pederson, Babigian, Izzo, & Trost, 1973), although it is not known whether peer judgments regarding the precise nature of these problems are likely to be accurate. Information obtained from siblings may also be important, in that many problem families are characterized by high rates of sibling conflict (Dunn & Munn, 1986). Studies with nonproblem families have suggested that children's views of their siblings are represented by patterns of positive and negative behaviors mixed with positive and negative feelings (Pepler, Corter, & Abramovitch, 1982). However, it may be that both perceptions and behaviors of siblings in problem families are more negatively toned (Patterson, 1982).

Structured Parental Reports about Child Behavior

In addition to unstructured interviews with parents, reports on child behavior and adjustment have also been obtained with more structured methods (Barkley, 1988; Kamphaus et al., 2000; McMahon, 1984). The most widely used methods have been global behavior rating scales requiring either binary judgments concerning the presence or absence of particular

child behaviors or ratings concerning the degree to which the behavior is present or perceived as a problem. These rating scales cover a wide range of presenting complaints and, to a somewhat lesser extent, child competencies, offer a degree of standardization that is uncharacteristic of clinical interviews, permit normative comparisons between children, are economical to administer and score, may be readily used as treatment outcome measures, and provide a rich source of information about parents' perceptions of their children's behavior, including discrepancies in parent perceptions in the same family, and the discrepancies between parent perceptions and data derived through other sources, such as reports by teachers (e.g., McDermott, 1993). On a cautionary note, data suggest that reading levels required for parents to read and understand several of the more commonly used behavior rating scales accurately often exceed parents' reading ability, a factor that has not been routinely considered in the use of rating scales with parents (Jensen, Fabiano, Lopez-Williams, & Chacko, 2006).

In the clinical context, behavior rating scales may serve as comprehensive but general screening instruments, most typically during the early phases of assessment. They provide a reasonable estimate of parental perceptions of a child's overall behavior and adjustment, as aggregated across a wide variety of situations. However, they fail to provide situation-specific information about behavior, or information that can be used to develop a program of intervention. Nevertheless, they may assist in identifying a specific problem, which, in combination with other diagnostic information, may suggest a specific form of evidence-based treatment. Most ratings scales have been used with parents of school-age children, but several checklists and rating scales have now been developed for use with toddlers and younger children (see, e.g., Brassard & Boehm, 2007; DelCarmen-Wiggins & Carter, 2004). For children younger than age 2, the most commonly used parent report measures have been subsumed under the general characteristic of infant temperament (e.g., Rothbart & Goldsmith, 1985; Slabach, Morrow, & Wachs, 1991; Stifter & Wiggins, 2004).

As we have noted, extensive multivariate analyses of parent-completed behavior rating scales have yielded consistent factors, although the factors that emerge vary with the age and sex of the child, the setting, and a variety of informant characteristics, including ethnicity, race, or income level (e.g., Gdowski, Lachar, & Kline, 1985; Gross et al., 2006). Within a DSA framework, such variations are consistent with the view that behaviors vary in degree and type across situations, and that different informants structure their views of the child in different ways. Although there is a need for more measures with situational norms, the likelihood that the most frequently used checklists will be modified in this direction seems quite low, in light of the large-scale empirical efforts that often go into establishing a sound normative database and psychometric characteristics for behavior rating scales.

One concern surrounding the use of parent behavior rating scales has been the degree of correspondence (or lack thereof) between reports by different informants, most commonly between mothers and fathers, parents and teachers, and, to a lesser extent, children and parents or teachers (e.g., Achenbach, Krukowski, Dumenci, & Ivanova, 2005; Achenbach, McConaughy, & Howell, 1987; De Los Reyes & Kazdin, 2004, 2005). Some researchers have reported high agreement (correlation of .69) between parents on global checklists for both narrow- and broad-band syndromes (Achenbach, 1985, p. 104). However, the degree of agreement or disagreement between parents likely depends on the types of measures being compared (e.g., narrow-band syndromes vs. profiles) and the type of agreement index that is used. Reports by mothers, compared to those by fathers, can lead to different profile interpretations and judgments of clinical significance (Hulbert, Gdowski, & Lachar, 1986). Furthermore, when different raters seeing children in different contexts are compared, interrater agreement tends to be quite low (Achenbach et al., 1987).

In addition to global rating scales and structured interviews, many parent-completed measures that focus on specific content areas or problems have also been developed. These include, for example, parental ratings of a child's overall development, ADHD, autism, self-control, psychopathy, or oppositional defiant disorder (e.g., Hommersen, Murray, Ohan, & Johnston, 2006).

Another type of parent report, used during initial assessments and to monitor changes during treatment, involves parent recording of targeted child behaviors. Typically, parents collect baseline data on one or two general (e.g., compliance) or specific (e.g., swearing) behaviors that may subsequently be targeted for modification. Less frequently, parents also collect systematic data about antecedent and consequent events to identify potentially important controlling variables to be utilized in treatment. Many different forms have been developed to assist parents in recording their children's behavior. Such forms are common fare in almost all manuals used in parent management training programs. Records kept by parents have the advantage of providing ongoing information in relevant settings, information about behaviors of interest that might not otherwise be accessible to observation in other contexts, and also secondary benefits not directly related to assessment. These include teaching parents better observation, tracking, and monitoring skills; assessing parental motivation; and providing parents with more realistic estimates of their children's rate of responding and feedback on the effects of treatment. On the negative side, there are many practical problems in getting parents to keep accurate records, and parental recordings of behavior may be reactive in the home situation, producing unrepresentative data. In addition, although parent recordings have been used extensively, there is little information available concerning their reliability or validity.

In most cases, parents are the primary informants in assessments of their children, because parental perceptions often determine what, if anything, will be done about their children's problems. Furthermore, professionals' judgments regarding childhood disorders may be influenced more by what parents say about their children than by observed child behavior. Because parent-completed checklists and rating scales provide more information more quickly than could otherwise be obtained through interviews, and are also much more economical with respect to cost, effort, and therapists' time, they are likely to continue to be widely used (Kamphaus et al., 2000).

Parent Self-Ratings

Recent approaches to DSA have increasingly emphasized the importance of assessing parents' self-reported perceptions, cognitions, and feelings (Mash & Terdal, 1997a). Earlier work tended to utilize parents' reports about themselves primarily in areas directly related to the children's problems (e.g., "How does it make you feel when he does not listen to you?"). Parents' feelings, attitudes, and cognitions were considered important variables, but usually in relation to their influences on how parents reacted to their children or as predictors of the likelihood that parents would involve themselves in treatment. Although these considerations continue, assessment of parents' reports about themselves has increasingly been viewed as important in understanding the nature of the families' problems and in determining potential targets for intervention. Although self-report information from both parents should be obtained, in practice, mothers more frequently provide information than do fathers.

Parent self-ratings have included a variety of procedures designed to assess parental behavior and disciplinary practices, parental cognitions, and parental affects. One type of self-rating concerns reported parenting practices, as assessed with questionnaires about parents' use of discipline (Arnold & O'Leary, 1993) or parents' brief written reports of what they would do in audiotaped or videotaped scenarios of child behavior or situations. Such analogue assessments are a reflection of how parents think they would respond, and the degree of correspondence between expressed intent and actual parent behavior in these situations has received little empirical investigation. Although potentially useful, these analogue self-reports have not been used routinely in clinical practice.

The increasing focus on cognitive variables in DSA, in cognitive-behavioral treatment, and in the study of parent–child relationships more generally, has led to the development of a host of self-report measures that describe different types of parental cognitions. Such measures have been used to assess constructs such as general attitudes about children and child rearing (e.g., Schaefer & Bell, 1958); implicit theories about discipline (e.g., Dix & Ruble, 1989); satisfaction in areas concerned with spouse support, the child–parent relationship, parent performance, family discipline, and control (e.g., Guidubaldi & Cleminshaw, 1985); parental self-esteem, as reflected in degree of comfort in the parenting role and perceived effectiveness as a parent (e.g., Johnston & Mash, 1989); expectations for development and developmentally appropriate behavior (e.g., Azar, Robinson, Hekemian, & Twentyman, 1984); parent attributional processes (Bugental, Johnston,

New, & Silvester, 1998), including those related to the causes of child behavior (e.g., Miller, 1995), childrearing outcomes (Bugental, 1993), or specific problems, such as enuresis (Butler, Brewin, & Forsythe, 1986) or ADHD (Johnston & Ohan, 2005); problem-solving skills in regard to commonly occurring child behaviors and childrearing situations (e.g., Holden, 1985a); empathy in general (e.g., Chlopan, McBain, Carbonell, & Hagen, 1985) and in the parenting domain (e.g., Newberger, 1978); and emotion recognition (e.g., Kropp & Haynes, 1987).

Studies of the cognitive and affective processes of parents have provided information about relationships between parental cognitions and behavior; possible differences in the cognitions of parents in disturbed versus nondisturbed families; and the ways in which parents process information about demanding childrearing situations, including their use of anticipatory or proactive strategies (Holden, 1985b), how anger influences thinking (Dix & Reinhold, 1990), and the effects of maternal mood on child evaluation and parent–child interaction (Jouriles, Murphy, & O'Leary, 1989; Jouriles & Thompson, 1993). Information concerning parents' decisional processes seems especially relevant to formulating treatment goals, because parents' problem solving styles may be directly targeted for treatment (e.g., Blechman, 1985). Many of the measures described have been used in a research context, and their potential utility in clinical assessment needs to be evaluated. Furthermore, a number of different cognitive dimensions have been assessed, and more work is needed to determine whether these are in fact independent dimensions.

An interest in how parents of problem and nonproblem children cope with the stresses surrounding child rearing has led to the development of measures designed to assess the stresses associated with being a parent (e.g., Abidin, 1995), the degree to which specific types of child behavior may be perceived as disturbing (e.g., Mooney & Algozzine, 1978), and the impact on parents of specific handicapping child conditions, such as hearing loss or intellectual disability. Similarly, growing interest in the social networks surrounding disturbed families has led to the development of measures of perceived social support and/or social isolation (e.g., Bristol, 1983; Dunst, Jenkins, & Trivette, 1984; Dunst & Trivett, 1985;

Salzinger, Kaplan, & Artemyeff, 1983; Wahler, Leske, & Rogers, 1979).

Much work has also been directed at parents' reports of their own mood states, particularly maternal anxiety and depression (e.g., Billings & Moos, 1986). A rapidly growing literature documents the profound impact of maternal depression on child functioning and family relationships, beginning in early infancy (Goodman & Gotlib, 2002). Although the prevalence of self-reported depression in mothers of problem children is high, the causal status surrounding this mood state as a determinant or outcome of disturbed family interactions is still under investigation. Likewise, research continues on whether feelings of depression may negatively color parent's views of their children (Richters, 1992).

In summary, parent self-ratings have been used to assess a variety of important characteristics that may contribute to how parents react to, and are affected by, their disturbed children. In addition, assessments of many of the cognitions and affects are likely to suggest important areas for needed interventions, such as when a parent is depressed. In consideration of the future use and development of such self-ratings, a number of evaluative criteria for selecting a self-report measure have been suggested, including whether it can be administered repeatedly as an outcome measure; whether it provides sufficient specificity; whether it is sensitive to treatment changes; whether it guards against common self-report biases, such as social desirability, acquiescence, demand characteristics, faking, or lying; and whether it possesses adequate reliability, validity, and norms (Hartmann, 1984). Many of the parent self-ratings used thus far in child and family DSA do not yet meet these criteria.

Child Self-Report

Concerns regarding the reliability, validity, and practical difficulties associated with obtaining self-report information from children, especially young children, resulted in a minimal reliance on such measures in early work in child and family DSA. Although interviews and checklists of the types administered to adults may not be very informative with preschool- or grade-school-age children, flexible interview formats that are consistent with a child's developmental level can provide important information about the child's behavior, thought

processes, affect, self-perceptions, and views of the environment (Greenspan & Greenspan, 2003; McConaughy, 2005).

The increased use of interviews and child-completed checklists and questionnaires, particularly with older children and adolescents (Bierman, 1983; Bierman & Schwartz, 1986; Reynolds, 1993), is related to a number of factors: (1) the growing recognition of children's unique position as observers of themselves and their social environment; (2) the accumulation of data in support of the notion that children's cognitions and emotions directly influence their behavior and often mediate the effects of intervention; (3) the increased emphasis on children's thoughts and feelings as potential targets for treatment, and the concomitant increase in the use of cognitively based therapy procedures (Kendall, 2006); (4) the growing concern for childhood internalizing disorders, such as depression (Rudolph & Lambert, Chapter 5, this volume) and anxiety (Southam-Gerow & Chorpita, Chapter 8, this volume), which require assessment of children's self-reported feelings; and (5) the development and widespread availability of a number of well-standardized, psychometrically sound structured and semistructured interview and questionnaire procedures.

Unstructured Interviews

The format and content of assessment interviews with children should vary in relation to the child's developmental status, the nature of the child's problem, and the interview purpose. Purposes vary but typically include attempts to elicit information regarding children's perceptions of themselves and their problems, and to obtain samples of how children handle themselves in social situations with adults or other children (Sattler, 1998). Children's views of the circumstances that have brought them to the clinic, expectations for improvement, and comprehension of the assessment situation are all important to assess, as is the manner in which the children interpret significant events in their lives, such as divorce (Kurdek, 1986) or sexual abuse (Wolfe, Chapter 15, this volume). In addition, children's perceptions of their parents, siblings, teachers, and peers likely influence their reactions to them, and are therefore especially important for understanding children's problems, designing interventions, and assessing the suitability of involving such individuals in intervention. Interviews may also focus on obtaining more specific types of information that children are in a unique position to report, such as their preferred activities and rewards.

Semistructured and Structured Interviews

Unstructured clinical interviews for the purpose of making a formal diagnosis can be extremely unreliable. There are several sources of unreliability, including a lack of clarity concerning decision rules, and the operation of confirmatory biases and other types of judgmental errors (Achenbach, 1985). As a result, structured interviews have been used extensively in research studies with a primary focus on identifying homogeneous populations of children conforming to particular diagnostic criteria. However, their use in clinical practice has been less common, mostly due to training requirements, time, and other resource demands.

A number of structured and semistructured diagnostic interviews for children and adolescents were developed in the late 1970s and early 1980s, for example, the Diagnostic Interview Schedule for Children and Adolescents (Costello, Edelbrock, & Costello, 1985; Costello, Edelbrock, Kalas, Kessler, & Klaric, 1982), the Child Assessment Schedule (Hodges, 1985), the Schedule for Affective Disorders and Schizophrenia for School-Age Children (Chambers et al., 1985; Puig-Antich & Chambers, 1978), and the Diagnostic Interview for Children and Adolescents (Herjanic & Reich, 1982). These interview schedules have undergone changes to accommodate subsequent revisions in DSM criteria, and the reader is referred to various chapters in this volume for discussions of the applicability of these interviews to specific childhood disorders.

Numerous empirical investigations with these interviews have produced interesting findings that have implications for the assessment of children more generally. For example, the reliability of the interview may interact with the particular dimension (e.g., affective, cognitive, behavioral) being evaluated. Edelbrock, Costello, Dulcan, Kalas. and Conover (1985) found that for descriptions of internal states, the reliability of the interview was related to the child's age; children under age 10 showed little consistency in their interview reports, even over periods as brief as 1 or 2 weeks. Young children showed a particular tendency to change their responses from affirmative during an initial interview to negative in a second interview several days later.

The potential utility of structured psychiatric interviews in clinical practice is not clear at this time. Certainly, the increased standardization and gains in reliability associated with use of these procedures provide some advantages. However, most of the structured interview formats tend to produce global indices concerning the presence or absence of a disorder rather than the more specific information needed to formulate a picture of a particular child, family, and peer group for the purposes of intervention. It is possible that more cost-effective methods (e.g., checklists and rating scales) can provide the necessary information concerning the presence of a disorder in a way that frees up time and resources to generate more useful information for treatment (cf. Pelham et al., 2005).

Few structured child interviews have been developed for purposes other than obtaining a formal diagnosis. Bierman (1983) presented some extremely useful guidelines as to how such interviews might be developed, illustrating how empirical information about developmental processes (e.g., person perception as related to age) may be used to determine the types of questions asked in an interview. The few structured formats for interviews with children have been developed primarily as research instruments. However, growing interest in children's perceptions and feelings in DSA suggests that greater standardization may be warranted in interview procedures with children for purposes other than formal diagnosis, particularly in interview procedures that are feasible in clinical practice. Presumably, such standardized instruments would examine children's reports in relation to a variety of commonly occurring situations in the home and classroom that are relevant for children with specific types of disorders.

Child-Completed Checklists and Questionnaires

The number and use of child-completed checklists and questionnaires in DSA have also increased (Reynolds, 1993). Although the content and response format for child-completed measures have varied with children's developmental status, these measures have for the most part been used with older children, and often as a measure of treatment outcome. A wide variety of self-report instruments have been developed for describing the cognitive, affective, and behavioral domains (Myers & Winters, 2002; Winters, Myers, & Proud, 2002). Although many of the early self-report measures were downward extensions of instruments initially developed for adults, current measures are based more directly on work with children. Some of the areas that have been assessed with child-completed checklists and questionnaires include general personality dimensions, such as introversion–extroversion; anxiety and depression; perceived locus of control; social competence; self-esteem and self-concept in general, and academic or social domains specifically; anxiety and depression; cognitive distortions; perceptions of family members and peers; and perceived behavior problems and competencies. A discussion of relevant child-completed checklists and questionnaires as used in the context of specific disorders is provided in each of the chapters that follow.

Self-Monitoring Procedures

A number of discussions of self-monitoring procedures in assessments with children, as well as related methodological issues, are available (e.g., Bornstein, Hamilton, & Bornstein, 1986; Shapiro & Cole, 1984). There is a long tradition of having children use self-monitoring procedures for behaviors such as attention in the classroom (Broden, Hall, & Mitts, 1971), academic responses (Lovitt, 1973), class attendance (McKenzie & Rushall, 1974), talking out in class (Broden et al., 1971), and aggression (Lovitt, 1973). In most instances, self-monitoring procedures with children have been undertaken as part of a larger set of self-assessment procedures (e.g., recording, evaluation) intended to modify the behavior being monitored. There are few descriptions of children self-monitoring their own behavior and life situations to provide diagnostic information for developing treatments or measuring treatment outcomes. Consequently, the assessment functions of self-monitoring procedures with children have not received much elaboration. In recent work, electronic diaries hold promise in providing the type of ongoing information about behavior in contexts that could be useful for developing a treatment plan and monitoring treatment progress and outcomes (Whalen et al., 2006).

Direct Observations of Behavior

Mash and Terdal (1976) have described a direct observational procedure as a method for obtaining samples of clinically important behaviors and settings (in relation to diagnosis, treatment design, prognosis, and evaluation), in a naturalistic or an analogue situation structured to provide information about behaviors and settings comparable to what would have been obtained *in situ*. Direct observational methods usually involve recording behavior when it occurs; using trained and impartial observers who follow clearly specified rules and procedures regarding the timing of observations and their context; using previously designated categories that require a minimal degree of inference; and using some procedure to assess reliability (Barrios, 1993; Cone & Foster, 1982; Hartmann, 1982; Reid et al., 1988).

It has been argued that direct observation is less subject to bias and distortion than are verbal reports from either children or parents and teachers. However, this question cannot really be addressed without considering the informant, the child or family behavior being described, and the context and purposes for assessment. Furthermore, support for this argument comes as much from studies demonstrating poor reliability and validity associated with verbal report as from studies directly demonstrating observational data to be accurate and unbiased. In fact, many studies have shown that observed behavior may be readily distorted by biases on the part of both observers and those being observed. For example, Johnson and Lobitz (1974) demonstrated that parents of nonproblem children can make their children look either good or bad when instructed to do so. However, it is possible that some types of problem families may find it difficult to make themselves "look good" to outside observers. For example, it has been reported that abusive mothers continue to behave in ways considered to be socially undesirable, even when they are being observed (Mash et al., 1983; Reid, Taplin, & Lorber, 1981). Nevertheless, in light of the demand characteristics of most observation situations (e.g., relating to diagnosis of the problem, eligibility for treatment, educational placement, legal adjudication, and evaluation of treatment change), it seems likely that observation likely influences the behavior of those being observed.

In discussing observational procedures, it should be noted that given the findings related to possible biases and reactivity in direct observation, the potential unrepresentativeness of observational data, the current conceptual emphasis on cognitive and affective variables in DSA, and particularly the many practical concerns and demands associated with observational procedures in clinical practice, the utility of direct observation as a clinical assessment procedure has yet to be established (Mash & Foster, 2001).

Observational Procedures with Children and Families

A wide range of observational procedures have been used to assess children and families, ranging from simple single-behavior or single-purpose recording schemes that can be conducted with a minimal amount of observer training to complex and exhaustive multi-behavior, multicontext interaction code systems (Reid et al., 1988). The numerous factors involved in selecting an appropriate observational procedure include the stage and purpose of the assessment, the behaviors of interest, the situation in which observation is to occur, observer characteristics, and technical resources (Mash & Terdal, 1981).

There are detailed discussions in the literature on direct observational assessment procedures, and the methodological and practical issues surrounding their use (e.g., Barrios, 1993; Foster & Cone, 1986; Hartmann, 1982). These issues are concerned with factors influencing the objectivity and reliability of observations, such as code system characteristics (e.g., number, complexity, and molecularity of categories); characteristics of the behaviors being observed (rate and complexity); methods of assessing reliability (e.g., awareness of reliability checks); observer characteristics (e.g., age, sex); methods of calculating reliability; sources of observer and observee bias under a range of conditions; reactivity to being observed; and ways in which observational data should be summarized and interpreted. An extensive discussion of these issues is beyond the scope of this chapter, but sensitivity to these methodological concerns is a necessary part of any observational assessment of children and families, because they have a direct bearing on the validity of the findings. A minimally acceptable set of criteria for any observational code would be that it is objective (e.g., two observers classify behavior in the same way), that it has mutually exclusive subcategories, and that it provides data that are amenable to objective analysis. Given these minimal requirements, further validation as to a wide range of goals and purposes is possible.

Selecting Code Categories

The use of observational codes requires decisions relating to both the content (e.g., what categories to include) and the structure (e.g., number of categories, temporal base, mechanics for observing and recording) of the code system (Hawkins, 1982). For the most part, content, code selection, and observational system construction have been carried out on a rational basis. Consistent with the view of maintaining low levels of inference, the family behaviors observed are often those directly reported as problematic by parents and teachers, or those that fit with the theories or experiences of the assessor. We believe that category and code system selection can be improved, with greater attention to the parameters associated with the specific populations of families being observed and the settings in which they function. Specialized observational assessment coding systems for specific childhood disorders are provided in some of the chapters of this volume. These systems reflect behaviors and setting variables shown to have empirical relevance for the disorders being assessed.

Recently, more attention has been given to observations that focus on not only molecular responses but also larger, more global units for describing family interaction. Implicit in this trend are the notions (1) that larger response chains have qualitative features of their own, and although molecular codes may not reveal these dimensions, subjective impressions by trained or "culturally sensitive" human observers may; and (2) that global ratings can provide a more efficiently obtained and equivalent integrative summary of the molecular responses. When Weiss and Chaffin (1986) compared two marital code systems based on either global ratings of communication or on many specific categories, they found that the degree of overlap was moderate and pointed out that the two systems might be useful for different purposes, and that in light of the high costs of using complex category systems, the use of more global ratings might be explored. Several researchers supplemented molecular observations with more global judgments and found that experienced raters whose global judgments are averaged and composited can often provide reliable and valid indices of psychologically complex behaviors (Moskowitz & Schwarz, 1982; Weinrott, Reid, Bauske, & Brummett, 1981). It would appear that there are assets and liabilities associated with the use of molar and molecular ratings, and that some combination of the two may be useful (Cairns & Green, 1979). If future empirical work can establish the utility, reliability, and validity of more global ratings for specific purposes, then the next step would be to promote the use of these procedures in the clinical context.

There has also been an increased interest in coding the affective qualities of interactions, in part as a result of the many studies that have found relationships between depression and behavior problems in families. Some code systems have superimposed a more subjectively based valence code over the behavioral dimension. It is possible, for example, to code compliant behavior that has either positive or negative accompanying affect (Dishion et al., 1984). Other observational systems code specific affects, such as anger, contempt, whining, sadness, or fear directly (Gottmann & Levenson, 1986), or code *categories* of affect, such as aversion, dysphoria, happiness, or caring (Hops & Davis, 1995). The work on affective coding in child and family behavioral assessment is relatively recent, and the empirical findings are sparse. In addition, most of this work has been conducted in a research context, and its direct applicability to clinical assessment and intervention is just now being explored. Nevertheless, it would appear that this promising trend in the observational assessment of children and families will likely continue.

Settings for Observation

Following from a situation-specific view of behavior, observational assessments with children have been carried out in a wide range of settings, the most common of which are the clinic, the home, and the classroom (Harris & Reid, 1981; Zangwill & Kniskern, 1982). Other examples of observational settings have included institutional environments, such as group homes for delinquent adolescents, living environments for intellectually disabled or autistic children, playgrounds, supermarkets, and children's groups. More specific situations within each of these global settings have also provided structure for observation—for example, free play versus command–compliance instructions in the clinic, or observation at mealtime versus bedtime in the home.

A major concern associated with the choice of observational settings has been the degree of control imposed on the situation by the assessor. Assessors have previously emphasized the importance of observation in the child and family's natural environment, imposing the least amount of structure as possible, to see things "as they typically occur." This emphasis has reflected a reaction against the nonrepresentative and exclusive clinic observations characteristic of many clinical child assessments. Although *in situ* assessment is still recognized as an important part of DSA with children, there is also an increased recognition that unstructured observations—in the home or preschool, for example—may not always be the most efficient or practical method for obtaining samples of the behaviors of interest.

Observation in natural environments may be especially unrevealing with behaviors that occur at a low rate or that are especially reactive to observation. Many nonstructured family and peer interactions consist of no interactions or low-rate "chatty" exchanges (Mash & Barkley, 1986). For example, in one study of nonproblem families, over one-third of the observations were characterized by mutual noninvolvement of family members (Baskett, 1985). In another study, in which dominance and dependent behaviors were observed in the preschool, almost 8 weeks of observation were required to obtain generalizable data (Moskowitz & Schwarz, 1982). Such findings suggest that, in some circumstances, the use of "evocative" situations to highlight infrequently occurring response systems may prove to be a more efficient and reliable assessment strategy than the use of unstructured naturalistic observations.

In further contrasting naturalistic and structured observations, the assumption that home observations are "natural" and that observations in the clinic or laboratory are "artificial" is an oversimplification. Home observations may at times provide us with artificial reactions to natural conditions, whereas clinic observations may provide us with natural reactions to artificial conditions. Which information is more meaningful depends a great deal on the purpose of the assessment. When cross-setting comparisons of behavior (e.g., home vs. clinic) do not agree, this cannot be assumed to be a function of the unrepresentativeness of behavior in the clinic, unless there is some independent verification of the representativeness of the home observation. In most instances there is no such verification; therefore, it is inaccurate to equate representativeness with the naturalness of the physical setting, as is often done.

When home or classroom observations have been neither feasible nor appropriate, a variety of structured laboratory or clinic observation settings for sampling the behaviors of interest may be utilized (Hughes & Haynes, 1978). Such analogue situations have provided a wide range of structures for assessing parent–child behaviors, including free-play interactions between parent and child; a variety of command–compliance situations, such as the parent having the child clean up or put away play materials, or occupy him- or herself while the parent is busy reading or talking on the telephone; academic task situations; problem-solving situations, such as figuring out how to play a game together; and highly structured observations of the social reinforcement properties or punishment styles of parents. The range of potentially relevant analogue situations to be used in assessment is restricted only by the ingenuity and physical resources of the assessor. The challenge, however, is for systematic assessments of reliability and validity that permit the use of more standardized, psychometrically well-developed, and practical analogues than have been the case to date (Mash & Foster, 2001).

Using and Interpreting Observational Data

Direct observational data are utilized for a number of assessment purposes: They can serve as a basis for making recommendations for treatment and be used to monitor treatment progress and outcomes. Perhaps the most frequent but least understood use is with respect to treatment, because the processes by which direct observations have been translated into clinical recommendations are often poorly defined, unspecified, or oversimplified. However, in practice, these types of observation-based treatment recommendations represent informal hypothesis testing rather than systematically or empirically derived outcomes. It is also not clear whether such recommendations represent the fitting of observations to preferred and/or common hypotheses, or the derivation of hypotheses that are genuinely based on what has been observed.

Interpretations of observational data have typically followed from summarizations of child behavior–adult response sequences over relatively brief time intervals. It is often the pattern of behavior based on interactional responses in immediately adjacent time intervals about which interpretations are made, with the assumption that immediate cues and reactions serve as major controlling events. For example, a mother's reaction to her child's behavior is assumed to follow from the child's response that preceded it. However, the causes for both child and adult behavior may emanate from more remote points in observational sequences than those immediately adjacent in time; there is a need for empirical and conceptual criteria that can be utilized to formulate interpretations of observational data based on stylistic patterns of responding, and in relation to more distal controlling events.

Perhaps the most recurrent issue in the use of observational assessment procedures has been their feasibility of use in clinical practice, including concerns related to cost. The latter has been noted as one factor in the lack of observational procedures use by clinicians. Interestingly, the cost (including dry runs, observer time, travel costs, and data summarization) of a comprehensive observational assessment can amount to less than the cost of a comprehensive personality assessment (Reid et al., 1988).

Family Assessment Methods

Consistent with the conceptualization and treatment of childhood disorders in the context of the family (Alexander & Parsons, 1982; Sroufe & Fleeson, 1986), many measures designed to tap family functioning have been developed. Many of these "family measures" are being incorporated into the DSA of children and families (e.g., Foster & Robin, 1997). Myriad tools have been created for assessing relational problems in the family (Mash & Johnston, 1996b). For example, in the *Handbook of Family Measurement Techniques* (Touliatos, Perlmutter, Straus, & Holden, 2001), well over 1,000 instruments are reviewed. For more specific information related to family assessment methods, the reader is referred to the comprehensive volumes on family assessment by Touliatos and colleagues (2001), Grotevant and Carlson (1989), Jacob and Tennenbaum (1988), and McCubbin and Thompson (1987).

Formal Testing with Children

The use of developmental scales, intelligence and achievement tests (Kamphaus, 2005), perceptual–motor tests, neuropsychological assessments (D'Amato, Fletcher-Janzen, & Reynolds, 2005; Yeates, Ris, & Taylor, 2000), personality tests, and many other instruments is common practice among clinicians who assess children and families (Kamphaus et al., 2000). The reader is referred to individual chapters in this volume for discussions of the utility of specific tests in DSA with specific populations of children, and to general resources describing the use of these other tests (e.g., Reynolds & Kamphaus, 2003a, 2003b; Sattler, 2001; Sattler & Hoge, 2006).

SUMMARY

In describing some of the more general issues characterizing the DSA of children and families in this introductory chapter, we have tried to set the stage for detailed discussions of the assessment of specific types of childhood disturbances in the chapters that follow. We have presented the view that DSA with children and families is best depicted as a problem-solving strategy for the clinical evaluation of disturbed children and families. This highly empirical approach to clinical child assessment uses theory and research to guide the selection of constructs to be assessed for a specific assessment purpose; the methods, informants, and measures to be used in the assessment; and the manner in which the assessment process unfolds. It involves the recognition that even with data from psychometrically strong measures, the assessment process is inherently a decision-making task in which the clinician must iteratively formulate and test hypotheses by integrating data that are often incomplete or inconsistent. Therefore, it is important to evaluate the accuracy and usefulness of this complex decision-making task in light of potential errors in data synthesis and interpretation, the costs associated with the assessment process

and, ultimately, the impact the assessment has on clinical outcomes for the children and families being assessed (Hunsley & Mash, 2007). Recent work in DSA has become increasingly systems oriented and sensitive to developmental parameters. A general theme we have emphasized in this introduction is that DSA of children and families is most meaningful when strategies are based on empirically established measurement principles and derived in relation to specific childhood disorders. This is the theme that underlies the chapters that follow.

REFERENCES

Abidin, R. R. (1995). *Parenting Stress Index professional manual* (3rd ed.). Odessa, FL: Psychological Assessment Resources.

Achenbach, T. M. (1985). *Assessment and taxonomy of child and adolescent psychopathology.* Beverly Hills, CA: Sage.

Achenbach, T. M. (1991). *Integrative guide for the 1991 CBCL/4–18, YSR and TRF profiles.* Burlington: University of Vermont, Department of Psychiatry.

Achenbach, T. M. (1993). *Empirically based taxonomy: How to use syndromes and profile types derived from the CBCL/4–18, TRF, and YSF.* Burlington: University of Vermont, Department of Psychiatry.

Achenbach, T. M. (2001). What are norms and why do we need valid ones? *Clinical Psychology: Science and Practice, 8,* 446–450.

Achenbach, T. M., & Edelbrock, C. S. (1978). The classification of child psychology: A review and analysis of empirical efforts. *Psychological Bulletin, 85,* 1275–1301.

Achenbach, T. M., & Edelbrock, C. S. (1981). Behavioral problems and competencies reported by parents of normal and disturbed children aged four through sixteen. *Monographs of the Society for Research in Child Development, 46*(1, Serial No. 188).

Achenbach, T. M., Howell, C. T., Quay, H. C., & Conners, C. K. (1991). National survey of problems and competencies among four- to sixteen-year-olds. *Monographs of the Society for Research in Child Development, 56*(3, Serial No. 225).

Achenbach, T. M., Krukowski, R. A., Dumenci, L., & Ivanova, M. Y. (2005). Assessment of adult psychopathology: Meta-analyses and implications of cross-informant correlations. *Psychological Bulletin, 131,* 361–382.

Achenbach, T. M., McConaughy, S. H., & Howell, C. T. (1987). Child/adolescent behavioral and emotional problems: Implications of cross-informant correlations for situational specificity. *Psychological Bulletin, 101,* 213–232.

Achenbach, T. M., & Rescorla, L. A. (2000). *Manual for the ASEBA preschool forms and profiles.*

Burlington: University of Vermont, Research Center for Children, Youth, and Families.

Achenbach, T. M., & Rescorla, L. A. (2001). *Manual for the ASEBA school-age forms and profiles.* Burlington: University of Vermont, Research Center for Children, Youth, and Families.

Achenbach, T. M., & Rescorla, L. A. (2006a). Developmental issues in assessment, taxonomy, and diagnosis of psychopathology: Life span and multicultural perspectives. In D. Cicchetti & D. J. Cohen (Eds.), *Developmental psychology: Vol. 1. Theory and method* (2nd ed., pp. 139–180). New York: Wiley.

Achenbach, T. M., & Rescorla, L. A. (2006b). *Multicultural understanding of child and adolescent psychopathology: Implications for mental health assessment.* New York: Guilford Press.

Adams, H. E., Doster, J. A., & Calhoun, K. S. (1977). A psychologically based system of response classification. In A. R. Ciminero, K. S. Calhoun, & H. E. Adams (Eds.), *Handbook of behavioral assessment* (pp. 47–78). New York: Wiley.

Adelman, H. S. (1995). Clinical psychology: Beyond psychopathology and clinical interventions. *Clinical Psychology: Science and Practice, 2,* 28–44.

Adelman, H. S., & Taylor, L. (1988). Clinical child psychology: Fundamental intervention questions and problems. *Clinical Psychology Review, 8,* 637–665.

Alexander, J. G., & Parsons, B. V. (1982). *Functional family therapy.* Monterey, CA: Brooks/Cole.

American Psychiatric Association. (1980). *Diagnostic and statistical manual of mental disorders* (3rd ed.). Washington, DC: Author.

American Psychiatric Association. (1987). *Diagnostic and statistical manual of mental disorders* (3rd ed., rev.). Washington, DC: Author.

American Psychiatric Association. (1994). *Diagnostic and statistical manual of mental disorders* (4th ed.). Washington, DC: Author.

American Psychiatric Association. (2000). *Diagnostic and statistical manual of mental disorders* (4th ed. text rev.). Washington, DC: Author.

Ancill, R. J., Carr, A. C., & Rogers, D. (1985). Comparing computerized self-rating scales for depression with conventional observer ratings. *Acta Psychiatrica Scandinavica, 71,* 315–317.

Angold, A., Costello, E., Farmer, E. M. Z., Burns, B. J., & Erkanli, A. (1999). Impaired but undiagnosed. *Journal of the American Academy of Child and Adolescent Psychiatry, 38,* 129–137.

Arnold, D. S., & O'Leary, S. G. (1993). The Parenting Scale: A measure of dysfunctional parenting in discipline situations. *Psychological Assessment, 5,* 137–144.

Atkins, D. C., Bedics, J. D., McGlinchey, J. B., & Beauchaine, T. P. (2005). Assessing clinical significance: Does it matter which method we use? *Journal of Consulting and Clinical Psychology, 73,* 982–989.

Azar, S. T., Robinson, D. R., Hekimian, E., & Twentyman, C. T. (1984). Unrealistic expectations and problem-solving ability in maltreating and comparison mothers. *Journal of Consulting and Clinical Psychology, 52,* 687–691.

Barkley, R. A. (1988). A review of child behavior rating scales and checklists for research in child psychopathology. In M. Rutter, A. H. Tuma, & I. S. Lann (Eds.), *Assessment and diagnosis in child psychopathology* (pp. 113–155). New York: Guilford Press.

Barkley, R. A. (2006). *Attention-deficit/hyperactivity disorder: A handbook for diagnosis and treatment* (3rd ed.). New York: Guilford Press.

Barkley, R. A., & Guevremont, D. C. (1992). A comparison of three family therapy programs for treating family conflicts in adolescents with attention-deficit hyperactivity disorder. *Journal of Consulting and Clinical Psychology, 60,* 450–462.

Barlow, D. H. (1986). In defense of panic disorder with agoraphobia and the behavioral treatment of panic: A comment on Kleiner. *Behavior Therapist, 9,* 99–100.

Barrett, P. M., & Ollendick, T. H. (2004). *Handbook of interventions that work with children and adolescents: Prevention and treatment.* New York: Wiley.

Barrios, B. A. (1993). Direct observation. In T. H. Ollendick & M. Hersen (Eds.), *Handbook of child and adolescent assessment* (pp. 140–164). Needham Heights, MA: Allyn & Bacon.

Baskett, L. M. (1985). Understanding family interactions: Most probable reactions by parents and siblings. *Child and Family Behavior Therapy, 7,* 41–50.

Bastiaansen, D., Koot, H. M., & Ferdinand, R. F. (2005). Determinants of quality of life in children with psychiatric disorders. *Quality of Life Research, 14,* 1599–1612.

Beach, S. R. H., Wamboldt, M. Z., Kaslow, N. J., Heyman, R. E., & Reiss, D. (2006). Describing relationship problems in DSM-V: Toward better guidance for research and clinical practice. *Journal of Family Psychology, 20,* 359–368.

Bell, D. J., Foster, S. L., & Mash, E. J. (2005). *Handbook of behavioral and emotional problems in girls.* New York: Kluwer Academic/Plenum Press.

Bell, R. Q., & Harper, L. V. (1977). *Child effects on adults.* Hillsdale, NJ: Erlbaum.

Bierman, K. L. (1983). Cognitive development and clinical interviews with children. In B. B. Lahey & A. E. Kazdin (Eds.), *Advances in clinical child psychology* (Vol. 6, pp. 217–250). New York: Plenum Press.

Bierman, K. L., & McCauley, E. (1987). Children's descriptions of their peer interactions: Useful information for clinical child assessment. *Journal of Clinical Child Psychology, 16,* 9–18.

Bierman, K. L., & Schwartz, L. A. (1986). Clinical child interviews: Approaches and developmental considerations. *Journal of Child and Adolescent Psychotherapy, 3,* 267–278.

Bierman, K. L., & Welsh, J. A. (1997). Social relationship deficits. In E. J. Mash & R. A. Barkley (Eds.), *Assessment of childhood disorders* (3rd ed., pp. 328–366). New York: Guilford Press.

Biglan, A., Mrazek, P., Carnine, D., & Flay, B. (2003).

The integration of research and practice in the prevention of youth behavior problems. *American Psychologist, 58*, 433–440.

Billings, A. G., & Moos, R. H. (1986). Children of parents with unipolar depression: A controlled l-year follow-up. *Journal of Abnormal Child Psychology, 14*, 149–166.

Blechman, E. A. (1985). *Solving child behavior problem at home and school.* Champaign, IL: Research Press.

Bongers, I. L., Koot, H. M., van der Ende, J., & Verhulst, F. C. (2003). The normative development of children and adolescent problem behavior. *Journal of Abnormal Psychology, 112*, 179–192.

Bornstein, P. H., Hamilton, S. B., & Bornstein, M. (1986). Self-monitoring procedures. In A. R. Ciminero, K. S. Calhoun, & H. E. Adams (Eds.), *Handbook of behavioral assessment* (2nd ed., pp. 176–222). New York: Wiley.

Bradbury, T. N., & Fincham, F. D. (1987). Affect and cognition in close relationships: Towards an integrative model. *Cognition and Emotion, 1*, 59–87.

Brassard, M. R., & Boehm, A. E. (2007). *Preschool assessment: Principles and practices.* New York: Guilford Press.

Bristol, M. M. (1983). Carolina Parent Support Scale. In M. Bristol, A. Donovan, & A. Harding (Eds.), *The broader impact of intervention: A workshop on measuring stress and support.* Chapel Hill, NC: Frank Porter Graham Child Development Center.

Broden, M., Hall, R. V., & Mitts, B. (1971). The effect of self-recording on the classroom behavior of two eighth grade students. *Journal of Applied Behavior Analysis, 4*, 191–199.

Bromfield, R., Weisz, J. R., & Messer, I. (1986). Children's judgments and attributions in response to the mental retarded label. *Journal of Abnormal Psychology, 95*, 81–87.

Bronfenbrenner, U. (1986). Ecology of the family as a context for human development: Research perspectives. *Developmental Psychology, 22*, 723–742.

Bugental, D. B. (1993). Communication in abusive relationships: Cognitive constructions of interpersonal power. *American Behavioral Scientist, 36*, 288–308.

Bugental, D. B., & Johnston, C. (2000). Parental and child cognitions in the context of the family. *Annual Review of Psychology, 51*, 315–344.

Bugental, D. B., Johnston, C., New, M., & Silvester, J. (1998). Measuring parental attributions: Conceptual and methodological issues. *Journal of Family Psychology, 12*, 459–480.

Burlingame, G. M., Wells, M. G., Lambert, M. J., & Cox, J. C. (2004). The Youth Outcome Questionnaire. In M. Maruish (Ed.), *The use of psychological tests for treatment planning and outcome assessment* (3rd ed., Vol. 2, pp. 235–274). Mahwah, NJ: Erlbaum.

Butler, R. J,. Brewin, C. R., & Forsythe, W. I. (1986). Maternal attributions and tolerance for nocturnal enuresis. *Behaviour Research and Therapy, 24*, 307–312.

Buysse, V., & Wesley, P. W. (Eds.). (2006). *Evidence-based practice in the early childhood field.* Washington, DC: Zero to Three Press.

Cairns, R. B., & Green, J. A. (1979). How to assess personality and social patterns: Observations or ratings? In R. B. Cairns (Ed.), *The analysis of social interactions: Methods, issues and illustrations* (pp. 209–226). Hillsdale, NJ: Erlbaum.

Cantor, N. (1982). "Everyday" versus normative models of clinical and social judgment. In G. Weary & H. L. Mirels (Eds.), *Integrations of clinical and social psychology* (pp. 27–47). New York: Oxford University Press.

Cantor, N., Smith, E. E., French, R. de S., & Mezzich, J. (1980). Psychiatric diagnosis as prototype categorization. *Journal of Abnormal Psychology, 89*, 181–193.

Caron, C., & Rutter, M. (1991). Comorbidity in child psychopathology: Concepts, issues, and research strategies. *Journal of Child Psychology and Psychiatry, 32*, 1063–1080.

Carr, E. G. (1994). Emerging themes in the functional analysis of problem behavior. *Journal of Applied Behavior Analysis, 27*, 393–399.

Carter, A. S., Marakovitz, S. E., & Sparrow, S. S. (2006). Comprehensive psychological assessment: A developmental psychopathology approach for clinical and applied research. In D. Cicchetti & D. J. Cohen (Eds.), *Developmental psychopathology: Vol. 1. Theory and method* (2nd ed., pp. 181–210). New York: Wiley.

Cattell, R. B. (1983). Let's end the duel. *American Psychologist, 38*, 769–776.

Chambers, W. J., Puig-Antich, J., Hirsch, M., Paez, P., Ambrosini, P. J., Tabrizi, M. A., et al. (1985). The assessment of affective disorders in children and adolescents by semi-structured interview: Test–retest reliability for school age children, present episode version. *Archives of General Psychiatry, 42*, 696–702.

Chlopan, B. E., McBain, M. L., Carbonell, J. L., & Hagen, R. L. (1985). Empathy: Review of available measures. *Journal of Personality and Social Psychology, 48*, 635–653.

Cicchetti, D. (2006). Development and psychopathology. In D. Cicchetti & D. J. Cohen (Eds.), *Developmental psychopathology: Vol. 1. Theory and method* (2nd ed., pp. 1–23). New York: Wiley.

Cicchetti, D., & Cohen, D. J. (2006a). *Developmental psychopathology: Vol. 1. Theory and method* (2nd ed.). New York: Wiley.

Cicchetti, D., & Cohen, D. J. (2006b). *Developmental psychopathology: Vol. 2. Developmental neuroscience* (2nd ed.). New York: Wiley.

Cicchetti, D., & Cohen, D. J. (2006c). *Developmental psychopathology: Vol. 3. Risk, disorder, and adaptation* (2nd ed.). New York: Wiley.

Cicchetti, D., & Curtis, W. J. (2006). The developing brain and neural plasticity: Implications for normality, psychopathology, and resilience. In D. Cicchetti

& D. J. Cohen (Eds.), *Developmental psychopathology: Vol. 2. Developmental neuroscience* (2nd ed., pp. 1–64). New York: Wiley.

Coie, J. D., & Pennington, B. F. (1976). Children's perceptions of deviance and disorder. *Child Development, 47,* 407–413.

Compas, B. E., Friedland-Bandes, R., Bastien, R., & Adelman, H. S. (1981). Parent and child causal attributions related to the child's clinical problem. *Journal of Abnormal Child Psychology, 9,* 389–397.

Cone, J. D., & Foster, S. L. (1982). Direct observation in clinical psychology. In P. C. Kendall & J. N. Butcher (Eds.), *Handbook of research methods in clinical psychology* (pp. 311–354). New York: Wiley.

Costello, E. J., Edelbrock, C., & Costello, A. J. (1985). Validity of the NIMH Diagnostic Interview Schedule for Children: A comparison between psychiatric and pediatric referrals. *Journal of Abnormal Child Psychology, 13,* 579–595.

Costello, A. J., Edelbrock, C., Kalas, R., Kessler, M. D., & Klaric, S. (1982). *The NIMH Diagnostic Interview Schedule for Children (DISC).* Pittsburgh, PA: Authors.

Cowan, P. A., & Cowan, C. P. (2006). Developmental psychopathology from family systems and family risk factors perspectives: Implications for family research, practice, and policy. In D. J. Cohen & D. Cicchetti (Eds.), *Developmental psychopathology: Vol. 1. Theory and method* (2nd ed., pp. 530–587). New York: Wiley.

Cowen, E. L., Pederson, A., Babigian, H., Izzo, L. D., & Trost, M. A. (1973). Long-term follow-up of early detected vulnerable children. *Journal of Consulting and Clinical Psychology, 41,* 438–445.

Cronbach, L. J. (1990). *Essentials of psychological testing* (5th ed.). New York: Harper & Row.

Daleiden, E. L., Chorpita, B. F., Donkervoet, C., Arensdorf, A. M., & Brogan, M. (2006). Getting better at getting them better: Health outcomes and evidence-based practice within a system of care. *American Journal of Child and Adolescent Psychiatry, 45,* 749–756.

D'Amato, R.C., Fletcher-Janzen, E., & Reynolds, C. R. (Eds.). (2005). *Handbook of school neuropsychology.* Hoboken, NJ: Wiley.

Davies, P. T., & Cummings, E. M. (2006). Interparental discord, family process, and developmental psychopathology. In D. Cicchetti & D. J. Cohen (Eds.), *Developmental psychopathology: Vol. 3. Risk, disorder, and adaptation* (2nd ed., pp. 86–128). New York: Wiley.

DC:0–3R Revision Task Force. (2005). DC:0–3R: *Diagnostic classification of mental health and developmental disorders of infancy and early childhood.* Washington, DC: Zero to Three Press.

DelCarmen-Wiggins, R., & Carter, A. (Eds.). (2004). *Handbook of infant, toddler, and preschool mental health assessment.* New York: Oxford University Press.

De Los Reyes, A., & Kazdin, A. E. (2004). Measuring informant discrepancies in clinical child research. *Psychological Assessment, 16,* 330–334.

De Los Reyes, A., & Kazdin, A. E. (2005). Informant discrepancies in the assessment of childhood psychopathology: A critical review, theoretical framework, and recommendations for further study. *Psychological Bulletin, 131,* 483–509.

Dishion, T., Gardner, K., Patterson, G. R., Reid, J., Spyrou, S., & Thibodeaux, S. (1984). *The Family Process Code: A multidimensional system for observing family interactions.* Unpublished manual, Oregon Social Learning Center, Eugene.

Dishion, T. J., & Patterson, G. R. (2006). The development and ecology of antisocial behavior in children. In D. Cicchetti & D. J. Cohen (Eds.), *Developmental psychopathology: Vol. 3. Risk, disorder, and adaptation* (2nd ed., pp. 503–541). New York: Wiley.

Dix, T. (1991). The affective organization of parenting: Adaptive and maladaptive processes. *Psychological Bulletin, 110,* 3–25.

Dix, T., & Reinhold, D. P. (1990). Mothers' judgment in moments of anger. *Merrill–Palmer Quarterly, 36,* 465–486.

Dix, T., & Ruble, D. N. (1989). Mothers' implicit theories of discipline: Child effects, parent effects, and the attribution process. *Child Development, 60,* 1373–1391.

Dodge, K. A., McClaskey, C. L., & Feldman, E. (1985). Situational approach to the assessment of social competence in children. *Journal of Consulting and Clinical Psychology, 53,* 344–353.

Dodge, K. A., & Pettit, G. S. (2003). A biopsychosocial model of the development of chronic conduct problems in adolescence. *Developmental Psychology, 39,* 349–371.

Dollinger, S. J., Thelan, M. H., & Walsh, M. L. (1980). Children's conceptions of psychological problems. *Journal of Clinical Child Psychology, 9,* 191–194.

Doucette, A. (2002). Child and adolescent diagnosis: The need for a model-based approach. In L. E. Beutler & M. L. Malik (Eds.), *Rethinking the DSM: A psychological perspective* (pp. 201–220). Washington, DC: American Psychological Association.

Dunn, J., & Munn, P. (1986). Sibling quarrels and maternal intervention: Individual differences in understanding and aggression. *Journal of Child Psychology and Psychiatry, 27,* 583–597.

Dunst, C. J., Jenkins, V., & Trivette, C. M. (1984). The Family Support Scale: Reliability and validity. *Journal of Individual, Family, and Community Wellness, 1,* 45–52.

Dunst, C. J., & Trivette, C. M. (1985). *A guide to measures of social support and family behavior* (Monograph of the Technical Assistance Development System, No. 1). Chapel Hill: University of North Carolina, Technical Assistance Development System.

Dunst, C. J., & Trivette, C. M. (1986). Looking beyond the parent–child dyad for the determinants of maternal styles of interaction. *Infant Mental Health Journal, 7,* 69–80.

DuPaul, G. J., & Barkley, R. A. (1992). Situational variability of attention problems: Psychometric properties of the Revised Home and School Situations Questionnaires. *Journal of Clinical Child Psychology*, *21*, 178–188.

Edelbrock, C. (1984). Developmental considerations. In T. H. Ollendick & M. Hersen (Eds.), *Child behavioral assessment: Principles and procedures* (pp. 20–37). New York: Pergamon Press.

Edelbrock, C., Costello, A. J., Dulcan, M. J., Conover, N. C., & Kalas, R. (1986). Parent–child agreement of child psychiatric symptoms assessed via structured interview. *Journal of Child Psychology and Psychiatry*, *27*, 181–190.

Edelbrock, C., Costello, A. J., Dulcan, M. J., Kalas, R., & Conover, N. C. (1985). Age differences in the reliability of the psychiatric interview of the child. *Child Development*, *56*, 265–275.

Eells, T. D. (Ed.). (2007). *Handbook of psychotherapy case formulation* (2nd ed.). New York: Guilford Press.

Egeland, B., & Sroufe, L. A. (1981). Attachment and early maltreatment. *Child Development*, *52*, 44–52.

Ellis, D., & DeKeseredy, W. (1994, March). *Pre-test report on the frequency, severity, and patterning of sibling violence in Canadian families: Causes and consequence* (Report to Family Violence Prevention Division). North York, Ontario: Health Canada, LaMarsh Centre on Violence and Conflict Resolution.

Emery, R. E., Binkoff, J. A., Houts, A. C., & Carr, E. G. (1983). Children as independent variables: Some clinical implications of child effects. *Behavioral Therapy*, *14*, 398–412.

Evans, I. M. (1985). Building systems models as a strategy for target behavior selection in clinical assessment. *Behavioral Assessment*, *7*, 21–32.

Evans, I. M., & Meyer, L. H. (1985). *An educative approach to behavior problems: A practical decision model for interventions with severely handicapped learners*. Baltimore: Brookes.

Evans, I. M., & Nelson, R. O. (1977). Assessment of child behavior problems. In A. R. Ciminero, K. S. Calhoun, & H. E. Adams (Eds.), *Handbook of behavioral assessment* (pp. 603–681). New York: Wiley.

Farrell, A. D. (1991). Computers and behavioral assessment: Current applications, future possibilities, and obstacles to routine use. *Behavioral Assessment*, *13*, 159–179.

First, M. B. (2005). Clinical utility: A prerequisite for the adoption of a dimensional approach in DSM. *Journal of Abnormal Psychology*, *114*, 560–564.

First, M. B. (2006). Beyond clinical utility: Broadening the DSM-V research appendix to include alternative diagnostic constructs. *American Journal of Psychiatry*, *163*, 1679–1681.

Forehand, R. (1977). Child noncompliance to parental requests: Behavioral analysis and treatment. In M. Hersen, R. M. Eisler, & P. M. Miller (Eds.), *Progress in behavior modification* (Vol. 5, pp. 111–147). New York: Academic Press.

Forehand, R., & Kotchick, B. A. (1996). Cultural diversity: A wake-up call for parent training. *Behavior Therapy*, *27*, 171–186.

Forehand, R., Long, N., Brody, G. H., & Fauber, R. (1986). Home predictors of young adolescents' school behavior and academic performance. *Child Development*, *57*, 1528–1533.

Forman, B. D., & Hagan, B. J. (1984). Measures for evaluating total family functioning. *Family Therapy*, *11*, 1–36.

Foster, S. L., & Cone, J. D. (1986). Design and use of direct observation procedures. In A. R. Ciminero, K. S. Calhoun, & H. E. Adams (Eds.), *Handbook of behavioral assessment* (2nd ed., pp. 253–324). New York: Wiley.

Foster, S. L., & Mash, E. J. (1999). Assessing social validity in clinical treatment research: Issues and procedures. *Journal of Consulting and Clinical Psychology*, *67*, 308–319.

Foster, S. L., & Robin, A. L. (1997). Family conflict and communication in adolescence. In E. J. Mash & L. G. Terdal (Eds.), *Assessment of childhood disorders* (3rd ed., pp. 627–682). New York: Guilford Press.

Frazier, T. W., & Youngstrom, E. A. (2006). Evidence-based assessment of attention-deficit/hyperactivity disorder: Using multiple sources of information. *Journal of the American Academy of Child and Adolescent Psychiatry*, *45*, 614–620.

Freeman, K. A., & Mash, E. J. (in press). Single case research. In M. Hersen & A. Gross (Eds.), *Handbook of clinical psychology: Vol. II. Children and adolescents*. Hoboken, NJ: Wiley.

Frick, P. J., & Lahey, B. B., Loeber, R., Stouthamer-Loeber, M., Christ, M. A. G., & Hanson, K. (1992). Familial risk factors to oppositional defiant disorder and conduct disorder: Parental psychopathology and maternal parenting. *Journal of Consulting and Clinical Psychology*, *60*, 49–55.

Garber, J. (1984). Classification of child psychopathology: A developmental perspective. *Child Development*, *55*, 30–48.

Gdowski, C. L., Lachar, D., & Kline, R. B. (1985). A PIC profile typology of children and adolescents: I. Empirically derived alternative to traditional diagnosis. *Journal of Abnormal Psychology*, *91*, 346–361.

Geffken, G. R., Keeley, M. L., Kellison, I., Storch, E. A., & Rodrigue, J. R. (2006). Parental adherence to child psychologists' recommendations from psychological testing. *Professional Psychology: Research and Practice*, *5*, 499–505.

Geller, J., & Johnston, C. (1995). Predictors of mothers' responses to child noncompliance: Attributions and attitudes. *Journal of Clinical Child Psychology*, *24*, 272–278.

Goldman, H. H., & Skodol, A. E. (1992). Revising Axis V for DSM-IV: A review of measures of social functioning. *American Journal of Psychiatry*, *149*, 1148–1156.

Goodman, S. H., & Gotlib, I. H. (Eds.). (2002). *Children of depressed parents: Mechanisms for risk and implications for treatment*. Washington, DC: American Psychological Association.

Gordon, M., Antshel, K., Faraone, S., Barkley, R., Lewandowski, L., Hudziak, J. J., et al. (2006). Symptoms versus impairment: The case for respecting DSM-IV's criterion D. *Journal of Attention Disorders, 9*, 465–475.

Gottman, J. M., Katz, L. F., & Hooven, C. (1996). Parental meta-emotion philosophy and the emotional life of families: Theoretical models and preliminary data. *Journal of Family Psychology, 10*, 243–268.

Gottman, J. M., & Levenson, R. W. (1986). Assessing the role of emotion in marriage. *Behavioral Assessment, 8*, 31–48.

Greenspan, S. I., & Greenspan, N. T. (2003). *The clinical interview of the child* (3rd ed.). Washington, DC: American Psychiatric Publishing.

Greenspan, S. I., & Porges, S. W. (1984). Psychopathology in infancy and early childhood: Clinical perspectives on the organization of sensory and affective thematic experience. *Child Development, 55*, 49–70.

Greenwood, C. R., Delquadri, J. C., Stanley, S. O., Terry, B., & Hall, R. V. (1985). Assessment of ecobehavioral interaction in school settings. *Behavioral Assessment, 7*, 331–348.

Gross, A. M., & Drabman, R. S. (1990). *Handbook of clinical behavioral pediatrics*. New York: Plenum Press.

Gross, D., Fogg, L., Young, M., Ridge, A., Cowell, J. M., Richardson, R., et al. (2006). The equivalence of the Child Behavior Checklist/11/2-5 across parent race/ethnicity, income level, and language. *Psychological Assessment, 18*, 313–323.

Grotevant, H. D., & Carlson, C. I. (1989). *Family assessment: A guide to methods and measures*. New York: Guilford Press.

Group for the Advancement of Psychiatry. (1974). *Psychopathological disorders in childhood: Theoretical considerations and a proposed classification*. New York: Aronson.

Guidubaldi, J., & Cleminshaw, H. K. (1985). The development of the Cleminshaw–Guidubaldi Parent Satisfaction Scale. *Journal of Clinical Child Psychology, 14*, 293–298.

Gunnar, M. R., & Vazquez, D. (2006). Stress neurobiology and developmental psychopathology. In D. Cicchetti & D. J. Cohen (Eds.), *Developmental psychopathology: Vol. 2. Developmental neuroscience* (2nd ed., pp. 533–577). New York: Wiley.

Guskin, S. L., Bartel, N. R., & MacMillan, D. L. (1975). Perspective of the labeled child. In N. Hobbs (Ed.), *Issues in the classification of children* (Vol. 2, pp. 185–212). San Francisco: Jossey-Bass.

Harris, A. M., & Reid, J. B. (1981). The consistency of a class of coercive child behavior across school settings for individual subjects. *Journal of Abnormal Child Psychology, 9*, 219–227.

Hartmann, D. P. (1982). *Using observers to study behavior*. San Francisco: Jossey-Bass.

Hartmann, D. P. (1984). Assessment strategies. In D. H. Barlow & M. Hersen (Eds.), *Single case experimental designs: Strategies for studying behavior change* (2nd ed., pp. 107–139). New York: Pergamon Press.

Hartmann, D. P., Roper, B. L., & Bradford, D. C. (1979). Some relationships between behavioral and traditional assessment. *Journal of Behavioral Assessment, 1*, 3–21.

Hartup, W. W. (1986). On relationships and development. In W. W. Hartup & Z. Rubin (Eds.), *Relationships and development* (pp. 1–26). Hillsdale, NJ: Erlbaum.

Hawkins, R. P. (1982). Developing a behavior code. In D. P. Hartmann (Ed.), *Using observers to study behavior* (pp. 21–35). San Francisco: Jossey-Bass.

Hayes, S. C. (1996). Creating the empirical clinician. *Clinical Psychology: Science and Practice, 3*, 179–181.

Hayes, S. C., & Follette, W. C. (1992). Can functional analysis provide a substitute for syndromal classification? *Behavioral Assessment, 14*, 345–365.

Hayes, S. C., Follette, W. C., Dawes, R. D., & Grady, K. (Eds.). (1995). *Scientific standards of psychological practice: Issues and recommendations*. Reno, NV: Context Press.

Hayes, S. C., & Nelson, R. O. (1987). The treatment utility of assessment: A functional approach to evaluating assessment quality. *American Psychologist, 42*, 963–974.

Hayes, S. C., & Nelson, R. O. (1989). The applicability of treatment utility. *American Psychologist, 44*, 1242–1243.

Haynes, S. N., & Jensen, B. J. (1979). The interview as a behavioral assessment instrument. *Behavioral Assessment, 1*, 97–106.

Herjanic, B., & Reich, W. (1982). Development of a structured psychiatric interview for children. *Journal of Abnormal Child Psychology, 10*, 307–324.

Hibbs, E. D., & Jensen, P. S. (Eds.). (2005). *Psychosocial treatments for child and adolescent disorders: Empirically based strategies for clinical practice* (2nd ed.). Washington, DC: American Psychological Association.

Hinshaw, S. P. (2006). Stigma and mental illness: Developmental issues and future prospects. In D. Cicchetti & D. J. Cohen (Eds.), *Developmental psychopathology: Vol. 3. Risk, disorder, and adaptation* (2nd ed., pp. 841–881). New York: Wiley.

Hoagwood, K., Jensen, P.S., Petti, T., & Burns, B. J. (1996). Outcomes of mental health care for children and adolescents: I. A comprehensive conceptual model. *Journal of the American Academy of Child and Adolescent Psychiatry, 35*, 1055–1063.

Hodges, K. (1985). *Manual for the Child Assessment Schedule (CAS)*. Durham, NC: Duke University Medical Center.

Holden, G. W. (1985a). Analyzing parental reasoning

with microcomputer-presented problems. *Simulation and Games, 16,* 203–210.

Holden, G. W. (1985b). How parents create a social environment via proactive behavior. In T. Garling & J. Valsiner (Eds.), *Children within environments* (pp. 193–215). New York: Plenum Press.

Holmbeck, G. N., Greenley, R. N., & Franks, E. A. (2003). Developmental issues and considerations in research and practice. In A. E. Kazdin & J. R. Weisz (Eds.), *Evidence-based psychotherapies for children and adolescents* (pp. 21–41). New York: Guilford Press.

Hommersen, P., Murray, C., Ohan, J. L., & Johnston, C. (2006). Oppositional defiant disorder rating scale: Preliminary evidence of reliability and validity. *Journal of Behavioral and Emotional Disorders, 14,* 118–125.

Hops, H., & Davis, B. (1995). Methodological issues in direct observation: Illustrations with the Living in Familial Environments (LIFE) coding system. *Journal of Clinical Child Psychology, 24,* 193–203.

Horowitz, L. M., Post, D. L., French, R. de S., Wallis, K. D., & Siegelman, E. Y. (1981). The prototype as a construct in abnormal psychology: 2. Clarifying disagreement in psychiatric judgments. *Journal of Abnormal Psychology, 90,* 575–585.

Horowitz, L. M., Wright, J. C., Lowenstein, E., & Parad, H. W. (1981). The prototype as a construct in abnormal psychology: 1. A method for deriving prototypes. *Journal of Abnormal Psychology, 90,* 568–574.

Hughes, H. M., & Haynes, S. N. (1978). Structured laboratory observation in the behavioral assessment of parent–child interactions: A methodological critique. *Behavior Therapy, 9,* 428–447.

Hulbert, T. A., Gdowski, C. L., & Lachar, D. (1986). Interparent agreement on the Personality Inventory for Children: Are substantial correlations sufficient? *Journal of Abnormal Child Psychology, 14,* 115–122.

Hunsley, J., & Mash, E. J. (2007). Evidence-based assessment. *Annual Review of Clinical Psychology, 3,* 57–79.

Hunsley, J., & Mash, E. J. (in press). *A guide to assessments that work.* New York: Oxford University Press.

Hunsley, J., & Meyer, G. J. (2003). The incremental validity of psychological testing and assessment: Conceptual, methodological, and statistical issues. *Psychological Assessment, 15,* 446–455.

Ialongo, N. S., Rogosch, F. A., Cicchetti, D., Toth, S. L., Buckley, J., Petras, H., et al. (2006). A developmental psychopathology approach to the prevention of mental health disorders. In D. Cicchetti & D. J. Cohen (Eds.), *Developmental psychopathology: Vol. 1. Theory and method* (2nd ed., pp. 968–1018). New York: Wiley.

Jacob, R. G., O'Leary, K. D., & Rosenblad, C. (1978). Formal and informal classroom settings: Effects on hyperactivity. *Journal of Abnormal Child Psychology, 6,* 47–59.

Jacob, T., & Tennenbaum, D. L. (1988). *Family assessment: Rationale, methods, and future directions.* New York: Plenum Press.

Jensen, P. S., Hoagwood, K., & Zitner, L. (2006). What's in a name?: Problems versus prospects in current diagnostic approaches. In D. Cicchetti & D. J. Cohen (Eds.), *Developmental psychopathology: Vol. 1. Theory and method* (2nd ed., pp. 24–40). New York: Wiley.

Jensen, P. S., Knapp, P., & Mrazek, D. A. (Eds.). (2006). *Toward a new diagnostic system for child psychopathology: Moving beyond the DSM.* New York: Guilford Press.

Jensen, S., Fabiano, G. A., Lopez-Williams, A., & Chacko, A. (2006). The reading grade level of common measures in child and adolescent clinical psychology. *Psychological Assessment, 18,* 346–352.

Johnson, S. M., & Lobitz, G. K. (1974). Parental manipulation of child behavior in home observations. *Journal of Applied Behavior Analysis, 7,* 23–32.

Johnston, C., & Mash, E. J. (1989). A measure of parenting satisfaction and efficacy. *Journal of Clinical Child Psychology, 18,* 167–175.

Johnston, C., & Murray, C. (2003). Incremental validity in the psychological assessment of children and adolescents. *Psychological Assessment, 15,* 496–507.

Johnston, C., & Ohan, J. L. (2005). The importance of parental attributions in families of children with attention-deficit/hyperactivity and disruptive behavior disorders. *Clinical Child and Family Psychology Review, 8,* 167–182.

Jouriles, E. N., Murphy, C. M., & O'Leary, K. D. (1989). Effects of maternal mood on mother–son interaction patterns. *Journal of Abnormal Child Psychology, 17,* 513–525.

Jouriles, E. N., & Thompson, S. M. (1993). Effects of mood on mothers' evaluations of children's behavior. *Journal of Family Psychology, 6,* 300–307.

Kagan, J. (1983). Classifications of the child. In W. Kessen (Ed.), *Handbook of child psychology: Vol. 1. History, theory, and methods* (pp. 527–560). New York: Wiley.

Kamphaus, R. W. (2005). *Clinical assessment of child and adolescent intelligence* (2nd ed.). New York: Springer.

Kamphaus, R. W., & Campbell, J. (2006). *Psychodiagnostic assessment of children: Dimensional and categorical approaches.* Hoboken, NJ: Wiley.

Kamphaus, R. W., & Frick, P. J. (2005). *Clinical assessment of child and adolescent personality and behavior.* New York: Springer.

Kamphaus, R. W., Petoskey, M. D., & Rowe, E. W. (2000). Current trends in psychological testing for children. *Professional Psychology, Research and Practice, 31,* 155–164.

Kanfer, F. H. (1979). A few comments on the current status of behavioral assessment. *Behavioral Assessment, 1,* 37–39.

Kanfer, F. H. (1985). Target selection for clinical change programs. *Behavioral Assessment, 7,* 7–20.

Kanfer, F. H., & Grimm, L. G. (1977). Behavioral analysis: Selecting target behaviors in the interview. *Behavior Modification, 1,* 7–28.

Kaye, K. (1984). Toward a developmental psychology of the family. In L. L'Abate (Ed.), *Handbook of family psychology and psychotherapy.* Homewood, IL: Dow Jones/Irwin.

Kazdin, A. E. (1977). Assessing the clinical or applied importance of behavior change through social validation. *Behavior Modification, 1,* 427–452.

Kazdin, A. E. (1981). Acceptability of child treatment techniques: The influence of treatment efficacy and adverse side effects. *Behavior Therapy, 12,* 493–506.

Kazdin, A. E. (1982). Symptom substitution, generalization, and response covariation: Implications for psychotherapy outcome. *Psychological Bulletin, 91,* 349–365.

Kazdin, A. E. (1983). Psychiatric diagnosis, dimensions of dysfunction and child behavior therapy. *Behavior Therapy, 14,* 73–99.

Kazdin, A. E. (1984). Acceptability of aversive procedures and medication as treatment alternatives for deviant child behavior. *Journal of Abnormal Child Psychology, 12,* 289–302.

Kazdin, A. E. (1985). Selection of target behaviors: The relationship of the treatment focus to clinical dysfunction. *Behavioral Assessment, 7,* 33–47.

Kazdin, A. E. (2005). Evidence-based assessment for children and adolescents: Issues in measurement development and clinical applications. *Journal of Clinical Child and Adolescent Psychology, 34,* 548–558.

Kazdin, A. E. (2006). Arbitrary metrics: Implications for identifying evidence-based treatment. *American Psychologist, 61,* 42–49.

Kazdin, A. E., & Esveldt-Dawson, K. (1987). Problem-solving skills training and relationship therapy in the treatment of antisocial child behavior. *Journal of Consulting and Clinical Psychology, 55,* 76–85.

Kazdin, A. E., & Kagan, J. (1994). Models of dysfunction in developmental psychopathology. *Clinical Psychology: Science and Practice, 1,* 35–52.

Kazdin, A. E., & Weisz, J. R. (Eds.). (2003). *Evidence-based psychotherapies for children and adolescents.* New York: Guilford Press.

Kendall, P. C. (Ed.). (1999). Clinical significance [Special section]. *Journal of Consulting and Clinical Psychology, 67,* 283–339.

Kendall, P. C. (Ed.). (2006). *Child and adolescent therapy: Cognitive-behavioral procedures* (3rd ed.). New York: Guilford Press.

Kendall, P. C., Hudson, J. L., Choudhury, M., Webb, A., & Pimentel, S. (2005). Cognitive-behavioral treatment for childhood anxiety disorders. In E.D. Hibbs & P. S. Jensen (Eds.), *Psychosocial treatments for child and adolescent disorders: Empirically based strategies for clinical practice* (2nd ed., pp. 47–73). Washington, DC: American Psychological Association.

Kendall, P.C., Lerner, R. M., & Craighead, W. E. (1984). Human development and intervention in child psychopathology. *Child Development, 55,* 71–82.

Kessler, J. W. (1971). Nosology in child psychopathology. In H. E. Rie (Ed.), *Perspectives in child psychopathology.* Chicago: Aldine–Atherton.

Kessler, R. C., Berglund, P., Demler, O., Jin, R., & Walters, M. S. (2005). Lifetime prevalence and age-of-onset distributions of DSM-IV disorders in the National Comorbidity Survey replication. *Archives of General Psychiatry, 62,* 593–602.

Kiesler, C. A. (1983). Social psychological issues in studying consumer satisfaction with behavior therapy. *Behavior Therapy, 14,* 226–236.

Kobak, R., Cassidy, J., Lyons-Ruth, K., & Ziv, Y. (2006). Attachment, stress, and psychopathology: A developmental pathways model. In D. Cicchetti & D. J. Cohen (Eds.), *Developmental psychopathology: Vol. 1. Theory and method* (2nd ed., pp. 333–369). New York: Wiley.

Koocher, G. P., & Rey-Casserly, C. M. (2003). Ethical issues in psychological assessment. In J. R. Graham & Naglieri, J. A. (Eds.), *Handbook of psychology: Assessment psychology* (Vol. 10, pp. 165–180). Hoboken, NJ: Wiley.

Kropp, J. P., & Haynes, O. M. (1987). Abusive and nonabusive mothers' ability to identify general and specific emotion signals of infants. *Child Development, 58,* 187–190.

Kupfer, D. A., First, M. B., & Regier, D. A. (Eds.). (2002). *A research agenda for DSM-V.* Washington, DC: American Psychiatric Association.

Kurdek, L. A. (1986). Children's reasoning about parental divorce. In R. D. Ashmore & D. M. Brodzinsky (Eds.), *Thinking about the family: Views of parents and children* (pp. 233–276). Hillsdale, NJ: Erlbaum.

Lambert, M. J., Whipple, J. L., Hawkins, E. J., Vermeersch, D. A., Nielsen, S. L., & Smart, D. W. (2003). Is it time for clinicians to routinely track patient outcome?: A meta-analysis. *Clinical Psychology: Science and Practice, 10,* 288–301.

Lapouse, R., & Monk, M. A. (1958). An epidemiologic study of behavior characteristic in children. *American Journal of Public Health, 48,* 1134–1144.

LeBow, J. (1982). Consumer satisfaction with mental health treatment. *Psychological Bulletin, 91,* 244–259.

LeBow, J., & Gordon, K. C. (2006). You cannot choose what is not on the menu—obstacles to and reasons for the inclusion of relational processes in the DSM-V: Comment on the Special Section. *Journal of Family Psychology, 20,* 432–437.

Lieberman, A. F., Barnard, K. E., & Wieder, S. (2004). Diagnosing infants, toddlers, and preschoolers: The Zero to Three diagnostic classification of early mental health disorders. In R. DelCarmen-Wiggins & A. Carter (Eds.), *Handbook of infant, toddler, and preschool mental health assessment* (pp. 141–160). New York: Oxford University Press.

Lorber, M. F., & Slep, A. M. (2005). Mothers' emotion dynamics and their relations with harsh and lax discipline: Microsocial time series analyses. *Journal of Clinical Child and Adolescent Psychology, 34,* 559–568.

Lovitt, T. C. (1973). Self-management projects with children with learning disabilities. *Journal of Learning Disabilities, 6,* 15–28.

Luby, J. L. (Ed.). (2006). *Handbook of preschool mental health: Development, disorders, and treatment.* New York: Guilford Press.

Luthar, S. S. (2006). Resilience in development: A synthesis of research across five decades. In D. Cicchetti & D. J. Cohen (Eds.), *Developmental psychopathology: Vol. 3. Risk, disorder, and adaptation* (2nd ed., pp. 739–795). New York: Wiley.

Lytton, H. (1979). Disciplinary encounters between young boys and their mothers and fathers: Is there a contingency system? *Developmental Psychology, 15,* 256–268.

Mace, F. C. (1994). The significance and future of functional analysis methodologies. *Journal of Applied Behavior Analysis, 27,* 385–392.

Martin, S. (2006). Youth and mental health stigma. *Trends and Tudes, 5*(8), 1–9.

Mash, E. J. (1985). Some comments on target selection in behavior therapy. *Behavioral Assessment, 7,* 63–78.

Mash, E. J., & Barkley, R. A. (1986). Assessment of family interaction with the Response-Class Matrix. In R. J. Prinz (Ed.), *Advances in the behavioral assessment of children and families* (pp. 29–67). Greenwich, CT: JAI Press.

Mash, E. J., & Barkley, R. A. (Eds.). (2003). *Child psychopathology* (2nd ed.). New York: Guilford Press.

Mash, E. J., & Barkley, R. A. (Eds.). (2006). *Treatment of childhood disorders* (3rd ed.). New York: Guilford Press.

Mash, E. J., & Dozois, D. J. A. (2003). Child psychopathology: A developmental-systems perspective. In E. J. Mash & R. A. Barkley (Eds.), *Child psychopathology* (2nd ed., pp. 3–71). New York: Guilford Press.

Mash, E. J., & Foster, S. L. (2001). Exporting analogue behavioral observation from research to clinical practice: Useful or cost-defective? *Psychological Assessment, 18,* 86–98.

Mash, E. J., & Hunsley, J. (1993). Behavior therapy and managed mental health care: Integrating effectiveness and economics in managed mental health care. *Behavior Therapy, 24,* 67–90.

Mash, E. J., & Hunsley, J. (2004). Behavioral assessment: Sometimes you get what you need. In M. Hersen, S. Haynes, & E. Heiby (Eds.), *The comprehensive handbook of psychological assessment: Vol. 3. Behavioral assessment* (pp. 489–501). New York: Wiley.

Mash, E. J., & Hunsley, J. (Eds.). (2005a). Developing guidelines for the evidence-based assessment of child and adolescent disorders [Special section]. *Journal of Clinical Child and Adolescent Psychology, 34,* 362–558.

Mash, E. J., & Hunsley, J. (2005b). Evidence-based assessment of child and adolescent disorders: Issues and challenges. *Journal of Clinical Child and Adolescent Psychology, 34,* 362–379.

Mash, E. J., & Johnston, C. (1983). A note on the prediction of mothers' behavior with their hyperactive children during play and task situations. *Child and Family Behavior Therapy, 5,* 1–14.

Mash, E. J., & Johnston, C. (1996a). Family relational problems. In V. E. Caballo, J. A. Carrobles, & G. Buela-Casal (Eds.), *Handbook of psychopathology and psychiatric disorders* (pp. 589–621). Madrid: Siglo XXI.

Mash, E. J., & Johnston, C. (1996b). Family relationship problems: Their place in the study of psychopathology. *Journal of Emotional and Behavioral Disorders, 4,* 240–254.

Mash, E. J., Johnston, C., & Kovitz, K. (1983). A comparison of the mother–child interactions of physically abused and non-abused children during play and task situations. *Journal of Clinical Child Psychology, 12,* 337–346.

Mash, E. J., & Terdal, L. G. (Eds.). (1976). *Behavior therapy assessment: Diagnosis, design, and evaluation.* New York: Springer.

Mash, E. J., & Terdal, L. G. (1980). Follow-up assessments in behavior therapy. In P. Karoly & J. J. Steffen (Eds.), *The long-range effects of psychotherapy: Models of durable outcome* (pp. 99–147). New York: Gardner Press.

Mash, E. J., & Terdal, L. G. (1981). Behavioral assessment of childhood disturbance. In E. J. Mash & L. G. Terdal (Eds.), *Behavioral assessment of childhood disorders* (pp. 3–76). New York: Guilford Press.

Mash, E. J., & Terdal, L. G. (1997a). Assessment of child and family disturbance: A behavioral–systems approach. In E. J. Mash & L. G. Terdal (Eds.), *Assessment of childhood disorders* (3rd ed., pp. 3–68). New York: Guilford Press.

Mash, E. J., & Terdal, L. G. (Eds.). (1997b). *Assessment of childhood disorders* (3rd ed.). New York: Guilford Press.

Masten, A. S., Burt, K. B., & Coatsworth, J. D. (2006). Competence and psychopathology in development. In D. Cicchetti & D. J. Cohen (Eds.), *Developmental psychopathology: Vol. 3. Risk, disorder, and adaptation* (2nd ed., pp. 696–738). New York: Wiley.

McConaughy, S. H. (2005). *Clinical interviews for children and adolescents: Assessment to intervention.* New York: Guilford Press.

McCubbin, H. I., & Thompson, A. I. (Eds.). (1987). *Family assessment inventories for research and practice.* Madison: University of Wisconsin–Madison, Family Stress Coping and Health Project.

McDermott, P. A. (1993). National standardization of uniform multisituational measures of child and adolescent behavior pathology. *Psychological Assessment, 5,* 413–424.

McDermott, P. A., & Weiss, R. V. (1995). A normative typology of healthy, subclinical, and clinical behavior styles among American children and adolescents. *Psychological Assessment, 7,* 162–170.

McFall, R. M. (1986). Theory and method in assessment: The vital link. *Behavioral Assessment, 8,* 3–10.

McGillicuddy-DeLisi, A. V. (1985). The relationship between parental beliefs and children's cognitive level. In I. Sigel (Ed.), *Parental belief systems: The psychological consequences for children* (pp. 7–24). Hillsdale, NJ: Erlbaum.

McGivern, J. E., & Marquart, A. M. (2000). Legal and ethical issues in child and adolescent assessment. In E. S. Shapiro & T. R. Kratochwill (Eds.), *Behavioral assessment in schools: Theory, research, and clinical foundations* (2nd ed., pp. 387–434). New York: Guilford Press.

McKenzie, T. L., & Rushall, B. S. (1974). Effects of self-recording on attendance and performance in a competitive swimming training environment. *Journal of Applied Behavior Analysis, 7,* 199–206.

McMahon, R. J. (1984). Self-report instruments. In T. H. Ollendick & M. Hersen (Eds.), *Child behavioral assessment: Principles and procedures* (pp. 80–105). New York: Pergamon Press.

McMahon, R. J., & Forehand, R. (1983). Consumer satisfaction in behavioral treatment of children: Types, issues, and recommendations. *Behavior Therapy, 14,* 209–225.

Melton, G. B., Ehrenreich, X., & Lyons, P. M., Jr. (2001). Ethical and legal issues. In C. E. Walker & M. C. Roberts (Eds.), *Handbook of clinical child psychology* (3rd ed., pp. 1074–1093). New York: Wiley.

Miller, S. A. (1995). Parents' attributions for their children's behavior. *Child Development, 66,* 1557–1584.

Mink, I. T., Meyers, C. E., & Nihara, K. (1984). Taxonomy of family life styles: II. Homes with slow-learning children. *American Journal of Mental Deficiency, 89,* 111–123.

Mink, I. T., Nihira, K., & Meyers, C. E. (1983). Taxonomy of family life styles: I. Homes with TMR children. *American Journal of Mental Deficiency, 87,* 484–497.

Mischel, W. (1973). Toward a cognitive social learning reconceptualization of personality. *Psychological Review, 80,* 252–283.

Mischel, W. (1977). The interaction of person and situation. In D. Magnusson & N. S. Endler (Eds.), *Personality at the crossroads: Current issues in interactional psychology* (pp. 333–352). Hillsdale, NJ: Erlbaum.

Mischel, W. (2004). Toward an integrative science of the person. *Annual Review of Psychology, 55,* 1–22.

Mischel, W., Shoda, Y., & Mendoza-Denton, R. (2002). Situation-behavior profiles as a locus of consistency in personality. *Current Directions in Psychological Science, 11,* 50–54.

Moffitt, T. E. (2006). Life-course persistent versus adolescent-limited antisocial behavior. In D. Cicchetti & D. J. Cohen (Eds.), *Developmental psychopathology: Vol. 3. Risk, disorder, and adaptation* (2nd ed., pp. 570–598). New York: Wiley.

Mooney, C., & Algozzine, B. (1978). A comparison of the disturbingness of behaviors related to learning disability and emotional disturbance. *Journal of Abnormal Child Psychology, 6,* 401–406.

Moos, R. H., & Trickett, E. J. (2002). *Classroom Environment Scale manual* (3rd ed.). Menlo Park, CA: Mind Garden.

Moskowitz, D. S., & Schwarz, J. C. (1982). Validity comparisons of behavior counts and ratings by knowledgeable informants. *Journal of Personality and Social Psychology, 42,* 518–528.

Mussen, P. H. (General Ed.). (1983). *Handbook of child psychology* (4th ed., 4 vols.). New York: Wiley.

Myers, K., & Winters, N. C. (2002). Ten-year review of rating scales: II. Scales for internalizing disorders. *Journal of the American Academy of Child and Adolescent Psychiatry, 41,* 634–659.

Nathan, P. E. (1986). [Review of R. K. Blashfield, *The classification of psychopathology*]. *Behavioral Assessment, 8,* 199–201.

Nelson-Gray, R. O. (1996). Treatment outcome measures: Nomothetic or idiographic? *Clinical Psychology: Science and Practice, 3,* 164–167.

Newberger, C. M. (1978). *Parental conceptions of children and child rearing: A structural developmental analysis.* Unpublished doctoral dissertation, Harvard University, Cambridge, MA.

Nezu, A. M., & Nezu, C. M. (1993). Identifying and selecting target problems for clinical interventions: A problem-solving model. *Psychological Assessment, 5,* 254–263.

Nisbett, R. E., Zukier, H., & Lemley, R. E. (1981). The dilution effect. Nondiagnostic information weakens the implications of diagnostic information. *Cognitive Psychology, 13,* 248–277.

Nordquist, V. M. (1971). The modification of a child's enuresis: Some response–response relationships. *Journal of Applied Behavior Analysis, 4,* 241–247.

Nunnally, J. C., & Bernstein, I. H. (1994). *Psychometric theory* (3rd ed.). New York: McGraw-Hill.

Nurcombe, B., Drell, M. J., Leonard, H. L., & McDermott, J. F. (2002). Clinical problem solving: The case of Matthew, Part I. *Journal of the American Academy of Child and Adolescent Psychiatry, 41,* 92–97.

Ogles, B. M., Lambert, M. J., & Masters, K. S. (1996). *Assessing outcome in clinical practice.* Needham Heights, MA: Allyn & Bacon.

Ollendick, T. H., & Hersen, M. (Eds.). (1993). *Handbook of child and adolescent assessment.* Needham Heights, MA: Allyn & Bacon.

Olweus, D. (1979). Stability of aggressive reaction patterns in males. *Psychological Bulletin, 86,* 852–875.

Ozonoff, S., Goodlin-Jones, B. L., & Solomon, M. (2005). Evidence-based assessment of autism spectrum disorders in children and adolescents. *Journal of Clinical Child and Adolescent Psychology, 34,* 523–540.

Parke, R. D., MacDonald, K. B., Beital, A., & Bhavnagri, N. (1988). The role of the family in the development of peer relationships. In R. DeV. Peters & R. J. McMahon (Eds.), *Social learning and systems approaches to marriage and the family* (pp. 17–44). Philadelphia: Brunner/Mazel.

Parker, S., Zucker, B., & Augustyn, M. (Eds.). (2005). *Developmental and behavioral pediatrics: A handbook for primary care*. Philadelphia: Lippincott/Williams & Wilkins.

Passman, R. H., & Mulhern, R. K. (1977). Maternal punitiveness as affected by situational stress: An experimental analogue of child abuse. *Journal of Abnormal Psychology, 86*, 565–569.

Patterson, G. R. (1982). *Coercive family process*. Eugene, OR: Castalia.

Patterson, G. R. (1986). Performance models for antisocial boys. *American Psychologist, 41*, 432–444.

Patterson, G. R., & Bank, L. (1986). Bootstrapping your way in the nomological thicket. *Behavioral Assessment, 8*, 49–73.

Patterson, G. R., & Bechtel, G. C. (1977). Formulating situational environment in relation to states and traits. In R. B. Cattell & R. M. Greger (Eds.), *Handbook of modern personality theory* (pp. 254–268). Washington, DC: Halstead.

Patterson, G. R., Reid, J. B., & Dishion, T. J. (1992). *Antisocial boys*. Eugene, OR: Castalia.

Pelham, W. E., Fabiano, G. A., & Massetti, G. M. (2005). Evidence-based assessment of attention deficit hyperactivity disorder in children and adolescents. *Journal of Clinical Child and Adolescent Psychology, 34*, 449–476.

Pepler, D. J., Corter, C., & Abramovitch, R. (1982, May). *Am I my brother's brother?: Sibling perceptions*. Paper presented at the Waterloo Conference on Child Development, Waterloo, Ontario, Canada.

Peterson, D. R. (1968). *The clinical study of social behavior*. New York: Appleton–Century–Crofts.

Peterson, L., Burbach, D. J., & Chaney, J. (1989). Developmental issues. In C. G. Last & M. Hersen (Eds.), *Handbook of child psychiatric diagnosis* (pp. 463–482). New York: Wiley-Interscience.

Pickles, A., & Angold, A. (2003). Natural categories or fundamental dimensions: On carving nature at the joints and the rearticulation of psychopathology. *Development and Psychopathology, 15*, 529–551.

Powers, M. D. (1984). Syndromal diagnosis and the behavioral assessment of childhood disorders. *Child and Family Behavior Therapy, 6*(3), 1–15.

Puig-Antich, J., & Chambers, W. (1978). *Schedule for Affective Disorders and Schizophrenia for School-Aged Children*. New York: New York State Psychiatric Institute.

Quintana, S. M., Aboud, F. E., Chao, R. K., Contreras-Grau, J., Cross, W. E., Jr., Hudley, C., et al. (2006). Race, ethnicity, and culture in child development: Contemporary research and future directions. *Child Development, 77*, 1129–1141.

Rae, W. A., Brunnquell, D., Sullivan, J. R. (2003). Ethical and legal issues in pediatric psychology. In M. C. Roberts (Ed.), *Handbook of pediatric psychology* (3rd ed., pp. 32–49). New York: Guilford Press.

Rains, P. M., Kitsuse, J. I., Duster, T., & Friedson, E. (1975). The labeling approach to deviance. In N. Hobbs (Ed.), *Issues in the classification of children* (Vol. 1, pp. 88–100). San Francisco: Jossey-Bass.

Reid, J. B., Patterson, G. R., Baldwin, D. V., & Dishion, T. J. (1988). Observations in the assessment of childhood disorders. In M. Rutter, A. H. Tuma, & I. S. Lann (Eds.), *Assessment and diagnosis in child psychopathology* (pp. 156–195). New York: Guilford Press.

Reid, J. B., Taplin, P. S., & Lorber, R. (1981). A social interactional approach to the treatment of abusive families. In R. B. Stuart (Ed.), *Violent behavior: Social learning approaches to prediction management and treatment* (pp. 83–101). New York: Brunner/Mazel.

Rende, R., & Waldman, I. (2006). Behavioral and molecular genetics and developmental psychopathology. In D. Cicchetti & D. J. Cohen (Eds.), *Developmental psychopathology: Vol. 2. Developmental neuroscience* (2nd ed., pp. 427–464). New York: Wiley.

Reynolds, C. R., & Kamphaus, R. W. (2002). *Clinician's guide to the Behavioral Assessment System for Children (BASC)*. New York: Guilford Press.

Reynolds, C. R., & Kamphaus, R. W. (Eds.). (2003a). *Handbook of psychological and educational assessment of children: Intelligence, aptitude, and achievement* (2nd ed.). New York: Guilford Press.

Reynolds, C. R., & Kamphaus, R. W. (Eds.). (2003b). *Handbook of psychological and educational assessment of children: Personality, behavior, and context* (2nd ed.). New York: Guilford Press.

Reynolds, C. R., & Kamphaus, R. W. (2004). *BASC-2: Behavior Assessment System for Children* (2nd ed.). Circle Pines, MN: AGS Publishing.

Reynolds, W. M. (1993). Self-report methodology. In T. H. Ollendick & M. Hersen (Eds.), *Handbook of child and adolescent assessment* (pp. 98–123). Needham Heights, MA: Allyn & Bacon.

Richters, J. E. (1992). Depressed mothers as informants about their children: A critical review of the evidence for distortion. *Psychological Bulletin, 112*, 485–499.

Roberts, M. C. (Ed.). (2005). *Handbook of pediatric psychology* (3rd ed.). New York: Guilford Press.

Rodick, J. D., Henggeler, S. W., & Hanson, C. L. (1986). An evaluation of the Family Adaptability and Cohesion Evaluation Scales and the Circumplex Model. *Journal of Abnormal Child Psychology, 14*, 77–87.

Rosch, E. (1978). Principles of categorization. In E. Rosch & B. B. Lloyd (Eds.), *Cognition and categorization* (pp. 27–48). Hillsdale, NJ: Erlbaum.

Rothbart, M. K., & Goldsmith, H. H. (1985). Three approaches to the study of infant temperament. *Developmental Review, 5*, 237–260.

Russell, M. B., & Bernal, M. E. (1977). Temporal and climatic variables in naturalistic observation. *Journal of Applied Behavior Analysis, 10*, 399–405.

Rutter, M. (1979). Maternal deprivation, 1972–1978: New findings, new concepts, new approaches. *Child Development, 50*, 283–305.

Sackett, D. L., Straus, S. E., Richardson, W. S., Rosenberg, W., & Haynes, R. B. (2000). *Evidence-based medicine: How to practice and teach EBM* (2nd ed.). London: Churchill Livingstone.

Salzinger, S., Kaplan, S., & Artemyeff, C. (1983). Mothers' personal social networks and child maltreatment. *Journal of Abnormal Psychology, 92,* 68–76.

Sanders, M. R., & Lawton, J. M. (1993). Discussing assessment findings with families: A guided participation model of information transfer. *Child and Family Behavior Therapy, 15,* 5–35.

Santostefano, S. (1978). *A biodevelopmental approach to clinical child psychology: Cognitive controls and cognitive control therapy.* New York: Wiley.

Sattler, J. M. (1998). *Clinical and forensic interviewing of children and families: Guidelines for the mental health, education, pediatric, and child maltreatment fields.* San Diego, CA: Author.

Sattler, J. M. (2001). *Assessment of children: Cognitive applications* (4th ed.). San Diego, CA: Author.

Sattler, J. M., & Hoge, R. D. (2006). *Assessment of children: Behavioral, social, and clinical foundations* (5th ed.). La Mesa, CA: Author.

Sattler, J. M., & Mash, E. J. (1998). Introduction to clinical assessment interviewing. In J. M. Sattler, *Clinical and forensic interviewing of children and families: Guidelines for the mental health, education, pediatric, and child maltreatment fields* (pp. 2–44). San Diego, CA: Author.

Schaefer, E. S., & Bell, R. Q. (1958). Development of a parent attitude research instrument. *Child Development, 9,* 339–361.

Schlundt, D. G., & McFall, R. M. (1987). Classifying social situations: A comparison of five methods. *Behavioral Assessments, 9,* 21–42.

Serafica, F. C., & Vargas, L. A. (2006). Cultural diversity in the development of child psychopathology. In D. Cicchetti & D. J. Cohen (Eds.), *Developmental psychopathology: Vol. 1. Theory and method* (2nd ed., pp. 588–626). New York: Wiley.

Shapiro, E. S., & Cole, C. L. (1984). Self-monitoring. In T. H. Ollendick & M. Hersen (Eds.), *Handbook of child and adolescent assessment* (pp. 124–139). Needham Heights, MA: Allyn & Bacon.

Sigel, I., McGillicuddy-DeLisi, A. V., & Goodnow, J. J. (Eds.). (1992). *Parental belief systems: The psychological consequences for children* (2nd ed.). Hillsdale, NJ: Erlbaum.

Silverman, W. K., & Ollendick, T. H. (2005). Evidence-based assessment of anxiety and its disorders in children and adolescents. *Journal of Clinical Child and Adolescent Psychology, 34,* 380–411.

Slabach, E. H., Morrow, J., & Wachs, T. (1991). Questionnaire measurement of infant and child temperament: Current status and future directions. In J. Strelau & A. Angleitner (Eds.), *Explorations in temperament: International perspectives on theory and measurement: Perspectives on individual differences* (pp. 205–234). New York: Plenum Press.

Sroufe, L. A., & Fleeson, J. (1986). Attachment and the construction of relationships. In W. Hartup & Z. Rubin (Eds.), *Relationships and development* (pp. 51–71). Hillsdale, NJ: Erlbaum.

Stifter, C. A., & Wiggins, C. N. (2004). Assessment of disturbances in emotion regulation and temperament. In R. DelCarmen-Wiggins & A. Carter (Eds.), *Handbook of infant, toddler, and preschool mental health assessment* (pp. 79–103). New York: Oxford University Press.

Strosahl, K. D. (1994). Entering the new frontier of managed mental health care: Gold mines and land mines. *Cognitive and Behavioral Practice, 1,* 5–23.

Tabachnik, N., & Alloy, L. B. (1988). Clinician and patient as aberrant actuaries: Expectation-based distortions in assessment of covariation. In L. Y. Abramson (Ed.), *Social cognition and clinical psychology: A synthesis* (pp. 295–365). New York: Guilford Press.

Tharp, R. G. (1991). Cultural diversity and treatment of children. *Journal of Consulting and Clinical Psychology, 59,* 799–812.

Touliatos, J., Perlmutter, B. F., Straus, M. A., & Holden, G. W. (Eds.). (2001). *Handbook of family measurement techniques* (Vols. 1–3). Thousand Oaks, CA: Sage.

Tronick, E. Q., & Gianino, A. (1986). Interactive mismatch and repair: Challenges to the coping infant. *Zero to Three, 6,* 1–6.

Tuma, F., Loeber, R., & Lochman, J. E. (2006). Introduction to special section on the National Institute of Health state of the science report on violence prevention. *Journal of Abnormal Child Psychology, 34,* 451–456.

Urbina, S. (2004). *Essentials of psychological testing.* Hoboken, NJ: Wiley.

U.S. Department of Health and Human Services. (1999). *Mental health: A report of the Surgeon General.* Rockville, MD: National Institutes of Health, National Institute of Mental Health.

Van Goor-Lambo, G. (1987). The reliability of Axis V of the multiaxial classification scheme. *Journal of Child Psychology and Psychiatry, 28,* 597–612.

Vincent, T. A., & Trickett, E. J. (1983). Preventive interventions and the human context: Ecological approaches to environmental assessment and change. In R. D. Felner, L. A. Jason, J. N. Moritsugu, & S. S. Farber (Eds.), *Preventive psychology: Theory research and practice* (pp. 67–86). New York: Pergamon Press.

Voeltz, L. M., & Evans, I. M. (1982). The assessment of behavioral interrelationships in child behavior therapy. *Behavioral Assessment, 4,* 131–165.

Wahler, R. G. (1975). Some structural aspects of deviant child behavior. *Journal of Applied Behavior Analysis, 8,* 27–42.

Wahler, R. G. (1980). The insular mother: Her problems in parent–child treatment. *Journal of Applied Behavior Analysis, 13,* 207–219.

Wahler, R. G., & Cormier, W. H. (1970). The ecological

interview: A first step in out-patient child behavior therapy. *Journal of Behavior Therapy and Experimental Psychiatry, 1,* 279–289.

Wahler, R. G., & Graves, M. G. (1983). Setting events in social networks: Ally or enemy in child behavior therapy? *Behavior Therapy, 14,* 19–36.

Wahler, R. G., Leske, G., & Rogers, E. D. (1979). The insular family: A deviance support system for oppositional children. In L. A. Hamerlynck (Ed.), *Behavioral systems for the developmentally disabled: Vol. 1. School and family environments* (pp. 102–127). New York: Brunner/Mazel.

Wahler, R. G., Sperling, K. A., Thomas, M. R., Teeter, N. C., & Luper, H. L. (1970). The modification of childhood stuttering: Some response–response relationships. *Journal of Experimental Child Psychology, 9,* 411–428.

Wasik, B. H. (1984). Clinical applications of direct behavioral observation: A look at the past and the future. In B. B. Lahey & A. E. Kazdin (Eds.), *Advances in clinical child psychology* (pp. 156–193). New York: Plenum Press.

Watson, D., & Clark, L. A. (2006). Clinical diagnosis at the crossroads. *Clinical Psychology: Science and Practice, 13,* 210–215.

Weinrott, M. R., Reid, J. B., Bauske, B. W., & Brummett, B. (1981). Supplementing naturalistic observations with observer impressions. *Behavioral Assessment, 3,* 151–159.

Weiss, R. L., & Chaffin, L. (1986, May). *Micro- and macro-coding of marital interactions.* Paper presented at the meeting of the Western Psychological Association, Seattle, WA.

Weiss, R. L., & Margolin, G. (1986). Assessment of marital conflict and accord. In A. R. Ciminero, K. S. Calhoun, & H. E. Adams (Eds.), *Handbook of behavioral assessment* (2nd ed., pp. 561–600). New York: Wiley.

Weisz, J. R., Chu, B. C., & Polo, A. J. (2004). Treatment dissemination and evidence-based practice: Strengthening intervention through clinician-research collaboration. *Clinical Psychology: Science and Practice, 11,* 300–307.

Whalen, C. K., Henker, B., Collins, B. E., Finck, D., & Dotemoto, S. (1979). A social ecology of hyperactive boys: Medication effects in structured classroom environments. *Journal of Applied Behavior Analysis, 12,* 65–81.

Whalen, C. K., Henker, B., Jamner, L. D., Ishikawa, S. S., Floro, J. N., Swindle, R., et al. (2006). Toward mapping daily challenges of living with ADHD: Maternal and child perspectives using electronic diaries. *Journal of Abnormal Child Psychology, 34,* 115–130.

Willems, E. P. (1973). Go ye into all the world and modify behavior: An ecologist's view. *Representative Research in Social Psychology, 4,* 93–105.

Willems, E. P. (1974). Behavioral technology and behavioral ecology. *Journal of Applied Behavior Analysis, 7,* 151–165.

Winters, N. C., Collett, B. R., & Myers, K. M. (2005). Ten-year review of rating scales, VII: Scales assessing functional impairment. *Journal of the American Academy of Child and Adolescent Psychiatry, 44,* 309–338.

Winters, N. C., Myers, K., & Proud, L. (2002). Ten-year review of rating scales: III. Scales assessing suicidality, cognitive style, and self-esteem. *Journal of the American Academy of Child and Adolescent Psychiatry, 41,* 1150–1181.

Wolf, M. M. (1978). Social validity: The case for subjective measurement or how applied behavior analysis is finding its heart. *Journal of Applied Behavior Analysis, 11,* 203–214.

World Health Organization. (1992). *The ICD-10 classification of mental and behavioral disorders: Clinical descriptions and diagnostic guidelines.* Geneva, Switzerland: Author.

Yarrow, M. R., Campbell, J. D., & Burton, R. V. (1970). Recollections of childhood: A study of the retrospective method. *Monographs of the Society for Research in Child Development* (Vol. 35, Serial No. 138).

Yeates, K. O., Ris, M. D., & Taylor, H. G. (Eds.). (2000). *Pediatric neuropsychology: Research, theory, and practice.* New York: Guilford Press.

Yeh, M., & Weisz, J. R. (2001). Why are we here at the clinic?: Parent–child (dis)agreement on referral problems at treatment entry. *Journal of Consulting and Clinical Psychology, 69,* 1018–1025.

Youngstrom, E. A., Findling, R. L., & Calabrese, J. R. (2003). Who are the comorbid adolescents?: Agreement between psychiatric diagnosis, youth, parent, and teacher report. *Journal of Abnormal Child Psychology, 31,* 231–245.

Yule, W. (1993). Developmental considerations in child assessment. In T. H. Ollendick & M. Hersen (Eds.), *Handbook of child and adolescent assessment* (pp. 15–25). Needham Heights, MA: Allyn & Bacon.

Zachary, R. A., Levin, B., Hargreaves, W. A., & Greene, J. A. (1981). *Trends in the use of psychiatric diagnoses for children: 1960–1979.* Unpublished manuscript, University of California at San Francisco.

Zangwill, W. M., & Kniskern, J. R. (1982). Comparison of problem families in the clinic and at home. *Behavior Therapy, 13,* 145–152.

Zero to Three/National Center for Clinical Infant Programs. (1994). *Diagnostic classification of mental health and developmental disorders of infancy and early childhood* (Diagnostic Classification: 0–3). Washington, DC: Author.

PART II

Behavior Disorders

CHAPTER 2

Attention-Deficit/Hyperactivity Disorder

Bradley H. Smith
Russell A. Barkley
Cheri J. Shapiro

Individuals with attention-deficit/hyperactivity disorder (ADHD), by definition, display difficulties with attention and/or impulse control and hyperactive behavior relative to most individuals of the same age and sex (American Psychiatric Association [APA], 2000). This is a prevalent disorder, with modern estimates indicating that at least 3.0 to 7.8% of the general population meet criteria for ADHD in studies in the United States and around the world (Biederman, 2005). Although ADHD is usually first diagnosed in childhood, it need not be so, with some cases not coming to clinical attention until adolescence or adulthood, if at all. Up to 67% of all cases arise in childhood, before 7 years of age (Applegate et al., 1997), with 98% or more developing by age 16 years (Barkley, Murphy, & Fischer, in press). ADHD typically persists into adulthood and is seen in 66% or more of cases diagnosed in childhood (Barkley, 2005).

ADHD causes significant impairment in the vast majority of major life domains, such as educational, family, and peer functioning, and may contribute to problems such as impaired personal safety, criminal behavior, and substance abuse (Barkley, Fischer, Smallish, & Fletcher, 2004, 2006; Molina & Pelham, 2003). The annual costs to society due to ADHD are estimated to be in the billions of dollars (Jensen et al., 2005). Thus, it is an important disorder to identify properly and treat effectively. Unfortunately, ADHD presents as a heterogeneous disorder, and response to treatment may be somewhat idiosyncratic. Fortunately, there are good methods for diagnosing and treating ADHD (Smith, Barkley, & Shapiro, 2006). The key elements of state-of-the-art procedures for diagnosis and monitoring treatment response are presented in this chapter, including, but not limited to, heavy reliance on collateral information, ability to account for variations in task and situation, and frequently repeated data collection.

This chapter focuses primarily on evaluation of children and adolescents with ADHD. We start with a brief discussion of background and theory related to ADHD, including a detailed critique of the current diagnostic criteria for ADHD. We then describe three levels of assessment for ADHD: (1) the minimally sufficient assessment; (2) the ADHD checkup, which combines assessment and intervention; and (3) the assessment of response to intervention. A more detailed presentation on assessing and treating ADHD, including information on evaluating adults with ADHD, is found in Barkley (2005).

This chapter extends its predecessor in the third edition in two important directions. First, by incorporating motivational interviewing into the assessment, it is reconceptualized as an intervention in part designed to motivate parents and individuals with ADHD to better adopt and comply with intervention recommendations. We call this the "ADHD checkup," or ACU, which is based on the "Family Checkup" (Dishion & Kavanagh, 2003) and the "drinker's checkup" (Miller & Rollnick, 2002).

The second new direction emphasizes assessment as an ongoing process. It is critically important to evaluate response to treatment repeatedly and on a case-by-case basis. This is necessary because response to treatment, although commonplace at the group level (e.g., 65–85% of cases respond to medications for ADHD), is hard to predict at the individual level of analysis; therefore, treatment is never guaranteed to work. Whether it does so should be specifically evaluated (Barkley, 2005). Thus, every case of ADHD should be approached as an individualized case study, yet be feasible for most families and clinicians.

This chapter makes an additional departure from previous editions by eschewing a compendium approach, in which all available measures receive notice and comment in favor of a focus on a reduced set of procedures that are feasible and clinically meaningful. It provides a new, dynamic, intervention-focused approach to evaluation of ADHD. For instance, even though the criteria for ADHD specified by the fourth edition of the *Diagnostic and Statistical Manual of Mental Disorders* (DSM-IV; APA, 1994) have merit, they also suffer from some significant limitations. A DSM-IV diagnosis of ADHD alone provides only the most basic information to guide selection and evaluation of treatment. It must be supplemented by a person × environment interaction, in which the symptoms of the disorder are conceded to have strong neurological and genetic underpinnings, whereas the extent of impairments in major life activities that arise from symptoms depend in large part on context and comorbidity. Therefore, we recommend that the scope of evaluation be expanded to include collecting data from multiple informants (e.g., parent and teacher knowledge of ADHD), assessing the extent of comorbid disorders and developmental/learning disabilities, comparing multiple environments associated with high and low func-

tioning, getting information on systemic factors that might influence diagnosis and treatment (e.g., marital discord, poor home–school communication, pertinent community resources), and assessing motivation or readiness to change. This is done with the ACU. Assessment should resemble not just a snapshot, but a dynamic video that informs treatment decisions by evaluating ongoing responses to intervention. Done efficiently, it can be acceptable, feasible, economical, and sustainable in settings in which the procedures are most needed, yet time and cost are crucial factors.

INCREMENTAL VALIDITY

A guiding principle in this chapter is the concept of incremental validity (Sechrest, 1963)— that purely redundant measures should be eliminated. This is especially true when the choice is between relatively inexpensive measures (e.g., standardized rating scales) and relatively expensive measures (e.g., structured interviews). The notion that "less is more" applied to redundant measures has both practical and scientific advantages (Cohen, 2003). Efficient nonredundant assessments place less of a burden on families, teachers, and practitioners, yet they achieve greater clarity and validity.

Unfortunately, many professionals use excessively lengthy, redundant assessment batteries or otherwise inefficient methods to seek unnecessary comprehensiveness (Pelham, Fabiano, & Massetti, 2005). This undermines the goal of making assessment feasible in most clinical settings. Practitioners should naturally make informed choices about assessment methods based on available evidence, allowing room for clinical judgment when such data are not available. We recommend that clinicians, and even researchers, should not waste their time routinely conducting structured diagnostic interviews for every child (e.g., Diagnostic Interview Schedule for Children [DISC]; Shaffer et al., 1996) because they add very little to clinical prediction or diagnostic accuracy beyond what is achieved with the far more efficient and cost-effective parent and teacher ratings scales (Pelham et al., 2005). Instead, we recommend a stepwise protocol in which symptom information is initially gained via rating scales, and screen-positive cases are further evaluated with semistructured interviews. Those interviews place emphasis on motivational interviewing techniques to enhance treatment adoption and adherence.

We appreciate that our recommendation is probably more rigorous than what is normally done in contemporary clinical practice. For instance, primary care clinicians often make diagnostic and treatment decisions based primarily on parent reports (Wolraich, 2002). Although sometimes "less is more," a multitude of biases exists in any single measure or source, giving a misleading view of the child. Instead, a multitrait–multimethod (MTMM; Campbell & Fiske, 1959) approach is indicated, but not slavishly so. It is surely expedient to rely on a simple, easy to collect measure, such as a parent rating scale, but it may be problematic for various reasons (i.e., parental bias due to maternal depression or anti-ADHD stories in the media). To paraphrase H. L. Menken, "For every complex problem, there is a simple solution—and it is wrong."

CHAPTER OVERVIEW

We begin with a brief overview of ADHD, covering the history, definition and primary problems, diagnostic criteria, onset and life course, prevalence, gender differences, etiologies, and predictors of outcomes. We then briefly review Barkley's theory of ADHD, because it can guide assessment and conceptualization of this disorder. We then describe the ACU. This approach includes "guided participation" or "motivational interviewing" that has a solid theoretical and empirical basis in other clinical populations (Dishion & Kavanagh, 2003; Miller & Rollnick, 2003; Sanders & Lawton, 1993). Thereafter, we make some recommendations for assessing adults with ADHD. The strong genetic basis to ADHD means that parents are likely to have the same disorder, so assessing adults may be a supplemental activity to the evaluation of the child. Also, because ADHD tends to be a chronic disorder, it seems important to take a lifespan perspective on its assessment. Finally, we provide some information on assessing response to treatment. For the specific details of treatment, we direct the interested reader to other volumes (e.g., Smith et al., 2006) and manuals or training materials (e.g., Barkley, 1997d) that have a strong evidence base (see Pelham, Wheeler, & Chronis, 1998).

The process of assessment typically changes the attributes being measured—what methodologists often call "reactivity," which is typically viewed as a negative confound in the evaluation process (Webb, Campbell, Schwartz, & Sechrest, 1966). Yet through the guided participation process, reactivity can be harnessed as a positive force in the therapeutic process. Thus, assessment should be regarded as the initial phase of intervention. Furthermore, good intervention includes continued assessment in an interactive or dialectical process.

OVERVIEW OF ADHD

Over the prior 25 years (Barkley, 1981) there has been tremendous change in the conceptualization of and criteria for diagnosing ADHD, with growing consensus that "ADHD" is heterogeneous, comprising a set of disorders or subtypes. Diagnosis involves looking at two sets of core symptoms (i.e., inattention and hyperactivity/impulsivity) and determining whether the disorder is predominately related to either set or to their combination. Yet future diagnostic criteria might need to consider a third set of core symptoms of ADHD, such as sluggish cognitive tempo, that may define a qualitatively different subset of children (Milich, Balentine, & Lynam, 2001; Todd, Rasmussen, Wood, Levy, & Hay, 2004).

History

A more extensive history can be found in the text by Barkley (2005). The first clinical description of children with symptoms of ADHD was published over 100 years ago. In a series of three lectures to the Royal College of Physicians in England, George Still described children in his clinical practice who were quite aggressive, defiant, resistant to discipline, highly emotional, poorly inhibited, and otherwise lacking in self-control (Still, 1902). Most were also excessively active and distractible, with poorly sustained attention to tasks. Such children would probably now be viewed as having not only ADHD but also oppositional defiant disorder (ODD) or even conduct disorder (CD) (APA, 2000).

During the next 35 years, few papers appeared on this subject in children, presumably as a consequence of two world wars. Papers that were published in relation to the disorder or its symptoms focused on either (1) the encephalitis epidemic of the early part of that century as causing such symptoms or (2) the motor restlessness that characterized these children (Childers, 1935; Levin, 1938). Scant attention was given to disturbances in self-regulation and social conduct.

More widespread interest in these children did not emerge until after World War II. At that time, the highly influential writings of Strauss and Lehtinen (1947) and their colleagues advocated that restless and inattentive behavior was de facto evidence of brain damage in children. The term "minimal brain damage" was coined to refer to these children, and strict guidelines were advocated for their education.

Conclusions concerning brain damage as a cause of hyperactivity became less frequent over time, though brain dysfunction was believed somehow to be related to the disorder. This resulted in a softening of the terminology for the disorder from "minimal brain damage" to "minimal brain dysfunction" (Wender, 1971). Eventually, the link with neurological damage was dropped from the diagnostic terminology. Nevertheless, the association of ADHD with abnormal brain functioning remained strong until the 1970s, when a series of publications disputed the relationship to brain damage (Rutter, 1977).

Increasing emphasis on excessive motor activity as the central symptom of the disorder arose from the 1950s through the 1970s. Some authors (Laufer, Denhoff, & Solomons, 1957) posited a possible defect in the filtering of stimuli in the central nervous system as the cause, allowing excessive stimulation to reach the cortex. Later, others viewed the disorder as simply a daily rate of motor activity significantly deviant from that of normal children (Chess, 1960; Werry & Sprague, 1970), without reference to its origins. The disorder began to be known by its behavioral symptoms instead, such as "hyperactive child syndrome" (Chess, 1960) or "hyperkinetic reaction of childhood" (APA, 1968).

By the mid-1970s, evidence suggested that hyperactive children also had major deficits with sustained attention and impulse control. Douglas and Peters (1979) argued that the disorder comprised impairments in (1) investment, organization, and maintenance of attention; (2) inhibition of impulsive responding; (3) modulation of arousal levels to meet situational demands; and (4) a strong tendency to seek immediate reinforcement. Excessive motor activity was viewed as being problematic, but the core deficit of the disorder was proposed to involve attention and inhibitory problems.

The APA (1980) eventually relabeled the disorder as "attention deficit disorder ([ADD] with or without hyperactivity)" in DSM-III, in part as a result of Douglas's (1983) influential reviews on the field. The change essentially demoted hyperactivity to an unnecessary or simply a related characteristic, yet one that could be used to create subtypes of the disorder based on its presence or absence (APA, 1980).

Later in the 1980s, the disorder was relabeled yet again as "attention-deficit/hyperactivity disorder" in DSM-III-R (APA, 1987), suggesting a reemergence of the importance of hyperactivity as one of the central features of the disorder, equal in import to the other features (i.e., inattention and impulsiveness). The subtyping scheme of "without hyperactivity" was demoted in this revision, not because children who are primarily inattentive do not exist, but because it was unclear at the time whether they represented a true subtype of this disorder or a separate diagnostic entity altogether (Barkley, 1990; Carlson, 1986). Clinicians could label such children as having "undifferentiated attention deficit disorder" but were provided no criteria for diagnosis, nor was the relationship of this disorder to ADHD clarified. More research was recommended before the answers to these issues could guide such a taxonomic enterprise.

Across the 1980s, many scientists came to posit that the central deficiency in ADD/ADHD children was poor executive functioning or poor self-regulation of behavior (Barkley, 1981, 1990; Douglas, 1983; Kendall & Braswell, 1985). This trend continues to the present (see below; Barkley & Murphy, 2006). It resembles in some respects a return to Still's (1902) earlier notions that deficits in volitional inhibition and moral regulation of behavior explain the disorder, if the moral regulation is taken to mean the selection of actions as a function of their future consequences for oneself and for others, as Still intended.

In 1994, when the DSM was once again revised (DSM-IV), several important changes were added to the diagnostic criteria. These are discussed in detail later in the chapter. Suffice it to say here that the option of diagnosing children with a subtype of the disorder characterized by primary attention problems without hyperactivity or impulsiveness has been restored to this taxonomy, despite continuing scientific uncertainty over whether children who are primarily inattentive actually represent a subtype of ADHD or an entirely separate disorder (Barkley, 2005; Barkley, Grodzinsky, & DuPaul, 1992; Lahey & Carlson, 1992; Milich et al., 2001).

In DSM-III-R (APA, 1987), an attempt was made to draw upon the results of factor-analytic studies of child behavior rating scales to aid expert opinion in the selection of symptoms (Spitzer, Davies, & Barkley, 1990). A small-scale field trial employing 500 children from multiple clinical sites was conducted to narrow down the potential list of symptoms and to specify a cutoff score on this list that best differentiated between children with ADHD and other diagnostic groups. In the most recent revision (APA, 2000), DSM-IV-TR criteria are based on a better field trial and more thorough analysis of its results (Applegate et al., 1997; Lahey et al., 1994). These DSM-IV-TR criteria appear in Table 2.1 and are discussed in detail in a separate section.

Definition and Primary Symptoms

The term "symptom" as used here refers to a behavior (e.g., skips from one uncompleted activity to another) or group of behaviors that covary (e.g., inattention) and are believed to represent a dimension of a mental disorder. We want to distinguish between the terms "symptom" and "impairment," because the two are often confused in clinical discussions of disorders. Impairments are consequences or outcomes of symptoms or symptom classes, such as retention in a grade; failure to graduate from high school; and proneness to vehicular crashes or license suspensions, teen pregnancy, or criminal arrests. In this section we describe the major symptom dimensions of ADHD. Related impairments are described elsewhere in the chapter.

There is strong consensus that ADHD is defined by two clusters of symptoms: inattention and hyperactivity–impulsivity (Barkley, 2005). These core symptoms of ADHD are correlated with each other, but growing information indicates that they are partially distinct, such that individuals having largely one set of symptoms (inattention, mainly) and not the other (hyperactive–impulsive behavior) may describe a qualitatively different group, and possibly a

different disorder (Diamond, 2005; Milich et al., 2001; Nigg et al., 2005). Thus, a person diagnosed with ADHD may have problems related to inattention or hyperactivity–impulsivity, or typically both. Available evidence indicates that by adulthood, this two-dimensional structure could evolve into a three-dimensional one, in that symptoms of largely verbal impulsiveness come to form a dimension separate from that of hyperactivity (Barkley et al., in press). Some have argued that other dimensions of ADHD may also exist (e.g., slowed cognitive tempo, discussed in more detail later). These dimensions have not yet been incorporated into the definition of ADHD. Therefore, this section focuses on the well-established core symptoms of inattention and hyperactivity–impulsivity.

Inattention

The construct of attention as studied in neuropsychology is multidimensional and may refer to alertness, arousal, selectivity, focus, encoding, sustained attention, distractibility, or span of apprehension, among others (Barkley, 1988; Hale & Lewis, 1979; Mirsky, 1996; Strauss, Thompson, Adams, Redline, & Burant, 2000). However, the number of distinct components identified in neuropsychological batteries remains unclear (Strauss et al., 2000). Research shows that those with ADHD do not have significant difficulties with automatically orienting to visual information, which may be mediated by posterior brain attention circuits (Nigg, 2006). Instead, they have their greatest difficulties with aspects of attention related to persistence of effort, or sustaining attention to tasks, sometimes called vigilance (Douglas, 1983; Newcorn et al., 2001; Swaab-Barneveld et al., 2000). These deficits are believed to be mediated through largely frontal brain attention circuits (Nigg, 2006).

Difficulties with persistence are sometimes apparent in free-play settings, as evidenced by shorter durations of play with each toy and frequent shifts in play across various toys (Barkley & Ullman, 1975; Routh & Schroeder, 1976; Zentall, 1985). However, inattention is most dramatically apparent in situations requiring the child to sustain attention to dull, boring, repetitive tasks (Barkley, DuPaul, & McMurray, 1990; Fischer, Barkley, Smallish, & Fletcher, 2005; Newcorn et al., 2001; Zentall, 1985). Examples of such tasks include independent

TABLE 2.1. DSM-IV-TR Criteria for ADHD

A. Either (1) or (2):
  (1) six (or more) of the following symptoms of **inattention** have persisted for at least 6 months to a degree that is maladaptive and inconsistent with developmental level:

  Inattention
  (a) often fails to give close attention to details or makes careless mistakes in schoolwork, work, or other activities
  (b) often has difficulty sustaining attention in tasks or play activities
  (c) often does not seem to listen when spoken to directly
  (d) often does not follow through on instructions and fails to finish schoolwork, chores, or duties in the workplace (not due to oppositional behavior or failure to understand instructions)
  (e) often has difficulty organizing tasks and activities
  (f) often avoids, dislikes, or is reluctant to engage in tasks that require sustained mental effort (such as school work or homework)
  (g) often loses things necessary for tasks or activities (e.g., toys, school assignments, pencils, books, or tools)
  (h) is often easily distracted by extraneous stimuli
  (i) is often forgetful in daily activities

  (2) six (or more) of the following symptoms of **hyperactivity–impulsivity** have persisted for at least 6 months to a degree that is maladaptive and inconsistent with developmental level:

  Hyperactivity
  (a) often fidgets with hands or feet or squirms in seat
  (b) often leaves seat in classroom or in other situations in which remaining seated is expected
  (c) often runs about or climbs excessively in situations in which it is inappropriate (in adolescents or adults, may be limited to subjective feelings of restlessness)
  (d) often has difficulty playing or engaging in leisure activities quietly
  (e) is often "on the go" or often acts as if "driven by a motor"
  (f) often talks excessively

  Impulsivity
  (g) often blurts out answers before the questions have been completed
  (h) often has difficulty awaiting turn
  (i) often interrupts or intrudes on others (e.g., butts into conversations or games)

B. Some hyperactive–impulsive or inattentive symptoms that caused impairment were present before age 7 years.

C. Some impairment from the symptoms is present in two or more settings (e.g., at school [or work] and at home).

D. There must be clear evidence of clinically significant impairment in social, academic, or occupational functioning.

E. The symptoms do not occur exclusively during the course of a Pervasive Developmental Disorder, Schizophrenia, or other Psychotic Disorder, and are not better accounted for by another mental disorder (e.g., Mood Disorder, Anxiety Disorder, Dissociative Disorder, or a Personality Disorder).

Code based on type:
  314.01 Attention-Deficit/Hyperactivity Disorder, Combined Type: if both Criteria A1 and A2 are met for the past 6 months.
  314.00 Attention-Deficit/Hyperactivity Disorder, Predominantly Inattentive Type: if Criterion A1 is met but Criterion A2 is not met for the past 6 months
  314.01 Attention-Deficit/Hyperactivity Disorder, Predominantly Hyperactive–Impulsive Type: if Criterion A2 is met but Criterion A1 is not met for the past 6 months.

Coding note: For individuals (especially adolescents and adults) who currently have symptoms that no longer meet full criteria, "In Partial Remission" should be specified.

Note. Reprinted with permission from the *Diagnostic and Statistical Manual of Mental Disorders.* Copyright 2000. American Psychiatric Association.

schoolwork (Hoza, Pelham, Waschbusch, Kipp, & Owens, 2001), homework or chore performance (Danforth, Barkley, & Stokes, 1991), and certain experimental lab tasks (Newcorn et al., 2001; Swaab-Barneveld et al., 2000).

Another problem is distractibility, or the likelihood that a child responds to the occurrence of extraneous events unrelated to the task. Parents and teachers often rate this symptom as significantly elevated among children with ADHD. The findings for such distracting irrelevant stimulation, however, appear to be a function of whether the distractors are contained within the task or outside of the task materials. Some researchers find that stimulation embedded in the task materials worsens the performance of children with ADHD (Barkley, Koplowitz, Anderson, & McMurray, 1997; Brodeur & Pond, 2001; Marzocchi, Lucangeli, De Meo, Fini, & Cornoldi, 2002; Rosenthal & Allen, 1980). This appears to be the case even with video games (Lawrence et al., 2002). Others find no such effect when studying teens with ADHD (Fischer, Barkley, Fletcher, & Smallish, 1993), suggesting a possible age-related improvement in this specific problem (Brodeur & Pond, 2001). One study found an enhancing effect on attention from intratask stimulation (Zentall, Falkenberg, & Smith, 1985). Thus, within-task cues appear to be key to engaging attention of children with ADHD.

Research supports the notion that impaired attention processes in individuals with ADHD are part of a larger domain of cognitive activities known as executive functioning (EF), and especially working memory (i.e., holding information in mind that one is using to guide performance toward a goal, or remembering to do so (Barkley, 1997b, 1997c; see Martinussen, Hayden, Hogg-Johnson, & Tannock, 2006, for a meta-analysis). Specifically, evidence from the development of rating scales indicates that the DSM items used to define the attention deficits in ADHD load on a larger dimension containing items reflecting EF and, specifically, working memory (Conners, Sitarenios, Parker, & Epstein, 1998; Gioia, Isquith, Guy, Kenworthy, & Baron, 2000). Such attention ratings also correlate significantly with neuropsychological tests of working memory and EF in contrast to those of hyperactive or impulsive behavior (Martinussen & Tannock, 2006). Thus, assess-

ment of ADHD might be improved by adding measures of EF (Jarratt, Riccio, & Siekierski, 2005), but the value of adding such measures has not been thoroughly evaluated.

Impulsivity

A second dimension of ADHD is a deficiency in inhibiting behavior. Usually it is strongly associated with hyperactivity and may be the source of it. Like attention, impulsivity is also multidimensional in nature (Nigg, 2006). Recent theories of impulsivity have focused on the capacity to inhibit or delay prepotent responses, particularly in settings in which those responses compete with rules (Barkley, 1997b). A prepotent response is one that gains the immediate reinforcement (i.e., reward or escape) available in a given context, or that has a strong history of such reinforcement in the past. Though symptoms of impulsivity intercorrelate with those of hyperactivity in childhood strongly enough to form a single dimension, by adulthood, symptoms related to verbal behavior become partially distinct from hyperactivity and motor impulsivity (Barkley et al., in press).

The combined type of ADHD may have several reward-related deficits (Luman, Oosterlaan, & Sergeant, 2005), including difficulties with sustained inhibition of such dominant responses over time (Nigg, 2006), poor delay of gratification (Rapport, Tucker, DuPaul, Merlo, & Stoner, 1986), a steeper discounting of the value of delayed over immediate rewards (Barkley, Edwards, Laneri, Fletcher, & Metevia, 2001), and impaired adherence to commands to inhibit behavior in social contexts (Danforth et al., 1991). This inhibitory deficit may also include difficulty interrupting an already ongoing response pattern (Schachar, Mota, Logan, Tannock, & Klim, 2000), particularly when given feedback about performance and errors. In the latter case, perseverative responding may be evident despite negative feedback concerning such responding, perhaps reflecting an insensitivity to errors (Wiersema, van der Meere, & Roeyers, 2005).

Children with ADHD tend to be more active, restless, and fidgety than their non-ADHD peers (Porrino et al., 1983; Teicher, Ito, Glod, & Barber, 1996). As with the other symptoms, there are significant situational fluctuations in this symptom class (Luk, 1985; Porrino et al., 1983). Level of activity does not always distinguish between ADHD and other clinic-referred groups of children (Werry, Reeves, & Elkind, 1987), though its pervasiveness across settings may do so (Taylor, 1986). Such hyperactivity declines significantly across the elementary school years, whereas problems with attention persist at relatively stable levels during this same period of development (Barkley, Fischer, Edelbrock, & Smallish, 1990; Hart, Lahey, Loeber, Applegate, & Frick, 1995; Wolraich et al., 2005). This implies that hyperactivity reflects an early developmental manifestation of a more central deficit in behavioral inhibition that may arise ahead of problems with attention, while declining more steeply with age. Studies that factor-analyze behavior ratings consistently show that hyperactivity and poor impulse control form a single dimension of behavior (DuPaul, 1991; Hinshaw, 1987; Molina, Smith, & Pelham, 2001), at least in children. As noted earlier, by adulthood, verbal impulsiveness may become partially decoupled from the former dimension (Barkley et al., in press). Accordingly, impulsivity and hyperactivity are currently collapsed into a single dimension in ADHD assessment with DSM-IV criteria. This deficit in inhibition, of which early hyperactivity is a part, may become increasingly reflected in poor self-regulation over various developmental stages, even though the difficulties with excessive activity level may wane with maturation (Barkley, 1997a; Barkley et al., in press).

Difficulties with adherence to rules and instructions are also evident in children with ADHD (APA, 2000; Barkley, 1997b). They typically have significant problems with compliance with parental and teacher commands (Danforth et al., 1991) and often do not follow experimental instructions in the absence of the experimenter (Draeger, Prior, & Sanson, 1986) or adhere to directives to defer gratification or resist temptations (Rapport et al., 1986). Like the other symptoms, rule-governed behavior is a multidimensional construct (Hayes, 1989). It remains to be shown which aspects of this construct are specifically impaired in ADHD and to what extent impairments in rule-governed behavior are secondary to the primary symptoms of ADHD (i.e., inattention and impulsivity).

Assessment Implications

The preceding brief review should make it clear that ADHD does not present as a unitary phenomenon. Assessors need to be prepared to deal with variability within and across persons. Yet it may be possible for a person with ADHD to appear focused, persistent, and well controlled in novel, stimulating, or highly rewarding activities or situations. Thus, being attentive and apparently self-disciplined on some occasions does not rule out a diagnosis of ADHD. Indeed, a comprehensive assessment of ADHD will identify situations in which there are few, if any, problems. These situations can be used to highlight positive influences on the behavior of the person with ADHD.

Diagnostic Criteria

DSM-IV criteria (see Table 2.1) are the most widely recognized and accepted criteria for diagnosing ADHD (Kupfer et al., 2000). Generally speaking, there is good support for most of these criteria, especially when they are applied to children (Barkley, 2005). But some significant problems that do exist argue for some latitude in adherence to DSM-IV criteria and anticipation of future refinements based on empirical evidence.

The key elements of the DSM-IV criteria for ADHD may be summarized by the following seven concepts.

1. Individuals with ADHD may have problems related to inattention, hyperactivity/impulsivity, or both.
2. These deficits are significantly inappropriate for the person's age.
3. The disorder should have an onset in childhood.
4. The condition is generally chronic or persistent over time.
5. The core symptoms are significantly pervasive or cross-situational in nature.
6. The deficits are not the direct result of severe language delay, deafness, blindness, or another psychiatric condition, such as autism, depression, or psychosis, that may better explain the symptoms.
7. The core symptoms of ADHD must be causally associated with significant impairment in major life activities, such as educational, familial, social, vocational, adaptive

(self-sufficiency), or other significant areas of life functioning.

DSM-IV Subtypes

The three subtypes set forth in DSM-IV are somewhat self-explanatory and comprise the predominately inattentive subtype (ADHD-I), the predominantly hyperactive–impulsive subtype (AH/HD-HI), and the combined subtype (ADHD-C). These subtypes are formed on the basis of the two symptom lists or dimensions presented in the criteria (Burns, Boe, Walsh, Sommers-Flanagan, & Teegarden, 2001; DuPaul et al., 1998; Gioia et al., 2000; Lahey et al., 1994). These dimensions have been replicated across various countries and ethnic groups, including Puerto Rico (Bauermeister et al., 1995); Native Americans (Beiser, Dion, & Gotowiec, 2000); U.S. ethnic groups (DuPaul et al., 1998); Australia: (Gomez, Harvey, Quick, Scharer, & Harris, 1999); Brazil (Rasmussen et al., 2002); and, Spain, Germany, and the United States (Wolraich et al., 2003).

Some researchers now find another construct or dimension of inattention symptoms that is not represented in the DSM-IV-TR inattention list. Indeed, the symptoms were eliminated as a result of a field trial that showed them to have low or weak association with the other inattention symptoms (see Lahey et al., 1994). Yet this subset of symptoms is becoming useful in identifying another subtype of inattentive children, and possibly adults. This dimension represents a sluggish cognitive tempo, or SCT, and its typical symptoms include children being more sluggish, passive, hypoactive, daydreamy, slow-moving, prone to stare, confused, and "in a fog" than are normal children or those with ADHD-C (McBurnett, Pfiffner, & Frick, 2001; Milich et al., 2001; Todd et al., 2004). Indeed, some of these symptoms are the very antithesis of ADHD (e.g., hypoactivity).

Given that SCT may be a valid and distinct dimension of inattention, evidence suggests that clinicians need to recognize one dimension of hyperactivity/impulsivity and two distinct dimensions of inattention. The first inattention dimension is the well-known and overwhelmingly established set of inattentive symptoms set forth in the DSM and in many child behavior rating scales. Children with these symptoms can be thought of as impersistent–distractible–forgetful. The second dimension of inattention

reflects a daydreamy–staring–confused quality that is more passive and lethargic in form and associated with slow–inaccurate information processing. This dimension of inattention is not currently addressed by DSM-IV-TR, requiring examiners to take care to evaluate its existence apart from DSM-IV-T– based rating scales and interviews.

Developmentally Inappropriate Behavior

Individuals with ADHD are certainly significantly different than their peers on measures of attention span, activity level, and impulse control (Barkley, 2005; Biederman, 2005; Fischer et al., 2005; Nigg, 2005; Wolraich et al., 2005). However, as mentioned previously, there are different types of inattention, overactivity, and impulsivity, and not all of the numerous ways to measure them have consistently revealed differences between individuals with and without ADHD (Firestone & Martin, 1979; Sandberg, Rutter, & Taylor, 1978). The inattention problems usually exhibited by persons with ADHD-C are the inability to sustain attention and to persist in responding to tasks or play activities for as long as other children of the same age (Barkley, 1997c, 2005; Hoza et al., 2001). An inability to follow through on rules and instructions is also evident. Among the most distinctive symptoms, however, is the proneness to distractibility (Barkley et al., in press; Milich, Widiger, & Landau, 1987). Another common manifestation of inattention is being more disorganized and forgetful than other children the same age (Barkley, DuPaul, & McMurray, 1990). Researchers employing objective measures corroborate their presence in persons with ADHD (Corkum & Siegel, 1993; Luk, 1985; Milich & Lorch, 1994; Schachar, Tannock, & Logan, 1993). These behaviors distinguish them from individuals with learning disabilities (Barkley, DuPaul, & McMurray, 1990) or other psychiatric disorders (Werry, Reeves, & Elkind, 1987). This symptom class correlates significantly with measures of working memory and EF; therefore, it likely represents a broader domain of cognitive impairment, most likely EF, than merely inattention (Barkley et al., in press; Gioia et al., 2000; Matinussen et al., 2006; Matinussen & Tannock, 2006).

Children with ADHD-HI or ADHD-C often exhibit difficulties with excessive activity level.

This is often manifested in greater fidgetiness; not staying seated when it is required; moving about, running, and climbing more than other children; playing noisily; talking excessively; often interrupting others' activities; and being less able than others to wait in line or take turns in games (APA, 1994). A problem with inhibition is also evident in many of these same complaints. Parents and teachers describe the children as being incessantly in motion and unable to wait for events to occur. As noted previously, research has objectively documented that they are more active than other children. Furthermore, children with ADHD-HI or ADHD-C come across as being relatively immature in controlling motor overflow movements (Denckla & Rudel, 1978); have considerable difficulties stopping an ongoing behavior (Hartung, Milich, Lynam, & Martin, 2002; Schachar et al., 1993); talk more than others (Barkley, Cunningham, & Karlsson, 1983); are less able to resist immediate temptations and delay gratification (Anderson, Hinshaw, & Simmel, 1994; Campbell, Pierce, March, Ewing, & Szumowski, 1994; Rapport et al., 1986); and tend to respond too quickly and too often when they are required to wait and watch for events to happen, as is often seen in impulsive errors on continuous performance tests (CPTs; Corkum & Siegel, 1993; Frazier, Demareem, & Youngstrom, 2004).

Although less frequently examined, differences in activity and impulsiveness have been found between children with ADHD and those with learning disabilities (Barkley, DuPaul, & McMurray, 1990) or other psychiatric disorders (Frazier et al., 2004; Halperin, Matier, Bedi, Sharma, & Newcorn, 1992; Werry, Reeves, & Elkind, 1987). Hyperactivity appears to diminish with advancing age; however, impulsivity and related impairments appear to persist for most individuals diagnosed with ADHD during childhood (Biederman et al., 2006; Wilens & Dodson, 2004).

Onset in Childhood

A formal diagnosis of ADHD by DSM-IV criteria requires documentation of early onset, arbitrarily defined as before age 7. There is minimal empirical justification for this cutoff (Applegate et al., 1997; Barkley & Biederman, 1997), with as many as 35% of children and 50% of adults with ADHD having onset of disorder after age 7 years (Barkley, Fischer, et al., 2006). We strongly encourage evaluators to use discretion regarding the onset prior to age 7 years requirement, preferring ourselves to use an onset of prior to 16 years of age to capture all legitimate cases of disorder (Barkley, Fischer, et al., 2006).

The key point of the early-onset requirement is that ADHD is usually a chronic disorder, with problems presumably having a biological basis that disrupts functioning in childhood. If inattention or impulsivity emerge suddenly or later in adulthood, then the assessor is advised to consider other disorders (e.g., depression) or to label the case as one of *acquired* ADHD secondary to (specify known etiology). Careful interviewing about the history of impairment is required if an older child or adolescent is presenting for treatment or for functional problems that have "sudden onset."

Studies of the developmental course and outcome of children with ADHD have been numerous and are only briefly summarized here. More detailed reviews are provided by others (Barkley, 2005; Biederman, 2005; Pelham, Fabiano, & Massetti, 2005; Weiss & Hechtman, 1993). Although some children with ADHD are reported to have been difficult in terms of their temperament since birth or early infancy (Barkley, DuPaul, & McMurray, 1990; Campbell et al., 1994), the majority appear to be identifiable as deviating from normal by their caregivers between 3 and 4 years of age (Lahey et al., 2004). However, for a variety of reasons, it may be several years before such children are brought to the attention of professionals (Foy & Earls, 2005).

A diagnosis of ADHD among preschoolers may be more difficult due to higher rates of disruptive behavior among the normal population at this age. Nevertheless, recent studies suggest that a reliable and valid diagnosis can be made for children as young as 3 years, 7 months old (Lahey et al., 2006). However, precision and reliability in diagnosis of subtypes of ADHD do not appear to stabilize until children are about 7 or 8 years old (Barkley, Fischer, et al., 1990; Lahey, Pelham, Loney, Lee, & Willcutt, 2005).

During their preschool years, children with ADHD are often excessively active, mischievous, noncompliant with parental requests, and difficult to toilet train (Campbell et al., 1994; Hartsough & Lambert, 1985; Mash &

Johnston, 1982). They may also already be manifesting some delays in academic readiness skills (Mariani & Barkley, 1997). Parental distress over child care and management is likely to reach its zenith when children are between 3 and 6 years of age, declining thereafter as the deficits in attention and rule-following improve (Barkley, Karlsson, & Pollard, 1985; Mash & Johnston, 1982).

Despite the decline from peak parenting distress in the later preschool years, the stress parents report in raising children with ADHD remains considerably higher than stress levels reported by parents of children in control groups (Anastopoulos, Guevremont, Shelton, & DuPaul, 1992; Bussing et al., 2003; Fischer, 1990). Likewise, parents of teenagers with ADHD report high levels of stress and family conflict with these youth, particularly if the youth carries a comorbid diagnosis of ODD (Barkley, Anastopoulos, Guevremont, & Fletcher, 1992; Barkley et al., 1991; Edwards, Barkley, Laneri, Fletcher, & Metevia, 2001).

By entry into formal schooling (i.e., 5 or 6 years of age), most children with ADHD have become recognizably deviant from normal peers due to poor sustained attention, impulsivity, or restlessness. Difficulties with aggression, defiance, or oppositional behavior may have emerged or will begin to emerge, if they did not manifest earlier in development (Barkley, Fischer, et al., 1990; Barkley et al., 1991). Children with ADHD who develop these oppositional or antisocial behaviors are likely to veer into a more severe path of maladjustment in later years than are children with ADHD who do not develop aggressive–defiant behaviors, or who do so only to a limited degree (Barkley et al., 2004). During these elementary school years, the majority of children with ADHD have varying degrees of poor school performance, usually related to failure to finish assigned tasks in school, relatively high rates of missing homework or long-term assignments, disruptive behavior during class activities, and increasingly poor peer relations. Learning disabilities in areas of reading, spelling, math, handwriting, and language, however, may also become manifest in a significant minority of children with ADHD, requiring additional evaluation and special educational assistance beyond that typically needed to manage the ADHD symptoms (Barkley, 2005; Tannock & Brown, 2000).

Persistent Life Course

Thirty years ago, there was a widespread belief that ADHD was a self-limiting disorder that typically remitted shortly after puberty (Brown & Borden, 1986). In the meantime, several well-conducted longitudinal studies have shown that 40–80% of children continue to have the disorder into adolescence (Barkley, Fischer, et al., 1990; Biederman, Faraone, Milberger, et al., 1996; Hinshaw, Owens, Sami, & Fargeon, 2006; Mannuzza et al., 1991; Weiss & Hechtman, 1993). Many children with ADHD who putatively "outgrow" their symptoms during adolescence may be borderline cases that switch back and forth between a diagnosed and a nondiagnosed status. Moreover, those who have subclinical levels of ADHD as adolescents are often significantly impaired relative to their peers (Molina & Pelham, 2003).

We believe that many of these borderline or impaired cases might be consistently diagnosed with ADHD if more developmentally appropriate diagnostic criteria were employed. Unfortunately, the DSM-IV-TR criteria were written primarily for children and field-tested primarily with elementary school–age students (age range, 4–16 years). As a consequence, some ADHD diagnostic criteria are less relevant to adolescents, who generally show a decline in hyperactive behavior (Barkley, 2005). For example, except in extremely rare cases, statements such as "Runs or climbs excessively" or "Cannot play quietly" no longer apply to postpubescent individuals with ADHD.

For adolescents with ADHD, family conflicts may continue or even increase (Barkley, Anastopoulos, et al., 1992; Fletcher, Fischer, Barkley, & Smallish, 1996) and may now center around failure of the teen to accept responsibility for performing routine tasks, difficulties with being trusted to obey rules when away from home, and impairments in problem-solving. Parents may try to compensate by adopting an authoritarian, highly emotional parenting style with an excessive use of ultimatums (Robin, 1990). This can result in a coercive interaction cycle that increases conflict and strains on the family.

Among the subset of teens with ADHD who have had significant problems with aggressive and oppositional behavior prior to being an adolescent, delinquency and conduct disorder are likely to emerge, if they have not done so already, because these adolescents spend greater amounts of unsupervised time in the community (Barkley, Fischer, et al., 1990; Satterfield & Schell, 1997; Weiss & Hechtman, 1993). Substance experimentation and abuse are more likely to occur within the adolescent years, mainly among youths diagnosed with ADHD and comorbid conduct disorder (Barkley, Fischer, et al., 1990; Barkley et al., 2004; Molina & Pelham, 2003; Thompson, Riggs, Mikulich, & Crowley, 1996) or bipolar disorder (Biederman, Faraone, Mick, et al., 1996). Thus, although there may not be a clear causal effect of ADHD on the development of alcohol and other drug problems, there does appear to be a clinically meaningful relationship between ADHD and substance use (Smith, Molina, & Pelham, 2002).

Another area of difficulty is increased risk-taking behavior (Flory, Molina, Pelham, Gnagy, & Smith, 2006). An increasing number of studies have replicated and extended the original report by Weiss and Hechtman (1993), suggesting that individuals diagnosed with ADHD in childhood followed into adolescence, and clinically referred teenagers (and adults) with ADHD have a greater number of automobile accidents and speeding citations than their peers (Barkley, Guevremont, Anastopoulos, DuPaul, & Shelton, 1993; Barkley, Murphy, DuPaul, & Bush, 2002).

Studies of other domains of major life activities have shown that teens with ADHD are at risk for a wide variety of impairments, including sexual intercourse at an earlier age, along with a greater risk of teenage pregnancy (Barkley, Fischer et al., 2006), and less likelihood of completing high school and college than their peers (Barkley, Fischer, et al., 2006; Biederman et al., 2006; Weiss & Hechtman, 1993). Even those who do make it to college appear to be more impaired than their peers (Barkley, in press, 2007; Heiligenstein, Guenther, Levy, Savino, & Fulwiler, 1999). Workplace problems include higher than expected unemployment and number of job changes, and elevated levels of ADHD and ODD symptoms, as rated by employers (Barkley, Fischer, et al., 2006; Biederman et al., 2006). People with ADHD also appear to have less stable relationships, including fewer long terms friends and more divorces (Barkley, Fischer, et al., 2006; Biederman et al., 2006; Weiss & Hechtman, 1993).

In contrast to the decline in hyperactivity with age noted earlier, DSM-IV-TR symptoms of inattention and EF appear to be very persistent. Adults with ADHD are highly likely to self-report many of the same symptoms of inattention from the DSM symptom list reported by parents of children having ADHD (Barkley et al., in press). Murphy and Barkley (1996a) found that 83% of adults diagnosed with ADHD reported having difficulties with sustaining attention (vs. 68% of a clinical control group and 10% of a normal sample); 94% reported being easily distracted (vs. 86% of clinical controls and 19% or normative controls); 90% claimed that they often do not listen to others (vs. 57 and 6%, respectively); 91% reported that they often fail to follow through on tasks or activities (vs. 78 and 6%, respectively); and 86% reported that they frequently shift from one uncompleted activity to another (vs. 75 and 12%, respectively). These self-reports are corroborated by others who know the subjects well, such as spouses ($r = .64$) or parents ($r = .75$), as is parents' recall of similar symptoms during their childhood years ($r = .74$ with parent reports) (Murphy & Barkley, 1996b).

Adults with ADHD appear to have many of the same attention problems as children who have the disorder (Barkley et al., in press), especially attention and EF problems (Barkley, Murphy, & Kwasnik, 1996; Epstein, Conners, Sitarenios, & Erhardt, 1998; Hervey, Epstein, & Curry, 2004; Murphy, Barkley, & Bush, 2001; Seidman, Biederman, Weber, Hatch, & Faraone, 1998). Also, results of direct behavioral observations of inattention in adults with ADHD parallel the previously cited research in children, indicating greater off-task behavior during task performance, including driving (Barkley, 2004; Fischer, Barkley, Smallish, & Fletcher, 2005).

Cross-Setting Pervasiveness of Symptoms

The DSM-IV requirement that the symptoms be demonstrated in at least two out of three environments to establish pervasiveness of symptoms is new to this edition of the DSM and potentially problematic. By stipulating that the symptoms must be present in at least two out of three contexts (home, school, work, in the case of DSM-IV; home, school, clinic, in the case of International Classification of Diseases [ICD-10]), the criteria now potentially confound settings with sources of information (parent, teacher, employer, clinician). Research shows that the degree of agreement between parents and teacher is modest for any dimension of psychological development, often ranging between .30 and .50 depending on the behavioral dimension being rated (Achenbach, McConaughy, & Howell, 1987; Mitsis, McKay, Schulz, Newcom, & Halperin, 2000). This low degree of agreement sets an upper limit on the extent to which parents and teachers can agree on the severity of ADHD symptoms and, thus, on whether the child has the disorder according to strict interpretation of DSM-IV criteria.

It is noteworthy that disagreements among sources presumably reflects some real differences in the child's behavior in these different settings, probably as a function of differences in situational demands. School, after all, involves quite different expectations, tasks, social context, and general demands for public self-regulation compared to the home environment. A more serious problem for assessment is that the disagreements may also reflect differences in the attitudes, experiences, and judgments between different people. Furthermore, because there is no scientific basis at this time to argue for one reporter's validity over another (e.g., teacher vs. parent), we believe that these views should be considered as providing information on the child in that particular context, from a particular adult's point of view, and nothing more. Cross-informant agreement is not critical for diagnosis. It may inappropriately confound the diagnosis with issues such as comorbid disorders and reporting source, severity, and subtype. For example, there may be a confounding of the ADHD with issues of comorbidity with ODD (Costello, Loeber, & Stouthamer-Loeber, 1991). Parent-identified children with ADHD may have predominantly ODD, with relatively milder ADHD, whereas teacher-identified children with ADHD may have chiefly ADHD and minimal or no ODD symptoms. Children identified by both parents and teachers as having ADHD may, therefore, have not only ADHD but also a higher likelihood of having ODD. Other research suggests that pervasiveness may measure a more severe condition of ADHD than do the home- or school-only cases, which differ in degree rather than in kind (Tripp & Luk, 1997). Furthermore, some studies suggest that the combined subtype (ADHD-C) may be more readily detected by pervasiveness criteria than the other hyperactive, impulsive, or inattentive subtypes (Gaub & Carlson, 1997). Children with defined pervasive ADHD (i.e., impairment at home and at school) may be more likely to have conduct disorder than ADHD identified only at home (Mannuzza, Klein, & Moulton, 2002). The results attest mainly to the validity of teacher reports in identifying a group of children with ADHD and severe behavior problems and, perhaps, a higher risk for adult antisocial disorder; however, it does not suggest that pervasiveness is necessary to diagnose ADHD. Indeed, this trend in the data suggests that pervasiveness is confounded with comorbidity. Clinicians need to keep in mind that DSM was constructed by blending the reports of parents and teachers, and they should do likewise. Thus, we recommend that symptoms reported by one source should be tallied; then, the number of additional symptoms identified by the other source should be added to the tally, totaling the number of different items endorsed across both sources.

Ruling Out Alternative Diagnoses

Many psychiatric disorders may be confused with ADHD. For instance, a depressed child may manifest symptoms of inattention (e.g., poor concentration), or a manic child may have increased activity levels. To clearly distinguish between ADHD and other disorders, examiners need to review with parents the problems that may exist in multiple developmental domains. A review of the following domains of functioning is recommended: motor, language, intellectual, academic, emotional, and social. Careful interviewing about symptom type, onset, duration, strength, and quality is also required to rule out alternative diagnoses. In addition, information about the social context and circumstances of the problem must be gathered (i.e., Can antecedent events such as a loss be identified?).

Accomplishing a differential diagnosis of ADHD versus another disorder requires that the examiner have an adequate knowledge of the diagnostic features of other childhood disorders. Questioning about inappropriate thinking, affect, social relations, and motor peculiarities may reveal another psychiatric or developmental disorder (e.g., Asperger syndrome). Family psychiatric history can provide information that increases or decreases the likelihood of certain disorders (i.e., bipolar disorder). Also, measures that screen for a wide variety of problems are helpful. We describe later a sample interview that we recommend for use with the parents of children with ADHD. An example of a detailed diagnostic interview for parents of children with ADHD may be found elsewhere (Barkley & Murphy, 2006). Regardless of the particular method chosen, some review of the major childhood disorders in DSM-IV (APA, 1994) is essential for a trustworthy diagnosis, because DSM-IV requires ruling out other diagnoses that most plausibly account for the current complaints. Usually a thoughtful semistructured interview will help with this task. Also, broad-based screening instruments, such as the Child Behavior Checklist (CBCL; Achenbach & Rescorla, 2001) and Behavioral Assessment System for Children, Second Edition (BASC-2; Reynolds & Kamphaus, 2005) may help with this important diagnostic consideration.

Over 80% of children with ADHD have a second disorder, and more than 60% have two or more additional disorders. These findings have major implications for both assessment and treatment. For example, the presence of high levels of anxiety specifically, and of internalizing symptoms more generally, has been shown in some instances to be a predictor of poorer responses to stimulant medication (Pliszka, 1989), thus indicating the need for more intensive psychosocial treatment with this population (Jensen et al., 2001). Similarly, the presence of high levels of hostile, defiant behavior or ODD has been shown to be a marker for greater family conflict (Barkley, Anastopoulos, et al., 1992; Barkley et al., 1991). In such cases, specialized and more intensive family-based interventions may be necessary (Barkley, Guevremont, Anastopoulos, & Fletcher, 1992). Also, ADHD has also been shown to be a predictor of risk for conduct disorder, antisocial behavior, and substance misuse (Barkley et al., 2004; Mannuzza, Klein, Bessler, Malloy, & LaPadula, 1998). The coexistence of major depressive disorder with ADHD increases the risk of suicidality two to four times, especially during high school, demanding much closer monitoring of such cases by clinicians and possibly the use of adjunctive antidepressant medications (Barkley & Fischer, 2005). Accordingly, treatment for ADHD should involve prevention of high-risk behavior. The foregoing data illustrate the impor-

tance of determining comorbidity as part of the evaluation of a child with ADHD, and its possible impact on treatment selection.

Parenting influences have been implicated as important mediators or moderators of internalizing problems experienced by adolescents with ADHD (Ostrander & Herman, 2006). This is also true for smoking tobacco (Molina, Marshal, Pelham, & Wirth, 2005). Therefore, the assessment of ADHD should also consider the parenting relationship and family-based prevention programs for high-risk adolescents (Dishion & Andrews, 1995; Farrington & Welsh, 2003; Sanders, 2000). Similarly, because peers may have a big influence on a child's conduct problems and substance use (Marshal, Molina, & Pelham, 2003), assessment of comorbid conditions should include an evaluation of the nature of the child's peer group and its level of deviant or antisocial behavior.

Documenting Impairment

Symptoms alone are not sufficient to make a diagnosis. Rather, a diagnosis of ADHD requires that (1) the person have clinically meaningful symptoms and (2) clinically meaningful impairment, and that (3) the symptoms seem to be the most likely cause of the impairment. A multiaxial assessment of ADHD with DSM-IV guidelines provides a Global Assessment of Functioning (GAF) that gives some information about impairment (APA, 2000). Some clinicians and researchers use the GAF (DSM-IV, Axis V) as an outcome measure in ADHD treatment. This type of assessment of functioning is useful but not as precise an index of impairment as we would like. Rather, we strongly recommend gathering specific data on functional impairments, quantifying them whenever possible (e.g., frequency counts or severity ratings), and making the functional impairments as much or more than the ADHD symptoms the target of intervention and outcome evaluation. This requires an individualized approach to assessment. It can be accomplished by instructing parents and/or teachers in the use of relatively straightforward behavioral methods of tracking problem behavior, such as frequency tallies, duration records, or time samples (Sanders, Markie-Dadds, & Turner, 2001; Sanders & Ralph, 2001). For example, a parent can record how long a child takes to complete homework each day (duration record) or the number of times a child is noncompliant with requests (frequency tally). How often a child fights with a sibling can be recorded during the most problematic times of the day, with a parent noting simply whether or not fighting occurred during half-hour increments in the morning and in the evening (time sample). These measures can begin with the initial assessment and be repeated throughout the treatment period, thus forming the data by which interventions can be evaluated. Another way parents and clinicians can obtain information about impairment is with rating scales that containing specific items on functioning in various major life activities (Pelham, Fabiano, & Massetti, 2005). These types of measures are discussed later in the chapter.

Prevalence Using Clinical Diagnostic Criteria

The only two studies to date reporting a U.S. prevalence rate using DSM-IV criteria found rates of 7.4 and 9.9% (see Barkley, 2005). These estimates of prevalence may be higher than the average for DSM-III-R, most likely due to the inclusion of the new ADHD-C subtype not recognized in DSM-III-R. Adding these subtypes, it would seem, nearly doubles the prevalence of disorder in the United States. In one study that reported the prevalence of ADHD in Australia using DSM-IV criteria by diagnostic interview (Gomez et al., 1999), the Australian prevalence estimate of 6.8% is comparable to those in the United States using these same DSM-IV criteria (Barkley, 2005). A Dutch study yielded a prevalence of 3.8% with children (i.e., 6–8 years old), which is approximately half the rate found in the United States and Australia (Kroes et al., 2001). The reasons for this discrepancy are not clear, but they may be due to methodological issues rather than cultural differences. A study in Brazil that used DSM-IV criteria yielded an ADHD prevalence estimate of 5.8% for a young adolescent age group (Rohde et al., 1999). The discrepancy between the Brazilian and United States/Australian studies may be due in part to the Brazilian study's use of early adolescents. As noted earlier, ADHD symptoms decline with age, thus driving a reduction in prevalence. There is no doubt that ADHD is a worldwide phenomenon. It has been found in every country in which it has been studied (see Barkley, 2005, for a review of 24 prevalence studies using earlier DSM editions).

A recent epidemiological study of U.S. adults has estimated a prevalence of 4.4% for adult ADHD using DSM-IV criteria (Kessler et al., 2006). This is similar to the figure obtained in an earlier study of adults in Massachusetts by Murphy and Barkley (1996a), who found a prevalence of 4.7% for all subtypes of ADHD, also using DSM-IV criteria.

Factors Affecting Rates of ADHD Diagnosis

Several factors affect reports of ADHD symptoms, including the source of information (e.g., parent, teacher, or self-reports), the version of DSM being used, the age and sex of the samples, and the country in which the study is conducted. However, after controlling for these factors, age and sex remain as clearly unique and important determinants of the prevalence of ADHD. Furthermore, socioeconomic status (SES) appears to affect prevalence estimates, but not as reliably as age and gender. More details on age, gender, source of information, and SES effects on ADHD prevalence estimates are given below.

ADHD is more common among males than among females. Epidemiological studies of ADHD typically find rates that are three to seven times greater among males than among females (Barkley, 2005). The discrepancy in clinical studies is even more pronounced, with males predominating by as much as a 9:1 (Barkley, 2005). Although ADHD is clearly more prevalent in boys than girls, the key clinical characteristics do not vary greatly by gender (Biederman et al., 2005).

Regarding SES, one study found that indicators of social class had a low but significant inverse relationship with rates of hyperactivity in a Canadian sample (Boyle & Lipman, 2002). Overall, the results indicated that being male, coming from a single-parent family or a smaller family with fewer children, and living in a disadvantaged neighborhood all significantly increased the likelihood of hyperactivity. Others have found that conditions associated with lower SES increase the risk for ADHD (Velez, Johnson, & Cohen, 1989). Important, however, was the additional finding by Szatmari, Offord, and Boyle (1989) that when comorbidity with other disorders was statistically controlled in the analyses (especially for ODD and CD), gender, family dysfunction, and low SES were no longer significantly associated with occurrence of the disorder. On the other hand, health problems, developmental impairment, young age, and urban living were uniquely associated with the occurrence of the disorder.

Base-Rate Considerations in Assessing ADHD

It has been known for about 50 years that diagnostic precision is heavily dependent on the base rate of the disorder (Meehl & Rosen, 1955). Three base rate considerations should be taken into account when diagnosing ADHD. The first is the base rate in the general population. Estimates presented previously in the chapter are that a small minority of children in the United States (i.e., about 7–9%) meet current diagnostic criteria for ADHD. Accordingly, when dealing with general populations, such as schools, the diagnosis should be approached with a high degree of scientific skepticism. In such cases, the odds are high that the child does not have ADHD. This consideration is highly relevant to screening or epidemiological studies to avoid false-positive "diagnoses."

Another base rate consideration is the local base rate among the children referred for evaluation. About half of the children referred to child mental health settings have ADHD (Barkley, 2005). We expect that similarly high base rates of ADHD are found in populations referred to school psychologists and similar professionals. Thus, the odds are pretty good that the child referred by a parent or teacher to a psychologist or psychiatrist due to problems of inattention or impulsivity actually has ADHD. In these situations (i.e., with a 50% base rate of ADHD), equal emphasis should be given to ruling in versus ruling out the disorder. For specialty ADHD clinics, the base rate would be expected to be even higher (80% or more in Barkley's experience); thus, referrals to such clinics would have a high probability of having the disorder.

A third base rate consideration is the rate of other disorders that might be confused with ADHD, such as major depression or bipolar disorder. Among populations referred for academic or behavior problems, it is very likely that ADHD is the most prevalent disorder. However, sometimes clinicians are swayed by the salience of a novel disorder, even though the base rate is much lower. For example, if the base rate of ADHD is 50% and the rate of bipolar disorder (BPD) (see Youngstrom, Chapter 6, this volume) is 2%, then it is much more likely that overactivity is due to ADHD rather than BPD. In this case, very strong data are needed to rule out ADHD and rule in BPD.

Implicit in these statistics is that preference in terms of selecting from a list of disorders with similar symptoms should be given to higher base rate disorders. Not clearly stated in DSM, but explicit in Meehl and Rosen (1955) and other noteworthy treatments of the base rate issue, is that professionals should collect data on local base rates to provide appropriate statistical guidance for making diagnostic decisions. This is simple to do. It merely involves keeping a running record of the diagnoses made by clinicians and their colleagues in a particular setting or referral stream over a period of time.

Gender Differences

Historically, so few girls were included in studies of ADHD that there was too little statistical power to examine gender differences. However, as larger scale studies have become available, it has become increasingly clear that a significant number of girls are affected by ADHD, and that many of the findings for boys replicate for girls (for reviews, see Gershon, 2002; Hinshaw & Blachman, 2005). For instance, Hinshaw and Blachman (2005) have undertaken a longitudinal study focusing on girls with ADHD. This program of research and other studies have shown that careful assessment can reliably differentiate between girls with and without ADHD. Also, consistent with research on boys diagnosed with ADHD, Hinshaw and colleagues (2006) have shown that ADHD in girls persists into adolescence.

Researchers have made some progress in understanding the extent to which gender is an important issue in diagnosing and treating ADHD. Indeed there have been enough studies that, if relatively lenient inclusion criteria are used, studies of gender differences and ADHD may be subjected to a quantitative (i.e., meta-analytic) review. The most recent of these reviews found that, in comparison to boys with ADHD, girls with ADHD tend to have lower ratings on hyperactivity, inattention, impulsivity, and externalizing problems. In addition, girls with ADHD appear to have greater intellectual impairments and more internalizing problems than boys with ADHD (Gershon, 2002). Furthermore, some researchers have found "masculine" and "feminine" clusters of symptoms to be valid characterizations of boys and girls with ADHD (Ohan & Johnston, 2005). Others have speculated that there are unique considerations in treating females with ADHD, for instance, when fluctuating hormones associated with menses might affect behavior (Quinn, 2005).

Taken together, the studies on girls with ADHD suggest a real difference in severity of symptoms and perhaps a different pattern of comorbidity, with more internalizing and learning problems experienced by girls relative to boys. The rate of ADHD is probably about four to nine times lower for girls than boys, and there may be a variety of biases that result in lower rates of identification of females with ADHD compared to males (Reid et al., 2000). Issues such as hormone effects and other gender-specific issues need to be subjected to more rigorous studies.

One possible explanation of differing rates of identification of ADHD in females may be that the ADHD-related problems experienced by girls may be less salient than those typically experienced by boys with ADHD. For instance, some studies indicate that girls with ADHD may employ more relational aggression than non-ADHD peers (Zalecki & Hinshaw, 2004). Relational aggression is more subtle than the overt aggression likely to be used by males, at least to adult observers; thus, it may possibly contribute to a referral bias.

Another consideration related to diagnostic biases is that the comorbidities experienced by girls with ADHD, such as depression, anxiety, and learning problems, may mask the symptoms of ADHD, or at least clinicians' recognition of it. This may lead to an erroneous primary diagnosis that overlooks ADHD, even though the stress of dealing with ADHD might be the reason the girl is anxious or depressed. To support this point, in Australia, the rate of service utilization for boys and girls with ADHD seems to be about the same, but girls were more likely to carry a primary diagnosis of an internalizing disorder (Graetz, Sawyer, Baghurst, & Hirte, 2006).

Yet some studies have found few, if any, clinically meaningful differences between males and females with ADHD. For instance, a classroom-based study of elementary-age students found higher rates of ADHD for boys than for girls, but no major clinical differences between the boys and girls with ADHD (DuPaul, Jitendra, Tresco, & Vile Junod, 2006). Similarly, in a study of adolescents with ADHD, Rucklidge (2006) found practically no gender-linked neuropsychological differences, with the possible exception that boys were more impulsive than girls. This gender difference in impulsivity is called into question by studies of adults that found no remarkable differences in neuropsychological functioning of men and women with ADHD, even though there were differences relative to normal controls (Barkley et al., in press; Seidman et al., 1998). Other studies have found no differences in functional impairments between boys and girls with ADHD, either at home or at school (Breen & Altepeter, 1990).

To summarize, with regard to assessment, assessors should be careful to avoid false negatives when evaluating girls for ADHD. And whereas the treatment implications for girls with uncomplicated ADHD appear to be similar to those for boys, one should be prepared to deal with a differing set of comorbid conditions and social relationship problems for girls and boys with ADHD. A key diagnostic consideration may be the decision to classify the comorbid condition as a primary disorder, or a secondary problem caused by ADHD. Whereas girls have historically been underidentified and treated, more recent studies suggest that there has been a substantial increase in the rate of treatment for girls with ADHD in the United States (Robison, Skaer, Sclar, & Galin, 2002).

Situational and Contextual Factors

As already noted, all the primary symptoms of ADHD show significant fluctuations across various settings and caregivers (Barkley, 2005). Playing alone, washing and bathing, and times when the father is at home are a few of the less troublesome situations for children with ADHD, whereas instances when children are asked to do chores, when parents are on the telephone, when visitors are in the home, or when children are in public places may be times of peak severity of their disorder. Significant fluctuations in activity are evident across these different contexts for children with ADHD and normal controls, with the differences becoming most evident during school classes in reading and math. Despite these situational fluctuations, children with ADHD appear to be more deviant in their primary symptoms than normal children in most settings, yet these differences can be exaggerated greatly as a function of several factors related to the settings and the tasks children perform in them (Luk, 1985; Zentall, 1985).

Other situational factors, such as the extent to which caregivers make demands on children with ADHD to restrict behavior, appear to affect the degree of deviance of the child's behavior from that of nondiagnosed children. In free-play or low-demand settings, where task complexity is low, children with ADHD are less distinguishable from normal children than in highly restrictive or task-demanding ones (Lawrence et al., 2002; Luk, 1985; Marzocchi et al., 2002). Children with ADHD often appear to be more compliant and less disruptive, and are rated as less symptomatic by fathers compared to mothers (DuPaul et al., 1998; Tallmadge & Barkley, 1983). Problems with sustained responding are also lessened on tasks in which instructions are repeated frequently to the child with ADHD (Douglas, 1980, 1983), at least by an experimenter. Yet parents and teachers frequently complain that repeating their commands and instructions to children with ADHD produces little change in compliance (Danforth et al., 1991). Children with ADHD display fewer behavioral problems in novel or unfamiliar surroundings, or when tasks are unusually novel, but their level of deviant behavior increases with familiarity with the setting (Barkley, 2005; Zentall, 1985). The degree of stimulation in the task also seems to be a factor in the performance of children with ADHD. Research suggests that colorful or highly stimulating educational materials are more likely to improve the attention of these children to such materials than are relatively low-stimulation or uncolored materials (Zentall, 1985). Interestingly, such differences may not affect the attention of typical children or may even worsen it. Activity levels may also be lower while watching television compared to more demanding academic work, such as in reading and math classes at school (Porrino et al., 1983). Yet even with high stimulation activities such as video games or TV, children with ADHD look away from displays more than do normal children, and may still have more problems with their performance than do normal children (Barkley & Ullman, 1975; Landau, Lorch, & Milich, 1992; Lawrence et al., 2002; Tannock, 1998).

Motivational factors also impact ADHD symptoms. Settings or tasks that involve a high rate of immediate reinforcement or punishment result in significant reductions in, or in some cases amelioration of, attention deficits (Barkley, 1997b; Barkley, Copeland, & Sivage, 1980; Douglas, 1983; Douglas & Parry, 1983). Or when children with ADHD are engaged in activities they find more enjoyable, they may even perform at normal or near-normal levels, perhaps because these children prefer immediate rather than delayed rewards (Barkley et al., 2001; Neef, Bicard, & Endo, 2001). When the schedule and magnitude of reinforcement are decreased, however, the behavior of children with ADHD may become readily distinguishable from non-ADHD peers (Barkley et al., 1980; Luman, Oosterlaan, & Sergeant, 2004). During one-to-one situations, children with ADHD may appear less active, inattentive, and impulsive, whereas in group situations, where there is little such attention, children with ADHD may appear at their worst. Clearly, rules and motivational factors in the setting have a significant impact on ADHD symptom severity (Draeger et al., 1986; Glow & Glow, 1979; Luman et al., 2005).

Fatigue or time of day (or both) may have an adverse impact on the degree of expression of children's ADHD symptoms (Zagar & Bowers, 1983) given that academic tasks are performed significantly better in the mornings but worsen in the afternoons more than is seen in normal children. This is not to say that differences between children with ADHD and normal controls do not exist in the early morning but emerge only as time of day advances, for this is not the case (Porrino et al., 1983). The findings so far suggest that educators would do well to schedule repetitive or difficult tasks that require the greatest powers of attention and behavioral restraint for morning periods, while placing recreational, entertaining, or physical activities in the afternoons (Zagar & Bowers, 1983).

Associated Problems and Impairments

Children with ADHD have a higher likelihood of having other medical, developmental, adaptive, behavioral, emotional, and academic difficulties than do peers who do not have ADHD. Delays in intelligence, academic achievement, and motor coordination are more prevalent in children with ADHD than in matched samples of normal children, or even in siblings (Barkley 2006), as are delays in adaptive functioning more generally (Greene et al., 1996; Roizen, Blondis, Irwin, & Stein, 1994; Stein,

Szumowski, & Blondis, & Roizen, 1995). Problems with peer acceptance and in peer interactions are commonly documented in children with ADHD (Bagwell, Molina, Pelham, & Hoza, 2001; Ernhardt & Hinshaw, 1994; Stroes, Alberts, & Van der Meere, 2003). These social impairments continue into adolescence and adulthood, possibly with escalating consequences that lead to progressively more serious problems, such as school dropout, vocational instability and underachievement, and unstable interpersonal relationships (Barkley, 2005).

As noted earlier, as many as 87% of clinically diagnosed children with ADHD may have at least one other disorder, and 67% may have at least two other disorders (Kadesjo & Gillberg, 2001). Children with ADHD are far more likely than children who do not have ADHD to have coexisting ODD and CD symptoms (Angold, Costello, & Erkanli, 1999). Depression, and possibly BPD, also may be more common in children with ADHD than would be expected in the general population (Biederman, Faraone, Mick, et al., 1996; Jensen, Shervette, Xenakis, & Richters, 1993), especially where CD is present with ADHD (Angold et al., 1999). There is a modest increase in risk for anxiety disorder as well, averaging 25% of clinical cases (Angold et al., 1999; Tannock, 2000). Severity of the ADHD symptoms may in part predict the severity of and risk for these comorbid conditions (Gabel, Schmidtz, & Fulker, 1996).

Children with ADHD appear to have more minor physical anomalies than do normal controls (Quinn & Rapoport, 1974) and may be physically smaller than normal children, at least during childhood (Spencer et al., 2006). They may also have more sleep difficulties than normal children (Ball & Koloian, 1995; Cortese, Lecendreux, Mouren, & Konofal, 2006). However, prior beliefs that ADHD may have a higher than normal association with either allergies or asthma have not been corroborated by research (Biederman, Milberger, Faraone, Guite, & Warburton, 1994; McGee, Stanton, & Sears, 1993; see also Pelham et al., 1998, for a brief review). Unfortunately, the well-meaning but ill-advised belief in putative food allergies may itself cause impairment due to restricted activities, social stigma, and escalated parent–child conflict.

ADHD symptoms produce significant alterations in family functioning, particularly in children who also display excessive opposition-

al and defiant behavior (Johnston & Mash, 2001). Children with ADHD have been shown to be less compliant, more negative, and less able to sustain compliance than normal children during task completion with their mothers (for a review, see Danforth et al., 1991). Their mothers are more directive and negative, more lax in their discipline, less rewarding and responsive to their children's behavior, and show lower levels of maternal coping than do mothers of normal children (Cunningham & Boyle, 2002; Keown & Woodward, 2002; McKee, Harvey, Danforth, Ulaszek, & Friedman, 2004). However, these problems also may be more closely aligned with the level of child conduct problems than just the severity of ADHD symptoms (Johnston, Murray, Hinshaw, Pelham, & Hoza, 2002; Kashdan et al., 2004). Although there is less conflict in the interactions of older children and teens with ADHD compared to younger age groups (Danforth et al., 1991), even they remain deviant in their parent–child conflicts (Barkley et al., 1991; Edwards et al., 2001; Fletcher et al., 1996), especially in those with both ADHD and ODD. The greater directive and negative behavior of the mothers of children with ADHD may be in part a reaction to their children's noncompliance and poor self-control rather than a cause of it (Danforth et al., 1991). Moreover, these conflicts in social interactions appear to exist in the relations of children with ADHD and their fathers (Edwards et al., 2001; Tallmadge & Barkley, 1983) and teachers (Cunningham & Boyle, 2002; Whalen, Henker, & Dotemoto, 1980). Yet both children and teens with ADHD do not perceive their relations with parents and teachers as being more problematic than do control children (Edwards et al., 2001; Gerdes, Hoza, & Pelham, 2003; Hoza et al., 2004). These results and others indicate a positive illusory bias associated with the disorder. Children with ADHD may have problems related to limited self-awareness, in which they perceive themselves as functioning as well as others, when clearly they are not.

Parents of children with ADHD report significantly greater stress in their parental roles and higher levels of depression than do parents of samples of normal children (Cunningham & Boyle, 2002; DuPaul, McGoey, Eckert, & VanBrakle, 2001; Harrison & Sofronoff, 2002; Johnston & Mash, 2001). Higher rates of maternal depression may contribute to a biased reporting of severity of children's ADHD symptoms as a function of depression-related distortions (Chi & Hinshaw, 2002). Parents of children with ADHD also have more ADHD, and if the child also manifests ODD or CD, parents may also manifest greater rates of mood, anxiety, and substance use disorders (Chronis et al., 2003).

Peer relations of children and teens with ADHD are typically problematic (Bagwell et al., 2001; Cunningham & Siegel, 1987) and involve more rejection and fewer close friendships, especially for the subset with ODD–CD (Bagwell et al., 2001; DuPaul et al., 2001; Mikami & Hinshaw, 2003). Children with ADHD exhibit more negative behavior (DuPaul et al., 2001) and are less socially involved with non-ADHD playmates during conversations. Yet children with ADHD may direct attention to their non-ADHD peers during play activities, receiving more structure in the form of praise and questions from peers during active play (Stroes et al., 2003). Children with ADHD also encode fewer social cues and generate fewer responses than normal children, whereas those with comorbid ODD–CD demonstrate a greater propensity for aggressive responses than do control children (Matthys, Cuperus, & Van Engeland, 1999).

The most reliably associated cognitive and psychomotor difficulties with ADHD include (1) motor coordination and sequencing (Barkley, 1997d; Barkley, DuPaul, & McMurray, 1990; Breen, 1989; Denckla & Rudel, 1978; Mariani & Barkley, 1997); (2) working memory and mental computation (Mariani & Barkley, 1997; Martinussen et al., 2006; Zentall & Smith, 1993); (3) planning and anticipation (Barkley, Grodzinsky, & DuPaul, 1992; Douglas, 1983; Grodzinsky & Diamond, 1992); (4) verbal fluency and confrontational communication (Grodzinsky & Diamond, 1992; Zentall, 1988); (5) effort allocation (Douglas, 1983; Voelker, Carter, Sprague, Gdowski, & Lachar, 1989); (6) application of organizational strategies (Hamlett, Pellegrini, & Conners, 1987; Voelker et al., 1989; Zentall, 1988); (7) internalization of self-directed speech (Berk & Potts, 1991; Copeland, 1979); (8) adherence to restrictive instructions (Danforth et al., 1991); (9) self-regulation of emotional arousal (Cole, Zahn-Waxler, & Smith, 1994; Douglas, 1983; Hinshaw, Buhrmeister, & Heller, 1989); and (10) less mature moral reasoning (Nucci & Herman, 1982). The commonality among most of these seemingly disparate abilities may be EF (Denckla,

1994; Torgesen, 1994) or "metacognition" (Torgesen, 1994; Welsh & Pennington, 1988). All may be mediated in part by the frontal cortex, particularly the prefrontal lobes (Fuster, 1989; Stuss & Benson, 1986)—brain regions implicated in ADHD.

Etiologies

The proposed etiologies for ADHD are too numerous to review here in any detail. Therefore, we concentrate on those for which there is substantial empirical support. More detailed information is available in the text by Nigg (2006). Although the definitive specific and most proximal causes of ADHD have not been established, the larger domains in which these precise causes exist have been much better clarified over the past decade. Substantial evidence points to both neurological and genetic contributions to this disorder, and even specific brain regions and specific genes are now being implicated as contributors. So although the exact neurochemical mechanisms remain to be established for the disorder, and the suites of genes contributing to its striking heritability have yet to be completely catalogued, there is no doubt that these etiological directions hold the greatest promise for understanding the causes of the disorder.

Purely social causes of ADHD can be largely ruled out as contributors to most forms of ADHD—a major advance in itself. Social factors surely moderate the types and degrees of impairments from the disorder, and possibly even risk for comorbid ODD, CD, depression, and anxiety. Social factors may play a role in biases against those having ADHD, as well as potentially moderate access to services for its management. However, social factors in and of themselves appear to have little research support as primary causes of the disorder.

Neurology

A large number of studies that have used neuropsychological tests of frontal lobe functions have detected deficits in children and adults with ADHD (Barkley, 1997d; Barkley, Edwards, et al., 2001; Murphy et al., 2001; Seidman et al., 1998; Seidman, Doyle, Fried, Valera, Crum, & Matthews, 2004), especially in response or "executive" inhibition (Nigg, 2006). The greatest support in meta-analyses of the burgeoning neuropsychological literature on ADHD is for difficulties with not only the cardinal domains of inattention and inhibition but also working memory (Frazier et al., 2004; Hervey et al., 2004). Less evidence exists for difficulties in other executive abilities, such as planning and verbal fluency, response perseveration, and emotional self-regulation, largely due to far fewer studies of these domains. Difficulties with sense of time have also been convincingly established (Barkley, Edwards, et al., 2001; Barkley, Murphy, & Bush, 2001). Moreover, research shows that not only do siblings of children with ADHD who themselves have ADHD show similar EF deficits, but also even siblings of children with ADHD who do not actually manifest ADHD appear to have milder yet significant EF impairments (Seidman et al., 1995). Such findings imply a phenotypic dimension to the disorder that is present, albeit in milder form, among genetically related individuals. Executive deficits in ADHD appear to arise from the same substantial shared genetic liability as do ADHD symptoms themselves (Coolidge, Thede, & Young, 2000).

Psychophysiological measures of nervous system (central and autonomic) electrical activity (galvanic skin responses, heart rate deceleration, etc.) have proven inconsistent in demonstrating group differences between children with ADHD and control children in resting arousal. Deviations from normal are found more consistently in diminished reactivity to stimulation, as in evoked responses (Beaucheine, Katkin, Strassberg, & Snarr, 2001; Borger & van der Meere, 2000; Herpertz et al., 2001). This may point to impaired right prefrontal mechanisms underlying response inhibition (Pliszka, Liotti, & Woldorff, 2000). Far more consistent have been the results of quantitative electroencephalograph (QEEG) and evoked response potential (ERP) measures, sometimes administered in conjunction with vigilance tests (El-Sayed, Larsson, Persson, & Rydelius, 2002; Monastra, Lubar, & Linden, 1999; see Loo & Barkley, 2005, for a review). Increased slow wave, or theta, activity, particularly in the frontal lobe, and excess beta activity the most common differences noted, are indicative of a pattern of underarousal and underreactivity in ADHD (Monastra, Lubar, & Linden, 2001). Children with ADHD have been found to have smaller amplitudes in the late positive and negative ERP components. These late components are believed to be a function of the prefrontal regions of the brain,

are related to poorer performances on inhibition and vigilance tests, and are corrected by stimulant medication (Johnstone, Barry, & Anderson, 2001; Pliszka, Liotti, et al., 2000). Improvements in these measures that result from stimulant medication may be partly a function of the human dopamine transporter (DAT1) gene allele, particularly in its 10-repeat form (Loo et al., 2003), a polymorphism that may be overrepresented in some forms of ADHD (Levy, Hay, McStephen, & Martin, 2001).

Several studies that have examined cerebral blood flow using single-photon emission computed tomography (SPECT) in children with ADHD and normal children (see Hendren, DeBacker, & Pandina, 2000, for a review) have consistently shown decreased blood flow to the prefrontal regions (particularly in the right frontal area) and pathways connecting these regions to the limbic system via the striatum, specifically, its anterior region known as the caudate, and the cerebellum. Degree of blood flow in the right frontal region has been correlated with behavioral severity of the disorder and with reduced EEG activity, whereas that in more posterior regions and the cerebellum seems related to degree of motor impairment (Gustafsson, Thernlund, Ryding, Rosen, & Ceterblad, 2000).

Studies using positron emission tomography (PET) to assess cerebral glucose metabolism have found diminished metabolism in adults with ADHD, particularly in the frontal region (Schweitzer et al., 2000; Zametkin et al., 1990) but have been far less consistent with teens and children (for reviews, see Ernst, 1996; Tannock, 1998). Using a radioactive tracer that indicates dopamine activity, Ernst and colleagues (1999) found abnormal dopamine activity in the right midbrain region of children with ADHD, with severity of symptoms correlated with degree of abnormality.

Studies using magnetic resonance imaging (MRI) find less brain volume in selected brain regions in those with ADHD relative to control groups (Tannock, 1998), particularly in the anterior right frontal region, caudate nucleus, and globus pallidus (Aylward et al., 1996; Castellanos et al., 2002; Filipek et al., 1997). Besides reduced size, there is some evidence of reduced neurometabolite activity in the right frontal region (Yeo et al., 2003), with degree of this activity associated with degree of attention problems on a CPT. The smaller size of the basal ganglia and right frontal lobe is correlated with a greater degree of impaired inhibition and attention in children with ADHD (Casey et al., 1997; Semrud-Clikeman et al., 2000). Numerous studies (Castellanos et al., 1996, 2001, 2002; Durston, Pol, et al., 2004) also found smaller cerebellar volume in those with ADHD, especially in a central region known as the vermis. The cerebellum plays a major role in EF and in the motor presetting aspects of sensory perception that derive from planning and other executive actions (Diamond, 2000), suggesting why these functions may be deficient in children with ADHD.

Studies using functional MRI find that children with ADHD have abnormal patterns of activation during attention and inhibition tasks in comparison to normal children, particularly in the right prefrontal region, basal ganglia (striatum and putamen), and cerebellum (Rubia et al., 1999; Teicher et al., 2000; Vaidya et al., 1998; Yeo et al., 2003). The demonstrated linkage between brain structure and function, and psychological measures of ADHD symptoms and executive deficits is exceptionally important and permits causal inferences about the role of these brain abnormalities in the cognitive and behavioral deficits comprising ADHD. Durston, Pol, and colleagues (2004) found that the reduced size of the brain (about 3–5%), particularly in the right frontal area, in children with ADHD may be evident as well in their non-ADHD siblings, which is perhaps consistent with the increased familial risk for the disorder and a spectrum of the phenotype for ADHD within these families. But the reduced volume of the cerebellum was found to be specific to the affected child with ADHD and was not evident in unaffected siblings, implying that this region may be directly related to the pathophysiology of the disorder.

Existence of possible neurotransmitter dysfunction or imbalances has been proposed in ADHD for quite some time (see Pliszka, McCracken, & Maas, 1996, for a review). Initially, this rested chiefly on the responses of children with ADHD to dopamine and norepinephrine reuptake inhibitors, such as methylphenidate and atomoxetine, respectively. Studies have used blood and urinary metabolites of brain neurotransmitters to infer deficiencies due to ADHD, largely related to dopamine regulation (Halperin et al., 1997). What limited evidence there is from this literature seems to point to a selective deficiency in the availability of both dopamine and norepinephrine.

Pregnancy and Birth Complications

Some studies have found a greater incidence of pregnancy or birth complications in children with ADHD compared to normal children (Claycomb, Ryan, Miller, & Schnakenberg-Ott, 2004). Prematurity has been associated with later risk for ADHD (Breslau et al., 1996; Schothorst & van Engeland, 1996). After controlling for other factors that may be associated with low birthweight and ADHD (maternal smoking, alcohol use, ADHD, social class, etc.), Mick, Biederman, Faraone, Sayer, and Kleinman (2002) continued to find low birthweight to be three times more common in children with ADHD than in control children, perhaps accounting for nearly 14% of all ADHD cases. Thus, low birthweight associated with prematurity may be a particularly salient marker for later ADHD. Furthermore, the extent of white matter abnormalities due to birth injuries, such as parenchymal lesions and/or ventricular enlargement, seems especially contributory to later ADHD among babies born prematurely (Whittaker, 1997). Mothers of children with ADHD are likely to be younger when they conceive than are mothers of control children, and such teen pregnancies may have a greater risk of adverse effects (Claycomb et al., 2004; Denson, Nanson, & McWatters, 1975; Hartsough & Lambert, 1985).

Genetics

Evidence for a genetic basis of ADHD is now overwhelming and comes from three sources: family studies, twin studies, and, most recently, molecular genetic studies identifying individual candidate genes. Nearly all of this research applies to ADHD-C, and most of it has occurred with children rather than adolescents. Between 10 and 35% of immediate family members of children with ADHD are also likely to have the disorder, with the risk to siblings of children with ADHD being approximately 32% (Levy & Hay, 2001). If a parent has ADHD, the risk to the offspring is 40–57% (Barkley et al., in press; Biederman, Faraone, Mick, et al., 1996). These elevated rates of the disorder also have been noted in African American ADHD samples (Samuel et al., 1999), as well as in girls compared to boys with ADHD (Faraone & Doyle, 2001). ADHD with CD may be a distinct familial subtype of ADHD (Faraone, Biederman, Mennin, Russell, & Tsuang, 1998; Smalley et al., 2000). Girls who manifest ADHD may have a greater genetic loading (higher family member prevalence) than do males with ADHD (Faraone & Doyle, 2001; Smalley et al., 2000).

Twin studies of ADHD and its behavioral dimensions have proven strikingly consistent. These studies have found a very high degree of heritability for ADHD, ranging from .70 to .97 (Coolidge et al., 2000; Kuntsi & Stevenson, 2000; for reviews, see Levy & Hay, 2001; Thapar et al., 2000). The average heritability of ADHD (degree of variance in the trait due to genetic effects) is at least .78. These studies consistently find little, if any, effect for shared (rearing) environment on the traits of ADHD, which refutes any effort to attribute ADHD to within-family factors such as poor parenting, family diet, household television exposure, or other popularly held causes of ADHD.

Approximately 9–20% of the variance in hyperactive–impulsive–inattentive behavior or ADHD symptoms can be attributed to such nonshared environmental (nongenetic) factors (Levy & Hay, 2001; Nigg, 2006). Factors in the nonshared environment include those events or conditions that have uniquely affected only one twin or child in a family and not others. Such unique factors include not only those typically thought of as involving the social environment (differing schools, peer groups, etc.) but also all biological factors that are nongenetic in origin (lead poisoning, head injury, etc.). Researchers who are interested in identifying environmental contributors to ADHD should focus on those biological, interactional, and social experiences that are specific and unique to the individual, and are not part of the common family environment to which other siblings have been exposed.

Multiple genes are likely to contribute to risk for the disorder given the complexity of the traits underlying ADHD and their dimensional nature. The dopamine transporter gene (DAT1) has been implicated repeatedly (Barkley, Smith, Fischer, & Navia, 2006; Cook, Stein, & Leventhal, 1997) but not universally (Swanson et al., 1998). The heterozygous 9/10 pairing of this gene has recently been shown to be associated substantially with degree of ADHD symp-

toms and related impairments as well as to response to methylphenidate and atomoxetine, both transporter reuptake inhibitors, relative to the homozygous 9/9 or 10/10 pairings (Barkley, Smith, et al., 2006; Gilbert et al., 2006). The DRD4 gene (dopamine D_4 receptor) has been the most reliably found in samples of children with ADHD (Faraone et al., 1999). The 7-repeat or longer forms (alleles) of this gene have been found to be overrepresented in children with ADHD (LaHoste et al., 1996). This gene has previously been associated with the personality trait of high novelty-seeking behavior, affects pharmacological responsiveness, and impacts on postsynaptic sensitivity primarily in frontal and prefrontal cortical regions (Swanson et al., 1998). More recently, the long allele of the dopamine beta-hydroxylase (DBH) gene has also been implicated in hyperactive children followed to adulthood (Mueller et al., 2003). Future research is likely to show distinct genetic subtypes of ADHD, differential associated risks for impairment and medication responding by genotype, and possibly some value of genetic testing to assist diagnosis.

Environmental Toxins

Apart from genetics, ADHD symptoms may be due to pre-, peri-, and postnatal complications, malnutrition, diseases, trauma, toxin exposure, and other neurologically compromising events that may occur during the development of the nervous system before and after birth. Such events are likely to happen to one child in a family but not to others, so they likely fall under the unique or nonshared variance found in twin studies associated with variation in ADHD symptoms in the population. Several of these biologically compromising events have been repeatedly linked to risk for inattention and hyperactive behavior. One such factor is exposure to environmental toxins, and one such toxin is lead (Needleman, Schell, Bellinger, Leviton, & Allred, 1990). An even stronger case for negative effects has been made for deliberately ingested toxins, such as tobacco (Maughan, Taylor, Caspi, & Moffitt, 2004; Mick et al., 2002; Milberger, Biederman, Faraone, Chen, & Jones, 1996; Streissguth, Bookstein, Sampson, & Parr, 1995). The relationship between maternal smoking during pregnancy and ADHD remains significant even after symptoms of ADHD are controlled in the parent (Mick et al., 2002; Milberger et al., 1996). Maternal alcohol consumption has been documented as a risk factor for ADHD (Nigg, 2006), albeit less consistently.

Predictors of Outcome

One key predictor of outcomes is comorbidity with other disorders, particularly ODD and CD. Those children with "pure" ADHD (i.e., ADHD that is not associated with significant aggressiveness, comorbid mood disorders, family adversity, or peer relationship problems) are likely to have problems primarily in school performance (Paternite & Loney, 1980); they are typically described as "underachieving." They may have a higher chance of early remission of the disorder (Biederman, Faraone, Milberger, et al., 1996). On the other hand, teenagers who had childhood ADHD that was associated with aggression and conduct problems apparently fare much worse than those with uncomplicated ADHD (Barkley, Fischer, et al., 1990; Barkley et al., 2004; Weiss & Hechtman, 1993). Not only are school performance problems significant, but difficulties with predelinquent or delinquent behavior in the community may also emerge, and peer relationship problems remain significant or increase in severity (Barkley, Fischer, et al., 1990; Fischer, Barkley, Edelbrock, & Smallish, 1990). Likewise, conflict with parents is elevated (Anastopoulos et al., 1992), which is of concern because it is a major predictor of outcomes for teenagers (Hinshaw et al., 2000; Ostrander & Herman, 2006; Reitz, Dekovic, & Meijer, 2006; Wills & Dishion, 2004).

With the exception of comorbid conduct problems, few other predictors are noteworthy. Even those that are statistically significant account for only a small percentage of the variance in outcome (Mannuzza & Klein, 1992). Some studies have identified low intelligence in childhood, poor peer acceptance, emotional instability, and extent of parental psychopathology as predictors of poorer outcomes (Barkley, Fischer, et al., 2006; Fischer, Barkley, Fletcher, & Smallish, 1993; Fischer, Barkley, Smallish, & Fletcher, 2005; Hechtman, Weiss, Perlmann, & Amsel, 1984; Loney, Kramer, & Milich, 1983; Paternite & Loney, 1980).

There is minimal evidence of positive effects of childhood treatment on the eventual adult health and functioning of individuals diagnosed with ADHD as children (Wilens & Dodson, 2004). Extensive, long-term treatment during adolescence may improve outcome somewhat (Satterfield, Satterfield, & Cantwell, 1981). However, lesser degrees of treatment limited to childhood provide no measurable benefits in later life (Barkley, Anastopoulos, et al., 1992; Barkley, Fischer, et al., 1990; Hechtman et al., 1984; Paternite & Loney, 1980; Weiss & Hechtman, 1993). Results of the Multimodal Treatment Study of Children with ADHD (MTA) study suggest that effects of intensive intervention, both pharmacological and psychosocial, fade when the treatments are withdrawn (Smith, Barkley, & Shapiro, 2006). Most children and teens therefore do not receive intensive or sustained treatment for ADHD across development, which may account for the lack of measurable treatment effects in adults (Barkley, 2005).

The long-term effects of stimulants have received some attention, but much research is still needed in this area, because high-quality longitudinal treatment studies are lacking (Kupfer et al., 2000). Thus, we are not aware of any conclusive effects of stimulant treatment on adult outcomes, such as ADHD symptoms, functioning, or health. For each report of deleterious effects there seems to be a report of no detrimental, long-term effect. For instance, some studies have reported growth suppression effects (Charach, Figueroa, Chen, Ickovicz, & Schachar, 2006; Jensen, Arnold, Severe, Vitiello, & Hoagwood, 2004), but these findings have been contradicted by other studies (Spencer et al., 2006). Likewise, for each report of positive effects, such as prevention of substance abuse (Wilens, Faraone, Biederman, & Gunawardene, 2003) there is a study that reports no effect of stimulant treatment on substance abuse (Fischer & Barkley, 2003). Thus, the long-term effect of treatment, for better or worse, remains unclear, and more research in this area is badly needed (Wilens & Dodson, 2004).

Yet the complete picture is not so bleak. As noted earlier, longitudinal studies to date that have followed children with ADHD into adulthood and examined them for stimulant-associated problems have, with one exception, not identified any long-term adverse events associated with such treatment. In the one study that claimed to have found such a link (Lambert & Hartsough, 1998), methodological problems were plentiful, and 12 other studies failed to replicate the linkage (Barkley et al., 2004; Wilens et al., 2003). Also worth noting is that stimulants have been on the market since the 1930s (amphetamines) to 1950s (methylphenidate), and millions of individuals have been treated with them, often over years. There is minimal or no evidence from postmarketing surveillance by the U.S. Food and Drug Administration (FDA) and pharmaceutical companies to indicate that significant health risks are convincingly associated with use of these medications over the short or long term. Recent media reports of suicidal thinking and attempts related to atomoxetine have not been shown to exceed the base rate for the ADHD population, despite the FDA black box warning in the package insert for the drug (Barkley & Fischer, 2005). And the black box warning for this medication concerning hepatotoxicity is based on one case in 3.4 million treated patients, illustrating how such warnings have become virtually meaningless in conveying a sense of risk to patient and clinician alike. Likewise, recent concern over the stimulant and cardiovascular risks and sudden death have been greatly exaggerated in media accounts of this story. Again, the adverse events have not been shown to exceed the base rates for sudden death in the population, thus calling into question any linkage between these events and stimulant treatment. Whereas caution is always in order with use of any medications, and clinical monitoring for such adverse events in treated cases is to be encouraged, especially if there are preexisting structural cardiac abnormalities, there is no evidence that common or widespread health risks are associated with ADHD medication management absent such abnormalities in the patient's history. Hence, whereas more rigorous long-term studies are to be encouraged, the limited number of such studies at present does not mean one cannot make legitimate inferences about long-term safety given these other sources of information that pertain to this issue.

CONCEPTUALIZATION OF THE DISORDER

Until recently, ADHD has lacked a reasonably credible scientific theory to explain its basic psychological nature and symptoms, and to link it with normal developmental processes. The field of ADHD treatment has reached a point, however, where the neuropsychological,

neuroimaging, and genetic studies cited earlier are setting clear limits on theorizing about not only the origins of ADHD but also theories about its nature. Any credible theory on the nature of ADHD must now posit neuropsychological constructs related to the normal development of inhibition, self-regulation, and executive functioning, and explain how they may go awry in ADHD. Such a theory will need to argue that these constructs arise from the functions of the prefrontal–striatal network and its interconnections with other brain regions, such as the cerebellum, that appear to underlie EFs and self-control. Those cognitive functions will be shown to have a substantial hereditary contribution to individual differences in the population according to the results of twin studies on the genetic contribution to variation in ADHD symptoms.

Barkley worked on just such a theoretical conceptualization of ADHD over the past 12 years (see Barkley, 1997b, 2006). It is briefly discussed below, followed by its implications for the management of ADHD. Research continues on the merits of this model for ADHD, but we include it here because of its far greater implications for evaluation with an eye toward treatment than any prior theories founded solely on ADHD arising from deficits in response inhibition (Quay, 1988), delay aversion (Solanto et al., 2001), or arousal and energetic pools (Sergeant & Van der Meere, 1989).

The model is founded on the premise that ADHD comprises mainly a developmental delay in or acquired impairment of the behavioral inhibition networks of the brain that disrupt self-regulation—an assertion for which there is substantial research support (see Barkley, 1997b; Nigg, 2006). This theory links behavioral inhibition to the EFs and shows them to provide for self-regulation. Behavioral inhibition occupies a foundation in relationship to self-control and four executive functions that are dependent upon it for their own effective execution. "Self-regulation" is defined as any self-directed action to change one's own behavior to alter the probability of a delayed (future) consequence. The EFs are forms of behavior-to-the-self—the actions one uses to change oneself so as to change their future.

Four executive functions are theorized to bring behavior progressively under the control of internally represented information (forms of self-directed action), time, and the probable future (delayed consequences), and wresting it from the control of the immediate external context and the prepotent responses it generates. Appropriate self-control functions to maximize future consequences for the individual over merely immediate ones. The model applies only to ADHD-C to date.

"Behavioral inhibition" involves the capacity to inhibit prepotent responses, creating a delay in the response to an event (response inhibition). There may be two other inhibitory processes related to it, at least for the moment, that Barkley has combined into a single construct concerning inhibition. These two other processes are (1) the capacity to interrupt ongoing responses, given feedback about performance, particularly those response patterns that are proving ineffective; and (2) the protection of this delay in responding, the self-directed actions occurring within it, and the goal-directed behaviors created from interference by competing events and their prepotent responses (interference control). Through the postponement of the prepotent response and the creation of this protected period of delay, the occasion is set for the four executive functions (covert, self-directed actions) to act effectively in modifying the individual's eventual response(s) to the event. The chain of goal-directed, temporally governed, and future-oriented behaviors set in motion by these acts of self-regulation are then protected during their performance by interference control. And even if disrupted, the individual retains the capacity or intention (via working memory) to return to the goal-directed actions, until the outcome is successfully achieved or judged to be no longer necessary. We list the four executive functions below, using both their more common label in the neuropsychological literature, followed by Barkley's redefinition of the self-directed action (in parentheses) that each comprises.

1. *Nonverbal working memory* (covert self-directed sensing). Nonverbal working memory is the ability to maintain nonverbal, largely visuospatial mental information online that is used subsequently to control a motor response toward a goal. These mental representations are achieved by the self covertly sensing (especially visual imagery) information that serves to recall past events for the sake of preparing a current response. They represent *hindsight* or the *retrospective function* of working memory (Fuster, 1999). Past events are retained in a

temporal sequence that contributes to the *subjective estimation of psychological time* (Michon, 1985). Analysis of these sequences for recurring patterns is used for conjecture about hypothetical future events—the individual's best guess as to what may happen next, or later in time, based on the detection of recurring patterns in past event sequences. This extension of hindsight forward into time also creates *forethought*, or the *prospective function* of working memory (Fuster, 1999). From this sense of the future arises anticipatory action in preparation for that future once it arrives. It likely explains the progressively greater valuation of future consequences over immediate ones that takes place throughout child development into young adult life (Green, Fry, & Meyerson, 1994). In so doing, individuals are then capable of the cross-temporal organization of behavior, that is, the linking of events, responses, and their eventual consequences via their representation in working memory despite what may be considerable gaps among them in real time.

2. *Verbal working memory (internalized, self-directed speech).* During the early preschool years, speech, once developed, is initially employed for communication with others. Language is a means of influencing the behavior of others. But around age 3 years, it becomes self-directed, thereby eventually providing a means of reflection (self-directed description), as well as a means for controlling one's own behavior (Berk & Potts, 1991). Self-directed speech progresses from being public, to being subvocal, to finally being private, all over the course of perhaps 6–10 years. With this progressive privatization of speech comes the increasing control it permits over behavior. Self-speech now provides a tremendously increased capacity for self-control, planning, and goal-directed behavior that further augments that being provided by the first EF, chiefly imagery.

3. *Self-regulation of affect–motivation–arousal (self-directed emotion).* The self-regulation of affect, motivation, and arousal can now develop through the use of the first two executive abilities (self-sensing and self-speech). Individuals now possess the capacity to present images (and other sensory information) along with words to themselves that can be used to manipulate emotional states. These images and other sensory information from the past come with emotional valences automati-

cally welded to them (how one felt about them) (Damasio, 1995). Yet it is not just one's affect that is being managed by the use of self-speech and self-sensing. Emotion is, by definition, a motivational state. And so this re-presenting of words and images to the self creates a capacity for self-motivation (Fuster, 1999) via self-emotion (Ekman & Davidson, 1994; Lang, 1995). By privately manipulating and modulating emotional and motivational states, the child can induce drive or motivational states that may be required for the initiation and maintenance of goal directed behavior (Barkley, 1997b).

4. *Planning or reconstitution (self-directed play).* Bronowski (1977) reasoned that the use of images and language to represent objects, actions, and their properties that exist in the world around us provides a means by which we can take the world apart. These pieces can then be combined to create novel recombinations, some of which yield truly innovative, functional response options. Internal speech and imagery permit *analysis* (taking apart), and out of this process comes its complement *synthesis* (recombination) to create entirely new ideas about the world (Bronowski, 1977), and entirely new responses to that world. It provides a means to synthesize novel behavioral sequences in the service of problem solving and goal-directed action, particularly when obstacles are encountered in pursuit of a goal and new behaviors must be generated to solve the problem (Barkley, 1997b; Fuster, 1999). Barkley has hypothesized that, like the other executive functions, this one is also a form of self-directed behavior that becomes turned on the self during development and eventually is privatized. That action-to-the-self is based on play in childhood that progresses from manual–verbal play to private mental manipulation of images and words that generates new ideas and related behavior to use in goal-directed problem solving.

Such internal control over behavior creates not only a greater purposefulness or intentionality to behavior but also a greater flexibility. The EFs grant behavior a more determined, persistent, reasoned, intentional, and purposive quality, while permitting greater shifting of behavior as needed to achieve one's goals— an appearance of volition, choice, and will arising from internally guided behavior (James, 1890).

The impairment in behavioral inhibition occurring in ADHD is hypothesized to disrupt the efficient performance of these EFs, thereby delimiting the capacity for self-regulation. The result is impairment in the cross-temporal organization of behavior, and in the guidance and control of behavior by internally represented information. This inevitably leads to a reduction in the maximization of long-term consequences for the individual. This theory, if correct, provides a much deeper insight into the nature of the disorder and a much broader perspective on its likely impairments, along with a litany of implications for its management (see below). In essence, ADHD is not so much an attention disorder as a disorder of executive functioning or of internally guided and regulated behavior across time and toward future events. This leaves the affected individual more controlled by external events in the moment and more governed by concerns for immediate than for delayed gratification.

Implications for Assessment

Several implications for assessment arise from Barkley's model of ADHD. First, a complete picture of ADHD and its impact on a child's functioning are difficult to capture in office evaluations. Some degree of inhibitory difficulties may be exhibited in an office setting, but not always, and not in most children presenting for evaluation of ADHD. The disruption in the four EFs prove even harder to pin down given that few psychological tests assess these functions, as described earlier, for clinical purposes, and few rating scales contain items focusing explicitly upon them. Compared to the clinician, caregivers have had far longer spans of time over which to evaluate the child's deficiencies in self-regulation, disorganization regarding time, ineffective cross-temporal organization of goal-directed behaviors, impersistence in task- or goal-directed behavior (inattention), and failure to defer gratification and to maximize longer-term consequences over short-term or immediate ones. Therefore, considerable weight should be given to parent and teacher opinions, initially via ratings, when assessing ADHD (Pelham et al., 2005).

Another important implication is that multiple observations of the child's behavior and task performance in natural settings may prove more informative about the presence and degree of ADHD than a brief office evaluation or psychological testing. Therefore, information provided by parents and teachers must also take into account variability due to setting, task, and time of day. When feasible, direct observations (e.g., classroom performance) as a part of school psychological evaluations are to be strongly encouraged so as to provide information collateral to that obtained via parent and teacher report.

To further encumber the assessment of ADHD, the complexity of ADHD is likely to increase over development given that the four EFs that are disrupted by the child's poor behavioral inhibition emerge in a staggered fashion across development. The older the child at the time of evaluation, the more likely the clinician is to find that caregivers are complaining about not only the child's hyperactivity or poor inhibition but about deficits in those EFs that normal children have recently developed. For instance, parents of 3- to 5-year-old children with ADHD are unlikely to complain about the children's poor sense of time, planning, and forethought, but parents of 10- to 16-year-olds with ADHD are far more likely to note such problems. This becomes especially problematic for the adult with the disorder (Barkley et al., in press). Thus, the scope and complexity of impairments broaden in children with ADHD as their development proceeds. This makes it essential for the clinician to ask the parents of an older child with ADHD about deficiencies in these EFs and their impact on the child's adaptive functioning at home and in school.

This model suggests that the full impact of ADHD on the child's adaptive functioning requires a longer span of time to appreciate than is likely to be evident in an initial evaluation of only a few hours. Using measures of adaptive functioning, besides the usual methods of interviewing and obtaining behavior ratings, will probably prove useful to some degree in capturing this impact of ADHD on the child's daily life. An evaluation of an individual with ADHD that appropriately documents the deficiencies in behavioral inhibition, EFs, and self-control is likely to lead to a number of suggestions for treatment, as discussed elsewhere (Barkley, 2005). These suggestions should be evaluated as part of an ongoing assessment process, because it is impossible to predict in advance precisely what treatments will work for an individual with ADHD, even though base rates of successful treatment are relatively high (i.e., 65–80% for medications, 35–75% for psychosocial treatments, etc.). Thus, state-of-the-art treatment for ADHD involves enlightened trial and error. The success of treatment must be documented as part of an ongoing assessment process, and lack of success should lead to a modification of the treatment plan.

Parents who bring their child for a clinical assessment of ADHD are often demoralized (Anastopoulos et al., 1992; Campbell et al., 1994; Hoza et al., 2000; Ostrander & Herman, 2006). They have usually been struggling with the child's impairments related to ADHD and associated problems for years, have tried multiple solutions without success, feel defensive about their role in their child's behavior, often have issues of their own (e.g., marital conflict), and are ambivalent about changing their own behavior (e.g., establishing and maintaining clear rules and consequences) even if it is clearly directed at the well-being of their child. Accordingly, a major consideration in assessment as a prelude to intervention should be the caregivers' knowledge about ADHD and effective interventions, and the caregivers' stage of readiness for change. This issue is addressed in our description of the ACU. Prior to that description, we provide guidelines for a minimally acceptable assessment of ADHD for diagnostic purposes.

RECOMMENDED ASSESSMENT PROCEDURES

In this section we describe (1) the state of assessment of ADHD, (2) methodological considerations in assessing ADHD, and (3) a checklist of considerations required to complete a minimally sufficient evaluation of ADHD. Finally, we briefly describe two promising approaches to evaluating ADHD that are based on motivational interviewing and response to intervention.

The State of ADHD Diagnosis

The "gold standard" diagnosis refers to accepted "proof" that the patient does or does not have the target disorder (Meehl & Rosen, 1955). Ideally, the "gold standard" provides objective criteria (e.g., a laboratory test not requiring interpretation) or a current clinical standard for diagnosis (e.g., an imaging technique that requires some interpretation, such as an MRI). Such "gold standards" do not exist for mental disorders, including ADHD (Kupfer et al., 2000), so diagnosis of this disorder is based on descriptions of behavior coupled with history, course, and knowledge of differential diagnosis. The current "silver standard" for diagnosis is DSM-IV.

A large gap exists between the assessment procedures used in research and in practice settings (Wolraich, 2002). Many of the procedures in research settings are not even remotely feasible in practice settings, because they are expensive, take hours or days to complete, and require specialized training not offered in most graduate education programs (e.g., coding of structured interviews or parent–child interactions). For instance, the initial assessment procedures for the Multimodal Treatment Study of Children with ADHD (MTA) occurred over several days and averaged 7–10 hours, during which the following data were gathered: rating scales from parents and teachers, clinical interviews with parents and children, structured diagnostic interviews covering a full range of disorders, intellectual and academic performance measures, measures of affective and social functioning, computerized assessments of attention, behavioral observations in clinic and school settings, and semistructured clinical interviews regarding parent psychopathology (MTA Collaborative Group, 1999). This is not acceptable or feasible in typical applied settings.

Despite the limitations in the current state of the art for assessment of ADHD, there is broad consensus that ADHD is a "real" disorder (Barkley, Cook, et al., 2002 [International Consensus Statement]; Kupfer et al., 2000). Dealing with uncertainty in diagnosis is not a unique problem. There are vagaries and disagreements even in most medical diagnoses (Kupfer et al., 2000). Nevertheless, as with other psychiatric disorders, there is consensus that it is possible to achieve a valid diagnosis of ADHD even though the diagnosis may be based on a variety of different procedures.

But one encounters some unique challenges when diagnosing ADHD. For instance, self-report of the core symptoms of ADHD (i.e., inattention, impulsivity, and hyperactivity) does not appear to be very dependable in children, even when followed to young adulthood (Barkley, Fischer, Smallish, & Fletcher, 2002; McCann & Roy-Byrne, 2004). The reports of clinic-referred adults diagnosed with ADHD,

however, are more reliable (Barkley et al., in press). A high degree of within-person variability is also endemic to ADHD and may indeed be one of the hallmarks of the disorder (Barkley, 2005). Still another challenge is the key informants' (i.e., teachers and parents) varying perspectives that are governed by a wide array of influences. All of these factors, and more, need to be considered to achieve a valid diagnosis of ADHD.

Measurement Theory Pertinent to ADHD

Classic true score theory divides variance into three major components (Lord, 1965). First is "true score variance," which is the variance of substantive interest (e.g., variance due to ADHD). Second is systematic error, the biases or irrelevant variance likely to be repeated across measurement occasions (e.g., an idiosyncratic teacher perspective, maternal depression, or unique setting effects). Third is random error, or psychometric noise in the assessment process (e.g., careless mistakes when filling out questionnaires, lapses by observers when coding behavior, or items that are so vague that they produce a broad range of responses). All three types of variance need to be considered when assessing ADHD.

Understanding Within-Subject Variability

A common mistake when measuring ADHD is to confuse the high within-subject variability typical of many persons with ADHD and random error, thus totally ignoring the potential information captured by within-subject variability. Unfortunately, most social scientists are trained to characterize groups using a measure of central tendency, usually the arithmetic average (i.e., group mean). Accordingly, assessment decisions are often based on comparing individuals to a group mean. In such comparisons, within-group variability is used to determine where an individual falls relative to his or her peer group. Commonly used statistics for diagnostic decisions, such as z-scores and T-scores, are based on central tendency and within-group variability. Such scores are the basis for cutoffs on standardized rating scales for ADHD (e.g., a T-score greater than 70).

The normative approach to evaluating ADHD has its place, especially when the items describe behavior over a broad range of situations (e.g., school and home) and a representative period of time (e.g., weeks or months). However, such assessments routinely fail to capture clinically and theoretically meaningful variance in within-person behavior. We are not aware of any scales that present data on deviant levels of variability in behavior, so this phenomenon is not well documented in the research literature, though it has been gleaned in laboratory tasks that use numerous repeated trials, such as reaction time tasks, CPTs, and even driving simulators.

In some instances it might be useful to understand the prognostic and treatment implications for within-subject variance. This issue has been explored in some behavior-analytic case studies, and within-subject variability has been used as an outcome variable in some treatment studies (Pelham, 1993). However, empirical investigation of the practical implications of within-subject variability has been neglected in the voluminous literature on ADHD. From a single-case standpoint, evaluating the existence and functional significance of fluctuations in performance can be critically important.

It is reasonable that treatment goals for ADHD address both central tendency and variability. Of interest should be (1) changes in variability of behavior and (2) moving averages or trends in behavior. Such an assessment requires much more frequent data gathering than the pre-, post-, and follow-up measure strategies that dominate the treatment literature on ADHD. Much more frequent data collection, such as daily or weekly intervals when feasible, is useful—a reasonable number of assessments (e.g., at least six occasions) can provide a decent moving picture of performance. The availability of online symptom and impairment tracking websites (e.g., *Symptomtracking.com* or *Myadhd.com*) that patients–parents, teachers, and clinicians can access and report on behavior repeatedly may go along way toward making such repeated measurements more feasible and cost-effective. The recent use of handheld personal data assistants for repeated measurement in home or school settings may eventually provide a similar advantage (Whalen et al., 2006).

Setting and Observer Influences on Scores

Research on interrater agreement in the child psychopathology literature has consistently found significant but relatively small correlations between informants. For example, in a classic review on the topic, Achenbach and colleagues (1987) found a correlation of only about .30 between parent and teacher ratings of child psychopathology. This means that studies were finding only about 10% shared variance in behavior ratings between key informants. The small, positive correlations between parent and teacher ratings on standardized child behavior scales have been replicated in research on ADHD (Andrews, Garrison, Jackson, Addy, & McKeown, 1993; Stranger & Lewis, 1993).

The low correlations between parent and teacher ratings of ADHD have been used (speciously) by some critics to question the validity of ADHD diagnoses (Barkley, Fischer, et al., 2002). However, we believe these correlational studies merely highlight the differences in child behavior at home compared to school, and the need for well-structured assessments of ADHD. Appropriately structured evaluations should account for major influences on behavior, including activity, setting, and rater effects. It is well known that persons with ADHD can focus nearly as well as persons without ADHD on activities that are intrinsically interesting. As reviewed previously in this chapter, setting effects such as structure, novelty, and behavioral contingencies have all been shown to have large effects on ADHD and related problems. Furthermore, rater effects, such as expectations of the use of the measure, knowledge of ADHD, wording of questions, and the rater's mood that day, can all have a large effect on assessment scores.

Given the strong influences on scores that can be directly attributed to activity, setting, and rater, it should not be surprising that there is wide variability in cross-informant ratings. Documenting activity, setting, and rater influences on scores can be tremendously informative (e.g., revealing why a student thrives in one class and languishes in another). Unfortunately, most assessments of ADHD do not systematically provide a mechanism for resolving cross-informant discrepancies, even though this information is critically important for (1) judging the validity of the ratings and (2) understanding the key influences on the behavior of the person being assessed for ADHD. Fortunately, some procedures can be added to an ADHD assessment to deal with these issues. These include (1) gathering data from multiple informants, (2) conducting structured interviews about reasons for cross-informant disagreement, and (3) observing standardized behavior samples where feasible.

One of the requirements for a minimally adequate assessment of ADHD is to gather data from multiple raters. This is often accomplished by obtaining information from at least one parent and one teacher. More raters are even better, especially if they sample unique settings, relationships, or perspectives. Thus, it is usually best to have each parent complete ratings when possible, and to have various teachers complete ratings, such as those teaching core subjects requiring protracted mental effort—English, math, and history. Understanding why the child does better with one parent compared to the other, or in one school activity compared to another, is important information that can usually be gleaned from a well-structured interview with parents.

The confounding influences of activity and setting effects can be untangled through several methods, including (1) structured interviewing, (2) direct observation, and (3) functional assessments when evaluating ADHD. We fully understand that most clinicians do not have time to engage in direct observation or to conduct functional assessments, so our focus here is primarily on interviewing. Questions about ADHD symptoms should be specifically designed to illuminate influences such as setting, activity, and raters. For instance, rater effects may be evident if one rater stands out as being much more negative than others. Diplomatically discussing the reason for such a discrepancy can illuminate whether the difference is due to setting or rater effects.

Another important way to reveal influences on behavior is to ask very specific questions. For instance, asking the global question, "Does the child have problems with sustained attention?" may lead to a variety of confusing answers. Respondents might say "no," if they were thinking about computer games, or "yes," if they were thinking about doing homework. Thus, it is best to ask for a range of behaviors:

"When does your child pay attention?"
"When does your child seem to have trouble paying attention?"
"Why do you think there is a difference across these activities?"

A proper interview about setting influences can also help to untangle some putative rater

influences on ratings. Toward this end, assessments of ADHD should include asking the rater to describe typical activities he or she shares or directs with the person being assessed. For example, one teacher may rate a child as more inattentive than another, because that teacher is leading the class through repetitive math drills, whereas the other teacher is leading the student through interactive, hands-on Web-based activities. Similarly, a mother might rate her child as problematic because she supervises all of the chores and homework, whereas the father might not see the child as problematic, because he is primarily involved in novel projects or leisure activities with the child.

Structured interviewing with a parent is a minimum condition for an adequate assessment of ADHD. In some cases, more interviewing may be necessary with a teacher. In others, such as interviewing school-based professionals, it might be worthwhile to supplement the interviewing with direct observation. This is a major assessment issue because (1) ADHD must be shown to be pervasive across settings and raters, and (2) interventions can target settings, activities, and raters.

Benchmark samples of behavior are important here and can be gathered from one informant and used as reference points with other informants who witness the behavior. For instance, a mother might be asked to describe a typical behavior related to ADHD, such as behavior when doing homework. Then, the father and teachers may be asked about their observations of homework completion or self-directed seat work. Probing the key informants about the degree of problems and success with the task, the influences on behavior in the task, and the developmental appropriateness of the behavior can be very informative. Of note, this approach to assessment is not only person-centered (e.g., what symptoms the child with ADHD exhibits) but also examines the person–environment fit (e.g., the influences on the person's behavior and how the person influences the environment).

After examining potential variation across settings, it is very important to consider the unique variance of the rater's knowledge, beliefs, and circumstances on the ratings. Unfortunately, despite widespread understanding that unique variance due to raters has a large effect on ratings, there is no widely agreed-upon procedure for controlling idiosyncratic rater variance in assessments of ADHD. Ideally, rating scales for ADHD should have correction factors that adjust for potentially biasing influences such as parental depression, knowledge of typical development, and understanding of ADHD. At best, the current state-of-the-art assessment involves a qualitative synthesis of such information, if it is collected at all. This can be ascertained in a well-constructed interview for ADHD, such as the ACU, described later.

In addition to controlling for rater bias, collecting information on parents' mood, knowledge, resources, social support, and motivation for change is critically important assessment information. What the parent chooses to do with the evaluation data is probably an important consideration when doing an assessment for ADHD. Therefore, such information is structured such that (1) the parent understands the conclusions, (2) understands how the recommendations arise from the conclusions, and (3) feels personally willing and able to carry out key recommendations arising from the evaluation. Unfortunately, many parents are informed that their child has a diagnosis, but they may not understand it (e.g., ADHD-C subtype) and may be told to pursue treatment they do not necessarily want (e.g., "parent training" or medication). Fortunately, there are ways to evaluate ADHD that overcome these common oversights in assessment and treatment recommendations.

Within-Person Variability

Assessment approaches that do not control for within-subject variability and systematic differences in ratings from multiple informants can yield assessment data that appear to be full of random error. With appropriate measurement procedures, however, it is possible to learn quite a bit of important information from these sources of information that appear to be random, if not approached properly. True random error, on the other hand, is pure noise, with no redeeming measurement value. Some studies suggest that self-report of ADHD may be essentially random noise. At the very least, it is not clear whether children with ADHD can provide useful information to the assessment of their symptoms or impairments beyond what is provided by collateral informants (e.g., parents). Self-reports may be more valid in clinic-referred adults (Barkley et al., in press). This

section briefly reviews the validity of self-report of ADHD.

Children under the ages 9–12 years are not especially reliable in reports of their own problems or those of other family members. Furthermore, developmentally appropriate threats to the validity of self-report of ADHD symptoms are compounded by the frequently diminished self-awareness and impulse control typical of children with ADHD (Hinshaw, 1994). Nevertheless, many self-report rating scales that address ADHD symptoms are normed on ages as young as 8 years. These include the widely used Youth Self-Report version of the CBCL (Achenbach, 2001) and BASC-2 (Reynolds & Kamphaus, 2005). Unfortunately, these and similar scales have significant limitations in assessing ADHD and until more compelling psychometric data are presented, they should not be used to rule in or rule out a diagnosis of ADHD. They may, however, reveal levels of insight or motivation to change. For instance, showing parents that their child has a low hyperactivity self-report score may help convince them that extrinsic motivators will be necessary to deal with this issue.

It is common practice to interview a child about ADHD. Unfortunately, children with ADHD often show little reflection about the examiner's questions and may lie or distort information in a socially pleasing direction. Despite evidence to the contrary, some children report having many friends and no interaction problems at home with their parents, and that they are doing well at school, in direct contrast to the extensive parental and teacher complaints about the inappropriate behavior of these children. The problem is so ubiquitous to children with ADHD that some have argued that a hallmark of ADHD is an inordinately large disparity between self-evaluations and actual functioning in that setting or task, most likely due to a positive illusory bias (Hoza et al., 2004). This has also been shown in adults with the disorder (Knouse, Bagwell, Barkley, & Murphy, 2005). Accordingly, there may be a fundamental deficit in self-evaluation of inattention or impulsivity and its consequences (Barkley, 2005). Thus, lengthy structured or semistructured interviews with children with ADHD symptoms is probably a waste of time. Brief interviews to establish rapport and cooperation with intervention, however, might be worthwhile.

Adolescent self-report may be more reliable and valid for assessing externalizing symptoms

(Smith, Pelham, Gnagy, Molina, & Evans, 2000). However, self-reports about external-izing symptoms by adolescents with ADHD add little incremental information beyond par-ent or teacher report. Nevertheless, adoles-cents' reports of their internalizing symptoms (e.g., anxiety and depression) do seem to con-tribute incrementally valid information to as-sessment and should therefore play an impor-tant role in the diagnosis of comorbid anxiety or mood disorders in adolescents with ADHD (Hinshaw, 1994).

Some studies have found that clinic-referred adults with ADHD report more symptoms of inattention and impulsivity than do compari-son groups. Although initial research on self-report of ADHD symptoms in adults was promising, more recent studies have raised questions about the validity of this source of in-formation, and the problem appears to be double-edged. On the one hand, there may be tendency of adults who do not have ADHD to overreport symptoms of ADHD. For instance, Murphy, Gordon, and Barkley (2002) found that 80% of a sample of 719 adults recruited from motor vehicle license renewal sites re-ported six symptoms of ADHD at least some-times during childhood, and this only dropped to 25% when more stringent criteria were im-posed. Clearly the term "often," as used in DSM-IV symptoms, needs to be emphasized to underscore the excessive, persistent, and devel-opmentally inappropriate nature of the behav-ior before it should be counted as a symptom. On the other hand, there appears to be a ten-dency for individuals diagnosed in childhood as having ADHD to underreport these symp-toms as adults. For example, in one study, 46% of the sample of young adults who had been followed for ADHD since childhood met crite-ria for ADHD based on parent or other collat-eral report, but only 5% met diagnostic criteria based on self-report (Barkley, Fischer, et al., 2002).

In a study of college students (Smith, Cole, Ingram, & Clement, 2004), low kappas for classification as ADHD for self-ratings and semistructured interviews suggested consider-able inconsistency in self-report of ADHD. In the same study, when parent report of diagno-sis of ADHD was used as a criterion, specificity of self-report and interview was .72 and .83, respectively. Sensitivity was .50 and .21, re-spectively. Such findings clearly emphasize a point we risk reiterating repeatedly here: the need for collateral information other than self-reports concerning symptoms and impairment.

Taken together, these findings suggest two major problems with self-reported symptoms of ADHD by adults. The first problem has to do with the patient source. Children with ADHD followed to adulthood may be under-reporting current ADHD symptoms relative to parent reports about their current functioning. Clinic-referred adults, in contrast, often report more symptoms than do others who know them well. The other problem is overreporting of retrospective (i.e., childhood) symptoms among those who do not have ADHD. Accord-ingly, adult self-report data should be used with some caution and should never be the sole source of information used in diagnosis.

To summarize, although research comparing self-report of ADHD symptoms among adults and objective measures is lacking, this type of research with children and adolescents shows that there is little or no incremental validity of self-report of externalizing symptoms by indi-viduals with ADHD. Self-report can add a large amount of error and, if taken too seri-ously, confusion to the assessment battery. Thus, self-report of ADHD symptoms by chil-dren can be detrimental to the assessment pro-cess, and clinicians should avoid wasting pre-cious time and energy on lengthy structured or semistructured interviews that focus on self-report of ADHD symptoms. On the other hand, brief interviews to build rapport or to examine other psychiatric conditions, such as anxiety or depression, are recommended. Therefore, assessment for ADHD should in-clude some self-report interviewing, but the de-cision about the diagnosis of ADHD in chil-dren should focus heavily on collateral report (e.g., parent ratings), and self-report should be viewed very cautiously.

Multimodal Assessment of ADHD

The purpose of this section is to provide our recommendations for completing an acceptable evaluation for ADHD. This includes describing assessment tools and the procedures for using those tools. In some cases we compare and con-trast various assessment options; however, this is not intended to be a comprehensive overview of a broad range of assessment options. Rather, we focus on specific methods that we believe are the best options available. As promised ear-lier, we provide empirical justification for our choices as often as possible and make it clear when our recommendations are based on consensus or professional experience.

Although we recommend collecting a significant amount of information, we have selected measures and procedures that should be feasible and clinically meaningful in the "real world." The procedures for the ACU should take about 4 hours of parent time, 30–45 minutes of teacher time, and 5 hours of clinician time. Parent time includes an hour for completing questionnaires and about 3 hours for meeting with the clinician. Teacher time is devoted to completing questionnaires. Clinician time includes helping the parents and teachers complete the ratings, collecting collateral information from the school (e.g., grades), scoring measures, conducting semistructured interviews, and providing feedback to the family. This level of assessment has been deemed to be reasonable in field trials in clinical settings (Foy & Earls, 2005).

Goals of Assessment

There are several goals to bear in mind in the evaluation of an individual suspected of having ADHD. One is determination of the presence or absence of ADHD, with careful attention to differential diagnosis of ADHD as opposed to other psychiatric disorders. This requires extensive clinical knowledge of these other psychiatric disorders. Pertinent information on other childhood disorders is found in other chapters of this volume. Also, more information on differentiating between ADHD and other disorders is found in DSM-IV and Barkley (2005).

A second goal of the evaluation is to begin delineating the types of interventions needed to address the psychiatric disorder(s) and psychological, academic, and social impairments identified in the course of assessment. As we note later, these may include individual counseling, parent training in behavior management, family therapy, classroom behavior modification, stimulant or antidepressant medications, and formal special educational services, to name just a few (see Smith et al., 2006, for a recent review of treatments for ADHD, and Barkley, 2005, for more extensive coverage of each).

Another important goal of the evaluation is determination of comorbid conditions and whether or not these may affect prognosis or decisions about treatment. For instance, the presence of high levels of anxiety specifically, and of internalizing symptoms more generally, has been shown in some instances to be a predictor of poorer responses to stimulant medication (DuPaul, Barkley, & McMurray, 1994; Jensen et al., 2001; Pliszka, 1989). Other studies, however, argue that this may not be the case, making this a current point of contention (Abikoff et al., 2005). Similarly, high levels of hostile, defiant behavior or ODD have been shown to be a marker for greater family conflict (Barkley, Anastopoulos, et al., 1992; Barkley et al., 1991) that may interfere with successful parent training or family therapy.

A further goal of the evaluation is to identify the pattern of the child's psychological strengths and weaknesses, and to consider how these may affect treatment planning. This may also include gaining some impression of the parents' own abilities to carry out the treatment program, as well as their social and economic circumstances, and the treatment resources that may (or may not) be available within their community and cultural group. The evaluation also usually needs to determine the child's potential eligibility for special educational services within the school district. Such eligibility has been granted to ADHD children under federal legislation over the past 20 years via the Individuals with Disabilities in Education Act and Section 504 of the Rehabilitation Act (DuPaul & Stoner, 1994; Latham & Latham, 1992), but particular state regulations that institute these federal policies in a child's home school district may vary.

A key issue in assessing ADHD, especially in children and adolescents, is evaluating the primary caregiver's knowledge of intervention options and motivation to change. Matching treatment options with the caregiver's level of readiness for change may make the difference between assessment that is an exercise in developing insight versus an experience that prompts effective behavior change. We think the emphasis should be on promoting the right kind of change when change is needed (Miller & Rollnick, 2002). Therefore, we recommend a guided participatory process that (1) matches information and strategies according to the caregiver's stage of readiness for change, and (2) provides ongoing tracking of target behaviors using individual case study methods designed to assess response to treatment. We review these two strategies following consideration of some basic issues in assessing ADHD.

Minimally Acceptable Evaluation of ADHD

There is consensus regarding the elements of a minimally acceptable evaluation of ADHD but there are several ways to accomplish such an assessment. Experts agree that the following data should be collected: (1) parent ratings of ADHD symptoms, other psychiatric disorders, and related impairment; (2) teacher ratings of ADHD symptoms and functioning at school; (3) a semistructured interview with a parent to ascertain influences on behavior, parental skills and knowledge, and the developmental history of ADHD-related impairment, comorbid conditions, and various treatments or efforts to change behavior; and (4) if the history so indicates, an examination by a physician to rule out plausible physical causes for putative ADHD symptoms (Foy & Earls, 2005; Pelham et al., 2005). In the following sections, we elaborate on these four cornerstones of ADHD assessment by recommending specific tools and the rationale for including those tools.

During the assessment process we ask parents to complete the measures listed in Table 2.2. It should take most parents less than an hour to complete these measures. Ideally, these

TABLE 2.2. Recommended Self-Report Measures to Be Completed by Parents

1. The Parent Rating Scale (PRS) of the Behavioral Assessment System for Children, Second Edition (BASC-2; Reynolds & Kamphaus, 2005).

2. A checklist of DSM-IV symptoms using the Disruptive Behavior Disorders Scale (Pelham, Fabiano, & Massetti, 2005).

3. The Home Situations Questionnaire (HSQ; Barkley & Murphy, 2006).

4. A brief ADHD scale such as the Conners Global Index (CGI; Conners, 1997) or ADHD Rating Scale–IV (DuPaul et al., 1998).

5. A brief index of impairment such as the Children's Impairment Rating Scale (CIRS; Fabiano et al., 2006).

6. The Beck Depression Inventory (BDI; Beck, Steer, & Brown, 1996) or Symptom Checklist–90—Revised (Derogatis, 1995).

7. The Alcohol Use Disorders Identification Test (AUDIT; Saunders, Aasland, Babor, Delafuente, & Grant, 1993).

8. Married or cohabitating caregivers should be asked to complete the Parenting Experiences Inventory (Sanders & Ralph, 2001). See Appendix 2.1.

may be mailed to parents before the assessment process starts, or parents may complete them between initial assessment meetings scheduled on two or more occasions. Because some parents will not complete these on their own, such as those with limited linguistic or intellectual competence, without some explanation, prompting, and support, it is often best to ask such parents to complete the measures between the first and second sessions or within the sessions.

The purpose of having the parent complete the Parent Rating Scale (PRS) of the BASC-2 is because it is important to use a standardized, well-normed, psychometrically sound instrument to conduct a broad screening for psychopathology and adaptation (Reynolds & Kamphaus, 2005). There are different versions of the PRS that allow the parent to provide developmentally appropriate information from preschool to college. The computerized scoring of the scale is readily interpreted and highly informative. The areas of psychopathology covered by the PRS vary with age group. For the child (ages 6–11) and adolescent versions (ages 12–21) the PRS provides the following clinical scales: aggression, anxiety, attention problems, atypicality, conduct problems, hyperactivity, somatization, and withdrawal. The PRS for these age groups also provides adaptive scales in the areas of activities of daily living, adaptability, functional communication, leadership, and social skills.

The major viable alternative to the PRS, the Child Behavior Checklist (CBCL; Achenbach, 1991, 2001; Achenbach & Rescorla, 2001), is probably the most widely used "broad-band" screening measure for child psychopathology. However, two studies by independent research groups have shown that the PRS is better than the CBCL at discriminating between children with and without ADHD (Ostrander, Weinfurt, Yarnold, & August, 1998; Vaughn, Riccio, Hynd, & Hall, 1997) . Moreover, the PRS provides information on adaptive functioning.

It is noteworthy that there have been revisions to the CBCL since the aforementioned studies were published. Currently, the CBCL provides normed scales for attention problems and attention deficit/hyperactivity problems, including hyperactivity/impulsivity and attention problems subscales (Reynolds & Kamphaus, 2005). In summary, the revised CBCL appears to be a good measure, but the PRS still has the advantage of providing adaptive functioning scales that are lacking in the CBCL.

The second measure we recommend, the Disruptive Behavior Disorders Scale (DBD), captures data specific to ADHD, ODD, and CD (Pelham et al., 2005). A very similar scale is provided in the clinical manual by Barkley and Murphy (2006). This scale rephrases symptom descriptions taken from DSM-IV and has the parent rate them on a 0- to 3-point scale (see Table 2.1 for ADHD symptoms; the DBD also measures ODD and CD symptoms). This type of rating scale is used widely in ADHD research and should be familiar to many clinicians who work with individuals with ADHD. Various cutoffs can be applied to the scores. In most applications, scores of 2 or 3 are considered to be clinically significant, whereas scores of 0 or 1 are not. Tallying these symptom counts can readily assist in evaluating DSM-IV diagnoses of ADHD, ODD, or CD. Psychometric data on the DBD supports its use (Pelham et al., 2005). Furthermore, mean item scores of less than 1 on the inattention, hyperactivity/impulsivity, and ODD scales have been used as a criterion for clinically significant change in major treatment studies of ADHD (Swanson et al., 2001).

The major alternatives to the DBD are (1) scales similar to the DBD that focus on ADHD symptoms from the DSM, but not ODD or CD, such as the ADHD Rating Scale–IV (DuPaul et al., 1998), and (2) scales that focus on ADHD symptoms and related problems, such as the various Conners ratings scales (Conners, 1997). We are not aware of studies that have compared directly the incremental validity or other psychometric considerations of the DBD-type scales relative to other "narrow-band" ADHD rating scales. They are likely to be equivalent in detecting ADHD at least, because norms are available from the ADHD Rating Scale–IV, which can be used to score the ADHD portion of the DBD scale by Barkley and Murphy (2006).

The pervasiveness of the child's behavior problems within the home and school settings should also be examined, as such measures of situational pervasiveness appear to have as much, if not more, stability over time as do the aforementioned scales (Fischer et al., 1993). The Home Situations Questionnaire (HSQ; Barkley & Murphy, 2006) requires parents to rate their child's behavior problems across 16 different home and public situations. Such in-formation may assist in planning behavioral interventions for children with ADHD and accounting for cross-informant discrepancies in ratings of ADHD symptoms and related problems. We are not aware of the development of any alternatives to the HSQ for the purpose of assessing situational pervasiveness of ADHD.

We recommend instituting some brief measures that are likely to be sensitive to response to treatment. For this reason, we ask parents to complete the Conners Global Index (CGI) and the Children's Impairment Rating Scale (CIRS) on a weekly basis. Along with tracking of specific problem behaviors, these brief rating scales provide important guidance in assessing intervention efforts.

The CGI, a 10-item scale with ratings on the familiar 0- to 3-point scale used by ADHD researchers (Pliszka, Liotti, et al., 2000), can be completed quickly and has been shown to be responsive to treatment (Pliszka, Liotti, et al., 2000). It is too much to ask parents to complete longer scales such as the BASC-2 on a weekly basis; furthermore, the validity of the broad-band scales (e.g., BASC-2) is unknown in the context of weekly administration. Other brief scales, such as the IOWA Conners (see Pelham et al., 2005), do not map directly onto DSM symptom lists and the research history seems to be stronger for the CGI. It might be reasonable to repeat DBD subscales (e.g., inattention symptoms) or items from the HSQ on a weekly basis, but when used repeatedly over short durations, the psychometrics of such measures need to be studied.

It is critically important to document impairment, which refers to the consequences of the ADHD symptoms for various domains of major life activities, such as home and school functioning, peer relations, and so on. We recommend the parent version of the CIRS. This scale covers key domains of impairment identified by parents, including relationship with peers, relationship with siblings, academic progress, effect on family, self-esteem, and overall functioning. Each area is rated on a 0- to 6-point scale (0, *no problem, no need for treatment*; 6, *severe problem, definite need for treatment*. This yields a clinically meaningful metric (i.e., scores less than 3 suggest that the child does not need intervention in that area). Recent validity studies support use of the CIRS with children with ADHD (Fabiano et al., 2006).

There are some alternatives to the CIRS. One approach is to use a single global measure, such as the Children's Global Assessment of Functioning Scale (C-GAS) described in DSM-IV. The C-GAS has been shown to be responsive to treatment and, like the CIRS, is brief enough to be given on a weekly basis. Although little research specifically supports this assumption, we hypothesize that the CIRS has greater clinical relevance and incremental validity over the C-GAS, so the CIRS is our measure of choice for impairment at this time. Another is to examine the adaptive functioning items from the CBCL individually for parent and teacher responses on items concerning home, school, and peer functioning.

Other alternatives to the CIRS are very detailed measures of adaptive functioning that are not usually clinically cost-effective. The Vineland Adaptive Behavior Scales (Sparrow, Balla, & Cicchetti, 1984) is probably the most commonly used measure for assessing adaptive functioning. The scales have been used in studies that identified impairment in children with ADHD relative to peers. Another option for assessing this domain is the Normative Adaptive Behavior Checklist (Adams, 1984), because of its greater ease of administration. Unfortunately, these detailed measures take a long time to complete (usually at least 40 minutes) and may add little important information beyond what is obtained from the CIRS as far as clinical diagnosis and treatment planning are concerned.

Of note, the BASC-2 provides Adaptive Functioning subscales, for example, in the areas of activities of daily living, adaptability, functional communication, leadership, and social skills. This portion of the BASC-2 is far shorter than the more extensive Adaptive Behavior scales noted earlier and is therefore more cost-effective. However, for initial evaluation of impairment, the CIRS seems most suitable. Such information can be incorporated into the assessment summary. Furthermore, we recommend using the CIRS in conjunction with the CGI, both of which can be completed daily to give an index of symptoms and impairment.

Asking caregivers to report on their own problems is a delicate issue, but one that must be explored to understand fully critical influences on child behavior and the ability of the parent to take a major role in the treatment of ADHD, whether providing medication or managing behavioral contingencies. We recommend having parents complete self-report measures that screen for the major dimensions of

psychopathology, such as the Symptom Checklist–90—Revised (SCL-90-R; Derogatis, 1995), and especially for major depression and alcohol use disorders. These prevalent disorders in the adult population have elevated rates in families of children with ADHD and are likely to impair caregiving (Barkley, 2005). Furthermore, treatment of depressed mothers appears to have a positive effect on childhood behavior disorders (Weissman et al., 2006). When parents have a partner in caregiving, measures of relationship satisfaction with parenting is an important issue to assess (Sanders, 1999).

In view of the high heritability of the disorder, we strongly recommend that biological parents of children with ADHD be screened for possible ADHD themselves. There is a nontrivial probability that one parent is likely to have the disorder (25–35%), and it can interfere with intervention for the child, as noted earlier. The easiest means for doing so is to employ an adult ADHD screening scale, such as that available in the manual by Barkley and Murphy (2006) or the lengthier Conners Adult ADHD Rating Scale (Conners, Erhardt, & Sparrow, 2001).

When screening for problems experienced by parents, it is important for parents to understand why information on their own functioning is important in the context of assessment of their child's behavior. The reason for such screening must be explained in a clear, supportive, and empathic manner prior to administration of these types of measures. Sending these measures without explanation in a screening packet might be off-putting for many parents. Rather, the rationale for collecting these data should be explained in person after some rapport has developed.

There are many options for screening for parental depression. A scale often used to provide a quick assessment of parental depression is the Beck Depression Inventory (BDI; Beck, Steer, & Brown, 1996). A more "broad-band" measure for assessing this area of parental difficulties, the SCL-90-R (Derogatis, 1995; Derogatis & Cleary, 1977), has not only a scale assessing depression in adults, but also contains scales measuring other dimensions of adult psychopathology and psychological distress. Parents of children with ADHD often have higher scores on the Depression, Hostility, Anxiety, and Interpersonal Difficulties subscales (Barkley, Anastopoulos, et al., 1992; Barkley et al., 1991; Murphy & Barkley, 1996b). However, the SCL-90-R may be measuring general distress, and may lack specificity for depression and other specific psychological conditions (Hafkenscheid, 1993). Therefore, we recommend that when depression is specifically of interest, use of shorter, more specific scales, such as the BDI, may be better.

As with depression measures, there are many choices for screening for alcohol use disorders. Research suggests that the Alcohol Use Disorders Identification Test (AUDIT) may be superior to other brief measures due to construct and external validity advantages (Bush et al., 2003; Cook, Chung, Kelly, & Clark, 2005; Knight, Sherritt, Harris, Gates, & Chang, 2003; MacKenzie, Langa, & Brown, 1996). Therefore, we recommend use of the AUDIT, a 10-item scale that measures alcohol consumption and alcohol-related problems. Cutoffs for the AUDIT have been published, with score of 8 or higher indicating a need for further evaluation of alcohol-related difficulties.

Next would be measures that assess the parent's interpersonal functioning. If the caregiver is married or cohabiting, completing the Dyadic Adjustment Scale (DAS) can provide important contextual information for assessment and treatment planning. Many instruments evaluate marital discord in parents. The one most often used in research on childhood disorders has been the Locke–Wallace Marital Adjustment Scale (Locke & Wallace, 1959). Research has indicated that parents of children with ADHD, regardless of child gender, have lower ratings of marital satisfaction than do parents of normal children (Breen & Barkley, 1988; Murphy & Barkley, 1996b), especially in the subgroup of children with ADHD and ODD or CD (Barkley, Anastopoulos, et al., 1992; Barkley et al., 1991; Befera & Barkley, 1985).

It is important to assess the level of discord between parenting partners, because it may play a role in how interventions are perceived and delivered. For example, a high degree of discord may portend significant disagreement between partners over the presence and/or management of behavioral problems in children. Depression, partner discord, and child behavioral problems are a common triad (Dawson et al., 2003; Low & Stocker, 2005; Sugawara et al., 2002). Moreover, it is possible that changes in one domain may result in changes in all three domains (DeGarmo, Patterson, & Forgatch, 2004; Sanders & McFarland, 2000).

Sanders and Ralph (2001) developed a brief index of marital satisfaction, called the Parenting Experiences Survey, that may be more amenable for screening purposes compared to some of the more detailed measures mentioned earlier. This 11-item scale provides a measure of the degree of success with parenting and comfort with coparenting (see Appendix 2.1). The first eight items focus on parenting satisfaction. The last three items assess the degree of comfort with coparenting. These items are taken from the DAS (Spanier & Cole, 1976) and have been shown to discriminate between distressed and nondistressed couples (Sharpley & Rogers, 1984).

It may be worthwhile to assess other areas of the parents' interpersonal functioning should time and resources permit (e.g., parent–child interactions). However, there is limited time and motivation to complete screening measures, especially about issues specific to the caregiver. Therefore, we relegate exploration of some issues of parental psychopathology and interpersonal functioning to the structured interview. The recommended foci of the parent self-report rating scales are ADHD, depression, alcohol use, and marital functioning.

TEACHER RATINGS

Obtaining information from teachers is crucially important for several reasons. First of all, a child who does not have any academic or behavioral problems at school most likely does not have ADHD. Second, teachers are probably better judges of developmentally appropriate behavior than parents, assuming it is not the first few days or weeks of school. This is matter of opportunity and experience, because teachers simply see more children. Third, teachers are likely to be involved in the intervention process, so engaging them early in the assessment phase and getting a solid baseline of behavior benefits later treatment plans.

The measures we recommend for teachers (see Table 2.3) parallel those for parents, with the same justification as was made for the parent measures. Thus, we ask teachers to complete the Teacher Rating Scale (TRS) of the BASC-2, a teacher version of the DBD, the School Situations Questionnaire (SSQ), the CGI, and the CIRS. Due to professional boundaries, we do not directly inquire about teacher

TABLE 2.3. Recommended Teacher Ratings

1. The Teacher Rating Scale (TRS) from the Behavioral Assessment System for Children, Second Edition (BASC-2)
2. The Disruptive Behavior Disorders checklist of DSM-IV symptoms (DBD)
3. The School Situations Questionnaire (SSQ)
4. The Conners Global Index (CGI)
5. The Children's Impairment Rating Scale (CIRS)

functioning (e.g., depression or substance use). Also, because of sensitivity to the response burden on teachers, every effort should be made to keep the data demands as slight as possible. Our clinical experience has been that this packet is very feasible for routine clinical use with teachers.

Elementary school teachers, who spend quite a bit of time with the child, can be key informants. However, as children get older, teachers may not know them as well, and teacher reports may be less reliable in middle and high school (Evans, Allen, Moore, & Strauss, 2005). Therefore, the evaluator should inquire how well the teacher knows the student prior to asking the teacher to complete the ratings. Even elementary school teachers may not know students very well in the first few weeks of the school year or shortly after moving to a new school.

As mentioned previously, cross-informant agreement may be low for parents and teachers, often because the parents and teachers observe different behaviors. Accordingly, the parent and teacher versions of the BASC-2 overlap on some scales and diverge on others. This is appropriate, considering that teachers and parents observe students in different contexts. Indeed, teachers often report difficulty in answering some questions. It is advisable to instruct teachers to make their best effort to answer questions and indicate "DK" (don't know) next to items that they do not have a basis for answering. Also, teachers might be advised that some items may seem shocking (e.g., "taking advantage of another sexually," which is a CD item on the DBD). They should be told that although such behavior is rare, its occurrence is so important that the clinician should know about it, so the item is included in the questionnaire.

The clinician directing the assessment usually has to take a very active role in getting in-

formation from teachers. Unless the parents have an exceptionally good relationship with teachers or a very organized and cooperative school, it is likely that the clinician will encounter many barriers when seeking ratings. Therefore, he or she should provide teachers with Health Insurance Portability and Accountability Act (HIPAA) compliant release of information forms, a note from the parent personally requesting the information, a note from the therapist explaining the scales and how they are used (including confidentiality considerations), very clear instructions, contact information, and a deadline for completion (usually 1 week), along with a self-addressed, stamped envelope. School visits and other direct contact bolster the chances for cooperation and allow the clinician to collect some incidental and qualitative information. When this is not possible, indirect contact by phone, mail, or the Internet is important.

CHILD SELF-REPORT MEASURES

As mentioned previously, we believe the research suggests that the incremental validity of child self-report measures of ADHD symptoms is questionable; therefore, self-report should receive minimal weight in an assessment of ADHD (Barkley, Fischer, et al., 2002; McCann & Roy-Byrne, 2004; Smith et al., 2000). However, child self-report of other areas, such as depression and anxiety, might provide unique and important information during the assessment process (Baxter & Rattan, 2004; Hope et al., 1999). Furthermore, having the child with ADHD provide input into the assessment process might make the child feel more involved or invested in the assessment, thus increasing the likelihood of cooperation with recommendations for intervention (Dishion & Kavanagh, 2003).

For individuals ages 8–21, we recommend using the Self-Report of Personality (SRP) from the BASC-2. The BASC-2 SRP includes self-report scales on inattention and hyperactivity. Factor-analytic studies apparently support the validity of these scales (Reynolds & Kamphaus, 2005), but the incremental and construct validity of self-reported attention problems and hyperactivity on the SRP have not yet been established. In contrast, evidence for the validity of the other BASC-2 self-report scales seems to be quite good (Reynolds & Kamphaus, 2005).

Another "broad-band" self-report measure, the Youth Self-Report (YSR; Achenbach, 1991, 2001), is designed and normed for children ages 11–18 years; thus, it has a restricted age range relative to the BASC SRP. Most items are similar to those on the parent- and the teacher-report form of the CBCL, except that they are worded in the first person. The Cross-Informant Version (Achenbach, 1991) permits direct comparisons of results among the parent, teacher, and youth versions of this popular rating scale. The BASC-2, on the other hand, does not have such complete overlap of scales. However, because evidence suggests that the BASC is superior to the CBCL for assessing ADHD, we advocate the use of the BASC scales.

THE ADHD CHECKUP

The semistructured interview we recommend is incorporated into a broader assessment framework of the ACU. Where time and resources permit, we recommend using the entire ACU protocol; otherwise, use of the aforementioned minimum assessment protocol is suggested when time is of the essence. The ACU is based on the Family Checkup (Dishion & Kavanagh, 2003), a parent-focused assessment process that we have modified in an effort to provide the best impact of a multimodal assessment of ADHD. The ACU comprises four phases: (1) telephone contact prior to the first session; (2) semistructured interview with the parent(s) to evaluate interpersonal functioning, major presenting problems, developmental history, and other background information; (3) videotaped interactions between the family members to assess parenting relationships; and (4) collaborative feedback with the parent(s) regarding diagnosis and treatment recommendations. Adolescents can be included in some or all of the feedback session, but it is probably best to work individually with the parent for some portions of the ACU, especially when there is a high degree of parent–child or parent–parent conflict. This section reviews the background and history, and the general procedures for conducting the ACU. More detailed descriptions of procedures pertinent to the ACU are found in Dishion and Kavanagh (2003), Miller and Rollnick (2002), and Sanders and Lawton (1993).

History and Background

The ACU is based on an earlier brief family intervention designed to prevent substance use and behavior problems among children and adolescents. The theory underlying the ACU, called "motivational interviewing" (Miller, 1998), is consistent with the principles of the "transtheoretical model of change" (Prochaska, DiClemente, & Norcross, 1992). This intervention theory is well established and empirically supported for problems related to substance abuse (Miller & Rollnick, 2002). The ACU represents the first application of this theory to family therapy (Dishion & Kavanagh, 2003). However, ACU procedures are consistent with the best applications of Behavioral Parent Training (Patterson & Forgatch, 1987; Sanders & Lawton, 1993) and the client-centered approach of Carl Rogers (1951). Thus, many ACU principles and procedures have been supported by a number of well-regarded experts who work with high-risk teenagers and their families. Nevertheless, we believe the reader will be impressed and agree that the proposed ACU is sufficiently novel to be called a unique approach.

A guiding principle in motivational interviewing, and hence in the ACU, is to expect ambivalence about change (Miller & Rollnick, 2002). In the context of family therapy, multiple levels of ambivalence are possible, because change can pertain to (1) the behavior of the target child, (2) the behavior of a parent, (3) the interactions between parent and child, (4) the interactions between siblings and the target child, and (5) the major interactions between the family and other systems (e.g., with a pediatrician or a school). Thus, during the phone contact process, the clinician should be on the alert to detect and deal with ambivalence about the change that is needed to solve problems related to ADHD.

Another important guiding principle in the ACU is to develop congruence between the family's expectations and the procedures in the assessment and recommendations. A theory supports this notion, the transtheoretical model of change proposed by Prochaska, DiClemente, and Norcross (1992). This theory, with its attendant stages and processes of change, is by now quite familiar to those who work in the field of addictions (Miller, 1998). Unfortunately, researchers have only begun to apply this very promising approach to problems other than addictive behaviors. Therefore, a brief introduction to this approach is warranted.

The roots of the transtheoretical model of change are found in the frequent result that promising treatments do not work equally well with all persons. Sometimes the poor outcomes are attributed to client factors; at other times, poor outcomes are attributed to therapist factors (Prochaska et al., 1992). Examples of patient factors associated with poor outcomes are lack of awareness, denial, inadequate motivation, and poor relational skills. Examples of therapist factors associated with poor outcomes are lack of empathy, inadequate diagnosis or treatment planning, and poorly implemented or otherwise inadequate techniques. However, there are many cases where therapy failed even though the client appeared to be engaged and the therapist seemed to be competent. The unique insight from the transtheoretical model of change is that therapy outcomes might be dependent on the match between stage of readiness for change, the treatment prescribed, and how the treatment is presented to the persons responsible for change. The five commonly accepted stages of readiness for change (Prochaska et al., 1992) are briefly described.

In the *precontemplative* stage, the person has no intention to change. This condition may be due to factors such as ignorance, denial, or hopelessness about the possibility of change. For example, someone might believe that hyperactivity is normal (e.g., "Boys will be boys, its not a problem") or that there is nothing that can be done about it (e.g., "All the boys in our family are rowdy, that's just the way we are").

In the *contemplation* stage, the person is aware of the problem and is seriously thinking about overcoming the problem but has not yet made a commitment to take action. This stage is characterized by knowing where one wants to go (i.e., to make changes) but not being quite ready to go there. A common phenomenon in the contemplation stage is weighing the pros and cons of the problem and the solution to the problem. A parent in the contemplation stage might say something like, "I know that inattention is a problem, but the things we have tried haven't worked and I don't know if it is worth trying something new."

In the *preparation* stage, the individual intends to take action or has been trying to take action. The person is beginning to make small behavioral changes, but nothing that would constitute effective action, such as abstinence from smoking. He or she intends, however, to take substantial action in the near future. A caregiver in the preparation stage may take some preliminary steps toward change, such as making an appointment for therapy or reading a book on ADHD and selecting some of the recommended techniques to try in the near future. Of note, many parents who schedule appointments for evaluations for ADHD are ready for their child's behavior to change, but they may not be in the preparation or action stage with regard to changing their own behavior. Other parents might be waiting for some revelation or insight that will provide a "magic bullet" to alleviate their child's problems. Such parents may engage in endless assessment and "doctor shopping" but never really implement any change strategies.

In the *action* stage, the person modifies his or her behavior or environment to overcome the problem. Modification of the target behavior or significant overt effort to change is the hallmark of the action stage. A caregiver who puts up a behavior chart and starts giving rewards based on the chart is in the action stage. The best-established interventions for ADHD involve behavioral intervention (Smith et al., 2006), and most assume that the parents are ready to put up a behavior chart after the first meeting (Sanders & Ralph, 2001). However, if the parent is not in the action stage, the behavioral instructions can create a mismatch or incongruence with the parent, thereby straining the rapport and threatening the viability of the intervention.

Maintenance is the stage in which a person works to consolidate gains attained during the action stage. The hallmarks of the maintenance stage are stabilizing behavior change and promoting generalization. For example, caregivers who achieve success with one particular task (e.g., independently completing academic tasks at home) start reinforcing the use of successful methods at other times, sometimes with the help of other caregivers (e.g., individual study time at school). Training in self-regulation, such as developing self-sufficiency, self-efficacy, and problem-solving skills that generalize to new issues and developmental levels, appear to be important goals for effective maintenance (Halford, Sanders, & Behrens, 1994).

Ordinarily, the more action that has been taken to change the problem, the better the prognosis (Prochaska et al., 1992). However, *the key and uniquely insightful contribution of the transtheoretical model of change is the attention to the match between therapist behavior and the client's stage of readiness for change.* Within this view, change is promoted by helping the individual advance from one stage to the next. A key task for the therapist is to sense the emotional, behavioral, and cognitive shifts that need to occur for the client to progress toward change (Miller, 1998). If a client is ready for action, the therapist may prescribe action-oriented therapy and the best outcomes are achieved. If a mismatch occurs, such as an action-oriented intervention prescribed to a client in the contemplation stage, results are expected to be poor. An ill-matched prescription may result in premature termination and loss of the therapist's opportunity to assist in the change process.

Telephone Contact

An important concept incorporated into the ACU is that treatment begins with the first phone contact between a family and a therapist (Coatsworth, Santisteban, McBride, & Szapocznik, 2001; Dakof et al., 2003; Santisteban, Suarez-Morales, Robbins, & Szapocznik, 2006). Thus, rather than viewing the initial phone call as a perfunctory exercise in scheduling, the initial phone call should be regarded at the start of the parent–therapist relationship. This early relationship can have a major effect on retention and engagement in therapy. Thus, one of the major goals of the ACU is to develop a positive relationship between the family and the therapist from the very beginning. A telephone call can create a positive relationship by increasing the congruence between a family's perspective on the ACU and the therapist's behavior. During a telephone call, a therapist can clearly define the process of obtaining services, invest the family in the help-seeking process, and explore any other barriers the family may be facing (McKay, McCadam, & Gonzales, 1996).

A recent review of the literature (Snell-Johns, Mendez, & Smith, 2004) identified three empirical studies that examined the effectiveness of telephone-based strategies (McKay et al.,

1996; Santisteban, Szapocznik, & Perez-Vidal, 1996; Szapocznik et al., 1988). The importance of phone contact can be summarized by the expression "Call early and often." Moreover, the quality and structure of the phone conversation can be very important. These calls are the first step in the change process. As such, phone contact should draw the family into the therapy process and socialize family members into behavior patterns that are productive in therapy and promote change. Thus, phone interactions should be guided by evidence-based procedures, especially those derived from motivational interviewing. Although these procedures have not yet been tested for specific relevance to ADHD, they are supposed to cut across disorders; therefore, they should be appropriate for use with families in which the target child has ADHD.

Overall, the key considerations in ACU phone contacts are to engage caregivers in the change process and to begin to develop a collaborative therapeutic relationship. Motivational interviewing techniques that apply here include (1) expressing empathy, and (2) rolling with resistance (Miller & Rollnick, 2002). Accordingly, the major goals of the ACU phone calls are to (1) communicate genuine interest and concern over the family's difficulties, (2) promote a positive therapeutic relationship by developing congruence between the family and the therapist's goals and procedures, (3) overcome ambivalence about change and engage the family in the ACU assessment process, and (4) begin to socialize family members toward the most effective interactions in assessment and therapy.

To prepare for the telephone contact, the clinician should review all available data previously completed by the family. Usually the call from the therapist is not the very first contact with the family, and some screening or background information on the reason for the referral should be available. In some settings, there may be intake forms, screening questionnaires, or records from previous contact with the clinic. Parents may be dismayed if the therapist is unaware of information they provided previously, so knowing information from prior contacts may help to build rapport.

The Semistructured Interview

To emphasize the importance of the caregiver in the evaluation and treatment process, we refer to the clinician directing the ACU as a parent consultant. However, we use the conventional term "therapist" in this chapter. The point is that in all meetings with caregivers, the therapist should promote self-regulation and promote the type of therapeutic relationship such that the parent is the primary decision maker.

Direct contact with the therapist occurs in three meetings. The getting-to-know-you (GTKY, which we pronounce "get key") session is the initial semistructured interview designed to get to know the family and to get key information. The goals of the GTKY meeting with the parent(s) arc to (1) develop rapport and trust with caregivers; (2) better understand the caregiver's interest and concerns as they apply to the target child and to the family in general; and (3) motivate interest in completing all three steps of the ACU. The steps of the GTKY session are described in the following section. The major activities of this first session of the ACU are given in Table 2.4. The second and third sessions, Family Assessment Task (FAST) and feedback sessions, are described in subsequent sections but are referred to several times in the GTKY session.

The GTKY session begins with setting an agenda and providing a rationale for completing three separate assessment sessions. It is crucially important, both during the initial phone call and early in the GTKY session, to create a link between concerns and assessment, thus engaging the caregiver in the evaluation process. Thus, immediately after setting the agenda, the

caregiver is asked to work with the therapist to complete a description of the parent's and child's social network. This combination of genogram and ecomap provides key information on social influences on behavior, caregiver social support and stressors, and family history of ADHD and other issues, including the parent's own past and present issues (Shapiro & Smith, 2002). A subtle implication of this phase of the assessment is to frame the behavior of the child with ADHD in a broader social context rather than as an individually based problem. Also, this discussion of social influences should draw on strengths, protective factors, and resources that will eventually be key considerations in suggesting interventions.

After spending 10 to 20 minutes on the social influences on the genogram and ecomap (longer with larger or complicated families), we ask the parent to complete a checklist of concerns, using a list based on surveys of parents regarding their top concerns about their adolescents (Sanders & Ralph, 2001). Other lists are available (see Dishion & Kavanagh, 2003), and a commonly used measure developed by Prinz, Foster, Kent, and O'Leary (1979) is available in Robin and Foster (1989). The most common problems include fighting with siblings, arguing with parents, noncompliance, failing to do homework, and behavior problems at school.

The next step in the GTKY session is to have the caregiver pick the top few problems, then, starting with the most distressing problem, conduct a detailed analysis of each (see Appendix 2.2). When multiple caregivers complete the GTKY checklist, they may disagree on some of the problems. Usually, the caregivers agree on at least one of the top three problems and, in such cases, agreed-upon problems should be discussed first. When caregivers completely disagree, the therapist can ask who owns the problem, and whether it is reasonable for that caregiver to work on the problem, separate from the other caregiver.

Problems should be discussed from an ABC (Antecedents–Behaviors–Consequences) framework, similar to the questioning described by Sanders and colleagues in the Triple-P Positive Parenting Program (Sanders, 1999; Sanders & Lawton, 1993; Sanders & Ralph, 2001) and other evidence-based parenting approaches based on social learning theory (Bank, Patterson, & Reid, 1987). This involves asking for the most recent example of the problem behav-

TABLE 2.4. Getting-to-Know-You (GTKY) Session with Parents

- Assessor meets with parents for up to 90 minutes, uses the "Getting to Know You" (GTKY) form.
- Complete a Problem Checklist.
- Complete a genogram and diagram of social supports.
- Rank-order the top problems.
- Complete a thorough discussion of top problems.
- Developmental and school history (emphasize influences on behavior).
- Confirm the appointment for the Family Assessment Task (FAST).
- Identify a conflict to discuss during the FAST.
- Identify a problem to discuss during the FAST.
- Explain the questionnaires that need to be completed prior to the FAST.

ior, inquiring whether it is typical of the problem being discussed, and, if so, finding out what happened before, during, and after the behavior. If the most recent example of the behavior is not typical, a more typical example is elicited for a discussion of the social context of the problem (i.e., antecedents and consequences). The discussion centers on the influences of the behavior, especially those that are modifiable and under the caregivers' control. Past attempts to change behavior are noted, and expectations about behavior change in the future are considered. After reviewing the problems, the therapist completes a brief school and developmental history with the caregivers (see Appendix 2.2).

The key function of the GTKY session (and the feedback session) is to help build a foundation for change. During these semistructured interviews, the caregiver and the therapist collaborate to establish a shared perspective on the child's behavior, and on the family situation as it applies to the child. The therapist is constantly evaluating the caregivers' stage of readiness for change and attempting to move them forward toward action, but in a gentle and subtle manner.

During the ACU it may become clear that some of the caregivers' outcome expectations are unrealistic (e.g., behavior therapy does not work, but sugar restriction does). Furthermore, there may be unrealistic self-efficacy expectations (e.g., "I can't be consistent with behavioral interventions, but I can control sugar intake"). Thus, it is important to instill a reasonable understanding of effective interventions and the expectation that caregivers can perform, or learn to perform, the desired behaviors. A person's belief in the possibility of changing ADHD-related behavior is an important motivator (Bor, Sanders, & Markie-Dadds, 2002).

Family Assessment Task

The second of the three meetings between the caregiver and the therapist is optional and is called the Family Assessment Task, or FAST. This session begins with setting the agenda, which includes making sure that the questionnaires given to the family at the end of the GTKY session have been completed (see Table 2.2). These questionnaires must be completed and scored prior to the feedback session, so it is important to spend the first part of the FAST

emphasizing the importance of completing these measures. This may be a delicate situation, because caregivers may feel embarrassed because they did not complete all of the measures recommended in Table 2.2. As was done in the GTKY session, the therapist should reward effort and link concerns with assessment.

When the caregivers have completed the forms, the family is asked to complete a series of standardized tasks, the FAST, while being videotaped. Basically, the therapist lets the family members interact among themselves without providing any immediate feedback. A brief outline of the current FAST is given in Table 2.5. The detailed version with verbatim instructions for the therapist and cue cards, as well as scoring instructions, may be obtained from Dr. Smith at *smithbrad@sc.edu*.

The FAST interactions are videotaped for later review by the therapist and discussion with the family. The use of the FAST makes the ACU overtly different

compared to many other assessments that do not include direct, structured observation of family management practices. Thus, many therapists may feel that they do not have the resources or expertise to code the FAST interactions. Furthermore, performing an unusual task in which family members are videotaped can strain subject families. Given that the incremental validity of the FAST in the ACU process has not been established, administering the FAST may not be necessary. Nevertheless, the use of structured videotaped interactions to assess close relationships builds on the vast literature of family and marital assessment (Granic, Hollenstein, Dishion, & Patterson, 2003).

We recognize that it takes considerable time and effort to conduct and code the FAST, and that it may not be feasibly implemented in many clinical settings, such as in primary care, family medicine, pediatric practices, or where case volume is high. The procedure may be more feasible as part of psychological evaluations, particularly those based in universities or medical schools. Yet there are some very important reasons to consider including the FAST in the ACU. First, one of the ACU goals is to promote self-regulatory skills that include self-awareness and self-sufficiency. Second, the FAST provides unique insights into family interaction patterns, especially the opportunity to compare family members' perceptions of interactions and management practices with directly observed interpersonal behavior. A third

TABLE 2.5. Family Assessment Task (FAST)

Part 1: For two parents or caregivers (skip if not applicable).

1. *Parenting discussion.* Discuss what you are currently trying to teach and how much you agree or disagree on these things.

Part 2: For parent(s) and target child.

1. *Encouraging growth.* In this interaction the therapist presents the area of growth to the parents that had been identified during the GTKY session.
2. *Monitoring and listening.* The adolescent describes a time when he or she spent 60 minutes or longer alone with peers without adult supervision. Adults listen, then ask questions and comment. This task is designed to have turn taking, with the adolescent speaking first, followed by comments and questioning by the parent.
3. *Family conflict.* Talk about a disagreement in the past month. This task is designed to be interactive, with the parent and adolescent contributing when they see fit.

Five-minute break (optional, decided by family)

Part 3: For the whole family.

1. *Problem solving.* Remind family of a problem discussed during the GTKY session. The family should talk about the problem and come up with at least one solution. This task should be interactive with family members contributing as they see fit.
2. *Substance use.* Parents talk about their beliefs about using tobacco, then alcohol, then marijuana and other drugs. They also talk about their specific drug-related expectations for the adolescent. Then siblings add their point of view. *This task is not appropriate for young children, so children younger than an adolescent should not be in the room for this task.* This is designed to have turn taking, with each family member stating his or her perspective starting with the parents, then the target child, then the sibling(s).
3. *Planning an activity.* Make detailed plans for a fun family activity. This task should be interactive with family members contributing as they see fit.
4. *Positive recognition.* Talk about what they like about the family and each other. This task should be interactive with family members contributing as they see fit.
5. *Debriefing.* The therapist asks two questions and gives the family time to answer them. This is the only task when the therapist is in the room. *During this task, and when administering all other family assessment tasks, the therapist should project neutral affect and body language, answer questions for clarification purposes only, and refrain from making any suggestions or evaluative statements.*

reason to use the FAST is to avoid false negatives in detection of families that need to improve family management skills. Due to factors such as denial, lack of information, and an effort to present the family in an overly positive light, self-report data in interviews and questionnaires can portray families as functioning very well, when actually they are struggling. In activities such as the FAST, it is much more difficult for a family in distress to "fake good" and very unlikely that a nondistressed family will "fake bad." A fourth reason to use FAST is to allow families an opportunity for self-reflection and self-discovery.

Consistent with these points, administration of the FAST should be as nondirective as possible. Before each task, when the therapist is reading the directions and soliciting questions about procedural issues, family members are likely to comment or offer opinions. When giving instructions and answering questions, the therapist should focus conversation on the procedural issues and avoid making any interpretive comments on the process or content revealed during the task. Nondirective techniques, such as restating, are acceptable. More directive techniques, such as reframing, should be avoided. Highly directive techniques, such as normalization, should be strenuously avoided. In general, the therapist should focus on providing instructions to the family for completing the task, with as little additional interaction as possible.

Of note, the ACU described in this section is for adolescents. Dishion and colleagues (Shaw, Dishion, Supplee, Gardner, & Arnds, 2006) have recently developed FAST procedures for preschool children and their mothers. No set protocol has been developed for elementary school–age students, but this is mostly relevant to the FAST. The GTKY and feedback sessions of the ACU should not vary much with age.

Pending development of a FAST specifically for elementary school–age children, the procedures described for adolescents will probably work for most children age 8 and older, as long as some developmentally appropriate considerations are implemented (e.g., eliminating the talk on substance use). For younger children (i.e., below age 8), the procedures described in Shaw and colleagues should be appropriate.

Feedback

The ACU includes 1 or 2 hours of therapist time used to gather collateral information, most notably teacher ratings and preparation for feedback. Preparation for feedback includes scoring questionnaires, evaluating the FAST, and the graphing this information. The therapist should bring these graphs, completed questionnaires, and markers (red, yellow, and green) to use on the Feedback from Family Checkup form (Appendix 2.3) to the feedback session. Providing feedback and discussing a menu for change are the primary considerations of the feedback meeting. The goal of this session is to put families in an active role, such that they take responsibility for change, without being blamed or left feeling helpless. Accordingly, the entire ACU should be presented as a collaborative effort, such that caregivers are the experts on their family and the therapist has a novel perspective that can be used to refresh caregivers' best efforts to address the needs of their children.

The feedback session begins with the caregivers providing a self-assessment. Then four areas of functioning are reviewed: (1) child strengths and need for improvement, (2) caregiver/family strengths and need for improvement, (3) contextual protective/risk factors, and (4) the menu of available resources. During the feedback discussion, the therapist must be sincere, credible, and highlight two or three areas of strength for every problem area. At the end of the feedback meeting, caregivers should commit to pursuing one or more items on the menu. The menu choices should match stages of readiness for change for each parent. For example, one caregiver might be at a precontemplative stage and require experiences that develop a realistic awareness of a problem, or awareness of their influence on the problem. The other caregiver might be in the action stage, so the appropriate recommendation would be to engage in a change process, such as

learning parenting skills and developing a new behavioral management system for the children.

The feedback session may be divided into four phases. The first phase, *self-assessment*, is an opportunity for parents to discuss their own self-assessment, based on their experiences in the assessment process. Parents' discussion of their self-assessment is an opportunity for the therapist to (1) appreciate the parents' approach to behavior change, (2) assess their level of insight, (3) learn more about the dynamics of the family, and (4) discover issues not covered in the assessment. In the second phase, *clarification and support*, the therapist uses empathic, reflective listening techniques to establish a clear understanding of the self-assessment. The third phase focuses on *summarizing feedback* to families, based on the information they have provided. During this phase, the therapist discusses the graphs prepared for the feedback session with the caregivers, soliciting reactions and opinions.

The feedback phases are repeated multiple times during the feedback process as each major issue is considered. We want to emphasize some general guiding principles that need to be addressed in the feedback process. The mnemonic FRAMES highlights six elements frequently present in effective, empirically supported brief interventions (Miller, 1998): Feedback on family status, emphasis on family Responsibility for change, Advice about change options listed on the menu, collaborative listing of change options or a Menu by which change might be achieved, an Empathic counseling style, and messages supporting Self-efficacy for change. Excellent considerations of the FRAMES approach are presented elsewhere, and we encourage the reader to review these resources, especially Miller and Rollnick (2002).

Symptoms of ADHD

First, the parents are asked to describe their understanding of ADHD and whether that diagnosis fits their child. Misunderstandings about ADHD need to be addressed as part of clarification and support from the therapist. Next, the caregivers are shown graphs summarizing the rating scales. We recommend using the BASC-2 ratings of inattention and hyperactivity for all respondents (i.e., parent, child, and teacher), all on one graph. There should be a similar graph for parent and teacher ratings on the DBD, but this can often be held in reserve and used primarily by the therapist to decide on the formal diagnosis of ADHD. Once the parents seem to understand the metric of the graph, the therapist should review the information portrayed on the graph with each family. Summarizing feedback and getting consensus from the parent(s) can lead directly into goal development.

After selecting the goal, the therapist and family members can "brainstorm" a list of intervention options. The role of the therapist is first to model brainstorming to generate options, then, in the final stages of the feedback session, to promote discussion of the pros and cons of each option. Options for menu items might include reading about an issue, getting a self-help book, consulting with a teacher, meeting with the school's intervention team, or receiving a referral for family or marital therapy. In building a viable menu, therapist knowledge of school and community resources is critical.

Feedback about Comorbid Conditions

More often than not, children diagnosed with ADHD also meet criteria for other mental health disorders that may affect parenting and response to treatment. These disorders are reviewed with the parent(s) and their implications are discussed. The therapist should follow the same four phases of feedback as with ADHD symptoms, including (1) caregivers' assessment, (2) clarification and support, (3) summarization of feedback, and (4) goal setting and methods for change.

Adult Functioning and Relationship Quality

The functioning of adult caregivers is crucially important to understand, because intervention for ADHD is usually heavily dependent on the adult caregiver. Therefore, is it important to provide feedback about how contextual factors in the form of adult mental illness, substance abuse, or marital problems might influence the child's behavior and efforts to change it. Every effort should be made to avoid having the parent feel blamed for the problems related to ADHD. Rather, it should be emphasized that the caregiver is an important part of the solution, and that it is legitimate to attend to the needs of the caregiver, as well as those of the child with ADHD.

The four-phase process of feedback regarding caregiver psychopatholology or substance use centers on the ADHD and depression rating scales and AUDIT. However, the GTKY should also address these and other psychopathology or substance abuse issues, especially during completion of the genogram. Other screening measures (e.g., anxiety scales) or semistructured interviews (e.g., for anxiety disorders) may be pursued as needed.

When conflict between caregivers is evident, or when the status of the relationship is unclear, there are often divergent viewpoints. It is usually surprising that partners disagree about the quality of their marriage, or at least the quality of certain aspects of the relationship. Ignoring a marital problem and the status of the parents' relationship may be tantamount to overlooking the source of family difficulty and may have long-term negative effects on a young child's positive adjustment. To prepare for this discussion, the therapist should score and summarize the DAS completed by both parents. Also, for parenting and other relationships, such as mother–grandmother, data from the GTKY session and the first FAST session interaction are very important.

It is important to frame the marital issues as contextual factors, but still focus parents' attention on their common goal of helping the child. Also, it is helpful to point out to parents that differences of opinion about parenting may occur for many reasons, including differences in relationships between families of origin, their own experience and education as parents, and the nature of their typical interactions with the child, which may be very different for fathers and mothers, or for custodial and noncustodial parents.

Parent–Child Interactions

Following the discussion of the marriage, it should seem logical to talk about the relationship between the parents and the child. After clarification and support, information on this issue can be taken from the CIRS, the BASC-2, and the FAST. With regard to the FAST, some of the interactions might be briefly reviewed to refresh caregivers' recall of the task and how it went. Because the CIRS and FAST scales have separate metrics, they need to be presented separately, with explanations of their metrics. After reviewing the parent–child relationships and parenting practices, the therapist should help caregivers identify goals, and methods for achieving these goals. Some of these goals should ideally be positive and support current activities.

Adjustment at School

After discussing parent management skills, it is helpful to transition into a discussion of relationships with teachers. This allows the therapist to draw parallels to other adults, thus generalizing findings and, in some cases, helping parents feel less blamed or defensive about their problematic dealings with their child. This also allows for reframes that highlight the influence of specific contexts or structures that positively influence the behavior of the child with ADHD. Data for discussing relationships with teachers can be taken from the appropriate CIRS and Teacher Report Form of the BASC-2.

Peer Relations

Peer functioning is a good concluding topic, because it almost always includes areas of strengths, as well as potential weaknesses. A variety of available multi-informant assessment data supports this discussion, including relevant BASC-2 scores (parent, child, and teachers), and the impairment rating scale (parent and teachers). In addition to talking about peers in general, it may be important to discuss best friends in terms of the depth and stability of the relationship.

Feedback with the Child or Adolescent

Following the feedback session with the caregivers, it is helpful to have a feedback session with the child, and especially with an adolescent. If the caregivers direct the feedback to the child, then this is an opportunity to reinforce caregivers' responsibility and knowledge in dealing with their child. The feedback to the child or adolescent should be an abbreviated version of the feedback given to the parents. Thus, it should have four phases: (1) self-assessment, (2) support and clarification, (3) feedback, and (4) selection of goals and change options. Parents who decide to give feedback themselves should be coached on these steps. In conjoint sessions, the therapist should allow the parents to give most of the feedback.

Finally, the child or adolescent should review the problems, goals, and options developed by the parents. Using his or her own feedback sheet, the child or adolescent should be allowed to add additional problems, state personal goals, and suggest his or her own solutions. Then, the therapist should discuss how the adolescent will communicate his or her own goals and menu of change options to the parents. The child or adolescent can rehearse this presentation with the therapist, self-evaluate the presentation, and receive feedback from the therapist regarding the rehearsal of the conversation with parents. Then, the therapist can support the child or adolescent by facilitating the presentation of what was rehearsed.

ADDITIONAL COMMENTS ON ASSESSMENT METHODS

In many cases, intelligence and achievement testing may already have been conducted by the child's public school. This information is important for review and when there are concerns about low IQ or significant learning disabilities. A psychoeducational evaluation may be one of the recommendations on the ACU menu. Brief screening tests are recommended as a first pass evaluation of the child. When evidence on the screen suggests deficiencies in the child's intelligence or achievement, more thorough testing may be conducted for these domains or the child may be referred to a professional more expert in such evaluations.

A more thorough discussion of useful psychological tests for ADHD may be found in Gordon, Barkley, and Lovett (2006). Although some of these methods may be valid, they are not practical for most applied settings, or they do not have demonstrated incremental or clinical utility in the context of the measures we do recommend (i.e., parent and teacher ratings, observation of brief structured family interactions, a structured interview with parents and, briefly, with children or adolescents, IQ screening and achievement testing, if not done previously, and a physical examination).

We do not recommend the routine use of CPTs as part of the standard evaluation for ADHD despite their popularity. Several of the CPTs available commercially to clinicians have norms that permit the clinical interpretation of their scores: the Conners Continuous Performance Test (Conners, 1995), the Gordon Diagnostic System (Gordon, 1983), and the Test of Variables of Attention (Greenberg & Kindschi, 1996), among others. CPTs are among the most reliable measures that discriminate between groups of individuals with ADHD and the general population (Barkley, 1991; Barkley, Grodzinsky, & DuPaul, 1992; Corkum & Siegel, 1993); are sensitive to stimulant drug effects (Barkley, 1997c; Rapport & Kelly, 1993); and correlate significantly with teacher ratings of inattention and hyperactivity, as well as other laboratory measures of attention and impulse control. However, the magnitude of these associations is low to moderate (typically .25–.35), suggesting limited ecological and construct validity for such instruments (Barkley, 1991). It is noteworthy that although these measures may be sensitive to the effects of stimulant medication on groups of children with ADHD, they are less sensitive to low doses of medication than are parent and teacher ratings (Barkley, Fischer, Newby, & Breen, 1988; Barkley, McMurray, Edelbrock, & Robbins, 1989). This means that using a CPT to titrate medication may result in overmedication, thus exposing children to greater risk for negative side effects. Furthermore, children with ADHD find this task to be very aversive. Given these results, it is not appropriate to use CPT as the basis for determining medication response. Also, because the incremental validity of the CPT for diagnostic purposes is questionable, we do not recommend use of the CPT in the routine assessment of ADHD.

A new addition to this chapter is the emphasis on evaluating the effectiveness of interventions, such that assessment becomes an ongoing process. This approach, often called response to intervention (RTI), is becoming the new standard for evaluating learning disabilities (Fuchs & Fuchs, 1998; Speece & Hines, Chapter 13, this volume). Although this type of assessment may be beyond the scope of practice for most clinicians, it is important for those who work with children with learning problems to be familiar with this growing movement in academic assessment. RTI is becoming common practice for assessing students who fall behind academically. Indeed, RTI is starting to replace traditional cognitive assessments (i.e., intelligence and achievement testing) for diagnosing learning disabilities. For a detailed description of RTI, the reader is referred to Speece and Hines, Chapter 13, this volume.

MENU OF TREATMENT OPTIONS

When a child is diagnosed with ADHD there is by definition at least one area of significantly impaired functioning related to ADHD. A well-conducted evaluation for ADHD provides a clear understanding of the functional impairment(s) and a sound basis for initiating treatment, including which problems to prioritize. Because response to treatment for ADHD is highly idiosyncratic (Pelham & Milich, 1991), competent intervention includes monitoring of the target problems and other relevant areas of functioning. Thus, each intervention needs to evaluate using appropriate case study methodology (Kazdin, 1990). For present purposes, we describe a menu of treatment options. Given the focus of this chapter on evaluation, this review of treatment is very succinct. More detailed reviews of our treatment may be found in Barkley (2006) and Smith and colleagues (2006).

Treatments abound for children with ADHD, but only a few have demonstrated efficacy (Kazdin, 1990; Pelham et al., 1998). Treatment recommendations may range from just parent counseling about the disorder in the case of children with few or no impairments, to residential treatment for children with ADHD and severe, chronic, or even dangerous forms of conduct problems or depression. Between these extremes, treatment recommendations may focus on reducing the primary ADHD symptoms through medication or classroom behavioral interventions; improving the oppositional behavior of children with ADHD through parent training in effective child management procedures; or addressing the conflicts of teenagers with ADHD and their parents through a behavioral problem-solving approach to family therapy. Many children with ADHD have peer relationship problems that may benefit from individual or group social skills training, provided that such training is implemented within the school or neighborhood settings in which such skills should be used, and that aggressive and nonaggressive children are not mixed into such groups (due to the side effect of deviancy training).

In most cases, evaluation will reveal the need for multiple interventions for a child and, in some cases, for other family members, to address fully the functional problems found during the evaluation. Thus, clinicians should approach intervention from the standpoint of a matrix of needs for intervention and prevention. When multimodal treatments are selected, they should be evidence-based and designed to complement each other by creating a synergy of effectiveness, or by targeting unique aspects of the disorder. Simply throwing myriad treatments at a problem has not been particularly effective. Moreover, it might not always be best to try to change everything at once, or to tackle the most difficult problem first.

When selecting treatment options, it is important to consider that using medication first might potentially lower parent motivation to get involved in behavioral interventions, thus leaving some important gaps in the matrix of needed interventions (Adelman & Taylor, 1998). In other cases, medication alone may be all that is required for relatively uncomplicated cases of ADHD, in which comorbidity is not an issue. Similarly, it is important to select treatment options that result in success and enhanced parent motivation and parenting efficacy (Sanders, 2000). Trying to deal with a complicated problem such as misbehavior in the classroom leaves parents dependent on factors beyond their control, which may be counterproductive. Therefore, if the goal is to engage parents productively in the change process, working on behavior that occurs at home may be the best way to start.

Medications

Two types of medications are FDA approved for use by children and adolescents with ADHD: stimulants (methylphenidate, amphetamines) and the nonstimulant, atomoxetine (Strattera). There is overwhelming evidence for the efficacy of these medications in the treatment of children and adolescents with ADHD (Barkley & Murphy, 2006; Pelham et al., 1998; Smith et al., 2000, 2006). However, these medications are neither necessary nor sufficient to treat ADHD because (1) at least 10–25% of children with ADHD do not benefit from treatment with stimulant medication (Smith et al., 2006), and (2) even among positive drug responders, stimulant drugs are not able to address all of the myriad difficulties of children and adolescents with ADHD. Nevertheless, medication can be an indispensable part of a total treatment program and often its most effective component.

The primary effects of the ADHD medications are improved attention span, decreased impulsivity, diminished task-irrelevant activity (especially in structured situations), and generally decreased disruptive behavior in social situations (see chapters by Conner for stimulants and Spencer for nonstimulants in the text by Barkley, 2005). Secondary effects of these changes appear to include increased compliance to commands and instructions; increased productivity on academic assignments; improved peer interactions and increased peer acceptance; and decreased parent and teacher reprimands, supervision, and punishment.

Although medication may appear to be equally effective compared to combined treatment (i.e., medication and intensive psychosocial interventions) in terms of reducing ADHD symptoms, the effects of combined treatment appear to be better than those for medicine alone in treating ancillary problems associated with ADHD (Smith et al., 2006). Thus, it is important for those concerned with children or adolescents with ADHD to be familiar with nonpharmacological treatments for ADHD. Of note, these may form a synergy with medication or treat problems not addressed by medication.

Parent Training in Contingency Management

The decision to employ parent training procedures should be based on the information obtained in the initial evaluation with respect to the child's primary symptoms of ADHD, as well as the level of noncompliant, oppositional, or defiant behaviors at home. Other key considerations are the parents' educational and intellectual level, the degree of motivation for training, and the absence of complicating factors, such as parental depression, stress, personal psychopathology, or sufficient marital discord to interfere with training.

There are several excellent parent training programs, and age of the child is a major factor in the choice of approach. Barkley (1997d) has developed a program specifically for parents of children ages 2 to 11 with ADHD. It includes sessions to provide information to families about ADHD; to train them in increasing attention and praise; to establish home token reinforcement systems; to implement time-out, response cost, and other mild disciplinary tactics; and to teach them to deal with misbehavior in public places.

Robin and Foster (1989; Robin, 1990) have designed a useful approach to resolving parent–adolescent conflicts in families with teenagers with ADHD that emphasizes negotiating with adolescents. The approach is often combined with advice to parents on contingency management methods appropriate to this age group (point systems, behavioral contracts, etc.; see also Barkley, Edwards, & Robin, 1999; Sanders & Ralph, 2001). Patterson and Forgatch (1987) designed a similar approach for addressing parent–teen conflicts. Another promising approach is the Triple P–Positive Parenting Program (Triple-P) recently developed by Sanders (1999).

Classroom Interventions

Given that the majority of children and adolescents with ADHD exhibit behavior problems in school, classroom interventions are likely to be employed. These may include training teachers in contingency management methods (see Pfiffner, Barkley, & DuPaul, 2006). Token reinforcement programs, home-based evaluation/reinforcement programs, increased attention to child compliance by teachers, in-class time-out procedures, and behavioral contracts may all be employed in the reduction of ADHD behaviors in the classroom. In extreme cases, some children or adolescents may need the intensive structure of special classrooms, afterschool programs, or therapeutic schools to succeed.

The choice and intensity of interventions should be based on a number of findings from the evaluation, including the level of the child's school behavior and performance problems, the degree of parent and teacher commitment to complying with these methods, the extent of previous school interventions, the degree to which stimulant medication may address these difficulties, and the eligibility of the child for special educational programs under federal and state statutes. Much evidence exists for the effectiveness of behavior modification techniques in reducing classroom behavior problems and improving the productivity of children with ADHD (DuPaul & Stoner, 2003). Less clear, however, is the extent to which these methods may normalize the behavior of children with ADHD, and the extent to which treatment gains persist once the behavioral techniques are withdrawn or the children move on to another grade, classroom, or teacher. Some evidence suggests that behavior, although improved, is not brought into the normal range of non-ADHD peers (Abikoff & Gittelman, 1984).

Summary of Treatments

This review has focused on the empirically supported treatments identified by numerous, high-profile reviews and treatment guidelines. some promising treatments mentioned in previous editions, such as self-control training, have not been well supported in recent research. Some new treatments that have emerged, such a neurofeedback, have not yet established a credible database. Other putative treatments for ADHD, such as dietary restriction of sugar or food additives, have not lived up to the expectations of anecdotes and do not appear to be effective for treating the typical child with ADHD (Pelham et al., 1998; Smith et al., 2006). Moreover, there is some risk of making ADHD-related problems worse, due to stigma and parent–child conflict. Thus, we strongly recommend that parents, teachers, and clinicians focus on mainstream treatments for ADHD that include parent training, classroom contingency management, and stimulant medication. Indeed, this combination of treatments may be the best (Smith et al., 2006).

EVALUATING INDIVIDUAL RESPONSES TO INTERVENTION

As with medication, children's responses to parenting interventions and classroom contingencies may be highly variable. The previously mentioned studies that provide empirical support for medication, parent training, and classroom management indicate that individuals with ADHD, as a group, tend to respond positively to these interventions. However, the intervention in many cases needs to be individualized, and some children may not respond (e.g., estimates of nonresponse to stimulant medication are usually around 30%). Therefore, treatment for ADHD must be evaluated on a case-by-case basis using individual case study methods. This is not as difficult as it may sound, because we are recommending (1) collection of data on a frequent basis, either daily or weekly, and (2) summarization of data with widely available graphing procedures. Some more detailed recommendations based on concepts previously introduced in this chapter are given below.

Individual Variability

Due to the high variability of children and adolescents with ADHD, individualized case studies may require long baselines and the use of moving averages or trend lines to summarize highly variable behavior. This issue is illustrated in Figure 2.1, which depicts hypothetical data from a child participating in a reversal study. In this example, the target behavior is interrupting a teacher, and the intervention is selective attention (i.e., ignoring inappropriate interruptions and attending to appropriate efforts to gain attention). The reversal design in this example, also known as an ABAB study, is appropriate for evaluating many behavioral or pharmacological interventions for ADHD.

What we intend to make clear in Figure 2.1 is that multiple data points are needed for each phase of individualized evaluation of response to treatment. This is contrasted with the pre- and posttest evaluations often conducted to evaluate response to treatment. To illustrate our point, one of the pairs of points selected in Figure 2.1 shows a favorable response; another

pair shows no response; and still another pair of points shows an adverse response. On the other hand, the trend lines in the data show a more coherent and dependable evaluation of response to treatment, a favorable response in this case.

Choice of Measures

A key consideration in repeatedly collecting data is to find measures that are sensitive to change, valid, and feasible to administer frequently. Rather than relying on self-report or laboratory measures, the evaluation must use collateral reports or objective measures of performance in the target setting. A collateral report usually comprises parent or teacher ratings on standardized measures. Objective measures may include direct observation of frequencies of behavior, often provided by parents, teachers, or schools. Institutional records, such daily homework completion, weekly grades, or disciplinary reports, can be good measures.

When measuring problems related to ADHD, particularly disruptive behaviors, the CGI has proven to be a sensitive and valid measure of change (Conners, 1997). This 10-item scale is easy to complete and may be administered on a daily or weekly basis. Another feasi-

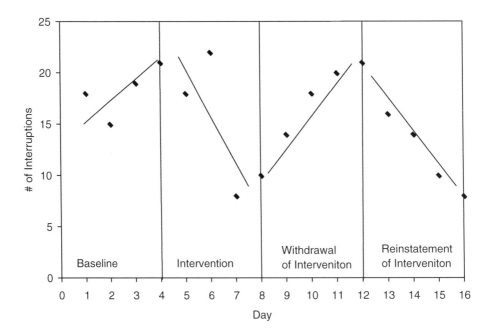

FIGURE 2.1. Number of interruptions per day.

ble and informative brief measure is behavioral tracking, such as frequency counts or duration records (also see one of the Triple P practitioner's manuals for an excellent description of several tracking procedures; e.g., Sanders & Ralph, 2001).

A detailed description of a protocol to assess response to treatment is provided in Smith and colleagues (2006). We should remind the reader that there need to be multiple repetitions of measurement in each treatment condition (see Figure 2.1). Also, double-blinds, or at least blinded raters, are helpful for controlling expectancy effects. Other methodological considerations, such as holding all but one variable as constant as possible, should allow for more confidence in the case study. Too often, multiple variables are changed at once (e.g., changing the dose of one medication while adding another), thus creating confusion about which variable produced the change. Although a "shotgun" approach of multiple changes at once may sometimes result in a quicker response, the resulting uncertainty about which intervention worked can hamper future management of ADHD.

LEGAL AND ETHICAL ISSUES

Several of the various legal and ethical issues involved in the general practice of providing mental health services to children may be more likely than usual to occur in the evaluation of children with ADHD. The first of these, the issue of custody or guardianship of a child who may have ADHD, pertains to who can request an evaluation of the child. Children with ADHD are more likely than those without the disorder to come from families in which the parents have separated or divorced, or in which significant marital discord may exist between the biological parents (DeGarmo, Patterson, & Forgatch, 2004; Sanders & McFarland, 2000; Sugawara et al., 2002). As a result, clinicians must take care at the point of first contact with such a family to determine who has legal custody of the child and, particularly, who has the right to request mental health services on behalf of the minor.

One must also determine in cases of joint custody (an increasingly common status in divorce/custody situations) whether the nonresident parent has the right to dispute the referral for the evaluation, consent to the evaluation, attend on the day of appointment, and/or have access to the final report. This right to review or dispute mental health services may also extend to the provision of treatment to the child with ADHD. Failing to attend to these issues before the evaluation can lead to great contentiousness, frustration, and even legal action among the parties to the evaluation, much or all of which could have been avoided had greater care been taken to resolve these issues beforehand.

A second issue that commonly arises in evaluations of children but may be more likely in cases involving ADHD is a clinician's duty to report to state agencies any suspicion of physical or sexual abuse, or neglect of a child that arises or is reported during an evaluation. *Before* starting formal evaluation procedures, clinicians should routinely forewarn parents of this duty to report as it applies in a particular state. In view of the greater stress that children with ADHD appear to cause for their parents, as well as the greater psychological distress their parents are likely to report, the risk for abuse of children with ADHD may be higher than average. The greater likelihood of parental ADHD or other psychiatric disorders may further contribute to this risk, resulting in a greater likelihood that evaluations of children with ADHD may involve suspicions of abuse. Understanding this legal duty as it applies in a given state or region, and taking care to exercise it properly yet with sensitivity to the larger clinical issues likely to be involved, are the responsibilities of any clinician involved in providing mental health services to children.

A third legal consideration is federal and state laws related to providing for children with disabilities. Increasingly over the past two decades, children with ADHD have gained access to government entitlements that make it necessary for clinicians to be well informed about these legal issues if they are to advise properly and correctly the parents and school staff involved in each case. For instance, children with ADHD are now entitled to formal special educational services in the United States under the "Other Health Impaired" category of the Individuals with Disabilities in Education Act, if their ADHD is sufficiently serious to interfere significantly with their academic performance. Less commonly understood is that such children also have legal protections and entitlements under Section 504 of the Rehabilitation Act of 1973, as it applies to the provision of an appropriate education to disabled children. Should children have sufficiently severe ADHD and reside in low-income families, they may also be eligible for financial assistance under the Social Security Act. Space precludes a more complete explication of these legal entitlements here; the reader is referred to the excellent texts by DuPaul and Stoner (2003) and Latham and Latham (1992) for fuller accounts of these matters. Suffice it to say here that clinicians working with children with ADHD need to familiarize themselves with these various rights and entitlements if they are to be effective advocates for the children they serve.

A final legal issue related to children with ADHD pertains to their legal accountability for their own actions in view of the argument made earlier that ADHD is a developmental disorder of self-control. Should children with ADHD be held legally responsible for the damage they may cause to property, the injury they may inflict on others, or the crimes they may commit? In short, is ADHD an excuse to behave irresponsibly, without being held accountable for the consequences of one's actions? The answer is unclear, and issues related to the legal status of an offender and competence to engage in legal proceedings may also be relevant. It has been the opinion of Barkley that ADHD provides an explanation for why certain impulsive acts may have been committed, but it does not constitute sufficient disturbance of mental faculties to serve as an excuse from legal accountability (e.g., as might occur under the insanity defense). Nor should it be permitted to serve as an extenuating factor in the determination of guilt or the sentencing of an individual involved in criminal activities, particularly violent crimes. This opinion is predicated on the fact that the vast majority of children with ADHD do not become involved in violent crimes as they grow up. Moreover, studies attempting to predict criminal conduct within samples of children with ADHD followed to adulthood have either not been able to find adequate predictors of such outcomes or have found them to be so weak as to account for a paltry amount of variance in such outcomes. Variables that may make a significant contribution to the prediction of criminal or delinquent behavior much more often involve parental and family dysfunction, as well as social disadvantage; they involve ADHD symptoms much less often, if at all. Until this matter receives

greater legal scrutiny, it seems wise to view ADHD as one of several explanations for impulsive conduct, but not as a direct, primary, or immediate cause of criminal conduct for which the individual should not be held accountable.

CONCLUSION

Our purpose in this current chapter has been to present a feasible and practical method for assessing ADHD. We have described several approaches depending on time and resources available to the clinician. The first is a minimally acceptable assessment for ADHD, which is appropriate when only a diagnosis is needed or when time is of the essence. The second approach, the ACU, is a more thorough method of assessment that engages caregivers in the ADHD treatment process. The third approach is evaluating response to treatment for ADHD. The resources and expertise to conduct such evaluations should be within the grasp of most mental heath professionals who are qualified to work with children.

The heterogeneous nature of ADHD and numerous additional problems that coexist with both types of ADHD make the assessment of the disorders a complex and challenging affair. The minimally acceptable assessment of ADHD in children includes (1) parent ratings of ADHD symptoms, other psychiatric disorders, and related impairment; (2) teacher ratings of ADHD symptoms and functioning at school; (3) a semistructured interview with a parent to ascertain influences on behavior, parental skills and knowledge, and the developmental history of ADHD-related impairment, comorbid conditions, and various treatments or efforts to change behavior; and (4) an examination by a physician to rule out plausible physical causes for putative ADHD symptoms (Barkley, 2005).

We should emphasize that even if the criteria for a minimally acceptable assessment for ADHD are met, one office visit and a discussion are hardly likely to change behavioral problems related to ADHD. Therefore, we recommend the ACU. The key consideration of the ACU is to provide an assessment experience that is imbued with motivational interviewing and to engage parents in the intervention process. This type of evaluation, coupled with appropriate ongoing evaluation of response to intervention, is the most promising approach to achieve therapeutic change related to ADHD. However, even when assessment and treatment are successful, it is important to note that the persistent nature of ADHD means that periodic assessment and intervention will be needed throughout the lifespan of individuals with the disorder.

REFERENCES

Abikoff, H., & Gittelman, R. (1984). Does behavior therapy normalize the classroom behavior of hyperactive children? *Archives of General Psychiatry*, *41*(5), 449–454.

Abikoff, A., McGough, J., Vitello, B., McCracken, J., Davies, M., Walkup, J., et al. (2005). Sequential pharmacotherapy for children with comorbid attention-deficit/hyperactivity and anxiety disorders. *Journal of the American Academy of Child and Adolescent Psychiatry*, *44*, 418–427.

Achenbach, T. M. (1991). *Manual for the Child Behavior Checklist/4–18 and 1991 profile*. Burlington: University of Vermont, Department of Psychiatry.

Achenbach, T. M. (2001). *Child Behavior Checklist—Cross-Informant Version*. (Available from Thomas Achenbach, PhD, Child and Adolescent Psychiatry, Department of Psychiatry, University of Vermont, 5 South Prospect Street, Burlington, VT 05401.)

Achenbach, T., McConaughy, S., & Howell, C. (1987). Child/adolescent behavioral and emotional problems: Implications of cross-informant correlations for situational specificity. *Psychological Bulletin*, *101*, 213–232.

Achenbach, T. M., & Rescorla, L. A. (2001). *Manual for the ASEBA school-age forms and profiles*. Burlington: University of Vermont, Research Center for Children, Youth, and Families.

Adams, G. L. (1984). *Normative Adaptive Behavior Checklist*. San Antonio, TX: Psychological Corporation.

Adelman, H. S., & Taylor, L. (1998). Reframing mental health in schools and expanding school reform. *Educational Psychology*, *33*, 135–153.

American Psychiatric Association (APA). (1968). *Diagnostic and statistical manual of mental disorders* (2nd ed.). Washington, DC: Author.

American Psychiatric Association (APA). (1980). *Diagnostic and statistical manual of mental disorders* (3rd ed.). New York: Author.

American Psychiatric Association (APA). (1987). *Diagnostic and statistical manual of mental disorders* (3rd ed., rev.). Washington, DC: Author.

American Psychiatric Association (APA). (1994). *Diagnostic and statistical manual of mental disorders* (4th ed.). Washington, DC: Author.

American Psychiatric Association (APA). (2000). *Diagnostic and statistical manual of mental disorders* (4th ed., text rev.). Washington, DC: Author.

Anastopoulos, A. D., Guevremont, D. C., Shelton, T. L., & DuPaul, G. J. (1992). Parenting stress among families of children with attention-deficit hyperactivity disorder. *Journal of Abnormal Child Psychology*, *20*, 503–520.

Anderson, C. A., Hinshaw, S. P., & Simmel, C. (1994). Mother–child interactions in ADHD and comparison boys: Relationships with overt and covert externalizing behavior. *Journal of Abnormal Child Psychology*, *22*(2), 247–265.

Andrews, V. C., Garrison, C. Z., Jackson, K. L., Addy, C. L., & McKeown, R. E. (1993). Mother–adolescent agreement on symptoms and diagnosis of adolescent depression and conduct disorders. *Journal of the American Academy of Child and Adolescent Psychiatry*, *32*, 731–738.

Angold, A., Costello, E. J., & Erkanli, A. (1999). Comorbidity. *Journal of Child Psychology and Psychiatry and Allied Disciplines*, *40*(1), 57–87.

Applegate, B., Lahey, B. B., Hart, E. L., Biederman, J., Hynd, G. W., Barkley, R. A., et al. (1997). Validity of the age-of-onset criterion for ADHD: A report from the DSM-IV field trials. *Journal of the American Academy of Child and Adolescent Psychiatry*, *36*(9), 1211–1221.

Aylward, E. H., Reiss, A. L., Reader, M. J., Singer, H. S., Brown, J. E., & Denckla, M. B. (1996). Basal ganglia volumes in children with attention-deficit hyperactivity disorder. *Journal of Child Neurology*, *11*(2), 112–115.

Bagwell, C. L., Molina, B. S. G., Pelham, W. E., & Hoza, B. (2001). Attention-deficit hyperactivity disorder and problems in peer relations: Predictions from childhood to adolescence. *Journal of the American Academy of Child and Adolescent Psychiatry*, *40*(11), 1285–1292.

Ball, J. D., & Koloian, B. (1995). Sleep patterns among ADHD children. *Clinical Psychology Review*, *15*(7), 681–691.

Bank, L., Patterson, G. R., & Reid, J. B. (1987). Delinquency prevention through training parents in family management. *Behavior Analyst*, *10*(1), 75–82.

Barkley, R. A. (1981). *Hyperactive children: A handbook for diagnosis and treatment*. New York: Guilford Press.

Barkley, R. A. (1988). Attention. In M. Tramontana & S. Hooper (Eds.), *Assessment issues in child neuropsychology* (pp. 145–176). New York: Plenum Press.

Barkley, R. A. (1990). *Attention-deficit hyperactivity disorder: A handbook for diagnosis and treatment*. New York: Guilford Press.

Barkley, R. A. (1991). The ecological validity of laboratory and analogue assessment methods of ADHD symptoms. *Journal of Abnormal Child Psychology*, *19*, 149–178.

Barkley, R. A. (1997a). Advancing age, declining ADHD. *American Journal of Psychiatry*, *154*(9), 1323–1324.

Barkley, R. A. (1997b). Attention-deficit/hyperactivity disorder, self-regulation, and time: Toward a more comprehensive theory. *Journal of Developmental and Behavioral Pediatrics, 18*(4), 271–279.

Barkley, R. A. (1997c). Behavioral inhibition, sustained attention, and executive functions: Constructing a unifying theory of ADHD. *Psychological Bulletin, 121*(1), 65–94.

Barkley, R. A. (1997d). *Defiant children: A clinician's manual for assessment and parent training* (2nd ed.). New York: Guilford Press.

Barkley, R. A. (2004). Driving impairments in teens and adults with attention-deficit/hyperactivity disorder. *Psychiatric Clinics of North America, 27,* 233–260.

Barkley, R. A. (2005). *Attention-deficit hyperactivity disorder: A handbook for diagnosis and treatment* (3rd ed.). New York: Guilford Press.

Barkley, R. A., Anastopoulos, A. D., Guevremont, D. C., & Fletcher, K. E. (1992). Adolescents with attention-deficit hyperactivity disorder: Mother–adolescent interactions, family beliefs and conflicts, and maternal psychopathology. *Journal of Abnormal Child Psychology, 20*(3), 263–288.

Barkley, R. A., & Biederman, J. (1997). Towards a broader definition of the age of onset criterion for attention deficit hyperactivity disorder. *Journal of the American Academy of Child and Adolescent Psychiatry, 36,* 1204–1210.

Barkley, R. A., Cook, E. H., Diamond, A., Zametkin, A., Thapar, A., Teeter, A., et al. (2002). International consensus statement on ADHD—January 2002. *Clinical Child and Family Psychology Review, 5*(2), 89–111.

Barkley, R. A., Copeland, A. P., & Sivage, C. (1980). A self-control classroom for hyperactive children. *Journal of Autism and Developmental Disorders, 10,* 75–89.

Barkley, R. A., Cunningham, C. E., & Karlsson, J. (1983). The speech of hyperactive children and their mothers: Comparison with normal children and stimulant drug effects. *Journal of Learning Disabilities, 16*(2), 105–110.

Barkley, R. A., DuPaul, G. J., & McMurray, M. B. (1990). Comprehensive evaluation of attention-deficit disorder with and without hyperactivity as defined by research criteria. *Journal of Consulting and Clinical Psychology, 58*(6), 775–789.

Barkley, R. A., Edwards, G., Laneri, M., Fletcher, K., & Metevia, L. (2001). Executive functioning, temporal discounting, and sense of time in adolescents with attention deficit hyperactivity disorder (ADHD) and oppositional defiant disorder (ODD). *Journal of Abnormal Child Psychology, 29*(6), 541–556.

Barkley, R. A., Edwards, G. H., & Robin, A. R. (1999). *Defiant teens: A clinician's manual for assessment and family intervention.* New York: Guilford Press.

Barkley, R. A., & Fischer, M. (2005). Suicidality in children with ADHD, grown up. *ADHD Report, 13*(6), 1–6.

Barkley, R. A., Fischer, M., Edelbrock, C. S., & Smallish, L. (1990). The adolescent outcome of hyperactive children diagnosed by research criteria: 1. An 8-year prospective follow-up study. *Journal of the American Academy of Child and Adolescent Psychiatry, 29*(4), 546–557.

Barkley, R. A., Fischer, M., Edelbrock, C., & Smallish, L. (1991). The adolescent outcome of hyperactive children diagnosed by research criteria: 3. Mother–child interactions, family conflicts and maternal psychopathology. *Journal of Child Psychology and Psychiatry and Allied Disciplines, 32*(2), 233–255.

Barkley, R. A., Fischer, M., Newby, R. F., & Breen, M. J. (1988). Development of a multimethod clinical protocol for assessing stimulant drug response in children with attention deficit disorder. *Journal of Clinical Child Psychology, 17*(1), 14–24.

Barkley, R. A., Fischer, M., Smallish, L., & Fletcher, K. (2002). The persistence of attention-deficit/hyperactivity disorder into young adulthood as a function of reporting source and definition of disorder. *Journal of Abnormal Psychology, 111,* 279–289.

Barkley, R. A., Fischer, M., Smallish, L., & Fletcher, K. (2004). Young adult follow-up of hyperactive children: Antisocial activities and drug use. *Journal of Child Psychology and Psychiatry, 45*(2), 195–211.

Barkley, R. A., Fischer, M., Smallish, L., & Fletcher, K. (2006). Young adult outcome of hyperactive children: Adaptive functioning in major life activities. *Journal of the American Academy of Child and Adolescent Psychiatry, 45*(2), 192–202.

Barkley, R. A., Grodzinsky, G., & DuPaul, G. J. (1992). Frontal-lobe functions in attention-deficit disorder with and without hyperactivity: A review and research report. *Journal of Abnormal Child Psychology, 20*(2), 163–188.

Barkley, R. A., Guevremont, D. C., Anastopoulos, A. D., DuPaul, G. J., & Shelton, T. L. (1993). Driving-related risks and outcomes of attention-deficit hyperactivity disorder in adolescents and young adults: A 3-year to 5-year follow-up survey. *Pediatrics, 92*(2), 212–218.

Barkley, R. A., Guevremont, D. C., Anastopoulos, A. D., & Fletcher, K. E. (1992). A comparison of three family therapy programs for treating family conflicts in adolescents with attention-deficit hyperactivity disorder. *Journal of Consulting and Clinical Psychology, 60*(3), 450–462.

Barkley, R. A., Karlsson, J., & Pollard, S. (1985). Effects of age on the mother–child interactions of ADD-H and normal boys. *Journal of Abnormal Child Psychology, 13*(4), 631–637.

Barkley, R. A., Koplowitz, S., Anderson, T., & McMurray, M. B. (1997). Sense of time in children with ADHD: Effects of duration, distraction, and stimulant medication. *Journal of the International Neuropsychological Society, 3,* 359–369.

Barkley, R. A., McMurray, M. B., Edelbrock, C. S., & Robbins, K. (1989). The response of aggressive and nonaggressive ADHD children to two doses of methylphenidate. *Journal of the American Academy of Child and Adolescent Psychiatry, 28*(6), 873–881.

Barkley, R. A., & Murphy, K. R. (2006). *Attention-*

deficit hyperactivity disorder: A clinical workbook. New York: Guilford Press.

Barkley, R. A., Murphy, K. R., & Bush, T. (2001). Time perception and reproduction in young adults with attention-deficit hyperactivity disorder. *Neuropsychology*, 15(3), 351–360.

Barkley, R. A., Murphy, K. R., DuPaul, G. J., & Bush, T. (2002). Driving in young adults with attention deficit hyperactivity disorder: Knowledge, performance, adverse outcomes, and the role of executive functioning. *Journal of the International Neuropsychological Society*, 8(5), 655–672.

Barkley, R. A., Murphy, K. R., & Fischer, M. (in press). *ADHD in adults: Original research and clinical implications.* New York: Guilford Press.

Barkley, R. A., Murphy, K. R., & Kwasnik, D. (1996). Motor vehicle driving competencies and risks in teens and young adults with attention deficit hyperactivity disorder. *Pediatrics*, 98, 1089–1095.

Barkley, R. A., Smith, K., Fischer, M., & Navia, B. (2006). An examination of the behavioral and neuropsychological correlates of three ADHD candidate gene polymorphisms (DRD4 7+, DBH TaqI A2, and DAT1 40bp VNTR) in hyperactive and normal children followed to adulthood. *American Journal of Medical Genetics: B. Neuropsychiatric Genetics*, 141(5), 487–498.

Barkley, R. A., & Ullman, D. G. (1975). Comparison of objective measures of activity and distractibility in hyperactive and non-hyperactive children. *Journal of Abnormal Child Psychology*, 3, 231–244.

Bauermeister, J. J., Bird, H. R., Canino, G., Rubiostipec, M., Bravo, M., & Alegria, M. (1995). Dimensions of attention-deficit hyperactivity disorder: Findings from teacher and parent reports in a community sample. *Journal of Clinical Child Psychology*, 24, 264–271.

Baxter, J., & Rattan, G. (2004). Attention deficit disorder and the internalizing dimension in males, ages 9-0 through 11-11. *International Journal of Neuroscience*, 114(7), 817–832.

Beauchaine, T. P., Katkin, E. S., Strassberg, Z., & Snarr, J. (2001). Disinhibitory psychopathology in male adolescents: Discriminating conduct disorder from attention-deficit/hyperactivity disorder through concurrent assessment of multiple autonomic states. *Journal of Abnormal Psychology*, 110, 610–624.

Beck, A. T., Steer, R. A., & Brown, G. K. (1996). *Manual for the Beck Depression Inventory—II.* San Antonio, TX: Psychological Corporation.

Befera, M. S., & Barkley, R. A. (1985). Hyperactive and normal girls and boys: Mother–child interaction, parent psychiatric status and child psychopathology. *Journal of Child Psychology and Psychiatry and Allied Disciplines*, 26(3), 439–452.

Beiser, M., Dion, R., & Gotowiec, A. (2000). The structure of attention-deficit and hyperactivity symptoms among Native and non-Native elementary school children. *Journal of Abnormal Child Psychology*, 28(5), 425–437.

Berk, L. E., & Potts, M. K. (1991). Development and functional significance of private speech among attention-deficit hyperactivity disordered and normal boys. *Journal of Abnormal Child Psychology*, 19(3), 357–377.

Biederman, J. (2005). Attention-deficit/hyperactivity disorder: A selective overview. *Biological Psychiatry*, 57(11), 1215–1220.

Biederman, J., Faraone, S. V., Mick, E., Wozniak, J., Chen, L., Ouellette, C., et al. (1996). Attention-deficit hyperactivity disorder and juvenile mania: An overlooked comorbidity. *Journal of the American Academy of Child Adolescent Psychiatry*, 35, 997–1008.

Biederman, J., Faraone, S. V., Milberger, S., Curtis, S., Chen, L., Marrs, A., et al. (1996). Predictors of persistence and remission of ADHD into adolescence: Results from a four-year prospective follow-up study. *Journal of the American Academy of Child and Adolescent Psychiatry*, 35(3), 343–351.

Biederman, J., Faraone, S. V., Spencer, T. J., Mick, E., Monuteaux, M. C., & Aleardi, M. (2006). Functional impairments in adults with self-reports of diagnosed ADHD: A controlled study of 1001 adults in the community. *Journal of Clinical Psychiatry*, 67(4), 524–540.

Biederman, J., Kwon, A., Aleardi, M., Chouinard, V. A., Marino, T., Cole, H., et al. (2005). Absence of gender effects on attention deficit hyperactivity disorder: Findings in nonreferred subjects. *American Journal of Psychiatry*, 162(6), 1083–1089.

Biederman, J., Milberger, S., Faraone, S. V., Guite, J., & Warburton, R. (1994). Associations between childhood asthma and ADHD: Issues of psychiatric comorbidity and familiality. *Journal of the American Academy of Child and Adolescent Psychiatry*, 33(6), 842–848.

Bor, W., Sanders, M. R., & Markie-Dadds, C. (2002). The effects of the Triple P–Positive Parenting Program on preschool children with co-occurring disruptive behavior and attentional/hyperactive difficulties. *Journal of Abnormal Child Psychology*, 30(6), 571–587.

Borger, N., & van der Meere, J. (2000). Motor control and state regulation in children with ADHD: A cardiac response study. *Biological Psychology*, 51(2–3), 247–267.

Boyle, M. H., & Lipman, E. L. (2002). Do places matter?: Socioeconomic disadvantage and behavioral problems of children in Canada. *Journal of Consulting and Clinical Psychology*, 70(2), 378–389.

Breen, M. J. (1989). Cognitive and behavioral differences in ADHD boys and girls. *Journal of Child Psychology and Psychiatry and Allied Disciplines*, 30(5), 711–716.

Breen, M. J., & Altepeter, T. S. (1990). Situational variability in boys and girls identified as ADHD. *Journal of Clinical Psychology*, 46(4), 486–490.

Breen, M. J., & Barkley, R. A. (1988). Child psychopathology and parenting stress in girls and boys having attention deficit disorder with hyperactivity. *Journal of Pediatric Psychology, 13*(2), 265–280.

Breslau, N., Brown, G. G., DelDotto, J. E., Kumar, S., Ezhuthachan, S., Andreski, P., et al. (1996). Psychiatric sequelae of low birth weight at 6 years of age. *Journal of Abnormal Child Psychology, 24*(3), 385–400.

Brodeur, D. A., & Pond, M. (2001). The development of selective attention in children with attention deficit hyperactivity disorder. *Journal of Abnormal Child Psychology, 29*(3), 229–239.

Bronowski, J. (1977). *A sense of the future.* Cambridge, MA: MIT Press.

Brown, R. T., & Borden, K. A. (1986). Hyperactivity at adolescence: Some misconceptions and new directions. *Journal of Clinical Child Psychology, 15*(3), 194–209.

Burns, G. L., Boe, B., Walsh, J. A., Sommers-Flanagan, R., & Teegarden, L. A. (2001). A confirmatory factor analysis on the DSM-IV ADHD and ODD symptoms: What is the best model for the organization of these symptoms? *Journal of Abnormal Child Psychology, 29*(4), 339–349.

Bush, K. R., Kivlahan, D. R., Davis, T. M., Dobie, D. J., Sporleder, J. L., Epler, A. J., et al. (2003). The TWEAK is weak for alcohol screening among female veterans affairs outpatients. *Alcoholism, Clinical and Experimental Research, 27*(12), 1971–1978.

Bussing, R., Gary, F. A., Mason, D. M., Leon, C. E., Sinha, K., & Garvan, C. W. (2003). Child temperament, ADHD, and caregiver strain: Exploring relationships in an epidemiological sample. *Journal of the American Academy of Child and Adolescent Psychiatry, 42*(2), 184–192.

Campbell, D. T., & Fiske, D. W. (1959). Convergent and discriminant validation by the multitrait–multimethod matrix. *Psychological Bulletin, 56*(2), 81–105.

Campbell, S. B., Pierce, E. W., March, C. L., Ewing, L. J., & Szumowski, E. K. (1994). Hard-to-manage preschool boys: Symptomatic behavior across contexts and time. *Child Development, 65*(3), 836–851.

Carlson, C. L. (1986). Attention-deficit disorder without hyperactivity: A review of preliminary experimental evidence. *Advances in Clinical Child Psychology, 9*, 153–175.

Casey, B. J., Castellanos, F. X., Giedd, J. N., Marsh, W. L., Hamburger, S. D., Schubert, A. B., et al. (1997). Implication of right frontostriatal circuitry in response inhibition and attention-deficit/hyperactivity disorder. *Journal of the American Academy of Child and Adolescent Psychiatry, 36*(3), 374–383.

Castellanos, F. X., Giedd, J. N., Jeffries, N. O., Sharp, W., Blumenthal, J., Clasen, L., et al. (2001). Longitudinal MRI in attention-deficit-hyperactivity disorder (ADHD): Effects of prior stimulant treatment in cerebellum and total brain. *Biological Psychiatry, 49*(8), 20S.

Castellanos, F. X., Giedd, J. N., Marsh, W. L., Hamburger, S. D., Vaituzis, A. C., Dickstein, D. P., et al. (1996). Quantitative brain magnetic resonance imaging in attention-deficit hyperactivity disorder. *Archives of General Psychiatry, 53*(7), 607–616.

Castellanos, F. X., Lee, P. P., Sharp, W., Jeffries, N. O., Greenstein, D. K., Clasen, L. S., et al. (2002). Developmental trajectories of brain volume abnormalities in children and adolescents with attention-deficit/hyperactivity disorder. *Journal of the American Medical Association, 288*(14), 1740–1748.

Charach, A., Figueroa, M., Chen, S., Ickovicz, A., & Schachar, R. (2006). Stimulant treatment over 5 years: Effects on growth. *Journal of the American Academy of Child and Adolescent Psychiatry, 45*(4), 415–421.

Chess, S. (1960). Diagnosis and treatment of the hyperactive child. *New York State Journal of Medicine, 17*, 371–391.

Chi, T. C., & Hinshaw, S. P. (2002). Mother–child relationships of children with ADHD: The role of maternal depressive symptoms and depression-related distortions. *Journal of Abnormal Child Psychology, 30*(4), 387–400.

Childers, A. T. (1935). Hyper-activity in children having behavior disorders. *American Journal of Orthopsychiatry, 5*, 227–243.

Chronis, A. M., Lahey, B. B., Pelham, W. E., Kipp, H. L., Baumann, B. L., & Lee, S. S. (2003). Psychopathology and substance abuse in parents of young children with attention-deficit/hyperactivity disorder. *Journal of the American Academy of Child and Adolescent Psychiatry, 42*(12), 1424–1432.

Claycomb, C. D., Ryan, J. J., Miller, L. J., & Schnakenberg-Ott, S. D. (2004). Relationships among attention deficit hyperactivity disorder, induced labor, and selected physiological and demographic variables. *Journal of Clinical Psychology, 60*(6), 689–693.

Coatsworth, J. D., Santisteban, D. A., McBride, C. K., & Szapocznik, J. (2001). Brief strategic family therapy versus community control: Engagement, retention, and an exploration of the moderating role of adolescent symptom severity. *Family Process, 40*, 313–332.

Cohen, J. (Ed.). (2003). *Things I have learned (so far).* Washington, DC: American Psychological Association.

Cole, P. M., Zahn-Waxler, C., & Smith, K. D. (1994). Expressive control during a disappointment: Variations related to preschoolers' behavior problems. *Developmental Psychology, 30*(6), 835–846.

Conners, C. K. (1995). *The Conners Continuous Performance Test.* North Tonowanda, NY: Multi-Health Systems.

Conners, C. K. (1997). *Conner's Rating Scales—Revised: User's manual.* Toronto: Multi-Health Systems.

Conners, C. K., Erhardt, D., & Sparrow, E. (2001). *Conners Adult ADHD Rating Scales (CAARS).* Toronto: Multi-Health Systems

Conners, C. K., Sitarenios, G., Parker, J. D. A., & Epstein, J. N. (1998). The revised Conners Parent Rating Scale (CPRS-R): Factor structure, reliability, and criterion validity. *Journal of Abnormal Child Psychology, 26*(4), 257–268.

Cook, E. H., Stein, M. A., & Leventhal, D. L. (1997). Family-based association of attention-deficit/hyperactivity disorder and the dopamine transporter. In K. Blum (Ed.), *Handbook of psychiatric genetics* (pp. 297–310). New York: CRC Press.

Cook, R. L., Chung, T., Kelly, T. M., & Clark, D. B. (2005). Alcohol screening in young persons attending a sexually transmitted disease clinic: Comparison of AUDIT, CRAFT, and CAGE instruments. *Journal of General Internal Medicine, 20*(1), 1–6.

Coolidge, F. L., Thede, L. L., & Young, S. F. (2000). Heritability and the comorbidity of attention deficit hyperactivity disorder with behavioral disorders and executive function deficits: A preliminary investigation. *Developmental Neuropsychology, 17*(3), 273–287.

Copeland, A. P. (1979). Types of private speech produced by hyperactive and non-hyperactive boys. *Journal of Abnormal Child Psychology, 7*(2), 169–177.

Corkum, P. V., & Siegel, L. S. (1993). Is the Continuous Performance Task a valuable research tool for use with children with attention-deficit-hyperactivity disorder? *Journal of Child Psychology and Psychiatry and Allied Disciplines, 34*(7), 1217–1239.

Cortese, S., Lecendreux, M., Mouren, M. C., & Konofal, E. (2006). ADHD and insomnia. *Journal of the American Academy of Child and Adolescent Psychiatry, 45*(4), 384–385.

Costello, E. J., Loeber, R., & Stouthamer-Loeber, M. (1991). Pervasive and situational hyperactivity—confounding effect of informant: A research note. *Journal of Child Psychology and Psychiatry, 32*, 367–376.

Cunningham, C. E., & Boyle, M. H. (2002). Preschoolers at risk for attention-deficit hyperactivity disorder and oppositional defiant disorder: Family, parenting, and behavioral correlates. *Journal of Abnormal Child Psychology, 30*(6), 555–569.

Cunningham, C. E., & Siegel, L. S. (1987). Peer interactions of normal and attention-deficit disordered boys during freeplay, cooperative task, and simulated classroom situations. *Journal of Abnormal Child Psychology, 15*, 247–268.

Dakof, G. A., Quille, T. J., Tejeda, M. J. K., Alberga, L. R., Bandstra, E., & Szapocznik, J. (2003). Enrolling and retaining mothers of substance-exposed infants in drug abuse treatment. *Journal of Consulting and Clinical Psychology, 71*(4), 764–772.

Damasio, A. R. (1995). On some functions of the human prefrontal cortex. *Annals of the New York Academy of Sciences, 769*, 241–251.

Danforth, J. S., Barkley, R. A., & Stokes, T. F. (1991). Observations of parent–child interactions with hyperactive children: Research and clinical implications. *Clinical Psychology Review, 11*(6), 703–727.

Dawson, G., Ashman, S. B., Panagiotides, H., Hessl, D., Self, J., Yamada, E., et al. (2003). Preschool outcomes of children of depressed mothers: Role of maternal behavior, contextual risk, and children's brain activity. *Child Development, 74*(4), 1158–1175.

DeGarmo, D. S., Patterson, G. R., & Forgatch, M. S. (2004). How do outcomes in a specified parent training intervention maintain or wane over time? *Prevention Science, 5*(2), 73–89.

Denckla, M. B. (1994). Measurement of executive function. In G. R. Lyon (Ed.), *Frames of reference for the assessment of learning disabilities: New views on measurement issues* (pp. 117–142). Baltimore: Brookes.

Denckla, M. B., & Rudel, R. G. (1978). Anomalies of motor development in hyperactive boys. *Annals of Neurology, 3*(3), 231–233.

Denson, R., Nanson, J. L., & McWatters, M. A. (1975). Hyperkinesis and maternal smoking. *Canadian Psychiatric Association Journal, 20*(3), 183–187.

Derogatis, L. R. (1995). *Manual for the Symptom Checklist 90—Revised (SCL-90-R)*. Dallas, TX: Psychological Corporation.

Derogatis, L. R., & Cleary, P. A. (1977). Confirmation of dimensional structure of SCL-90: A study in construct validation. *Journal of Clinical Psychology, 33*, 981–989.

Diamond, A. (2000). Close interrelation of motor development and cognitive development and of the cerebellum and prefrontal cortex. *Child Development, 71*, 44–56.

Diamond, A. (2005). Attention-deficit disorder (attention-deficit/hyperactivity disorder without hyperactivity): A neurobiologically and behaviorally distinct disorder from attention-deficit/hyperactivity disorder (with hyperactivity). *Development and Psychopathology, 17*, 807–825.

Dishion, T. J., & Andrews, D. W. (1995). Preventing escalation in problem behaviors with high-risk young adolescents: Immediate and 1-year outcomes. *Journal of Consulting and Clinical Psychology, 63*(4), 538–548.

Dishion, T. J., & Kavanagh, K. (2003). *Intervening in adolescent problem behavior: A family-centered approach*. New York: Guilford Press.

Douglas, V. I. (1980). Higher mental processes in hyperactive children: Implications for training. In R. Knights & D. Bakker (Eds.), *Treatment of hyperactive and learning disordered children: Current research* (pp. 65–92). Baltimore: University Park Press.

Douglas, V. I. (1983). Attention and cognitive problems. In M. Rutter (Ed.), *Developmental neuropsychiatry* (pp. 280–329). New York: Guilford Press.

Douglas, V. I., & Parry, P. A. (1983). Effects of reward on delayed-reaction time task performance of hyperactive children. *Journal of Abnormal Child Psychology, 11*(2), 313–326.

Douglas, V. I., & Peters, K. G. (1979). Toward a clearer definition of the attention deficit of hyperactive children. In G. A. Hale & M. Lewis (Eds.), *Attention and the development of cognitive skills.* New York: Plenum Press.

Draeger, S., Prior, M., & Sanson, A. (1986). Visual and auditory attention performance in hyperactive children: Competence or compliance. *Journal of Abnormal Child Psychology, 14*(3), 411–424.

DuPaul, G. J. (1991). Parent and teacher ratings of ADHD symptoms: Psychometric properties in a community-based sample. *Journal of Clinical Child Psychology, 20*(3), 245–253.

DuPaul, G. J., Anastopoulos, A. D., Power, T. J., Reid, R., Ikeda, M. J., & McGoey, K. E. (1998). Parent ratings of attention-deficit/hyperactivity disorder symptoms: Factor structure and normative data. *Journal of Psychopathology and Behavioral Assessment, 20*(1), 83–102.

DuPaul, G. J., & Barkley, R. A. (1992). Situational variability of attention problems: Psychometric properties of the Revised Home and School Situations Questionnaires. *Journal of Clinical Child Psychology, 21*(2), 178–188.

DuPaul, G. J., Barkley, R. A., & McMurray, M. B. (1994). Response of children with ADHD to methylphenidate: Interaction with internalizing symptoms. *Journal of the American Academy of Child and Adolescent Psychiatry, 93,* 894–903.

DuPaul, G. J., Jitendra, A. K., Tresco, K. E., & Vile Junod, R. E. (2006). Children with attention deficit hyperactivity disorder: Are there gender differences in school functioning? *School Psychology Review, 35,* 292–308.

DuPaul, G. J., McGoey, K. E., Eckert, T. L., & VanBrakle, J. (2001). Preschool children with attention-deficit/hyperactivity disorder: Impairments in behavioral, social, and school functioning. *Journal of the American Academy of Child and Adolescent Psychiatry, 40*(5), 508–515.

DuPaul, G. J., & Stoner, G. (1994). *ADHD in the schools: Assessment and intervention strategies.* New York: Guilford Press.

DuPaul, G. J., & Stoner, G. (2003). *ADHD in the schools: Assessment and intervention strategies* (2nd ed.). New York: Guilford Press.

Durston, S., Pol, H. E., Schnack, H. G., Buitelaar, J. K., Steenhuis, M. P., Minderaa, R. B., et al.(2004). Magnetic resonance imaging of boys with attention-deficit/hyperactivity disorder and their unaffected siblings. *Journal of the American Academy of Child and Adolescent Psychiatry, 43,* 332–340.

Edwards, G., Barkley, R. A., Laneri, M., Fletcher, K., & Metevia, L. (2001). Parent–adolescent conflict in teenagers with ADHD and ODD. *Journal of Abnormal Child Psychology, 29*(6), 557–572.

Ekman, P., & Davidson, R. J. (1994). *The nature of emotion: Fundamental questions.* New York: Oxford University Press.

El-Sayed, E., Larsson, J. O., Persson, H. E., & Rydelius, P. A. (2002). Altered cortical activity in children with attention-deficit/hyperactivity disorder during attentional load task. *Journal of the American Academy of Child and Adolescent Psychiatry, 41*(7), 811–819.

Epstein, J. N., Conners, C. K., Sitarenios, G., & Erhardt, D. (1998). Continuous performance test results of adults with attention deficit hyperactivity disorder. *Clinical Neuropsychologist, 12*(2), 155–168.

Erhardt, D., & Hinshaw, S. P. (1994). Initial sociometric impressions of attention-deficit hyperactivity disorder and comparison boys: Predictions from social behaviors and from nonbehavioral variables. *Journal of Consulting and Clinical Psychology, 62*(4), 833–842.

Ernst, M, (1996). Neuroimaging in attention-deficit/hyperactivity disorder. In G. R. Lyon & J. M. Rumsey (Eds.), *Neuroimaging: A window to the neurological foundations of learning and behavior in children* (pp. 95–118). Baltimore: Brookes.

Ernst, M., Zametkin, A. J., Matochik, J. A., Pascualvaca, D., Jons, P. H., & Cohen, R. M. (1999). High midbrain [F-18]DOPA accumulation in children with attention deficit hyperactivity disorder. *American Journal of Psychiatry, 156*(8), 1209–1215.

Evans, S. W., Allen, J., Moore, S., & Strauss, V. (2005). Measuring symptoms and functioning of youth with ADHD in middle schools. *Journal of Abnormal Child Psychology, 33*(6), 695–706.

Fabiano, G. A., Pelham, W. E., Waschbusch, D. A., Gnagy, E. M., Lahey, B. B., Chronis, A. M., et al. (2006). A practical measure of impairment: Psychometric properties of the impairment rating scale in samples of children with attention-deficit hyperactivity disorder and two school-based samples. *Journal of Clinical Child and Adolescent Psychology, 35*(3), 369–385.

Faraone, S. V., Biederman, J., Mennin, D., Russell, R., & Tsuang, M. T. (1998). Familial subtypes of attention deficit hyperactivity disorder: A 4-year follow-up study of children from antisocial-ADHD families. *Journal of Child Psychology and Psychiatry and Allied Disciplines, 39*(7), 1045–1053.

Faraone, S. V., Biederman, J., Weiffenbach, B., Keith, T., Chu, M. P., Weaver, A., et al. (1999). Dopamine D-4 gene 7-repeat allele and attention deficit hyperactivity disorder. *American Journal of Psychiatry, 156*(5), 768–770.

Faraone, S. V., & Doyle, A. E. (2001). The nature and heritability of attention-deficit/hyperactivity disorder. *Child and Adolescent Psychiatric Clinics of North America, 10*(2), 299–316.

Farrington, D. P., & Welsh, B. C. (2003). Family-based prevention of offending: A meta-analysis. *Australian and New Zealand Journal of Criminology, 36*(2), 127–151.

Filipek, P. A., Semrud-Clikeman, M., Steingard, R. J., Renshaw, P. F., Kennedy, D. N., & Biederman, J. (1997). Volumetric MRI analysis comparing subjects having attention-deficit hyperactivity disorder with normal controls. *Neurology, 48*(3), 589–601.

Firestone, P., & Martin, J. E. (1979). Analysis of the hyperactive syndrome: Comparison of hyperactive, behavior-problem, asthmatic, and normal children. *Journal of Abnormal Child Psychology, 7*(3), 261–273.

Fischer, M. (1990). Parenting stress and the child with attention deficit hyperactivity disorder. *Journal of Child Psychology, 7,* 261–273.

Fischer, M., & Barkley, R. A. (2003). Childhood stimulant treatment and risk for later substance abuse. *Journal of Clinical Psychiatry, 64,* 19–23.

Fischer, M., Barkley, R. A., Edelbrock, C. S., & Smallish, L. (1990). The adolescent outcome of hyperactive children diagnosed by research criteria: 2. Academic, attentional, and neuropsychological status. *Journal of Consulting and Clinical Psychology, 58*(5), 580–588.

Fischer, M., Barkley, R. A., Fletcher, K. E., & Smallish, L. (1993). The adolescent outcome of hyperactive children: Predictors of psychiatric, academic, social, and emotional adjustment. *Journal of the American Academy of Child and Adolescent Psychiatry, 32*(2), 324–332.

Fischer, M., Barkley, R. A., Smallish, L., & Fletcher, K. (2005). Executive functioning in hyperactive children as young adults: Attention, inhibition, response perseveration, and the impact of comorbidity. *Developmental Neuropsychology, 27*(1), 107–133.

Fischer, M., Barkley, R. A., Smallish, L., Fletcher, K. (2007). Hyperactive children as young adults: Driving behavior, safe driving abilities, and adverse driving outcomes. *Accident Analysis and Prevention, 39,* 94–105.

Fletcher, K. E., Fischer, M., Barkley, R. A., & Smallish, L. (1996). A sequential analysis of the mother–adolescent interactions of ADHD, ADHD/ODD, and normal teenagers during neutral and conflict discussions. *Journal of Abnormal Child Psychology, 24*(3), 271–297.

Flory, K., Molina, B. S. G., Pelham, W., Gnagy, B., & Smith, B. H. (2006). ADHD and risky behavior. *Journal of Clinical Child and Adolescent Psychology, 53,* 571–577.

Foy, J. M., & Earls, M. F. (2005). Process for developing community consensus regarding the diagnosis and management of attention-deficit/hyperactivity disorder. *Pediatrics, 115*(1), E97–E104.

Frazier, T. W., Demareem, H. A., & Youngstrom, E. A. (2004). Meta-analysis of intellectual and neuropsychological test performance in attention-deficit/hyperactivity disorder. *Neuropsychology, 18,* 543–555.

Fuchs, L. S., & Fuchs, D. (1998). Treatment validity: A unifying concept for reconceptualizing the identification of learning disabilities. *Learning Disabilities Research and Practice, 13,* 204–219.

Fuster, J. M. (1989). *The prefrontal cortex.* New York: Raven Press.

Fuster, J. M. (1999). Cognitive functions of the frontal lobes. In B. L. Miller & J. L. Cummings (Eds.), *The human frontal lobes: Functions and disorders.* New York: Guilford Press.

Gabel, S., Schmitz, S., & Fulker, D. W. (1996). Comorbidity in hyperactive children: Issues related to selection bias, gender, severity, and internalizing symptoms. *Child Psychiatry and Human Development, 27*(1), 15–28.

Gaub, M., & Carlson, C. L. (1997). Behavioral characteristics of DSM-IV ADHD subtypes in a school-based population. *Journal of Abnormal Child Psychology, 25,* 103–111.

Gerdes, A. C., Hoza, B., & Pelham, W. E. (2003). Attention-deficit/hyperactivity disordered boys' relationships with their mothers and fathers: Child, mother, and father perceptions. *Development and Psychopathology, 15*(2), 363–382.

Gershon, J. (2002). A meta-analytic review of gender differences in ADHD. *Journal of Attention Disorders, 5,* 134–154.

Gilbert, D. L., Wang, Z., Sallee, F. R., Ridel, K. R., Merhar, S., Zhang, J., et al. (2006). Dopamine transporter genotype influences the physiological response to medication in ADHD. *Brain, 129,* 2038–2046.

Gioia, G. A., Isquith, P. K., Guy, S. C., Kenworthy, L., & Baron, I. S. (2000). Test review: Behavior rating inventory of executive function. *Child Neuropsychology, 6*(3), 235–238.

Glow, P. H., & Glow, R. A. (1979). Hyperkinetic impulse disorder: Developmental defect of motivation. *Genetic Psychology Monographs, 100*(2), 159–231.

Gomez, R., Harvey, J., Quick, C., Scharer, I., & Harris, G. (1999). DSM-IV ADHD: Confirmatory factor models, prevalence, and gender and age differences based on parent and teacher ratings of Australian primary school children. *Journal of Child Psychology and Psychiatry and Allied Disciplines, 40*(2), 265–274.

Gordon, M. (1983). *The Gordon Diagnostic System.* DeWitt, NY: Gordon Systems.

Gordon, M., Barkley, R. A., & Lovett, B. J. (2006). Tests and observational measures. In R. A. Barkley, *Attention-deficit hyperactivity disorder: A handbook for diagnosis and treatment* (3rd ed., pp. 369–388). New York: Guilford Press.

Graetz, B. W., Sawyer, M. G., Baghurst, P., & Hirte, C. (2006). Gender comparisons of service use among youth with attention-deficit/hyperactivity disorder. *Journal of Emotional and Behavioral Disorders, 14,* 2–11.

Granic, I., Hollenstein, T., Dishion, T. J., & Patterson, G. R. (2003). Longitudinal analysis of flexibility and reorganization in early adolescence: A dynamic systems study of family interactions. *Developmental Psychology, 39*(3), 606–617.

Green, L., Fry, A. F., & Meyerson, J. (1994). Discounting of delayed rewards: A life-span comparison. *Psychological Science, 5,* 33–36.

Greenberg, L. M., & Kindschi, C. L. (1996). *T.O.V.A. Test of Variables of Attention: Clinical guide.* St. Paul, MN: TOVA Research Foundation.

Greene, R. W., Biederman, J., Faraone, S. V., Ouellette, C. A., Penn, C., & Griffin, S. M. (1996). Toward a psychometric definition of social disability in children with attention-deficit hyperactivity disorder. *Journal of the American Academy of Child and Adolescent Psychiatry, 35,* 571–578.

Grodzinsky, G. M., & Diamond, R. (1992). Frontal-lobe functioning in boys with attention-deficit hyperactivity disorder. *Developmental Neuropsychology,* 8(4), 427–445.

Gustafsson, P., Thernlund, G., Ryding, E., Rosen, I., & Cederblad, M. (2000). Associations between cerebral blood-flow measured by single photon emission computed tomography (SPECT), electro-encephalogram (EEG), behaviour symptoms, cognition and neurological soft signs in children with attention-deficit hyperactivity disorder (ADHD). *Acta Paediatrica,* 89(7), 830–835.

Hafkenscheid, A. (1993). Psychometric evaluation of the Symptom Checklist (SCL-90) in psychiatric inpatients. *Personality and Individual Differences,* 14(6), 751–756.

Hale, G. A., & Lewis, M. (1979). *Attention and cognitive development.* New York: Plenum Press.

Halford, W. K., Sanders, M. R., & Behrens, B. C. (1994). Self-regulation in behavioral couples therapy. *Behavior Therapy,* 25(3), 431–452.

Halperin, J. M., Matier, K., Bedi, G., Sharma, V., & Newcorn, J. H. (1992). Specificity of inattention, impulsivity, and hyperactivity to the diagnosis of attention-deficit hyperactivity disorder. *Journal of the American Academy of Child and Adolescent Psychiatry,* 31(2), 190–196.

Halperin, J. M., Newcorn, J. H., Koda, V. H., Pick, L., McKay, K. E., & Knott, P. (1997). Noradrenergic mechanisms in ADHD children with and without reading disabilities: A replication and extension. *Journal of the American Academy of Child and Adolescent Psychiatry,* 36(12), 1688–1697.

Hamlett, K. W., Pellegrini, D. S., & Conners, C. K. (1987). An investigation of executive processes in the problem-solving of attention-deficit disorder hyperactive children. *Journal of Pediatric Psychology,* 12(2), 227–240.

Harrison, C., & Sofronoff, K. (2002). ADHD and parental psychological distress: Role of demographics, child behavioral characteristics, and parental cognitions. *Journal of the American Academy of Child and Adolescent Psychiatry,* 41(6), 703–711.

Hart, E. L., Lahey, B. B., Loeber, R., Applegate, B., & Frick, P. J. (1995). Developmental change in attention-deficit hyperactivity disorder in boys: A 4-year longitudinal study. *Journal of Abnormal Child Psychology,* 23(6), 729–749.

Hartsough, C. S., & Lambert, N. M. (1985). Medical factors in hyperactive and normal children: Prenatal, developmental, and health history findings. *American Journal of Orthopsychiatry,* 55(2), 190–201.

Hartung, C. M., Milich, G., Lynam, D. R., & Martin, C. A. (2002). Understanding the relations among gender, disinhibition, and disruptive behavior in adolescents. *Journal of Abnormal Psychology,* 111(4), 659–664.

Hayes, S. (1989). *Rule-governed behavior.* New York: Plenum Press.

Hechtman, L., Weiss, G., Perlman, T., & Amsel, R. (1984). Hyperactives as young adults: Initial predictors of adult outcome. *Journal of the American Acad-*

emy of Child and Adolescent Psychiatry, 23, 250–260.

Heiligenstein, E., Guenther, G., Levy, A., Savino, F., & Fulwiler, J. (1999). Psychological and academic functioning in college students with attention deficit hyperactivity disorder. *Journal of American College Health,* 47, 181–185.

Hendren, R. L., DeBacker, I., & Pandina, G. J. (2000, July). Review of neuroimaging studies of child and adolescent psychiatric disorders from the past 10 years. *Journal of the American Academy of Child and Adolescent Psychiatry,* 39(1), 815–828.

Herpertz, S. C., Wenning, B., Mueller, B., Qunaibi, M., Sass, H., & Herpertz-Dahlmann, B. (2001). Psychophysiological responses in ADHD boys with and without conduct disorder: Implications for adult antisocial behavior. *Journal of the American Academy of Child and Adolescent Psychiatry,* 40(10), 1222–1230.

Hervey, A. S., Epstein, J. N., & Curry, J. F. (2004). Neuropsychology of adults with attention-deficit/hyperactivity disorder: A meta-analytic review. *Neuropsychology,* 18, 495–503.

Hinshaw, S. P. (1987). On the distinction between attentional deficits/hyperactivity and conduct problems/aggression in child psychopathology. *Psychological Bulletin,* 101(3), 443–463.

Hinshaw, S. P. (1994). *Attention deficits and hyperactivity in children.* Thousand Oaks, CA: Sage.

Hinshaw, S. P., & Blachman, D. R. (2005). Attention-deficit/hyperactivity disorder. In D. Bell, S. Foster, & E. J. Mash (Eds.), *Handbook of behavioral and emotional problems in girls* (pp. 117–147). New York: Kluwer Academic/Plenum Press.

Hinshaw, S. P., Buhrmester, D., & Heller, T. (1989). Anger control in response to verbal provocation: Effects of stimulant medication for boys with ADHD. *Journal of Abnormal Child Psychology,* 17(4), 393–407.

Hinshaw, S. P., Owens, E. B., Sami, N., & Fargeon, S. (2006). Prospective follow-up of girls with attention-deficit/hyperactivity disorder into adolescence: Evidence for continuing cross-domain impairment. *Journal of Consulting and Clinical Psychology,* 74, 489–499.

Hinshaw, S. P., Owens, E. B., Wells, K. C., Kraemer, H. C., Abikoff, H. B., Arnold, L. E., et al. (2000). Family processes and treatment outcome in the MTA: Negative/ineffective parenting practices in relation to multimodal treatment. *Journal of Abnormal Child Psychology,* 28(6), 555–568.

Hope, T. L., Adams, C., Reynolds, L., Powers, D., Perez, R. A., & Kelley, M. L. (1999). Parent vs. self-report: Contributions toward diagnosis of adolescent psychopathology. *Journal of Psychopathology and Behavioral Assessment,* 21(4), 349–363.

Hoza, B., Gerdes, A. C., Hinshaw, S. P., Arnold, L. E., Pelham, W. E., Molina, B. S. G., et al. (2004). Self-perceptions of competence in children with ADHD and comparison children. *Journal of Consulting and Clinical Psychology,* 72(3), 382–391.

Hoza, B., Owens, J. S., Pelham, W. E., Swanson, J. M., Conners, C. K., Hinshaw, S. P., et al. (2000). Parent cognitions as predictors of child treatment response in attention-deficit/hyperactivity disorder. *Journal of Abnormal Child Psychology, 28,* 569–583.

Hoza, B., Pelham, W. E., Waschbusch, D. A., Kipp, H., & Owens, J. S. (2001). Academic task persistence of normally achieving ADHD and control boys: Performance, self-evaluations, and attributions. *Journal of Consulting and Clinical Psychology, 69,* 271–283.

James, W. (1890). *The principles of psychology* (2 vols.). New York: Holt.

Jarratt, K. P., Riccio, C. A., & Siekierski, B. M. (2005). Assessment of attention deficit hyperactivity disorder (ADHD) using the BASC and BRIEF. *Applied Neuropsychology, 12,* 83–93.

Jensen, P. S., Arnold, L. E., Severe, J. B., Vitiello, B., & Hoagwood, K. (2004). National Institute of Mental Health Multimodal Treatment Study of ADHD follow-up: Changes in effectiveness and growth after the end of treatment. *Pediatrics, 113*(4), 762–769.

Jensen, P. S., Garcia, J. A., Glied, S., Crowe, M., Foster, M., Schlander, M., et al. (2005). Cost-effectiveness of ADHD treatments: Findings from the multimodal treatment study of children with ADHD. *American Journal of Psychiatry, 162*(9), 1628–1636.

Jensen, P. S., Hinshaw, S. P., Kraemer, H. C., Lenora, N., Newcorn, J. H., Abikoff, H. B., et al. (2001). ADHD comorbidity findings from the MTA study: Comparing comorbid subgroups. *Journal of the American Academy of Child and Adolescent Psychiatry, 40*(2), 147–158.

Jensen, P. S., Shervette, R. E., Xenakis, S. N., & Richters, J. (1993). Anxiety and depressive disorders in attention-deficit disorder with hyperactivity: New findings. *American Journal of Psychiatry, 150*(8), 1203–1209.

Johnston, C., & Mash, E. J. (2001). Families of children with attention-deficit/hyperactivity disorder: Review and recommendations for future research. *Clinical Child and Family Psychology Review, 4*(3), 183–207.

Johnston, C., Murray, C., Hinshaw, S. P., Pelham, W. E., & Hoza, B. (2002). Responsiveness in interactions of mothers and sons with ADHD: Relations to maternal and child characteristics. *Journal of Abnormal Child Psychology, 30*(1), 77–88.

Johnstone, S. J., Barry, R. J., & Anderson, J. W. (2001). Topographic distribution and developmental time-course of auditory event-related potentials in two subtypes of attention-deficit hyperactivity disorder. *International Journal of Psychophysiology, 42*(1), 73–94.

Kadesjo, B., & Gillberg, C. (2001). The comorbidity of ADHD in the general population of Swedish school-age children. *Journal of Child Psychology and Psychiatry and Allied Disciplines, 42*(4), 487–492.

Kashdan, T. B., Jacob, R. G., Pelham, W. E., Lang, A. R., Hoza, B., Blumenthal, J. D., et al. (2004). Depression and anxiety in parents of children with ADHD and varying levels of oppositional defiant behaviors:

Modeling relationships with family functioning. *Journal of Clinical Child and Adolescent Psychology, 33*(1), 169–181.

Kazdin, A. E. (1990). Psychotherapy for children and adolescents. *Annual Review of Psychology, 41,* 21–54.

Kendall, P. C., & Braswell, L. (1985). *Cognitive-behavioral therapy for impulsive children.* New York: Guilford Press.

Keown, L. J., & Woodward, L. J. (2002). Early parent–child relations and family functioning of preschool boys with pervasive hyperactivity. *Journal of Abnormal Child Psychology, 30*(6), 541–553.

Kessler, R. C., Adler, L., Barkley, R. A., Biederman, J., Conners, C. K., Demler, O., et al. (2006). The prevalence and correlates of adult ADHD in the United States: Results from the National Comorbidity Survey Replication. *American Journal of Psychiatry, 163,* 716–723.

Knight, J. R., Sherritt, L., Harris, S. K., Gates, E. C., & Chang, G. (2003). Validity of brief alcohol screening tests among adolescents: A comparison of the AUDIT, POSIT, CAGE, and CRAFFT. *Alcoholism, Clinical and Experimental Research, 27*(1), 67–73.

Knouse, L. E., Bagwell, C. L., Barkley, R. A., & Murphy, K. R. (2005). Accuracy of self-evaluation in adults with attention-deficit hyperactivity disorder. *Journal of Attention Disorders, 8,* 221–234.

Kroes, M., Kalff, A. C., Kessels, A. G. H., Steyaert, J., Feron, F. J. M., van Someren, A., et al. (2001). Child psychiatric diagnoses in a population of Dutch schoolchildren aged 6 to 8 years. *Journal of the American Academy of Child and Adolescent Psychiatry, 40*(12), 1401–1409.

Kuntsi, J., & Stevenson, J. (2001). Psychological mechanisms in hyperactivity: II. The role of genetic factors. *Journal of Child Psychology and Psychiatry and Allied Disciplines, 42,* 211–219.

Kupfer, D. J., Baltimore, R. S., Berry, D. A., Breslau, N., Ellinwood, E. H., Ferre, J., et al. (2000). National Institutes of Health Consensus Development Conference Statement: Diagnosis and treatment of attention-deficit/hyperactivity disorder (ADHD). *Journal of the American Academy of Child and Adolescent Psychiatry, 39*(2), 182–193.

Lahey, B. B., Applegate, B., McBurnett, K., Biederman, J., Greenhill, L., Hynd, G. W., et al. (1994). DSM-IV field trials for attention-deficit hyperactivity disorder in children and adolescents. *American Journal of Psychiatry, 151*(11), 1673–1685.

Lahey, B. B., & Carlson, C. L. (1992). Validity of the diagnostic category of attention deficit disorder without hyperactivity: A review of the literature. In S. E. Shaywitz & B. B. Shaywitz (Eds.), *Attention-deficit disorder comes of age: Toward the twenty-first century* (pp. 119–144). Austin, TX: PRO-ED.

Lahey, B. B., Pelham, W. E., Chronis, A., Massetti, G., Kipp, H., Ehrhardt, A., et al. (2006). Predictive validity of ICD-10 hyperkinetic disorder relative to DSM-IV attention-deficit/hyperactivity disorder among younger children. *Journal of Child Psychology and Psychiatry, 47*(5), 472–479.

Lahey, B. B., Pelham, W. E., Loney, J., Kipp, H., Ehrhardt, A., Lee, S. S., et al. (2004). Three-year predictive validity of DSM-IV attention deficit hyperactivity disorder in children diagnosed at 4–6 years of age. *American Journal of Psychiatry, 161*(11), 2014–2020.

Lahey, B. B., Pelham, W. E., Loney, J., Lee, S. S., & Willcutt, E. (2005). Instability of the DSM-IV subtypes of ADHD from preschool through elementary school. *Archives of General Psychiatry, 62*(8), 896–902.

LaHoste, G. J., Swanson, J. M., Wigal, S. B., Glabe, C., Wigal, T., King, N., et al. (1996). Dopamine D4 receptor gene polymorphism is associated with attention deficit hyperactivity disorder. *Molecular Psychiatry, 1*(2), 121–124.

Lambert, N. M., & Hartsough, C. S. (1998). Prospective study of tobacco smoking and substance dependence among samples of ADHD and non ADHD students. *Journal of Learning Disabilities, 31*, 533–544.

Landau, S., Lorch, E. P., & Milich, R. (1992). Visual attention to and comprehension of television in attention-deficit hyperactivity disordered and normal boys. *Child Development, 63*(4), 928–937.

Lang, P. J. (1995). The emotion probe: Studies of motivation and attention. *American Psychologist, 50*(5), 372–385.

Latham, P., & Latham, R. (1992). *ADD and the law.* Washington, DC: JKL Communications.

Laufer, M. W., Denhoff, E., & Solomons, G. (1957). Hyperkinetic impulse disorder in children's behavior problems. *Psychosomatic Medicine, 19*(1), 38–49.

Lawrence, V., Houghton, S., Tannock, R., Douglas, G., Durkin, K., & Whiting, K. (2002). ADHD outside the laboratory: Boys' executive function performance on tasks in videogame play and on a visit to the zoo. *Journal of Abnormal Child Psychology, 30*(5), 447–462.

Levin, P. M. (1938). Restlessness in children. *Archives of Neurological Psychiatry, 39*, 764–770.

Levy, F., & Hay, D. A. (Eds.). (2001). *Attention genes and ADHD.* Philadelphia: Brunner–Routledge.

Levy, F., Hay, D. A., McStephen, M., & Martin, N. G. (2001). Intergenerational transmission of ADHD and associated psychopathologies. *Behavior Genetics, 31*(5), 459–459.

Locke, H. J., & Wallace, K. M. (1959). Short marital adjustment and prediction tests: Their reliability and validity. *Marriage and Family Living, 21*(3), 251–255.

Loney, J., Kramer, J., & Milich, R. (1981). The hyperkinetic child grows up: Predictors of symptoms, delinquency, and achievement at follow-up. In K. Gadow & J. Loney (Eds.), *Psychosocial aspects of drug treatment for hyperactivity.* Boulder, CO: Westview Press.

Loo, S. K., & Barkley, R. A. (2005). Clinical utility of EEG in attention deficit hyperactivity disorder. *Applied Neuropsychology, 12*(2), 64–76.

Loo, S. K., Specter, E., Smolen, A., Hopfer, C., Teale, P. D., & Reite, M. L. (2003). Functional effects of the DAT1 polymorphism on EEG measures in ADHD. *Journal of the American Academy of Child and Adolescent Psychiatry, 42*(8), 986–993.

Lord, F. M. (1965). A strong true-score theory, with applications. *Psychometrika, 30*(3), 239–270.

Low, S. A., & Stocker, C. (2005). Family functioning and children's adjustment: Associations among parents' depressed mood, marital hostility, parent–child hostility, and children's adjustment. *Journal of Family Psychology, 19*(3), 394–403.

Luk, S. L. (1985). Direct observation studies of hyperactive behaviors. *Journal of the American Academy of Child and Adolescent Psychiatry, 24*(3), 338–344.

Luman, M., Oosterlaan, J., & Sergeant, J. A. (2005). The impact of reinforcement contingencies on ADHD: A review and theoretical appraisal. *Clinical Psychology Review, 25*, 183–213.

MacKenzie, D. M., Langa, A., & Brown, T. M. (1996). Identifying hazardous or harmful alcohol use in medical admissions: A comparison of AUDIT, CAGE and brief MAST. *Alcohol and Alcoholism, 31*(6), 591–599.

Mannuzza, S., & Klein, R. (1992). Predictors of outcome of children with attention-deficit hyperactivity disorder. *Child and Adolescent Psychiatric Clinics of North America, 1*(2), 567–578.

Mannuzza, S., Klein, R. G., Bessler, A., Malloy, P., & LaPadula, M. (1998). Adult psychiatric status of hyperactive boys grown up. *American Journal of Psychiatry, 155*, 493–498.

Mannuzza, S., Klein, R. G., Bonagura, N., Malloy, P., Giampino, T. L., & Addalli, K. A. (1991). Hyperactive boys almost grown up. *Archives of General Psychiatry, 48*, 77–83.

Mannuzza, S., Klein, R. G., & Moulton, J. L. (2002). Young adult outcome of children with "situational" hyperactivity: A prospective, controlled follow-up study. *Journal of Abnormal Child Psychology, 30*(2), 191–198.

Mariani, M. A., & Barkley, R. A. (1997). Neuropsychological and academic functioning in preschool boys with attention deficit hyperactivity disorder. *Developmental Neuropsychology, 13*(1), 111–129.

Marshal, M. P., Molina, B. S. G., & Pelham, W. E. (2003). Childhood ADHD and adolescent substance use: An examination of deviant peer group affiliation as a risk factor. *Psychology of Addictive Behaviors, 17*(4), 293–302.

Martinussen, R., Hayden, J., Hogg-Johnson, S., & Tannock, R. (2006). A meta-analysis of working memory impairments in children with attention-deficit/hyperactivity disorder. *Journal of the American Academy of Child and Adolescent Psychiatry, 44*, 377–384.

Martinussen, R., & Tannock, R. (2006). Working memory impairments in children with attention-deficit/hyperactivity disorder with and without comorbid language learning disorders. *Journal of*

Clinical and Experimental Neuropsychology, 28, 1073–1094.

Marzocchi, G. M., Lucangeli, D., De Meo, T., Fini, F., & Cornoldi, C. (2002). The disturbing effect of irrelevant information on arithmetic problem solving in inattentive children. *Developmental Neuropsychology, 21*(1), 73–92.

Mash, E. J., & Johnston, C. (1982). A Comparison of the mother–child interactions of younger and older hyperactive and normal children. *Child Development, 53*(5), 1371–1381.

Matthys, W., Cuperus, J. M., & Van Engeland, M. (1999). Deficient social problem-solving in boys with ODD/CD, with ADHD, and with both disorders. *Journal of the American Academy of Child and Adolescent Psychiatry, 38*(3), 311–321.

Maughan, B., Taylor, A., Caspi, A., & Moffitt, T. E. (2004). Prenatal smoking and early childhood conduct problems: Testing genetic and environmental explanations of the association. *Archives of General Psychiatry, 61*(8), 836–843.

McBurnett, K., Pfiffner, L. J., & Frick, P. J. (2001). Symptom properties as a function of ADHD type: An argument for continued study of sluggish cognitive tempo. *Journal of Abnormal Child Psychology, 29,* 207–213.

McCann, B. S., & Roy-Byrne, P. (2004). Screening and diagnostic utility of self-report attention deficit hyperactivity disorder scales in adults. *Comprehensive Psychiatry, 45,* 175–183.

McGee, R., Stanton, W. R., & Sears, M. R. (1993). Allergic disorders and attention-deficit disorder in children. *Journal of Abnormal Child Psychology, 21*(1), 79–88.

McKay, M. M., McCadam, K., & Gonzales, J. J. (1996). Addressing the barriers to mental health services for inner city children and their caretakers. *Community Mental Health Journal, 32*(4), 353–361.

McKee, T. E., Harvey, E., Danforth, J. S., Ulaszek, W. R., & Friedman, J. L. (2004). The relation between parental coping styles and parent–child interactions before and after treatment for children with ADHD and oppositional behavior. *Journal of Clinical Child and Adolescent Psychology, 33*(1), 158–168.

Meehl, P. E., & Rosen, A. (1955). Antecedent probability and the efficiency of psychometric signs, patterns, and cutting scores. *Psychological Bulletin, 52,* 194–216.

Michon, J. (1985). Introduction. In J. Michon & T. Jackson (Eds.), *Time, mind, and behavior* (pp. 27–37). Berlin: Springer-Verlag.

Mick, E., Biederman, J., Faraone, S. V., Sayer, J., & Kleinman, S. (2002). Case–control study of attention-deficit hyperactivity disorder and maternal smoking, alcohol use, and drug use during pregnancy. *Journal of the American Academy of Child and Adolescent Psychiatry, 41*(4), 378–385.

Mikami, A. Y., & Hinshaw, S. P. (2003). Buffers of peer rejection among girls with and without ADHD: The role of popularity with adults and goal-directed soli-

tary play. *Journal of Abnormal Child Psychology, 31*(4), 381–397.

Milberger, S., Biederman, J., Faraone, S. V., Chen, L., & Jones, J. (1996). Maternal smoking during pregnancy a risk factor for attention deficit hyperactivity disorder in children? *American Journal of Psychiatry, 153*(9), 1138–1142.

Milich, R., Balentine, A. C., & Lynam, D. R. (2001). ADHD combined type and ADHD predominantly inattentive type are distinct and unrelated disorders. *Clinical Psychology: Science and Practice, 8,* 463–488.

Milich, R., & Lorch, E. P. (1994). Television viewing methodology to understand cognitive processing of ADHD children. *Advances in Clinical Child Psychology, 16,* 177–201.

Milich, R., Widiger, T. A., & Landau, S. (1987). Differential diagnosis of attention deficit and conduct disorders using conditional probabilities. *Journal of Consulting and Clinical Psychology, 55,* 762–767.

Miller, W. R. (1998). Why do people change addictive behavior?: The 1996 H. David Archibald Lecture. *Addiction, 93*(2), 163–172.

Miller, W. R., & Rollnick, S. (2002). *Motivational interviewing: Preparing people for change* (2nd ed.). New York: Guilford Press.

Miller, W. R., & Rollnick, S. (2003). Motivational interviewing: Preparing people for change. *American Journal of Forensic Psychology, 21*(1), 83–85.

Mirsky, A. F. (1996). Disorders of attention: A neuropsychological perspective. In R. G. Lyon & N. A. Krasnegor (Eds.), *Attention, memory, and executive function* (pp. 71–96). Baltimore: Brookes.

Mitsis, E. M., McKay, K. E., Schulz, K. P., Newcorn, J. H., & Halperin, J. M. (2000). Parent–teacher concordance for DSM-IV attention-deficit/hyperactivity disorder in a clinic-referred sample. *Journal of the American Academy of Child and Adolescent Psychiatry, 39,* 308–313.

Molina, B. S. G., Marshal, M. P., Pelham, W. E., & Wirth, R. J. (2005). Coping skills and parent support mediate the association between childhood attention-deficit/hyperactivity disorder and adolescent cigarette use. *Journal of Pediatric Psychology, 30*(4), 345–357.

Molina, B. S. G., & Pelham, W. E., Jr. (2003). Childhood predictors of adolescent substance use in a longitudinal study of children with ADHD. *Journal of Abnormal Psychology, 112*(3), 497–507.

Molina, B. S. G., Smith, B. H., & Pelham, W. E. (2001). Factor structure and criterion validity of secondary school teacher ratings of ADHD and ODD. *Journal of Abnormal Child Psychology, 29*(1), 71–82.

Monastra, V. J., Lubar, J. F., & Linden, M. (1999). Assessing ADHD via quantitative electro-encephalography: Test validation and reliability studies. *Clinical Neuropsychologist, 13*(2), 227–227.

Monastra, V. J., Lubar, J. F., & Linden, M. (2001). The development of a quantitative electroencephalographic scanning process for attention deficit-hyperactivity disorder: Reliability and validity studies. *Neuropsychology*, 15(1), 136–144.

MTA Collaborative Group. (1999). A 14-month randomized clinical trial of treatment strategies for attention-deficit/hyperactivity disorder. *Archives of General Psychiatry*, 56, 1073–1086.

Mueller, K., Daly, M., Fischer, M., Yiannoutsos, C. T., Bauer, L., Barkley, R. A., et al. (2003). Association of the dopamine beta hydroxylase gene with attention deficit hyperactivity disorder: Genetic analysis of the Milwaukee longitudinal study. *American Journal of Medical Genetics*, 119B, 77–85.

Murphy, K., & Barkley, R. A. (1996a). Attention-deficit hyperactivity disorder adults: Comorbidities and adaptive impairments. *Comprehensive Psychiatry*, 37(6), 393–401.

Murphy, K. R., & Barkley, R. A. (1996b). Parents of children with attention-deficit hyperactivity disorder: Psychological and attentional impairment. *American Journal of Orthopsychiatry*, 66(1), 93–102.

Murphy, K. R., Barkley, R. A., & Bush, T. (2001). Executive functioning and olfactory identification in young adults with attention deficit-hyperactivity disorder. *Neuropsychology*, 15(2), 211–220.

Murphy, K. R., Gordon, M., & Barkley, R. A. (2002). To what extent are ADHD symptoms common?: A reanalysis of standardization data from a DSM-IV checklist. *ADHD Report*, 8(3), 1–5.

Needleman, H. L., Schell, A., Bellinger, D., Leviton, A., & Allred, E. N. (1990). The long-term effects of exposure to low doses of lead in childhood: An 11-year follow-up report. *New England Journal of Medicine*, 322(2), 83–88.

Neef, N. A., Bicard, D. F., & Endo, S. (2001). Assessment of impulsivity and the development of self-control in students with attention deficit hyperactivity disorder. *Journal of Applied Behavior Analysis*, 34(4), 397–408.

Newcorn, J. H., Halperin, J. M., Jensen, P. S., Abikoff, H. B., Arnold, L. E., Cantwell, D. P., et al. (2001). Symptom profiles in children with ADHD: Effects of comorbidity and gender. *Journal of the American Academy of Child and Adolescent Psychiatry*, 40(2), 137–146.

Nigg, J. T. (2005). Neuropsychologic theory and findings in attention-deficit/hyperactivity disorder: The state of the field and salient challenges for the coming decade. *Biological Psychiatry*, 57(11), 1424–1435.

Nigg, J. T. (2006). *What causes ADHD?: Understanding what goes wrong and why.* New York: Guilford Press.

Nigg, J. T., Stavro, G., Ettenhofer, M., Hambrick, D. Z., Miller, T., & Henderson, J. M. (2005). Executive functions and ADHD in adults: Evidence for selective effects on ADHD symptom domains. *Journal of Abnormal Psychology*, 114(4), 706–717.

Nucci, L. P., & Herman, S. (1982). Behavioral disordered children's conceptions of moral, conventional, and personal Issues. *Journal of Abnormal Child Psychology*, 10(3), 411–425.

Ohan, J. L., & Johnston, C. (2005). Gender appropriateness of symptom criteria for attention-deficit/hyperactivity disorder, oppositional-defiant disorder, and conduct disorder. *Child Psychiatry and Human Development*, 35(4), 359–381.

Ostrander, R., & Herman, K. C. (2006). Potential cognitive, parenting, and developmental mediators of the relationship between ADHD and depression. *Journal of Consulting and Clinical Psychology*, 74(1), 89–98.

Ostrander, R., Weinfurt, K. P., Yarnold, P. R., & August, G. J. (1998). Diagnosing attention deficit disorders with the Behavioral Assessment System for Children and the Child Behavior Checklist: Test and construct validity analyses using optimal discriminant classification trees. *Journal of Consulting and Clinical Psychology*, 66(4), 660–672.

Paternite, C., & Loney, J. (1980). Childhood hyperkinesis: Relationships between symptomatology and home environment. In C. K. Whalen & B. Henker (Eds.), *Hyperactive children: The social ecology of identification and treatment* (pp. 105–141). New York: Academic Press.

Patterson, G. R., & Forgatch, M. (1987). *Parents and adolescents living together: Part 1. The basics.* Eugene, OR: Castalia Press.

Pelham, W. E., Jr. (1993). Pharmacotherapy for children with attention-deficit hyperactivity disorder. *School Psychology Review*, 22(2), 199–227.

Pelham, W. E., Jr., Fabiano, G. A., & Massetti, G. M. (2005). Evidence-based assessment of attention deficit hyperactivity disorder in children and adolescents. *Journal of Clinical Child and Adolescent Psychology*, 34, 449–476.

Pelham, W. E., Jr., & Milich, R. (1991). Individual differences in response to Ritalin in classwork and social behavior. In L. Greenhill & B. P. Osman (Eds.), *Ritalin: Theory and patient management* (pp. 203–221). New York: MaryAnn Libert, Inc.

Pelham, W. E., Jr., Wheeler, T., & Chronis, A. (1998). Empirically supported psychosocial treatments for attention deficit hyperactivity disorder. *Journal of Clinical Child Psychology*, 27(2), 190–205.

Pfiffner, L. J., Barkley, R. A., & DuPaul, G. J. (2006). Treatment of ADHD in school settings. In R. A. Barkley, *Attention-deficit hyperactivity disorder: A handbook for diagnosis and treatment* (3rd ed., pp. 547–589). New York: Guilford Press.

Pliszka, S. R. (1989). Effects of anxiety on cognition, behaviour, and stimulant response in ADHD. *Journal of the American Academy of Child and Adolescent Psychiatry*, 28, 882–887.

Pliszka, S. R., Liotti, M., & Woldorff, M. G. (2000). Inhibitory control in children with attention-deficit/hyperactivity disorder: Event-related potentials identify the processing component and timing of an impaired right-frontal response-inhibition mechanism. *Biological Psychiatry*, 48(3), 238–246.

Pliszka, S. R., McCracken, J. T., & Maas, J. W. (1996). Catecholamines in attention-deficit hyperactivity disorder: Current perspectives. *Journal of the American Academy of Child and Adolescent Psychiatry, 35,* 264–272.

Porrino, L. J., Rapoport, J. L., Behar, D., Sceery, W., Ismond, D. R., & Bunney, W. E. (1983). A naturalistic assessment of the motor activity of hyperactive boys: 1. Comparison with normal controls. *Archives of General Psychiatry, 40*(6), 681–687.

Prinz, R. J., Foster, S., Kent, R. N., & O'Leary, K. D. (1979). Multivariate assessment of conflict in distressed and non-distressed mother–adolescent dyads. *Journal of Applied Behavior Analysis, 12*(4), 691–700.

Prochaska, J. O., DiClemente, C. C., & Norcross, J. C. (1992). In search of how people change: Application to addictive behaviors. *American Psychologist, 47*(9), 107–116.

Quinn, P. O. (2005). Treating adolescent girls and women with ADHD: Gender-specific issues. *Journal of Clinical Psychology, 61*(5), 579–587.

Quinn, P. O., & Rapoport, J. L. (1974). Minor physical anomalies and neurologic status in hyperactive boys. *Pediatrics, 53*(5), 742–747.

Rapport, M. D., & Kelly, K. L. (1993). Psychostimulant effects on learning and cognitive function in children with attention deficit hyperactivity disorder: Findings and implications. In J. L. Matson (Ed.), *Hyperactivity in children: A handbook* (pp. 97–136). Elmsford, NY: Pergamon Press.

Rapport, M. D., Tucker, S. B., DuPaul, G. J., Merlo, M., & Stoner, G. (1986). Hyperactivity and frustration: The influence of control over and size of rewards in delaying gratification. *Journal of Abnormal Child Psychology, 14*(2), 191–204.

Rasmussen, E. R., Todd, R. D., Neuman, R. J., Heath, A. C., Reich, W., & Rohde, L. A. (2002). Comparison of male adolescent report of attention-deficit/hyperactivity disorder (ADHD) symptoms across two cultures using latent class and principal components analysis. *Journal of Child Psychology and Psychiatry and Allied Disciplines, 43*(6), 797–805.

Reid, R., Riccio, C. A., Kessler, R. H., DuPaul, G. J., Power, T. J., Anastopoulos, A. D., et al. (2000). Gender and ethnic differences in ADHD as assessed by behavior ratings. *Journal of Emotional and Behavioral Disorders, 8*(1), 38–48.

Reitz, E., Dekovic, M., & Meijer, A. M. (2006). Relations between parenting and externalizing and internalizing problem behaviour in early adolescence: Child behaviour as moderator and predictor. *Journal of Adolescence, 29*(3), 419–436.

Reynolds, C. R., & Kamphaus, R. W. (2005). *Behavioral Assessment System for Children, Second Edition.* Bloomington, MN: Pearson Assessments.

Robin, A. R. (1990). Training families with ADHD adolescents. In R. A. Barkley, *Attention-deficit hyperactivity disorder: A handbook for diagnosis and treatment* (pp. 462–497). New York: Guilford Press.

Robin, A. L., & Foster, S. L. (1989). *Negotiating parent–adolescent conflict: A behavioral–family systems approach.* New York: Guilford Press.

Robison, L. M., Skaer, T. L., Sclar, D. A., & Galin, R. S. (2002). Is attention deficit hyperactivity disorder increasing among girls in the US?: Trends in diagnosis and the prescribing of stimulants. *CNS Drugs, 16*(2), 129–137.

Rogers, C. R. (1951). *Client-centered therapy.* Boston: Houghton Mifflin.

Rohde, L. A., Biederman, J., Busnello, E. A., Zimmermann, H., Schmitz, M., Martins, S., et al. (1999). ADHD in a school sample of Brazilian adolescents: A study of prevalence, comorbid conditions, and impairments. *Journal of the American Academy of Child and Adolescent Psychiatry, 38*(6), 716–722.

Roizen, N. J., Blondis, T. A., Irwin, M., & Stein, M. (1994). Adaptive functioning in children with attention-deficit hyperactivity disorder. *Archives of Pediatrics and Adolescent Medicine, 148*(11), 1137–1142.

Rosenthal, R. H., & Allen, T. W. (1980). Intratask distractibility in hyperkinetic and non-hyperkinetic children. *Journal of Abnormal Child Psychology, 8*(2), 175–187.

Routh, D. K., & Schroeder, C. S. (1976). Standardized playroom measures as indexes of hyperactivity. *Journal of Abnormal Child Psychology, 4*(2), 199–207.

Rubia, K., Overmeyer, S., Taylor, E., Brammer, M., Williams, S. C., Simmons, A., et al. (1999). Hypofrontality in attention deficit hyperactivity disorder during higher-order motor control: A study with functional MRI. *American Journal of Psychiatry, 156*(6), 891–896.

Rucklidge, J. (2006). Gender differences in neuropsychological functioning of New Zealand adolescents with and without attention deficit hyperactivity disorder. *International Journal of Disability, Development and Education, 53,* 47–66.

Rutter, M. (1977). Brain damage syndromes in childhood: Concepts and findings. *Journal of Child Psychology and Psychiatry, 18,* 1–21.

Samuel, V. J., George, P., Thornell, A., Curtis, S., Taylor, A., Brome, D., et al. (1999). A pilot controlled family study of DSM-III-R and DSM-IV ADHD in African-American children. *Journal of the American Academy of Child and Adolescent Psychiatry, 38*(1), 34–39.

Sandberg, S. T., Rutter, M., & Taylor, E. (1978). Hyperkinetic disorder in psychiatric clinic attenders. *Developmental Medicine and Child Neurology, 20*(3), 279–299.

Sanders, M. (1999). Triple-P Positive Parenting Program: Towards an empirically validated multi-level parenting and family support strategy for the prevention of behavioral and emotional problems in children. *Clinical Child and Family Psychology Review, 2,* 71–90.

Sanders, M. R. (2000). Community-based parenting and family support interventions and the prevention of drug abuse. *Addictive Behaviors, 25*, 929–942.

Sanders, M. R., & Lawton, J. M. (1993). Discussing assessment findings with families: A guided participatory model of information transfer. *Child and Family Behavior Therapy, 15*, 5–35.

Sanders, M. R., Markie-Dadds, C., & Turner, K. (2001). *Practitioner's manual for Standard Triple-P.* Brisbane: Families International.

Sanders, M. R., & McFarland, M. (2000). Treatment of depressed mothers with disruptive children: A controlled evaluation of cognitive behavioral family intervention. *Behavior Therapy, 31*, 89–112.

Sanders, M. R., & Ralph, A. (2001). *Practitioner's manual for primary care Teen Triple P.* Milton, Brisbane: Families International.

Santisteban, D. A., Suarez-Morales, L., Robbins, M. S., & Szapocznik, J. (2006). Brief strategic family therapy: Lessons learned in efficacy research and challenges to blending research and practice. *Family Process, 45*, 259–271.

Santisteban, D. A., Szapocznik, J., & Perez-Vidal, A. (1996). Efficacy of intervention for engaging youth and families into treatment and some variables that may contribute to differential effectiveness. *Journal of Family Psychology, 10*(1), 35–44.

Satterfield, J. H., Satterfield, B. T., & Cantwell, D. P. (1981). Three-year multimodality treatment study of 100 hyperactive boys. *Journal of Pediatrics, 98*, 650–655.

Satterfield, J. H., & Schell, A. (1997). A prospective study of hyperactive boys with conduct problems and normal boys: Adolescent and adult criminality. *Journal of the American Academy of Child and Adolescent Psychiatry, 36*, 1726–1735.

Saunders, J. B., Aasland, O. G., Babor, T. F., Delafuente, J. R., & Grant, M. (1993). Development of the Alcohol-Use Disorders Identification Test (AUDIT): WHO collaborative project on early detection of persons with harmful alcohol consumption—II. *Addiction, 88*(6), 791–804.

Schachar, R. J., Mota, V. L., Logan, G. D., Tannock, R., & Klim, P. (2000). Confirmation of an inhibitory control deficit in attention-deficit/hyperactivity disorder. *Journal of Abnormal Child Psychology, 28*(3), 227–235.

Schachar, R. J., Tannock, R., & Logan, G. (1993). Inhibitory control, impulsiveness, and attention-deficit hyperactivity disorder. *Clinical Psychology Review, 13*(8), 721–739.

Schothorst, P. F., & van Engeland, H. (1996). Long-term behavioral sequelae of prematurity. *Journal of the American Academy of Child and Adolescent Psychiatry, 35*(2), 175–183.

Schweitzer, J. B., Faber, T. L., Grafton, S. T., Tune, L. E., Hoffman, J. M., & Kilts, C. D. (2000). Alterations in the functional anatomy of working memory in adult attention deficit hyperactivity disorder. *American Journal of Psychiatry, 157*(2), 278–280.

Sechrest, L. (1963). Incremental validity: A recommendation. *Educational and Psychological Measurement, 23*(1), 153–158.

Seidman, L. J., Benedict, K. B., Biederman, J., Bernstein, J. H., Seiverd, K., Milberger, S., et al. (1995). Performance of children with ADHD on the Rey-Osterrieth, complex figure: A pilot neuropsychological study. *Journal of Child Psychology and Psychiatry and Allied Disciplines, 38*(8), 1459–1473.

Seidman, L. J., Biederman, J., Weber, W., Hatch, M., & Faraone, S. V. (1998). Neuropsychological function in adults with attention-deficit hyperactivity disorder. *Biological Psychiatry, 44*(4), 260–268.

Seidman, L. J., Doyle, A., Fried, R., Valera, E., Crum, K., & Matthews, L. (2004). Neuropsychological function in adults with attention-deficit/hyperactivity disorder. *Psychiatric Clinics of North America, 27*(2), 261–282.

Semrud-Clikeman, M., Steingard, R. J., Filipek, P., Biederman, J., Bekken, K., & Renshaw, P. F. (2000). Using MRI to examine brain–behavior relationships in males with attention deficit disorder with hyperactivity. *Journal of the American Academy of Child and Adolescent Psychiatry, 39*(4), 477–484.

Sergeant, J., & Van der Meere, J. J. (1989). The diagnostic significance of attentional processing: Its significance for ADDH classification in a future DSM. In T. Sagvolden & T. Archer (Eds.), *Attention deficit disorder: Clinical and basic research* (pp. 151–166). Hillsdale, NJ: Erlbaum.

Shaffer, D., Fisher, P., Dulcan, M. K., Davies, M., Piacentini, J., Schwab-Stone, M. E., et al. (1996). The NIMH Diagnostic Interview Schedule for Children Version 2.3 (DISC-2.3): Description, acceptability, prevalence rates, and performance in the MECA study. *Journal of the American Academy of Child and Adolescent Psychiatry, 35*(7), 865–877.

Shapiro, C. J., & Smith, B. H. (2002). Parent guidance and consultation. In D. Kaye, M. Montgomery, & S. Munson (Eds.), *Child and adolescent mental health* (pp. 18–30). Philadelphia: Lippincott, Williams & Wilkins.

Sharpley, C. F., & Rogers, H. J. (1984). Preliminary validation of the Abbreviated Spanier Dyadic Adjustment Scale: Some psychometric data regarding a screening test of marital adjustment. *Educational and Psychological Measurement, 44*(4), 1045–1050.

Shaw, D. S., Dishion, T. J., Supplee, L., Gardner, F., & Arnds, K. (2006). Randomized trial of a family-centered approach to the prevention of early conduct problems: Two-year effects of the family check-up in early childhood. *Journal of Consulting and Clinical Psychology, 74*, 1–9.

Smalley, S. L., McGough, J. J., Del'Homme, M., Newdelman, J., Gordon, E., Kim, T., et al. (2000). Familial clustering of symptoms and disruptive behaviors in multiplex families with attention-deficit/hyperactivity disorder. *Journal of the American Academy of Child and Adolescent Psychiatry, 39*(9), 1135–1143.

Smith, B. H. (2006). Rear end validity: A caution. In R. R. Bootzin & P. E. McNight (Eds.), *Strengthening research methodology: Psychological measurement and evaluation* (pp. 233–248). Washington, DC: American Psychological Association.

Smith, B. H., Barkley, R. A., & Shapiro, C. J. (2006). Attention-deficit/hyperactivity disorder. In E. J. Mash & R. A. Barkley (Eds.), *Treatment of childhood disorders* (3rd ed., pp. 65–136). New York: Guilford Press.

Smith, B. H., Cole, W., Ingram, A. D., & Clement, K. (2004). Screening for ADHD among first-year college students: Psychometrics and implications for early intervention programs. *ADHD Report, 12*, 6–10.

Smith, B. H., Molina, B. S. G., & Pelham, W. E. J. (2002). The clinically meaningful link between ADHD and Alcohol. *Alcohol Research and Health, 26*, 122–129.

Smith, B. H., Pelham, W. E., Gnagy, E., Molina, B., & Evans, S. (2000). The reliability, validity, and unique contributions of self-report by adolescents receiving treatment for attention-deficit/hyperactivity disorder. *Journal of Consulting and Clinical Psychology, 68*(3), 489–499.

Snell-Johns, J., Mendez, J., & Smith, B. H. (2004). Evidence-based solutions for overcoming access barriers, decreasing attrition, and promoting change with under-served families. *Journal of Family Psychology, 18*, 19–35.

Solanto, M. V., Abikoff, H., Sonuga-Barke, E., Schachar, R., Logan, G. D., Wigal, T., et al. (2001). The ecological validity of delay aversion and response inhibition as measures of impulsivity in ADHD: A supplement to the NIMH multimodal treatment study of ADHD. *Journal of Abnormal Child Psychology, 29*(3), 215–228.

Spanier, G. B., & Cole, C. L. (1976). Toward clarification and investigation of marital adjustment. *International Journal of Sociology of the Family, 6*(1), 121–146.

Sparrow, S. S., Balla, D. A., & Cicchetti, D. (1984). *Vineland Adaptive Behavior Scales*. Bloomington, MN: Pearson Assessments.

Spencer, T. J., Faraone, S. V., Biederman, J., Lerner, M., Cooper, K. M., & Zimmerman, B. (2006). Does prolonged therapy with a long-acting stimulant suppress growth in children with ADHD? *Journal of the American Academy of Child and Adolescent Psychiatry, 45*(5), 527–537.

Spitzer, R. L., Davies, M., & Barkley, R. A. (1990). The DSM-III-R field trial of disruptive behavior disorders. *Journal of the American Academy of Child and Adolescent Psychiatry, 29*(5), 690–697.

Stein, M. A., Szumowski, E., Blondis, T. A., & Roizen, N. J. (1995). Adaptive skills dysfunction in ADD and ADHD children. *Journal of Child Psychology and Psychiatry and Allied Disciplines, 36*(4), 663–670.

Still, G. F. (1902). Some abnormal psychical conditions in children. *Lancet, 1*, 1008–1012, 1077–1082, 1163–1168.

Stranger, C., & Lewis, M. (1993). Agreement among parents, teachers, and children on internalizing and externalizing behavior problems. *Journal of Consulting and Clinical Psychology, 22*, 107–115.

Strauss, A. A., & Lehtinen, L. E. (1947). *Psychopathology and education of the brain-injured child*. New York: Grune & Stratton.

Strauss, M. E., Thompson, P., Adams, N. L., Redline, S., & Burant, C. (2000). Evaluation of a model of attention with confirmatory factor analysis. *Neuropsychology, 14*, 210–208.

Streissguth, A. P., Bookstein, F. L., Sampson, P. D., & Parr, H. M. (1995). Attention: Prenatal alcohol and continuities of vigilance and attentional problems from 4 through 14 years. *Development and Psychopathology, 7*(3), 419–446.

Stroes, A. D., Alberts, E., & Van der Meere, J. J. (2003). Boys with ADHD in social interaction with a nonfamiliar adult: An observational study. *Journal of the American Academy of Child and Adolescent Psychiatry, 42*(3), 295–302.

Stuss, D. T., & Benson, D. F. (1986). *The frontal lobes*. New York: Raven Press.

Sugawara, M., Yagishita, A., Takuma, N., Koizumi, T., Sechiyama, H., Sugawara, K., et al. (2002). Marital relations and depression in school-age children: Links with family functioning and parental attitudes toward child rearing. *Japanese Journal of Educational Psychology, 50*(2), 129–140.

Swaab-Barneveld, H., de Sonneville, L., Cohen-Kettenis, P., Gielen, A., Buitelaar, J., & van Engeland, H. (2000). Visual sustained attention in a child psychiatric population. *Journal of the American Academy of Child and Adolescent Psychiatry, 39*(5), 651–659.

Swanson, J. M., Kraemer, H. C., Hinshaw, S. P., Arnold, L. E., Conners, C. K., Abikoff, H. B., et al. (2001). Clinical relevance of the primary findings of the MTA: Success rates based on severity of ADHD and ODD symptoms at the end of treatment. *Journal of the American Academy of Child and Adolescent Psychiatry, 40*(2), 168–179.

Swanson, J. M., Sunohara, G. A., Kennedy, J. L., Regino, R., Fineberg, E., Wigal, T., et al. (1998). Association of the dopamine receptor D4 (DRD4) gene with a refined phenotype of attention deficit hyperactivity disorder (ADHD): A family-based approach. *Molecular Psychiatry, 3*(1), 38–41.

Szapocznik, J., Perezvidal, A., Brickman, A. L., Foote, F. H., Santisteban, D., Hervis, O., et al. (1988). Engaging adolescent drug abusers and their families in treatment: A strategic structural systems approach. *Journal of Consulting and Clinical Psychology, 56*(4), 552–557.

Szatmari, P., Offord, D. R., & Boyle, M. H. (1989). Correlates, associated impairments and patterns of service utilization of children with attention deficit disorder: Findings from the Ontario Child Health

Study. *Journal of Child Psychology and Psychiatry and Allied Disciplines, 30*(2), 205–217.

Tallmadge, J., & Barkley, R. A. (1983). The interactions of hyperactive and normal boys with their fathers and mothers. *Journal of Abnormal Child Psychology, 11*(4), 565–580.

Tannock, R. (1998). Attention deficit hyperactivity disorder: Advances in cognitive, neurobiological, and genetic research. *Journal of Child Psychology and Psychiatry, 39*(1), 65–99.

Tannock, R. (2000). Attention deficit disorders with anxiety disorders. In T. E. Brown (Ed.), *Subtypes of attention deficit disorders in children, adolescents, and adults.* Washington, DC: American Psychiatric Press.

Tannock, R., & Brown, T. (2000). Attention-deficit disorders with learning disorders in children and adolescents. In T. Brown (Ed.), *Attention-deficit disorders and comorbidities in children, adolescents, and adults* (pp. 231–296). Washington, DC: American Psychiatric Press.

Taylor, E. (1986). *The overactive child.* Philadelphia: Lippincott.

Teicher, M. H., Anderson, C. M., Polcari, A., Glod, C. A., Maas, L. C., & Renshaw, P. F. (2000). Functional deficits in basal ganglia of children with attention-deficit/hyperactivity disorder shown with functional magnetic resonance imaging relaxometry. *Nature Medicine, 6,* 470–473.

Teicher, M. H., Ito, Y., Glod, C. A., & Barber, N. I. (1996). Objective measurement of hyperactivity and attentional problems in ADHD. *Journal of the American Academy of Child and Adolescent Psychiatry, 35,* 334–342.

Thompson, L. L., Riggs, P. D., Mikulich, S. K., & Crowley, T. J. (1996). Contribution of ADHD symptoms to substance problems and delinquency in conduct-disordered adolescents. *Journal of Abnormal Child Psychology, 24*(3), 325–347.

Todd, R. D., Rasmussen, E. R., Wood, C., Levy, F., & Hay, D. A. (2004). Should sluggish cognitive tempo symptoms be included in the diagnosis of attention-deficit/hyperactivity disorder? *Journal of the American Academy of Child and Adolescent Psychiatry, 43*(5), 588–597.

Torgesen, J. K. (1994). Issues in the assessment of executive function: An information-processing perspective. In G. R. Lyon (Ed.), *Frames of reference for the assessment of learning disabilities: New views on measurement issues* (pp. 143–162). Baltimore: Brookes.

Tripp, G., & Luk, S. L. (1997). The identification of pervasive hyperactivity: Is clinic observation necessary? *Journal of Child Psychology and Psychiatry and Allied Disciplines, 38*(2), 219–234.

Vaidya, C. J., Austin, G., Kirkorian, G., Ridlehuber, H. W., Desmond, J. E., Glover, G. H., et al. (1998). Selective effects of methylphenidate in attention deficit hyperactivity disorder: A functional magnetic resonance study. *Proceedings of the National Academy of*

Sciences of the United States of America, 95, 14494–14499.

Vaughn, M. L., Riccio, C. A., Hynd, G. W., & Hall, J. (1997). Diagnosing ADHD (predominantly inattentive and combined type subtypes): Discriminant validity of the Behavior Assessment System for Children and the Achenbach Parent and Teacher Rating Scales. *Journal of Clinical Child Psychology, 26*(4), 349–357.

Velez, C. N., Johnson, J., & Cohen, P. (1989). A longitudinal analysis of selected risk factors for childhood psychopathology. *Journal of the American Academy of Child and Adolescent Psychiatry, 28*(6), 861–864.

Voelker, S. L., Carter, R. A., Sprague, D. J., Gdowski, C. L., & Lachar, D. (1989). Developmental trends in memory and metamemory in children with attention deficit disorder. *Journal of Pediatric Psychology, 14*(1), 75–88.

Webb, E. J., Campbell, D. T., Schwartz, R. D., & Sechrest, L. (1966). *Unobtrusive measures: Nonreactive research in the social sciences.* Oxford, UK: Rand McNally.

Welsh, M. C., & Pennington, B. F. (1988). Assessing frontal lobe functioning in children: Views from developmental psychology. *Developmental Neuropsychology, 4,* 199–230.

Weiss, G., & Hechtman, L. T. (1993). *Hyperactive children grown up: ADHD in children, adolescents, and adults* (2nd ed.). New York: Guilford Press.

Weissman, M. M., Pilowsky, D. J., Wickramaratne, P. J., Talati, A., Wisniewski, S. R., Fava, M., et al. (2006). Remissions in maternal depression and child psychopathology—A STAR*D-Child report. *Journal of the American Medical Association, 295*(12), 1389–1398.

Wender, P. H. (1971). *Minimal brain dysfunction in children.* New York: Wiley.

Werry, J. S., Reeves, J. C., & Elkind, G. S. (1987). Attention-deficit, conduct, oppositional, and anxiety disorders in children: 1. A review of research on differentiating characteristics. *Journal of the American Academy of Child and Adolescent Psychiatry, 26*(2), 133–143.

Werry, J. S., & Sprague, R. L. (1970). Hyperactivity. In C. G. Costello (Ed.), *Symptoms of psychopathology* (pp. 397–417). New York: Wiley.

Whalen, C. K., Henker, B., & Dotemoto, S. (1980). Methylphenidate and hyperactivity: Effects on teacher behaviors. *Science, 208,* 1280–1282.

Whalen, C. L., Henker, B., Ishikawa, S. S., Jamner, L. D., Floro, J. N., Jophnston, J. A., et al. (2006). An electronic diary study of contextual triggers and ADHD: Get ready, get set, get mad. *Journal of the American Academy of Child and Adolescent Psychiatry, 45,* 166–174.

Whittaker, J. (1997). *Developmental neuropsychiatry, Volume 1. Fundamentals. Volume 2, Assessment, diagnosis and treatment of developmental disorders* by J. C. Harris [Book review]. *Psychological Medicine, 27*(5), 1235–1236.

Wiersema, J. R., van der Meere, J. J., & Roeyers, H. (2005). ERP correlates of impaired error monitoring in children with ADHD. *Journal of Neural Transmission, 112*(10), 1417–1430.

Wilens, T. E., & Dodson, W. (2004). A clinical perspective of attention-deficit/hyperactivity disorder into adulthood. *Journal of Clinical Psychiatry, 65*(10), 1301–1313.

Wilens, T. E., Faraone, S. V., Biederman, J., & Gunawardene, S. (2003). Does stimulant therapy of attention-deficit/hyperactivity disorder beget later substance abuse?: A meta-analytic review of the literature. *Pediatrics, 111*(1), 179–185.

Wills, T. A., & Dishion, T. J. (2004). Temperament and adolescent substance use: A transactional analysis of emerging self-control. *Journal of Clinical Child and Adolescent Psychology, 33*(1), 69–81.

Wolraich, M. L. (Ed.). (2002). *Current assessment and treatment practices in ADHD.* Kingston, NJ: Civic Research Institute.

Wolraich, M. L., Lambert, E. W., Baumgaertel, A., Garcia-Tornel, S., Feurer, I. D., Bickman, L., et al. (2003). Teachers' screening for attention deficit/hyperactivity disorder: Comparing multinational samples on teacher ratings of ADHD. *Journal of Abnormal Child Psychology, 31*(4), 445–455.

Wolraich, M. L., Wibbelsman, C. J., Brown, T. E., Evans, S. W., Gotlieb, E. M., Knight, J. R., et al. (2005). Attention-deficit/hyperactivity disorder among adolescents: A review of the diagnosis, treatment, and clinical implications. *Pediatrics, 115*(6), 1734–1746.

Yeo, R. A., Hill, D. E., Campbell, R. A., Vigil, J., Petropoulos, H., Hart, B., et al. (2003). Proton magnetic resonance spectroscopy investigation of the right frontal lobe in children with attention-deficit/hyperactivity disorder. *Journal of the American Academy of Child and Adolescent Psychiatry, 42*(3), 303–310.

Zagar, R., & Bowers, N. (1983). The effect of time of day on problem solving and classroom behavior. *Psychology in the Schools, 20,* 337–345.

Zalecki, C. A., & Hinshaw, S. P. (2004). Overt and relational aggression in girls with attention deficit hyperactivity disorder. *Journal of Clinical Child and Adolescent Psychology, 33*(1), 125–137.

Zametkin, A. J., Nordahl, T. E., Gross, M., King, A. C., Semple, W. E., Rumsey, J., et al. (1990). Cerebral glucose metabolism in adults with hyperactivity of childhood onset. *New England Journal of Medicine, 323*(20), 1361–1366.

Zentall, S. S. (1985). Stimulus-control factors in search performance of hyperactive children. *Journal of Learning Disabilities, 18*(8), 480–485.

Zentall, S. S. (1988). Production deficiencies in elicited language but not in the spontaneous verbalizations of hyperactive children. *Journal of Abnormal Child Psychology, 16*(6), 657–673.

Zentall, S. S., Falkenberg, S. D., & Smith, L. B. (1985). Effects of color stimulation and information on the copying performance of attention-problem adolescents. *Journal of Abnormal Child Psychology, 13,* 501–511.

Zentall, S. S., & Smith, Y. N. (1993). Mathematical performance and behavior of children with hyperactivity with and without coexisting aggression. *Behaviour Research and Therapy, 31*(7), 701–710.

APPENDIX 2.1. Parenting Experiences Inventory

Below is a list of issues related to being a parent. Please circle the number describing the response that best describes how you honestly feel.

1. In an overall sense, how difficult has your teenager's behavior been over the past 6 weeks?

Not at All	Slightly	Moderately	Very	Extremely
1	2	3	4	5

2. To what extent do the following statements describe your experiences as a parent in the last 6 weeks?

	Not at All	Slightly	Moderately	Very	Extremely
Parenting is rewarding	1	2	3	4	5
Parenting is demanding	1	2	3	4	5
Parenting is stressful	1	2	3	4	5
Parenting is fulfilling	1	2	3	4	5
Parenting is depressing	1	2	3	4	5

3. In the past 6 weeks, how confident have you felt to undertake your responsibilities as a parent?

Not at All	Slightly	Moderately	Very	Extremely
1	2	3	4	5

4. How supported have you felt in your role as a parent over the past 6 weeks?

Not at All	Slightly	Moderately	Very	Extremely
1	2	3	4	5

If you have a partner, please complete the following items:

5. To what extent do you both agree over methods of disciplining your child?

Not at All	Slightly	Moderately	Very	Extremely
1	2	3	4	5

6. How supportive has your partner been toward you in your role as a parent over the past 6 weeks?

Not at All	Slightly	Moderately	Very	Extremely
1	2	3	4	5

7. In an overall sense, how happy are you with your relationship with your partner?

Not at All	Slightly	Moderately	Very	Extremely
1	2	3	4	5

APPENDIX 2.2. Getting to Know You

Parent Name: _____

Child Name: _____

Instructions: Here is a variety of questions regarding your child's peer relationships, school preferences, family interactions, support networks, involvement in community activities, and hobbies. Please answer each question as completely as possible. When asked to provide a number of hours spent on an activity, please give your best guess. It is acceptable to give a range or provide more information on the back of this sheet.

PEERS

1. My child has a best friend.   ☐ Yes   ☐ No

2. My child makes friends easily.   ☐ Yes   ☐ No

3. My child shows strong leadership skills most of the time.   ☐ Yes   ☐ No

4. My child enjoys organized youth activities   ☐ Yes   ☐ No
   (e.g., sports, scouts, church activities).

5. My child is good at sports (e.g., is athletic).   ☐ Yes   ☐ No

6. My child's favorite sports are _____
   _____.

7. My child spends an average of ____ hours exercising each week.

SCHOOL

8. My child's best academic subjects are _____ and
   _____.

9. My child's favorite part about school is _____
   _____.

10. My child spends ____ hours on homework each night.

FAMILY

11. My child has regular contact with extended family

12. My child has contact with the following adults on a regular basis (include parents in list, and list relationship of each person to your child; do not include teachers unless your child sees them regularly outside of school):
    _____
    _____
    _____

RELIGION

13. My child is active in the church community.   ☐ Yes   ☐ No

14. My child attends church regularly   ☐ Yes   ☐ No

ACTIVITIES

14. My child enjoys the following pastimes/hobbies: _____, _____,
    and _____.

15. If your child was not attending CHP, what would they be doing or where would they be going instead? _____
    _____
    _____

16. My child uses the computer for ____ hours a day during the week and ____ hours a day on weekends.

17. My child watches TV for ____ hours a day during the week and ____ hours a day on weekends.

18. My child plays videogames for ____ hours a day during the week and ____ hours a day on weekends.

19. My child listens to music for ____ hours a day during the week and ____ hours a day on weekends.

20. My child does chores for ____ hours a day during the week and ____ hours a day on weekends.

20. My child spends ____ hours doing _____ each weekday and ____ hours doing that activity on the weekends (please list any other activity not mentioned that your child engages in regularly, excluding necessary activities like eating, sleeping, or showering).

21. Please list any other information you feel we should know about your child:

_____

_____

_____

Getting to Know You Form

Practitioner: _____

Client number: _____ Date: _____

1. Teenager Behavior—Female Guardian's Ratings

Please rate your teenager's behavior by checking "Yes" or "No" next to each issue to indicate if it is a main concern for your family.

	Yes	No			Yes	No	
1.	☐	☐	Arguing with or talking back to adults	15.	☐	☐	Sulking
2.	☐	☐	Screaming, yelling, or shouting	16.	☐	☐	Lack of physical activity
3.	☐	☐	Fighting with siblings	17.	☐	☐	Unhappy with school
4.	☐	☐	Physically fighting	18.	☐	☐	Fearful or anxious
5.	☐	☐	Too much television or video games	19.	☐	☐	Sleeping problems
6.	☐	☐	Not doing homework	20.	☐	☐	Eating problems
7.	☐	☐	Not minding; deliberate disobedience	21.	☐	☐	Hyperactivity or attention problems
8.	☐	☐	Lying	22.	☐	☐	Family responsibilities
9.	☐	☐	Stealing	23.	☐	☐	Negative attitude, overly pessimistic
10.	☐	☐	Moodiness or irritability	24.	☐	☐	Rebellious
11.	☐	☐	Swearing; abusive/offensive language	25.	☐	☐	Crying or emotional distress
12.	☐	☐	Physically fighting	26.	☐	☐	Throwing tantrums
13.	☐	☐	Teasing	27.	☐	☐	Shyness
14.	☐	☐	Overly influenced by friends	28.	☐	☐	Finding school difficult or not trying hard enough

Other concerns not listed above:

2. Family Stresses

Please identify any stressors (issues or events) over the past year in the family that relate to the presenting problems or get in the way of making changes.

☐ Parent has health problem	☐ Parent not in home, uncooperative or unavailable
☐ Parent work schedule	☐ Unstable home situation
☐ Stress between home and school	☐ Parent has mental health problem
☐ Child has reading problems	☐ Separation/divorce
☐ Domestic violence	☐ Recent remarriage
☐ High-crime neighborhood	☐ Other stressors _____
☐ Spending time with friends	_____
☐ Death in the family	_____
☐ Past traumatic experience (abuse or other event)	_____
☐ Drug use by parent	_____
☐ Drug use by sibling	_____
☐ Ongoing conflict between caretakers	

Getting to Know You Form

Practitioner: _____

Client number: _____ Date: _____

1. Teenager Behavior—Male Guardian's Ratings

Please rate your teenager's behavior by checking "Yes" or "No" next to each issue to indicate if it is a main concern for your family.

	Yes	No				Yes	No	
1.	☐	☐	Arguing with or talking back to adults		15.	☐	☐	Sulking
2.	☐	☐	Screaming, yelling, or shouting		16.	☐	☐	Lack of physical activity
3.	☐	☐	Fighting with siblings		17.	☐	☐	Unhappy with school
4.	☐	☐	Physically fighting		18.	☐	☐	Fearful or anxious
5.	☐	☐	Too much television or video games		19.	☐	☐	Sleeping problems
6.	☐	☐	Not doing homework		20.	☐	☐	Eating problems
7.	☐	☐	Not minding; deliberate disobedience		21.	☐	☐	Hyperactivity or attention problems
8.	☐	☐	Lying		22.	☐	☐	Family responsibilities
9.	☐	☐	Stealing		23.	☐	☐	Negative attitude, overly pessimistic
10.	☐	☐	Moodiness or irritability		24.	☐	☐	Rebellious
11.	☐	☐	Swearing; abusive/offensive language		25.	☐	☐	Crying or emotional distress
12.	☐	☐	Physically fighting		26.	☐	☐	Throwing tantrums
13.	☐	☐	Teasing		27.	☐	☐	Shyness
14.	☐	☐	Overly influenced by friends		28.	☐	☐	Finding school difficult or not trying hard enough

Other concerns not listed above:

2. Family Stresses

Please identify any stressors (issues or events) over the past year in the family that relate to the presenting problems or get in the way of making changes.

☐ Parent has health problem	☐ Parent not in home, uncooperative or unavailable
☐ Parent work schedule	
☐ Stress between home and school	☐ Unstable home situation
☐ Child has reading problems	☐ Parent has mental health problem
☐ Domestic violence	☐ Separation/divorce
☐ High-crime neighborhood	☐ Recent remarriage
☐ Spending time with friends	☐ Other stressors _____
☐ Death in the family	_____
☐ Past traumatic experience (abuse or other event)	_____
☐ Drug use by parent	_____
☐ Drug use by sibling	_____
☐ Ongoing conflict between caretakers	

Now that the guardian(s) have completed their ratings independently, have them each choose the three most troubling teenager behaviors out of those they identified as problematic or "of concern."

Female guardian's choices:

_____

_____

Male guardian's choices:

_____

_____

Establish approximate frequency of each of those problem behaviors (per minute, hour, or month).

_____

_____

_____

_____

Establish approximate duration of each occurrence of problem behavior.

_____

_____

_____

_____

_____

Note other relevant information (date of onset of the problem behavior, changes over time, how the behavior is dealt with by other caretakers).

_____

_____

_____

_____

_____

3. Developmental History
Note any significant deviations from normal developmental milestones and any factors that may affect the teenager's development.

_____

_____

_____

_____

4. Health Status
Note general information regarding health status that may influence the teenager's behavior and/or the parent's/s' ability to implement a parenting plan (e.g., current medical conditions or disabilities; significant previous illness, operations, or hospitalizations; medication).

_____

_____

_____

_____

Is a medical examination indicated? (Yes/No)

_____

If so, why?

_____

5. Educational History
List any significant events relating to school that may have a bearing on the teenager's present problems. Explore academic performance, behavior at school, and peer relationships.

_____

_____

_____

_____

_____

6. **Family Relationships and Interactions**

Explore the teenager's family unit and living arrangements (e.g., family members, caregivers). Explore the nature of parent–teenager relationships and the teenager's relationships with other family members. Check for any other family issues that may create obstacles to therapeutic change (e.g., parental adjustment problems, financial concerns, other stressors).

_____

_____

_____

_____

_____

7. **Observation of Parent–Teenager Interaction (where appropriate)**

Note any significant observations about parent–teenager interaction in the session or in the waiting room, such as praise comments (descriptive vs. general), instructions (specific vs. vague), accidental rewards for problem behavior, and discipline strategies used. Try to note strengths and weaknesses, and record specific examples of interactions.

_____

_____

_____

_____

_____

APPENDIX 2.3. Feedback from Family Checkup

ADHD Symptoms ⊘	Related Strengths	Related Challenges
Inattention ◯		
Impulsivity ◯		
Hyperactivity ◯		

Comorbid Conditions	Related Strengths	Related Challenges
ODD ◯		
CD ◯		
Depression ◯		
Anxiety ◯		
Other ◯		

Parent's Agreement	Strengths	Challenges
Relationship Quality ◯		
Problem Definition ◯		
Problem Solution ◯		
Other issues ◯		

Interactions with Parents	Strengths	Challenges
Mother ◯		
Father ◯		
Others ◯		

Interactions with Teachers	Strengths	Challenges
Teacher ○		
Name:		
Teacher ○		
Name:		
Teacher ○		
Name:		

Academic Progress	Strengths	Challenges
In General ○		
School Behavior ○		
Ability ○		
Other ○		

Relationship with Peers	Strengths	Challenges
Friends ○		
Siblings ○		
Peers at School ○		
Other Peers ○		

Menu

Area of Change (red)	Goal	Options

CHAPTER 3

Conduct and Oppositional Disorders

Robert J. McMahon
Paul J. Frick

Conduct problems (CPs) in youth have been a major focus of research and practice in child psychology for a number of reasons. CPs are some of the most common reasons that children and adolescents are referred to mental health clinics (Frick & Silverthorn, 2001), cause significant disruptions for the child at home (Frick, 1998) and school (Gottfredson & Gottfredson, 2001), and are the form of psychopathology most strongly associated with delinquency (Moffitt, 1993). An extensive body of research has led to an increased understanding of the many processes that may be involved in the development of severe CPs (Dodge & Pettit, 2003; Frick, 1998; Loeber & Farrington, 2000; Raine, 2002) with important implications for designing more effective interventions to prevent or treat these problems (Conduct Problems Prevention Research Group, 2000; Frick, 1998, 2001, 2006).

Unfortunately, little attention has been paid to the implications that this research may have for improving the methods for assessing children and adolescents with severe CPs (McMahon & Frick, 2005). However, if the field is to continue to improve its intervention technology by being guided by advances in research, it is critical that assessment strategies used in practice also be informed by research findings.

An exhaustive review of recent research on CPs and their implications for the clinical assessment of antisocial youth is not possible within the space limitations of this chapter. However, in the next section we provide an overview of four sets of findings from research that have clear and important implications for the evidence-based assessment of children with CPs: (1) heterogeneity in the types and severity of CPs, (2) CPs and comorbid problems in adjustment, (3) the multiple risks associated with CPs, and (4) the multiple developmental pathways of CPs. This is followed by an overview of assessment issues and a more extended discussion of the implications of the research on CPs for guiding clinical assessments within each of the four areas. We also identify key measures that we believe have potential for contributing to the evidence-based assessment of CPs. We conclude with a summary and recommendations for future research.

KEY FINDINGS FROM RESEARCH ON CHILDHOOD CPs

Heterogeneity in the Types and Severity of CPs

CPs constitute a broad spectrum of "acting-out" behaviors, ranging from relatively minor oppositional behaviors, such as yelling and temper tantrums, to more serious forms of antisocial behavior, such as aggression, physical destructiveness, and stealing. When displayed as a cluster, these behaviors have been referred to as "oppositional," "antisocial," "conduct-disordered," and "delinquent" (see Hinshaw & Lee [2003] for a thorough discussion of terminology). Our conceptualization of CPs is consistent, but not isomorphic, with the *Diagnostic and Statistical Manual of Mental Disorders* (4th edition, text revision [DSM-IV-TR]; American Psychiatric Association [APA], 2000) diagnostic categories of oppositional defiant disorder (ODD) and conduct disorder (CD). ODD is a pattern of negativistic (e.g., deliberately doing things that annoy other people, blaming others for one's own mistakes), disobedient (e.g., defying or not complying with grownups' rules or requests), and hostile behaviors (e.g., losing one's temper). CD consists of more severe antisocial and aggressive behavior that involves serious violations of others' rights or deviations from major age-appropriate norms. The behaviors are categorized into four groups: aggressiveness to people and animals (e.g., bullying, fighting); property destruction (e.g., firesetting, other destruction of property); deceptiveness or theft (e.g., breaking and entering, stealing without confronting the victim); and serious rule violations (e.g., running away from home, being truant from school before age 13).

In addition to the DSM-IV-TR distinction between ODD and CD, other methods have been used to separate different types of CP behaviors. Frick and colleagues (1993) conducted a meta-analysis of over 60 published factor analyses on more than 28,401 children and adolescents. They found that CPs may be described by two bipolar dimensions. In the first, an overt–covert dimension, the overt pole comprises directly confrontational behaviors such as oppositional defiant behaviors and aggression. In contrast, the covert pole comprises behaviors that are nonconfrontational in nature (e.g., stealing, lying) (see also Patterson & Yoerger, 2002; Tiet, Wasserman, Loeber, Larken, & Miller, 2001; Tolan, Gorman-Smith, & Loeber, 2000; Willoughby, Kupersmidt, & Bryant, 2001). However, a second dimension also seemed to be important for explaining the covariation of CPs. This destructive–nondestructive dimension divides the overt behaviors into those that are overt–destructive (aggression) and those that are overt–

nondestructive (oppositional), and it divides the covert behaviors into those that are covert–destructive (property violations) and those that are covert–nondestructive (status offenses; i.e., behaviors that are illegal because of the child's or adolescent's age).

The clustering of CPs into these four symptom patterns has proven to be useful for three purposes. First, this division of CPs is fairly consistent with the distinctions made in many legal systems for differentiating types of delinquent behaviors, which generally distinguish between violent offenses (overt–destructive), status offenses (covert–nondestructive), and property offenses (covert–destructive; e.g., Office of Juvenile Justice and Delinquency Prevention, 1995). Second, this grouping of CPs can aid in distinguishing between youth who show a single type of CP (e.g., aggressive behavior only) and those who show a more varied pattern of CP behavior (e.g., both aggression and status offenses) (see Christian, Frick, Hill, Tyler, & Frazer, 1997). This distinction is important, because the more varied pattern of CP is associated with a poorer outcome (Frick & Loney, 1999; Loeber et al., 1993). Third, there may be differences in the etiology of different types of CP. For example, a twin study found that genetic factors seem to play a greater role in the development of the destructive behaviors (i.e., property violations and aggression) than in the development of the nondestructive behaviors (i.e., oppositional, status offenses) (Simonoff, Pickles, Meyer, Silberg, & Maes, 1998).

Two specific forms of CP behavior—noncompliance and aggression—deserve additional attention. Noncompliance (i.e., excessive disobedience to adults) appears to be a keystone behavior in the development of CPs. It appears early in the progression of CPs and continues to be manifested in subsequent developmental periods (e.g., Chamberlain & Patterson, 1995; Loeber et al., 1993; McMahon & Forehand, 2003), playing a role in subsequent academic and peer relationship problems. Low levels of compliance are also associated with referral for services in young children with CPs (Dumas, 1996). Furthermore, intervention research has shown that when child noncompliance is targeted, there is often concomitant improvement in other CP behaviors as well (Russo, Cataldo, & Cushing, 1981; Wells, Forehand, & Griest, 1980).

The importance of aggression as a CP dimension is supported by research showing that aggressive behavior in children and adolescents is often quite stable and very difficult to treat (Broidy et al., 2003). Importantly, there appear to be several different forms of aggressive behavior (Crick & Dodge, 1996; Poulin & Boivin, 2000). The first type of aggression, often referred to as retaliatory, hostile, or reactive aggression, is viewed as a defensive reaction to a perceived threat and is characterized by anger and hostility (Crick & Dodge, 1996). The second type of aggressive behavior is generally unprovoked, and is used for personal gain (instrumental) or to influence and coerce others (bullying and dominance). This type of aggressive behavior is referred to as instrumental, premeditated, or proactive aggression (Poulin & Boivin, 2000).

These different types of aggression often co-occur, with correlations ranging from $r = .40–.70$ in school-age samples (Frick & Marsee, 2006). Despite this high degree of association, many studies have documented different correlates to the two forms of aggression. For example, reactive aggression has been associated with higher risk for social isolation and social rejection by peers (Dodge & Pettit, 2003), and a temperamental propensity for angry reactivity and emotional dysregulation (Hubbard et al., 2002). Reactively aggressive youth also show a number of deficits in their social information processing, such as difficulty employing effective problem-solving skills in social situations and a hostile attributional bias to ambiguous provocation situations (Crick & Dodge, 1996). Proactively aggressive youth, on the other hand, associate more positive outcomes with their aggressive behavior and report significantly fewer symptoms related to anxiety than do reactively aggressive youth (Schwartz et al., 1998). In addition to proactive and reactive forms of aggression, both of which are overt in nature, Crick and colleagues have identified a form of indirect aggression, called "relational aggression," that involves strategies such as social isolation and exclusion, and behaviors that include slandering, rumor spreading, and manipulating friendships (e.g., Crick & Grotpeter, 1995). Evidence suggests that relational aggression occurs more frequently in girls (Underwood, 2003), and it may be possible to divide it into instrumental and reactive forms as well (Little, Jones, Henrich, & Hawley, 2003).

CP and Comorbid Problems in Adjustment

Another important finding from research is that youth with CPs are at increased risk for manifesting a variety of other adjustment problems as well. There are a number of possible reasons for this high rate of comorbidity. It is possible that the CP behaviors disrupt the child's or adolescent's psychosocial context, resulting in other problems in adjustment, such as anxiety and depression (Capaldi, 1992; Frick, Lilienfeld, Ellis, Loney, & Silverthorn, 1999). It is also possible that the CP itself is a result of the comorbid conditions, such as the result of impulsivity associated with attention-deficit/hyperactivity disorder (ADHD) (Burns & Walsh, 2002). Finally, it is also possible that the same risk factors (e.g., deficits in social cognition) may lead to the CPs and co-occurring problems in adjustment, such as peer rejection (Dodge & Pettit, 2003). Whatever the reason, understanding the common comorbid problems has proven to be very important for understanding and treating children and adolescents with CPs.

ADHD, the comorbid condition most commonly associated with CPs, is thought to precede the development of CPs in the majority of cases. In a meta-analytic study, Waschbush (2002) reported that 36% of boys and 57% of girls with CPs had comorbid ADHD. Some investigators consider ADHD (or, more specifically, the impulsivity or hyperactivity components of ADHD) to be the "motor" that drives the development of early-onset CPs, especially for boys (e.g., Burns & Walsh, 2002; Moffitt, 1993). Importantly, the presence of ADHD usually signals the presence of a more severe and more chronic form of CPs in children (see Waschbush, 2002). For example, children with both ADHD and CD seem to show a greater variety of delinquent (Loeber, Brinthaupt, & Green, 1990) and aggressive (Moffitt, 1993) behaviors in adolescence, and more violent offending in adulthood (Klinteberg, Andersson, Magnusson, & Stattin, 1993).

Internalizing disorders, such as depression and anxiety, also co-occur with CPs at rates higher than expected by chance (Zoccolillo, 1992). In most cases, CPs precede the onset of depressive and anxiety symptoms (Loeber & Keenan, 1994), although in a minority of cases depression may precede CP behavior (e.g., Kovacs, Paulauskas, Gatsonis, & Richards, 1988). However, this relationship between CPs and depression may be due to common risk factors as opposed to a causal relationship (Fergusson, Lynskey, & Horwood, 1996). Also, the relationship appears to differ for boys and girls, at least during middle to late adolescence. Wiesner (2003) found a reciprocal relationship between delinquent behaviors and depressive symptoms for girls, whereas for boys, the effect of delinquent behavior on depressive symptoms was unidirectional. Regardless of the temporal sequencing, the co-occurrence of CPs and depression appears to increase the risk for suicide in youth (e.g., Capaldi, 1991, 1992), and this risk appears to be higher for girls than for boys (Loeber & Keenan, 1994).

Additionally, Loeber and Keenan (1994) indicated that the co-occurrence of anxiety disorders with CPs is also especially likely for girls. The implications of comorbid anxiety have been unclear. In some studies, youth with CPs and a comorbid anxiety disorder are less seriously impaired than are youth with CPs alone (e.g., Walker et al., 1991); in other studies, the presence of a comorbid anxiety disorder has not been shown to have a differential effect (e.g., Campbell & Ewing, 1990); still other studies indicate that comorbid anxiety is associated with increased impairment (e.g., Serbin, Moskowitz, Schwartzman, & Ledingham, 1991). In trying to explain these inconsistent findings, Frick, Lilienfeld, and colleagues (1999) demonstrated that low levels of anxiety in some children with CPs may be a sign of a more severe type of disturbance, in which the child is not distressed by the consequences of his or her behavior whereas, in other children with CPs, higher levels of anxiety may be due to the greater levels of impairment and stress caused by more severe behavioral problems.

Both longitudinal and cross-sectional studies have documented that having CPs constitutes a significant risk factor for substance use (e.g., Hawkins, Catalano, & Miller, 1992). The comorbidity between CPs and substance abuse is important, because when youths with CPs also abuse substances, they tend to show an early onset of substance use and are more likely to abuse multiple substances (Lynskey & Fergusson, 1995). Although most of the research on the association between CPs and substance abuse prior to adulthood has been conducted with adolescents, the association between CPs and substance use may begin much earlier in development (Van Kammen, Loeber, & Stouthamer-Loeber, 1991).

With preschool-age children, language impairment may be associated with increased levels of CPs. Wakschlag and Danis (2004) suggest that if the CPs appear to result primarily as a reaction to frustration, or if the child's noncompliance appears to be due to a failure to understand directions from parents or teachers, then a language impairment may be implicated. An association between CPs and academic underachievement has also been documented in research. Approximately 20–25% of youth with CD underachieve in school relative to a level predicted by their age and intellectual abilities (Frick et al., 1991). In a comprehensive review, Hinshaw (1992) concluded that during preadolescence, this relationship is actually a function of comorbid ADHD rather than of CPs per se. In adolescence, the relationship is more complex, with preexisting ADHD (and perhaps other neuropsychological deficits), a history of academic difficulty and failure, and long-standing socialization difficulties with family and peers all playing interacting roles.

Multiple Risks Associated with CPs

Most researchers agree that CPs are the result of a complex interaction of multiple causal factors (Frick, 2006; Hinshaw & Lee, 2003; McMahon, Wells, & Kotler, 2006). Identifying the important causal agents and how they interact to cause CPs is an area in need of more research. Past research has uncovered a large number of factors *associated* with CP and that *may* a play a role in their development and/or maintenance. These factors may be summarized in five categories: biological factors, cognitive correlates, family context, peers, and the broader social ecology.

As noted earlier, a number of researchers have proposed that early hyperactivity is a significant (and perhaps necessary) risk factor for development of CPs (e.g., Loeber & Keenan, 1994; Moffitt, 1993). Moffitt has suggested that subtle neuropsychological variations in the central nervous system increase the likelihood that an infant will display characteristics such as irritability, hyperactivity, impulsivity, and negative emotionality. These temperamental dimensions measured early in life have proven to predict CPs later in preschool (Keenan, Shaw, Delliquadri, Giovannelli, & Walsh, 1998), in childhood (Raine, Reynolds, Venables, & Mednick, 1997), and even into adolescence (Caspi, Henry, Moffitt, & Silva, 1995). There are a number of other biological correlates (e.g., neurochemical and autonomic irregularities) of CPs in children and adolescents (see Dodge & Pettit, 2003; Raine, 2002) that, although crucial for developing causal theories, are not reviewed here, because the current state of knowledge is not sufficiently developed to have clear implications for assessment.

In contrast, several aspects of a youth's cognitive and learning styles that have been associated with CPs may be important to the assessment process (see Frick & Loney, 2000). First, in general, youth with CPs tend to score lower on intelligence tests, especially in the area of verbal intelligence (Loney, Frick, Ellis, & McCoy, 1998; Moffitt, 1993). Furthermore, these scores are predictive of the persistence of childhood-onset CD and of engagement in delinquent behaviors during adolescence (Frick & Loney, 1999). Second, many children and adolescents with serious CPs tend to show a learning style that is more sensitive to rewards than punishments. This has been labeled as a reward-dominant response style, and may explain why many of these youth persist in their maladaptive behaviors despite the threat of serious potential consequences (Frick, Cornell, Bodin, et al., 2003; O'Brien & Frick, 1996). Third, many youth with CPs show a variety of deficits in social cognition, which is the way they interpret and use social cues to respond in social situations (Crick & Dodge, 1994; Webster-Stratton & Lindsay, 1999). For example, children and adolescents with CPs have been shown to have deficits in encoding (e.g., lack of attention to relevant social cues, hypervigilant biases), to make more hostile attributional biases and errors in the interpretation of social cues, to have deficient quantity and quality of generated solutions to social situations, to evaluate aggressive solutions more positively, and to be more likely to engage in aggressive behavior (Dodge & Petit, 2003).

These dispositional characteristics (i.e., difficult temperamental style and deficits in social information processing) may then place the youth at risk for developing an insecure attachment to his or her parent (Greenberg, Speltz, & DeKlyen, 1993) and/or a coercive style of parent–child interaction (Patterson, Reid, & Dishion, 1992). Both of these problems in the parent–child relationship have been implicated in the development of CPs, although the relationship between insecure patterns of attachment in infancy and later CPs is probably mediated or moderated by other risk or protective factors (e.g., parenting practices, maternal depression, family adversity) over time (e.g., Greenberg et al., 1993; Lyons-Ruth, 1996). The critical role of parenting practices in the development and maintenance of CPs has been well established (e.g., Chamberlain & Patterson, 1995; Loeber & Stouthamer-Loeber, 1986). Types of parenting practices that have been closely associated with the development of CPs include inconsistent or irritable, explosive discipline; low supervision and involvement; and inflexible, rigid discipline (Chamberlain, Reid, Ray, Capaldi, & Fisher, 1997).

In addition to parenting practices, various other risk factors may have an impact on the family and serve to precipitate or maintain CPs. These include familial factors such as parental social cognitions (e.g., perceptions of the child), parental personal and marital adjustment, and parental stress, as well as parental functioning in extrafamilial social contexts (McMahon & Estes, 1997). Less clear are the mechanisms by which these factors exert their effects on CPs. For example, these risk factors may have a direct effect on CPs or they may exert their effects by disrupting parenting practices (Patterson et al., 1992). Furthermore, in some cases, the familial "risk" factor may be a *result* of CPs, rather than a potential cause, such as a child or adolescent with CPs being more difficult to monitor and supervise (Stattin & Kerr, 2000). With these caveats in mind, we note some of the relationships of these factors to CPs.

Parents of children with CPs display more maladaptive social cognitions and experience more personal (e.g., depression, antisocial behavior) and interparental (e.g., marital problems) distress, and greater social isolation (e.g., insularity) than do parents of nonreferred youth. Parents of clinic-referred children with CPs more likely misperceive their children's behaviors (e.g., Holleran, Littman, Freund, & Schmaling, 1982; Wahler & Sansbury, 1990), have fewer positive and more negative family-referent cognitions (Sanders & Dadds, 1992), and perceive CP behaviors as intentional and attribute them to stable and global causes (Baden & Howe, 1992). Sense of parenting efficacy has been shown to relate negatively to

CPs in both clinic-referred and nonreferred samples (e.g., Johnston & Mash, 1989; Roberts, Joe, & Rowe-Hallbert, 1992).

Parental personal adjustment has been implicated in the development of CPs. Maternal depression may adversely affect parenting behavior and may also negatively bias maternal perceptions of children and adolescents with CPs (e.g., Dumas & Serketich, 1994; Fergusson, Lynskey, & Horwood, 1993). Mothers of youth presenting with comorbid CPs and ADHD have been shown to be at increased risk for a history of childhood ADHD themselves (Chronis et al., 2003). Parental antisocial behavior has received increasing attention as both a direct and an indirect influence on the development and maintenance of CPs. Links between parental criminality, aggressive behavior, and a diagnosis of antisocial personality disorder (APD), and childhood delinquency, aggression, and CD/ODD diagnoses have been reported by a number of investigators (see Frick & Loney, 2002, for a review). Some evidence suggests that parental antisocial behavior may play a more central role than other risk factors in its effect on parenting practices and CPs (e.g., Frick & Loney, 2002; Patterson & Capaldi, 1991). For example, parenting and marital status were not associated with CPs independently of parental APD (Frick et al., 1992).

Similarly, parental substance abuse has been associated with children's CPs, at least in part, because of its association with disrupted parenting practices (Patterson et al., 1992; Wills, Schreibman, Benson, & Vaccaro, 1994). In families with parental alcohol problems, the parents are less able to engage their children and are less congenial (Jacob, Krahn, & Leonard, 1991; Whipple, Fitzgerald, & Zucker, 1995). In addition, children's inappropriate behavior increases parental alcohol consumption (for parents with a positive family history of alcohol problems) and distress (for all parents) (Pelham & Lang, 1993).

Marital distress and conflict have been shown to be associated with CPs, negative parenting behavior, and parental perceptions of youth maladjustment (Amato & Keith, 1991; Cummings & Davies, 1994). The most commonly offered hypothesis for the relationship has been that marital distress and conflict interfere with the parents' ability to engage in appropriate parenting practices, which then leads

to CPs.[1] More narrowly focused constructs that relate directly to parenting, such as disagreement over childrearing practices, marital conflict in a child's presence, or the strength of the parenting alliance, may demonstrate stronger relationships to CPs than many broader constructs, such as marital distress (e.g., Abidin & Brunner, 1995; Jouriles et al., 1991; Porter & O'Leary, 1980).

Parents of children or adolescents with CPs also appear to experience higher frequencies of stressful events, both minor ones (e.g., daily hassles) and those of a more significant nature (e.g., unemployment, major transitions) (Patterson, 1983; Webster-Stratton, 1990). The effects of stress on the development of CPs may be mediated through parenting practices such as disrupted parental discipline (e.g., Snyder, 1991) and maladaptive parental social cognitions (e.g., Johnston, 1996a).

In addition to the family context, the child's or adolescent's relationship with peers plays a significant role in the development, maintenance, and escalation of CPs. Research has documented a relationship between peer rejection in elementary school and the later development of CPs (Roff & Wirt, 1984). In addition, peer rejection in elementary school is predictive of an association with a deviant peer group (i.e., one that shows a high rate of antisocial behavior and substance abuse) in early adolescence (e.g., Fergusson, Swain, & Horwood, 2002). This relationship is important, because association with a deviant peer group leads to an increase in the frequency and severity of CPs (Patterson & Dishion, 1985), and it has proven to be a strong predictor of later delinquency (Patterson, Capaldi, & Bank, 1991) and other negative outcomes, such as substance abuse (Dishion, Capaldi, Spracklen, & Li, 1995; Fergusson et al., 2002). Therefore, peer rejection may not only be directly related to the development of CPs but it also may indirectly influence CPs by increasing the child's or adolescent's chance of associating with a deviant peer group.

---

[1]However, other explanations are possible (see Rutter, 1994), including direct modeling of aggressive and coercive behavior, and the cumulative stressful effects of such conflict (e.g., maternal depression). It has been suggested that both youth CPs and parental marital distress/conflict may be the result of parental antisocial behavior in some cases (Frick & Jackson, 1993).

Finally, factors within a youth's larger social ecology may play a causal role in the development of CPs. One of the most consistently documented of these correlates has been low socioeconomic status (SES) (Frick, Lahey, Hartdagen, & Hynd, 1989). However, several other ecological factors, many of which are related to low SES, such as poor housing, poor schools, and disadvantaged neighborhoods, have also been linked to the development of CPs (see Frick, 1998; Peeples & Loeber, 1994). In addition, the high rate of violence witnessed by youth who live in impoverished, inner-city neighborhoods has also been linked to the development of CPs (Osofsky, Wewers, Hann, & Fick, 1993).

Some parents of children with CPs may be quite isolated from friends, neighbors, and the community. Wahler and his colleagues have developed a construct called *insularity*, which is defined as a "specific pattern of social contacts within the community that is characterized by a high level of negatively perceived coercive interchanges with relatives and/or helping agency representatives and by a low level of positively perceived supportive interchanges with friends" (Wahler & Dumas, 1984, p. 387). Insularity is positively related to negative parent behavior directed toward children and oppositional child behavior directed toward parents (Dumas & Wahler, 1985; Wahler, 1980). It has also been associated with poor maintenance of parent management training effects (e.g., Dumas & Wahler, 1983). Thus, when a mother has a large proportion of aversive interactions outside the home, interactions between mother and child within the home are likely to be negative as well.

Multiple Developmental Pathways to CPs

One final area of research that is critical for understanding children and adolescents with CPs has focused on the many different causal pathways through which youth may develop these behaviors, each involving different constellations of risk factors and somewhat different causal processes (Frick, Cornell, Bodin, et al., 2003; Frick & Morris, 2004; Lahey, Moffitt, & Caspi, 2003; Thornberry & Krohn, 2003). This area of research may be most important for developing guidelines for assessment for at least two reasons. First, the different developmental mechanisms that operate in specific subgroups of youth with CPs may help to explain some of the differences in the type and severity of CPs, the presence of comorbid conditions, and the operation of multiple causal factors (Frick, 2006; Frick & Morris, 2004). Second, this area of research suggests that treatments likely need to be tailored to the youth's specific needs, which necessitates an adequate assessment to implement such individualized interventions (Frick, 1998, 2006).

The most widely accepted model for delineating distinct pathways in the development of CPs distinguishes between childhood- and adolescent-onset subtypes of CPs; that is, the DSM-IV-TR (APA, 2000) makes the distinction between youth who begin showing severe CP behaviors before age 10 (i.e., childhood onset) and those who do not show severe CP behaviors before age 10 (i.e., adolescent onset). This distinction is supported by substantial research documenting important differences between these two groups of youth with CP (see Moffitt, 2003, for a review). Specifically, youth in the childhood-onset group show more severe CPs in childhood and adolescence, and are more likely to continue to show antisocial and criminal behavior into adulthood (Frick & Loney, 1999; Moffitt & Caspi, 2001). More relevant to causal theory, most of the dispositional (e.g., temperamental risk, low intelligence) and contextual (e.g., family dysfunction) correlates associated with CPs are more strongly associated with the childhood-onset subtype. In contrast, the youth in the adolescent-onset subtype do not consistently show these same risk factors. If they do differ from other youth, then it is primarily in showing greater affiliation with delinquent peers and scoring higher on measures of rebelliousness and authority conflict (Moffitt & Caspi, 2001; Moffitt, Caspi, Dickson, Silva, & Stanton, 1996).

The different characteristics of youth in the two CP subtypes have led to theoretical models that propose very different causal mechanisms operating across the two groups. For example, Moffitt (1993, 2003) has proposed that youth in the childhood-onset group develop CP behavior through a transactional process involving a difficult and vulnerable child (e.g., impulsive, with verbal deficits, with a difficult temperament) who experiences an inadequate rearing environment (e.g., poor parental supervision, poor quality schools). This dysfunctional transactional process disrupts the child's socialization, leading to poor social relations with persons both inside (i.e., parents and siblings) and outside (i.e., peers and teachers) the family, which further disrupts the child's socialization. These disruptions lead to enduring vulnerabilities that may negatively affect the child's psychosocial adjustment across multiple developmental stages. In contrast, Moffitt views youth in the adolescent-onset pathway as showing an exaggeration of the normative developmental process of identity formation that takes place in adolescence. Their engagement in antisocial and delinquent behaviors is conceptualized as a misguided attempt to obtain a subjective sense of maturity and adult status in a way that is maladaptive (e.g., breaking societal norms) but encouraged by an antisocial peer group. Given that their behavior is viewed as an exaggeration of a process specific to the adolescent developmental stage, and not due to enduring vulnerabilities, their CPs are less likely to persist beyond adolescence. However, they may still have impairments that persist into adulthood as a consequence of their CPs (e.g., a criminal record, dropping out of school, substance abuse) (Moffitt & Caspi, 2001).

This distinction between childhood- and adolescent-onset trajectories to severe CPs has been very influential for delineating different pathways through which youth develop CPs, although it is important to note that clear differences between the pathways are not always found (Lahey et al., 2000) and the applicability of this model to girls requires further testing (Silverthorn & Frick, 1999). Researchers have begun extending this conceptualization in a number of important ways. Specifically, they have begun to test whether additional distinctions can be made in youth who follow the childhood-onset pathway to (1) identify groups based on the severity, type, and stability of CPs exhibited; (2) identify groups that have distinct vulnerabilities that can make them more difficult to socialize by parents, teachers, and other important socializing agents; and (3) more clearly specify the developmental processes that can be disrupted by the transactional process that takes place between a vulnerable child and a nonoptimal socializing environment.

For example, research has identified a subgroup of youth that shows high rates of callous and unemotional (CU) traits (e.g., lacking empathy and guilt). Importantly, Frick and Dickens (2006) reviewed 22 published studies, showing that CU traits either co-occurred with ($n = 10$) or predicted ($n = 12$) serious antisocial and aggressive behavior, and five studies showing that CU traits were related to poorer treatment response among youth with CPs. There is also evidence that the CP subgroup of youth with CU traits also exhibits a temperamental style distinct from other youth with CPs (for reviews, see Blair, Peschardt, Budhani, Mitchell, & Pine, 2006; Frick & Morris, 2004). Specifically, compared to other antisocial youth, youth with CU traits are more likely to show deficits in their processing of negative emotional stimuli (Blair, 1999; Blair, Colledge, Murray, & Mitchell, 2001; Kimonis, Frick, Fazekas, & Loney, 2006; Loney, Frick, Clements, Ellis, & Kerlin, 2003), to show low levels of fearful inhibitions and anxiety (Frick, Cornell, Bodin, et al., 2003; Frick, Lilienfeld, et al., 1999; Lynam et al., 2005) and to show decreased sensitivity to punishment cues, especially when a reward-oriented response set is primed (Barry et al., 2000; Fisher & Blair, 1998).

These characteristics are all consistent with a temperamental style that has been variously labeled as low fearfulness (Rothbart & Bates, 1998) or low behavioral inhibition (Kagan & Snidman, 1991). This temperamental style could place a young child at risk for missing some of the early precursors to empathetic concern that involve emotional arousal evoked by the misfortune and distress of others (Blair, 1995), make the child less responsive than other youth to typical parental socialization practices (Oxford, Cavell, & Hughes, 2003; Wootton, Frick, Shelton, & Silverthorn, 1997), and lead to impairments in moral reasoning and empathic concern toward others (Blair, 1999; Pardini, Lochman, & Frick, 2003).

The few studies that have identified youth within the childhood-onset group who differ relative to the presence of CU traits also provide some clues as to the mechanisms that may be involved in the development of CPs in children and adolescents without these traits. These youth with CPs who do not have elevated CU traits are less likely to be aggressive than those who have elevated CU traits and who, when they do act aggressively, are more likely to be reactive (Frick, Cornell, Barry, Bodin, & Dane, 2003) in response to real or perceived provocation by others (Frick, Cornell, Bodin, et al., 2003). Also, CPs of antisocial youth who do not show CU traits are more strongly associated with dysfunctional parenting practices (Oxford et al., 2003; Wootton et al., 1997) and with deficits in verbal intelligence (Loney et al., 1998). Finally, youth with CPs who do not show CU traits exhibit high levels of emotional distress (Frick, Cornell, Bodin, et al., 2003; Frick, Lilienfeld, et al., 1999), are more reactive to the distress of others in social situations (Pardini et al., 2003), and are highly reactive to negative emotional stimuli (Kimonis et al., 2006; Loney et al., 2003).

Overall, these findings suggest that a large number of children and adolescents with CPs but without CU traits have problems regulating their emotions (Frick & Morris, 2004). These problems in emotion regulation can lead to very impulsive, unplanned, aggressive and antisocial acts for which the child or adolescent may be remorseful afterwards but may still have difficulty controlling in the future (Pardini et al., 2003). The problems in emotion regulation can also make a youth particularly susceptible to becoming angry due to perceived provocations from peers, leading to violent and aggressive acts within the context of high emotional arousal (Hubbard et al., 2002; Loney et al., 2003).

CONDUCTING AN EVIDENCE-BASED ASSESSMENT OF CPs

Overview

Evidence-based assessment is necessarily evolving; as research accumulates to guide these assessments, these recommendations should change to incorporate new findings. Furthermore, in many areas of assessment, available measures with demonstrated adequate psychometric properties are quite limited, making the scientific basis stronger for some recommendations than for others. With these caveats in mind, we hope that the following guidelines (McMahon & Frick, 2005) are of practical use to practitioners and researchers as a way to translate the currently available research into practice recommendations and to stimulate further clinically based research in this area.

When a child or adolescent is referred for CP assessment, the first order of business is to ascertain whether the youth is in fact demonstrating significant CP levels. Most child referrals for mental health evaluation and services are initiated by individuals and entities other than the child, such as parents, teachers, and the juvenile justice system. This is especially true for children with CPs, whose behavior is inherently distressing to others. Thus, it is important to rule out the possibility of the occasional inappropriate referral due, for example, to unrealistic parental or teacher expectations. After the appropriateness of the referral is determined, the primary tasks are to (1) identify the type and severity of the youth's CPs and determine the degree and types of impairment associated with them; (2) determine whether the youth is also experiencing significant levels of impairment related to other disorders and associated conditions; (3) determine what risk factors may have led to the development of the youth's CPs and/or more importantly, contribute to the continuation of these problems; and (4) determine which developmental pathway is most consistent with the youth's CP pattern, comorbid conditions, and risk factors.

As we detail below, knowledge concerning the particular developmental pathway that best fits the youth's clinical presentation is key to conducting an evidence-based assessment. It can provide a set of working hypotheses on the nature of the CP behavior, comorbid conditions, and salient risk factors. Determination of the likely developmental pathway guides the structure and focus of other areas of the assessment. For example, based on the available literature, one would hypothesize that a youth with adolescent-onset CPs would be less likely to be aggressive and to have intellectual deficits, temperamental vulnerabilities, and comorbid ADHD. However, association with a deviant peer group, and factors that may contribute to this deviant peer group affiliation (e.g., lack of parental monitoring and supervision), would be especially important to assess in youth on this pathway. In contrast, for a youth whose serious CPs began prior to adolescence, one would expect more cognitive and temperamental vulnerabilities, comorbid ADHD, and more serious problems in family functioning. For youth in this childhood-onset CP group who do not show CU traits, the cognitive deficits would more likely be verbal deficits, and the temperamental vulnerabilities would more likely be problems regulating emotions, leading to higher levels of anxiety, depression, and aggression involving anger. In contrast, for youth in the childhood-onset CP group who show high levels of CU traits, the cognitive deficits more likely involve a lack of sensitivity to punishment, and the temperamental vulnerabilities more likely involve a preference for dangerous and novel activities, and a failure to experience many types of emotion (e.g., guilt and empathy). Furthermore, assessing the level and severity of aggressive behavior, especially the presence of instrumental aggression, would be critical for youth in this group.

As most clinicians recognize, people do not often fall neatly into the prototypes suggested by research. Therefore, these descriptions are meant to serve as hypotheses around which to organize an evidence-based assessment. Furthermore, to test these hypotheses adequately and determine how well a youth might fit into the prototypical descriptions of these developmental pathways, it is often necessary to conduct a comprehensive assessment. Finally, all of the constructs that are necessary to determine which of these developmental pathways might best describe the youth should be assessed by multiple assessment techniques and by measures that provide information on the youth in multiple contexts, further adding to the comprehensive nature of the assessment.

Therefore, a multistage assessment strategy is typically recommended (McMahon & Estes, 1997; McMahon & Frick, 2005; Nock & Kurtz, 2005). At the first stage, developmentally appropriate, broad-band screening instruments and unstructured clinical interviews should be employed initially to identify the relevant CP behaviors, as well as likely comorbid conditions. At the second stage, more focused and/or labor-intensive measures are administered to provide more detailed information concerning the youth's CP behavior, to assess factors that could help to identify the youth's most likely developmental trajectory (e.g., age of onset of the CPs, level of CU traits, problems in emotional regulation), and to assess associated conditions in multiple settings (e.g., home, school) based on the results of this initial assessment. Also, at this second stage, it is essential that the level of functional impairment or adaptive disability associated with the youth's CPs be determined. At the third stage, an array of risk factors needs to be assessed, guided by the information obtained at the first two stages of assessment as to the most likely developmental pathway that the youth may be following, and guided by the prototypical descriptions of these pathways provided earlier.

These recommendations are influenced by a number of issues related to the developmental level of the child. First, the issue of whether the youth's CPs represent a clinically significant phenomenon or are a temporary developmental perturbation is especially salient for preschool-age children and for adolescents. Research suggests that some level of CP behavior in both of these developmental stages is normative (Keenan et al., 1998; Moffitt, 1993). Second, youth generally do not become reliable reporters of their CP behaviors until they are approximately 9 years of age (Kamphaus & Frick, 2005). Thus, reliance on self-report in the assessment battery may be more limited in the assessment of very young children. Third, with preschool-age children, assessment of language functioning and noncompliance is particularly important, and the use of structured laboratory observation analogues of parent–child interaction is important for the assessment of child noncompliance (McMahon & Forehand, 2003). Fourth, the number and breadth of salient domains of risk tend to increase with the youth's age, as a result of the broader social milieu in which he or she functions (Dodge & Pettit, 2003). Thus, whereas assessment of the youth's functioning in the family context is important across all ages, assessments of school and peer contexts become increasingly important in middle childhood and adolescence.

With respect to assessing CPs in girls, there is a relative dearth of information to guide clinicians in gender-specific issues, with two exceptions. A measure of relational aggression should be included in clinical or research settings that include girls with CPs. Also, because girls with CPs appear to be at increased risk for presenting with comorbid anxiety and depression, careful assessment of such conditions is especially warranted. Fortunately, a recent proliferation of research on CPs concerning girls (e.g., Moretti, Odgers, & Jackson, 2004; Pepler, Madsen, Webster, & Levene, 2005; Putallaz & Bierman, 2004; Silverthorn & Frick, 1999; Underwood, 2003) should in the near future facilitate the development of evidence-based guidelines that are applicable to girls with CPs.

These broad guidelines follow from the CP research. Importantly, there are many different ways to follow these recommendations in the various settings in which children with CPs may be assessed. Furthermore, given the length limitations of this chapter, it is impossible to provide an exhaustive discussion of all of the different measures that might be used to follow these recommendations. In the following sections, we provide examples of selected relevant measures that both have empirical support and are feasible for clinicians to implement in their practice.

Heterogeneity of CPs: Implications for Assessment

Based on the research showing the heterogeneity of CP behavior, a primary goal of assessment is to assess carefully and thoroughly the number, type, and severity of the CPs and the level of impairment they cause for the child or adolescent (e.g., school suspensions, police contacts, peer rejection). This is essential not only for diagnosis and screening but also to determine the validity of the initial referral, so that primary diagnoses of other disorders and the occasional referral due to inappropriate parent or teacher expectations can be identified (i.e., case conceptualization/planning). To obtain an accurate representation of the referred youth's CP behavior, it is important to use multiple assessment methods. Several methods are especially helpful in this respect, including interviews with the parents, youth, and other relevant parties (e.g., teachers); behavior rating scales; and behavioral observations in the clinic, home, and/or school settings. The first section of Table 3.1 lists instruments that may be used to assess CPs.

Interviews

Interviews may be divided into two general categories: clinical interviews and structured diagnostic interviews. The clinical interview with the parent is of major importance. Besides providing a method for assessing the type, severity, and impairment associated with the CPs, the clinical interview with the parent helps to assess typical parent–child interactions that may be contributing to the CPs, the antecedent stimulus conditions under which the CP behaviors occur, and the consequences that accompany such behaviors. A number of interview formats are available to aid the clinician in structuring the information from the parents about their child's behavior and about parent–child interactions (e.g., McMahon & Forehand, 2003; Patterson, Reid, Jones, & Conger, 1975; Wahler & Cormier, 1970). An individual interview with the child or adolescent may or may not provide useful, content-oriented information depending on the age and/or developmental level of the child and the nature of the specific behaviors. As noted earlier, it has been difficult to obtain reliable self-report information from interviews with children younger than age 9 (Kamphaus & Frick, 2005). However, even with younger children, informal interviews may be extremely useful, in that they can provide the therapist an opportunity to assess the child's perception of why he or she has been brought to the clinic, and a subjective evaluation of the child's cognitive, affective, and behavioral characteristics (e.g., Bierman, 1983). Furthermore, when assessing overt types of CPs, Loeber and Schmaling (1985) have suggested that maternal and teacher reports may be preferable to youth reports, because youth often underestimate or minimize their own aggressive behavior (see also David & Kistner, 2000; Edens, 1998). However, when assessing covert types of CPs, more valid reports are likely to be obtained from the child or adolescent.[2]

When the presenting problems include classroom behavior or academic underachievement, an interview with the youth's teachers is also appropriate. Breen and Altepeter (1990) have provided an outline for a brief interview with the teacher, which can be conducted at the school or by telephone. Situationally formatted interview guides based on Barkley's (1987, 1997) School Situations Questionnaire or Wahler and Cormier's (1970) preinterview checklists may be employed in conjunction with specific questions related to the child's problem behaviors. Contextual factors, such as classroom rules of conduct, teacher expectations, and the behavior of other children in the classroom, are important as well. (For additional discussions of teacher interviewing procedures, see McMahon & Forehand, 2003; Walker, 1995.)

Researchers and practitioners increasingly are using functional behavioral assessment (FBA) methods to assess children's needs in school and to match intervention strategies and behavioral functions to enhance treatment effectiveness (LaRue & Handleman, 2006; Walker, Ramsey, & Gresham, 2004). This is in part due to changes in the Individuals with Disabilities Education Act (IDEA; 1997), which now mandates an FBA for all students who have been suspended from school for at least

---

[2]However, given the strong positive correlations between stealing and lying, youth who steal may not be veridical in their self-reports.

TABLE 3.1. Implications of Research for the Assessment of Children and Adolescents with Conduct Problems

Assessment focus	Selected measures
Heterogeneity in types and severity of CPs	
Screen broadly for CP behaviors	ASEBA, BASC-2; DISC/DICA, CI
Focused assessments ODD/CD diagnosis	DISC/DICA, ASEBA (DSM scales); Child Symptom Inventories
Overt/covert CPs	ASEBA (Aggressive Behavior vs. Rule-Breaking Behavior); BASC-2 (Aggression vs. Conduct Problems); RBPC (Conduct Disorder vs. Social Aggression); ECBI/SESBI-R; SRD; Parent Daily Report; DISC/DICA, CI
Overt CPs only	Conner's Rating Scales; Problem-Solving Discussion
Covert CPs only	Firesetting History Screen/Firesetting Risk Interview/Children's Firesetting Interview; Lying Scale; Temptation provocation tasks (stealing/property destruction, firesetting); TIROSSA
Noncompliance	Child's Game/Parent's Game/Clean Up (BCS, DPICS); Compliance Test; REDSOCS
Reactive/proactive aggression	Parent Checklist; Teacher Checklist; Aggressive Behavior Rating Scale; Reactive–Proactive Aggression Questionnaire
Relational aggression	Ratings of Children's Social Behavior; peer nominations
Delinquency	SRD
Functional impairment/adaptive disability	C-GAS; CIS; CAFAS; NABC
Comorbid adjustment problems	
Screen broadly for comorbid disorders/conditions	ASEBA, BASC-2; DISC/DICA, CI
Focused assessments (as needed) ADHD[a] Depression[a] Anxiety[a] Substance use[a] Academic underachievement[a] Language impairment	 CBCL/1½–5 Language Development Survey; BASC-2 Functional Communication
Functional impairment/adaptive disability	See above
Multiple risks	
Biological factors Temperament	 Children's Behavior Questionnaire
Cognitive correlates Social-information processing	 Intention–Cue Detection Task; Problem-Solving Measure for Conflict; WALLY Game; SCAP
Peers Peer interaction problems	 ASEBA; BASC-2; SNAP!
Family Parenting practices	 Child's Game/Parent's Game/Clean Up (BCS, DPICS); Problem-Solving Discussion; Parenting Scale; Alabama Parenting Questionnaire
Parenting cognitions	ECBI (Problem vs. Intensity); video-mediated recall; Parenting Sense of Competenc Scale; Parenting Locus of Control Scale

(continued)

TABLE 3.1. *(continued)*

Assessment focus	Selected measures
Parental personal/marital adjustment	Beck Depression Inventory–II Antisocial Behavior Checklist SMAST/DAST/AUDIT DSM-IV ADHD Rating Scale; Dyadic Adjustment Scale; Marital Adjustment Test; O'Leary–Porter Scale; Conflict Tactics Scales—Partner; Parenting Alliance Measure; Child-Rearing Disagreements; Parent Problem Checklist
Parenting stress	Life Experiences Survey; Family Events List; Daily Hassles; Parenting Stress Index
Functioning in extrafamilial contexts	Neighborhood Questionnaire; Things I Have Seen and Heard; Community Interaction Checklist
Parental satisfaction with treatment	Therapy Attitude Inventory; Parent's Consumer Satisfaction Questionnaire
Multiple developmental pathways	
Age of onset of CP behaviors	DISC/DICA, CI
Callous–unemotional traits	Antisocial Process Screening Device

Note. ASEBA, Achenbach System of Empirically Based Assessment; BASC-2, Behavior Assessment System for Children, Second Edition; DISC/DICA, Diagnostic Interview Schedule for Children/Diagnostic Interview for Children and Adolescents; CI, clinical interview; RBPC, Revised Behavior Problem Checklist; ECBI/SESBI-R, Eyberg Child Behavior Inventory/Sutter–Eyberg Child Behavior Inventory—Revised; SRD, Self-Report Delinquency Scale; TIROSSA, Telephone Interview Report on Stealing and Social Aggression; BCS, Behavioral Coding System; DPICS, Dyadic Parent–Child Interaction Coding System; REDSOCS, Revised Edition of the School Observation Coding System; C-GAS, Children's Global Assessment Scale; CIS, Columbia Impairment Scale; CAFAS, Child and Adolescent Functional Assessment Scale; NABC, Normative Adaptive Behavior Checklist; SCAP, Social-Cognitive Assessment Profile; SMAST/DAST/AUDIT, Short Michigan Alcoholism Screening Test/Drug Abuse Screening Test/Alcohol Use Disorders Identification Test. Adapted from McMahon and Frick (2005). Copyright 2005 by Lawrence Erlbaum Associates, Inc. Adapted by permission.
[a]See relevant chapters in this volume for appropriate measures.

10 days for exhibiting CP types of behavior. FBA involves specification of problem behaviors in school in operational terms (e.g., what types of CPs are being exhibited in the classroom), as well as identification of events that reliably predict and control behavior through an examination of antecedents and consequences. For example, an FBA would determine whether the child's CPs are occurring only in certain classes or situations (e.g., during class change, at lunch), and whether certain factors reliably lead to the CPs (e.g., teasing by peers, disciplinary confrontations with teachers). It would also determine the consequences associated with the CPs that may contribute to their likelihood of occurring in the future (e.g., getting sent home from school; preventing further teasing). Information relevant to an FBA is gathered through both interviews and direct observation of classroom behavior by teachers or school psychologists. Use of these methods has been shown to contribute to beneficial outcomes for children and adolescents in school (Walker et al., 2004).

One criticism of the unstructured interview has been the difficulty in obtaining reliable information in this format. Structured interviews have been used in efforts to improve the reliability and validity of the information that is obtained. Two frequently used structured diagnostic interviews in the assessment of children with CPs are the Diagnostic Interview Schedule for Children (DISC; Shaffer, Fisher, Lucas, Dulcan, & Schwab-Stone, 2000) and the Diagnostic Interview for Children and Adolescents (DICA; Reich, 2000). For reviews of these and other structured diagnostic interviews, see Loney and Frick (2003) and McClellan and Werry (2000). Most of these interviews provide a structured format for obtaining parent and youth reports on symptoms that comprise the criteria for ODD and CD according to DSM-IV-TR (APA, 2000). Also, such interviews provide a structured method to assess how much these symptoms impair a child's or adolescent's social and academic functioning.

There are a number of limitations in the information provided by structured interviews, however (see Loney & Frick, 2003). The interviews are time-consuming to administer (often taking over 2 hours for youth with many problems in adjustment) and often do not contain information that can be compared to a normative comparison group. Furthermore, most structured interviews do not have formats for obtaining teacher information, and obtaining reliable information from young children (below age 9) has been problematic. Thus, it is difficult to obtain multi-informant assessments for many youth using structured interviews. Perhaps one of the major limitations in the use of structured interviews, however, is the evidence that the number of reported symptoms declines within an interview schedule; that is, parents and youth tend to report more symptoms for diagnoses assessed early in the interview, regardless of which diagnoses are assessed first (Jensen, Watanabe, & Richters, 1999), calling into question the validity of diagnoses assessed later in the interview.

An alternative approach to interviewing youth, developed by McConaughy and Achenbach (2001), the Semistructured Clinical Interview for Children and Adolescents (SCICA) is a broad interview administered to youth (ages 6–18) that employs a protocol of open-ended questions to assess a variety of areas of youth functioning. Dimensional scores similar to those obtained from various instruments in the Achenbach System of Empirically Based Assessment (ASEBA; Achenbach & Rescorla, 2000, 2001; see below) can also be derived from these items. Kolko and colleagues have developed several semistructured interviews for parents and children that have been used to assess various aspects of firesetting and matchplay in inpatient, outpatient, and community samples of children, including the Firesetting History Screen, the Firesetting Risk Interview, and the Children's Firesetting Interview (Kolko, Nishi-Strattner, Wilcox, & Kopet, 2002; Wilcox & Kolko, 2002). Evidence for the reliability and validity of these interviews is encouraging. For example, there is relatively good agreement between parent and child reporters on the Firesetting History Screen, and it is related to other measures of firesetting involvement. Both the Firesetting Risk Interview

and the Children's Firesetting Interview have adequate internal consistency, differentiate between firesetters and nonfiresetters, and predict recidivism.

The interview as an assessment tool does not end with the first contact with the youth, but continues throughout treatment formulation and implementation. It is used to obtain information necessary for the development of interventions, to assess the effectiveness of the intervention and its implementation, and to alter the intervention, if necessary (Breen & Altepeter, 1990).

Behavior Rating Scales

Behavior rating scales completed by adults (i.e., parents, teachers) or by the youth him- or herself are very useful as screening devices that cover a broad range of CP behaviors and assess other problems in adjustment that may be used to evaluate the level of CP-associated impairment. For example, many rating scales contain items assessing the child's or adolescent's peer relations and academic performance, both of which are important areas of impairment experienced by many youth with CPs (e.g., Reynolds & Kamphaus, 2004). More importantly, these rating scales often provide the best norm-referenced assessment concerning the child's or adolescent's CPs. Specifically, these scales often have large normative bases from which the scores obtained (e.g., *T*-scores) compare the child's CP level to a reference group of youth of the same age and gender. Although there are many behavior rating scales, several have been used extensively in clinical practice and research with children and adolescents with CPs (Kamphaus & Frick, 2005; McMahon & Frick, 2005). These scales, which are summarized in Table 3.2, include the ASEBA (Achenbach & Rescorla, 2000, 2001), the Behavior Assessment System for Children—Second Edition (BASC-2; Reynolds & Kamphaus, 2004), the Conners Rating Scales (Conners, 1997), the Revised Behavior Problem Checklist (RBPC; Quay & Peterson, 1996), and the Child Symptom Inventories (e.g., Gadow & Sprafkin, 1998). See Kamphaus and Frick (2005) for a more comprehensive summary of the strengths and weaknesses of each of these scales.

Most of the scales listed in Table 3.2 cover the same age range and have parallel forms for

TABLE 3.2. Summary of Selected Comprehensive Behavior Rating Scales Used in the Assessment of Conduct Problems

Scale/authors	Publisher	Age range	CP assessed	Domains assessed	Informant
Achenbach System of Empirically Based Assessment (ASEBA; Achenbach & Rescorla, 2000, 2001)	Author, University of Vermont	1.5–18	*Aggressive behavior*—overt conduct problems including arguing, bragging, and being mean. *Rule-breaking behavior*—covert conduct problems such as lying, cheating, stealing, and truancy (6–18 only).	6–18: withdrawn, somatic complaints, anxious/depressed, social problems, thought problems, attention problems (hyperactivity-impulsivity—Teacher's Report Form only), competence DSM scales: Affective Problems, Anxiety Problems, Somatic Problems, Attention Deficit/Hyperactivity Problems, Oppositional Defiant Problems, Conduct Problems 1.5–5: emotionally reactive, anxious/depressed, somatic complaints, withdrawn, sleep problems, attention problems, aggressive behavior, language development survey (1.5–5) DSM scales: Affective Problems, Anxiety Problems, Pervasive Developmental Problems, Attention Deficit/Hyperactivity Problems, Oppositional Defiant Problems	Parent, teacher, and child (ages 11–18)
Behavior Assessment System for Children, Second Edition (BASC-2; Reynolds & Kamphaus, 2004)	American Guidance Service	2–21	*Aggression*—overt conduct problems including oppositional behavior, arguing, and hitting. *Conduct problems*—covert conduct problems, including lying and stealing.	Adaptability, anxiety, attention problems, atypicality, depression, hyperactivity, leadership, learning problems, functional communication, social skills, somatization, study skills, withdrawal, activities of daily living, attitude to school, attitude to teachers,	Parent, teacher, and child (ages 8–21)

				interpersonal relations, locus of control, relations with parents, self-esteem, self-reliance, sensation seeking, sense of inadequacy, social stress	
Child Symptom Inventory (e.g., Gadow & Sprafkin, 1998).	Checkmate Plus	3–18	Oppositional defiant disorder—angry, hostile, and defiant behaviors; Conduct disorder—violations of the rights of others or age-appropriate norms.	Attention-deficit/hyperactivity disorder, generalized anxiety disorder, social phobia, separation anxiety disorder, major depressive disorder, dysthymic disorder, pervasive developmental disorder, autistic disorder, schizophrenia, tic disorder	Parent, teacher, and child (ages 12–18)
Conners Rating Scales (Conners, 1997)	Multi-Health Systems	3–17	Oppositional—overt behaviors such as being angry and hostile, losing temper, and arguing with adults.	Cognitive problems, hyperactivity, anxious–shy, perfectionism, social problems, psychosomatic, family problems, anger control problems	Parent, teacher, and child (ages 12–18)
Revised Behavior Problem Checklist (Quay & Peterson, 1996)	PAR	5–18	Conduct disorder—overt behaviors such as anger, fighting, and disobedience. Socialized aggression—covert conduct problems such as stealing, substance use, lying, and truancy.	Attention problems, immaturity, anxiety–withdrawal, psychotic behavior, motor tension–excess	Parent and teacher

Note. From McMahon and Frick (2005). Copyright 2005 by Lawrence Erlbaum Associates, Inc. Reprinted by permission.

parent, teacher, and youth reports. The exception, the BASC-2 (Reynolds & Kamphaus, 2004), includes CPs only on their parent and teacher versions. Also, most of these scales divide CP assessment into scales that assess overt and covert CP. Exceptions are the Child Symptom Inventories (e.g., Gadow & Sprafkin, 1995), whose items correspond to the DSM-IV-TR symptom list for ODD and CD.

We provide an overview of the ASEBA family of instruments (Achenbach & Rescorla, 2000, 2001) because of their widespread adoption in both research and clinical settings. A number of instruments in the ASEBA are applicable for use with children and adolescents. There are parallel forms for parents (Child Behavior Checklist; CBCL/1½–5, CBCL/6–18), teachers (Caregiver-Teacher Report Form for Ages 1½–5, C-TRF; Teacher's Report Form, TRF/6–18), youth (Youth Self-Report; YSR/11–18), and observers (Direct Observation Form; DOF/5–14; described below). These instruments are similar in terms of structure, items, scoring, and interpretation. They are designed to be self-administered, and each can usually be completed in 10 to 20 minutes. The instruments include sections concerning Competence and Problem items (the CBCL/1½–5 includes Problem items and a Language Development Survey; the DOF includes only Problem items). Competence scales include items related to various activities, social relationships, and success in school. With respect to the Problem items, the various ASEBA instruments typically yield Total, Internalizing, and Externalizing broad-band scales, and a number of narrow-band scales. With respect to CPs, narrow-band scales comprising the Externalizing scale (e.g., Rule-Breaking Behavior and Aggressive Behavior on the CBCL/6–18) are of particular interest. The ASEBA now also includes DSM-oriented scales, such as Oppositional Defiant Problems and Conduct Problems on the CBCL/6–18 (Achenbach, Dumenci, & Rescorla, 2003), and parent ratings on a Dutch version of the CBCL have been shown to predict DSM-IV diagnoses (Krol, De Bruyn, Coolen, & van Aarle, 2006).

The normative samples collected for the components of the ASEBA are generally quite extensive and representative of the 48 contiguous United States for SES, ethnicity, region, and urban–suburban–rural residence (Achenbach & Rescorla, 2000, 2001). Importantly, the samples generally excluded children referred for mental health or special education services within the past year, which makes them normal rather than normative samples. However, the large samples allow for norm-referenced scores that can be age- and gender-specific. These extensive normative samples also provided extensive factor support for the various ASEBA scales, and the factor structure has been replicated extensively not only in the United States but also in many other countries (Achenbach, Rescorla, & Ivanova, 2005). These studies have provided strong support for the reliability of both the global composites and, with only a few exceptions, the narrow-band scales (Achenbach & Rescorla, 2001). Finally, the extensive research on the rating scale component of the ASEBA has provided strong support for the validity of the scales in differentiating between children with CP and normally developing children, and in documenting the effects of treatment for children with CPs (e.g., DeGarmo, Patterson, & Forgatch, 2004; Eisenstadt, Eyberg, McNeil, Newcomb, & Funderburk, 1993; Kazdin, Bass, Siegel, & Thomas, 1989; Kendall, Reber, McLeer, Epps, & Ronan, 1990; Scott, Spender, Doolan, Jacobs, & Aspland, 2001). Thus, the ASEBA instruments may be used for both general and more specific purposes, including classification, screening, diagnosis, and treatment evaluation. With children with CPs, its comprehensive coverage can be useful in screening for some of the disorders that are often comorbid with CPs (see below).

The primary limitations in the ASEBA scales involve the narrow-band scales. The content, by being broad in coverage, sometimes does not allow for adequate assessment of specific domains that may be important for some evaluations. For example, there is no separate depression scale or a scale assessing hyperactivity. Furthermore, the sole reliance on factor analysis in developing scales led to some heterogeneity in the content of some of the narrow-band scales (Kamphaus & Frick, 2005). For example, the Attention Problems scales on the parent and teacher measures include items related to attention (e.g., "can't concentrate," "can't pay attention for long"), as well as items such as "acts too young for his or her age" and "nervous or high strung" that are not specific to inattention. This scale heterogeneity needs to be considered when interpreting the narrow-band scales.

The scales summarized in Table 3.2 are broad rating scales that cover many dimensions of child and adolescent adjustment, not just CPs. Also, due to the need to cover a large number of domains, they often include only a limited number of CP behaviors. Several rating scales, however, focus solely on CPs and provide a more comprehensive coverage of various CP types. Two examples of parent and teacher report measures are the Eyberg Child Behavior Inventory and the Sutter–Eyberg Student Behavior Inventory—Revised (ECBI and SESBI-R, respectively; Eyberg & Pincus, 1999). The ECBI is completed by parents and is intended for use with children ages 2–16. It takes approximately 10 minutes to administer and score. The 36 items describe specific CP behaviors (primarily overt) and are scored on both a frequency-of-occurrence (Intensity) scale and a yes–no problem identification (Problem) scale. Both scales have been shown to discriminate between children with CPs and other, clinic-referred children and nonreferred children (e.g., Burns & Patterson, 1990, 2001; Burns, Patterson, Nussbaum, & Parker, 1991; Eyberg, 1992; Eyberg & Colvin, 1994; Rich & Eyberg, 2001), and to be sensitive to treatment effects from parent management training interventions with young children (e.g., Eisenstadt et al., 1993; McNeil, Eyberg, Eisenstadt, Newcomb, & Funderburk, 1991; Nixon, Sweeney, Erickson, & Touyz, 2003; Webster-Stratton & Hammond, 1997).

The original normative data for the ECBI (Eyberg & Robinson, 1983; Robinson, Eyberg, & Ross, 1980) were limited in sample size and age range. Based on a larger and more demographically representative sample (Colvin, Eyberg, & Adams, 1999; Eyberg & Pincus, 1999), currently recommended cutoff points for the Intensity and Problem scales have been revised, resulting in improved sensitivity, specificity, and predictive power (Rich & Eyberg, 2001). There have not been meaningful gender or ethnic differences (Burns & Patterson, 2001; Eyberg & Colvin, 1994), although Burns and Patterson (2001) found that scores tended to decrease with children's age increases, especially for the Intensity score.

With respect to other psychometric considerations, adequate test–retest, split-half, and internal consistency reliabilities have been reported (e.g., Burns & Patterson, 1990; Burns et al., 1991; Eyberg, 1992; Eyberg & Colvin, 1994; Funderburk, Eyberg, Rich, & Behar, 2003). Mean levels of scores are stable across time as well (Eyberg, 1992; Funderburk et al., 2003), and evidence for longer-term (10-month) test–retest reliability has also been obtained (Funderburk et al., 2003). Interparent agreement on the ECBI is moderate to strong for both Intensity ($r = .69$) and Problem ($r = .61$) scales (e.g., Eisenstadt, McElreath, Eyberg, & McNeil, 1994). The ECBI is significantly correlated with the Externalizing broad-band scale of the CBCL (Boggs, Eyberg, & Reynolds, 1990), with other rating scales (e.g., Funderburk et al., 2003), and with various clinic-based observational coding systems (e.g., Robinson & Eyberg, 1981; Webster-Stratton, 1985). Responses on the ECBI have been shown to be independent of social desirability factors (Robinson & Anderson, 1983).

The original SESBI is identical in format to the ECBI, with 36 items rated on both Intensity and Problem scales, although items on the ECBI that were not relevant to the school setting were replaced by 13 new items. Standardization studies have been done on the SESBI, with samples ranging from preschoolers through high school students (e.g., Burns & Patterson, 2001; Burns, Sosna, & Ladish, 1992; Floyd, Rayfield, Eyberg, & Riley, 2004; Funderburk et al., 2003). The SESBI has also been shown to be sensitive to the effects of a parent management training intervention (McNeil et al., 1991). Eyberg and colleagues have begun to evaluate a revised version of the SESBI (SESBI-R; Eyberg & Pincus, 1999) that includes additional items derived from the disruptive behavior categories of DSM-IV (APA, 1994) and deletion of infrequently occurring items. The SESBI-R, which comprises 38 items, appears to have adequate psychometric properties (Querido & Eyberg, 2003; Rayfield, Eyberg, & Foote, 1998) and discriminates between children referred for CPs and nonreferred children (Querido & Eyberg, 2003).

Children whose scores exceed the cutoff points on the ECBI or the SESBI-R are probably a heterogeneous group that may present with ADHD, as well as ODD or CD (McMahon & Estes, 1997), because the items that comprise the ECBI and SESBI-R are consistent with the DSM diagnostic categories of ODD, CD, and ADHD (Burns & Patterson, 1991). Given the increasing attention paid to comorbidity of ADHD and CPs, this represents a potentially serious limitation of these instruments. However, the ECBI and SESBI-R show promise as useful rating scales in clinical settings, where they can be employed as screening instruments and as treatment outcome measures for disruptive behavior (broadly defined), as rated by parents and teachers.

To begin to address limitations resulting from the unidimensional nature of the ECBI and SESBI-R, researchers have conducted factor analyses, resulting in a three-factor solution for the ECBI (Oppositional Defiant Behavior toward Adults, Inattentive Behavior, and Conduct Problem Behavior) (Burns & Patterson, 2000; Weis, Lovejoy, & Lundahl, 2005) and a two-factor solution for the SESBI and SESBI-R (Oppositional Behavior and Attentional Difficulties) (Floyd et al., 2004; Rayfield, Eyberg, & Foote, 2003). This additional information on the factor structure of the ECBI and SESBI-R may increase their utility as screening instruments. However, for situations in which a broader screening is desired, or when information pertinent to differential diagnosis is sought, the CBCL, TRF, and related ASEBA instruments are recommended.

The Intensity and Problem scales on the ECBI and SESBI-R may also provide useful information concerning the role of parental perceptions of a child in the rating process (Robinson et al., 1980). Eyberg (1992) has suggested that a low Intensity score in conjunction with a high Problem score may indicate that the parent (or teacher) is intolerant or personally distressed. On the other hand, a high Intensity score and a low Problem score may occur when a parent (or teacher) has a very high tolerance level or is reluctant to admit that the child is a behavior problem.

Another rating scale that focuses specifically on CPs, the Self-Report Delinquency Scale (SRD; Elliott, Huizinga, & Ageton, 1985), is probably the most widely used self-report measure of CP behavior. It comprises 47 items derived from offenses listed in the *Uniform Crime Reports* (Federal Bureau of Investigation, 2004), and covers Property Offenses (e.g., "Have you ever purposely damaged or destroyed property belonging to school?"), Status Offenses (e.g., "Have you ever taken a vehicle for a ride without the owners' permission?"), Drug Offenses (e.g., "Have you ever sold hard drugs such as heroin, cocaine, and LSD?"), and Violent Offenses ("Have you ever been involved in gang fights?"). Importantly, the Violent Offenses scale includes threats of physical violence, as well as actual violence (e.g., "Have you ever hit [or threatened to hit] a teacher or other adult at school?"). The SRD is intended

for use by 11- to 19-year-olds, who report on the frequency of engagement in each behavior over the past year. It has been employed primarily in epidemiological and community samples to assess prevalence of delinquent behaviors (e.g., Elliott et al., 1985; Loeber, Stouthamer-Loeber, Van Kammen, & Farrington, 1989), as an outcome measure in longitudinal studies (Frick, Stickle, Dandreaux, Farrell, & Kimonis, 2005), and as a measure of intervention outcome (e.g., Kazdin, Mazurick, & Siegel, 1994; Kazdin, Siegel, & Bass, 1992; Scherer, Brondino, Henggeler, Melton, & Hanley, 1994).

The Parent Checklist and the Teacher Checklist (Conduct Problems Prevention Research Group, 1999; Dodge & Coie, 1987), the Reactive–Proactive Aggression Questionnaire (Brown, Atkins, Osborne, & Milnamow, 1996), and the Aggressive Behavior Rating Scale (Raine et al., 2006) were developed to distinguish between reactive and proactive forms of aggression. The Ratings of Children's Social Behavior (RCSB; Crick, 1996), a 17-item rating scale, assesses relational aggression, using item content analogous to the peer-nomination procedure used in past studies of relational aggression (Crick & Grotpeter, 1995). Little and colleagues (2003) recently developed a scale that is unique in assessing reactive and proactive forms of aggression for both relational and overt aggression. These authors reported that these different forms of aggression could be distinguished in a factor analysis, and that reactive forms of relational aggression (but not proactive forms) were positively associated with low frustration tolerance and a measure of hostility. The Lying Scale is a brief (12 items), parent-completed scale to assess parental perceptions of lying in their adolescent children (Engels, Finkenauer, & van Kooten, 2006). Psychometric analyses indicate that it taps into a single factor, and possesses adequate reliability and concurrent validity.

Behavioral Observations

Behavioral observations provide a third common way to assess CP behaviors. Behavioral observations in a child's or adolescent's natural setting (e.g., home, school, playground) can make a unique contribution by providing an assessment of the youth's behavior that is not filtered through the perceptions of an informant and an assessment of the immediate environmental context of the youth's behavior that, as noted earlier, can be critical for conducting an FBA. In some cases, observational CP data have been stronger predictors of adolescent arrest rates and incarceration than were parent-reported data (Patterson & Forgatch, 1995). Because such naturalistic observations can be quite time-consuming and expensive, a variety of clinic- and laboratory-based analogues have been developed, many of which have evidence to support their clinical utility and sensitivity to intervention effects (for reviews, see Frick & Loney, 2000; Roberts, 2001).

Two widely used structured, microanalytic observation procedures available for assessing parental interactions with younger children (3–8 years) in the clinic and the home are the Behavioral Coding System (BCS; Forehand & McMahon, 1981) and the Dyadic Parent–Child Interaction Coding System (DPICS; Eyberg, Nelson, Duke, & Boggs, 2005). The BCS and the DPICS are modifications of the assessment procedure developed by Hanf (1970) for the observation of parent–child interactions in the clinic. As employed in clinic settings, both the BCS and DPICS place the parent–child dyad in standard situations that vary in the degree to which parental control is required, ranging from a free-play situation (i.e., Child's Game, Child-Directed Interaction) to one in which the parent directs the child's activity, either in the context of parent-directed play (i.e., Parent's Game, Parent-Directed Interaction) and/or in cleaning up the toys (i.e., Clean Up). Each task typically lasts 5 to 10 minutes. In the home setting, observations usually occur in a less structured manner (e.g., the parent and child are instructed to "do whatever you would normally do together"). In each coding system, a variety of parent and child behaviors are scored, many of which emphasize parental antecedents (e.g., commands) and consequences (e.g., praise, time out) for child compliance–noncompliance and other CP behaviors. The BCS comprises six parent behaviors and three child behaviors; the DPICS comprises 12 parent and 14 child behaviors. Interobserver agreement for both coding systems is adequate (e.g., Eyberg et al., 2005; Forehand & Peed, 1979); they discriminate between referred and nonreferred samples of parents and children (e.g., Eyberg et al., 2005; Griest, Forehand, Wells, & McMahon, 1980); and they have been employed successfully as intervention outcome measures for parent management train-ing (e.g., Eisenstadt et al., 1993; McMahon, Forehand, & Griest, 1981; Peed, Roberts, & Forehand, 1977; Webster-Stratton & Hammond, 1997). In addition, both the BCS and the DPICS are used to determine movement from one set of parenting skills to the next in parent management training interventions (e.g., Herschell, Calzada, Eyberg, & McNeil, 2002; McMahon & Forehand, 2003). The BCS is available in Forehand and McMahon (1981) and the DPICS is available online at *www.pcit.org*. Simplified versions of both the DPICS and the BCS have been developed (Eyberg, Bessmer, Newcomb, Edwards, & Robinson, 1994; McMahon & Estes, 1994). These adaptations are designed to reduce training demands, and may ultimately prove to be more useful to clinicians.

A direct observational assessment of child compliance–noncompliance can also be obtained in the clinic with the Compliance Test (CT; Roberts & Powers, 1988), in which the parent issues a series of structured commands to the child. The parent is instructed to give a series of 30 standard commands without helping or following up on the commands with other verbalizations or nonverbal cues. In one version of the CT, two-part commands are given (e.g., "(Child's name), put the (toy) in the (container)"). In another version, the commands are separated into two codeable units (e.g., "(Child's name), pick up the (toy). Put it in the (container)"). The CT takes between 5 and 15 minutes to complete.

Roberts (2001; Roberts & Powers, 1988) presents evidence for the reliability and validity of the CT. For example, there is high interobserver agreement (97%), adequate test–retest reliability ($r = .73$ over 12 days), and convergent validity with other home and clinic observational measures. The CT appears to be a useful measure in identifying noncompliant children in research and clinical settings (Roberts & Powers, 1990), and there is preliminary evidence to support its discriminant, convergent, and divergent validity in a preschool setting (Filcheck, Berry, & McNeil, 2004). Because the CT does not measure parental instruction giving, Roberts (2001; Roberts & Powers, 1988) recommends that it be used in conjunction with a parent-directed chore analogue that allows coding of parental behavior, such as Clean Up (Eyberg et al., 2005).

For older children and adolescents, structured clinical observational paradigms have been developed for the direct assessment of parent–child communication and problem solving (see Foster & Robin, 1997, for a review). For example, Martinez and Forgatch (2001) employed a series of tasks that included a parent–child problem-solving discussion and teaching tasks with elementary school-age children. They coded these tasks for various parenting practices, and child aversive behavior and noncompliance, using both microanalytic and global rating systems.

Many common CP behaviors are by nature covert (e.g., lying, stealing, firesetting), which makes them more difficult to capture through observational techniques. However, Hinshaw and colleagues have developed and evaluated an analogue observational procedure to assess stealing, property destruction, and cheating in children ages 6 to 12 years (Hinshaw, Heller, & McHale, 1992; Hinshaw, Simmel, & Heller, 1995; Hinshaw, Zupan, Simmel, Nigg, & Melnick, 1997). Samples of boys (ages 6–12) with ADHD (most of whom also had ODD or CD) and a comparison group were asked to complete an academic worksheet alone in a room that contained a completed answer sheet, money, and toys. Stealing was measured by counting objects in the room immediately following the work session, whereas property destruction and cheating were assessed by ratings derived from observing the child's behavior during the session. Each of these observational measures of child covert CPs was correlated with parental ratings of covert CPs. When the boys with ADHD were treated with methylphenidate, stealing and property destruction, which were also associated with staff ratings of potential for covert behavior, decreased to a level similar to that displayed by boys in the comparison condition. None of the three measures of covert CP correlated significantly with each other.

Kolko, Watson, and Faust (1991) employed a very brief (1-minute) observation to assess children's preference for fire-related stimuli (e.g., a simulated book of matches) over toys in a play setting. Interobserver agreement for percentage of time in contact with fire-related stimuli, picking up the matchbook, or attempting to strike a match, ranged from 93 to 100%. All three indices demonstrated significant decreases from pretreatment to posttreatment in an inpatient sample of children with disruptive behavior disorders who also engaged in matchplay or firesetting.

In general, we recommend the use of structured clinical observations such as those described here to assess parent–child interactions. If there is a discrepancy between the clinic observations and the parent reports of interactions at home, then home observation may be necessary. The use of a coding system in the home setting instead of the clinic requires changes in the structure of the observation, transportation time, and scheduling flexibility (if home observations are planned to coincide with the times when the problem child behaviors are more likely to occur) (McMahon & Estes, 1997). Drotar and Crawford (1987) discuss many of the issues for clinicians involved in conducting home observations.

Although home observations are designed to record social interactions among family members in their "natural" environment (the home), the sessions are not completely unstructured. For example, prior to the observation, members of the family are typically given instructions such as the following: (1) Everyone in the family must be present; (2) no guests should be present during observations; (3) the family is limited to two rooms; (4) no telephone calls are to be made, and incoming calls must be answered briefly; (5) no television viewing is permitted; (6) no conversations may be held with observers while they are coding; and (7) therapy-related issues are not to be discussed with the observer (Reid, 1978).

The BCS (Forehand & McMahon, 1981) and DPICS (Eyberg et al., 2005) have been used in both the home and the clinic. For example, when employed in the home setting, the BCS is used to collect data in blocks of four 40-minute observations. The observations are conducted on different days and may be done at different times of the day. As noted earlier, McMahon and Estes (1994) developed a simplified version of the BCS that has been used in structured observations in the home. It has fewer codes to maximize reliability and to minimize training time, while retaining important treatment outcome information about parent–child interaction. Observers use a standardized set of toys and give standardized instructions to the parents before the interaction begins. The structure of the session includes Child's Game (5 minutes), Parent's Game (5 minutes), a Lego Task (in which the child is told to construct a developmentally challenging Lego figure and the parent is instructed to give only verbal aid; 5 minutes), and Clean Up (3 minutes).

Throughout each task, three parent and three child behaviors are recorded in 30-second intervals.

Behavioral observation systems designed specifically for assessing CP types of behavior in the school setting have received relatively less attention. Direct observations in the school have the same practical problems as those previously mentioned for home observations. The necessity of training reliable observers and the lengthy observation time are similar. Unfortunately, unlike the case with home observation, the clinician does not have the option of observing teacher–child interactions in the clinic. Therefore, if the presenting problems concern behavior at school (whether in the classroom or on the playground), observation in that setting may be necessary.

Nock and Kurtz (2005) have presented an excellent guide for clinicians on how to conduct direct observations in school settings. They provide information concerning formulation of the primary question(s) to be addressed in the observation, collaboration with school psychologists and teachers, description of the school/classroom context, and the selection and implementation of the actual observational procedures. Their recommendations about the key questions to be addressed by clinicians are presented in Table 3.3.

To aid in the observation of a child's behavior in the classroom, several of the rating scales systems reviewed previously include observational systems designed to be used in conjunction with parent-, teacher-, and self-report ratings. For example, the BASC-2 (Reynolds & Kamphaus, 2004) includes a Student Observation System (SOS), in which one can observe children's behavior in the classroom using a momentary time-sampling procedure. The SOS specifies 65 common behaviors in classrooms settings and includes both adaptive (e.g., "follows directions," "returns material used in class") and maladaptive (e.g., "fidgets in seat," "teases others") behaviors. The observation period in the classroom involves 15 minutes, divided into 30 intervals of 30 seconds each. The child's behavior is observed for 3 seconds at the end of each interval, and the observer codes all behaviors observed during this time window. Unfortunately, there has been minimal empirical testing of the BASC-SOS, although scores from this observation system did differentiate between students with and without disruptive

behavior disorders in one sample of schoolchildren (Lett & Kamphaus, 1997).

A similar observational system can be used as part of the ASEBA assessment system. The DOF/5–14 (Achenbach & Rescorla, 2001) was designed to observe students, ages 5–14, for 10-minute periods in the classroom. Following this period, the observer writes a narrative of the child's behavior and rates 96 behaviors on a 4-point scale (0, *Behavior was not observed*, through 3, *Definite occurrence of behavior with severe intensity or for greater than 3 minutes duration*). Like the ASEBA rating scales, these ratings can be summed into Total Problem, Internalizing, and Externalizing behavior composites. The DOF has been shown to discriminate between referred and nonreferred children in the classroom (e.g., Reed & Edelbrock, 1983), as well as between children with externalizing and other behavior problems (e.g., McConaughey, Achenbach, & Gent, 1988).

The BCS (Forehand & McMahon, 1981) has been modified for use in the classroom to assess teacher–child interactions, both alone (e.g., Breiner & Forehand, 1981) and in combination with a measure of academic engaged time (AET) (McNeil et al., 1991). AET, the amount of time that a child or adolescent is appropriately engaged in on-task behavior during class time, is assessed with a simple stopwatch recording procedure (Walker, Colvin, & Ramsey, 1995). Walker and colleagues (1995) recommend observing children during two 15-minute periods. AET has been shown to correlate positively with academic performance and to discriminate between boys at risk for CPs and those not at risk (e.g., Walker, Shinn, O'Neill, & Ramsey, 1987). The Revised Edition of the School Observation Coding System (REDSOCS; Jacobs et al., 2000), which has been used with 3- to 6-year-old clinic-referred children with ODD and nonreferred children in preschool and kindergarten classrooms (e.g., Filcheck et al., 2004), may be particularly appropriate for classroom observations of young, noncompliant children.

There are surprisingly few data to guide pragmatic decisions concerning the number and length of observation sessions needed to obtain reliable and valid information. Although potentially very useful, as noted earlier, observational assessment methods may be expensive in terms of time and personnel, especially if multiple observation sessions are

TABLE 3.3. Major Questions Guiding the School Observation Report

Descriptive information

What is the child's name, date of birth, parents' names, and contact information?
Who is the referring clinician?
What is the location, date and time of the actual observation?
What is the name of the teacher or any other staff involved with the child?

Reason for observation

Who requested the observation?
What are the goals of the observation?
What are the primary referral questions?
What are the specific target behaviors (both adaptive and maladaptive)?
Were any previous observations performed? What were the results?

Teacher interview

What problem behaviors are reported by teacher?
What academic difficulties are reported by teacher?
In what settings do the problem behaviors most frequently occur?
What are the suspected triggers of the problem behaviors?
What are the current consequences of the problem behaviors?
What past or current interventions were implemented by the teacher or other professionals? How effective
    were they?

Classroom environment

What is the number of students and staff in the classroom?
What is the size and shape of the classroom?
What is the location of furniture/equipment, seating arrangements and placement of the child?
Are there distracting stimuli, background noises, or outside-class interruptions?
Are the traffic patterns well defined and safe?
Are there established routines for toileting, drinks, snack time, etc.?
Are the class rules and consequences posted in a visible location? Are the rules reinforced?

Child observation

What classes, lessons, or tasks occurred during the observation period?
What evaluation procedures were used and are they described?
What were the results of the observation?
Describe the severity, frequency, and duration of the target behaviors
Describe the antecedents and consequences of the observed behaviors
Support all statements with data from the observation
Are the results of the observation reliable and valid?
Was the child's behavior during the observation representative of this child's behavior in this context more
    generally?

Recommendations

Based on the results, what should the teachers and school personnel do to effectively modify the child's
    behavior?
Based on the results, what can the parents do to effectively modify the child's behavior?
What implications do the results have for the therapist treating the child?
Is a follow-up school observation warranted? If so, when?

Note. From Nock and Kurtz (2005). Copyright 2005 by the Association for Advancement of Behavior Therapy. Reprinted by permission.

conducted to enhance sensitivity to treatment effects (Aspland & Gardner, 2003). Reactivity to being observed does not appear to be a significant problem for most young children and their parents, especially if clinicians and researchers provide the opportunity for them to become familiar with the observation procedures, use the same observer across multiple sessions, and minimize the obtrusiveness of recording equipment (Aspland & Gardner, 2003).

An alternative to observations by independent observers in the natural setting is to train significant adults in the child's or adolescent's environment to observe and record certain types of behavior. The most widely used procedure of this type, the Parent Daily Report (PDR; Chamberlain & Reid, 1987), is a parent observation measure that is typically administered during brief (5- to 10-minute) telephone interviews. Parents are asked which of a number of overt and covert behaviors have occurred in the past 24 hours. The PDR can be employed on a pretreatment basis to assess the magnitude of behavior problems and as a check on information presented by the parents in the initial interview. It can also be used during intervention to monitor the progress of the family. Finally, the PDR has been employed extensively as a measure of parent management training outcome (e.g., Bank, Marlowe, Reid, Patterson, & Weinrott, 1991; Chamberlain & Reid, 1991; Webster-Stratton & Hammond, 1997). It has the added advantages of being brief and, because of the 24-hour reporting frame, of perhaps providing more objective data than that obtained from behavior rating scales or interviews.

Reviews of the psychometric characteristics of the PDR are presented by Patterson (1982) and Chamberlain and Reid (1987). The PDR possesses adequate intercaller and interparent reliability, as well as internal consistency and temporal stability. With respect to stability, Chamberlain and Reid noted that, at least with nonreferred families, PDR scores tend to be inflated on the first day but stable thereafter. It may be advisable to discard data from the first telephone interview with the PDR. Normative data are presented by Chamberlain and Reid for parents of children ages 4–10. The PDR has been shown to correlate significantly with direct observation measures in populations of socially aggressive, stealing, and normal children

(Patterson, 1982; Webster-Stratton & Spitzer, 1991). The PDR has shown moderate convergent validity with other parent report measures of child behavior and parental adjustment (Chamberlain & Reid, 1987; Webster-Stratton & Spitzer, 1991). Chamberlain and Reid reported that social desirability factors seem to exert minimal influence on PDR scores, at least with nonreferred families.

For the occurrence of certain low-rate covert behaviors, such as stealing, firesetting, and truancy, parent- and/or teacher-collected data may be the only sources of information. Patterson and his colleagues (1975) developed specific techniques for the assessment and treatment of children who steal. Because behaviors such as stealing are rarely observed, the target behavior is redefined as "the child's taking, or being in possession of, anything that does not clearly belong to him" or the parent's "receiving a report or complaint by a reliable informant" (Patterson et al., 1975, p. 137). Jones (1974) developed a brief daily interview similar to the PDR for collecting parent report data on stealing by children between ages 5 and 15. The parent is queried as to whether stealing took place, and, if so, the item(s) stolen and their value, the location and social context of the theft, how the parent learned of the theft, and the parent's response to the theft. The Telephone Interview Report on Stealing and Social Aggression (TIROSSA) has adequate test–retest reliability and is sensitive to the effects of treatment procedures designed to reduce stealing (Reid, Hinojosa Rivera, & Lorber, 1980).

Functional Impairment

It is increasingly being recognized that the child's or adolescent's level of functional impairment, over and above the level of CP symptomatology, is critical to determining whether the youth needs treatment and the intensity of treatment that may be required (Bird, 1999; Bloomquist & Schnell, 2002). Furthermore, degree of impairment may vary across domains of functioning, so it is important that multiple domains be assessed, and by multiple informants when possible. As noted earlier, structured interviews based on the DSM allow for the assessment of impairment. There are also a number of measures designed specifically to assess the youth's level of impairment, including the Children's Global Assessment Scale (C-GAS;

Shaffer et al., 1983), the Columbia Impairment Scale (CIS; Bird et al., 1993), and the Child and Adolescent Functional Assessment Scale (CAFAS; Hodges, 2000). Also, several of the broad rating scales summarized in Table 3.2 include subscales that assess important areas of potential impairment of children with CPs. For example, the BASC-2 (Reynolds & Kamphaus, 2004) contains scales that assess the child's academic adjustment (e.g., learning problems, attitude toward school and teacher, study skills), social adjustment (e.g., social stress, interpersonal relations), and self-concept (e.g., self-concept, sense of inadequacy).

Knowledge of impairment is important for a number of reasons. First, it can determine how intensive and restrictive an intervention may need to be (Frick, 2004), it can provide useful information to the clinician concerning possible intervention targets (Frick, 2006), and it may also serve as an important indicator of intervention outcome (Hodges, Xue, & Wotring, 2004). A related construct, adaptive disability, is based on the degree of discrepancy between the child's or adolescent's adaptive functioning and IQ level (Barkley et al., 2002). Using the parent-completed Normative Adaptive Behavior Checklist (NABC; Adams, 1984) to assess adaptive functioning in samples of normal and behaviorally disruptive preschool-age children, Barkley and colleagues (2002) found adaptive disability to be an independent predictor of negative outcomes, over and above initial levels of disruptive behavior.

Summary

Because of the heterogeneity in CP behaviors, it is essential to assess levels and types of these behaviors. Developmentally appropriate, broad-based behavior rating scales may be completed by multiple informants in relatively brief time periods and provide good, norm-referenced information on the child's or adolescent's behaviors. Structured diagnostic interviews may also be employed, although they are usually much more time-consuming. Noncompliance is best assessed through structured clinical interviews and observation of parent–child interaction (e.g., McMahon & Forehand, 2003). A number of clinic-based analogues to assess CPs (especially in the context of parent–child interaction) demonstrate sensitivity to treatment effects. Other forms of aggression (e.g., reactive, proactive, relational) may be assessed through youth, parent, and teacher rating scales. Covert CP behaviors, because of their clandestine nature, are extremely difficult to assess. At present, clinicians are forced to rely primarily on reports from multiple informants on behavior rating scales (or in the case of stealing, on brief phone interviews) as to whether, and to what extent, such behaviors are occurring. Innovative observational paradigms to assess covert behaviors such as stealing, property destruction, and firesetting behaviors (e.g., Hinshaw et al., 1992; Kolko et al., 1991) are promising, but their clinical utility has yet to be demonstrated. A major task for the field is to develop valid and clinically useful instruments for the assessment of covert CPs.

Comorbidity: Implications for Assessment

The large number of co-occurring conditions that are often present in youth with CPs suggest that assessment must be comprehensive and cover a large number of adjustment areas, and not focus solely on CPs (see Table 3.1). As illustrated in Table 3.2, many behavior rating scales provide information on a number of important areas of adjustment; thus, they have utility as screening instruments. As mentioned previously, these often include forms for parents, teachers, and the youth to complete, providing information from multiple informants in a time-efficient manner. Furthermore, most scales provide good, norm-referenced scores to compare the child's or adolescent's score to a reference group. However, to assess many of the comorbid conditions, more detailed information on the history of symptoms and the level of impairment they cause for the child or adolescent may be important. This typically requires a clinical and/or a structured interview, perhaps in conjunction with a rating scale designed to assess functional impairment or adaptive functioning, to make the diagnosis adequately. If CPs occur in the context of a language impairment, then a developmental assessment is warranted (Wakschlag & Danis, 2004). The CBCL/1½–5 (Achenbach & Rescorla, 2000) incorporates the Language Development Survey, and the BASC-2 (Reynolds & Kamphaus, 2004) includes a Functional Communication subscale, both of which assess risk factors for language delays and parental report of the young child's expressive vocabulary and word combinations.

Space limitations preclude discussion of the assessment of the various conditions that co-occur with CPs. Instead, we refer the reader to Chapters 2, 4, 5, 8, and 13, this volume, on ADHD, substance use, depression, anxiety, and learning disabilities, respectively.

Summary

Comorbid disorders that are most likely to be encountered in youth referred for CPs include ADHD, depressive and anxiety disorders, substance use problems, language impairment, and learning difficulties. As a result, most assessments of children and adolescents with CPs need to be comprehensive, covering many domains of psychological functioning. Most of the same broad-band measures recommended for initial use in identifying the range of CP behaviors may also be used as general screens for the identification of comorbid disorders and conditions. Disorder-specific behavior rating scales, interviews, and other, more intensive assessment procedures (e.g., intelligence and achievement testing) should then be conducted as needed for the comorbid disorders.

Multiple Risks: Implications for Assessment

Research clearly documents myriad factors in various domains, both internal and external to the child or adolescent, associated with CPs. The availability of instruments to assess these many factors is quite variable. In this section, we note those that seem most salient and potentially appropriate for use in applied settings, although the clinical utility of many of these instruments has yet to be adequately tested. (See Table 3.1 for a list of representative measures.)

One should obtain a brief developmental and medical history of the child or adolescent to determine whether any medical factors might be associated with the development or maintenance of the CP behaviors, and whether the youth's early temperament may have contributed to the development of a coercive style of parent–child interaction. A number of standardized ratings of temperament may have utility in assessing youth with CPs (Frick, 2004), such as the Children's Behavior Questionnaire (Rothbart & Jones, 1998).

One class of potentially important correlates to severe CPs is specific cognitive deficits and learning styles. As discussed earlier, because deficits in intelligence, especially verbal intelli-

gence, have been associated with CPs, a standard intellectual evaluation should be part of most assessment batteries for CPs. There are also computerized tasks that assess the characteristic learning style of many youth with CPs (e.g., heightened sensitivity to rewards compared to punishments). However, some major limitations in the development of these tasks make their usefulness in many clinical assessments somewhat limited at the present time (see Frick & Loney, 2000, for a review). There are also research-based measures, typically involving a child or adolescent being provided a hypothetical vignette of a social situation and asked to state how he or she would respond if the situation were real, that assess several deficits in social cognition associated with CPs, such as a hostile attributional bias. Examples include the Intention–Cue Detection Task, the Problem-Solving Measure for Conflict, and the Wally Child Social Problem-Solving Detective (WALLY) Game (Conduct Problems Prevention Research Group, 1999; Dodge & Coie, 1987; Webster-Stratton & Lindsay, 1999). Although these measures are also not without limitations in their clinical usefulness (Frick & Loney, 2000), interventions for the deficits assessed by these measures are part of many treatment programs for CPs; therefore, the information they provide may be useful in treatment planning (Lochman & Wells, 1996). The recently developed Social-Cognitive Assessment Profile (SCAP; Hughes, Meehan, & Cavell, 2004), which shows promise as a brief (15- to 20-minute), clinically useful interview with elementary school–age children, is designed to assess social-cognitive deficits associated with CPs.

As noted earlier, children and adolescents with CPs frequently have problems with peer interactions (e.g., peer rejection, association with a deviant peer group). If the information from behavioral interviews, behavior rating scales (e.g., the Social Competence scales of the CBCL/6–18; Achenbach & Rescorla, 2001), and/or observations indicate that this is a problem area for a particular youth, additional assessment of his or her social skills is necessary. The assessment should examine not only the behavioral aspects of the social skills difficulties but also cognitive and affective dimensions. Traditionally, assessment of social skills has involved behavioral observations, sociometric measures, and questionnaires. Bierman and Welsh (1997) provided strategies for the assessment of social relationship problems, and Demaray and colleagues (1995) reviewed several behavior rating scales for the assessment of social competence. Although a number of strategies have been developed to assess social functioning, some of the measures (e.g., sociometrics) have minimal clinical utility, because these data are extremely time-consuming to collect (Kamphaus & Frick, 2005). However, a brief (5- to 10-minute) observation analogue procedure for assessing young children's CPs with peers in a rigged card game (SNAP!— Hughes, Cutting, & Dunn, 2001; Hughes et al., 2002) shows promise, because it differentiates between children with CP and control children, and is associated with parent and teacher CP ratings. Similarly, clinically useful measures to assess associations with a deviant peer group are limited currently to youth or parent reports, although a structured observational paradigm developed for research purposes may prove to be adaptable to the clinical setting (e.g., Dishion, Andrews, & Crosby, 1995).

McMahon and Estes (1997) delineated six areas that are relevant to the assessment of familial and extrafamilial factors in youth with CPs: parenting practices; parents' perceptions of the youth and social cognitions; parents' perceptions of their own personal and marital adjustment; parental stress; parental functioning in extrafamilial social contexts; and parental satisfaction with treatment. The first area, *parenting practices*, has been assessed through clinical interviews, behavioral observation of parent–child interactions, and parent and youth reports on behavior rating scales. As noted earlier, direct behavioral observation has long been a critical component of the assessment of youth with CPs and their families, both for delineating specific patterns of maladaptive parent–child interaction and for assessing change in those interactions as a function of treatment. Observational data can be compared with data gathered via other methods to assist the clinician in determining whether the focus of treatment should be on the parent–child interaction or on parental perceptual and/ or personal adjustment issues. For example, congruence between observational data and a parent-completed behavior rating scale would be consistent with the former focus, whereas normal levels of youth behavior in the observed interaction might suggest that the focus of intervention be on parental perceptual issues. The observation procedures and coding sys-

tems described earlier for assessing CPs in the context of parent–child interactions (e.g., BCS, DPICS) also provide important information concerning parent behavior.

Several questionnaires designed specifically to assess parenting practices may potentially be quite useful as adjuncts to behavioral observations and/or to assess parental behaviors that either occur infrequently or are otherwise difficult to observe (e.g., physical discipline, parental monitoring practices), as screening instruments, and to measure the effects of parent management training interventions. Two examples that have significant psychometric support are the Parenting Scale (Arnold, O'Leary, Wolff, & Acker, 1993) and the Alabama Parenting Questionnaire (Shelton, Frick, & Wootton, 1996). (See Morsbach & Prinz, 2006, for a summary of parent report measures of parenting practices and suggestions for improving their validity.)

The Parenting Scale (Arnold et al., 1993) comprises 30 items that describe parental discipline practices in response to child misbehavior. Each item has a 7-point rating scale anchored by statements of the effective and ineffective forms of a particular parenting behavior (e.g., "I coax or beg my child to stop" and "I firmly tell my child to stop"). Items are worded at a sixth-grade level or below, and the measure takes 5–10 minutes to complete.

The original factor analysis of the Parenting Scale conducted with parents of 2- to 3-year-old children indicated that three factors accounted for 37% of the variance: Laxness, Overreactivity, and Verbosity (Arnold et al., 1993). However, subsequent research with more ethnically diverse samples and broader age ranges have generally found a two-factor solution, with factors that resemble the original Laxness and Overactivity factors. The Verbosity factor has not been replicated in these subsequent studies. The two-factor solution has been identified in samples of European American 2- to 12 year-old children (Collett, Gimpel, Greenson, & Gunderson, 2001) and middle school students (Irvine, Biglan, Smolkowski, & Ary, 1999), as well as in preschool-age (Reitman et al., 2001) and elementary school–age (Steele, Nesbitt-Daly, Daniel, & Forehand, 2005) African American samples. In addition, these studies have generally found that 5- to 6-item solutions for each factor are sufficient, thus suggesting that the original 30-item Parenting Scale can be shortened considerably.

These studies have documented that the Parenting Scale has reasonable properties with respect to reliability and validity, and that it is sensitive to intervention effects (e.g., Gardner, Burton, & Klimes, 2006; Irvine et al., 1999; Nixon et al., 2003; Sanders, Markie-Dadds, Tully, & Bor, 2000).

The Alabama Parenting Questionnaire (APQ; Frick, 1991) was developed for use with parents of elementary school–age children and adolescents (6–17 years old), although it has been used in samples as young as age 4 (e.g., Dadds, Maujean, & Fraser, 2003). It comprises 42 items that have been divided into five a priori constructs—Involvement, Positive Parenting, Poor Monitoring/Supervision, Inconsistent Discipline, and Corporal Punishment. It also includes several other items assessing "other discipline practices," such as use of time out or taking away privileges. The items are presented in both global report (i.e., questionnaire) and telephone interview formats, and there are separate versions of each format for parents and children. Thus, there are currently four different versions of the APQ. The questionnaire format employs a 5-point Likert-type frequency scale and asks the informant how frequently each of the various parenting practices typically occurs. Four telephone interviews are conducted, and the informant is asked to report the frequency with which each parenting practice has occurred over the previous 3 days.

Most of the published research using the APQ to date has utilized the global report formats of the scale, with the exception of Shelton and colleagues (1996). Two studies now provide support for the five-factor structure of the parent global report format of the APQ, which corresponds to the five dimensions around which the scale was developed. The first study was conducted with 1,402 children, ages 4–9, in Australia (Elgar, Waschbusch, Dadds, & Sigvaldason, 2007), and the second study, with 1,219 German schoolchildren, ages 10–12 (Essau, Sasagawa, & Frick, 2006). Importantly, one study has also shown that parent ratings on the APQ are significantly associated with observations of parenting behavior in 4- to 8-year-old boys (Hawes & Dadds, 2006). A number of studies have shown that the APQ scales are associated with CPs in children in community (Dadds et al., 2003), clinic-referred (Frick, Christian, & Wootton, 1999; Hawes & Dadds, 2006), and inpatient samples (Blader, 2004), as well as in families with deaf children

(Brubaker & Szakowski, 2000) and with substance-abusing parents (Stanger, Dumenci, Kamon, & Burstein, 2004). Also, these studies have documented this relationship in samples as young as age 4 (Dadds et al., 2003; Hawes & Dadds, 2006) and as old as age 17 (Frick, Christian, & Wootton, 1999). However, Frick, Christian, and Wootton (1999) did demonstrate some differences in which dimensions of parenting were most strongly associated with CPs at different ages: Inconsistent Discipline was most strongly associated with CPs in young children (ages 6–8); Corporal Punishment was most strongly associated with CPs in older children (ages 9–12), and Involvement and Poor Monitoring/Supervision were most strongly related to CPs in adolescents (ages 13–17). Also, this study raised concerns about the reliability of the child report format in very young children (under age 9) (see also Shelton et al., 1996). Finally, several studies have used the APQ scales to test changes in parenting behaviors following interventions with children with CPs (e.g., August, Lee, Bloomquist, Realmuto, & Hektner, 2003; Feinfield & Baker, 2004; Hawes & Dadds, 2006).

Parental perceptions of the youth and social cognitions are a second important area to be assessed. Parental perception of a child is a strong predictor of referral for CP types of behavior, perhaps even more so than the child's behavior (e.g., Griest et al., 1980). In an analogue study, Johnston and Patenaude (1994) reported that parents of children with ADHD perceived children who displayed oppositional behavior as having more control over their behavior than did children who displayed inattentive/overactive behavior, and they reported more negative affective responses to the oppositional children. As noted earlier, studies with parents of clinic-referred children have shown that they are more likely to misperceive child behaviors than are parents of nonreferred children (e.g., Holleran et al., 1982; Wahler & Sansbury, 1990).

These findings suggest that some measure of significant adults' perceptions of the child is an essential component of the assessment process. The behavior rating scales described earlier are the most ready sources of such data. As noted, comparisons of the ECBI Problem and Intensity scores may be especially useful with respect to parent tolerance for child behavior. (This also applies to the SESBI-R with teachers.) When examined in the context of behavioral observation data and the clinician's own impressions, these behavior rating scales can be important indicators of whether the informants (parents, teachers) appear to have a perceptual bias in their assessment of the referred child's behavior.

An alternative methodology for assessing potential perceptual biases in the parents of children with CPs is the use of brief written, audiotaped, or videotaped scenarios or vignettes describing parent–child interactions in which a child displays a variety of inappropriate, neutral, and positive behaviors (e.g., Holleran et al., 1982; Wahler & Sansbury, 1990). Although such methods have been employed on a limited basis in the research literature, their validity and utility in clinical settings have yet to be examined. A more clinically relevant method for assessing parent and child perceptions of self and each other was developed by Sanders and Dadds (1992). In their video-mediated recall procedure, the parent views a videotape of a previously recorded problem-solving discussion with his or her child. The videotape is stopped every 20 seconds, and the parent describes what he or she was thinking at that point in the interaction. Sanders and Dadds demonstrated that this procedure discriminated between clinic-referred families whose child has CPs and nonreferred families. The clinic-referred parents stated fewer self- and family-referent positive cognitions and more family-referent negative cognitions than did the nonreferred parents. Furthermore, the video-mediated recall procedure was superior to an alternative thought-listing procedure.

Two measures that assess aspects of parental self-esteem (e.g., satisfaction, self-efficacy, and locus of control with the parenting role) are the Parenting Sense of Competence Scale (PSOC; as adapted by Johnston & Mash, 1989) and the Parental Locus of Control Scale (PLOC; Campis, Lyman, & Prentice-Dunn, 1986). The PSOC comprises 16 items that typically load on two factors: Satisfaction, which refers to the extent to which the parent reports satisfaction with the parenting role, and Efficacy, which reflects the parent's self-report of skill and familiarity with the parenting role (Johnston & Mash, 1989; Ohan, Leung, & Johnston, 2000; Rogers & Matthews, 2004), although Rogers and Matthews also found support for a third factor of parental Interest. Adequate internal consistency reliabilities for the total, Satisfaction, and Efficacy scales have been reported

(e.g., r's = .79, .75, and .76, respectively) by Johnston and Mash (1989). The Satisfaction score was consistently more highly correlated with measures of child behavior and parental adjustment than was the Efficacy score (Johnston & Mash, 1989; Ohan et al., 2000; Rogers & Matthews, 2004). The Efficacy score was positively correlated with social desirability in a nonreferred sample (Lovejoy, Verda, & Hays, 1997). There are minimal effects of child age or gender on PSOC scores.

The PSOC has been employed with several clinic-referred populations, including children with CPs (Gardner et al., 2006), physically abused children (Mash, Johnston, & Kovitz, 1983), and children with ADHD (e.g., Mash & Johnston, 1983) and ADHD plus CPs (Johnston, 1996b). Johnston reported that the total PSOC score distinguished among parents (mothers and fathers) of nonreferred children, children with ADHD plus low levels of oppositional behavior, and children with ADHD plus high levels of oppositional behavior. The PSOC has been shown to be sensitive to the effects of parent management training in samples of children with CPs (Gardner et al., 2006) and ADHD (Pisterman et al., 1992).

The PLOC comprises 47 items that load on five factors: Parental Efficacy, Parental Responsibility, Child Control of Parent's Life, Parental Belief in Fate/Chance, and Parental Control of Child's Behavior. Adequate internal consistency and test–retest reliabilities have been demonstrated (Campis et al., 1986; Roberts et al., 1992). Parents of clinic-referred children have a more external locus of control than do parents of nonreferred children (Campis et al., 1986; Mouton & Tuma, 1988; Roberts et al., 1992). Scores on the PLOC have been shown to be affected by social desirability (Campis et al., 1986; Lovejoy et al., 1997). The total score on the PLOC is correlated with the PSOC (Lovejoy et al., 1997) and the Parenting Stress Index (Mouton & Tuma, 1988), but not with observed parent behavior (Roberts et al., 1992). It is associated with observed severity of child oppositional behavior on the CT (Roberts et al., 1992). Parents who completed a parent management training program had a more internal locus of control by the end of treatment (e.g., Eyberg, Boggs, & Algina, 1995; Nixon et al., 2003; Roberts et al., 1992). Roberts and colleagues (1992) also reported that parental locus of control was not associated with treatment dropout.

To assess the extent to which *parents' personal and marital adjustment problems* may be playing a role in the youth's CPs, a set of screening procedures that includes brief questions in the initial interviews with the parents and certain parental self-report measures can be utilized. Exposition and discussion of a thorough assessment of various personal (e.g., depression, antisocial behavior, substance abuse) and marital adjustment problems that may occur in parents of children with CPs are beyond the scope of this chapter. Instead, a set of brief screening procedures is needed to ascertain whether a more complete and thorough assessment for a particular problem, or group of problems, is required. Questions related to these issues can best be incorporated into the initial interview with the parents. In some cases, the youth may also be asked for his or her perceptions (e.g., "Does your dad ever seem to have too much to drink?" "How do your mom and dad get along with each other?"). In conjunction with the judicious use of the various self-report measures described below, the clinician should be able to make a decision as to the necessity of pursuing any of these areas in greater detail. Should that be the case, then the Special Section, "Developing Guidelines for the Evidence-Based Assessment (EBA) of Adult Disorders" in the journal *Psychological Assessment* (2005, Volume 17) is a useful resource. Additional sources are cited in the relevant sections below.

The Beck Depression Inventory (BDI; Beck, Rush, Shaw, & Emery, 1979) (and its successor, the BDI-II [Beck, Steer, & Brown, 1996], which was modified to make it more consistent with the DSM-IV criteria) has been the most frequently employed measure of maternal depression with mothers of children with CPs. The BDI-II comprises 21 items that assess sadness, anhedonia, and suicidal ideation. Each item is scored on a 4-point scale, with higher scores indicating greater depression. It is typically self-administered and can be completed in 5–10 minutes. Psychometric data on the BDI and BDI-II with various populations are quite extensive and supportive of their validity for assessing clinically significant levels of distress (e.g., Beck et al., 1996; Beck, Steer, & Garbin, 1988). With respect to its use with parents of children with CPs, most of the extant research has used the BDI rather than the BDI-II. The BDI differentiates between mothers of non-referred children and mothers of clinic-referred

children with CPs (e.g., Griest et al., 1980), and relative to other types of measures (e.g., behavioral observations of child behavior), has been found to be the best predictor of maternal perceptions of clinic-referred children with CPs (Forehand, Wells, McMahon, Griest, & Rogers, 1982; Webster-Stratton, 1988). It has been shown to change in a positive direction following parents' completion of a parent management training program and/or a child's cognitive-behavioral therapy intervention (e.g., Forehand, Wells, & Griest, 1980; Kazdin et al., 1992; Webster-Stratton, 1994), and to predict dropout and response to treatment (e.g., Kazdin 1995; McMahon, Forehand, Griest, & Wells, 1981).

It should be noted that the BDI/BDI-II is not intended for diagnosing depression; rather, it is a measure of the severity of various depressive symptoms (which cluster into cognitive and somatic–affective dimensions of depression; e.g., Steer, Ball, Ranieri, & Beck, 1999). Thus, when used with parents of children with CPs, the BDI/BDI-II is probably best regarded as an indicator of parental personal distress and of the need for more in-depth assessment of depression, rather than of depression per se (McMahon & Estes, 1997).

Parental antisocial behavior can be assessed with structured diagnostic interviews or the Minnesota Multiphasic Personality Inventory (MMPI), although time considerations may make these options less feasible. The Antisocial Behavior Checklist (ASB Checklist; Zucker & Noll, 1980) is a self-report instrument that comprises 46 items describing a variety of overt and covert antisocial activities that may have occurred from adolescence through adulthood. Each item is rated on a 4-point scale for frequency of occurrence. A cutoff score of 24 or higher is considered indicative of antisocial behavior and is consistent with DSM-III-R criteria for APD (with a sensitivity of .85 and specificity of .83). The ASB Checklist has reasonable psychometric properties when assessed in samples from prison populations, court offenders, community-based alcoholics, court-referred alcoholics, university students, and community dwellers (Ham, Zucker, & Fitzgerald, 1993). Scores on the ASB Checklist were negatively correlated with SES and education, and positively correlated with measures of hostility, depression, family conflict, and alcohol-related problems (e.g., Ham et al., 1993; Loukas, Fitzgerald, Zucker, & von Eye, 2001).

In a sample of families with alcoholic fathers, scores on the ASB Checklist were significantly higher for both the alcoholic fathers and their spouses than for fathers and mothers in comparison families (Fitzgerald et al., 1993). However, neither paternal nor maternal ASB Checklist scores were significant predictors of child behavior problems (externalizing or internalizing) in 3-year-old sons. In a subsequent report, both the alcoholic fathers and the mothers of 3- to 5-year-old boys who scored above the clinical cutoff on the CBCL Total Behavior Problems scale had higher scores on the ASB Checklist than the parents of boys who scored below the CBCL cutoff (Jansen, Fitzgerald, Ham, & Zucker, 1995). Both maternal and paternal scores on the ASB Checklist contributed to the prediction of CBCL scores for the total sample. To our knowledge, this measure has not been used with samples of parents whose children have CPs. However, given the findings we described with alcoholic families, its use as a measure of parental ASB appears promising.

Because antisocial fathers are often absent or uninvolved, clinicians are often forced to rely on these men's female partners for reports about the fathers' antisocial behavior, and this seems especially to be the case in families of children with CPs (Tapscott, Frick, Wootton, & Kruh, 1996). Tapscott and colleagues (1996) reported significant correlations between mothers' and fathers' report of fathers' history of antisocial behavior in a clinical referred sample of children. Similarly, Caspi and colleagues (2001) demonstrated that women's and men's reports about the men's antisocial behavior were highly correlated. However, in this latter study, the women's reports underestimated the absolute level of the antisocial behavior. Thus, whereas a mother's report may be a reasonably accurate proxy of a father's relative level of antisocial behavior, reliance on this information is not sufficient to determine the true frequency of antisocial behavior in fathers.

With respect to substance use, some of the more frequently employed screening instruments that may prove useful in working with parents of youth with CPs include the Short Michigan Alcoholism Screening Test (SMAST; Selzer, Vinokur, & van Rooijen, 1975), the Drug Abuse Screening Test (DAST; Skinner, 1982), and the Alcohol Use Disorders Identification Test (AUDIT; Saunders, Aasland, Babor, de la Fuente, & Grant, 1993).

Parents also should be screened for both lifetime and current ADHD if the youth presents with comorbid CP and ADHD. The DSM-IV ADHD Rating Scale is a screening device that can be used for this purpose (Murphy & Gordon, 1998).

With respect to marital discord, the Marital Adjustment Test (MAT; Locke & Wallace, 1959) and the Dyadic Adjustment Scale (DAS; Spanier, 1976) have been the most widely used instruments with parents of children with CPs. The MAT has been shown to discriminate between distressed and nondistressed couples (Locke & Wallace, 1959) and to correlate with children's CPs (e.g., Forehand & Brody, 1985; Frick et al., 1989). The MAT has shown high levels of reliability, stability (i.e., 2 years; Kimmel & van der Veen, 1974), and validity (Burgess, Locke, & Thomes, 1971). It has shown convergent validity with independent observations of marital interaction (Julien, Markman, & Lindahl, 1989) and with scores on the DAS (Busby, Christensen, Crane, & Larson, 1995). Webster-Stratton (1988) found that marital distress measured by the MAT contributed to negative perceptions of child behavior and to increased negative maternal behavior.

The DAS (Spanier, 1976), a 32-item self-report inventory, contains four subscales of marital adjustment: Dyadic Consensus (spouses' agreement regarding various marital issues), Dyadic Cohesion (extent to which partners involve themselves in joint activities), Dyadic Satisfaction (overall evaluation of the marital relationship and level of commitment to the relationship), and Affectional Expression (degree of affection and sexual involvement in the relationship). The DAS has been found to possess adequate reliability (e.g., Carey, Spector, Lantinga, & Krauss, 1993; Spanier, 1976) and validity (e.g., Crane, Allgood, Larson, & Griffin, 1990). Marital dissatisfaction, as measured by the DAS, has been shown to relate to greater oppositional behavior in elementary school–age boys through the indirect pathway of rejection by fathers (Mann & MacKenzie, 1996).

Two questionnaires are often used to assess general marital conflict: the O'Leary–Porter Scale (OPS; Porter & O'Leary, 1980), and the Conflict Tactics Scales—Partner (CTS-Partner; Straus, 1979, 1990). The OPS, a 10-item parent-completed questionnaire, is designed to assess the frequency of various forms of overt marital hostility (e.g., quarrels, sarcasm, and physical abuse) that are witnessed by the child. There is some evidence that this scale is more strongly associated than the MAT with parental ratings of CP behavior (Porter & O'Leary, 1980). Conflict, as measured by the OPS, is related to increased oppositional behavior in boys through disruptions in maternal discipline (Mann & MacKenzie, 1996) and to adolescent overt and covert CP behavior (Forehand, Long, & Hedrick, 1987).

The CTS-Partner, a 38-item parent-report questionnaire, assesses the strategies couples use to resolve conflict. It includes a range of strategies, from discussion to yelling, pushing, threatening or beating up the partner. Straus (1979, 1990) reported adequate reliability, validity, and norms to use in interpreting scores on the CTS-Partner. O'Leary, Vivian and Malone (1992) suggest that the CTS-Partner may be a particularly accurate method for obtaining reports of physical aggression, because wives tend to underreport aggression in written self-reports and interviews. Marital physical and nonphysical aggression as measured by the CTS-Partner, has been shown to be positively correlated with children's CPs (Jouriles, Norwood, McDonald, Vincent, & Mahoney, 1996). The CTS-Partner has been revised extensively. Psychometric properties of the CTS2 are presented in Straus, Hamby, Boney-McCoy, and Sugarman (1996).

In addition, instruments that have been designed to measure parenting-related conflict include the Parenting Alliance Inventory (Abidin & Brunner, 1995) (now called the Parenting Alliance Measure; Abidin & Konold, 1999), Child-Rearing Disagreements (Jouriles et al., 1991), and the Parent Problem Checklist (Dadds & Powell, 1991). There is some evidence to suggest that these more specific measures may account for additional explanatory variance over measures of marital satisfaction. For example, Jouriles and colleagues (1991) reported that Child-Rearing Disagreements significantly predicted CPs even after general marital dissatisfaction, as measured by the MAT, was controlled.

The fourth area, *parenting stress*, includes both general measures of stress (e.g., life event scales) and specific measures of parenting-related stress. Examples of the former include the Life Experiences Survey (Sarason, Johnson,

& Siegel, 1978) and the Family Events List (Patterson, 1982). The Life Experiences Survey, a 47-item, self-report measure, has been shown to be a moderately reliable instrument. Parents of children with ADHD and CPs have been shown to have higher scores on the Life Experiences Survey (Johnston, 1996b), and in families whose children have CPs, the measure has discriminated between abusive and nonabusive parents (Whipple & Webster-Stratton, 1991). The Family Events List (Patterson, 1982) is a self-report measure with 46 minor but "hassling" events that may occur in daily living (e.g., child care problems, car problems, work-related problems). Snyder (1991) reported that when mothers of children with CPs experienced frequent hassles and negative mood, they tend to respond to their children's negative behavior in a more coercive manner. The types of stressors and the time frame for reporting on these life event scales vary. This is important, because it may be that proximal "hassle" stressors, such as those on the Family Events List, have a different relationship to family functioning, parenting behavior, and CPs than the distal stressors on the Life Experiences Survey.

Measures specific to parenting-related stress include Parenting Daily Hassles (Crnic & Greenberg, 1990) and the Parenting Stress Index (PSI; Abidin, 1995). Parenting Daily Hassles, a 20-item self-report questionnaire, measures events in parenting and parent–child interactions (Crnic & Greenberg, 1990). Parents rate the frequency, the degree of hassle, and the intensity of each hassle. In a non-referred sample, Crnic and Greenberg found that the cumulative effects of relatively minor stresses related to parenting are important predictors of parent and child behaviors, and that daily hassles are more predictive of children's CPs than scores on the Life Experiences Survey. Greater mother-reported daily hassles are positively correlated with CBCL/1½–5 Externalizing scores in 1-, 2-, and 3-year-olds (van Zeijl et al., 2006) and greater trouble managing toddlers' behavior (Belsky, Woodworth, & Crnic, 1996).

The PSI (Abidin, 1995) was designed as a screening instrument for assessing relative levels of stress in the early parent–child system (0–3 years), although it has been used with children up to 12 years of age. There is also a version for parents of youth ages 11–19—the

Stress Index for Parents of Adolescents (Sheras, Abidin, & Konold, 1998). The design of the PSI was theoretically derived and includes domains related to stress and coping in parent and child temperament. The PSI comprises 120 items, requires approximately 20 minutes to complete, and yields a total score and two scale scores: Child and Parent. The Child domain includes six subscales concerning the child's Adaptability, Reinforcing Qualities, Demandingness, Distractibility/Hyperactivity, Mood, and Acceptability to the parent. The Parent domain includes subscales related to Depression, Attachment to the Child, Spousal and Social System Support, Parental Health, Perceived Restrictions of Role, and Parent's Sense of Competence. High total scores may indicate risk for problems in development; low scores may also be a reason for concern, either because of a "fake good" response set or indications of lack of parental involvement with the child. A high score in the Parent domain may indicate difficulty with parental functioning. High scores in the Child domain may indicate that a child has difficult characteristics (i.e., "temperamentally difficult"). Webster-Stratton (1990) reported that the mean Child domain score in a sample of 120 children with CPs was above the 95th percentile. (See Abidin, Flens, & Austin [2006] for a summary of research on the PSI.)

The PSI has been used extensively with parents of children with CPs. Scores on the PSI obtained in infancy have been used to predict child CPs 4½ years later in nonclinical samples (Abidin, Jenkins, & McGaughey, 1992). Higher PSI scores have been related to CPs in several samples (e.g., Cuccaro, Holmes, & Wright, 1993; Eyberg, Boggs, & Rodriguez, 1992; Webster-Stratton, 1990). Webster-Stratton and Hammond (1988) found that the Parent domain score on the PSI, in combination with the Life Experiences Survey Negative Change score, discriminated between depressed and nondepressed mothers in families with children with CPs. Parent management training outcome in families with children with CPs has been evaluated with the PSI (e.g., Eisenstadt et al., 1993; Nixon et al., 2003; Webster-Stratton & Hammond, 1997), and higher scores on the Child and Parent domains of the PSI have been linked with premature termination of treatment for CPs (e.g., Kazdin, 1990).

The PSI Short Form (PSI/SF; Abidin, 1995) comprises 36 items from the PSI and can be administered in less than 10 minutes. In addition to a total score, there are three factor-analytically derived subscales (Parental Distress, Parent–Child Dysfunctional Interaction, Difficult Child). The PSI/SF subscales correlate with the full-length PSI in the expected pattern, and have shown adequate internal consistency and test–retest (6 month) reliability. However, other researchers (e.g., Haskett, Ahern, Ward, & Allaire, 2006) have identified a two-factor solution that appears similar to the two conceptually derived scales in the original PSI.

The youth's broader social ecology (i.e., extrafamilial functioning) is often crucial for understanding the development of CPs in many cases. Therefore, it is important to assess variables such as the economic situation of the family, the level of social and community support provided to the youth and his or her family, and other aspects of the youth's social climate (e.g., neighborhood, quality of school, and degree of exposure to violence). The Neighborhood Questionnaire (Greenberg, Lengua, Coie, Pinderhughes, & the Conduct Problems Prevention Research Group, 1999), a brief parent report measure, assesses the parent's perception of the family's neighborhood in terms of safety, violence, drug traffic, satisfaction, and stability. Things That I Have Seen and Heard (Richters & Martinez, 1990) is an example of an interview that focuses on the youth's exposure to violence.

The Community Interaction Checklist (CIC; Wahler, Leske, & Rogers, 1979), a brief interview that is usually administered on multiple occasions, has been used extensively in research with children with CPs and their families to assess maternal insularity. On the basis of maternal reports of extrafamily contacts over several previous 24-hour periods, mothers are categorized as insular if they report at least twice as many daily contacts with relatives and/or helping agency representatives as with friends, and if at least one-third of the daily contacts are reported as neutral or aversive (Dumas & Wahler, 1983, 1985). These mothers are more aversive and indiscriminate than noninsular mothers in the use of aversive consequences with their children, their children are more aversive, and coercive exchanges between insular mothers and their children are of longer duration than those involving noninsular mother–child dyads (Dumas & Wahler, 1985; Wahler, Hughey, & Gordon, 1981). Aversive maternal contacts with adults, as measured on the CIC, are associated with mothers' aversive behavior toward their children on the same day (Wahler, 1980; Wahler & Graves, 1983). Finally, classification as insular on the CIC is a strong predictor of poor maintenance of the effects of parent management training interventions for children with CPs (e.g., Dumas & Wahler, 1983; Wahler, 1980). None of the mothers who were both insular and socioeconomically disadvantaged had a favorable outcome over the 1-year period.

Finally, it is important to evaluate *parental satisfaction with treatment*, which is a form of social validity that may be assessed in terms of satisfaction with the outcome of treatment, therapists, treatment procedures, and teaching format (McMahon & Forehand, 1983). At present, no single consumer satisfaction measure is appropriate for use with all types of interventions for youth with CPs and their families. In fact, most assessments of treatment satisfaction have focused on parents involved in parent management training interventions, although teachers have occasionally been assessed. The children and adolescents themselves have rarely been asked about their satisfaction with treatment, with the exception of some evaluations of multisystemic therapy with adolescents (e.g., Henggeler et al., 1999). The Therapy Attitude Inventory (TAI—Brestan, Jacobs, Rayfield, & Eyberg, 1999; Eyberg, 1993) and the Parent's Consumer Satisfaction Questionnaire (PCSQ—McMahon & Forehand, 2003; McMahon, Tiedemann, Forehand, & Griest, 1984) are examples of measures designed to evaluate parental satisfaction with parent management training programs (e.g., Brinkmeyer & Eyberg, 2003; McMahon & Forehand, 2003). Both the TAI and the PCSQ have data supporting their reliability and validity (e.g., Baum & Forehand, 1981; Eisenstadt et al., 1993; McMahon et al., 1981, 1984; Webster-Stratton, 1989; Webster-Stratton & Hammond, 1997).

Summary

CPs are associated with a wide variety of risk factors, both internal and external to the child. A correspondingly large array of measures have been developed to measure these various factors, although the clinical utility of many of the measures requires further testing. Assessment of youth social-cognitive processing difficulties is beginning to make its way into more applied settings, but assessments of peer rejection processes and associations with deviant peer groups that are appropriate for the clinical setting are less well developed. Assessment of family-related factors is essential, and includes, at a minimum, measurement of parenting practices, parents' cognitions about their children and about their parenting, parental personal and marital adjustment, parental stress, parental functioning in extrafamilial contexts, and parental satisfaction with treatment. Although these constructs have most typically been assessed by behavior rating scales, it is imperative to assess parent–child interaction via observational methods whenever possible. A number of structured observational analogue tasks have a successful history of clinical utility and have been shown to be sensitive to treatment effects (e.g., McMahon & Estes, 1997; Roberts, 2001).

Multiple Developmental Pathways: Implications for Assessment

The key implication of the research base for the assessment of youth with CPs is that it is imperative for the clinician to be aware of the various potential developmental pathways to CPs. Knowledge of the different pathways can serve as a guide for structuring and conducting the assessment with respect to the CP behaviors themselves, the most likely candidates for comorbid disorders and conditions, and the most clinically salient risk factors (McMahon & Frick, 2005). Also, different intervention strategies can be designed for youth in these different developmental pathways (Frick, 1998, 2006).

One of the most critical pieces of information in guiding assessment, and perhaps ultimately intervention, is the age at which various CP behaviors began, which provides some indication of whether the youth may be on the childhood-onset pathway. An important advantage of many structured interviews over behavior rating scales (and behavioral observations) is that they provide a structured method for assessing when a youth first began showing serious CP behaviors, thereby providing an important source of information about the developmental trajectory. For example, in the DISC-IV (Shaffer et al., 2000), following any question related to the presence of a CD symptom that is answered affirmatively, the parent or youth is asked to estimate at what age the first occurrence of the behavior took place. Obviously, such questions can also be integrated into an unstructured interview format.

In either case, however, there is always some concern about how accurately the parent or youth reports the timing of specific behaviors. Three findings from research can help in interpreting such reports. First, the longer the time frame involved in the retrospective report (e.g., a parent of a 17-year-old vs. a parent of a 6-year-old reporting on preschool behavior), the less accurate the report is likely to be (Green, Loeber, & Lahey, 1991). Second, although a parental report of the exact age of onset may not be very reliable over time, typical variations in years are usually small, and the relative rankings within symptoms (e.g., which symptom began first) and within a sample (e.g., which children exhibited the earliest onset of behavior) seem to be fairly stable (Green et al., 1991). As a result, these reports should be viewed as rough estimates of the timing of onset and not as exact dating procedures. Third, there is evidence that combining informants (e.g., such as a parent or youth) or combining sources of information (e.g., self-report and record of police contact), and taking the earliest reported onset from any source, provides an estimate that shows somewhat greater validity than any single source of information alone (Lahey et al., 1999).

If the youth's history of CPs is consistent with the childhood-onset pathway, then additional assessment to examine the extent to which CU traits may also be present is important. The Antisocial Process Screening Device (Frick & Hare, 2001), a behavior rating scale completed by parents and teachers, can be used to identify children with CPs who also exhibit CU traits (Christian et al., 1997; Frick, Bodin, & Barry, 2000; Frick, O'Brien, Wootton, & McBurnett, 1994). A self-report version of this scale is also available for older children and adolescents, and although it has been validated in a number of studies (Munoz & Frick, in press), it lacks normative data from which to make interpretations. If the presenting child is preschool age, then one assessment goal is to attempt to determine whether the child's behavior is indicative of the childhood-onset pathway or a less serious manifestation of CP. Although there are no clear-cut algorithms for making this determination, a broad assessment of overall risk is called for (see Wakschlag & Danis, 2004). Also, with preschool-age chil-

dren, a more extensive assessment of noncompliance is warranted given its centrality to early CPs and its amenability to intervention at that age (McMahon & Forehand, 2003).

Finally, because much of the current knowledge about developmental pathways to CPs has been based on longitudinal samples of boys, many questions about onset and development of CP behavior in girls remain unanswered (Silverthorn & Frick, 1999). At present, with few exceptions (e.g., relational aggression), there is a paucity of information to guide the development of evidence-based assessment of CPs in girls. There is even less information with respect to evidence-based assessment of CPs with ethnically diverse youth. Prinz and Miller (1991) noted that, in general, the validity of various methods to assess CPs has not been examined in specific cultural groups. They stressed the importance of ensuring that assessment methods are interpreted within the cultural context of the child with a CP. Others have noted the importance of assessing the acceptability of various intervention procedures (e.g., parenting skills taught in parent management training interventions) across different ethnic groups (Forehand & Kotchick, 1996). Based on accumulating evidence, we recommend that clinicians use these developmental pathways constructs (albeit cautiously) to guide their assessments of girls and ethnically diverse youth with CPs until research suggests otherwise.

Summary

Knowledge about the multiple developmental pathways of CPs is extremely important for assessment practice, in that it can guide the structure and focus of clinicians' assessment. At present, the most well-established pathways are the childhood- and adolescent-onset pathways, although others will likely be identified by future research. Thus, establishing age of onset of CPs is a critical and relatively straightforward step in the assessment of youth. Furthermore, given the growing body of evidence that youth with high levels of both CP and CU traits show many distinct risk factors compared to youth with CP who do not also display elevated levels of CU traits, determination of the extent to which the child or adolescent also displays CU traits is indicated. With preschool-age children who display CPs, the most critical issue is to determine whether their behavior indicates the early stages of the childhood-onset pathway of CPs or a more temporary developmental perturbation. Finally, the applicability of these pathways to girls and ethnically diverse youth is less well established.

CONCLUSIONS

In this chapter, we have summarized four areas of research that we feel have direct and important implications for assessing youth with CPs: (1) the heterogeneity in the types and severity of CPs, (2) the presence of multiple comorbid conditions, (3) the multiple risk factors associated with CPs, and (4) the multiple developmental pathways to CPs. For each of these domains, we discussed the implications for assessment and presented examples of specific measures that can aid in assessments. We also provided recommendations for evidence-based assessment of CPs based on this research. In this final section of the chapter, we identify (1) some overarching issues in applying this knowledge to clinical assessments and (2) areas that we believe are in greatest need of attention for advancing evidence-based assessments of CPs.

The first overarching issue in most cases of youth with CPs is the need for a comprehensive assessment. We have emphasized throughout this chapter that adequate assessment of a youth with CPs must make use of multiple methods (e.g., interviews, behavior rating scales, observation) completed by multiple informants (parents, teacher, youth) and concern multiple aspects of the child's or adolescent's adjustment (e.g., CPs, anxiety, learning problems) in multiple settings (e.g., home, school) (Kamphaus & Frick, 2005; McMahon & Estes, 1997; McMahon & Frick, 2005). However, because of issues of time, expense, and practicality, how best to acquire and interpret this large array of information become important issues. As described earlier, a multistage approach may prove to be cost-effective in conducting such comprehensive assessments, which start with more time-efficient measures (e.g., broad-band behavior rating scales, unstructured clinical interviews) and are then followed by more time-intensive measures (e.g., structured interviews, behavioral observations) when indicated (McMahon & Estes, 1997; McMahon & Frick, 2005; Nock & Kurtz, 2005).

However, once these assessment data are collected, few guidelines are available to guide clinicians in integrating and synthesizing the multiple pieces of information to make important clinical decisions at each stage of the assessment process. This endeavor is complicated by the fact that data from different informants (Achenbach, McConaughy, & Howell, 1987; De Los Reyes & Kazdin, 2005) and different methods (Barkley, 1991) often show only modest correlations with each other. As a result, after collecting multiple sources of information on a youth's adjustment, the assessor often must make sense of an array of often conflicting information.

Several clinically oriented strategies for integrating and interpreting information from comprehensive assessments have been proposed elsewhere (Breen & Altepeter, 1990; Kamphaus & Frick, 2005; McMahon & Forehand, 2003; Sanders & Lawton, 1993; Wakschlag & Danis, 2004). The continued development and refinement of the ASEBA (Achenbach & Rescorla, 2000, 2001) have been particularly noteworthy for their emphases on integrating and interpreting data from parents, teachers, youth, direct observations, and clinical interviews from this family of instruments. Others have suggested that incorporation of a functional-analytic approach into more traditional assessment practices will facilitate integration of information from multiple sources and the selection of appropriate treatments (e.g., Reitman, 2006; Scotti, Morris, McNeil, & Hawkins, 1996). Such functional-analytic approaches are quite compatible with research on the different developmental pathways to CPs and emphasize the need to understand the specific causal processes that lead to or maintain each child's or adolescent's CPs, in order to guide more individualized interventions. Regardless of the approach, much more research is needed to guide this process of integrating data from comprehensive assessments.

Another issue that requires further attention is the great need to enhance the clinical utility of evidence-based assessment tools (Frick, 2000; Hodges, 2004). As noted throughout this chapter, many of the recommended assessment measures have been developed and employed in research as opposed to applied settings. Progress toward the development of brief, clinically useful assessment methods has occurred, but in a limited way. On one front, there have been attempts to simplify well validated but complex observational systems such as the DPICS and the BCS. On another front has been the development of structured laboratory analogue tasks to assess the child's or adolescent's behavior under standardized conditions (Frick & Loney, 2000; Roberts, 2001). Especially encouraging have been the attempts to develop methods for assessing covert types of CP behavior (e.g., Hinshaw et al., 1992; Kolko et al., 1991). Although the clinical utility of these methods has yet to be demonstrated, clinicians at least now have a number of brief assessment methods with some empirical support from which to choose.

There is still somewhat of a disconnect between assessment concerning case conceptualization and treatment planning on the one hand, and the availability of evidence-based interventions that map onto those assessment findings. For example, interventions are much less developed for youth engaging primarily in covert forms of CPs (e.g., stealing, firesetting) than for youth involved in more overt CP behaviors such as noncompliance and aggression (McMahon et al., 2006). Similarly, subtype-specific interventions for reactive and proactive aggression, for relational aggression (e.g., Leff, Angelucci, Grabowski, & Weil, 2004; Levene, Walsh, Augimeri, & Pepler, 2004) and for the treatment of youth with and without CU traits (e.g., Frick, 1998, 2001, 2006) are in relatively early stages of development. On the other hand, high levels of noncompliance in a preschool-age child suggest selection of one of several well-validated parent management training interventions (McMahon et al., 2006).

Another area that requires additional investigation is testing the sensitivity of measures to change. Many of the applications of research to the assessment process have focused on making diagnostic decisions (e.g., determining whether CPs should be the primary source of concern, and whether they are severe and impairing enough to warrant treatment) and on treatment planning (e.g., determine what types of treatment the child may need). However, an important third goal of the assessment process is intervention monitoring and evaluating treatment outcome. Evidence-based assessments should provide a means for testing whether interventions have brought about meaningful changes in the child's or adolescent's adjustment for better or worse (i.e., an iatrogenic effect). As noted throughout this chapter, many behavior rating scales and observational measures have demonstrated sensitivity to intervention outcomes. Unfortunately, there is very little evidence to date of the successful use of assessment measures to monitor the effects of *ongoing* intervention for CPs. Exceptions to this are the structured observational analogues employed in some parent management training programs for young oppositional children (Herschell et al., 2002; McMahon & Forehand, 2003). These analogues (e.g., Child's Game, Parent's Game, Clean Up) are employed repeatedly throughout the course of treatment not only to monitor progress but also to determine whether the parent has met specific behavioral performance criteria necessary for progression to the next step of the parent management training program.

An assessment domain that is related to outcome evaluation is satisfaction with treatment. As noted earlier, assessment of this domain has been limited largely to parental satisfaction with parent management training (and, in the case of multisystemic therapy, youth satisfaction also). Areas for future research include the development and evaluation of similar satisfaction measures for other interventions employed with youth with CPs, and the development of such measures to assess youth satisfaction. Similarly, there is a need for research examining the treatment acceptability of, and satisfaction with, assessment procedures and measures themselves (e.g., Kazdin, 2005; Rhule, McMahon, & Vando, 2005).

Several important issues are involved in developing measures suitable for treatment monitoring and outcome evaluation (McMahon & Metzler, 1998). First, the way questions on an interview or rating scale are framed may affect its sensitivity to change. For example, the response scale on a parent report behavior rating scale may be too general (e.g., *Never* vs. *Sometimes* vs. *Always*) or the time interval for reporting the frequency of a parent behavior (e.g., the past 6 months) may not be discrete enough to detect changes brought about by treatment. Second, the degree to which the behaviors measured in assessment match the behaviors targeted in intervention can greatly affect sensitivity to change. For example, if major parenting constructs addressed by an intervention (e.g., limit setting, positive reinforcement, monitoring) are measured weakly or not at all in the assessment, then changes in these constructs as a function of intervention are not likely to be captured. Finally, assessment × intervention interactions may occur. For example, as a function of intervention, parents may learn to become more effective monitors of their youths' behavior. As a consequence, they may become more aware of their children's CP behaviors. Comparison of parent reports of their children's behavior prior to and after the intervention may actually suggest that parents perceive deterioration in their children's behavior (i.e., a false iatrogenic effect), when in reality the parents have simply become more accurate reporters of such behavior (Dishion & McMahon, 1998).

Perhaps the most central issue for advancing evidence-based assessment is the need to focus assessment around the emerging research on the different developmental pathways to CPs. As noted previously, this research may be the most important area for understanding youth with CPs, because it might explain many of the variations in severity, the multiple co-occurring conditions, and the many different risk factors associated with CPs. This research may also be very important for designing more individualized treatments for youth with CPs, especially older children and adolescents with more severe antisocial behaviors (Frick, 1998, 2001, 2006). However, for research on developmental pathways to be translated into practice, it is critical that better assessment methods for reliably and validly designating youth in these pathways be developed. This is especially the case for girls and for ethnically diverse youth. Furthermore, the different causal processes and developmental mechanisms (e.g., lack of empathy and guilt, poor emotion regulation) that may be involved in the different pathways need to be assessed, and this typically involves translating measures that have been used in developmental research into forms that are appropriate for clinical practice (Frick & Morris, 2004; Lahey, 2004). This is perhaps the best illustration of the role that evidence-based assessment can play in translating research into practice.

REFERENCES

Abidin, R. R. (1995). *Parenting Stress Index— Professional manual* (3rd ed.). Odessa, FL: Psychological Assessment Resources.

Abidin, R. R., & Brunner, J. F. (1995). Development of a parenting alliance inventory. *Journal of Clinical Child Psychology, 24,* 31–40.

Abidin, R. R., Flens, J. R., & Austin, W. G. (2006). The Parenting Stress Index: Forensic use and limitations. In R. P. Archer (Ed.), *Forensic uses of clinical assessment instruments* (pp. 297–328). Mahwah, NJ: Erlbaum.

Abidin, R. R., Jenkins, C. L., & McGaughey, M. C. (1992). The relationship of early family variables to children's subsequent behavioral adjustment. *Journal of Clinical Child Psychology, 21,* 60–69.

Abidin, R. R., & Konold, T. R. (1999). *Parenting Alliance Measure: Professional manual.* Sarasota, FL: Psychological Assessment Resources.

Achenbach, T. M., Dumenci, L., & Rescorla, L. A. (2003). DSM-oriented and empirically based approaches to constructing scales from the same item pools. *Journal of Clinical Child and Adolescent Psychology, 32,* 328–340.

Achenbach, T. M., McConaughy, S. H., & Howell, C. T. (1987). Child–adolescent behavioral and emotional problems: Implications of cross-informant correlations for situational specificity. *Psychological Bulletin, 101,* 213–232.

Achenbach, T. M., & Rescorla, L. A. (2000). *Manual for the ASEBA preschool forms and profiles.* Burlington: University of Vermont, Department of Psychiatry.

Achenbach, T. M., & Rescorla, L. A. (2001). *Manual for the ASEBA school-age forms and profiles.* Burlington: University of Vermont, Research Center for Children, Youth, and Families.

Achenbach, T. M., Rescorla, L. A., & Ivanova, M. Y. (2005). International cross-cultural consistencies and variations in child and adolescent psychopathology. In C. L. Frisby & C. R. Reynolds (Eds.), *Comprehensive handbook of multicultural school psychology* (pp. 674–709). Hoboken, NJ: Wiley.

Adams, G. L. (1984). *Normative Adaptive Behavior Checklist (NABC).* San Antonio, TX: Psychological Corporation.

Amato, P. R., & Keith, B. (1991). Parental divorce and the well-being of children: A meta analysis. *Psychological Bulletin, 110,* 26–46.

American Psychiatric Association (APA). (1994). *The diagnostic and statistical manual of mental disorders* (4th ed.). Washington, DC: Author.

American Psychiatric Association (APA). (2000). *The diagnostic and statistical manual of mental disorders* (4th ed., text rev.). Washington, DC: Author.

Arnold, D. S., O'Leary, S. G., Wolff, L. S., & Acker, M. M. (1993). The Parenting Scale: A measure of dysfunctional parenting in discipline situations. *Psychological Assessment, 5,* 137–144.

Aspland, H., & Gardner, F. (2003). Observational measures of parent–child interaction: An introductory review. *Child and Adolescent Mental Health, 8,* 136–143.

August, G. J., Lee, S. S., Bloomquist, M. L., Realmuto, G. M., & Hektner, J. M. (2003). Dissemination of an evidence-based prevention innovation for aggressive children living in culturally diverse, urban neighborhoods: The Early Risers effectiveness study. *Prevention Science, 4*, 271–286.

Baden, A. D., & Howe, G. W. (1992). Mothers' attributions and expectancies regarding their conduct-disordered children. *Journal of Abnormal Child Psychology, 20*, 467–485.

Bank, L., Marlowe, J. H., Reid, J. B., Patterson, G. R., & Weinrott, M. R. (1991). A comparative evaluation of parent training interventions for families of chronic delinquents. *Journal of Abnormal Child Psychology, 19*, 15–33.

Barkley, R. A. (1987). *Defiant children: A clinician's manual for parent training.* New York: Guilford Press.

Barkley, R. A. (1991). The ecological validity of laboratory and analogue assessment methods of ADHD. *Journal of Abnormal Child Psychology, 19*, 149–178.

Barkley, R. A. (1997). *Defiant children: A clinician's manual for assessment and parent training* (2nd ed.). New York: Guilford Press.

Barkley, R. A., Shelton, T. L., Crosswait, C., Moorehouse, M., Fletcher, K., Barrett, S., et al. (2002). Preschool children with disruptive behavior: Three-year outcome as a function of adaptive disability. *Development and Psychopathology, 14*, 45–67.

Barry, C. T., Frick, P. J., Grooms, T., McCoy, M. G., Ellis, M. L., & Loney, B. R. (2000). The importance of callous–unemotional traits for extending the concept of psychopathy to children. *Journal of Abnormal Psychology, 109*, 335–340.

Baum, C. G., & Forehand, R. (1981). Long-term follow-up assessment of parent training by use of multiple-outcome measures. *Behavior Therapy, 12*, 643–652.

Beck, A. T., Rush, A. J., Shaw, B. F., & Emery, G. (1979). *Cognitive therapy of depression.* New York: Guilford Press.

Beck, A. T., Steer, R. A., & Brown, G. K. (1996). *Manual for the Beck Depression Inventory–II.* San Antonio, TX: Psychological Corporation.

Beck, A. T., Steer, R. A., & Garbin, M. G. (1988). Psychometric properties of the Beck Depression Inventory: Twenty-five years of evaluation. *Clinical Psychology Review, 8*, 77–100.

Belsky, J., Woodworth, S., & Crnic, K. (1996). Trouble in the second year: Three questions about family interaction. *Child Development, 67*, 556–578.

Bierman, K. L. (1983). Cognitive development and clinical interviews with children. In B. B. Lahey & A. E. Kazdin (Eds.), *Advances in clinical child psychology* (Vol. 6, pp. 217–250). New York: Plenum Press.

Bierman, K. L., & Welsh, J. A. (1997). Social relationship deficits. In E. J. Mash & L. G. Terdal (Eds.), *Assessment of childhood disorders* (3rd ed., pp. 328–365). New York: Guilford Press.

Bird, H. R. (1999). The assessment of functional impairment. In D. Shaffer, C. P. Lucas, & J. E. Richters (Eds.), *Diagnostic assessment in child and adolescent psychopathology* (pp. 209–229). New York: Guilford Press.

Bird, H. R., Shaffer, D., Fisher, P., Gould, M. S., Staghezza, B., Chen, J., et al. (1993). The Columbia Impairment Scale (CIS): Pilot findings on a measure of global impairment for children and adolescents. *International Journal of Methods in Psychiatric Research, 3*, 167–176.

Blader, J. C. (2004). Symptom, family, and service predictors of children's psychiatric rehospitalization within one year of discharge. *Journal of the American Academy of Child and Adolescent Psychiatry, 43*, 440–451.

Blair, R. J. R. (1995). A cognitive developmental approach to morality: Investigating the psychopath. *Cognition, 57*, 1–29.

Blair, R. J. R. (1999). Responsiveness to distress cues in the child with psychopathic tendencies. *Personality and Individual Differences, 27*, 135–145.

Blair, R. J. R., Colledge, E., Murray, L., & Mitchell, D. G. V. (2001). A selective impairment in the processing of sad and fearful expressions in children with psychopathic tendencies. *Journal of Abnormal Child Psychology, 29*, 491–498.

Blair, R. J. R., Peschardt, K. S., Budhani, S., Mitchell, D. G. V., & Pine, D. S. (2006). The development of psychopathy. *Journal of Child Psychology and Psychiatry, 47*, 262–275.

Bloomquist, M. L., & Schnell, S. V. (2002). *Helping children with aggression and conduct problems: Best practices for intervention.* New York: Guilford Press.

Boggs, S. R., Eyberg, S., & Reynolds, L. A. (1990). Concurrent validity of the Eyberg Child Behavior Inventory. *Journal of Clinical Child Psychology, 19*, 75–78.

Breen, M. J., & Altepeter, T. S. (1990). *Disruptive behavior disorders in children: Treatment-focused assessment.* New York: Guilford Press.

Breiner, J. L., & Forehand, R. (1981). An assessment of the effects of parent training on clinic-referred children's school behavior. *Behavioral Assessment, 3*, 31–42.

Brestan, E. V., Jacobs, J. R., Rayfield, A. D., & Eyberg, S. M. (1999). A consumer satisfaction measure for parent–child treatments and its relation to measures of child behavior change. *Behavior Therapy, 30*, 17–30.

Brinkmeyer, M., & Eyberg, S. M. (2003). Parent–child interaction therapy for oppositional children. In A. E. Kazdin & J. R. Weisz (Eds.), *Evidence-based psychotherapies for children and adolescents* (pp. 204–223). New York: Guilford Press.

Broidy, L. M., Nagin, D. S., Tremblay, R. E., Bates, J. E., Brame, B. U., Dodge, K. A., et al. (2003). Developmental trajectories of childhood disruptive behaviors and adolescent delinquency: A six-site, cross-national study. *Developmental Psychology, 39*, 222–245.

Brown, K., Atkins, M. S., Osborne, M. L., & Milnamow, M. (1996). A revised teacher rating scale for reactive and proactive aggression. *Journal of Abnormal Child Psychology, 24,* 473–480.

Brubaker, R. G., & Szakowski, A. (2000). Parenting practices and behavior problems among deaf children. *Child and Family Behavior Therapy, 22*(4), 13–28.

Burgess, E. W., Locke, H. J., & Thomes, M. M. (1971). *The family.* New York: Van Nostrand Reinhold.

Burns, G. L., & Patterson, D. R. (1990). Conduct problem behaviors in a stratified random sample of children and adolescents: New standardization data on the Eyberg Child Behavior Inventory. *Psychological Assessment, 2,* 391–397.

Burns, G. L., & Patterson, D. R. (1991). Factor structure of the Eyberg Child Behavior Inventory: Unidimensional or multidimensional measure of disruptive behavior? *Journal of Clinical Child Psychology, 20,* 439–444.

Burns, G. L., & Patterson, D. R. (2000). Factor structure of the Eyberg Child Behavior Inventory: A parent rating scale of oppositional defiant behavior toward adults, inattentive behavior, and conduct problem behavior. *Journal of Clinical Child Psychology, 29,* 569–577.

Burns, G. L., & Patterson, D. R. (2001). Normative data on the Eyberg Child Behavior Inventory and Sutter–Eyberg Student Behavior Inventory: Parent and teacher rating scales of disruptive behavior problems in children and adolescents. *Child and Family Behavior Therapy, 23*(1), 15–28.

Burns, G. L., Patterson, D. R., Nussbaum, B. R., & Parker, C. M. (1991). Disruptive behaviors in an outpatient pediatric population: Additional standardization data on the Eyberg Child Behavior Inventory. *Psychological Assessment, 3,* 202–207.

Burns, G. L., Sosna, T. D., & Ladish, C. (1992). Distinction between well-standardized norms and the psychometric properties of a measure: Measurement of disruptive behaviors with the Sutter–Eyberg Student Behavior Inventory. *Child and Family Behavior Therapy, 14*(4), 43–54.

Burns, G. L., & Walsh, J. A. (2002). The influence of ADHD-hyperactivity/impulsivity symptoms on the development of oppositional defiant disorder symptoms in a 2-year longitudinal study. *Journal of Abnormal Child Psychology, 30,* 245–256.

Busby, D. M., Christensen, C., Crane, D. R., & Larson, J. H. (1995). A revision of the Dyadic Adjustment Scale for use with distressed and nondistressed couples: Construct hierarchy and multidimensional scales. *Journal of Marital and Family Therapy, 21,* 289–308.

Campbell, S. B., & Ewing, L. J. (1990). Follow up of hard to manage preschoolers: Adjustment at age 9 and predictors of continuing symptoms. *Journal of Child Psychology and Psychiatry and Allied Disciplines, 31,* 871–889.

Campis, L. K., Lyman, R. D., & Prentice-Dunn, S. (1986). The Parental Locus of Control Scale: Development and validation. *Journal of Clinical Child Psychology, 15,* 260–267.

Capaldi, D. M. (1991). Co-occurrence of conduct problems and depressive symptoms in early adolescent boys: I. Familial factors and general adjustment at age 6. *Development and Psychopathology, 3,* 277–300.

Capaldi, D. M. (1992). The co-occurrence of conduct problems and depressive symptoms in early adolescent boys: II. A 2-year follow-up at grade 8. *Development and Psychopathology, 4,* 125–144.

Carey, M. P., Spector, I. P., Lantinga, L. J., & Krauss, D. J. (1993). Reliability of the Dyadic Adjustment Scale. *Psychological Assessment, 5,* 238–240.

Caspi, A., Henry, B., Moffitt, T. E., & Silva, P. A. (1995). Temperamental origins of child and adolescent behavior problems: From age 3 to age 15. *Child Development, 66,* 55–68.

Caspi, A., Taylor, A., Smart, M., Jackson, J., Tagami, S., & Moffitt, T. E. (2001). Can women provide reliable information about their children's fathers?: Cross-informant agreement about men's lifetime antisocial behaviour. *Journal of Child Psychology and Psychiatry, 42,* 915–920.

Chamberlain, P., & Patterson, G. R. (1995). Discipline and child compliance in parenting. In M. H. Bornstein (Ed.), *Handbook of parenting: Vol. 4. Applied and practical parenting* (pp. 205–225). Hillsdale, NJ: Erlbaum.

Chamberlain, P., & Reid, J. B. (1987). Parent observation and report of child symptoms. *Behavioral Assessment, 9,* 97–109.

Chamberlain, P., & Reid, J. B. (1991). Using a specialized foster care community treatment model for children and adolescents leaving the state mental health hospital. *Journal of Community Psychology, 19,* 266–276.

Chamberlain, P., Reid, J. B., Ray, J., Capaldi, D. M., & Fisher, P. (1997). Parent inadequate discipline (PID). In T. A. Widiger, A. J. Frances, H. A. Pincus, R. Ross, M. B. First, & W. Davis (Eds.), *DSM-IV sourcebook* (Vol. 3, pp. 569–629). Washington, DC: American Psychiatric Association.

Christian, R. E., Frick, P. J., Hill, N. L., Tyler, L., & Frazer, D. R. (1997). Psychopathy and conduct problems in children: II. Implications for subtyping children with conduct problems. *Journal of the American Academy of Child and Adolescent Psychiatry, 36,* 233–241.

Chronis, A. M., Lahey, B. B., Pelham, W. E., Kipp, H. L., Baumann, B. L., & Lee, S. S. (2003). Psychopathology and substance use in parents of young children with attention-deficit/hyperactivity disorder. *Journal of the American Academy of Child and Adolescent Psychiatry, 42,* 1424–1432.

Collett, B. R., Gimpel, G. A., Greenson, J. N., & Gunderson, T. L. (2001). Assessment of discipline styles among parents of preschool through school-age children. *Journal of Psychopathology and Behavioral Assessment, 23,* 163–170.

Colvin, A., Eyberg, S. M., & Adams, C. D. (1999).

Restandardization of the Eyberg Child Behavior Inventory. Unpublished manuscript, University of Florida, Gainesville.

Conduct Problems Prevention Research Group. (1999). Initial impact of the Fast Track prevention trial for conduct problems: I. The high-risk sample. *Journal of Consulting and Clinical Psychology, 67,* 631–647.

Conduct Problems Prevention Research Group. (2000). Merging universal and indicated prevention programs: The Fast Track model. *Addictive Behaviors, 25,* 913–927.

Conners, C. K. (1997). *Conners Rating Scales—Revised manual.* North Tonawanda, NY: Multi-Health Systems.

Crane, D. R., Allgood, S. M., Larson, J. H., & Griffin, W. (1990). Assessing marital quality with distressed and nondistressed couples: A comparison and equivalency table for three frequently used measures. *Journal of Marriage and the Family, 52,* 87–93.

Crick, N. R. (1996). The role of overt aggression, relational aggression, and prosocial behavior in the prediction of children's future social adjustment. *Child Development, 67,* 2317–2327.

Crick, N. R., & Dodge, K. A. (1994). A review and reformulation of social information-processing mechanisms in children's social adjustment. *Psychological Bulletin, 115,* 74–101.

Crick, N. R., & Dodge, K. A. (1996). Social information-processing mechanisms in reactive and proactive aggression. *Child Development, 67,* 993–1002.

Crick, N. R., & Grotpeter, J. K. (1995). Relational aggression, gender, and social-psychological adjustment. *Child Development, 66,* 710–722.

Crnic, K. A., & Greenberg, M. T. (1990). Minor parenting stresses with young children. *Child Development, 61,* 1628–1637.

Cuccaro, M. L., Holmes, G. R., & Wright, H. H. (1993). Behavior problems in preschool children: A pilot study. *Psychological Reports, 72,* 121–122.

Cummings, E. M., & Davies, P. T. (1994). *Children and marital conflict: The impact of family dispute resolution.* New York: Guilford Press.

Dadds, M. R., Maujean, A., & Fraser, J. A. (2003). Parenting and conduct problems in children: Australian data and psychometric properties of the Alabama Parenting Questionnaire. *Australian Psychologist, 38,* 238–241.

Dadds, M. R., & Powell, M. B. (1991). The relationship of interparental conflict and global marital adjustment to aggression, anxiety, and immaturity in aggressive and nonclinic children. *Journal of Abnormal Child Psychology, 19,* 553–567.

David, C. F., & Kistner, J. A. (2000). Do positive self-perceptions have a "dark side"? Examination of the link between perceptual bias and aggression. *Journal of Abnormal Child Psychology, 28,* 327–337.

DeGarmo, D. S., Patterson, G. R., & Forgatch, M. S. (2004). How do outcomes in a specified parent training intervention maintain or wane over time? *Prevention Science, 5,* 73–89.

De Los Reyes, A., & Kazdin, A. E. (2005). Informant discrepancies in the assessment of childhood psychology: A critical review, theoretical framework, and recommendations for further study. *Psychological Bulletin, 131,* 483–509.

Demaray, M. K., Ruffalo, S. L., Carlson, J., Busse, R. T., Olson, A. E., McManus, S. M., et al. (1995). Social skills assessment: A comparative evaluation of six published rating scales. *School Psychology Review, 24,* 648–671.

Dishion, T. J., Andrews, D. W., & Crosby, L. (1995). Antisocial boys and their friends in early adolescence: Relationship characteristics, quality, and interactional process. *Child Development, 66,* 139–151.

Dishion, T. J., Capaldi, D., Spracklen, K. M., & Li, F. (1995). Peer ecology of male adolescent drug use. *Development and Psychopathology, 7,* 803–824.

Dishion, T. J., & McMahon, R. J. (1998). Parental monitoring and the prevention of child and adolescent problem behavior: A conceptual and empirical formulation. *Clinical Child and Family Psychology Review, 1,* 61–75.

Dodge, K. A., & Coie, J. D. (1987). Social-information processing factors in reactive and proactive aggression in children's peer groups. *Journal of Personality and Social Psychology, 53,* 1146–1158.

Dodge, K. A., & Pettit, G. S. (2003). A biopsychosocial model of the development of chronic conduct problems in adolescence. *Developmental Psychology, 39,* 349–371.

Drotar, D., & Crawford, P. (1987). Using home observation in the clinical assessment of children. *Journal of Clinical Child Psychology, 16,* 342–349.

Dumas, J. E. (1996). Why was this child referred?: Interactional correlates of referral status in families of children with disruptive behavior problems. *Journal of Clinical Child Psychology, 25,* 106–115.

Dumas, J. E., & Serketich, W. J. (1994). Maternal depressive symptomatology and child maladjustment: A comparison of three process models. *Behavior Therapy, 25,* 161–181.

Dumas, J. E., & Wahler, R. G. (1983). Predictors of treatment outcome in parent training: Mother insularity and socioeconomic disadvantage. *Behavioral Assessment, 5,* 301–313.

Dumas, J. E., & Wahler, R. G. (1985). Indiscriminate mothering as a contextual factor in aggressive–oppositional child behavior: "Damned if you do and damned if you don't." *Journal of Abnormal Child Psychology, 13,* 1–17.

Edens, J. F. (1998). Aggressive children's self-systems and the quality of their relationships with significant others. *Aggression and Violent Behavior, 4,* 151–177.

Eisenstadt, T. H., Eyberg, S., McNeil, C. B., Newcomb, K., & Funderburk, B. (1993). Parent–child interaction therapy with behavior problem children: Relative effectiveness of two stages and overall treatment outcome. *Journal of Clinical Child Psychology, 22,* 42–51.

Eisenstadt, T. H., McElreath, L. H., Eyberg, S. M., & McNeil, C. B. (1994). Interparent agreement on the Eyberg Child Behavior Inventory. *Child and Family Behavior Therapy, 16*(1), 21–27.

Elgar, F. J., Waschbusch, D. A., Dadds, M. R., & Sigvaldason, N. (2007). Development and validation of a short form of the Alabama Parenting Questionnaire. *Journal of Child and Family Studies, 16,* 243–259.

Elliott, D. S., Huizinga, D., & Ageton, S. S. (1985). *Explaining delinquency and drug use.* Beverly Hills, CA: Sage.

Engels, R. C. M. E., Finkenauer, C., & van Kooten, D. C. (2006). Lying behavior, family functioning and adjustment in early adolescence. *Journal of Youth and Adolescence, 35,* 949–958.

Essau, C. A., Sasagawa, S., & Frick, P. J. (2006). Psychometric properties of the Alabama Parenting Questionnaire. *Journal of Child and Family Studies, 15,* 597–616.

Eyberg, S. (1992). Parent and teacher behavior inventories for the assessment of conduct problem behaviors in children. In L. VandeCreek, S. Knapp, & T. L. Jackson (Eds.), *Innovations in clinical practice: A source book* (Vol. 11, pp. 261–270). Sarasota, FL: Professional Resource Press.

Eyberg, S. (1993). Consumer satisfaction measures for assessing parent training programs. In L. VandeCreek, S. Knapp, & T. L. Jackson (Eds.), *Innovations in clinical practice: A source book* (Vol. 12, pp. 377–382). Sarasota, FL: Professional Resource Press.

Eyberg, S., Bessmer, J., Newcomb, K., Edwards, D., & Robinson, E. (1994). *Dyadic Parent–Child Interaction Coding System II: A manual.* Unpublished manuscript, University of Florida, Gainesville.

Eyberg, S., & Colvin, A. (1994, August). *Restandardization of the Eyberg Child Behavior Inventory.* Paper presented at the annual meeting of the American Psychological Association, Los Angeles.

Eyberg, S. M., Boggs, S. R., & Algina, J. (1995). Parent–child interaction therapy: A psychosocial model for the treatment of young children with conduct problem behavior and their families. *Psychopharmacology Bulletin, 31,* 83–91.

Eyberg, S. M., Boggs, S. R., & Rodriguez, C. M. (1992). Relationships between maternal parenting stress and child disruptive behavior. *Child and Family Behavior Therapy, 14*(4), 1–9.

Eyberg, S. M., Nelson, M. M., Duke, M., & Boggs, S. R. (2005). *Manual for the Dyadic Parent–Child Interaction Coding System* (3rd ed.). Available online at *www.pcit.org.*

Eyberg, S. M., & Pincus, D. (1999). *The Eyberg Child Behavior Inventory and Sutter–Eyberg Student Behavior Inventory: Professional manual.* Lutz, FL: Psychological Assessment Resources.

Eyberg, S. M., & Robinson, E. A. (1983). Conduct problem behavior: Standardization of a behavioral rating scale with adolescents. *Journal of Clinical Child Psychology, 12,* 347–357.

Federal Bureau of Investigation. (2004). *Uniform crime reports, 2003.* Washington, DC: Author.

Feinfield, K. A., & Baker, B. L. (2004). Empirical support for a treatment program for families of young children with externalizing problems. *Journal of Clinical Child and Adolescent Psychology, 33,* 182–195.

Fergusson, D. M., Lynskey, M. T., & Horwood, L. J. (1993). The effect of maternal depression on maternal ratings of child behavior. *Journal of Abnormal Child Psychology, 21,* 245–269.

Fergusson, D. M., Lynskey, M. T., & Horwood, L. J. (1996). Origins of comorbidity between conduct and affective disorders. *Journal of the American Academy of Child and Adolescent Psychiatry, 35,* 451–460.

Fergusson, D. M., Swain, N. R., & Horwood, L. J. (2002). Deviant peer affiliations, crime and substance use: A fixed effects regression analysis. *Journal of Abnormal Child Psychology, 30,* 419–430.

Filcheck, H. A., Berry, T. A., & McNeil, C. B. (2004). Preliminary investigation examining the validity of the Compliance Test and a brief behavioral observation measure for identifying children with disruptive behavior. *Child Study Journal, 34,* 1–12.

Fisher, L., & Blair, R. J. R. (1998). Cognitive impairment and its relationship to psychopathic tendencies in children with emotional and behavioral difficulties. *Journal of Abnormal Child Psychology, 26,* 511–519.

Fitzgerald, H. E., Sullivan, L. A., Ham, H. P., Zucker, R. A., Bruckel, S., Schneider, A. M., et al. (1993). Predictors of behavior problems in three-year-old sons of alcoholics: Early evidence for the onset of risk. *Child Development, 64,* 110–123.

Floyd, E. M., Rayfield, A., Eyberg, S. M., & Riley, J. L. (2004). Psychometric properties of the Sutter–Eyberg Student Behavior Inventory with rural middle school and high school children. *Assessment, 11,* 64–72.

Forehand, R., & Brody, G. (1985). The association between parental personal/marital adjustment and parent–child interactions in a clinic sample. *Behaviour Research and Therapy, 23,* 211–212.

Forehand, R., & Kotchick, B. A. (1996). Cultural diversity: A wake-up call for parent training. *Behavior Therapy, 27,* 187–206.

Forehand, R., Long, N., & Hedrick, M. (1987). Family characteristics of adolescents who display overt and covert behavior problems. *Journal of Behavior Therapy and Experimental Psychiatry, 18,* 325–328.

Forehand, R. L., & McMahon, R. J. (1981). *Helping the noncompliant child: A clinician's guide to parent training.* New York: Guilford Press.

Forehand, R., & Peed, S. (1979). Training parents to modify noncompliant behavior of their children. In A. J. Finch, Jr. & P. C. Kendall (Eds.), *Treatment and research in child psychopathology* (pp. 159–184). New York: Spectrum.

Forehand, R., Wells, K. C., & Griest, D. L. (1980). An

examination of the social validity of a parent training program. *Behavior Therapy*, 11, 488–502.

Forehand, R., Wells, K. C., McMahon, R. J., Griest, D. L., & Rogers, T. (1982). Maternal perceptions of maladjustment in clinic-referred children: An extension of earlier research. *Journal of Behavioral Assessment*, 4, 145–151.

Foster, S. L., & Robin, A. L. (1997). Family conflict and communication in adolescence. In E. J. Mash & L. G. Terdal (Eds.), *Assessment of childhood disorders* (3rd ed., pp. 627–682). New York: Guilford Press.

Frick, P. J. (1991). *The Alabama Parenting Questionnaire*. Unpublished rating scale, University of Alabama, Tuscaloosa.

Frick, P. J. (1998). *Conduct disorders and severe antisocial behavior*. New York: Plenum Press.

Frick, P. J. (2000). Laboratory and performance-based measures of childhood disorders. *Journal of Clinical Child Psychology*, 29, 475–478.

Frick, P. J. (2001). Effective interventions for children and adolescents with conduct disorder. *Canadian Journal of Psychiatry*, 46, 26–37.

Frick, P. J. (2004). Integrating research on temperament and childhood psychopathology: Its pitfalls and promise. *Journal of Clinical Child and Adolescent Psychology*, 33, 2–7.

Frick, P. J. (2006). Developmental pathways to conduct disorder. *Child and Adolescent Psychiatric Clinics of North America*, 15, 311–331.

Frick, P. J., Bodin, S. D., & Barry, C. T. (2000). Psychopathic traits and conduct problems in community and clinic-referred samples of children: Further development of the Psychopathy Screening Device. *Psychological Assessment*, 12, 382–393.

Frick, P. J., Christian, R. E., & Wootton, J. M. (1999). Age trends in the association between parenting practices and conduct problems. *Behavior Modification*, 23, 106–128.

Frick, P. J., Cornell, A. H., Barry, C. T., Bodin, S. D., & Dane, H. A. (2003). Callous–unemotional traits and conduct problems in the prediction of conduct problem severity, aggression, and self-report of delinquency. *Journal of Abnormal Child Psychology*, 31, 457–470.

Frick, P. J., Cornell, A. H., Bodin, S. D., Dane, H. A., Barry, C. T., & Loney, B. R. (2003). Callous–unemotional traits and developmental pathways to severe conduct problems. *Developmental Psychology*, 39, 246–260.

Frick, P. J., & Dickens, C. (2006). Current perspectives on conduct disorder. *Current Psychiatry Reports*, 8, 59–72.

Frick, P. J., & Hare, R. D. (2001). *The Antisocial Process Screening Device* (APSD). Toronto: Multi-Health Systems.

Frick, P. J., & Jackson, Y. K. (1993). Family functioning and childhood antisocial behavior: Yet another reinterpretation. *Journal of Clinical Child Psychology*, 22, 410–419.

Frick, P. J., Kamphaus, R. W., Lahey, B. B., Loeber, R., Christ, M. A. G., Hart, E. L., et al. (1991). Academic underachievement and the disruptive behavior disorders. *Journal of Consulting and Clinical Psychology*, 59, 289–294.

Frick, P. J., Lahey, B. B., Hartdagen, S. E., & Hynd, G. W. (1989). Conduct problems in boys: Relations to maternal personality, marital satisfaction, and socioeconomic status. *Journal of Clinical Child Psychology*, 18, 114–120.

Frick, P. J., Lahey, B. B., Loeber, R., Stouthamer-Loeber, M., Christ, M. A. G., & Hanson, K. (1992). Familial risk factors to conduct disorder and oppositional defiant disorder: Parental psychopathology and maternal parenting. *Journal of Consulting and Clinical Psychology*, 60, 49–55.

Frick, P. J., Lahey, B. B., Loeber, R., Tannenbaum, L. E., Van Horn, Y., Christ, M. A. G., et al. (1993). Oppositional defiant disorder and conduct disorder: A meta-analytic review of factor analyses and cross-validation in a clinic sample. *Clinical Psychology Review*, 13, 319–340.

Frick, P. J., Lilienfeld, S. O., Ellis, M. L., Loney, B. R., & Silverthorn, P. (1999). The association between anxiety and psychopathy dimensions in children. *Journal of Abnormal Child Psychology*, 27, 381–390.

Frick, P. J., & Loney, B. R. (1999). Outcomes of children and adolescents with conduct disorder and oppositional defiant disorder. In H. C. Quay & A. Hogan (Eds.), *Handbook of disruptive behavior disorders* (pp. 507–524). New York: Plenum Press.

Frick, P. J., & Loney, B. R. (2000). The use of laboratory and performance-based measures in the assessment of children and adolescents with conduct disorders. *Journal of Clinical Child Psychology*, 29, 540–554.

Frick, P. J., & Loney, B. R. (2002). Understanding the association between parent and child antisocial behavior. In R. J. McMahon & R. D. Peters (Eds.), *The effects of parental dysfunction on children* (pp. 105–126). New York: Kluwer Academic/Plenum Press.

Frick, P. J., & Marsee, M. A. (2006). Psychopathy traits and developmental pathways to antisocial behavior in youth. In C. J. Patrick (Ed.), *Handbook of psychopathy* (pp. 355–374). New York: Guilford Press.

Frick, P. J., & Morris, A. S. (2004). Temperament and developmental pathways to conduct problems. *Journal of Clinical Child and Adolescent Psychology*, 33, 54–68.

Frick, P. J., O'Brien, B. S., Wootton, J. M., & McBurnett, K. (1994). Psychopathy and conduct problems in children. *Journal of Abnormal Psychology*, 103, 700–707.

Frick, P. J., & Silverthorn, P. (2001). Psychopathology in children. In P. B. Sutker & H. E. Adams (Eds.), *Comprehensive handbook of psychopathology* (3rd ed., pp. 881–920). New York: Kluwer Academic/Plenum Press.

Frick, P. J., Stickle, T. R., Dandreaux, D. M., Farrell, J. M., & Kimonis, E. R. (2005). Callous–unemotional traits in predicting the severity and stability of conduct problems and delinquency. *Journal of Abnormal Child Psychology, 33,* 471–487.

Funderburk, B. W., Eyberg, S. M., Rich, B. A., & Behar, L. (2003). Further psychometric evaluation of the Eyberg and Behar rating scales for parents and teachers of preschoolers. *Early Education and Development, 14,* 67–79.

Gadow, K. D., & Sprafkin, J. (1998). *CSI-4 screening manual.* Stony Brook, NY: Checkmate Plus.

Gardner, F., Burton, J., & Klimes, I. (2006). Randomised controlled trial of a parenting intervention in the voluntary sector for reducing child conduct problems: Outcomes and mechanisms of change. *Journal of Child Psychology and Psychiatry and Allied Disciplines, 47,* 1123–1132.

Gottfredson, G. D., & Gottfredson, D. C. (2001). What schools do to prevent problem behavior and promote safe environments. *Journal of Educational and Psychological Consultation, 12,* 313–344.

Green, S. M., Loeber, R., & Lahey, B. B. (1991). Stability of mothers' recall of the age of onset of their child's attention and hyperactivity problems. *Journal of the American Academy of Child and Adolescent Psychiatry, 30,* 135–137.

Greenberg, M. T., Lengua, L. J., Coie, J., Pinderhughes, E., & the Conduct Problems Prevention Research Group. (1999). Predicting developmental outcomes at school entry using a multiple-risk model: Four American communities. *Developmental Psychology, 35,* 403–417.

Greenberg, M. T., Speltz, M. L., & DeKlyen, M. (1993). The role of attachment in the early development of disruptive behavior problems. *Development and Psychopathology, 5,* 191–213.

Griest, D. L., Forehand, R., Wells, K. C., & McMahon, R. J. (1980). An examination of differences between nonclinic and behavior problem clinic-referred children. *Journal of Abnormal Psychology, 89,* 497–500.

Ham, H. P., Zucker, R. A., & Fitzgerald, H. E. (1993, June). *Assessing antisocial behavior with the Antisocial Behavior Checklist: Reliability and validity studies.* Paper presented at the annual meeting of the American Psychological Society, Chicago.

Hanf, C. (1970). *Shaping mothers to shape their children's behavior.* Unpublished manuscript, University of Oregon Medical School, Portland.

Haskett, M. E., Ahern, L. S., Ward, C. S., & Allaire, J. C. (2006). Factor structure and validity of the Parenting Stress Index—Short Form. *Journal of Clinical Child and Adolescent Psychology, 35,* 302–312.

Hawes, D. J., & Dadds, M. R. (2006). Assessing parenting practices through parent report and direct observation during parenting training. *Journal of Child and Family Studies, 15,* 555–568.

Hawkins, J. D., Catalano, R. F., & Miller, J. Y. (1992). Risk and protective factors for alcohol and other drug problems in adolescence and early adulthood: Implications for substance abuse prevention. *Psychological Bulletin, 112,* 64–105.

Henggeler, S. W., Rowland, M. D., Randall, J., Ward, D. M., Pickrel, S. G., Cunningham, P. B., et al. (1999). Home-based multisystemic therapy as an alternative to the hospitalization of youths in psychiatric crisis: Clinical outcomes. *Journal of the American Academy of Child and Adolescent Psychiatry, 38,* 1331–1339.

Herschell, A., Calzada, E., Eyberg, S. M., & McNeil, C. B. (2002). Clinical issues in parent–child interaction therapy: Clinical past and future. *Cognitive and Behavioral Practice, 9,* 16–27.

Hinshaw, S. P. (1992). Externalizing behavior problems and academic underachievement in childhood and adolescence: Causal relationships and underlying mechanisms. *Psychological Bulletin, 111,* 127–155.

Hinshaw, S. P., Heller, T., & McHale, J. P. (1992). Covert antisocial behavior in boys with attention-deficit hyperactivity disorder: External validation and effects of methylphenidate. *Journal of Consulting and Clinical Psychology, 60,* 274–281.

Hinshaw, S. P., & Lee, S. S. (2003). Conduct and oppositional defiant disorders. In E. J. Mash & R. A. Barkley (Eds.), *Child psychopathology* (2nd ed., pp. 144–198). New York: Guilford Press.

Hinshaw, S. P., Simmel, C., & Heller, T. L. (1995). Multimethod assessment of covert antisocial behavior in children: Laboratory observation, adult ratings, and child self-report. *Psychological Assessment, 7,* 209–219.

Hinshaw, S. P., Zupan, B. A., Simmel, C., Nigg, J. T., & Melnick, S. (1997). Peer status in boys with and without attention-deficit hyperactivity disorder: Predictions from overt and covert antisocial behavior, social isolation, and authoritative parenting beliefs. *Child Development, 68,* 880–896.

Hodges, K. (2000). *Child and Adolescent Functional Assessment Scale* (2nd rev.). Ypsilanti: Eastern Michigan University.

Hodges, K. (2004). Using assessment in everyday practice for the benefit of families and practitioners. *Professional Psychology: Research and Practice, 35,* 449–456.

Hodges, K., Xue, Y., & Wotring, J. (2004). Use of the CAFAS to evaluate outcomes for youths with severe emotional disturbance served by public mental health. *Journal of Child and Family Studies, 13,* 325–339.

Holleran, P. A., Littman, D. C., Freund, R. D., & Schmaling, K. B. (1982). A signal detection approach to social perception: Identification of negative and positive behaviors by parents of normal and problem children. *Journal of Abnormal Child Psychology, 10,* 547–557.

Hubbard, J. A., Smithmyer, C. M., Ramsden, S. R., Parker, E. H., Flanagan, K. D., Dearing, K. F., et al. (2002). Observational, physiological, and self-report measures of children's anger: Relations to reactive versus proactive aggression. *Child Development, 73,* 1101–1118.

Hughes, C., Cutting, A. L., & Dunn, J. (2001). Acting nasty in the face of failure?: Longitudinal observations of "hard-to-manage" children playing a rigged competitive game with a friend. *Journal of Abnormal Child Psychology, 29*, 403–416.

Hughes, C., Oksanen, H., Taylor, A., Jackson, J., Murray, L., Caspi, A., et al. (2002). "I'm gonna beat you!" SNAP!: An observational paradigm for assessing young children's disruptive behaviour in competitive play. *Journal of Child Psychology and Psychiatry and Allied Disciplines, 43*, 507–516.

Hughes, J. N., Meehan, B. T., & Cavell, T. A. (2004). Development and validation of a gender-balanced measure of aggression-relevant social cognition. *Journal of Clinical Child and Adolescent Psychology, 33*, 292–302.

Individuals with Disabilities Education Act Amendments of 1997 (Pub. L. No. 105-17), 20 U.S.C. §1400 *et seq.*

Irvine, A. B., Biglan, A., Smolkowski, K., & Ary, D. V. (1999). The value of the Parenting Scale for measuring the discipline practices of parents of middle school children. *Behaviour Research and Therapy, 37*, 127–142.

Jacob, T., Krahn, G. L., & Leonard, K. (1991). Parent–child interactions in families with alcoholic fathers. *Journal of Consulting and Clinical Psychology, 59*, 176–181.

Jacobs, J. R., Boggs, S. R., Eyberg, S. M., Edwards, D., Durning, P., Querido, J. G., et al. (2000). Psychometric properties and reference point data for the Revised Edition of the School Observation Coding System. *Behavior Therapy, 31*, 695–712.

Jansen, R. E., Fitzgerald, H. E., Ham, H. P., & Zucker, R. A. (1995). Pathways into risk: Temperament and behavior problems in three-to five-year-old sons of alcoholics. *Alcoholism, Clinical and Experimental Research, 19*, 501–509.

Jensen, P. S., Watanabe, H. K., & Richters, J. E. (1999). Who's up first?: Testing for order effects in structured interviews using a counterbalanced experimental design. *Journal of Abnormal Child Psychology, 27*, 439–445.

Johnston, C. (1996a). Addressing parent cognitions in interventions with families of disruptive children. In K. S. Dobson & K. D. Craig (Eds.), *Advances in cognitive-behavioral therapy* (pp. 193–209). Thousand Oaks, CA: Sage.

Johnston, C. (1996b). Parent characteristics and parent–child interactions in families of nonproblem children and ADHD children with higher and lower levels of oppositional-defiant behavior. *Journal of Abnormal Child Psychology, 24*, 85–104.

Johnston, C., & Mash, E. J. (1989). A measure of parenting satisfaction and efficacy. *Journal of Clinical Child Psychology, 18*, 167–175.

Johnston, C., & Patenaude, R. (1994). Parent attributions of inattentive-overactive and oppositional-defiant child behaviors. *Cognitive Therapy and Research, 18*, 261–275.

Jones, R. R. (1974). "*Observation*" *by telephone: An economical behavior sampling technique* (Oregon Research Institute Technical Report No. 1411). Eugene: Oregon Research Institute.

Jouriles, E. N., Murphy, C. M., Farris, A. M., Smith, D. A., Richters, J. E., & Waters, E. (1991). Marital adjustment, parental disagreements about child rearing, and behavior problems in boys: Increasing the specificity of the marital assessment. *Child Development, 62*, 1424–1433.

Jouriles, E. N., Norwood, W. D., McDonald, R., Vincent, J. P., & Mahoney, A. (1996). Physical violence and other forms of marital aggression: Links with children's behavior problems. *Journal of Family Psychology, 10*, 223–234.

Julien, D., Markman, H. J., & Lindahl, K. M. (1989). A comparison of a global and a microanalytic coding system: Implications for future trends in studying interactions. *Behavioral Assessment, 11*, 81–100.

Kagan, J., & Snidman, N. (1991). Temperamental factors in human development. *American Psychologist, 46*, 856–862.

Kamphaus, R. W., & Frick, P. J. (2005). *Clinical assessment of child and adolescent personality and behavior* (2nd ed.). New York: Springer.

Kazdin, A. E. (1990). Premature termination from treatment among children referred for antisocial behavior. *Journal of Child Psychology and Psychiatry and Allied Disciplines, 31*, 415–425.

Kazdin, A. E. (1995). Child, parent and family dysfunction as predictors of outcome in cognitive-behavioral treatment of antisocial children. *Behaviour Research and Therapy, 33*, 271–281.

Kazdin, A. E. (2005). Evidence-based assessment for children and adolescents: Issues in measurement development and clinical application. *Journal of Clinical Child and Adolescent Psychology, 34*, 548–558.

Kazdin, A. E., Bass, D., Siegel, T., & Thomas, C. (1989). Cognitive-behavioral therapy and relationship therapy in the treatment of children referred for antisocial behavior. *Journal of Consulting and Clinical Psychology, 57*, 522–535.

Kazdin, A. E., Mazurick, J. L., & Siegel, T. C. (1994). Treatment outcome among children with externalizing disorder who terminate prematurely versus those who complete psychotherapy. *Journal of the American Academy of Child and Adolescent Psychiatry, 33*, 549–557.

Kazdin, A. E., Siegel, T. C., & Bass, D. (1992). Cognitive problem-solving skills training and parent management training in the treatment of antisocial behavior in children. *Journal of Consulting and Clinical Psychology, 60*, 733–747.

Keenan, K., Shaw, D., Delliquadri, E., Giovannelli, J., & Walsh, B. (1998). Evidence for the continuity of early problem behaviors: Application of a developmental model. *Journal of Abnormal Child Psychology, 26*, 441–452.

Kendall, P. C., Reber, M., McLeer, S., Epps, J., & Ronan, K. R. (1990). Cognitive-behavioral treatment of conduct-disordered children. *Cognitive Therapy and Research*, 14, 279–297.

Kimmel, D. C., & van der Veen, F. (1974). Factors of marital adjustment in Locke's Marital Adjustment Test. *Journal of Marriage and the Family*, 36, 57–63.

Kimonis, E. R., Frick, P. J., Fazekas, H., & Loney, B. R. (2006). Psychopathic traits, aggression, and the processing of emotional stimuli in non-referred children. *Behavioral Sciences and the Law*, 24, 21–37.

Klinteberg, B. A., Andersson, T., Magnusson, D., & Stattin, H. (1993). Hyperactive behavior in childhood as related to subsequent alcohol problems and violent offending: A longitudinal study of male subjects. *Personality and Individual Differences*, 15, 381–388.

Kolko, D. J., Nishi-Strattner, L., Wilcox, D. K., & Kopet, T. (2002). Clinical assessment of juvenile firesetters and their families: Tools and tips. In D. J. Kolko (Ed.), *Handbook on firesetting in children and youth* (pp. 177–212). San Diego, CA: Academic Press.

Kolko, D. J., Watson, S., & Faust, J. (1991). Fire safety/prevention skills training to reduce involvement with fire in young psychiatric inpatients: Preliminary findings. *Behavior Therapy*, 22, 269–284.

Kovacs, M., Paulauskas, S., Gatsonis, C., & Richards, C. (1988). Depressive disorders in childhood. *Journal of Affective Disorders*, 15, 205–217.

Krol, N. P. C. M., De Bruyn, E. E. J., Coolen, J. C., & van Aarle, E. J. M. (2006). From CBCL to DSM: A comparison of two methods to screen for DSM-IV diagnoses using CBCL data. *Journal of Clinical Child and Adolescent Psychology*, 35, 127–135.

Lahey, B. B. (2004). Commentary: Role of temperament in developmental models of psychopathology. *Journal of Clinical Child and Adolescent Psychology*, 33, 88–93.

Lahey, B. B., Goodman, S. H., Waldman, I. D., Bird, H., Canino, G., Jensen, P., et al. (1999). Relation of age of onset to the type and severity of child and adolescent conduct problems. *Journal of Abnormal Child Psychology*, 27, 247–260.

Lahey, B. B., Moffitt, T. E., & Caspi, A. (Eds.). (2003). *Causes of conduct disorder and juvenile delinquency.* New York: Guilford Press.

Lahey, B. B., Schwab-Stone, M., Goodman, S. H., Waldman, I. D., Canino, G., Rathouz, P. J., et al. (2000). Age and gender differences in oppositional behavior and conduct problems: A cross-sectional household study of middle childhood and adolescence. *Journal of Abnormal Psychology*, 109, 488–503.

LaRue, R. H., & Handleman, J. (2006). A primer on school-based functional assessment. *Behavior Therapist*, 29, 48–52.

Leff, S. S., Angelucci, J., Grabowski, L., & Weil, J. (2004, July). Using school and community partners to design, implement, and evaluate a group intervention for relationally aggressive girls. In S. S. Leff (Chair), *Using partnerships to design, implement, and evaluate aggression prevention programs.* Symposium conducted at the annual meeting of the American Psychological Association, Honolulu, HI.

Lett, N. J., & Kamphaus, R. W. (1997). Differential validity of the BASC Student Observation System and the BASC Teacher Rating Scale. *Canadian Journal of School Psychology*, 13, 1–14.

Levene, K. S., Walsh, M. M., Augimeri, L. K., & Pepler, D. J. (2004). Linking identification and treatment of early risk factors for female delinquency. In M. M. Moretti, C. L. Odgers, & M. A. Jackson (Eds.), *Girls and aggression: Contributing factors and intervention principles* (pp. 147–163). New York: Kluwer Academic/Plenum Press.

Little, T. D., Jones, S. M., Henrich, C. C., & Hawley, P. H. (2003). Disentangling the "whys" from the "whats" of aggressive behavior. *International Journal of Behavioural Development*, 27, 122–133.

Lochman, J. E., & Wells, K. C. (1996). A social-cognitive intervention with aggressive children: Prevention effects and contextual implementation issues. In R. D. Peters & R. J. McMahon (Eds.), *Preventing childhood disorders, substance abuse, and delinquency* (pp. 111–143). Thousand Oaks, CA: Sage.

Locke, H. J., & Wallace, K. M. (1959). Short marital adjustment and prediction tests: Their reliability and validity. *Marriage and Family Living*, 21, 251–255.

Loeber, R., Brinthaupt, V. P., & Green, S. M. (1990). Attention deficits, impulsivity, and hyperactivity with or without conduct problems: Relationships to delinquency and unique contextual factors. In R. J. McMahon & R. D. Peters (Eds.), *Behavior disorders of adolescence: Research, intervention, and policy in clinical and school setting* (pp. 39–61). New York: Plenum Press.

Loeber, R., & Farrington, D. P. (2000). Young children who commit crime: Epidemiology, developmental origins, risk factors, early interventions, and policy implications. *Development and Psychopathology*, 12, 737–762.

Loeber, R., & Keenan, K. (1994). Interaction between conduct disorder and its comorbid conditions: Effects of age and gender. *Clinical Psychology Review*, 14, 497–523.

Loeber, R., & Schmaling, K. B. (1985). The utility of differentiating between mixed and pure forms of antisocial child behavior. *Journal of Abnormal Child Psychology*, 13, 315–336.

Loeber, R., & Stouthamer-Loeber, M. (1986). Family factors as correlates and predictors of juvenile conduct problems and delinquency. In M. Tonry & N. Morris (Eds.), *Crime and justice* (Vol. 7, pp. 29–149). Chicago: University of Chicago Press.

Loeber, R., Stouthamer-Loeber, M., Van Kammen, W. B., & Farrington, D. P. (1989). Development of a new measure of self-reported antisocial behavior for young children: Prevalence and reliability. In M. W. Klein (Ed.), *Cross national research and self-reported crime and delinquency* (pp. 203–225). Dordrecht, the Netherlands: Kluwer-Nijhoff.

Loeber, R., Wung, P., Keenan, K., Giroux, B., Stouthamer-Loeber, M., Van Kammen, W. B., et al. (1993). Developmental pathways in disruptive child behavior. *Development and Psychopathology, 5,* 101–131.

Loney, B. R., & Frick, P. J. (2003). Structured diagnostic interviewing. In C. R. Reynolds & R. W. Kamphaus (Eds.), *Handbook of psychological and educational assessment of children: Personality, behavior, and context* (2nd ed., pp. 235–247). New York: Guilford Press.

Loney, B. R., Frick, P. J., Clements, C. B., Ellis, M. L., & Kerlin, K. (2003). Callous-unemotional traits, impulsivity, and emotional processing in antisocial adolescents. *Journal of Clinical Child and Adolescent Psychology, 32,* 139–152.

Loney, B. R., Frick, P. J., Ellis, M., & McCoy, M. G. (1998). Intelligence, psychopathy, and antisocial behavior. *Journal of Psychopathology and Behavioral Assessment, 20,* 231–247.

Loukas, A., Fitzgerald, H. E., Zucker, R. A., & von Eye, A. (2001). Parental alcoholism and co-occurring antisocial behavior: Prospective relationships to externalizing behavior problems in their young sons. *Journal of Abnormal Child Psychology, 29,* 91–106.

Lovejoy, M. C., Verda, M. R., & Hays, C. E. (1997). Convergent and discriminant validity of measures of parenting efficacy and control. *Journal of Clinical Child Psychology, 26,* 366–376.

Lynam, D. R., Caspi, A., Moffitt, T. E., Raine, A., Loeber, R., & Stouthamer-Loeber, M. (2005). Adolescent psychopathy and the Big Five: Results from two samples. *Journal of Abnormal Child Psychology, 33,* 431–443.

Lynskey, M. T., & Fergusson, D. M. (1995). Childhood conduct problems, attention deficit behaviors, and adolescent alcohol, tobacco, and illicit drug use. *Journal of Abnormal Child Psychology, 23,* 281–302.

Lyons-Ruth, K. (1996). Attachment relationships among children with aggressive behavior problems: The role of disorganized early attachment patterns. *Journal of Consulting and Clinical Psychology, 64,* 64–73.

Mann, B. J., & MacKenzie, E. P. (1996). Pathways among marital functioning, parental behaviors, and child behavior problems in school-age boys. *Journal of Clinical Child Psychology, 25,* 183–191.

Martinez, C. R., & Forgatch, M. S. (2001). Preventing problems with boys' noncompliance: Effects of a parent training intervention for divorcing mothers. *Journal of Consulting and Clinical Psychology, 69,* 416–428.

Mash, E. J., & Johnston, C. (1983). Sibling interactions of hyperactive and normal children and their relationship to reports of maternal stress and self-esteem. *Journal of Clinical Child Psychology, 12,* 91–99.

Mash, E. J., Johnston, C., & Kovitz, K. (1983). A com-

parison of the mother–child interactions of physically abused and non-abused children during play and task situations. *Journal of Clinical Child Psychology, 12,* 337–346.

McClellan, J., & Werry, J. S. (2000). Introduction to special section: Research psychiatric diagnostic interviews for children and adolescents. *Journal of the American Academy of Child and Adolescent Psychiatry, 39,* 19–27.

McConaughy, S. H., & Achenbach, T. M. (2001). *Manual for the Semistructured Clinical Interview for Children and Adolescents* (2nd ed.). Burlington: University of Vermont, Center for Children, Youth, and Families.

McConaughy, S. H., Achenbach, T. M., & Gent, C. L. (1988). Multiaxial empirically based assessment: Parent, teacher, observational, cognitive, and personality correlates of Child Behavior Profile types for 6- to 11-year-old boys. *Journal of Abnormal Child Psychology, 16,* 485–509.

McMahon, R. J., & Estes, A. (1994). *Fast Track parent–child interaction task: Observational data collection manuals.* Unpublished manuscript, University of Washington, Seattle.

McMahon, R. J., & Estes, A. M. (1997). Conduct problems. In E. J. Mash & L. G. Terdal (Eds.), *Assessment of childhood disorders* (3rd ed., pp. 130–193). New York: Guilford Press.

McMahon, R. J., & Forehand, R. (1983). Consumer satisfaction in behavioral treatment of children: Types issues, and recommendations. *Behavior Therapy, 14,* 209–225.

McMahon, R. J., & Forehand, R. L. (2003). *Helping the noncompliant child: Family-based treatment for oppositional behavior* (2nd ed.). New York: Guilford Press.

McMahon, R. J., Forehand, R., & Griest, D. L. (1981). Effects of knowledge of social learning principles on enhancing treatment outcome and generalization in a parent training program. *Journal of Consulting and Clinical Psychology, 49,* 526–532.

McMahon, R. J., Forehand, R., Griest, D. L., & Wells, K. C. (1981). Who drops out of treatment during parent behavioral training? *Behavioral Counseling Quarterly, 1,* 79–85.

McMahon, R. J., & Frick, P. J. (2005). Evidence-based assessment of conduct problems in children and adolescents. *Journal of Clinical Child and Adolescent Psychology, 34,* 477–505.

McMahon, R. J., & Metzler, C. W. (1998). Selecting parenting measures for assessing family-based preventive interventions. In R. S. Ashery, E. B. Robertson, & K. L. Kumpfer (Eds.), *Drug abuse prevention through family interventions* (NIDA Research Monograph No. 177, pp. 294–323). Rockville, MD: National Institute on Drug Abuse.

McMahon, R. J., Tiedemann, G. L., Forehand, R., & Griest, D. L. (1984). Parental satisfaction with parent training to modify child noncompliance. *Behavior Therapy, 15,* 295–303.

McMahon, R. J., Wells, K. C., & Kotler, J. S. (2006). Conduct problems. In E. J. Mash & R. A. Barkley (Eds.), *Treatment of childhood disorders* (3rd ed., pp. 137–268). New York: Guilford Press.

McNeil, C. B., Eyberg, S., Eisenstadt, T. H., Newcomb, K., & Funderburk, B. (1991). Parent–Child Interaction Therapy with behavior problem children: Generalization of treatment effects to the school setting. *Journal of Clinical Child Psychology, 20,* 140–151.

Moffitt, T. E. (1993). Adolescence-limited and life-course persistent antisocial behavior: A developmental taxonomy. *Psychological Review, 100,* 674–701.

Moffitt, T. E. (2003). Life-course persistent and adolescence-limited antisocial behavior: A ten-year research review and a research agenda. In B. B. Lahey, T. E. Moffitt, & A. Caspi (Eds.), *Causes of conduct disorder and juvenile delinquency* (pp. 49–75). New York: Guilford Press.

Moffitt, T. E., & Caspi, A. (2001). Childhood predictors differentiate life-course persistent and adolescence-limited antisocial pathways in males and females. *Development and Psychopathology, 13,* 355–376.

Moffitt, T. E., Caspi, A., Dickson, N., Silva, P., & Stanton, W. (1996). Childhood-onset versus adolescent-onset antisocial conduct problems in males: Natural history from ages 3 to 18 years. *Development and Psychopathology, 8,* 399–424.

Moretti, M. M., Odgers, C. L., & Jackson, M. A. (Eds.). (2004). *Girls and aggression: Contributing factors and intervention principles.* New York: Kluwer Academic/Plenum Press.

Morsbach, S. K., & Prinz, R. J. (2006). Understanding and improving the validity of self-report of parenting. *Clinical Child and Family Psychology Review, 9,* 1–21.

Mouton, P. Y., & Tuma, J. M. (1988). Stress, locus of control, and role satisfaction in clinic and control mothers. *Journal of Clinical Child Psychology, 17,* 217–224.

Munoz, L. C., & Frick, P. J. (in press). The reliability, stability, and predictive utility of the self-report version of the Antisocial Process Screening Device. *Scandinavian Journal of Psychology.*

Murphy, K. R., & Gordon, M. (1998). Assessment of adults with ADHD. In R. A. Barkley, *Attention-deficit hyperactivity disorder: A handbook for diagnosis and treatment* (2nd ed., pp. 345–369). New York: Guilford Press.

Nixon, R. D. V., Sweeney, L., Erickson, D. B., & Touyz, S. W. (2003). Parent–child interaction therapy: A comparison of standard and abbreviated treatments for oppositional defiant preschoolers. *Journal of Consulting and Clinical Psychology, 71,* 251–260.

Nock, M. K., & Kurtz, S. M. S. (2005). Direct behavioral observation in school settings: Bringing science to practice. *Cognitive and Behavioral Practice, 12,* 359–370.

O'Brien, B. S., & Frick, P. J. (1996). Reward dominance: Associations with anxiety, conduct problems, and

psychopathy in children. *Journal of Abnormal Child Psychology, 24,* 223–240.

Office of Juvenile Justice and Delinquency Prevention. (1995). *Juvenile offenders and victims: A focus on violence.* Pittsburgh, PA: National Center for Juvenile Justice.

Ohan, J. L., Leung, D. W., & Johnston, C. (2000). The Parenting Sense of Competence Scale: Evidence of a stable factor structure and validity. *Canadian Journal of Behavioural Science, 32,* 251–261.

O'Leary, K. D., Vivian, D., & Malone, J. (1992). Assessment of physical aggression against women in marriage: The need for multimodal assessment. *Behavioral Assessment, 14,* 5–14.

Osofsky, J. D., Wewers, S., Hann, D. M., & Fick, A. C. (1993). Chronic community violence: What is happening to our children? *Psychiatry, 56,* 36–45.

Oxford, M., Cavell, T. A., & Hughes, J. N. (2003). Callous-unemotional traits moderate the relation between ineffective parenting and child externalizing problems: A partial replication and extension. *Journal of Clinical Child and Adolescent Psychology, 32,* 577–585.

Pardini, D. A., Lochman, J. E., & Frick, P. J. (2003). Callous/unemotional traits and social cognitive processes in adjudicated youth. *Journal of the American Academy of Child and Adolescent Psychiatry, 42,* 364–371.

Patterson, G. R. (1982). *Coercive family process.* Eugene, OR: Castalia.

Patterson, G. R. (1983). Stress: A change agent for family process. In N. Garmezy & M. Rutter (Eds.), *Stress, coping and development in children* (pp. 235–264). New York: McGraw-Hill.

Patterson, G. R., & Capaldi, D. M. (1991). Antisocial parents: Unskilled and vulnerable. In P. A. Cowan & E. M. Hetherington (Eds.), *Family transitions* (pp. 195–218). Hillsdale, NJ: Erlbaum.

Patterson, G. R., Capaldi, D., & Bank, L. (1991). An early starter model for predicting delinquency. In D. J. Pepler & K. H. Rubin (Eds.), *The development and treatment of childhood aggression* (pp. 139–168). Hillsdale, NJ: Erlbaum.

Patterson, G. R., & Dishion, T. J. (1985). Contributions of family and peers to delinquency. *Criminology, 23,* 63–79.

Patterson, G. R., & Forgatch, M. S. (1995). Predicting future clinical adjustment from treatment outcome and process variables. *Psychological Assessment, 7,* 275–285.

Patterson, G. R., Reid, J. B., & Dishion, T. J. (1992). *Antisocial boys.* Eugene, OR: Castalia.

Patterson, G. R., Reid, J. B., Jones, R. R., & Conger, R. E. (1975). *A social learning approach to family intervention: Vol. 1. Families with aggressive children.* Eugene, OR: Castalia.

Patterson, G. R., & Yoerger, K. (2002). A developmental model for early and late-onset delinquency. In J. B. Reid, G. R. Patterson, & J. Snyder (Eds.), *Antisocial behavior in children and adolescents: A developmen-*

tal analysis and model for intervention (pp. 147–172). Washington, DC: American Psychological Association.

Peed, S., Roberts, M., & Forehand, R. (1977). Evaluation of the effectiveness of a standardized parent training program in altering the interaction of mothers and their noncompliant children. *Behavior Modification, 1,* 323–350.

Peeples, F., & Loeber, R. (1994). Do individual factors and neighborhood context explain ethnic differences in juvenile delinquency? *Journal of Quantitative Criminology, 10,* 141–158.

Pelham, W. E., & Lang, A. R. (1993). Parental alcohol consumption and deviant child behavior: Laboratory studies of reciprocal effects. *Clinical Psychology Review, 13,* 763–784.

Pepler, D. J., Madsen, K. C., Webster, C., & Levene, K. S. (Eds.). (2005). *The development and treatment of girlhood aggression.* Mahwah, NJ: Erlbaum.

Pisterman, S., Firestone, P., McGrath, P., Goodman, J. T., Webster, I., Mallory, R., et al. (1992). The effects of parent training on parenting stress and sense of competence. *Canadian Journal of Behavioural Science, 24,* 41–58.

Porter, B., & O'Leary, K. D. (1980). Marital discord and childhood behavior problems. *Journal of Abnormal Child Psychology, 8,* 287–295.

Poulin, F., & Boivin, M. (2000). Reactive and proactive aggression: Evidence of a two-factor model. *Psychological Assessment, 12,* 115–122.

Prinz, R. J., & Miller, G. E. (1991). Issues in understanding and treating childhood conduct problems in disadvantaged populations. *Journal of Clinical Child Psychology, 20,* 379–385.

Putallaz, M., & Bierman, K. L. (Eds.). (2004). *Aggression, antisocial behavior, and violence among girls: A developmental perspective.* New York: Guilford Press.

Quay, H. C., & Peterson, D. (1996). *Revised Behavior Problem Checklist, PAR Edition: Professional manual.* Odessa, FL: Psychological Assessment Resources.

Querido, J. G., & Eyberg, S. M. (2003). Psychometric properties of the Sutter–Eyberg Student Behavior Inventory—Revised with preschool children. *Behavior Therapy, 34,* 1–15.

Raine, A. (2002). Biosocial studies of antisocial and violent behavior in children and adults: A review. *Journal of Abnormal Child Psychology, 30,* 311–326.

Raine, A., Dodge, K., Loeber, R., Gatzke-Kopp, L., Lynam, D., Reynolds, C., et al. (2006). The Reactive–Proactive Aggression Questionnaire: Differential correlates of reactive and proactive aggression in adolescent boys. *Aggressive Behavior, 32,* 159–171.

Raine, A., Reynolds, C., Venables, P. H., & Mednick, S. A. (1997). Biosocial bases of aggressive behavior in childhood. In A. Raine, P. A. Brennan, D. P. Farrington, & S. A. Mednick (Eds.), *Biosocial bases of violence* (pp. 107–126). New York: Plenum Press.

Rayfield, A., Eyberg, S. M., & Foote, R. (1998). Revision of the Sutter–Eyberg Student Behavior Inventory: Teacher ratings of conduct problem behavior. *Educational and Psychological Measurement, 58,* 88–99.

Reed, M. L., & Edelbrock, C. (1983). Reliability and validity of the Direct Observation Form of the Child Behavior Checklist. *Journal of Abnormal Child Psychology, 11,* 521–530.

Reich, W. (2000). Diagnostic Interview for Children and Adolescents (DICA). *Journal of the American Academy of Child and Adolescent Psychiatry, 39,* 59–66.

Reid, J. B. (Ed.). (1978). *A social learning approach to family intervention: Vol. 2. Observation in home settings.* Eugene, OR: Castalia.

Reid, J. B., Hinojosa Rivera, G., & Lorber, R. (1980). *A social learning approach to the outpatient treatment of children who steal.* Unpublished manuscript, Oregon Social Learning Center, Eugene.

Reitman, D. (2006). Overview of child behavioral assessment. In M. Hersen (Ed.), *Clinician's handbook of child behavioral assessment* (pp. 3–24). New York: Elsevier.

Reitman, D., Currier, R. O., Hupp, S. D. A., Rhode, P. C., Murphy, M. A., & O'Callaghan, P. M. (2001). Psychometric characteristics of the Parenting Scale in a Head Start population. *Journal of Clinical Child Psychology, 30,* 514–524.

Reynolds, C. R., & Kamphaus, R. W. (2004). *Behavior Assessment System for Children–2 (BASC-2).* Bloomington, MN: Pearson Assessments.

Rhule, D. M., McMahon, R. J., & Vando, J. (2005, November). The social validity of standardized parent–child interaction task analogues. In M. Nock (Chair), *Building bridges into behavior therapy: Improving engagement in child and adolescent treatments.* Symposium presented at the annual meeting of the Association for Advancement of Behavior Therapy, Washington, DC.

Rich, B. A., & Eyberg, S. M. (2001). Accuracy of assessment: The discriminative and predictive power of the Eyberg Child Behavior Inventory. *Ambulatory Child Heath, 7,* 249–257.

Richters, J. E., & Martinez, P. (1990). *Things I Have Seen and Heard: An interview for young children about exposure to violence.* Rockville, MD: National Institute of Mental Health.

Roberts, M. W. (2001). Clinic observations of structured parent–child interaction designed to evaluate externalizing problems. *Psychological Assessment, 13,* 46–58.

Roberts, M. W., Joe, V. C., & Rowe-Hallbert, A. (1992). Oppositional child behavior and parental locus of control. *Journal of Clinical Child Psychology, 21,* 170–177.

Roberts, M. W., & Powers, S. W. (1988). The Compliance Test. *Behavioral Assessment, 10,* 375–398.

Roberts, M. W., & Powers, S. W. (1990). Adjusting chair timeout enforcement procedures for oppositional children. *Behavior Therapy, 21,* 257–271.

Robinson, E. A., & Anderson, L. L. (1983). Family adjustment, parental attitudes, and social desirability. *Journal of Abnormal Child Psychology, 11,* 247–256.

Robinson, E. A., & Eyberg, S. M. (1981). The Dyadic Parent–Child Interaction Coding System: Standardization and validation. *Journal of Consulting and Clinical Psychology, 49,* 245–250.

Robinson, E. A., Eyberg, S. M., & Ross, A. W. (1980). The standardization of an inventory of child conduct problem behaviors. *Journal of Clinical Child Psychology, 9,* 22–29.

Roff, J. D., & Wirt, R. D. (1984). Childhood aggression and social adjustment as antecedents of delinquency. *Journal of Abnormal Child Psychology, 12,* 111–126.

Rogers, H., & Matthews, J. (2004). The Parenting Sense of Competence Scale: Investigation of the factor structure, reliability, and validity for an Australian sample. *Australian Psychologist, 39,* 88–96.

Rothbart, M. K., & Bates, J. E. (1998). Temperament. In W. Damon (Ed.), *Handbook of child psychology: Vol. 3. Social, emotional, and personality development* (pp. 105–176). New York: Wiley.

Rothbart, M. K., & Jones, L. B. (1998). Temperament, self-regulation, and education. *School Psychology Review, 27,* 479–491.

Russo, D. C., Cataldo, M. F., & Cushing, P. J. (1981). Compliance training and behavioral covariation in the treatment of multiple behavior problems. *Journal of Applied Behavior Analysis, 14,* 209–222.

Rutter, M. (1994). Family discord and conduct disorder: Cause, consequence, or correlate? *Journal of Family Psychology, 8,* 170–186.

Sanders, M. R., & Dadds, M. R. (1992). Children's and parents' cognitions about family interaction: An evaluation of video-mediated recall and thought listing procedures in the assessment of conduct-disordered children. *Journal of Clinical Child Psychology, 21,* 371–379.

Sanders, M. R., & Lawton, J. M. (1993). Discussing assessment findings with families: A guided participation model of information transfer. *Child and Family Behavior Therapy, 15*(2), 5–35.

Sanders, M. R., Markie-Dadds, C., Tully, L. A., & Bor, W. (2000). The Triple P-Positive Parenting Program: A comparison of enhanced, standard, and self-directed behavioral family intervention for parents of children with early onset conduct problems. *Journal of Consulting and Clinical Psychology, 68,* 624–640.

Sarason, I. G., Johnson, J. H., & Siegel, J. M. (1978). Assessing the impact of life changes: Development of the Life Experiences Survey. *Journal of Consulting and Clinical Psychology, 46,* 932–946.

Saunders, J. D., Aasland, O. G., Babor, T. F., de la Fuente, J. R., & Grant, M. (1993). Development of the Alcohol Use Disorders Identification Test (AUDIT): WHO collaborative project on early detection of persons with harmful alcohol consumption—II. *Addiction, 88,* 791–804.

Scherer, D. G., Brondino, M. J., Henggeler, S. W., Melton, G. B., & Hanley, J. H. (1994). Multisystemic family preservation therapy: Preliminary findings from a study of rural and minority serious adolescent offenders. *Journal of Emotional and Behavioral Disorders, 2,* 198–206.

Schwartz, D., Dodge, K. A., Coie, J. D., Hubbard, J. A., Cillessen, A. H. N., Lemerise, E. A., et al. (1998). Social-cognitive and behavioral correlates of aggression and victimization in boys' play groups. *Journal of Abnormal Child Psychology, 26,* 431–440.

Scott, S., Spender, Q., Doolan, M., Jacobs, B., & Aspland, H. (2001). Multicentre controlled trial of parenting groups for child antisocial behaviour in clinical practice. *British Medical Journal, 323,* 1–7.

Scotti, J. R., Morris, T. L., McNeil, C. B., & Hawkins, R. P. (1996). DSM-IV and disorders of childhood and adolescence: Can structural criteria be functional? *Journal of Consulting and Clinical Psychology, 64,* 1177–1191.

Selzer, M. L., Vinokur, A., & van Rooijen, L. (1975). A self-administered short Michigan Alcoholism Screening Test. *Journal of Studies on Alcohol, 36,* 117–126.

Serbin, L. A., Moskowitz, K. S., Schwartzman, A. E., & Ledingham, J. E. (1991). Aggressive, withdrawn, and aggressive/withdrawn children in adolescence: Into the next generation. In D. J. Pepler & K. H. Rubin (Eds.), *The development and treatment of childhood aggression* (pp. 55–70). Hillsdale, NJ: Erlbaum.

Shaffer, D., Fisher, P., Lucas, C. P., Dulcan, M. K., & Schwab-Stone, M. E. (2000). NIMH Diagnostic Interview Schedule for Children Version IV (NIMH DISC-IV): Description, differences from previous versions, and reliability of some common diagnoses. *Journal of the American Academy of Child and Adolescent Psychiatry, 39,* 28–38.

Shaffer, D., Gould, M. S., Brasic, J., Ambrosini, P., Fisher, P., Bird, H., et al. (1983). A Children's Global Assessment Scale (CGAS). *Archives of General Psychiatry, 40,* 1228–1231.

Shelton, K. K., Frick, P. J., & Wootton, J. M. (1996). Assessment of parenting practices in families of elementary school-age children. *Journal of Clinical Child Psychology, 25,* 317–329.

Sheras, P. L., Abidin, R. R., & Konold, T. R. (1998). *Stress Index for Parents of Adolescents, professional manual.* Lutz, FL: Psychological Assessment Resources.

Silverthorn, P., & Frick, P. J. (1999). Developmental pathways to antisocial behavior: The delayed-onset pathway in girls. *Development and Psychopathology, 11,* 101–126.

Simonoff, E., Pickles, A., Meyer, J., Silberg, J., & Maes, H. (1998). Genetic and environmental influences on subtypes of conduct disorder behavior in boys. *Journal of Abnormal Child Psychology, 26,* 495–510.

Skinner, H. A. (1982). The Drug Abuse Screening Test. *Addictive Behaviors, 7,* 363–371.

Snyder, J. (1991). Discipline as a mediator of the impact

of maternal stress and mood on child conduct problems. *Development and Psychopathology, 3,* 263–276.

Spanier, G. B. (1976). Measuring dyadic adjustment: New scales for assessing the quality of marriage and similar dyads. *Journal of Marriage and the Family, 38,* 15–28.

Stanger, C., Dumenci, L., Kamon, J., & Burstein, M. (2004). Parenting and children's externalizing problems in substance-abusing families. *Journal of Clinical Child and Adolescent Psychology, 33,* 590–600.

Stattin, H., & Kerr, M. (2000). Parental monitoring: A reinterpretation. *Child Development, 71,* 1072–1085.

Steele, R. G., Nesbitt-Daly, J. S., Daniel, R. C., & Forehand, R. (2005). Factor structure of the Parenting Scale in a low-income African American sample. *Journal of Child and Family Studies, 14,* 535–549.

Steer, R. A., Ball, R., Ranieri, W. F., & Beck, A. T. (1999). Dimensions of Beck Depression Inventory–II in clinically depressed outpatients. *Journal of Clinical Psychology, 55,* 117–28.

Straus, M. A. (1979). Measuring intrafamily conflict and violence: The Conflict Tactics (CT) Scales. *Journal of Marriage and the Family, 41,* 75–88.

Straus, M. A. (1990). The Conflict Tactics Scales and its critics: An evaluation and new data on validity and reliability. In M. A. Straus & R. J. Gelles (Eds.), *Physical violence in American families: Risk factors and adaptations to violence in 8,145 families* (pp. 49–73). New Brunswick, NJ: Transaction.

Straus, M. A., Hamby, S. L., Boney-McCoy, S., & Sugarman, D. B. (1996). The Revised Conflict Tactics Scales (CTS2): Development and preliminary psychometric data. *Journal of Family Issues, 17,* 283–316.

Tapscott, M., Frick, P. J., Wootton, J., & Kruh, I. (1996). The intergenerational link to antisocial behavior: Effects of paternal contact. *Journal of Child and Family Studies, 5,* 229–240.

Thornberry, T. P., & Krohn, M. D. (Eds.). (2003). *Taking stock of delinquency: An overview of findings from contemporary longitudinal studies.* New York: Kluwer Academic/Plenum Press.

Tiet, Q. Q., Wasserman, G. A., Loeber, R., Larken, S. M., & Miller, L. S. (2001). Developmental and sex differences in types of conduct problems. *Journal of Child and Family Studies, 10,* 181–197.

Tolan, P. H., Gorman-Smith, D., & Loeber, R. (2000). Developmental timing of onsets of disruptive behaviors and later delinquency of inner-city youth. *Journal of Child and Family Studies, 9,* 203–220.

Underwood, M. K. (2003). *Social aggression among girls.* New York: Guilford Press.

Van Kammen, W. B., Loeber, R., & Stouthamer-Loeber, M. (1991). Substance use and its relationship to conduct problems and delinquency in young boys. *Journal of Youth and Adolescence, 20,* 399–413.

van Zeijl, J., Mesman, J., Stolk, M. N., Alink, L. R. A.,

van IJzendoorn, M. H., Bakermans-Kranenburg, M. J., et al. (2006). Terrible ones?: Assessment of externalizing behaviors in infancy with the Child Behavior Checklist. *Journal of Child Psychology and Psychiatry, 47,* 801–810.

Wahler, R. G. (1980). The insular mother: Her problems in parent–child treatment. *Journal of Applied Behavior Analysis, 13,* 207–219.

Wahler, R. G., & Cormier, W. H. (1970). The ecological interview: A first step in out-patient child behavior therapy. *Journal of Behavior Therapy and Experimental Psychiatry, 1,* 279–289.

Wahler, R. G., & Dumas, J. E. (1984). Changing the observational coding styles of insular and noninsular mothers: A step toward maintenance of parent training effects. In R. F. Dangel & R. A. Polster (Eds.), *Parent training: Foundations of research and practice* (pp. 379–416). New York: Guilford Press.

Wahler, R. G., & Graves, M. G. (1983). Setting events in social networks: Ally or enemy in child behavior therapy? *Behavior Therapy, 14,* 19–36.

Wahler, R. G., Hughey, J. B., & Gordon, J. S. (1981). Chronic patterns of mother–child coercion: Some differences between insular and noninsular families. *Analysis and Intervention in Developmental Disabilities, 1,* 145–156.

Wahler, R. G., Leske, G., & Rogers, E. S. (1979). The insular family: A deviance support system for oppositional children. In L. A. Hamerlynck (Ed.), *Behavioral systems for the developmentally disabled: Vol. 1. School and family environments* (pp. 102–127). New York: Brunner/Mazel.

Wahler, R. G., & Sansbury, L. E. (1990). The monitoring skills of troubled mothers: Their problems in defining child deviance. *Journal of Abnormal Child Psychology, 18,* 577–589.

Wakschlag, L. S., & Danis, B. (2004). Assessment of disruptive behaviors in young children: A clinical–developmental framework. In R. Del Carmen & A. Carter (Eds.), *Handbook of infant and toddler mental health assessment* (pp. 421–440). New York: Oxford University Press.

Walker, H. M. (1995). *The acting-out child: Coping with classroom disruption* (2nd ed.). Longmont, CO: Sopris West.

Walker, H. M., Colvin, G., & Ramsey, E. (1995). *Antisocial behavior in school: Strategies and best practices.* Pacific Grove, CA: Brooks/Cole.

Walker, H. M., Ramsey, E., & Gresham, F. M. (2004). *Antisocial behavior in school: Evidence-based practice.* Belmont, CA: Wadsworth/Thomas Learning.

Walker, H. M., Shinn, M. R., O'Neill, R. E., & Ramsey, E. (1987). A longitudinal assessment of the development of antisocial behavior in boys: Rationale, methodology, and first-year results. *RASE: Remedial and Special Education, 8,* 7–16, 27.

Walker, J. L., Lahey, B. B., Russo, M. F., Frick, P. J., Christ, M. A., McBurnett, K., et al. (1991). Anxiety, inhibition, and conduct disorder in children: I. Relations to social impairment. *Journal of the American Academy of Child and Adolescent Psychiatry, 30,* 187–191.

Waschbusch, D. A. (2002). A meta-analytic examination of comorbid hyperactive–impulsive–attention problems and conduct problems. *Psychological Bulletin, 128,* 118–50.

Webster-Stratton, C. (1985). Comparisons of behavior transactions between conduct-disordered children and their mothers in the clinic and at home. *Journal of Abnormal Child Psychology, 13,* 169–184.

Webster-Stratton, C. (1988). Mothers' and fathers' perceptions of child deviance: Roles of parent and child behaviors and parent adjustment. *Journal of Consulting and Clinical Psychology, 56,* 909–915.

Webster-Stratton, C. (1989). Systematic comparison of consumer satisfaction of three cost-effective parent training programs for conduct problem children. *Behavior Therapy, 20,* 103–115.

Webster-Stratton, C. (1990). Stress: A potential disruptor of parent perceptions and family interactions. *Journal of Clinical Child Psychology, 19,* 302–312.

Webster-Stratton, C. (1994). Advancing videotape parent training: A comparison study. *Journal of Consulting and Clinical Psychology, 62,* 583–593.

Webster-Stratton, C., & Hammond, M. (1988). Maternal depression and its relationship to life stress, perceptions of child behavior problems, parenting behaviors, and child conduct problems. *Journal of Abnormal Child Psychology, 16,* 299–315.

Webster-Stratton, C., & Hammond, M. (1997). Treating children with early-onset conduct problems: A comparison of child and parent training programs. *Journal of Consulting and Clinical Psychology, 65,* 93–109.

Webster-Stratton, C., & Lindsay, D. W. (1999). Social competence and conduct problems in young children: Issues in assessment. *Journal of Clinical Child Psychology, 28,* 25–43.

Webster-Stratton, C., & Spitzer, A. (1991). Development, reliability, and validity of the Daily Telephone Discipline Interview. *Behavioral Assessment, 13,* 221–239.

Weis, R., Lovejoy, M. C., & Lundahl, B. W. (2005). Factor structure and discriminative validity of the Eyberg Child Behavior Inventory with young children. *Journal of Psychopathology and Behavioral Assessment, 27,* 269–278.

Wells, K. C., Forehand, R., & Griest, D. L. (1980). Generality of treatment effects from treated to untreated behaviors resulting from a parent training program. *Journal of Clinical Child Psychology, 8,* 217–219.

Whipple, E. E., Fitzgerald, H. E., & Zucker, R. A. (1995). Parent–child interactions in alcoholic and nonalcoholic families. *American Journal of Orthopsychiatry, 65,* 153–159.

Whipple, E. E., & Webster-Stratton, C. (1991). The role of parental stress in physically abusive families. *Child Abuse and Neglect, 15,* 279–291.

Wiesner, M. (2003). A longitudinal latent variable analysis of reciprocal relations between depressive symptoms and delinquency during adolescence. *Journal of Abnormal Psychology, 112,* 633–645.

Wilcox, D. K., & Kolko, D. J. (2002). Assessing recent firesetting behavior and taking a firesetting history. In D. J. Kolko (Ed.), *Handbook on firesetting in children and youth* (pp. 161–175). San Diego, CA: Academic Press.

Willoughby, M., Kupersmidt, J., & Bryant, D. (2001). Overt and covert dimensions of antisocial behavior in early childhood. *Journal of Abnormal Child Psychology, 29,* 177–187.

Wills, T. A., Schreibman, D., Benson, G., & Vaccaro, D. (1994). Impact of parental substance use on adolescents: A test of a mediational model. *Journal of Pediatric Psychology, 19,* 537–555.

Wootton, J. M., Frick, P. J., Shelton, K. K., & Silverthorn, P. (1997). Ineffective parenting and childhood conduct problems: The moderating role of callous–unemotional traits. *Journal of Consulting and Clinical Psychology, 65,* 301–308.

Zoccolillo, M. (1992). Co-occurrence of conduct disorder and its adult outcomes with depressive and anxiety disorders: A review. *Journal of the American Academy of Child and Adolescent Psychiatry, 31,* 547–556.

Zucker, R. A., & Noll, R. B. (1980). *The Antisocial Behavior Checklist.* Unpublished instrument, Michigan State University, Department of Psychology, East Lansing.

CHAPTER 4

Adolescent Substance Use and Abuse

Ken C. Winters
Tamara Fahnhorst
Andria Botzet

The use of alcohol and other drugs (hereafter referred to simply as "drugs") among adolescents remains a public health threat within U.S. society. From an epidemiological standpoint, drug use by teenagers is relatively common. According to a recent nationwide survey, Monitoring the Future (Johnston, O'Malley, Bachman, & Schulenberg, 2005), over half (51%) of 12th graders have used an illicit drug in their lifetime, and nearly one-fourth (23.4%) reported use of an illicit drug within the prior month. Lifetime alcohol use was reported by 12th-grade students as over three-fourths (76.8%), and nearly half (48.0%) of the senior class had used alcohol within the past month. Thirty percent of eighth graders have used illicit drugs (including inhalants) in their lifetime, and almost half (44%) have used alcohol in their lifetime. In the prior month, usage of any illicit drug was reported at 8%, and alcohol was used by approximately 19% of eighth graders.

Certainly, not all adolescents who use drugs become dependent. Drug use is often best conceptualized along a continuum that starts with *abstinence* and is followed by several stages (see Figure 4.1): *experimental use*, which reflects minimal use (typically limited to alcohol) in social settings; *early abuse*, in which individuals often use more than one drug, use relatively frequently, and begin to face negative consequences; *abuse*, which reflects more regular and frequent drug use in the presence of social and personal negative consequences; and *dependence*, which marks the most severe end of the continuum and is characterized by signs of tolerance to the drug, continued use despite adverse consequences, and frequent failed attempts to reduce or quit using.

Though there is controversy about the applicability of abuse and dependence diagnostic criteria among adolescents (see "Developmental Considerations in Drug Use Assessment"),

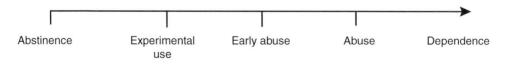

FIGURE 4.1. Continuum of alcohol and drug use.

youth who display abuse and dependence symptoms are still a cause for concern within the public health area. According to a national survey of representative youth in 2004 in the United States (Substance Abuse and Mental Health Services Administration [SAMHSA], 2005), 5.2% of 12- to 18-year-olds met current (prior year) criteria of a substance dependence disorder for at least one drug, and an additional 5.8% met current criteria for an abuse disorder for at least one drug (excluding those that met criteria for a dependence disorder; Winters, Leitten, Wagner, & O'Leary Tevyaw, 2007). In other words, approximately 11% of U.S. adolescents likely fall in the severe end of the drug use continuum.

With such a large base of the adolescent population using substances, and an appreciable percent that may meet abuse or dependence criteria, there are several health and societal implications to consider, including school failure, risky sexual behavior (Jainchill, Yagelka, Hawke, & DeLeon, 1999; MacKenzie, 1993), delinquency, incarceration, suicidality (Bolognini, Plancherel, Laget, & Halfon, 2003; Kaminer, 1994), motor vehicle injuries–fatalities (Kokotailo, 1995), and significant medical health care costs (Drug Abuse Warning Network [DAWN], 1996; King, Gaines, Lambert, Summerfelt, & Bickman, 2000).

Thus, precise assessment of adolescent drug use is essential if we are to gain an accurate understanding of the prevalence and health significance of adolescent drug use. We discuss several issues surrounding assessment in this chapter, including the clinical content, developmental considerations, types of instruments used to assess drug use, and other issues related to methods and sources for assessment of adolescent drug use.

CLINICAL CONTENT

Substance Use Disorders

Drug use that goes beyond experimentation and progresses into problematic involvement is formally delineated by various classification systems: Primary systems include the fourth edition of the *Diagnostic and Statistical Manual of Mental Disorders* (DSM-IV; American Psychiatric Association [APA], 1994) and the 10th revision of *International Classification of Diseases* (ICD-10; World Health Organization [WHO], 1992).

In the DSM-IV diagnostic system, problematic drug use is separated into categories of *abuse* or *dependence*, as shown in Table 4.1. Abuse symptoms reflect drug involvement that increases risk for or results in negative health and social consequences. Indicators of abuse include role impairment, physically hazardous use, recurrent substance-related legal problems, and *drug*-related social and interpersonal difficulties. Abuse symptoms, although associated with clinically significant impairment or distress, are expected to fall short of dependence symptoms on a severity spectrum. Accordingly, an individual must have met at least one of the abuse criteria within the prior 12 months, without obtaining a dependence diagnosis, to receive an abuse diagnosis. DSM-based dependence, on the other hand, requires the positive endorsement of at least three out of seven symptoms defined by psychological and physiological dimensions. Items indicating psychological dependence refer to continued and compulsive use in the face of negative consequences, such as continuing drug use despite recognition of drug-induced depression or quitting important social or occupational activities because of drug use. Items indicating physiological dependence refer to tolerance (i.e., the need for increased drug amounts to achieve intoxication) and withdrawal (i.e., the development of symptoms such as nausea, anxiety, increased pulse rate, or insomnia due to the cessation of heavy or prolonged drug use). In DSM-IV, substance abuse and dependence criteria are the same for all substances, are mutually exclusive, and the diagnoses of abuse and dependence are hierarchically arranged (i.e., a dependence diagnosis precludes an abuse diagnosis). One or two dependence symptoms without abuse symptoms results in the individual not meeting any diagnostic criteria for a substance use disorder (SUD); individuals falling into this category have been described as "diagnostic orphans" (Pollock & Martin, 1999) and are further discussed in the "Applicability of SUD Criteria" section.

It is noteworthy that ICD-10 (WHO, 1992) also identifies two subgroups of problematic drug use: harmful use and dependence. These two ICD-10 groups are defined similarly to the abuse and dependence groups of DSM-IV, and their applicability to youth has been supported (Pollock, Martin, & Langenbucher, 2000). However, most research on adolescent SUDs has focused almost exclusively on the applica-

TABLE 4.1. DSM-IV-TR Criteria for Substance Abuse and Dependence Disorders

Abuse criteria (must endorse at least one item in past 12 months and have no dependence diagnosis)	Dependence driteria (must endorse at least three items in past 12 months)
1. Failure to fulfill role obligations at work, school, or home, such as: • Absences from work/school due to use • Avoiding family activities due to use	1. Tolerance, defined by: • Need for larger amounts of the drug to achieve intoxication • Current effect of drug is diminished compared to previous use of same drug
2. Use in physically hazardous situations, such as: • Driving • Operating a machine • Participating in dangerous activities	2. Withdrawal, defined by: • Two or more symptoms that occur as a result of diminished regular or heavy use, such as increased pulse rate, nausea, anxiety, hand tremors, hallucinations, insomnia • Use of same or similar drug to avoid symptoms mentioned above
3. Substance-related legal problems, such as: • Possession of an illegal substance • Selling or distribution of an illegal substance • Minor consumption	3. Using more than intended, such as: • Using for a longer period than intended • Using a larger quantity than planned
4. Continued use despite social or interpersonal problems, such as: • Physical fights • Arguments with loved ones regarding consequences of drug use	4. Desire to cut down or control use, defined by: • Repeated efforts to cut back or quit using substance • Efforts to cut back or control use were considered "unsuccessful"
	5. Excessive time spent in obtaining or using the drug, such as: • Driving long distances to obtain drug • Spending significant portions of the day using the drug • Spending significant portions of the day recovering from use
	6. Activities given up or reduced due to use, such as: • Quitting social or recreational activities • Missing appointments or meetings to use the drug or recover from its use
	7. Continued use despite physical or psychological problems, such as: • Continuing to use drugs even though person has drug-induced depression • Continuing to use drugs even though person suffers from a physical ailment, such as an ulcer, that can be aggravated by drug use

Note Reprinted with permission from the *Diagnostic and Statistical Manual of Mental Disorders*. Copyright 2000. American Psychiatric Association.

tion of DSM-based criteria, making DSM-IV diagnosis more readily recognized in the field; therefore, it is the only classification system discussed in this chapter.

Diagnostic categories are intended to capture and describe a cluster of associated behaviors and symptoms, thus complementing dimensional approaches by providing categorical groupings. Theoretically, these features should represent core pathological processes and follow a distinctive course (Millon, 1991). Functions of a diagnosis include the ability to identify cases for clinical intervention, convey information about prognosis, facilitate communication among clinicians and researchers, increase the homogeneity of research samples, and provide phenotypes for genetic research (McGue, 1999).

To achieve an accurate diagnosis, a thorough assessment of SUDs should include reliable precursors of the SUD, such as onset prior to age 12 (Henly & Winters, 1988), preadolescent tobacco use (Clark, Kirisci, & Moss, 1998), and polydrug use (Winters, 1994). All of these drug use behaviors have been associated with an increased likelihood of developing an SUD. Though reported levels of substance use are not significantly correlated with the presence of an SUD, especially in the case of alcohol (Pollock & Martin, 1999), quantity and frequency variables can produce important information, particularly when data are compared with regularly updated norms of use; thus, they should also be considered during an assessment of SUDs.

Course of SUDs

The clinical course of an SUD indicates both the changes and expression of an SUD, and the associated functioning over time (Brown, 1993). Understanding the course of adolescent SUDs is essential in determining the etiology and prognosis; as previously mentioned, some adolescent drug use occurs within an experimentation phase that is quite normal within adolescent development (Kandel, 1975), whereas other adolescent drug use is at a level more indicative of abuse or dependence. Multiple studies that have examined developmental trajectories of adolescent drug use (Lewinsohn, Rohde, & Seeley, 1996; Schulenberg, O'Malley, Bachman, Wadsworth, & Johnson, 1996) have found results that support the notion of separate experimental and SUD paths. Devel-

opmental trajectories have been characterized as *developmentally limited* or *intermittent*, as would be expected in an experimental case, as well as *persistent* or *relatively continuous*, suggestive of an SUD. One such trajectory by Lewinsohn and colleagues found gender differences in alcohol use within a community sample; females had an earlier age of onset for an alcohol use disorder (AUD) compared to males (14.6 vs. 16.1 years old, respectively), though males developed alcohol-related problems at a faster rate between ages 18 and 19. The same sample provided evidence that the average duration of an AUD was about 52 weeks for the community sample of adolescents (Lewinsohn et al., 1996).

Certain populations of adolescents tend to have higher rates of SUDs, such as homeless youth, those in the juvenile justice system, and those in psychiatric settings. In one study of homeless youth, nearly half met criteria for alcohol dependence (45%; Baer, Ginzler, & Peterson, 2003), and almost one-third (32%) of youth in the juvenile justice system are estimated to have an SUD (Bilchik, 1998). In addition, approximately 41% of teenagers in a study of adolescent psychiatric inpatients met DSM criteria for an AUD (Grilo, Fehon, Walker, & Martino, 1996). These data suggest that the course of SUDs among certain populations of youth is more acute and calls for a heightened awareness of SUD assessment by treatment providers within these settings.

Some variables have been found to predict the course of SUDs among adolescents in a chemical dependence treatment setting. Pretreatment characteristics associated with more favorable substance use outcomes include a lower severity level of substance use at admission (Maisto, Pollock, Lynch, Martin, & Ammerman, 2001), greater readiness to change (Kelly, Myers, & Brown, 2000), and fewer conduct problems or other co-occurring psychopathology (Grella, Hser, Joshi, & Rounds-Bryant, 2001; Winters, Stinchfield, Opland, Weller, & Latimer, 2000). Factors influencing better outcomes during treatment include a longer length of treatment (Hser et al., 2001) and family involvement in treatment (Liddle & Dakof, 1995). Posttreatment predictors of better outcome include participation in aftercare (Winters, Stinchfield, et al., 2000), low levels of peer substance use (Winters, Stinchfield, et al., 2000), ability to use coping skills (Myers, Brown, & Mott, 1993), and continued commitment to abstain (Kelly et al., 2000). Of all these factors, the posttreatment predictors accounted for more variance in the teenagers' outcomes 1 year after treatment than did the pretreatment and during-treatment variables. However, it is important to recognize that the predictors may change over time, just as the impact of the predictor on the course of SUD may change. For example, sibling drug use is associated with more frequent drug use during the first 6 months posttreatment, but as time passes, peer drug use becomes a stronger predictor of SUD course than does family environment, including sibling drug use (Latimer, Winters, Stinchfield, & Traver, 2000).

Psychosocial Factors

An accurate and detailed assessment of the adolescent's psychosocial functioning is additionally important. Measurement of the various psychosocial dimensions provides beneficial information regarding the extent of the drug use, aids in treatment planning, and yields data to monitor treatment efficacy. Dimensions that should be included in the assessment protocol include the deterioration of interpersonal relationships, school and employment problems, history of legal problems, the discontinuation (or significant change) of recreational activities, and the extent of sexual promiscuity. Two salient psychosocial factors merit additional discussion and are addressed in the following paragraphs: peer factors and family environment.

Peer Factors

The assessment protocol needs to examine the role of peer influence within the adolescent's drug use behaviors. Multiple research studies have found evidence that peer issues comprise one of the most prominent factors contributing to the onset and maintenance of drug use. For example, Chilcoat and Breslau (1999) found that youth who associate with peers who use drugs were six times as likely to use drugs as those who did not associate with drug-using peers. Similar results were found by Farrell and Danish (1993) and Winters, Latimer, Stinchfield, and Henly (1999). A parallel finding by Guo, Hill, Hawkins, Catalano, and Abbott (2002) revealed that adolescents involved with peers exhibiting antisocial behaviors were at a higher risk of initiating illicit

drug use. Understanding the intricacies of peer relationships is complex, to say the least. The nature of this association between drug use and peers may be due to pressure to use drugs exerted by drug-using friends, or to the increased likelihood that drug-using individuals seek out other drug-using peers. Peer influences may also impact a youth's attitudes and expectancies regarding drug use, as well as his or her access to drugs (Dishion, Capaldi, Spracklen, & Fuzhong, 1995; Hawkins, Catalano, & Miller, 1992; Patterson, Forgatch, Yoerger & Stoolmiller, 1998).

Family Factors

Family influences encompass several variables, including familial genetic risk and parenting practices. Children with parents who have an SUD have been shown to be at increased risk for the development of a SUD (McGue, 1999). Parent SUDs constitute both genetic liability and environmental influences for drug involvement and SUDs in the child. Also, other psychopathology in family members, particularly a history of parental antisocial behavior, is relevant in offspring SUD liability (Clark, Moss, et al., 1997; Earls, Reich, Jung, & Cloninger, 1988; Hill & Muka, 1996; Zucker, Fitzgerald, & Moses, 1995). Results from twin and family studies provide additional insight into the role of family genetics and home environment on youth drug use. There is converging evidence that the initiation of alcohol use in midadolescence is predominantly influenced by factors such as parental monitoring and the father's drinking level rather than genetic factors (e.g., Heath & Martin, 1988; Iacono, Carlson, Taylor, Elkins, & McGue, 1999; Koopmans & Boomsma, 1996), but once drinking is initiated, it appears that genetic factors increasingly influence the frequency of alcohol and other drug use, as well as the prevalence of SUDs (e.g., Rose, Dick, Viken, Pulkkinen, & Kaprio, 2001). Of course, it is important to keep in mind that normative developmental outcomes are more common among youth than a disordered developmental course in the face of presumed SUD heritable liability (Clark & Winters, 2002).

Parenting factors are strongly associated with adolescent risk for drug involvement, especially factors such as closeness or warmth and control or monitoring. These aspects of parenting reflect characteristics of affection, nurturance, and acceptance of the child by the parent, and of supervision of the child's activities and firmness in setting limits (Clark, Thatcher, & Maisto, 2005; Kandel, 1990). Several researchers have found increased drug use among adolescents in families that lack closeness or affection, effective discipline, and supervision; that have excessive or weak parental control and inconsistent parenting (Cleveland, Gibbons, Gerrard, Pomery, & Brody, 2005; Dishion, Patterson, & Reid, 1988; Kandel, 1990; Kosterman, Hawkins, Guo, Catalano, & Abbott, 2000; Patock-Peckham, Cheong, Balhorn, & Nagoshi, 2001; Zucker & Noll, 1987).

Psychological Benefits

In spite of the detrimental effects incurred by drug use, many adolescents are driven by psychological benefits from such use (Shaffer, 1997). Psychological advantages of adolescent drug use include mood enhancement, stress reduction, and relief from boredom (Petraitis, Flay, & Miller, 1995). In one study, mood enhancement played a more central role in drug use among youth with an SUD, whereas these psychological benefits were not as important to youth who use drugs infrequently (Henly & Winters, 1988). Because these psychological benefits play such an important role in the attraction and exacerbation of drug use among adolescents, prevention and early intervention efforts must underscore the harmful implications to outweigh the perceived benefits.

Coexisting Mental Health Disorders

Numerous clinical and epidemiological studies have demonstrated that adolescents who are involved with drugs often have coexisting psychological disorders (Boys et al., 2003; Clark & Bukstein, 1998; Kandel et al., 1999). Rohde, Lewinsohn, and Sealy (1996) reported that among adolescents who either abused or were dependent on alcohol, 80% also had some other form of psychopathology. The most common types of comorbid psychiatric conditions include externalizing disorders (i.e., conduct disorder [CD], oppositional defiant disorder [ODD], and attention-deficit/hyperactivity disorder [ADHD]) and internalizing disorders (i.e., depression and anxiety disorders—primarily posttraumatic stress disorder [PTSD]). Comprehensive drug use assessment should

therefore not only ascertain information regarding problems the adolescent is experiencing with alcohol and other drugs but also thoroughly identify comorbid psychiatric symptomatology. Doing so may be a key element in the projected success of an SUD intervention and subsequent relapse prevention. In addition, the knowledge obtained from these comprehensive assessments may facilitate more effective drug abuse prevention initiatives.

Comorbid Externalizing Disorders

Childhood aggression, rebelliousness, theft, and destructiveness, along with related externalizing disorders such as CD and ODD, are common among youth with SUDs, as well as among children of parents with SUDs (Clark, Moss, et al., 1997; Earls et al., 1988; Zucker et al., 1995). Prospective research reveals that antisocial behaviors in late childhood and the initiation of drug use in early adolescence predict later drug involvement (Boyle et al., 1992; Clark, Parker, & Lynch, 1999). The exact relationship between externalizing behavior and SUDs is complex. Three theories have been outlined regarding their potential association (Clark & Bukstein, 1998). First, CD has been found to predate or contribute to the development of an SUD (Clark et al., 1998), whereby poor behavioral inhibition or increased novelty seeking may lead to increased substance use. Second, other researchers have found that SUDs precede CD. For example, Clark and Bukstein (1998) reported that factors coinciding with an SUD, such as poor judgment and association with delinquent peers, may act as a catalyst for antisocial behavior and subsequent ODD or CD. Finally, in a third perspective, CD and substance use may occur concurrently, for they may share common environmental and personal risk factors (e.g., socioeconomic status, family problems, low academic achievement, association with deviant peer group). These risk factors may act independently or synergistically to impact the severity of the substance use and antisocial behavior (Clark & Bukstein, 1998; Donovan & Jessor, 1985). Barkley, Fischer, Smallish, and Fletcher (2004) showed that both CD and drug use interact over time to escalate the severity of the other set of symptoms.

The relationship between ADHD and SUDs is equally complex despite the significant literature that has explored the association. Some studies have found that individuals with a history of ADHD, compared with controls, are more likely to develop substance use and substance-related problems (Barkley et al., 2004; Mannuzza, Klein, Bessler, Malloy, & LaPadula, 1993; Milberger, Biederman, Faraone, Chen, & Jones, 1997). Other studies have not found similar relationships (Biederman et al., 1997; Hechtman & Weiss, 1986). Some researchers have found that the association between ADHD and drug use problems is mediated by CD (August et al., 2006; Biederman et al., 1997; Clark et al., 1999; Lynskey & Fergusson, 1995), whereas others have revealed an independent association beyond that explained by CD (Thompson, Riggs, Mikulich, & Crowley, 1996). For example, Barkley and colleagues (2004) found that ADHD is related to some forms of drug use and nonviolent, drug-related illegal activities, independent of CD. Another study found that by examining ADHD symptomatology dimensionally rather than categorically, level of attention predicted subsequent substance use beyond that of CD symptomatology (Tapert, Baratta, Abrantes, & Brown, 2002). With regard to tobacco, a commonly cited gateway drug, ADHD has also been linked to its early initiation and increased use (Milberger et al., 1997). Other researchers who have studied specific ADHD symptomatology found that inattention (Burke, Loeber, & Lahey, 2001) or impulsivity–hyperactivity (Molina, Smith, & Pelham, 1999) accounts for an association between tobacco use and ADHD, even after they controlled for CD.

Comorbid Internalizing Disorders

Internalizing disorders such as anxiety disorders (e.g., PTSD) and mood disorders (e.g., major depression) may be another pathway associated with SUDs (Clark & Miller, 1998; Clark & Sayette, 1993). Children of parents with SUDs have been found to have increased rates of internalizing disorders and related symptoms (Clark, Moss, et al., 1997; Earls et al., 1988; Hill & Muka, 1996). Among adolescents with SUDs, elevated rates of internalizing disorders and related symptoms have been reported, especially among female compared to male adolescents with SUDs (Deykin, Levy, & Wells, 1987; Martin, Lynch, Pollock, & Clark, 2000). Childhood major depression was more common in individuals with adolescent-onset

rather than adult-onset SUDs (Clark & Bukstein, 1998). These associations do not, however, establish a causal pathway between childhood internalizing disorders and later SUDs. Similar to the "chicken and egg" conundrum that exists with SUDs and externalizing disorders, the specific association between internalizing disorders and SUDs remains indistinct. Some researchers have found that symptoms of anxiety and depression may be produced by alcohol or other substances (Clark & Sayette, 1993; Schuckit & Hesselbrock, 1994), whereas others have demonstrated that an AUD may exacerbate symptoms of PTSD (Stewart, 1996).

Another complicating feature is that data from adolescents with SUDs indicate that both CDs and major depression may coexist in some individuals (Clark, Pollock, et al., 1997). Prospective longitudinal research that integrates findings for antisocial disorders and those for internalizing disorders that begin in preadolescence, and assesses the sequencing of these characteristics for specific developmental periods (i.e., early adolescence, middle adolescence) is needed to clarify these relationships (Clark et al., 1999).

Other psychiatric disturbances have also been shown to correlate with SUDs in adolescents though at a lower rate. A number of individuals with eating disorders such as bulimia nervosa also have been shown to abuse substances or to have an SUD (Lewinsohn, Hops, Roberts, Seeley, & Andrews, 1993). In addition, adverse life events, including childhood maltreatment (i.e., physical abuse, sexual abuse, neglect), are also associated with the development of an SUD (Stewart, 1996). Finally, some researchers have suggested that efforts be extended to study the possible co-occurrence of learning and language disabilities, and SUDs in adolescents (Weinberg, Rahdert, Colliver, & Glantz, 1998).

DEVELOPMENTAL CONSIDERATIONS IN DRUG USE ASSESSMENT

Categories Reflecting Use

Of great importance in assessing adolescent drug use is differentiation among normative use, abuse, and dependence. It can be difficult to determine when adolescent drug use will have short-term, minimal health effects, and when it may escalate, with negative, long-term repercussions. As previously noted, its popularity among youth places drug use within a normative developmental phase for adolescents. Most often, drug use among youth occurs within a social context of legal drug use, namely, alcohol or tobacco (Kandel, 1975; SAMHSA, 2005). These so-called *gateway drugs* are readily accessible to minors due to their legality and general availability. Though the large majority of youth do not progress beyond the use of these gateway drugs, some progress to more serious levels of drug use that result in abuse or dependence. As already noted, national estimates indicate that about 11% of youth use drugs to the point of meeting criteria for either a substance abuse or substance dependence disorder during the teenage years (Winters et al., 2007).

Applicability of SUD Criteria

The applicability of DSM criteria to adolescents' use of alcohol and other drugs (AOD) has aroused researchers' reservations for several reasons (Martin & Winters, 1998). The first such reason, previously mentioned in the "Substance Use Disorders" section, concerns the distinction between abuse and dependence criterion sets, which are not well supported by research. The abuse diagnosis has low concordance across different classification systems (Pollock et al., 2000), and abuse criteria cover symptoms that are conceptually less severe that some dependence criteria (Pollock & Martin, 1999). Similarly, some studies have found a higher prevalence of the more severe dependence diagnosis in relation to the more moderate abuse diagnosis (Chung, Martin, Armstrong, & Labouvie, 2002).

Second, other reservations exist at the criterion level; certain criteria have limited utility among adolescents. For example, tolerance, an important criterion for dependence, has low diagnostic specificity among adolescents, because tolerance for drugs is likely a normal physiological phenomenon that can take extended lengths of time to develop; most adolescents have not been using drugs for a long enough period for this criterion to develop. This is particularly the case for alcohol (Chung, Martin, Winters, & Langenbucher, 2001). The definition of "tolerance" also imparts concern, because it is characterized as a marked increase in quantity used, so a tolerance symptom may be overassigned to those who report low initial

quantities, and underassigned to those who report high initial quantities, regardless of the physical effect on the individual. Another important diagnostic criterion, withdrawal, has limited utility for adolescents because it occurs at very low base rates even in clinical samples (Martin, Kaczynski, Maisto, Bukstein, & Moss, 1995; Winters, Latimer, & Stinchfield, 1999).

A third criterion issue concerns the interpretation or meaning of the symptom for adolescents. For example, "drinking more than intended" may be endorsed more frequently among teenagers not because of a compulsive pattern of use, but rather because of poor judgment, inexperience with the effects of the drug, or social pressures to use. Specific interview probes, such as motivation to use, perceived ability to control use, and reasons for limiting use, are more beneficial in discerning a clinical phenomenon of impaired control in adolescents.

A final word regarding the applicability of SUD criteria for adolescents pertains to the heterogeneity of the DSM-IV substance abuse criteria. The abuse symptoms cover a broad range of problems, yet only one symptom is required to meet the criteria. In addition, symptoms of abuse do not always precede symptoms of dependence, contrary to the notion that abuse should be a precursory condition to dependence (Martin, Kaczynski, Maisto, & Tarter, 1996). For these reasons, adolescents can more easily "fall through the cracks" of the DSM-IV system; that is, individuals who meet criteria only for one or two dependence symptoms, and no abuse symptoms, therefore do not qualify for any diagnosis (Hasin & Paykin, 1998; Pollock & Martin, 1999). Approximately 10–30% of adolescents in clinical settings fall into this "crack" of the diagnostic system (Harrison, Fulkerson, & Beebe, 1998; Lewinsohn et al., 1996; Pollock & Martin, 1999).

Differences with Adults

The groundwork for adolescent drug assessment and treatment procedures is largely based on theory and experience with adult drug use, with little or no modification of the criteria or diagnostic thresholds. Thus, the applicability of current assessment procedures to adolescents is uncertain (Martin & Winters, 1998; Tarter, 1990). Research has shown that adolescents exhibit behavioral, psychological, and physiological characteristics differently than do adults (Kaminer, 1991). For example, alcohol is rarely the sole substance abused among adolescents; rather, they are likely also to abuse marijuana and other drugs concurrently with alcohol (SAMHSA, 1999). However, adults in treatment for substance problems frequently report alcohol as the primary substance abused. These drug use patterns in the two age groups probably reflect differences between generations, as well as the effects of age and age-related responsibility.

Another example illustrating the differences between adult and adolescent drug assessment pertains to the rate at which SUDs progress. Martin and colleagues (1995) found that drug use can progress from experimentation to abuse or dependence much more rapidly for adolescents than it can for adults. Adolescents are often diagnosed with SUDs within a year of their initial use, whereas adults generally use drugs for several years before progressing to dependence.

Neurobiology

Recent research has indicated that the brain does not fully develop until early adulthood (Giedd, 2004). In some regions of the brain, particularly the prefrontal cortical region associated with judgment (resisting impulses and other executive functioning), nearly 50% of the neurons undergo "pruning" and transformation during adolescence. Because of this immaturity, there is speculation that the developing adolescent brain may be highly vulnerable to the effects of drug use. Studies with laboratory animals have provided evidence that adolescents differ significantly from adults in their receptivity to the effects of alcohol (Spear, 2000). Adolescent rats show decreased sensitivity to the unpleasant effects of alcohol (i.e., vomiting, hangovers) and increased sensitivity to the social benefits of alcohol compared to older rats. Adolescent rats also require a larger amount of alcohol to reduce anxiety than do older rats (Varlinskaya & Spear, 2002). These findings suggest that adolescents may be less capable than adults of moderating their alcohol intake.

Laboratory animals also provide evidence that exposure to drugs during adolescence influences later neural functioning. Rats that were chronically exposed to alcohol during adolescence exhibited greater cognitive difficulties than rats exposed to the same amount of alcohol in adulthood (Markwiese, Acheson, Levin, Wilson, & Swartzwelder, 1998). In regards to human subjects, Tapert and Schweinsburg (2005) reported that adolescents with a history of heavy alcohol use had smaller hippocampi compared to those of a matched control sample; the hippocampus is the area of the brain responsible for creating memories. The same adolescents revealed memory and other neuropsychological impairment during recall tasks, due to reduced brain activation. These findings are only suggestive because brain functioning prior to alcohol use was not measured, but they emphasize the importance of further study on the possible deleterious effects of alcohol use on the developing brain.

Gender

Although some exceptions exist, prevalence studies generally indicate that boys are at a greater risk than girls for drug use and drug problems (Kahler, Read, Wood, & Palfai, 2003). This pattern was emphasized in a recent national report of drug use among Americans. Adolescent boys reported higher rates on nearly every drug use variable, including early (prior to age 12) onset of drug use, binge drinking, illicit drug use, and SUDs (SAMHSA, 2005). Cigarette use is roughly the same across genders, however (Johnston et al., 2005).

Clinical studies have revealed both gender differences and similarities with regard to possible psychosocial determinants of drug use. Opland, Winters, and Stinchfield (1995) found that girls' drug use is a coping mechanism in response to stress, whereas boys tend to use drugs for the pleasurable effects. In a cross-sectional study of drug-abusing youth assessed in clinical settings, Winters, Latimer, Stinchfield, and Henly (1999) found that scales measuring delinquency and peer drug involvement were most highly correlated with overall drug use in both girls and boys. However, girls, compared to boys, tended to have higher associations between drug involvement and psychological distress. A related question is the relative severity of reported psychosocial problems. Hsieh and Hollister (2004) found that female subjects who were entering a substance abuse treatment program exhibited more severe psychological difficulties, poorer self-image, increased family problems, and more exposure to sexual abuse than did their male counterparts. However, boys, compared to girls, in the same study exhibited higher rates of conduct problems related to school difficulties and legal problems. Dakof, Tejeda, and Liddle (2000) found similar results in their clinical sample, namely, that drug-abusing girls exhibited much higher levels of internalizing symptoms and higher levels of family dysfunction, even though they used drugs just as extensively as the boys.

Other Factors

Other developmental issues are relevant with respect to assessing adolescent drug use. Delays in social and emotional functioning (Noam & Houlihan, 1990), diminished respect toward authority, and the tendency to be egocentric (Erikson, 1968) and to minimize negative consequences (Lewinsohn et al., 1996) may contribute to inaccurate reporting of personal drug use behaviors and to poor motivation to change (Cady, Winters, Jordan, Solberg, & Stinchfield, 1996).

THE ASSESSMENT PROCESS

When an adolescent is suspected of using drugs, the assessment process should begin with screening questions about recent drug use quantity and frequency (e.g., "How often did you use drugs in the past 6 months?"), the presence of adverse consequences of use (e.g., "Has your drug use led to problems with your parents?"), and situations in which drug use is common (e.g., "Do you use drugs before or during school?"). Several psychometrically sound screening instruments help to guide the screening process (a summary of screeners is provided in the next section).

If the screening suggests a possible drug use problem, the clinician should conduct a more comprehensive assessment to determine details of drug use quantity and frequency, consequences of such use, whether the teenager meets criteria for an SUD, and what other behavioral and mental comorbid problems may exist. Numerous examples of comprehensive instruments with established psychometric properties, including interviews and paper-and-pencil questionnaires, are available in the literature (these tools are summarized in the next section).

A thorough assessment of the adolescent's drug use should include detailed inquiry into the age of onset and progression of use for specific substances, circumstances, frequency and variability of use, and types of drugs used. The assessor should also inquire about the context of use, which should include the usual times and places of drug use, the attitudes and use patterns of the adolescent's peers, and typical behavioral and social triggers, and antecedents associated with drug use. The clinician should also ask about direct and indirect consequences of use in the domains of school, social, family, psychological functioning, and physical/medical problems. Finally, the assessor should evaluate the adolescent's problem recognition and readiness for treatment. These questions may help to determine the initial treatment goals.

The determination of an SUD requires that the assessor review the criteria for substance abuse and dependence for specific substances. As previously mentioned, abuse criteria focus on negative social and personal consequences as a result of repetitive use; dependence criteria address symptoms associated with the continued use of drugs in the face of negative consequences (see Table 4.1). The differential diagnosis of adolescent SUDs requires consideration that the symptoms of drug use are not due to premorbid or concurrent problems, such as CD or family issues. Given the frequent comorbidity of SUDs and other psychiatric disorders, it is important that the assessor comprehensively review in timeline fashion the past and present history of psychiatric symptoms. Such a timeline approach can help the assessor sort out the interrelationship between drug use and comorbid psychopathology (Riggs & Davies, 2002).

OVERVIEW OF INSTRUMENTS FOR ASSESSING ADOLESCENT DRUG USE AND RELATED PROBLEMS

Significant contributions by researchers over the past decade have provided clinicians and researchers with numerous instruments to assist in the assessment of adolescent drug use behaviors (Leccese & Waldron, 1994; Winters, 2001). Many measures have been normed for adolescents of varying ages and written to be conducive to young people's comprehension levels. Some tools are designed to identify quickly youth at risk for drug problems, whereas other measures provide extensive, diagnostically related information.

Several summaries of adolescent screening and comprehensive assessments exist, including two by the federal government—*Screening Assessment of Adolescents with a Substance Use Disorder* (Center for Substance Abuse Treatment, 1999) and the second edition of *Assessing Alcohol Problems: A Guide for Clinicians and Researchers* (National Institute on Alcohol Abuse and Alcoholism [NIAAA], 2003)—and others in journal articles (Leccese & Waldron, 1994; Martin & Winters, 1998) and chapters in handbooks (Winters, 2001). We provide our own summary below. Inclusion in our overview required that the instrument be developed specifically for adolescents, with its psychometric properties reported in a peer-reviewed publication, user information available in print (e.g., manual, scoring information), and the instrument's author or publisher easily accessible to answer user questions. Thus, the reviewed measures are both scientifically rigorous and have high clinical utility.

Screening Instruments

Clinicians and researchers working with adolescents have access to a wide range of screening instruments, most commonly self-report questionnaires, to describe the possible or probable presence of a drug problem (see Table 4.2 for a listing). We review four categories of screening tools: alcohol, all drugs (including alcohol), nonalcohol drugs, and multiscreens.

Alcohol Screens

Two contemporary screening tools focus exclusively on alcohol use. The 24-item Adolescent Drinking Inventory (Harrell & Wirtz, 1989) examines adolescent problem drinking by measuring psychological symptoms, physical symptoms, social symptoms, and loss of control. Written at a fifth-grade reading level, it yields a single score with cutoffs, as well as two research subscale scores (Self-Medicating Drinking and Rebellious Drinking). The Adolescent Drinking Inventory yields high internal consistency reliability (coefficient alpha, .93–.95), and has demonstrated validity in measuring the severity of adolescent drinking problems (e.g., it has revealed a very favorable hit rate of 82% in classification accuracy). The second measure in this group, the 23-item Rutgers Alcohol Problem Index (RAPI; White & Labouvie, 1989), measures consequences of alcohol use pertaining to family life, social relations, psychological functioning, delinquency, physical problems, and neuropsychological functioning. Based on a large general population sample, the RAPI was found to have high internal consistency (.92), and, among heavy alcohol users, a strong correlation with DSM-III-R criteria for substance use disorders (.75–.95) (White & Labouvie, 1989).

Screens for All Drugs

Another group of screening tools comprise the relatively short measures that nonspecifically cover all drug categories, including alcohol. Examples of these measures are the Adolescent Alcohol and Drug Involvement Scale (AADIS; Moberg, 2003), CRAFFT (Knight, Sherritt, Harris, Gates, & Chang, 2003; Knight, Sherritt, Shrier, Harris, & Chang, 2002), Personal Experience Screening Questionnaire (PESQ; Winters, 1992), and the Substance Abuse Subtle Screening Inventory—Adolescents (SASSI-A; Miller, 1985). The 14-item AADIS includes a drug abuse problem severity scale; a range of reliability and validity evidence for this screen has been reported (Moberg, 2003). The CRAFFT is a specialized, six-item screen designed to be administered verbally during a primary care interview to address both alcohol and drug use. Its name is a mnemonic device to help physicians incorporate six questions into their primary care exams. Based on a study in a large, hospital-based adolescent clinic, scores from the CRAFFT were found to be highly correlated with scores from several existing and valid measures, and a cutoff score of 2 has been found to be highly predictive of a drug problem (Knight et al., 2002, 2003). The 40-item PESQ comprises a problem severity scale (coefficient alpha, .91–.95), drug use history, select psychosocial problems, and response distortion tendencies ("faking good" and "faking bad"). Norms for normal, juvenile offender, and drug abusing populations are available. The PESQ is estimated to have an accuracy rate of 87% in predicting the need for further drug abuse assessment (Winters, 1992). The 81-item SASSI-A yields scores for several scales, including face-valid alcohol, face-valid other drug, obvious attributes, subtle attributes, and defensiveness. Validity data indicate that SASSI-A scale scores are highly correlated with Minnesota Multiphasic Personality Inventory (MMPI) scales, and that its cutoff score for "chemical de-

TABLE 4.2. Screening Instruments

Instrument	Purpose	Source	Group used	Norms	Normed groups	Format	Time (min)
Adolescent Alcohol and Drug Involvement Scale (AADIS)	Screen for drug abuse problem severity	Moberg (2003)	Adolescents referred for emotional or behavioral disorders	Yes	Substance abusers	14 items, questionnaire	5
Adolescent Drinking Inventory	Screen for alcohol use problem severity	Harrell & Wirtz (1989)	Adolescents suspected of alcohol use problems	Yes	Normals; substance abusers	24 items, questionnaire	5
CRAFFT	Screen for drug use problem severity	Knight, Sherritt, Harris, Gates, & Chang (2003)	Adolescents referred for emotional or behavioral disorders	Yes	Normals; substance abusers	6 items, questionnaire	5
Drug Abuse Screening Test—Adolescents (DAST-A)	Screen for drug use problem severity	Martino, Grilo, & Fehon (2000)	Adolescents referred for emotional or behavioral disorders	Yes	Substance abusers	27 items, questionnaire	5
Drug Use Screening Inventory—Revised (DUSI-R)	Screen for substance use problem severity and related problems	Kirisci, Mezzich, & Tarter (1995)	Adolescents referred for emotional or behavioral disorders	Yes	Substance abusers	159 items, questionnaire	20
Personal Experience screening Questionnaire (PESQ)	Screen for substance use problem severity	Winters (1992)	Adolescents referred for emotional or behavioral disorders	Yes	Normals; substance abusers	40 items, questionnaire	10
Problem Oriented Screening Instrument for Teenagers (POSIT)	Multiscreen for substance use problem severity and related problems	Latimer, Winters, & Stinchfield (1997); Rahdert (1991)	Adolescents referred for emotional or behavioral disorders	Yes	Normals; substance abusers	139 items, questionnaire	20–25
Rutgers Alcohol Problem Index (RAPI)	Screen for alcohol use problem severity	White & Labouvie (1989)	Adolescents at risk for alcohol use problems	Yes	Normals; substance abusers	23 items, questionnaire	10
Substance Abuse Subtle Screening Inventory—Adolescents (SASSI-A)	Screen for substance use problem severity and related problems	Miller (1985)	Adolescents referred for emotional or behavioral disorders	Yes	Normals; substance abusers	81 items, questionnaire	10–15

pendency" corresponds highly with intake diagnoses of substance use disorders (Risberg, Stevens, & Graybill, 1995). However, claims that the SASSI-A is valid in detecting *unreported* drug use and related problems have not been empirically justified (Rogers, Cashel, Johansen, Sewell, & Gonzalez, 1997).

Screens for Nonalcohol Drugs

The third category of screening tools pertains to those that screen only nonalcohol drugs. Only one screen falls into this group: the Drug Abuse Screening Test for Adolescents (DAST-A; Martino, Grilo, & Fehon, 2000), adapted from Skinner's (1982) adult tool, the Drug Abuse Screening Test. This 27-item questionnaire is associated with favorable reliability data and is highly predictive of DSM-IV drug-related disorders when tested among adolescent psychiatric inpatients.

Multiproblem Screens

The final group of screening measures comprise two "multiscreen" instruments that examine several domains, in addition to drug involvement. The 139-item Problem Oriented Screening Instrument for Teenagers (POSIT; Rahdert, 1991) is part of the Adolescent Assessment and Referral System developed by the National Institute on Drug Abuse (NIDA). It tests for 10 functional adolescent problem areas: substance use, physical health, mental health, family relations, peer relationships, educational status, vocational status, social skills, leisure and recreation, and aggressive behavior/delinquency. Cutoff scores for determining the need for further assessment have been rationally established, and some have been confirmed with empirical procedures (Latimer, Winters, & Stinchfield, 1997). Convergent and discriminant evidence for the POSIT have been reported by several investigators (e.g., Dembo, Schmeidler, Borden, Chin-Sue, & Manning, 1997; McLaney, Del-Boca, & Babor, 1994). The Drug Use Screening Inventory—Revised (DUSI-R), a 159-item instrument that describes drug use problem severity and related problems, produces scores on 10 subscales, as well as one Lie Scale. Domain scores were related to DSM-III-R substance use disorder criteria in a sample of adolescent substance abusers (Tarter, Laird, Bukstein, & Kaminer, 1992). An additional psychometric report provides norms and

evidence of scale sensitivity (Kirisci, Mezzich, & Tarter, 1995).

Comprehensive Assessment Instruments

If an initial screening indicates the need for further assessment, clinicians and researchers can employ various diagnostic interviews, problem-focused interviews, and multiscale questionnaires (see Table 4.3 for a list). These instruments yield information that can more definitively assess the nature and severity of the drug involvement, typically assign an SUD diagnosis, and identify the psychosocial factors that may predispose, perpetuate, and maintain the drug involvement.

Diagnostic Interviews

Diagnostic interviews, which focus on DSM-based criteria for SUDs, include both general *psychiatric* interviews that address all psychiatric disorders and SUD interviews that focus primarily on drug use and related domains of functioning. The majority of the diagnostic interviews are structured; that is, the format directs the interviewer to read verbatim a series of questions in a decision-tree format, and the answers to these questions are restricted to a few predefined alternatives. The respondent is assigned the principal responsibility of interpreting the question and deciding on a reply.

Two well-researched *psychiatric* diagnostic interviews address SUDs, as well as the full range of child and adolescent psychiatric disorders. The Diagnostic Interview for Children and Adolescents—Revised (DICA-R; Reich, Shayla, & Taibelson, 1992), a structured interview, is used widely among researchers and clinicians. Psychometric evidence specific to SUDs has not been published on the DICA-R, but some of the other sections have been evaluated for reliability and validity (Welner, Reich, Herjanic, Jung, & Amado, 1987). An instrument that has undergone several adaptations is the Diagnostic Interview Schedule for Children (DISC-C; Costello, Edelbrock, & Costello, 1985; Shaffer et al., 1993). Its revised DSM-IV version is the DISC-R (Shaffer, Fisher, & Dulcan, 1996; Shaffer, Fisher, Lucas, Dulcan, & Schwab-Stone, 2000). Separate forms of the interview exist for the child and the parent. As part of a larger study focusing on several diagnoses, Fisher and colleagues (1993) found the DSM-IV-based DISC-C to be highly sensitive in

TABLE 4.3. Comprehensive Assessment Instruments

Instrument	Purpose	Source	Examples of group used	Norms	Normed groups	Format	Time (min)
Diagnostic interviews							
Adolescent Diagnostic Interview (ADI)	Assess DSM-IV substance use disorders and problems	Winters & Henly (1993)	Adolescents suspected of drug use problems	NA	NA	Structured interview	45
Customary Drinking and Drug Use Record (CDDR)	Assess DSM-IV substance use disorders and problems	Brown et al. (1998)	Adolescents suspected of drug use problems	NA	NA	Structured interview	10–30
Diagnostic Interview for Children and Adolescents—Revised (DICA-R)	Assess DSM-IV child/adolescent disorders	Reich, Shayla, & Taibelson (1992)	Youth suspected mental, behavioral problems	NA	NA	Structured interview	45–60
Diagnostic Interview Schedule for Children—Revised (DISC-R)	Assess DSM-IV child/adolescent disorders	Shaffer, Fisher, & Dulcan (1996)	Youth suspected mental, behavioral problems	NA	NA	Structured interview	45–60
Problem-focused interviews							
Comprehensive Adolescent Severity Inventory (CASI)	Assess drug use and other life problems	Meyers, McLellan, Jaeger, & Pettinati (1995)	Adolescents suspected of drug use problems	NA	NA	Semistructured interview	45–55
Teen Addiction Severity Index (T-ASI)	Assess drug use and other life problems	Kaminer, Bukstein, & Tarter (1991)	Adolescents at risk for drug use problems	NA	NA	Semistructured interview	20–45
Multiscale questionnaires							
Adolescent Self-Assessment Profile (ASAP)	Multiscale measure of drug use and related problems	Wanberg (1992)	Adolescents suspected of substance use problems	Yes	Normals; substance abusers	225 items, questionnaire	45–60
Hilson Adolescent Profile (HAP)	Multiscale measure of drug use and related problems	Inwald, Brobst, & Morissey (1986)	Adolescents suspected of substance use and related problems	Yes	Normals; substance abusers	310 items, questionnaire	45
Juvenile Automated Substance Abuse Evaluation (JASAE)	Multiscale measure of drug use and related problems	Ellis (1987)	Adolescents suspected of substance use problems	Yes	Normals; substance abusers	108 items	20
Personal Experience Inventory (PEI)	Multiscale measure of drug use and related problems	Winters, Stinchfield, & Henly (1996)	Adolescents suspected of substance use problems	Yes	Normals; substance abusers	276 items, questionnaire	45–60

correctly identifying youth who had received a hospital diagnosis of any SUD ($n = 8$). Both interview forms (parent and child) had a sensitivity of 75%. For the one parent–child disagreement case, the parent indicated not knowing any details about the child's substance use.

The second subgroup of diagnostic interviews primarily focuses on *diagnostic criteria for SUDs*. The Adolescent Diagnostic Interview (ADI; Winters & Henly 1993) assesses diagnostic symptoms associated with psychoactive SUDs. Other sections provide an assessment of substance use consumption history, psychosocial stressors, and level of functioning. Also, screens for several adolescent psychiatric disorders are provided. The authors have developed a revised DSM-IV version of the ADI (ADI-R). Evidence that supports the interview's psychometric properties has been reported (Winters & Henly, 1993; Winters, Latimer, & Stinchfield, 1999; Winters, Stinchfield, Fulkerson, & Henly, 1993; Winters, Latimer, & Stinchfield, 1999). A second SUD-focused interview, the Customary Drinking and Drug Use Record (CDDR; Brown et al., 1998), measures alcohol and other drug use consumption, DSM-IV substance dependence symptoms (including a detailed assessment of withdrawal symptoms), and several types of consequences of drug involvement. There are both lifetime and prior-2-years versions of the CDDR. Psychometric studies provide supporting evidence for this instrument's reliability and validity (Brown et al., 1998). The third instrument in this subgroup, the Global Assessment of Individual Needs (GAIN; Dennis, 1999), is a semistructured interview that covers recent and lifetime functioning in several areas, including substance use, legal and school functioning, and psychiatric symptoms. Very favorable reliability and validity data are associated with the GAIN, including data for the SUDs section when administered to a treatment-seeking adolescent population (Buchan, Dennis, Tims, & Diamond, 2002; Dennis, Funk, Godley, Godley, & Waldron, 2004). A shortened version of the GAIN is under development.

Problem-Focused Interviews

The second major group of comprehensive instruments—problem-focused interviews—measure several problem areas associated with adolescent drug involvement but do not provide a means to obtain a formal diagnosis of an SUD. The interviews summarized here are adapted from the well-known adult tool, the Addiction Severity Index (ASI; McLellan, Luborsky, Woody, & O'Brien, 1980). Thus, these interviews assess drug use history and related consequences, as well as several functioning difficulties often experienced by drug-abusing adolescents.

The Comprehensive Adolescent Severity Inventory (CASI; Meyers, McLellan, Jaeger, & Pettinati, 1995) measures education, substance use, use of free time, leisure activities, peer relationships, family (including family history and intrafamilial abuse), psychiatric status, and legal history. At the end of several major topics, space is provided for the assessor's comments, severity ratings, and quality ratings of the respondent's answers. An interesting feature of this interview is that it incorporates results from a urine drug screen and observations from the assessor. Psychometric studies on the CASI support the instrument's reliability and validity (Meyers et al., 1995). The other ASI-adapted interview of note, the Teen Addiction Severity Index (T-ASI; Kaminer, Bukstein, & Tarter, 1991), has seven content areas: chemical use, school status, employment–support status, family relationships, legal status, peer–social relationships, and psychiatric status. A medical status section was not included, because it was deemed to be less relevant to adolescent drug abusers. Adolescent and interviewer severity ratings are elicited on a 5-point scale for each of the content areas. Psychometric data indicate favorable interrater agreement and validity evidence (Kaminer, Wagner, Plummer, & Seifer, 1993). Kaminer, Blitz, Burleson, and Sussman (1998) also developed a health service utilization tool that complements the T-ASI, named the Teen Treatment Services Review (T-TSR). This interview examines the type and number of services that the youth received during the treatment episode.

Multiscale Questionnaires

The third group of comprehensive instruments comprise the self-administered multiscale questionnaires. These instruments range considerably in terms of length; some can be administered in less than 20 minutes, whereas others may take a full hour to administer. Yet, as a group, many of them share several characteristics: measures of both drug use problem severity and psychosocial risk factors are provided; strategies are included for detecting response distortion tendencies; the scales are standardized to a clinical sample; and the option of computer administration and scoring is available. Four examples of instruments in this group are briefly summarized. The Adolescent Self-Assessment Profile (ASAP) was developed on the basis of a series of multivariate research studies by Wanberg (1992). The 225-item instrument provides an in-depth assessment of drug involvement, including drug use frequency, drug use consequences and benefits, and major risk factors associated with such involvement (e.g., deviance, peer influence). Supplemental scales, which are based on common factors found within the specific psychosocial and problem severity domains, can be scored as well. Extensive reliability and validity data based on several normative groups are provided in the manual. The Hilson Adolescent Profile (HAP; Inwald, Brobst, & Morissey, 1986), a 310-item questionnaire (true–false) has 16 scales, two of which measure alcohol and drug use. The other content scales correspond to characteristics found in psychiatric diagnostic categories (e.g., antisocial behavior, depression) and psychosocial problems (e.g., home life conflicts). Normative data have been collected from clinical patients, juvenile offenders, and normal adolescents (Inwald et al., 1986). Another true–false questionnaire, the 108-item Juvenile Automated Substance Abuse Evaluation (JASAE; Ellis, 1987) is a computer-assisted instrument that produces a five-category score, ranging from *No use* to *Drug abuse* (including a suggested DSM-IV classification), as well as a summary of drug use history, measure of life stress, and a scale for test-taking attitude. The JASAE has been shown to discriminate between clinical and nonclinical groups. The Personal Experience Inventory (PEI; Winters & Henly, 1989) comprises several scales that measure chemical involvement problem severity, psychosocial risk, and response distortion tendencies. Supplemental problem screens measure eating disorders, suicide potential, physical–sexual abuse, and parental history of drug abuse. The scoring program provides a computerized report that includes narratives and standardized scores for each scale, as well as other clinical information. Normative and psychometric data are available (Winters & Henly, 1989; Winters, Stinchfield, & Henly, 1996).

METHODS OF DATA COLLECTION AND SOURCES OF INFORMATION

Several types of data collection, when combined, can provided a thorough and accurate account of a young person's drug use history. Parents, peers, professionals, and adolescents themselves can all contribute important information that assists in determining the nature and extent of the drug involvement.

Self-Report

The utilization of a self-report format has been nearly universal throughout clinical and epidemiological studies. Convenience, comprehensiveness, low cost, ease of administration, and the perception that the individual is the most knowledgeable reporter have encouraged the use of this method. Self-report formats include the *self-administered questionnaire* (SAQ), *diagnostic interview, timeline followback* (TLFB; Sobell & Sobell, 1992), and *computer-assisted interview* (CAI). SAQs are completed independently by an individual, traditionally via paper-and-pencil format. An interview is completed by a trained individual and often yields specific diagnostic data related to SUDs and psychiatric comorbidity. Research on the concordance of SAQ and interview format in clinical and epidemiological samples has varied but for the most part reveals similar levels of disclosure (Stone & Latimer, 2005). The TLFB is a calendar-based tool that compiles a history of drug use over a specified time. The TLFB method uses specific dates and events (e.g., birthdays, holidays, and vacations) to enhance interviewee recollection to elicit a detailed pattern of recent drug use. Research on the psychometric properties of this method indicates favorable reliability and validity evidence (Sobell & Sobell, 1992), including that with adolescents (Dillon, Turner, Robbins, & Szapocznik, 2005). The CAI method has been utilized with drug-abusing adolescent populations (Williams et al., 2000). With this method, the respondent completes an interview independently on a computer, with the questions delivered audibly via headphones. This approach may promote a greater sense of privacy, while the subject responds to potentially sensitive questions. Research comparing CAI to in-person interviews has revealed mixed results. Some studies indicate that the CAI format is associated with higher rates of endorsement of drug use (e.g., Lapham, Henley, & Kleyboecker, 1993; Turner et al., 1998), yet other studies have found no difference between the methods (Sarrazin, Hall, Richards, & Carswell, 2002). The CAI method, despite the uncertainty of its relative validity compared to other methods, has several advantages: Minimal training of interviewers is needed; many individuals can be assessed at a given time; the sense of privacy for the interviewee is enhanced; and data can be directly entered into a database upon completion of the interview.

The overall validity and reliability of the self-report method of assessment for adolescent drug use remains somewhat ambiguous. Stinchfield (1997) found that adolescents attending a treatment program for drug dependence generally reported notably more past drug use and consequences compared to disclosures at the start of intervention. In other studies, underreporting occurred more frequently with less socially acceptable drugs, such as cocaine or opiates, compared to marijuana (Harrison, 1995; Williams & Nowatzki, 2005). Improved urinalysis techniques (immunoassays), and the more recent sophistication of examining hair strands, are being used to corroborate adolescent self-report of drug use (Dolan, Rouen, & Kimber, 2004). Williams and Nowatzki (2005) reported that some adolescents disclosed drug use in an interview, though the urinalysis conducted immediately after the interview showed a negative finding. Some of this discrepancy was accounted for by limitations in the urinalysis "detection window" for different drugs and individuals' varying metabolic rates, but the authors hypothesized that deliberate fabrication, poor memory, and boastfulness may also have been contributing factors (Williams & Nowatzki, 2005). These findings are not surprising given the circumstances under which an adolescent assessment may be conducted. Defiance, fear, and apprehension can influence the results of an assessment. In addition, youth may see the assessment as an opportunity to "cry for help" and exaggerate their responses. Despite possible limitations, the validity of self-report for adolescent drug use has been supported by several lines of evidence: Only a small percentage of youth endorse improbable questions; adolescent self-reports agree with corroborating sources of information, such as archival records, and for the most part, urinalyses; and the base rate of elevations on

"faking good" and "faking bad" scales are relatively low (Johnston & O'Malley, 1997; Maisto, Connors, & Allen, 1995; Winters, Anderson, Bengston, Stinchfield, & Latimer, 2000; Winters, Stinchfield, Henly, & Schwartz, 1990–1991).

Drug Testing

Four biologically based tests (urine, hair, saliva, and sweat) are currently utilized to detect drugs in the body (Dolan et al., 2004). The main aspect that distinguishes these specimens is the period or window of time for which the drug can be detected. In addition, cost, access, tampering vulnerability, invasiveness, and reliability–validity are other factors that differentiate these biological sampling procedures. Urinalysis is the most commonly used procedure to detect drug use and to validate self-report. The window of detection varies considerably for illicit drugs; the detection period for alcohol is only about 8 hours. Tampering can be minimized by directly monitoring collection of the urine. Hair analysis has been utilized more commonly to detect exposure to drugs over a longer period of time than that afforded by urine testing (Dolan et al, 2004). A hair sample of approximately pencil width in size is necessary for accurate testing. However, significant limitations in hair analysis exist. Chemical processing, differences in hair structure, growth, porosity, and hygiene, along with exposure to drugs in the air (e.g., marijuana smoke) have all been shown significantly to impact the concentrations of drugs in the hair (see Kidwell & Blank, 1996; Kidwell, Lee, & DeLauder, 2000; Reid, O'Connor, Deakin, Ivery, & Crayton, 1996; Sachs, 1995; Rohrich, Zorntlein, Pötsch, Skopp, & Becker, 2000). The testing of saliva to detect drug exposure is still being refined. Advantages of this method include a noninvasive collection and the detection of very recent drug use (12–24 hours). However, the cost of saliva analysis is greater than that for urinalysis, and several collection requirements may be difficult to enforce (e.g., individual must refrain from eating, drinking, or smoking up to 30 minutes prior to sample collection). A final biological assay to detect illicit drugs is sweat. A sweat patch provides an estimate of drug exposure over several days (Dolan et al., 2004). Disadvantages with this technique include accidental or purposeful removal of the patch during the evaluation period and the lack of validation of this technology.

Clinical Observation

In addition to self-report and biological tests, direct observation by the assessor for behavioral and psychological symptomatology may be an objective and useful supplement to adolescent drug use assessment. A simple checklist of items, such as the presence of needle marks, unsteady gait, slurred or incoherent speech, shaking of hands or twitching of eyelids, and so forth, can indicate problematic use. A 14-item checklist of observable signs that may indicate a drug problem is contained in the Simple Screening Instrument for AOD Abuse (SAMHSA, 1994).

Parent Report

Although parent report is relatively valid in the identification of many mental health problems, such as ADHD and conduct problems, it is unlikely that parents can provide detailed reports about the types, frequency, and quantity of drug use by their son or daughter. Winters, Stinchfield, Opland, Weller, and Latimer (2000) found that parents tend to underreport the extent to which their adolescent experiments with drugs. Parental reports may be helpful, however, in providing valuable information on risk and protective factors associated with drug use.

Peer Report

Collecting information from an adolescent's friends may prove to be a valuable resource, especially if the peers are not currently using drugs or are in recovery. Peers may be able to detail a change in an adolescent's recent behavior or provide information substantiating drug use behaviors they witnessed or in which they collaboratively participated.

Archival Records

Data collected from sources other than family and friends may help to document the severity of an adolescent's drug use and identify resulting consequences. Archival records include information from school reports, police reports, and medical records.

ASSESSMENT FOR TREATMENT PLANNING AND OUTCOME EVALUATION

Treatment Planning

The primary goal of assessment is to establish client characteristics that may influence treatment planning and ultimately contribute to the success of treatment (Donovan, 2003). Treatment planning involves the integration of the client's drug use involvement, drug-related problems, and other areas of psychosocial functioning to assist in developing and prioritizing short- and long-term goals for treatment, selecting the most appropriate treatment approaches to address the identified problems, identifying perceived barriers to treatment engagement and compliance, and monitoring progress toward the specified treatment goals (Allen, 1991). As an example of how assessment may inform treatment referral decisions, we propose a general referral model for matching level of treatment, and severity of drug involvement and related problems (see Table 4.4). The model presents three levels of treatment: brief intervention, nonintensive drug treatment, and intensive drug treatment. Brief interventions are appropriate responses for adolescents with relatively mild drug involvement problems, such as when an individual meets a diagnosis for a substance abuse disorder (Winters et al., 2007). On the other hand, nonintensive and intensive drug treatments are more specialized; thus, they are more appropriate for youth who meet criteria for a substance dependence disorder. The referral model becomes more complex as more client characteristics are included in the decision-making process. For example, an adolescent with a mild drug use problem who also has ADHD may require more treatment than a brief intervention.

Evaluating Outcome

Quality drug use assessment tools are not only crucial in the identification of youth who abuse drugs but also invaluable in the multifaceted evaluation of drug treatment programs. These instruments help to identify the types of clients the centers are serving (e.g., type of substance abused; gender, ethnic, and racial information), determine the efficacy of a program, including distinct intervention strategies; provide data for a cost–benefit analysis; and document areas for necessary program enhancement. Treat-

TABLE 4.4. Guidelines for Drug Abuse Treatment Placement along a Continuum of Care

Level of intervention or treatment	Suggested characteristics
Brief intervention (2–4 sessions)	Mild-to-moderate drug use: absence of dependence disorder, polydrug use pattern, abuse coexisting with psychiatric disorder, relatively supportive and stable home life.
Low-intensive treatment (e.g., 7–20 days or sessions)	Substance abuse disorder(s), or a single substance dependence disorder with recent onset; if a coexisting disorder is present, then mild symptoms; relatively supportive and stable home life.
Intensive treatment (e.g., 21 or more days or sessions)	Substance dependence disorder; severe coexisting disorder present; relatively unsupportive and unstable home life.

ment outcome information is useful to treatment providers not only in terms of outcomes but also to obtain an overview of the clientele coming for treatment and to improve treatment and obtain improved outcomes. Therefore, treatment program staff need scientifically valid information about the effectiveness of their treatment programs.

Researchers have outlined parameters for selecting treatment outcome evaluation tools (Newman, Ciarlo, & Carpenter, 1999). Some of the guidelines are related to the need to develop a sound and valid evaluation plan, such as gathering input from multiple respondents (e.g., youth and parent) and using measures that are relevant to the target group and associated with objective referents and adequate psychometric properties. Other guidelines are important in the context of developing a useful evaluation of the program, such as including measures that assess extent of engagement by the client in treatment, and other treatment process variables and perceived satisfaction with clinical services. We are familiar with three treatment evaluation tools that are generally consistent with these outcome instrumentation guidelines. Each represents an evaluation version of their intake assessment "cousin": the ADI (Winters & Henly, 1993), the CASI (Meyers et al., 1995), and the GAIN (Dennis, 1999). These three instruments were reviewed in an earlier section, "Comprehensive Assessment Instruments."

SUMMARY

Drugs are prevalent among teenagers in the United States; nearly half of American eighth graders reported having already used alcohol (Johnston et al., 2005). To complicate the issue, researchers have found that drug use frequently co-occurs with psychological disorders (Clark & Bukstein, 1998; Rhode et al., 1996), making the assessment process even more complex. In addition, new research on neurobiology has revealed differences in the adolescent brain that bring to light the importance of distinguishing between "normal" use and an SUD. Given this large proportion of drug-using youth, along with these other commonly mitigating factors, the need for efficient, easily administered, and psychometrically sound assessment tools is even more imperative.

The evaluation of adolescent drug use has evolved over the past 15 years, with methodology becoming more distinct from adult procedures and taking into account numerous developmental considerations. Multiple valid, reliable screening and comprehensive measures are available to assess not only level but also patterns of use accompanying drug use behaviors, comorbidity, and outcome. The continued development of new and improved biological assays is a welcome accompaniment to methods of self-report. Valid and reliable adolescent drug assessment is key to understanding the true scope of adolescent drug involvement, identifying biological indicators and behavior patterns associated with risk for the development of an SUD, obtaining a more thorough and ongoing understanding of the costs to society, and evaluating short- and long-term outcomes.

Nonetheless, future research is needed to fill important measurement gaps. Many tests do not report validity evidence among subpopulations of young people defined by age, race, and type of setting (e.g., juvenile detention program, treatment program). And most measures have not been formally tested to determine their adequacy as a measure of change (Stinchfield & Winters, 1997). A good measure of change should meet the condition that its standard error of measurement is sufficiently minimal to permit its use in detecting small to medium change over time (Jacobson & Truax, 1991). As we have already noted, it is unclear whether the distinction between substance abuse and dependence is diagnostically meaningful when applied to adolescents, and there is a need to improve our measurement of individual abuse and dependence criteria for youth, given that some criteria appear to have questionable relevance when applied to young people (Martin & Winters, 1998). A related unresolved area is the need for more precise identification of related psychosocial problems that may contribute to the onset and maintenance of drug involvement. Many existing tools assess psychosocial risk factors historically, which does not permit an understanding of the extent to which risk factors may precede the drug use or be a consequence of it.

REFERENCES

Allen, J. P. (1991). The interrelationship of alcoholism assessment and treatment. *Alcohol Health Research World*, *15*, 178–185.

American Psychiatric Association (APA). (1994). *Diagnostic and statistical manual of mental disorders* (4th ed.). Washington, DC: Author.

American Psychiatric Association (APA). (2000). *Diagnostic and statistical manual of mental disorders* (4th ed., text rev.). Washington, DC: Author.

August, G. J., Winters, K. C., Realmuto, G. M., Fahnhorst, T., Botzet, A. M., & Lee, S. (2006). Prospective longitudinal study of adolescent drug abuse among community samples of ADHD and non-ADHD participants. *Journal of the American Academy of Child and Adolescent Psychiatry*, *45*, 824–832.

Baer, J. S., Ginzler, J. A., & Peterson, P. L. (2003). DSM-IV alcohol and substance abuse and dependence in homeless youth. *Journal of Studies on Alcohol*, *64*(1), 5–14.

Barkley, R. A., Fischer, M., Smallish, L., & Fletcher, K. (2004). Young adult follow-up of hyperactive children: Antisocial activities and drug use. *Journal of Child Psychology and Psychiatry*, *45*, 195–211.

Biederman, J., Wilens, T., Mick, E., Farone, S. V., Weber, W., Curtis, S., et al. (1997). Is ADHD a risk factor for psychoactive substance use disorders?: Findings from a four-year prospective follow-up study. *Journal of the American Academy of Child and Adolescent Psychiatry*, *36*, 21–29.

Bilchik, S. (1998). A juvenile justice system for the 21st century. *Crime and Delinquency*, *44*(1), 89–102.

Bolognini, M., Plancherel, B., Laget, J., & Halfon, O. (2003). Adolescent's suicide attempts: Populations at risk, vulnerability, and substance use. *Substance Use and Misuse*, *38*(11–13), 1651–1669.

Boyle, M. H., Offord, D. R., Racine, Y. A., Szatmari, P., Fleming, J. E., & Links, P. (1992). Predicting substance use in late adolescence: Results of the Ontario Child Health Study follow-up. *American Journal of Psychiatry*, *149*, 761–767.

Boys, A., Farrell, C., Taylor, J., Marsden, R., Goodman, T., Brugha, P., et al. (2003). Psychiatric morbidity and substance use in young people aged 13–15 years: Results from the child and adolescent survey of mental health. *British Journal of Psychiatry*, *182*, 509–517.

Brown, S. A. (1993). Drug expectancies and addictive behavior change. *Experimental and Clinical Psychopharmacology*, *1*, 55–67.

Brown, S. A., Myers, M. G., Lippke, L., Tapert, S. F., Stewart, D. G., & Vik, P. W. (1998). Psychometric evaluation of the Customary Drinking and Drug Use Record (CDDR): A measure of adolescent alcohol and drug involvement. *Journal of Studies on Alcohol*, *59*, 427–438.

Buchan, B., Dennis, M. L., Tims, F., & Diamond, G. S. (2002). Cannabis use: Consistency and validity of self-report, on-site testing and laboratory testing. *Addiction*, *97*(Suppl. 1), 98–108.

Burke, J. D., Loeber, R., & Lahey, B. B. (2001). Which aspects of ADHD are associated with tobacco use in early adolescence? *Journal of Child Psychology and Psychiatry*, *42*, 493–502.

Cady, M., Winters, K. C., Jordan, D. A., Solberg, K. R., & Stinchfield, R. D. (1996). Measuring treatment readiness for adolescent drug abusers. *Journal of Child and Adolescent Substance Abuse*, *5*, 73–91.

Center for Substance Abuse Treatment. (1999). *Screening and assessing adolescents for substance use disorders* (Treatment Improvement Protocol (TIP) Series 31). Rockville, MD: Substance Abuse and Mental Health Services Administration.

Chilcoat, H., & Breslau, N. (1999). Pathways from ADHD to early drug use. *Journal of the American Academy of Child and Adolescent Psychiatry*, *38*(11), 1347–1354.

Chung, T., Martin, C. S., Armstrong, T. D., & Labouvie, E. W. (2002). Prevalence of DSM-IV alcohol diagnoses and symptoms in adolescent community and clinical samples. *Journal of the American Academy of Child and Adolescent Psychiatry*, *41*(5), 546–554.

Chung, T., Martin, C. S., Winters, K. C., & Langenbucher, J. W. (2001). Assessment of alcohol tolerance in adolescents. *Journal of Studies on Alcohol*, *62*, 687–695.

Clark, D., & Winters, K. C. (2002). Measuring risks and outcomes in substance use disorders prevention research. *Journal of Consulting and Clinical Psychology*, *70*, 1207–1223.

Clark, D. B., & Bukstein, O. G. (1998). Psychopathology in adolescent alcohol abuse and dependence. *Alcohol Health and Research World*, 22(2), 117–121.

Clark, D. B., Kirisci, L., & Moss, H. B. (1998). Early adolescent gateway drug use in sons of fathers with substance use disorders. *Addictive Behaviors*, 23(4), 561–566.

Clark, D. B., & Miller, T. W. (1998). Stress adaptation in children: Theoretical models. In T. W. Miller (Ed.), *Stressful life events: Children and trauma* (pp. 3–27). Madison, CT: International Universities Press.

Clark, D. B., Moss, H., Kirisci, L., Mezzich, A. C., Miles, R., & Ott, P. (1997). Psychopathology in preadolescent sons of substance abusers. *Journal of the American Academy of Child and Adolescent Psychiatry*, 36, 495–502.

Clark, D. B., Parker, A., & Lynch, K. (1999). Psychopathology and substance-related problems during early adolescence: A survival analysis. *Journal of Clinical Child Psychology*, 28, 333–341.

Clark, D. B., Pollock, N. A., Bromberger, J. T., Bukstein, O. G., Mezzich, A. C., & Donovan, J. E. (1997). Gender and comorbid psychopathology in adolescents with alcohol use disorders. *Journal of the American Academy of Child and Adolescent Psychiatry*, 36(9), 1195–1203.

Clark, D. B., & Sayette, M. A. (1993). Anxiety and the development of alcoholism: Clinical and scientific issues. *American Journal on Addictions*, 2, 59–76.

Clark, D. B., Thatcher, D. L., & Maisto, S. A. (2005). Supervisory neglect and adolescent alcohol use disorders: Effects on AOD onset and treatment outcome. *Addictive Behaviors*, 30(9), 1737–1750.

Cleveland, M. J., Gibbons, F. X., Gerrard, M., Pomery, E. A., & Brody, G. H. (2005). The impact of parenting on risk cognitions and risk behavior: A study of mediation and moderation in a panel of African American adolescents. *Child Development*, 76(4), 900–916.

Costello, E. J., Edelbrock, C., & Costello, A. J. (1985). Validity of the NIMH Diagnostic Interview Schedule for Children: A comparison between psychiatric and pediatric referrals. *Journal of Abnormal Child Psychology*, 13, 570–595.

Dakof, G., Tejeda, M., & Liddle, H. (2000). Predictors of engagement in adolescent drug abuse treatment. *Journal of the American Academy of Child and Adolescent Psychiatry*, 40, 274–281.

DAWN (Drug Abuse Warning Network). (1996). *1996 DAWN report*. Washington, DC: Substance Abuse and Mental Health Services Administration.

Dembo, R., Schmeidler, J., Borden, P., Chin Sue, C., & Manning, D. (1997). Use of the POSIT among arrested youths entering a juvenile assessment center: A replication and update. *Journal of Child and Adolescent Substance Abuse*, 6, 19–42.

Dennis, M. L. (1999). *Global Appraisal of Individual Needs (GAIN): Administration guide for the GAIN and related measures*. Bloomington, IL: Lighthouse.

Dennis, M. L., Funk, R., Godley, S. H., Godley, M. D., & Waldron, H. (2004). Cross-validation of the alcohol and cannabis use measures in the Global Appraisal of Individual Needs (GAIN) and Timeline Followback (TLFB; Form 90) among adolescents in substance abuse treatment. *Addiction*, 99(Suppl. 2), 120–128.

Deykin, E. Y., Levy, J. C., & Wells, V. (1987). Adolescent depression, alcohol and drug abuse. *American Journal of Public Health*, 77, 178–182.

Dillon, F., Turner, C., Robbins, M., & Szapocznik, J. (2005). Concordance among biological, interview, and self-report measures of drug use among African American and Hispanic adolescents referred for drug abuse treatment. *Psychology of Addictive Medicine*, 19(4), 404–413.

Dishion, T. J., Capaldi, D., Spracklen, K. M., & Fuzhong, L. (1995). Peer ecology and male adolescent drug use. *Development and Psychopathology*, 7, 803–824.

Dishion, T. J., Patterson, G. R., & Reid, J. R. (1988). Parent and peer factors associated with drug sampling in early adolescence. In E. R. Rahdert & J. Grabowski (Eds.), *Adolescent drug abuse: Analyses of treatment research*. Rockville, MD: National Institute on Drug Abuse.

Dolan, K., Rouen, D., & Kimber, J. (2004). An overview of the use of urine, hair, sweat, and saliva to detect drug use. *Drug and Alcohol Review*, 23, 213–217.

Donovan, D. M. (2003). Assessment to aid in the treatment planning process. In J. Allen & M. Colombus (Eds.), *Assessing alcohol problems: A guide for clinicians and researchers* (2nd ed., pp. 125–177). Rockville, MD: National Institute on Alcohol Abuse and Alcoholism.

Donovan, J. E., & Jessor, R. (1985). Structure of problem behavior in adolescence and young adulthood. *Journal of Consulting and Clinical Psychology*, 53(6), 890–904.

Earls, F., Reich, W., Jung, K. G., & Cloninger, C. R. (1988). Psychopathology in children of alcoholic and antisocial parents. *Alcoholism, Clinical and Experimental Research*, 12, 481–487.

Ellis, B. R. (1987). *Juvenile Automated Substance Abuse Evaluation (JASAE)*. Clarkston, MI: ADE Incorporated.

Erikson, E. H. (1968). *Identity, youth and crisis*. New York: Norton.

Farrell, A. D., & Danish, S. J. (1993). Peer drug associations and emotional restraint: Causes and consequences of adolescents' drug use? *Journal of Consulting and Clinical Psychology*, 61, 327–334.

Fisher, P., Shaffer, D., Piacentini, J. C., Lapkin, J., Kafantaris, V., Leonard, H., et al. (1993). Sensitivity of the Diagnostic Interview Schedule for Children, 2nd edition (DISC-2.1) for specific diagnoses of children and adolescents. *Journal of the American Academy of Child and Adolescent Psychiatry*, 32, 666–673.

Giedd, J. (2004). Structural magnetic resonance imaging

of the adolescent brain. In R. E. Dahl & L. P. Spear (Eds.), *Adolescent brain development: Vulnerabilities and opportunities* (pp. 77–85). New York: New York Academy of Sciences.

Grella, C., Hser, Y.-I., Joshi, V., & Rounds-Bryant, J. (2001). Drug treatment outcomes for adolescents with comorbid mental and substance use disorders. *Journal of Nervous and Mental Disease, 189,* 384–392.

Grilo, C. M., Fehon, D. C., Walker, M., & Martino, S. (1996). A comparison of adolescent inpatients with and without substance abuse using the Millon Adolescent Clinical Inventory. *Journal of Youth and Adolescence, 25(3),* 379–388.

Guo, J., Hill, K. G., Hawkins, J. D., Catalano, R. F., & Abbott, R. D. (2002). A developmental analysis of sociodemographic, family, and peer effects on adolescent illicit drug initiation. *Journal of the American Academy of Child and Adolescent Psychiatry, 41,* 838–845.

Harrell, A., & Wirtz, P. M. (1989). Screening for adolescent problem drinking: Validation of a multidimensional instrument for case identification. *Psychological Assessment, 1,* 61–63.

Harrison, L. D. (1995). The validity of self-reported data on drug use. *Journal of Drug Issues, 25,* 91–111.

Harrison, P. A., Fulkerson, J. A., & Beebe, T. J. (1998). DSM-IV substance use disorder criteria for adolescents: A critical examination based on a statewide school survey. *American Journal of Psychiatry, 155,* 486–492.

Hasin, D., & Paykin, A. (1998). Dependence symptoms but no diagnosis: Diagnostic orphans in a community sample. *Drug and Alcohol Dependence, 50,* 19–26.

Hawkins, J. D., Catalano, R. F., & Miller, J. Y. (1992). Risk and protective factors for alcohol and other drug problems in adolescence and early adulthood: Implications for substance abuse prevention. *Psychological Bulletin, 112,* 64–105.

Heath, A. C., & Martin, N. G. (1988). Teenage alcohol use in the Australian Twin Register: Genetic and social determinants of starting to drink. *Alcoholism: Clinical and Experimental Research, 12,* 735–741.

Hechtman, L., & Weiss, G. (1986). Controlled prospective fifteen-year follow-up of hyperactives as adults: Non-medical drug and alcohol use and anti-social behavior. *Canadian Journal of Psychiatry, 31,* 557–567.

Henly, G. A., & Winters, K. C. (1988). Development of problem severity scales for the assessment of adolescent alcohol and drug abuse. *International Journal of the Addictions, 23,* 65–85.

Hill, S. Y., & Muka, D. (1996). Childhood psychopathology in children from families of alcoholic female probands. *Journal of the American Academy of Child and Adolescent Psychiatry, 31,* 1024–1030.

Hser, Y.-I., Grella, C. E., Hubbard, R. L., Hsieh, S.-C., Fletcher, B. W., Brown, B. S., et al. (2001). An evaluation of drug treatments for adolescents in four US cities. *Archives of General Psychiatry, 58(7),* 689–695.

Hsieh, S., & Hollister, C. D. (2004). Examining gender differences in adolescent substance abuse behavior: Comparison and implications for treatment. *Journal of Child and Adolescent Substance Abuse, 13,* 53–70.

Iacono, W. G., Carlson, S. R., Taylor, J., Elkins, I. J., & McGue, M. (1999). Behavioral disinhibition and the development of substance-use disorders: Findings from the Minnesota Twin Family Study. *Developmental Psychopathology, 11(4),* 869–900.

Inwald, R. E., Brobst, M. A., & Morissey, R. F. (1986). Identifying and predicting adolescent behavioral problems by using a new profile. *Juvenile Justice Digest, 14,* 1–9.

Jacobson, N. S., & Truax, P. (1991). Clinical significance: A statistical approach to defining meaningful change in psychotherapy research. *Journal of Consulting and Clinical Psychology, 59,* 12–19.

Jainchill, N., Yagelka, J., Hawke, J., & De Leon, G. (1999). Adolescent admissions to residential drug treatment: HIV risk behaviors pre- and post-treatment. *Psychology of Addictive Behaviors, 13(3),* 163–173.

Johnston, L. D., & O'Malley, P. M. (1997). The recanting of earlier reported drug use by young adults. *NIDA Research Monograph, 167,* 59–80.

Johnston, L. D., O'Malley, P. M., Bachman, J. G., & Schulenberg, J. E. (2005). *Monitoring the future national survey results on drug use, 1975–2004. Volume I: Secondary school students* (NIH Publication No. 05-5727). Bethesda, MD: National Institute on Drug Abuse.

Kahler, C., Read, J., Wood, M., & Palfai, T. (2003). Social environmental selection as a mediator of gender, ethnic, and personality effects on college student drinking. *Psychology of Addictive Behaviors, 17,* 226–234.

Kaminer, Y. (1991). Adolescent substance abuse. In R. J. Frances & S. I. Miller (Eds.), *The clinical textbook of addictive disorders* (pp. 320–346). New York: Guilford Press.

Kaminer, Y. (1994). *Adolescent substance abuse.* New York: Plenum Press.

Kaminer, Y., Blitz, C., Burleson, J. A., & Sussman, J. (1998). The Teen Treatment Services Review (T-TSR). *Journal of Substance Abuse Treatment, 15,* 291–300.

Kaminer, Y., Bukstein, O. G., & Tarter, T. E. (1991). The Teen Addiction Severity Index (T-ASI): Rationale and reliability. *International Journal of Addiction, 26,* 219–226.

Kaminer, Y., Wagner, E., Plummer, B., & Seifer, R. (1993). Validation of the Teen Addiction Severity Index (T-ASI): Preliminary findings. *American Journal on Addiction, 2,* 221–224.

Kandel, D. B. (1975). Stages in adolescent involvement in drug use. *Science, 90,* 912–914.

Kandel, D. B. (1990). Parenting styles, drug use, and children's adjustment in families of young adults. *Journal of Marriage and the Family, 52(1),* 183–196.

Kandel, D. B., Johnson, J. G., Bird, H. R., Weissman, M., Goodman, S. H., Lahey, B. B., et al. (1999). Psychiatric comorbidity among adolescents with substance use disorders: Findings from the MECA study. *Journal of the American Academy of Child and Adolescent Psychiatry, 38*(6), 693–699.

Kelly, J. F., Myers, M. G., & Brown, S. A. (2000). A multivariate process model of adolescent 12-step attendance and substance use outcome following inpatient treatment. *Psychology of Addictive Behaviors, 4,* 376–389.

Kidwell, D. A., & Blank, D. L. (1996). Environmental exposure: The stumbling block of hair testing. In P. Kintz (Ed.), *Drug testing in hair* (pp. 17–68). Boca Raton, FL: CRC Press.

Kidwell, D. A., Lee, E. H., & DeLauder, S. F. (2000). Evidence for bias on hair testing and procedures to correct bias. *Forensic Science International, 107,* 39–61.

King, R. D., Gaines, L. S., Lambert, E. W., Summerfelt, W. T., & Bickman, L. (2000). The co-occurrence of psychiatric substance use diagnoses in adolescents in different service systems: Frequency, recognition, cost, and outcomes. *Journal of Behavioral Health Services and Research, 27*(4), 417–430.

Kirisci, L., Mezzich, A., & Tarter, R. (1995). Norms and sensitivity of the adolescent version of the Drug Use Screening Inventory. *Addictive Behaviors, 20,* 149–157.

Knight, J., Sherritt, L., Harris, S. K., Gates, E., & Chang, G. (2003). Validity of brief alcohol screening tests among adolescents: A comparison of the AUDIT, POSIT, CAGE and CRAFFT. *Alcoholism: Clinical and Experimental Research, 27,* 67–73.

Knight, J. R., Sherritt, L., Shrier, L. A., Harris, S. K., & Chang, G. (2002). Validity of the CRAFFT substance abuse screening test among adolescent clinic patients. *Archives of Adolescent Medicine, 156,* 607–614.

Kokotailo, P. (1995). Physical health problems associated with adolescent substance abuse. In E. Rahdert & D. Czechowicz (Eds.), *Adolescent drug abuse: Clinical assessment and therapeutic interventions* (pp. 112–129, NIDA Research Monograph No. 156, NIH Publication No. 95-3908). Rockville, MD: National Institute on Drug Abuse.

Koopmans, J. R., & Boomsma, D. I. (1996). Familial resemblances in alcohol use: Genetic or cultural transmission? *Journal of Studies on Alcohol, 57,* 19–28.

Kosterman, R., Hawkins, J., Guo, J., Catalano, R. F., & Abbott, R. D. (2000). The dynamics of alcohol and marijuana initiation: Patterns and predictors of first use in adolescence. *American Journal of Public Health, 90,* 360–366.

Lapham, S. C., Henley, E., & Kleyboecker, K. (1993). Prenatal behavioral risk screening by computer among Native Americans. *Family Medicine, 25,* 197–202.

Latimer, W. W., Winters, K. C., & Stinchfield, R. D. (1997). Screening for drug abuse among adolescents in clinical and correctional settings using the Problem Oriented Screening Instrument for Teenagers. *American Journal of Drug and Alcohol Abuse, 23,* 79–98.

Latimer, W. W., Winters, K. C., Stinchfield, R. D., & Traver, R. E. (2000). Demographic, individual and interpersonal predictors of adolescent alcohol and marijuana use following treatment. *Psychology of Addictive Behaviors, 14,* 162–173.

Leccese, M., & Waldron, H. B. (1994). Assessing adolescent substance use: A critique of current measurement instruments. *Journal of Substance Abuse Treatment, 11,* 553–563.

Lewinsohn, P. M., Hops, H., Roberts, R. E., Seeley, J. R., & Andrews, J. A. (1993). Adolescent psychopathology: 1. Prevalence and incidence of depression and other DSM-III R disorders in high school students. *Journal of Abnormal Psychology, 102,* 133–144.

Lewinsohn, P. M., Rohde, P., & Seeley, J. R. (1996). Alcohol consumption in high school adolescents: Frequency of use and dimensional structure of associated problems. *Addiction, 91,* 375–390.

Liddle, H. A., & Dakof, G. A. (1995). Family-based treatment for adolescent drug use: State of the science. In E. Rahdert & D. Czechowicz (Eds.), *Adolescent drug abuse: Clinical assessment and therapeutic interventions* (pp. 218–254). Rockville, MD: National Institute on Drug Abuse.

Lynskey, M. T., & Fergusson, D. M. (1995). Childhood conduct problems, attention deficit behaviors, and adolescent alcohol, tobacco, and illicit drug use. *Journal of Abnormal Child Psychology, 23*(3), 281–302.

MacKenzie, R. G. (1993). Influence of drug use on adolescent sexual activity. *Adolescent Medicine, 4*(2), 417–422.

Maisto, S. A., Connors, G. J., & Allen, J. P. (1995). Contrasting self-report screens for alcohol problems: A review. *Alcoholism, Clinical and Experimental Research, 19,* 1510–1516.

Maisto, S. A., Pollock, N. K., Lynch, K. G., Martin, C. S., & Ammerman, R. (2001). Course of functioning in adolescents 1 year after alcohol and other drug treatment. *Psychology of Addictive Behaviors, 15,* 68–76.

Mannuzza, S., Klein, R. G., Bessler, A., Malloy, P., & LaPadula, M. (1993). Adult outcome of hyperactive boys' educational achievement, occupational rank, and psychiatric status. *Archives of General Psychiatry, 50,* 565–576.

Markwiese, B. J., Acheson, S. K., Levin, E. D., Wilson, W. A., & Swartzwelder, H. S. (1998). Differential effects of ethanol on memory in adolescent and adults rats. *Alcoholism, Clinical and Experimental Research, 22,* 416–421.

Martin, C. S., Kaczynski, N. A., Maisto, S. A., Buckstein, O. M., & Moss, H. B. (1995). Patterns of DSM-IV alcohol abuse and dependence symptoms in adolescent drinkers. *Journal of Studies on Alcohol, 56,* 672–680.

Martin, C. S., Kaczynski, N. A., Maisto, S. A., & Tarter, R. E. (1996). Polydrug use in adolescent drinkers with and without DSM-IV alcohol abuse and dependence. *Alcoholism, Clinical and Experimental Research, 20,* 1099–1108.

Martin, C. S., Lynch, K. G., Pollock, N. K., & Clark, D. B. (2000). Gender differences and similarities in the personality correlates of adolescent alcohol problems. *Psychology of Addictive Behaviors, 14*, 121–133.

Martin, C. S., & Winters, K. C. (1998). Diagnosis and assessment of alcohol use disorders among adolescents. *Alcohol Health and Research World, 22*(2), 95–105.

Martino, S., Grilo, C. M., & Fehon, D. C. (2000). The development of the Drug Abuse Screening Test for Adolescents (DAST-A). *Addictive Behaviors, 25*, 57–70.

McGue, M. (1999). Behavioral genetics models of alcoholism and drinking. In K. E. Leonard & H. T. Blane (Eds.), *Psychological theories of drinking and alcoholism* (2nd ed., pp. 372–421). New York: Guilford Press.

McLaney, M. A., Del-Boca, F., & Babor, T. (1994). A validation study of the Problem Oriented Screening Instrument for Teenagers (POSIT). *Journal of Mental Health, 3*, 363–376.

McLellan, A. T., Luborsky, L., Woody, G. E., & O'Brien, C. P. (1980). An improved diagnostic evaluation instrument for substance abuse patients: The Addiction Severity Index. *Journal of Nervous and Mental Disease, 186*, 26–33.

Meyers, K., McLellan, A. T., Jaeger, J. L., & Pettinati, H. M. (1995). The development of the Comprehensive Addiction Severity Index for Adolescents (CASI-A): An interview for assessing multiple problems of adolescents. *Journal of Substance Abuse Treatment, 12*, 181–193.

Milberger, S., Biederman, J., Faraone, S. V., Chen, L., & Jones, J. (1997). ADHD is associated with early initiation of cigarette smoking in children and adolescents. *Journal of the American Academy of Child and Adolescent Psychiatry, 36*, 37–44.

Miller, G. (1985). *The Substance Abuse Subtle Screening Inventory—Adolescent Version.* Bloomington, IN: SASSI Institute.

Millon, T. (1991). Classification in psychopathology: Rationale, alternatives, and standards. *Journal of Abnormal Psychology, 100*(3), 245–261.

Moberg, D. P. (1983). Identifying adolescents with alcohol problems: A field test of the Adolescent Alcohol Involvement Scale. *Journal of Studies on Alcohol, 44*, 701–721.

Moberg, D. P. (2003). *Screening for alcohol and other drug problems using the Adolescent Alcohol and Drug Involvement Scale (AADIS).* Madison: Center for Health Policy and Program Evaluation, University of Wisconsin.

Molina, B. S. G., Smith, B. H., & Pelham, W. E. (1999). Interactive effects of attention deficit hyperactivity disorder and conduct disorder on early adolescent substance use. *Psychology of Addictive Behaviors, 13*, 348–358.

Myers, M. G., Brown, S. A., & Mott, M. A. (1993). Coping as a predictor of adolescent substance abuse treatment outcome. *Journal of Substance Abuse, 5*, 15–29.

National Institute on Alcohol Abuse and Alcoholism (NIAAA). (2003). *Assessing alcohol problems: A guide for clinicians and researchers* (NIH Publication No. 03-3745). Retrieved February 3, 2006, from *pubs.niaaa.nih.gov/ publications/assessing%20alcohol/index.htm*

Newman, F. L., Ciarlo, J. A., & Carpenter, D. (1999). Guidelines for selecting psychological instruments for treatment planning and outcome. In M. E. Maruish (Ed.), *The use of psychological testing and treatment planning for outcomes and assessment, second edition* (pp. 153–170). Mahwah, NJ: Erlbaum.

Noam, G. G., & Houlihan, J. (1990). Developmental dimensions of DSM-III diagnoses in adolescent psychiatric patients. *American Journal of Orthopsychiatry, 60*, 371–378.

Opland, E., Winters, K. C., & Stinchfield, R. (1995). Examining gender differences in drug-abusing adolescents. *Psychology of Addictive Behaviors, 9*, 167–175.

Patock-Peckham, J. A., Cheong, J., Balhorn, M. E., & Nagoshi, C. T. (2001). A social learning perspective: A model of parenting styles, self-regulation, perceived drinking control, and alcohol use and problems. *Alcoholism: Clinical and Experimental Research, 25*, 1284–1292.

Patterson, G. R., Forgatch, M. S., Yoerger, K. L., & Stoolmiller, M. (1998). Variables that initiate and maintain an early-onset trajectory for juvenile offending. *Development and Psychopathology, 10*, 531–548.

Petraitis, J., Flay, B. R., & Miller, T. Q. (1995). Reviewing theories of adolescent substance abuse: Organizing pieces in the puzzle. *Psychological Bulletin, 117*, 67–86.

Pollock, N. K., & Martin, C. S. (1999). Diagnostic orphans: Adolescents with alcohol symptoms who do not qualify for DSM-IV abuse or dependence diagnoses. *American Journal of Psychiatry, 156*, 897–901.

Pollock, N. K., Martin, C. S., & Langenbucher, J. W. (2000). Diagnostic concordance of DSM-III, DSM-III-R, DSM-IV, and ICD-10 alcohol diagnoses in adolescents. *Journal of Studies on Alcohol, 61*(3), 439–446.

Rahdert, E. (Ed.). (1991). *The Adolescent Assessment/Referral System manual* (DHHS Publication No. [ADM] 91-1735). Rockville, MD: U.S. Department of Health and Human Services, ADAMHA, National Institute on Drug Abuse.

Reich, W., Shayla, J. J., & Taibelson, C. (1992). *The Diagnostic Interview for Children and Adolescents—Revised (DICA-R).* St. Louis, MO: Washington University.

Reid, R. W., O'Connor, F. L., Deakin, A. G., Ivery, D. M., & Crayton, J. W. (1996). Cocaine and metabolites in human graying hair: Pigmentary relationship. *Journal of Toxicology: Clinical Toxicology, 34*, 685–690.

Riggs, P. D., & Davies, R. (2002). A clinical approach to treatment of depression in adolescents with substance use disorders and conduct disorder. *Journal of the American Academy of Child and Adolescent Psychiatry, 41,* 1253–1255.

Risberg, R. A., Stevens, M. J., & Graybill, D. F. (1995). Validating the adolescent form of the Substance Abuse Subtle Screening Inventory. *Journal of Child and Adolescent Substance Abuse, 4,* 25–41.

Rogers, R., Cashel, M. L., Johansen, J., Sewell, K. S., & Gonzalez, C. (1997). Evaluation of adolescent offenders with substance abuse: Validation of the SASSI with conduct-disordered youth. *Criminal Justice and Behavior, 24,* 114–128.

Rohde, P., Lewinsohn, P. M., & Seely, J. R. (1996). Psychiatric comorbidity with problematic alcohol use in high school students. *Journal of the American Academy of Child and Adolescent Psychiatry, 35*(1), 101–109.

Rohrich, J., Zorntlein, S., Pötsch, L., Skopp, G., & Becker, J. (2000). Effect of the shampoo Ultra Clean on drug concentrations. *International Journal of Legal Medicine, 113,* 102–106.

Rose, R. J., Dick, D. M., Viken, R. J., Pulkkinen, L., & Kaprio, J. (2001). Drinking or abstaining at age 14?: A genetic epidemiological study. *Alcoholism: Clinical and Experimental Research, 25,* 1594–1604.

Sachs, H. (1995). Theoretical limits of the evaluation of drug concentrations in hair due to irregular hair growth. *Forensic Science International, 70,* 53–61.

Sarrazin, M. S., Hall, J. A., Richards, C., & Carswell, C. (2002). The comparison of computer-based versus pencil-and-paper assessment of drug use. *Research on Social Work Practice, 12*(5), 669–683.

Schuckit, M. A., & Hesselbrock, V. (1994). Alcohol dependence and anxiety disorders: What is the relationship? *American Journal of Psychiatry, 151,* 1723–1734.

Schulenberg, J., O'Malley, P. M., Bachman, J. G., Wadsworth, K. N., & Johnston, L. D. (1996) Getting drunk and growing up: Trajectories of frequent binge drinking during the transition to young adulthood. *Journal of Studies on Alcohol, 57,* 289–304.

Shaffer, D., Fisher, P., & Dulcan, M. (1996). The NIMH Diagnostic Interview Schedule for Children (DISC 2.3): Description, acceptability, prevalence, and performance in the MECA study. *Journal of the American Academy of Child and Adolescent Psychiatry, 35,* 865–877.

Shaffer, D., Fisher, P., Lucas, C. P., Dulcan, M. K., & Schwab-Stone, M. E. (2000). NIMH Diagnostic Interview Schedule for Children Version IV (NIMH DISC-IV): Description, differences from previous versions, and reliability of some common diagnoses. *Journal of the American Academy of Child and Adolescent Psychiatry, 39,* 28–38.

Shaffer, D., Schwab-Stone, M., Fisher, P., Cohen, P., Piacentini, J., Davies, M., et al. (1993). Revised version of the Diagnostic Interview Schedule for Children (DISC-R): Preparation, field-testing, and acceptability. *Journal of the American Academy of Child and Adolescent Psychiatry, 32,* 643–650.

Shaffer, H. J. (1997). The psychology of change. In J. Lowinson, P. Ruiz, R. B. Millman, & J. G. Langrod (Eds.), *Substance abuse: A comprehensive textbook* (pp. 100–106). Baltimore: Williams & Wilkins.

Skinner, H. (1982). *Development and validation of a lifetime Alcohol consumption assessment procedure: Substudy No. 1248.* Toronto: Addiction Research Foundation.

Sobell, L. C., & Sobell, M. B. (1992). Timeline followback: A technique for assessing self-reported alcohol consumption. In R. Z. Litten & J. P. Allen (Eds.), *Measuring alcohol consumption* (pp. 73–98). Totowa, NJ: Humana Press.

Spear, L. P. (2000). The adolescent brain and age-related behavioral manifestations. *Neuroscience and Biobehavioral Reviews, 24,* 417–463.

Stewart, S. H. (1996). Alcohol abuse in individuals exposed to trauma: A critical review. *Psychological Bulletin, 120*(1), 83–112.

Stinchfield, R. D. (1997). Reliability of adolescent self-reported pretreatment alcohol and other drug use. *Substance Use and Misuse, 32,* 63–76.

Stinchfield, R. D., & Winters, K. C. (1997). Measuring change in adolescent drug misuse with the Personal Experience Inventory (PEI). *Substance Use and Misuse, 32,* 63–76.

Stone, A., & Latimer, W. (2005). Adolescent substance use assessment: Concordance between tools using self-administered and interview formats. *Substance Use and Misuse, 40,* 1865–1874.

Substance Abuse and Mental Health Services Administration (SAMHSA). (1994). *Simple screening for infectious diseases and drug abuse (Treatment Improvement Protocol Series #11).* Rockville, MD: Center for Substance Abuse Treatment.

Substance Abuse and Mental Health Services Administration (SAMHSA). (1999). *Youth substance use: State estimates from the 1999 National Household Survey on Drug Abuse.* Retrieved December 14, 2005, from *www.oas.samhsa.gov/nhsda/99youthstate/toc.htm*

Substance Abuse and Mental Health Services Administration (SAMHSA). (2005). *Results from the 2004 National Survey on Drug Use and Health: National Findings* (Office of Applied Studies, NDSDUH Series H-28, DHHS Publication No. SMA 05-4062). Rockville, MD: Author.

Tapert, S. F., Baratta, M. V., Abrantes, A. M., & Brown, S. A. (2002). Attention dysfunction predicts substance involvement in community youths. *Journal of the American Academy of Child and Adolescent Psychiatry, 41,* 680–686.

Tapert, S. F., & Schweinsburg, A. D. (2005). The human adolescent brain and alcohol use disorders. In M. Galanter (Ed.), *Recent developments in alcoholism: Vol. 17. Alcohol problems in adolescents and young adults: Epidemiology, neurobiology, prevention, treatment* (pp. 177–197). New York: Springer.

Tarter, R. E. (1990). Evaluation and treatment of adolescent substance abuse: A decision tree model.

American Journal of Drug and Alcohol Abuse, 16, 1–46.

Tarter, R. E., Laird, S. B., Bukstein, O., & Kaminer, Y. (1992). Validation of the adolescent drug use screening inventory: Preliminary findings. *Psychology of Addictive Behaviors, 6,* 322–236.

Thompson, L. L., Riggs, P. D., Mikulich, S. K., & Crowley, T. J. (1996). Contribution of ADHD symptoms to substance problems and delinquency in conduct-disordered adolescents. *Journal of Abnormal Child Psychology, 24*(3), 325–347.

Turner, C. F., Ku, L., Rogers, S. M., Lindberg, L. D., & Pleck, J. H. (1998). Adolescent sexual behavior, drug use, and violence: Increased reporting with computer survey technology. *Science, 280,* 867–873.

Varlinskaya, E. I., & Spear, L. P. (2002). Acute effects of ethanol on social behavior and adults rats: Role of familiarity of the test situation. *Alcoholism: Clinical and Experimental Research, 26,* 1502–1511.

Wanberg, K. (1992). *Adolescent Self-Assessment Profile (ASAP).* Arvada, CO: Center for Addictions Research and Evaluation.

Weinberg, N. Z., Rahdert, E., Colliver, J., & Glantz, M. D. (1998). Adolescent substance abuse: A review of the past 10 years. *Journal of the American Academy of Child and Adolescent Psychiatry, 37*(3), 252–261.

Welner, Z., Reich, W., Herjanic, B., Jung, K., & Amado, K. (1987). Reliability, validity and parent–child agreement studies of the Diagnostic Interview for Children and Adolescents (DICA). *Journal of American Academy of Child Psychiatry, 26,* 649–653.

White, H. R., & Labouvie, E. W. (1989). Towards the assessment of adolescent problem drinking. *Journal of Studies on Alcohol, 50,* 30–37.

Williams, M. L., Freeman, R. C., Bowen, A. M., Zhao, Z., Elwood, W. N., & Gordon, C., et al. (2000). A comparison of the reliability of self-reported drug use and sexual behaviors using computer assisted versus face-to-face interviewing. *AIDS Education and Prevention, 12*(3), 199–213.

Williams, R., & Nowatzki, N. (2005). Validity of adolescent self-report of substance use. *Substance Use and Misuse, 40,* 299–311.

Winters, K. C. (1992). Development of an adolescent alcohol and other drug abuse screening scale: Personal Experience Screening Questionnaire. *Addictive Behaviors, 17,* 479–490.

Winters, K. C. (1994). *Assessment of adolescent drug abuse: A handbook.* Los Angeles: Western Psychological Services.

Winters, K. C. (2001). Adolescent assessment of alcohol and other drug use behaviors. In J. P. Allen & V. Wilson (Eds.), *Assessing alcohol problems: A guide for clinicians and researchers* (2nd ed.). Rockville, MD: National Institute on Alcohol Abuse and Alcoholism.

Winters, K. C., Anderson, N., Bengston, P., Stinchfield, R. D., & Latimer, W. W. (2000). Development of a parent questionnaire for the assessment of adolescent drug abuse. *Journal of Psychoactive Drugs, 32,* 3–13.

Winters, K. C., & Henly, G. A. (1989). *Personal Experience Inventory and manual.* Los Angeles: Western Psychological Services.

Winters, K. C., & Henly, G. A. (1993). *Adolescent Diagnostic Interview Schedule and manual.* Los Angeles: Western Psychological Services.

Winters, K. C., Latimer, W., & Stinchfield, R. D. (1999). The DSM-IV criteria for adolescent alcohol and cannabis use disorders. *Journal of Studies on Alcohol, 60*(3), 337–344.

Winters, K. C., Latimer, W. W., Stinchfield, R. D., & Henly, G. A. (1999). Examining psychosocial correlates of drug involvement among drug clinic-referred youth. *Journal of Child and Adolescent Substance Abuse, 9*(1), 1–17.

Winters, K. C., Leitten, W., Wagner, E., & O'Leary Tevyaw, T. (2007). Use of brief interventions in a middle and high school setting. *Journal of School Health, 77,* 196–206.

Winters, K. C., Stinchfield, R. D., Fulkerson, J., & Henly, G. A. (1993). Measuring alcohol and cannabis use disorders in an adolescent clinical sample. *Psychology of Addictive Behaviors, 7*(3), 185–196.

Winters, K. C., Stinchfield, R. D., & Henly, G. A. (1996). Convergent and predictive validity of the Personal Experience Inventory. *Journal of Child and Adolescent Substance Abuse, 5,* 37–55.

Winters, K. C., Stinchfield, R. D., Henly, G. A., & Schwartz, R. (1990–1991). Validity of adolescent self report of substance involvement. *International Journal of the Addictions, 25,* 1379–1395.

Winters, K. C., Stinchfield, R. D., Opland, E., Weller, C., & Latimer, W. W. (2000). The effectiveness of the Minnesota Model for treating adolescent drug abusers. *Addiction, 95,* 601–612.

World Health Organization. (1992). *The ICD-10 classification of mental and behavioural disorders: Diagnostic criteria for research* (10th rev.). Geneva: Author.

Zucker, R. A., Fitzgerald, H. E., & Moses, H. D. (1995). Emergence of alcohol problems and the several alcoholisms: A developmental perspective on etiologic theory and life course trajectory. In D. Cicchetti & D. J. Cohen (Eds.), *Developmental psychopathology: Vol. 2. Risk, disorder, and adaptation* (pp. 677–711). New York: Wiley.

Zucker, R. A., & Noll, R. A. (1987). The interaction of child and environment in the early development of drug involvement: A far ranging review and a planned very early intervention. *Drugs and Society, 1,* 57–97.

PART III

Mood Disorders and Suicide Risk

CHAPTER 5

Child and Adolescent Depression

Karen D. Rudolph
Sharon F. Lambert

Depression strikes a significant minority of youth during critical stages of development, with a particularly high prevalence during adolescence (for reviews, see Lewinsohn & Essau, 2002; Rudolph, Hammen, & Daley, 2006). Moreover, depression frequently follows a pernicious course across development and creates impairment in many spheres of youths' lives. Given these features of depression, there is a great need for assessment methods that allow for the accurate identification of depression, and for the evaluation of prevention and intervention efforts with depressed youth. Determining the most appropriate assessment strategy is a complicated endeavor that requires both a thorough understanding of the heterogeneous nature and causes of depression, and a careful consideration of the goals and targets of assessment.

This chapter presents an overview of contemporary issues and methods in the assessment of youth with depression. To provide a background for evaluating various assessment approaches, we first summarize the basic features and causes of youth depression. This discussion emphasizes the need to consider developmental aspects of the disorder and to place our understanding of depression within the context of emerging knowledge about gender, ethnic, and cultural differences in the phenomenology and etiology of depression. Second, we discuss major considerations that arise in determining the optimal approach for assessing youth with depression. Third, we provide a critical, selective review of the predominant methods of assessment, with a focus on those that have established reliability, validity, and clinical utility.

DESCRIPTION OF YOUTH DEPRESSION AND DIAGNOSTIC ISSUES

Developing a comprehensive base of knowledge about depression in young people has been complicated by the heterogeneous taxonomic systems that psychologists use to conceptualize depression. This heterogeneity creates a challenge for psychologists in several areas: delineating basic clinical characteristics of depression (e.g., prevalence, course), determining the etiology of depression, selecting appropriate assessment approaches, and evaluating the efficacy and effectiveness of prevention and intervention efforts. Here we present a brief summary of taxonomic issues relevant to depression (for comprehensive reviews, see Compas, Ey, & Grant, 1993; Klein, Dougherty, & Olino, 2005).

Taxonomy of Depression

Psychologists use three different broad approaches to define depression (Compas et al., 1993). The first approach, which focuses on depressed *mood*, views depression as an individual symptom of unhappiness. Depressed mood is most often assessed via self-report on checklists. The second approach, which focuses on the depressive *syndrome* (i.e., an empirically derived constellation of behaviors and emotions that cluster together in multivariate analyses), views depression in terms of quantitative deviations in levels of symptoms that vary along a continuum. Although the most widespread application of this approach suggests that depressive symptoms cluster together with anxiety symptoms into an anxious–depressive syndrome in youth (e.g., Achenbach, Connors, Quay, Verhulst, & Howell, 1989), researchers also have established validity for a cluster of pure depressive symptoms (e.g., Lengua, Sadowski, Friedrich, & Fisher, 2001). The depressive (or anxious–depressive) syndrome most often is assessed via multi-informant (e.g., youth, parent, teacher) report on behavior checklists. The third approach, which focuses on depression as a *diagnosis*, views depression as a categorical disorder that is distinguished along quantitative (e.g., number of symptoms) and qualitative (e.g., change from prior functioning, significant levels of distress and impairment) dimensions. According to this approach, most commonly reflected in the *Diagnostic and Statistical Manual of Mental Disorders*, fourth edition, text revision (DSM-IV-TR; American Psychiatric Association, 2000) and the International Classification of Diseases (ICD-10; World Health Organization, 1993), depression is characterized by features such as number and configuration of symptoms, frequency, severity, duration, and associated disability. Diagnoses of depression are assessed through structured, clinician-administered interviews. Although there is some overlap among these three conceptualizations of depression (e.g., the presence of negative affectivity), there also are distinct characteristics (e.g., the depressive syndrome often includes symptoms other than depression, such as anxiety; somatic and vegetative symptoms are not well represented in the mood or syndrome definitions). Which conceptualization of depression is applied greatly influences the selection of assessment approaches, the information derived from assessment, and the implications of this information for treatment planning and evaluation.

A related, long-standing debate concerns whether depression is best conceptualized as a discrete category or as a continuum of symptoms (Klein et al., 2005). On the one hand, it has been argued that subsyndromal symptoms and clinical depression represent qualitatively different phenomena. On the other hand, research indicates that subsyndromal forms of disorder are associated with significant functional impairment and future risk for major depression (Angst, Sellaro, & Merikangas, 2000; Pine, Cohen, Cohen, & Brook, 1999). Recent taxometric analysis reveals that depression in youth is better conceptualized along a continuum than as a discrete entity (Hankin, Fraley, Lahey, & Waldman, 2005). This evidence, combined with the impairment associated with subsyndromal depression, suggests that it is important to assess not only clinical depression but also the presence of mild, enduring symptoms that might portend functional impairment and a more severe disorder in the future. This is especially important in youth, because even mild depressive symptoms may interrupt normative developmental trajectories, potentially resulting in impairment that persists beyond the symptoms.

Diagnostic Criteria and Associated Features

In a categorical approach, depressive disorders are a subset of the mood disorders. In this chapter, we focus on the description and assessment of unipolar depression (see Youngstrom, Chapter 6, this volume, for a discussion of pediatric bipolar disorder). DSM-IV-TR criteria for a major depressive episode (MDE) are depressed or irritable mood and/or loss of pleasure, combined with at least four somatic or cognitive symptoms (see Table 5.1). Symptoms must persist at least 2 weeks and cause impaired functioning or significant distress. Criteria for dysthymic disorder are chronic mood symptoms, combined with at least two somatic or cognitive symptoms (see Table 5.1). Symptoms must persist at least 1 year. Some researchers have questioned whether the distinction between major depressive disorder (MDD) and dysthymia is meaningful, although data indicating more significant impairment in youth with "double depression" (both MDD and dysthymia; Goodman, Schwab-Stone, Lahey, Shaffer, & Jensen, 2000) suggest that indepen-

TABLE 5.1. DSM-IV-TR Diagnostic Criteria for Depressive Disorders

Major Depressive Disorder

A. Five (or more) of the following symptoms during the same 2-week period; at least one of the symptoms is either (1) depressed mood or (2) loss of interest or pleasure.

   (1) depressed mood most of the day, nearly every day, as indicated by either subjective report or observation made by others. Note: In children and adolescents, can be irritable mood.
   (2) markedly diminished interest or pleasure in all, or almost all, activities most of the day, nearly every day (as indicated by either subjective account or observation made by others)
   (3) significant weight loss when not dieting or weight gain (e.g., a change of more than 5% of body weight in a month), or decrease or increase in appetite nearly every day. Note: In children, consider failure to make expected weight gains.
   (4) insomnia or hypersomnia nearly every day
   (5) psychomotor agitation or retardation nearly every day (observable by others)
   (6) fatigue or loss of energy nearly every day
   (7) feelings of worthlessness or excessive or inappropriate guilt nearly every day
   (8) diminished ability to think or concentrate, or indecisiveness, nearly every day (either by subjective account or as observed by others)
   (9) recurrent thoughts of death (not just fear of dying), recurrent suicidal ideation without a specific plan, or a suicide attempt or a specific plan for committing suicide

Major Depressive Episode (unipolar) can be further specified as mild, moderate, severe (based on functional impairment and severity of symptoms), with or without psychotic features, with or without melancholic features, whether or not recurrent, or chronic.

Dysthymic Disorder

A. Depressed mood for most of the day, for more days than not, as indicated either by subjective account or observation by others, for at least 2 years. Note: In children and adolescents, mood can be irritable and duration must be at least 1 year.

B. Presence, while depressed, of two (or more) of the following:

   (1) poor appetite or overeating
   (2) insomnia or hypersomnia
   (3) low energy or fatigue
   (4) low self-esteem
   (5) poor concentration or difficulty making decisions
   (6) feelings of hopelessness

C. During the 2-year period (1 year for children or adolescents) of the disturbance, the person has never been without symptoms in Criteria A and B for more than 2 months at a time.

D. No Major Depressive Episode during the first 2 years of the disturbance (1 year for children and adolescents); i.e., the disturbance is not better accounted for by chronic Major Depressive Disorder, or Major Depressive Disorder, In Partial Remission).

Note Reprinted with permission from the *Diagnostic and Statistical Manual of Mental Disorders.* Copyright 2000. American Psychiatric Association.

dent assessment of the two conditions is worthwhile.

Youth depression also might include psychotic symptoms (Mitchell, McCauley, Burke, & Moss, 1988) and endogenous features, such as lack of reactivity, distinct quality of mood, and diurnal variation (McCauley et al., 1993). In addition to the core diagnostic criteria, depression in youth frequently is associated with social withdrawal (Bell-Dolan, Reaven, & Peterson, 1993; Puura et al., 1998), somatic complaints (Puura et al., 1998; Ryan et al., 1987), and body image dissatisfaction, particularly in adolescent girls (Wichstrom, 1999).

Epidemiology of Depression

Prevalence

Prevalence estimates vary according to the conceptualization of depression (i.e., as a mood, syndrome, or disorder). In community samples, epidemiological surveys reveal lifetime depressive disorders prevalence rates of less than 3% in preadolescents and 15–20% in adolescents (for reviews, see Kessler, Avenevoli, & Merikangas, 2001; Lewinsohn & Essau, 2002). A growing body of research indicates that the prevalence of depression has increased in recent birth cohorts (Kessler et al., 2001).

In addition to diagnosable depression, a significant minority of youth experience depressed mood, subsyndromal symptoms, and minor depression. Depending on the informant (e.g., youth vs. parent), age, and gender, 10–40% of youth experience an unhappy, sad, or depressed mood (Achenbach, 1991; Compas et al., 1993). Use of formal diagnostic criteria indicates that 10–20% of youth experience subsyndromal levels of symptoms or minor depression (e.g., Kessler & Walters, 1998; Roberts, Lewinsohn, & Seeley, 1991), whereas self-reports of symptoms indicate that 20–50% of youth exceed conventional cutoffs for clinically significant levels of depression (Kessler et al., 2001). As discussed earlier, these elevated levels of symptoms are meaningful and may forecast more severe disorders in the future.

Age of Onset, Clinical Features, and Developmental Course

Retrospective studies of depressed adults and prospective studies of youth suggest that major depression is most likely to emerge during the midadolescent years (about ages 13—15), with a somewhat younger age of onset for dysthymia (e.g., Burke, Burke, Regier, & Rae, 1990; Hankin et al., 1998; Lewinsohn & Essau, 2002). In community samples of untreated youth, MDEs have a median duration of about 8 weeks (Lewinsohn, Rohde, & Seeley, 1994). Longer mean durations (e.g., 7 to 9 months) generally are found in clinical versus community samples (e.g., Birmaher, Arbeleaz, & Brent, 2002; Kovacs, 1996). Dysthymic disorder has a mean duration of 4 years, and many youth with dysthymia eventually experience MDEs (for a review, see Birmaher et al., 1996).

Although the majority of MDEs remit within a few months, with almost all remitting within 2 years (for a review, see Birmaher et al., 1996), depression frequently has a recurrent or chronic course, with continuity across time and developmental periods (Birmaher et al., 2002; Kessler et al., 2001). Self-reported symptoms also show significant stability over several years (Verhulst & van der Ende, 1992). Risk for chronicity and recurrence is predicted by a variety of factors, such as severity, personal or family history of MDD, suicidality, comorbidity, negative beliefs, and family adversity (Birmaher et al., 2002; Rohde, Lewinsohn, Klein, & Seeley, 2005).

Research suggests that adolescent-onset depression is likely to portend depression in adulthood. Large-scale studies of community samples (e.g., Lewinsohn, Rohde, Klein, & Seeley, 1999; Pine, Cohen, Gurley, Brook, & Ma, 1998) and studies of clinical samples (Birmaher et al., 2002; Weissman, Wolk, Goldstein, et al., 1999) demonstrate significant continuity in depressive diagnoses from adolescence through young adulthood. Continuity of depression from childhood to adulthood is less clear. Although a subgroup of youth with childhood-onset symptoms and disorders go on to experience depression in adulthood (i.e., *disorder-specific continuity*), particularly those with recurrent childhood depression and family histories of depression (Weissman, Wolk, Wickramaratne, et al., 1999), a significant majority, particularly those with comorbid disruptive behavior disorders, demonstrate *disorder-nonspecific continuity*, that is, high rates of psychological disorders and adjustment difficulties other than depression at later developmental stages (Harrington, Fudge, Rutter, Pickles, & Hill, 1990). This pattern suggests that certain childhood-onset depressive disorders might be a different form of depression than those with an onset in adolescence or adulthood. However, more research is needed to clarify dimensions on which the forms of disorder might differ across developmental stages.

In summary, depression often emerges during adolescence and follows a recurrent course, with a great deal of associated impairment. However, most depressive episodes do remit naturally. These characteristics of depression have important implications for the selection and implementation of assessment strategies in the context of treatment planning and evaluation. For example, assessment protocols need to account for the fact that improvement might be expected over time even in nontreated youth, but recurrence is the rule rather than the exception.

Associated Comorbid Disorders

Research reveals high rates of co-occurrence between depression and other symptoms and disorders in youth. A meta-analysis by Angold, Costello, and Erkanli (1999), using a categorical approach, revealed significant comorbidity between depression and anxiety disorders (odds ratio [OR] = 8.2), conduct/oppositional defiant disorders (OR = 6.6), and attention-deficit/hyperactivity disorder (OR = 5.5). Depression also co-occurs frequently (rate of 20%) with substance use disorders in adolescents (Lewinsohn, Hops, Roberts, Seeley, & Andrews, 1993). Research that uses a continuous approach also reveals significant covariation between depression and other forms of internalizing distress (e.g., anxiety, somatic problems), as well as externalizing behavior problems (e.g., aggression, oppositionality).

A variety of explanations might account for these high rates of co-occurrence. "Artifactual" comorbidity might reflect problems with the specificity of assessment tools, or with the taxonomic systems on which diagnostic categories are based (Angold et al., 1999). True comorbidity might result from the presence of shared risk factors (e.g., genetic liability for depression and anxiety), co-occurring risk factors (e.g., co-occurring parental depression and family discord, creating a risk for both youth depression and youth conduct disorder), or a causal relation between two disorders (e.g., disruptions in social and academic functioning associated

with behavior disorders, creating a risk for depression). Distinguishing between artifactual and true comorbidity is a crucial goal for the development and application of valid assessment approaches. Knowledge about functional relations between other disorders and subsequent depression can guide early identification of youth who may be at risk for depression due to the disruptive influence of earlier anxiety or behavior problems. Unfortunately, as we discuss later, because many assessment instruments show poor specificity for depression, it is difficult to distinguish between artifactual and true sources of comorbidity.

Progress has been made in understanding the high rates of co-occurrence between depression and anxiety (Watson et al., 1995). Historically, the high co-occurrence between these disorders led psychologists to question their distinctiveness. However, contemporary conceptualizations and assessment instruments emphasize both shared and unique components of the two disorders. For example, the tripartite model (Watson et al., 1995) distinguishes among three major clusters of affective symptoms: negative affect or general emotional distress (common to anxiety and depression), physiological arousal or somatic tension (unique to anxiety), and anhedonia or lack of positive affect (unique to depression). Preliminary research supports the tripartite model in youth, with some differences across age and gender (e.g., Chorpita, Daleiden, Moffitt, Yim, & Umemoto, 2000; Jacques & Mash, 2004; for a review, see Laurent & Ettelson, 2001). Additional research is needed to develop assessment instruments that identify overlapping and distinct features of depression and disorders that frequently co-occur with depression.

Developmental Features

Diagnostic criteria are the same in youth and adults, except for the inclusion of irritability as one of the mood disturbances and a shorter duration criterion for dysthymia in youth. However, there are some developmental differences in the expression of symptoms and in the structure of the depressive syndrome (for reviews, see Hammen & Rudolph, 2003; Weiss & Garber, 2003). With regard to symptom expression, depressed young children show more depressed appearance, somatic complaints, and irritability, whereas depressed adolescents show more anhedonia, vegetative symptoms (e.g., eating and sleeping difficulties), and diurnal variation of mood. With regard to the structure of symptoms, factor analysis reveals that vegetative symptoms, affective symptoms, and concerns about the future are more a part of depression in adolescents, whereas cognitive symptoms and externalizing behavior are more a part of depression in preadolescents. Patterns of comorbidity also differ somewhat by age. For example, depressed preadolescents are more likely to display separation anxiety, whereas depressed adolescents are more likely to display eating disorders (particularly females) and substance use disorders (particularly males) (e.g., Lewinsohn et al., 1993). These developmental patterns can inform decisions about which associated disorders should be thoroughly assessed.

Gender Differences

One of the best established findings in depression research concerns the emergence of higher rates of depression in girls than in boys at about 13–15 years of age (Hankin et al., 1998; Wichstrom, 1999; for a review, see Hankin & Abramson, 2001). This sex difference is robust across conceptualizations of depression as a mood, syndrome, and disorder, although the difference is more consistent in referred than in nonreferred samples (Compas et al., 1997).

Several models that have been proposed to explain the origins of sex differences in depression focus on the role of hormonal changes and pubertal maturation, stress and coping, and interpersonal processes that characterize the adolescent transition (for reviews, see Hankin & Abramson, 2001; Nolen-Hoeksema, 2002; Rudolph et al., 2006). Collectively, these theories and supportive evidence suggest that heightened risk for depression in adolescent girls is driven by interactions among biological and social aspects of puberty; an interpersonal orientation that emphasizes affiliation and social approval; heightened exposure and sensitivity to interpersonal stress; and a ruminative style of responding to depressive symptoms and stressors. Moreover, girls experience more adverse interpersonal consequences of depression, such as deterioration in close friendships (for a review, see Rudolph, Flynn, & Abaied, in press). Appreciation for this backdrop of risk in adolescent girls can guide early identification of youth who are likely to be vulnerable during the adolescent transition, as well as highlight

potential disruptions that might emerge following the onset of a depressive episode in girls. Assessment efforts can then be directed toward the appropriate domains of vulnerability and disruption.

Ethnic and Cultural Considerations

Few epidemiological studies include samples with sufficient ethnic diversity to compare rates of depression in youth from different ethnic backgrounds, and findings are mixed. Some research indicates no differences in rates of depression across ethnic groups (e.g., Costello et al., 1996; Kandel & Davies, 1982; Manson, Ackerson, Dick, Baron, & Fleming, 1990), whereas other research suggests that ethnic/minority youth have higher rates of depression. For example, in a large epidemiological survey examining differences in rates of adolescent depressive symptoms, African American, Hispanic, and Asian adolescents reported significantly more depressive symptoms than did white adolescents (Rushton, Forcier, & Schectman, 2002), but specific differences between groups were not described. In another large study using an ethnically diverse sample, adolescents reported few differences in the prevalence of MDD across nine ethnic groups, with the exception of higher rates for Mexican American youth (Roberts, Roberts, & Chen, 1997), after adjustment for age, gender, and socioeconomic status. Similarly, Latino adolescents reported greater depressed mood than did African American, Asian American, and white adolescents, independent of socioeconomic status (Siegel, Aneshensel, Taub, Cantwell, & Driscoll, 1998). Unfortunately, it is difficult to draw firm conclusions about differences in the prevalence of depression due to different methods for assessing depression, inclusion of different racial and ethnic groups across studies, and examination of racial groups without attention to ethnicity (Chang, 2002). In addition, findings may vary depending on whether socioeconomic status is taken into account (e.g., Doi, Roberts, Takeuchi, & Suzuki, 2001).

There is some evidence that correlates and predictors of depressive symptoms vary across ethnic groups. For example, Hayward, Gotlib, Schraedley, and Litt (1999) found that pubertal status was a better predictor of depressive symptoms than chronological age in white adolescents as compared to African American and Hispanic adolescents. Dolan, Lacey, and Evans

(1990) reported that disordered eating and depression were correlated for white but not Afro-Caribbean adolescents. There also is evidence to suggest that youth of different ethnicities experience depression differently. In one study comparing the factor structure of the Children's Depression Inventory in African American and white inpatient youth, African American youth were less suicidal but scored higher on behavioral dimensions of depression, whereas white youth scored higher on affective dimensions (Politano, Nelson, Evans, Sorenson, & Zelman, 1986).

It is important to note that sole reliance on race or ethnic status to examine group differences in youth depression can be problematic. Conceptions of depression might vary across cultures, having implications for whether or not youth are referred for treatment, how symptoms manifest, and how individuals describe their symptoms (Choi, 2002; Okazaki, 2000). Culture also might influence the behaviors that clinicians observe during an assessment. For example, in some cultures, youth are socialized to display deferential behavior to authority figures (Yee, Huang, & Lew, 1998), which may include limited eye contact and limited initiation of verbal interaction. Similarly, youth whose cultural norms include suppressing emotions and keeping problems in the family might limit self-disclosure of their own difficulties and restrict their display of emotions with the clinician (Yeh & Yeh, 2002). Because some correlates of depression might indicate positive adjustment in certain cultures, it is important for clinicians to consider cultural factors when interpreting data obtained from depression assessment measures.

Culture also has important implications for the validity and utility of measures to assess depression. A scale developed and normed in one cultural group might not assess the same construct or have the same psychometric properties in another group (Arnold & Matus, 2000). Cross-cultural differences in language used to describe depression also are important to consider. For example, whereas psychological and physical symptoms typically are considered separate entities in mainstream American culture, these two sets of concerns are integrated in many Asian cultures (Ying, 2002); thus, youth from these cultures might describe their depressive symptoms in terms of somatic rather than affective concerns. Relatedly, linguistic issues, such as language proficiency and ethnic language variations, might affect the assessment of depression in diverse youth (Choi, 2002). Linguistic concerns are not addressed by translation alone, because translation does not necessarily indicate cultural equivalence of constructs assessed.

Research is needed to examine the validity of instruments to assess depression in youth from different racial, ethnic, cultural, and linguistic backgrounds, as well as the strength of their psychometric properties across diverse groups. In addition, assessments with diverse youth must include an evaluation of other factors with particular relevance to depression that vary across racial and ethnic groups, including ethnic identity (e.g., Roberts et al., 1999), acculturation and acculturative stress (Hovey & King, 1996), immigration history, and experiences with racism and discrimination (Hammack, 2003; Nyborg & Curry, 2003), each of which has been linked to depression in ethnic minority youth. Because ethnicity and culture can have a significant impact on both the assessment process and the interpretation of assessment results, a comprehensive evaluation of depression should consider these factors.

Domains of Impairment

Youth depression is associated with impairment in several key life domains. Depressed youth demonstrate compromised academic performance, interpersonal difficulties (e.g., social withdrawal, conflict in relationships), negative self-perceptions, and disruptions in important social roles, as reflected in problems such as school dropout and early pregnancy (for reviews, see Garber & Horowitz, 2002; Hammen & Rudolph, 2003; Rudolph et al., 2006). A particularly dangerous correlate of depression is suicidal ideation and attempts (see Goldston & Compton, Chapter 7, this volume, for a discussion of suicidal behavior). Although research is inconsistent regarding the stability of impairment and its endurance beyond acute depressive episodes, a growing body of evidence suggests that depression predicts subsequent difficulties in the psychological, academic, and social realms (e.g., Cole, Martin, Peeke, Seroczynski, & Hoffman, 1998; Ialongo, Edelsohn, Werthamer-Larsson, Crockett, & Kellam, 1993; Pomerantz & Rudolph, 2003), and that depressed youth experience some ongoing impairment even following remission or successful treatment of depression (Puig-Antich et al., 1985; Rao et al., 1995). Youth with depression also often develop new comorbid disorders, including substance use, anxiety, and personality disorders (e.g., Lewinsohn et al., 1999; Weissman, Wolk, Goldstein, et al., 1999). Moreover, depression early in life predicts impairment into adulthood (Lewinsohn, Rohde, Seeley, Klein, & Gotlib, 2003; Weissman, Wolk, Goldstein, et al., 1999). These correlates and consequences of depression indicate the need to assess multiple domains of functioning along with the core symptoms.

ETIOLOGY OF YOUTH DEPRESSION

Contemporary conceptualizations of youth depression have two defining characteristics with implications for assessment (for reviews, see Cicchetti & Toth, 1998; Garber & Horowitz, 2002; Hankin & Abramson, 2001; Rudolph et al., 2006). First, recent perspectives focus on interactional and transactional influences among biological, cognitive, interpersonal, and contextual factors in the onset and maintenance of depression. This integrative focus highlights the need to evaluate diverse areas of impairment in addition to formal diagnostic criteria and related symptoms. Assessing these areas of impairment can (1) facilitate the identification of youth at particular risk for depression, (2) guide predictions about the course of depression, (3) help determine collateral targets for intervention (e.g., family adversity, interpersonal difficulties, academic deficits), and (4) provide information about potential processes of change over the course of treatment (e.g., whether improvement in social-cognitive processes predicts declines in depressive symptoms). Second, recent perspectives emphasize a developmental approach to understanding youth depression, with an elaboration of both similarities and differences in the nature, course, risk factors, and consequences of depression across the lifespan. This developmental focus highlights the need to consider the developmental stage of youth in selection of appropriate assessment strategies and formulation of hypotheses about potential causes and consequences of depression. Here we provide a brief overview of the major components of integrative models of youth depression. Later in the chapter, we provide a more detailed review

of key constructs and measures that assess different aspects of these models.

Genetic Influences

Research using a variety of methods establishes a strong aggregation of depression in families. Indeed, a family history of depression, particularly in a parent, is one of the best predictors of depression, especially recurrent depression (Klein, Lewinsohn, Rohde, Seeley, & Durbin, 2002) in youth (for a review, see Goodman & Gotlib, 1999). Moreover, biometric modeling studies that provide direct assessments of heritability reveal a significant genetic component to depression (estimates of 20–45% for milder forms and 40–70% for severe forms); heritability seems to be particularly high during adolescence (for reviews, see Sullivan, Neale, & Kendler, 2000; Wallace, Schneider, & McGuffin, 2002). Genetic liability may be coupled with environmental risks linked to parental depression, such as family adversity and problematic parenting styles (Kessler et al., 2001). This consistent evidence for the family transmission of risk indicates that a comprehensive evaluation of youth depression should include a thorough assessment of current symptoms and past history of parental affective disorder.

Biological Influences

Research examining biological vulnerability to depression focuses primarily on four areas: dysregulation of neuroendocrine systems; disruptions in neurotransmitter processes; dysregulation of biological rhythms, as reflected in sleep patterns; and atypical activation of particular brain regions, especially the left frontal cortex. Studies of these biological processes reveal somewhat inconsistent evidence regarding patterns of dysregulation in depressed youth.

Adult depressives demonstrate consistent abnormalities in the hypothalamic–pituitary–adrenal (HPA) axis, suggesting dysregulation of the stress response system (for a review, see Thase, Jindal, & Howland, 2002). Specifically, depression in adults is associated with higher levels of basal cortisol, abnormal responses to the dexamethasone suppression test (DST; used to measure the response of the adrenal glands to adrenocorticotropic hormone [ACTH]), and abnormalities in corticotropin-releasing factor (CRF). Differences in basal cortisol and responses to CRF infusion are not apparent in depressed youth (Kaufman, Martin, King, & Charney, 2001; Kutcher et al., 1991). Although depressed children, and adolescents to a lesser extent, do demonstrate nonsuppression of cortisol on the DST at rates similar to those of depressed adults, the specificity of this index to youth depression is unclear (Kaufman et al., 2001). Depressed preadolescents also show blunted growth hormone responses to pharmacological stimulation (Dahl et al., 2000). This atypical response persists following remission of depression (Dahl et al., 2000) and is present in high-risk youth with no personal history of depression (i.e., those with depressed parents; Birmaher et al., 2000), suggesting that it might be an important marker of a predisposition to depression (for a review, see Kaufman et al., 2001).

Some research indicates abnormalities of the serotonergic neurotransmitter system in depressed youth. For example, both high-risk and currently depressed youth demonstrate atypical responses (blunted cortisol and increased prolactin) to a pharmacological challenge, namely administration of L-5-hydroxytryptophan (L-5HTP) (Birmaher et al., 1997). Moreover, recent research suggests that a polymorphism in the serotonin transporter (5-HTT) gene serves as a vulnerability to depression in the face of life stress (Caspi et al., 2003). Efficacy of antidepressants that target serotonergic systems (selective serotonin reuptake inhibitors [SSRIs]) also indirectly implicates disrupted neurotransmitter systems in depressed youth (e.g., Emslie et al., 1997).

Research on sleep abnormalities in depressed youth yields mixed findings. Depressed adolescents show some similar patterns of disruption to those of adults, including reduced rapid-eye-movement (REM) latency and increased REM density, although conflicting results emerge for other sleep disturbances. Moreover, studies of sleep behavior and neurophysiology in younger depressed children do not reveal similar abnormalities (Birmaher et al., 1996; Kaufman et al., 2001). Inconsistent findings across studies and developmental differences in the nature and function of sleep suggest that measures of sleep abnormalities are not likely to be useful diagnostic tools for youth depression (Emslie, Rush, Weinberg, Rintelmann, & Roffwarg, 1994).

Both structural and functional brain abnormalities have been linked to depression in adults, including reduced blood flow and metabolism in the prefrontal cortex, reductions in amygdala volume, and hippocampal abnormalities (for a review, see Davidson, Pizzagalli, & Nitschke, 2002). Moreover, electrophysiological research in adults with depression reveals relative hypoactivation in the left frontal cortex, suggesting possible underactivation of brain systems that drive the experience of pleasure and positive engagement (Davidson et al., 2002). Few studies have been conducted with youth; thus, little is known about the relevance of these findings for youth depression. However, research does reveal similar patterns of asymmetry (i.e., relative left frontal hypoactivation) in the infants and toddlers of depressed mothers (Dawson, Frey, Panagiotides, Osterling, & Hessl, 1997), suggesting possible links to early risk for depression.

Social-Cognitive Influences

Social-cognitive theories focus on the role of maladaptive thought processes and negative belief systems as risk factors for depression. Specifically, negative appraisals of the self and the world are hypothesized to heighten vulnerability to depression, particularly in the face of stressful life experiences. Variants of these theories focus on different aspects of social-cognitive processes, including self-schemas; beliefs and attitudes about the self and others; inferences about the causes and consequences of life events; and perceptions of control and competence.

Consistent with Beck's (1967) pioneering information-processing theory of depression, research reveals that depressed youth show idiosyncratic processing of self- and other-relevant information (Cole & Jordan, 1995; Rudolph, Hammen, & Burge, 1997; Shirk, Van Horn, & Leber, 1997), and endorse statements that reflect low self-worth, irrational beliefs, and dysfunctional attitudes (for reviews, see Garber & Horowitz, 2002; Hankin & Abramson, 2001; Kaslow, Adamson, & Collins, 2000; Rudolph et al., 2006). Moreover, consistent with helplessness–hopelessness (Abramson, Metalsky, & Alloy, 1989) and self-regulation (Cole, Martin, & Powers, 1997; Weisz, Southam-Gerow, & McCarty, 2001) theories of depression, research links youth depression with a negative attributional style (i.e., a tendency to make internal, global, and stable attributions for negative experiences), hopelessness, and low perceptions of control and competence (for reviews, see Garber & Horowitz, 2002; Hankin & Abramson, 2001; Kaslow et al., 2000; Rudolph et al., 2006).

Despite evidence for the role of maladaptive social-cognitive processes in depression, research reveals that certain aspects of cognitive vulnerability do not emerge until adolescence (Abela, 2001; Cole & Jordan, 1995; Weisz et al., 2001). These developmental changes in vulnerability suggest that supplementing assessments of depression with an evaluation of particular social-cognitive processes should be guided by the developmental stage of the child.

Interpersonal Influences

According to interpersonal models that emphasize the social context of depression, depressed individuals both react to and contribute to disruption in their close relationships (Gotlib & Hammen, 1992; Joiner, Coyne, & Blalock, 1999). These models emphasize the ongoing transactions between individuals and their social environments. Specifically, particular interpersonal styles and social deficits of depressed youth elicit negative responses from others. These negative interpersonal experiences maintain or exacerbate depression.

Within the family, disturbances that disrupt early social bonds and undermine the achievement of key developmental tasks (e.g., creation of a healthy sense of self, acquisition of emotion regulation and coping skills) are believed to create a vulnerability to depression. Theory and research implicate various forms of family adversity, including the loss of a caregiver, maltreatment, insecure parent–child attachment, family discord, and parenting styles characterized by low levels of warmth, heightened rejection, and overcontrolling behavior. Such disruption in the family environment might account in part for the intergenerational transmission of depression. Depressed youth in turn show less effective communication, problem solving, and support during interactions with their parents than do nondepressed youth (for reviews, see Garber & Horowitz, 2002; Goodman & Gotlib, 1999; Rudolph et al., in press).

Depressed youth also show significant social-behavioral deficits and impairment in their peer relationships, friendships, and romantic relationships. For example, compared to nondepressed youth, depressed youth are more aggressive and less prosocial with peers; engage in more excessive reassurance seeking; and demonstrate less active, assertive, and problem-focused, and more passive, avoidant, ruminative, and helpless responses to challenges, including interpersonal problems and conflict. Not surprisingly, given these deficits, depressed youth experience higher levels of rejection by familiar and unfamiliar peers, less stable friendships, and poorer friendship and romantic relationship quality than do nondepressed youth. This interpersonal disruption appears to be both an antecedent and a consequence of depression, particularly in adolescent girls (for a review, see Rudolph et al., in press).

Collectively, research suggests a transactional relation between youth and their social contexts, such that depressed youth are exposed to higher levels of interpersonal adversity and create more adverse relationship contexts. Thus, assessing interpersonal relationships might provide information about not only possible risk factors for depression but also the social difficulties that depression creates in youths' lives.

Contextual Influences

Theory and research implicate several types of environmental adversity as triggers of depression in vulnerable individuals, including acute negative life events, chronic stressors and daily hassles, and broader stressful conditions, such as socioeconomic disadvantage, parental unemployment, and low levels of parental education. Consistent with these perspectives, a significant amount of research reveals an association between contextual stressors and depression in youth (for reviews, see Garber & Horowitz, 2002; Rudolph et al., 2006).

Although early life stress models viewed stress as a contributor to depression, more recent perspectives emphasize the transactional nature of stress and depression (Hammen, 1992). Research supports the idea that depressed youth both react (Garber, Keiley, & Martin, 2002) and contribute (Rudolph et al., 2000) to life stress. In fact, genetic liability to depression might be expressed in part as heightened exposure to self-generated life stress (Rice, Harold, & Thapar, 2003). Stress within close relationships is an especially salient predictor and consequence of depression, particularly in adolescent girls (Hankin & Abramson, 2001; Rudolph, 2002). Researchers have proposed a variety of personal attributes and environmental conditions that either dampen or enhance stress reactivity, including genetic liability, physiological reactivity, cognitive appraisals, emotion regulation and coping responses, and external resources (for reviews, see Garber & Horowitz, 2002; Hankin & Abramson, 2001; Rudolph et al., 2006).

ASSESSMENT CONSIDERATIONS

Selecting and implementing appropriate assessment approaches has implications for both research and clinical practice with depressed youth. In research settings, accurate assessment of depression is required for establishing relatively homogeneous subgroups of youth in an effort to determine the phenomenology, course, and etiology of depression. In clinical settings, comprehensive assessments are essential for formulating diagnoses and prognoses, determining the appropriate type and setting of treatment, monitoring treatment progress, and evaluating treatment effectiveness (Klein et al., 2005). Despite this integral role of assessment in clinical practice, few formal guidelines exist to assist in decision making during the assessment process. In recent years, however, efforts have been made to articulate evidence-based guidelines for the assessment of psychological symptoms and disorders in youth (Mash & Hunsley, 2005). These guidelines integrate standard psychometric information about the reliability and validity of assessment methods derived from scientific research, with pragmatic considerations regarding the utility of particular assessment approaches in applied settings. Evidence-based guidelines for the assessment of depression are discussed in detail elsewhere (Klein et al., 2005). Here we highlight a few key considerations relevant to the assessment of youth with depression.

Identifying the Purpose of Assessment

Determining the optimal assessment approach is contingent on the goals of the assessment. These goals likely vary across research and clinical practice, as well as across different clinical settings (Mash & Foster, 2001). At a broad level, there are several purposes of clinical assessment (Mash & Hunsley, 2005): (1) diagnosis and case formulation; (2) screening; (3) prognosis; (4) treatment design and planning;

(5) treatment monitoring; and (6) treatment evaluation. The specific purpose of the assessment might in part determine the most appropriate methods due either to differing psychometric strengths of the methods (e.g., the relative balance of sensitivity and specificity) or to pragmatic concerns (e.g., the intensiveness of the method or the implications of making a misdiagnosis). For example, for screening purposes (e.g., detecting youth who might benefit from further in-depth assessment), researchers or clinicians might be most interested in minimizing false negatives—that is, ensuring that they do not misidentify a child who is depressed. Thus, they might be interested in a measure that casts a wide net and "catches" most possible cases of depression (Angold, Costello, et al., 1995). In contrast, researchers or clinicians who are selecting youth to participate in an intensive intervention might be most interested in minimizing false positives—that is, ensuring that they do not provide intensive services to a child who is not depressed. More intensive assessment methods that might be useful for initial diagnosis and treatment planning are less practical for weekly monitoring of progress. Indeed, assessing treatment effectiveness requires methods that are sensitive to change (Mash & Hunsley, 2005). Unfortunately, relatively little is known about this characteristic of assessment methods for depression. Furthermore, assessment methods need to be sensitive to context-specific symptoms (e.g., social withdrawal at school vs. at home). Because assessment goals also might vary depending on the stage of assessment and the results of prior assessment, selection of the most appropriate strategy might involve delineating a sequence of methods rather than an individual method or instrument (Klein et al., 2005).

Determining the Target of Assessment

As discussed earlier, it also is important to consider the level of depression—mood, syndrome, or disorder—that is being targeted. Analyses of item overlap among commonly used youth- and other-report checklists, which tap depressed mood and the depressive syndrome, and formal diagnostic criteria (assessed with clinical interviews), as well as empirical analyses of the correspondence among data derived from these three methods, reveal only moderate correspondence (Compas, 1997; Compas et al., 1993). Thus, different information is gathered with each method, and careful thought must be given to which level of depression is of interest. If the goal is to evaluate the severity of depressive symptoms, self-report questionnaires, behavior checklists, or clinician-rated depression scales might be sufficient, but if the goal is to determine a formal clinical diagnosis, then an interview-based method is required. Questionnaires might be useful for screening purposes, but because they often yield a high false-positive rate, they are typically followed up with a clinical interview (Angold, Costello, et al., 1995; Klein et al., 2005; Reynolds, 1994).

Integrating Information across Informants and Methods

A major challenge in the assessment of youth depression is the selection of informants and methods of assessment. Comprehensive assessments involve gathering information from multiple sources (e.g., youth, parents, teacher), methods (e.g., questionnaires, interviews, observations), and contexts (e.g., clinician's office, home, school). However, much evidence suggests a lack of convergence in data obtained across informants, methods, and contexts (Jensen et al., 1999; Kazdin, 1994). Moreover, few formal guidelines are available to determine the relative validity of these different types of information or to guide the integration of information. A few assessment methods (e.g., structured clinical interviews) have established algorithms for integrating information. For semistructured diagnostic interviews, one common solution is a clinician-driven "best estimate" approach (Klein, Ouimette, Kelly, Ferro, & Riso, 1994), wherein information from parent and youth interviews is integrated and weighted based on clinical judgment regarding the validity of the information. Some guidelines (e.g., giving preference to adults' report of depressive symptoms in young children) are available to increase the reliability of this "best estimate" method and to reduce idiosyncrasies in clinician decision making (Jensen et al., 1999). However, these decisions are still quite subjective; thus, this process might be variable across interviewers. Some interviewers might rely on the "or" rule (assuming that a symptom is present if at least one informant reports it), whereas others might rely on the "and" rule (assuming that a symptom is pres-

ent only if it is reported by multiple informants) (Klein et al., 2005). Moreover, structured and semistructured interviews rarely are used in clinical practice. Information from multiple sources also might be combined according to statistical algorithms to optimize prediction (e.g., Rubio-Stipec et al., 1994). However, prediction rules from statistical equations do not necessarily or easily translate into practice, and might not provide an advantage over other methods (Bird, Gould, & Staghezza, 1992).

Additional informal guidelines have been proposed to reconcile cross-informant data. For example, one might take into account both the subjective nature of many depressive symptoms and the developmental stage of the child. Self-report typically is useful for assessing internal experiences, such as feelings of sadness and low self-worth. However, because very young children have difficulty reflecting on their internal experiences, information from adults is essential. In contrast, adolescents possess the cognitive and linguistic ability to reflect on their experiences, and can provide essential information about subjective symptoms that might be difficult to observe (Edelbrock, Costello, Dulcan, Kalas, & Conover, 1985; Jensen et al., 1999). However, even adolescents might have difficulty placing their experiences in the context of typical norms for youth, and reporting on the timing and duration of symptoms. Parent and teacher perspectives might therefore still provide critical information about observable symptoms, and about the onset, course, severity, and prior history of symptoms even in adolescents.

Although discrepancies across informants clearly complicate the assessment process and often are viewed as evidence for poor reliability or validity of the methods, these discrepancies might be meaningful and worthy of attention. Discrepancies might be driven by systematic rater biases, such that they provide important information about characteristics of the informant. For example, depressed mothers may overestimate depressive symptoms in their offspring, resulting in low parent–child agreement (Boyle & Pickles, 1997; Youngstrom, Izard, & Ackerman, 1999). Alternatively, discrepancies might reflect cross-situational specificity in behavior, such as differences across home versus school (Clarizio, 1994). Therefore, rather than dismissing lack of convergence as "noise" in the assessment process, it might be important to consider these inconsistencies as useful data that can help guide case formulation and treatment planning.

Given the possibility that different informants might provide useful information about different aspects of depression and associated impairment, it is important to consider the incremental validity of various measures, namely, the degree to which the measure adds data that improve the outcome of the assessment (e.g., increasing diagnostic accuracy). Surprisingly little research has examined whether different informants and methods provide incremental validity in the assessment of depression. Among the few available studies that examine the incremental validity of multi-informant data, results are mixed. Some research suggests that parent and teacher ratings, and clinician judgments of emotional and behavioral problems contribute uniquely to the prediction of poor outcomes, such as receipt of mental health services and school difficulties (Ferdinand et al., 2003). However, few studies examine the relative contribution of different informants to the assessment of depression specifically, rather than more global ratings of emotion and behavior. One study (Hope et al., 1999) did reveal that adolescent reports of internalizing problems on the Youth Self-Report (Achenbach, 1991) accounted for a significant increment in variance over parent reports on the Child Behavior Checklist (Achenbach, 1991) when predicting the number of internalizing symptoms endorsed by parents on the Diagnostic Interview for Children and Adolescents (Reich, Shayka, & Taibleson, 1991). Although depression and anxiety were not examined separately, these results suggest that parents and youth likely contribute unique sources of information to the assessment of depression.

Although the incremental validity of self-report versus interview methods has not been examined directly, one might assume that diagnostic interviews provide important incremental information necessary for making a diagnosis, such as data about the frequency, severity, and duration of each symptom. Diagnostic interviews also provide important data necessary for making a differential diagnosis, such as information about exclusionary criteria (e.g., the presence of a medical disorder associated with depression), and about other types of psychopathology. Other information often gathered from such interviews, such as family history of psychopathology and depression-related impairment, also may aid in making a differential diagnosis and in distinguishing between normative levels of sad mood and clinical depression. Research has not examined the incremental validity of methods other than rating scales and interviews (e.g., behavior observations) in the assessment of depression, possibly as a result of their limited use due to costs associated with training, accessibility of observation techniques and settings, and time to conduct and code the observations (Garber & Kaminski, 2000).

Clearly, more research is needed to establish the incremental validity of assessment measures for depression, although this endeavor is challenging. The incremental validity of a measure depends on the quality of other measures included in the assessment; thus, incremental validity is difficult to demonstrate for any one measure when other valid measures are part of the assessment. Incremental validity of youth depression measures also depends on other factors, such as developmental status (e.g., parent reports might add significant information that young children are not able to provide) and culture (e.g., given cultural norms about self-disclosure, youth may be reluctant to disclose information that might be obtained from other informants).

Establishing the Clinical Utility of Assessment Approaches

Typically, systematic evaluations of assessment methods for depression focus on traditional psychometric properties (e.g., reliability, convergence with other methods). Far less is known about the utility of various methods for clinical application. Clinical utility includes features such as usefulness for monitoring treatment progress, incremental validity, and prognostic utility (e.g., ability to predict treatment outcome) (Klein et al., 2005; Mash & Hunsley, 2005). Determining the clinical utility of different methods depends on the specific purpose of assessment. For example, the clinical utility of an assessment method for diagnosis depends on its ability to maximize the accuracy of diagnostic classification; thus, the focus is on the positive and negative predictive power of the measure. The clinical utility of a method for evaluating treatment progress and outcome depends on its sensitivity to change and the feasibility of repeated administrations. In many cases, practical considerations might outweigh scientific evidence regarding the strength of different assessment approaches.

Considering Developmental Factors

Although similar methods are used to assess depression at different ages, developmentally sensitive assessment approaches require a consideration of developmental factors that might complicate assessment of depression in youth. As noted earlier, there are some developmental differences in the expression of depression, such that young children might not articulate a depressed or anhedonic mood, and might not experience typical vegetative symptoms of depression. Moreover, because irritability rather than sadness might be the predominant mood, depressive symptoms might be mistaken for other forms of psychopathology. Distinguishing between normative fluctuations in mood and clinically meaningful depression in youth also might be difficult due to ongoing developmental changes in the expression and regulation of mood. Despite the fact that many early myths about depression in youth (e.g., depression in young children is "masked" in the form of other disturbances; depression in adolescents just reflects normative "storm and stress") have been dispelled, significant others in their lives might still misattribute symptoms to normative developmental experiences and disruptions. Thus, assessment of depression requires a careful consideration of developmental norms in emotions and behavior.

A developmental perspective also can inform which domains of impairment to target in a comprehensive assessment. Depression is likely to interfere with developmentally salient tasks (Garber, 1984), such as academic achievement and success with peers during middle to late childhood, and the formation of romantic relationships during adolescence. Thus, assessments should target particular domains of functioning during particular life stages.

A final developmental issue is whether certain assessment methods are most valid and useful at certain stages of maturation. For the most part, similar methods have been used across a wide age span. For example, the same or slightly modified self-report questionnaires and clinical interviews often are used across developmental levels (e.g., ages 8–18). The relative validity and clinical utility of these methods at different ages have not been systematically evaluated.

Assessing Associated Symptoms and Characteristics

A comprehensive assessment of youth with depression involves an evaluation of co-occurring psychopathology and depression-related impairment. We noted earlier the high co-occurrence between depression and other forms of psychopathology, including anxiety disorders, disruptive behavior disorders, substance abuse disorders, eating disorders, and somatic problems. Moreover, depressed youth with comorbid disorders experience more impairment than those with depression alone (Marmorstein & Iacono, 2003; Rudolph, Hammen, & Burge, 1994; Rudolph et al., 2000), and are at risk for a more severe and persistent course of depression (Birmaher et al., 1996; Lewinsohn, Rohde, Seeley, Klein, & Gotlib, 2000). Thus, assessing associated disorders is essential for accurate diagnosis (e.g., making a differential diagnosis or determining whether depression or a comorbid disorder should be the primary diagnosis), case conceptualization (e.g., understanding the complex pattern of symptoms in youth with comorbid disorders and how other symptoms may interact with depression in the expression of dysfunction), and treatment planning (e.g., decision making regarding appropriate treatment options and needs given the presence of comorbid disorders). Assessment of co-occurring problems should include an evaluation of developmental and medical conditions associated with depression and specific features of depression that might have implications for prognosis, treatment planning, and monitoring (e.g., suicidal ideation, psychotic symptoms, hypomania).

Because depressed youth experience disruptions in multiple psychological and life domains, including biological dysregulation, maladaptive social-cognitive processes, academic performance deficits, family conflict, and peer stress (see earlier sections), the assessment process should include an evaluation of other relevant domains. Indeed, as discussed earlier, even youth with subclinical levels of symptoms demonstrate significant psychosocial impairment and often go on to experience more severe depression (Angst et al., 2000; Pine et al., 1999), suggesting that impairment and subjective distress are important targets of assessment beyond formal diagnosis (Mash & Hunsley, 2005). Gathering information about depression-related impairment is critical not only for case formulation and treatment planning, but also for determining prognosis and assessing processes of change during treatment. For example, assessments in youth might include evaluating whether negative cognitive style or maladaptive responses to stress improve over the course of treatment. Unfortunately, because many of the methods used to assess these domains lack normative information or evaluation of their clinical utility, it is difficult to develop specific criteria for inclusion in an assessment battery.

Finally, an essential part of assessment is the evaluation of clinical and family characteristics that predict the course of depression and have implications for treatment planning. As discussed earlier, continuity of depression across developmental stages is high. Moreover, research indicates a significant family aggregation of depression. In fact, a prior history of recurrent depression in youth or their families is a strong predictor of recurrence (Birmaher et al., 2002; Rohde et al., 2005), suggesting that a thorough assessment of personal and family history of depression is critical. Of course, given limited resources, decisions need to be made regarding the most relevant areas to target. Unfortunately, at present, few criteria are available to guide this decision-making process.

Interpreting Changes in Depression

Because a key goal of assessment is to evaluate treatment progress and effectiveness, assessments must be sensitive to changes over time. Two important considerations complicate efforts to evaluate this aspect of clinical utility. First, the majority of MDEs remit naturally over time. Second, reported levels of depressive symptoms tend to decrease across repeated assessments (Twenge & Nolen-Hoeksema, 2002). Thus, tracking the course of disorder during treatment requires an awareness of the possibility that apparent, treatment-related improvement is due to natural remission of symptoms or to artifacts resulting from an attenuation effect.

OVERVIEW OF ASSESSMENT METHODS

In this section, we provide a selective review of assessment methods for depression. When evaluating the measures, we consider standard psychometric indexes of reliability (internal consistency, test–retest reliability, interrater reliability) and validity (content, convergent, discriminant, and incremental validity; sensitivity and specificity), as well as clinical utility (sensitivity to change, prognostic utility, feasibility for use in a clinical setting).

It is difficult to establish strict criteria for evaluating the psychometric properties of youth depression measures. Depressive syndromes in youth tend to fluctuate naturally over time, possibly reducing stability estimates (Kovacs, 1992). Similarly, normative developmental changes (e.g., intellectual, affective) may lower stability estimates (Flannery, 1990) and result in varying levels of validity at different ages (Kessler et al., 2001). Estimates of test–retest reliability that use structured interviews might be lower than those with other assessment measures (e.g., rating scales), because a change in a single response can change diagnostic status and lower reliability estimates. Continuous measures are less sensitive to such small differences in ratings. An additional challenge in evaluating test–retest reliability coefficients is the attenuation effect. Moreover, establishing the validity of measures is difficult given the absence of a "gold standard." Specifically, many evaluations of validity compare information from diagnostic interviews and information from rating scales, which leads to some circularity in determining the strength of each method. Consideration of alternative forms of validity and utility (e.g., prognostic utility), can help to circumvent these complications.

Standard assessment approaches for youth depression fall broadly into two major categories: diagnostic interviews and rating scales. Although physiological, performance-based, and observational measures of depression and related constructs have been developed (for a review, see Garber & Kaminski, 2000), insufficient normative information, idiosyncratic aspects of these assessments (e.g., investigator-specific coding systems), and lack of feasibility (e.g., time intensiveness, cost, training requirements) prevent their standard application in clinical settings. Thus, we provide only a brief review of these types of measures.

Diagnostic Interviews

Diagnostic interviews are used to determine depression diagnoses, as well as to rule out alternative diagnoses. These interviews are classified as unstructured or structured. The content and format of unstructured diagnostic assessments vary by clinician; therefore, these interviews vary in the amount and type of information elicited. Thus, diagnoses based solely on unstructured interviews might fail to consider all necessary diagnostic criteria. Unstructured interviews also might be subject to a number of biases, such as the tendency to collect information selectively to confirm or rule out a particular diagnosis (Angold, 2002; Jensen & Weisz, 2002).

Structured interviews are standardized interviews in which the interviewer determines the presence or absence of diagnostic criteria and associated clinical features, including duration and past history, using a prescribed set of probes. Structured interviews also are useful for differential diagnosis and assessment of comorbid conditions. Parallel child and parent versions often are available (Hodges, 1994). The primary benefit of structured compared to unstructured interviews is standardization in terms of format, language, sequencing of inquiries, methods for rating severity and impairment, and criteria for assigning a diagnosis (Rogers, 2003).

Structured interviews may be classified further as either fully structured, respondent-based or semistructured, interviewer-based (Rogers, 2003). Respondent-based interviews require adherence to a prescribed set of probes; diagnoses are based solely on respondents' answers. Interviewer-based interviews permit the interviewer to supplement a prescribed set of inquiries with additional probes. As a result, respondent-based interviews may be administered by well-trained laypeople, whereas interviewer-based interviews can only be administered by interviewers trained in clinical diagnosis.

In terms of validity, it is increasingly recognized that diagnostic assessments guided solely by clinical judgment may be less accurate than evidence-based diagnoses informed by standard assessment procedures with established reliability and validity, such as structured diagnostic interviews (Doss, 2005). The selection of a fully structured or semistructured interview depends in part on the availability of trained mental health professionals to conduct interviews. Fully structured interviews are preferred when the costs associated with training and administration are prohibitive, such as in large epidemiological studies. When trained interviewers are available, the flexibility of semistructured interviews may yield greater validity (Kessler et al., 2001). Another consideration is whether respondents are deemed able to make judgments about symptom presence or absence without any interviewer input. In cases in which respondents may have difficulty understanding or evaluating interview probes, an interviewer-based interview may increase diagnostic accuracy.

Rating Scales

Depression rating scales and behavior checklists assess depressive mood and symptoms. Symptoms might be rated by the youth, clinicians, or others familiar with the youth (e.g., parents, teachers). Respondents typically rate the extent to which each symptom applies, using Likert scales to select among response options that vary in symptom frequency or severity. Summary scores are created by aggregating across symptoms. These scores do not provide information about the duration of symptoms or about specific configurations of symptoms required for a diagnosis (e.g., a youth might score high on a rating scale despite the absence of depressed mood or anhedonia). Moreover, many items on standard rating scales are not core symptoms of depression but are associated features (e.g., behavior problems, academic impairment). Thus, rating scales do not provide sufficient information to inform diagnoses.

Rating scales are widely used because of their convenience, ease of administration, and low cost. Self-report scales are well suited to assess symptoms that are not observable by others, such as feelings of hopelessness and guilt (Reynolds, 1994). However, these scales share problems characteristic of self-report in general. Youth might be reluctant to disclose depressive symptoms due to social desirability or concern about others' reactions. Alternatively, depressed youth might overestimate their difficulties (Garber & Kaminski, 2000). Also, self-report scales often do not discriminate between depression and other types of negative affect, particularly anxiety. In addition, these measures require a certain level of reading and comprehension, and youth must rate the frequency, intensity, and duration of multiple symptoms. Reports from other informants address these limitations (Clarizio, 1994) but also are subject to biases. Unfortunately, little empirical evidence documents the added value of obtaining information about depression from different sources (Johnston & Murray, 2003), making it difficult to evaluate the relative costs and benefits associated with a multi-informant assessment approach.

Alternative Methods: Observational, Performance-Based, and Physiological Methods

Several laboratory and performance-based methods are available to assess depression and its correlates. For example, observations in laboratory settings may provide useful information about symptoms such as depressive affect, psychomotor abnormalities, and sleep difficulties, as well as correlates of depression, such as interpersonal difficulties. Such methods have several benefits. First, performance-based methods and analogue behavior observations (i.e., structured observations designed to parallel situations encountered in natural settings) (Mash & Foster, 2001) are less subject to difficulties associated with interviews and rating scales, such as self-presentation demands or limited self-reflection capability. Second, these methods provide a means of systematically eliciting and observing responses or behaviors of interest, thereby allowing for the assessment of low base-rate or situation-specific behaviors (Mash & Foster, 2001). Thus, these methods may provide an important supplement to traditional methods.

Unfortunately, several issues limit the utility of these methods in applied settings. One concern is their lack of ecological validity, namely, that the situations and observed behaviors do not accurately reflect real-world experiences (Sanders, Dadds, Johnston, & Cash, 1992). However, these methods may be useful for certain clinical assessment purposes even in the absence of ecological validity (Mash & Foster, 2001). For example, a clinician may wish to evaluate youth behavior in a specific, structured situation (e.g., a problem-solving discussion between a depressed youth and parent) as a step in determining whether an intermediate treatment goal has been met (e.g., whether the family has learned certain communication skills), even though the conditions and behaviors do not mirror those in natural settings. Pragmatic constraints (e.g., cost, training, and time requirements) also may limit the utility of these methods in clinical settings. Moreover, because these methods were designed for use in research, their focus is on differentiating between groups of relatively homogeneous youth rather than providing idiographic information about an individual youth and the complexity of his or her presenting problems (Mash & Foster, 2001). Even within research settings, the psychometric adequacy of these measures is not always sufficiently established, and idiosyncratic administration and coding procedures are used; this lack of standardization makes it difficult to transport these methods into clinical settings (Mash & Foster, 2001). In addition, many constructs assessed with these methods (e.g., social interaction) are characteristic of not only depression but also other disorders, resulting in limited discriminant validity. Evidence is limited concerning the clinical utility and incremental validity of laboratory and performance-based measures (Johnston & Murray, 2003; Mash & Foster, 2001), although these methods may provide information about targets for treatment (Garber & Kaminski, 2000). Given the time and cost necessary to use these methods, it is important to determine whether they provide information that other methods do not, and whether inclusion of these methods in an assessment battery significantly aids in diagnosis and case formulation, prognosis, treatment planning, or treatment outcome.

Review of Diagnostic Interviews

Schedule for Affective Disorders and Schizophrenia for School-Age Children

The Schedule for Affective Disorders and Schizophrenia for School-Age Children (K-SADS; Kaufman et al., 1997; Puig-Antich & Chambers, 1978), an interviewer-based schedule to assess psychopathology in youth ages 6 to 18, is designed for use by mental health professionals trained to make psychiatric diagnoses. Parent and child are interviewed separately; major discrepancies are resolved through a joint interview. Three versions are compatible with the DSM-IV. The K-SADS-P assesses current and past year diagnoses only. The K-SADS-E (epidemiological version) and

K-SADS-P/L assess lifetime and current diagnoses, and the K-SADS-P/L includes an 82-item screening interview. Although both the K-SADS-P/L and K-SADS-P include a global assessment scale, the K-SADS-P also includes clinical severity and improvement ratings, and the Hamilton Depression Rating Scale, making it more sensitive to treatment effects. Administration of the K-SADS ranges between 1.5 and 3 hours (Ambrosini, 2000).

Preliminary data for the K-SADS-P IV-R, the DSM-IV version of the K-SADS-P, indicate excellent agreement for current (kappa = .90) and lifetime (kappa = 1.00) MDD diagnoses (Ambrosini, 2000; Kaufman et al., 1997). Studies that use the K-SADS as the *criterion* for establishing validity reveal that scores from self-report, parent-report, and clinician rating scales distinguish between youth with MDD and nondepressed youth (Kaufman et al., 1997). Moreover, youth who met criteria for depression on the K-SADS at age 9 reported more depressive symptoms on the Diagnostic Interview Schedule for Children at ages 11 and 13 (McGee & Williams, 1988).

Child and Adolescent Psychiatric Assessment

The Child and Adolescent Psychiatric Assessment (CAPA; Angold & Costello, 1995) is a semistructured interview designed to assess psychiatric diagnoses occurring in the past 3 months in youth ages 9 to 17. Administration time is 1 to 2 hours. The interview includes an assessment of psychosocial impairment and clinician ratings of behaviors observed in the interview. The CAPA includes a glossary with operational definitions of symptoms, facilitating its use by not only clinicians but also highly trained lay interviewers. The CAPA is appropriate for use in clinical and epidemiological research (Angold & Costello, 2000).

Test–retest reliability of CAPA depression diagnoses is high for MDD (kappa = .90) and dysthymia (kappa = .85). Interrater reliability of MDD diagnoses also is high (intraclass correlation coefficient [ICC] = .88; Angold & Costello, 1995). There are limited data on the association of the CAPA with other depression measures. In one study, adolescents with a CAPA MDD diagnosis scored higher on the Mood and Feelings Questionnaire than youth without an MDD diagnosis (Thapar & McGuffin, 1998). Other support for the validity of CAPA depression diagnoses includes

higher prevalence of MDD diagnoses in adolescent girls than in boys (Angold, Costello, & Worthman, 1998), and higher concordance of MDD diagnoses in monozygotic than in dizygotic twins (Eaves et al., 1997).

Diagnostic Interview for Children and Adolescents

The most recent version of the Diagnostic Interview for Children and Adolescents (DICA), the DICA-IV (Reich, 2000), is a semistructured interview designed to assess lifetime psychiatric diagnoses in youth ages 6 to 17. This version of the DICA assesses DSM-III-R and DSM-IV criteria. Separate interviews are available for children (ages 6–12) and adolescents (ages 13–17). The DICA can be administered by laypeople after 2 to 4 weeks of training; the computer version may be self-administered. Administration time is typically 1 to 2 hours.

One week test–retest reliability for the DICA-IV is high for adolescents (kappa = .80) but lower for children (kappa = .55). In one community sample using the DICA-R (revised version), interrater agreement was poor for interviews of children (kappa = .00) and moderate for interviews of adolescents (kappa = .45); agreement between child and parent reports was better than that between adolescent and parent reports (kappa = .77 and .31, respectively) (Boyle et al., 1993). Low to moderate agreement between clinicians also has been obtained in outpatient samples of youth (Ezpeleta et al., 1997). Youth diagnosed with MDD using the DICA score higher on the Depression Self-Rating Scale (McClure, Rogeness, & Thompson, 1997), the Beck Depression Inventory (Beck & Steer, 1993), and the Center for Epidemiologic Studies Depression Scale (Olsson & von Knorring, 1997) than do youth without a diagnosis.

Diagnostic Interview Schedule for Children

The Diagnostic Interview Schedule for Children (DISC; Shaffer, Fisher, Lucas, Dulcan, & Schwab-Stone, 2000) is a structured, respondent-based interview for children, with content corresponding to the adult Diagnostic Interview Schedule (Robins, Helzer, Croughan, & Ratcliff, 1981). The DISC-IV assesses diagnoses in the past year and in the past 4 weeks, as well as lifetime diagnoses. The DISC and its revisions, the most recent of which is the DISC-IV (Shaffer et al., 2000), can be administered by lay interviewers after training. Child (DISC-C) and parent (DISC-P) versions are available. In the C-DISC-4.0, the computerized version of the DISC-IV, the computerized format aids in standardization of assessment, which is useful for research studies. However, because the C-DISC-4.0 is a structured interview, it is not possible to address problems such as misinterpretation of probes. Administration time is 1 to 2 hours.

Test–retest reliability of DISC-IV past-year MDD diagnoses was moderate for parent report ($r = .66$) and high for child report ($r = .92$) in a clinic sample. Estimates of diagnostic agreement in a community sample were low for child report (kappa = .37) and moderate for parent report (kappa = .55). Use of symptom counts to assess reliability in the same sample yielded higher reliability estimates (ICCs = .52 for child report and .79 for parent report). Validity information is not available for the DISC-IV affective disorder scales. Earlier versions of the DISC showed low correlations with the Children's Depression Inventory (Angold, Prendergast, et al., 1995) and low concordance between DISC depression diagnoses and clinician diagnoses (e.g., Pellegrino, Singh, & Carmanico, 1999). Earlier versions of the DISC yielded high numbers of false-positive depression diagnoses.

Review of Self-Report Rating Scales

Beck Depression Inventory

Although designed for adults, the Beck Depression Inventory (BDI; Beck & Steer, 1993) is the rating scale most often used with adolescents. For each of the 21 items, respondents indicate which of four statements varying in severity best describes how they have been feeling for the past week. Scores range from 0 to 63. The BDI can be completed in less than 10 minutes. A 13-item short form is available (Bennett, Ambrosini, et al., 1997). The BDI for Primary Care (BDI-PC; Beck, Guth, Steer, & Ball, 1997), a 7-item scale, has been used successfully with adolescents in medical settings (e.g., Winter, Steer, Jones-Hicks, & Beck, 1999).

Internal consistency of the BDI in adolescent samples generally is high (e.g., Ambrosini, Metz, Bianchi, Rabinovich, & Undie, 1991), and the BDI has demonstrated validity in adolescent samples, as evidenced by correlations with other depression self-report measures

(e.g., Roberts et al., 1991). A comparison of the BDI and the Reynolds Adolescent Depression Scale (RADS) revealed that the BDI was more sensitive to changes in severity of depression due to treatment (Reynolds & Coats, 1986). The BDI discriminates between depressed and nondepressed adolescents in hospital (Carter & Dacey, 1996) and outpatient (Ambrosini et al., 1991) settings. However, some research shows that elevated scores on the BDI yield a high number of false-positive cases—that is, adolescents with elevated BDI scores who do not meet diagnostic criteria for depression—and few true-positive cases of depression (Roberts et al., 1991). Also, some research suggests that high scores on the BDI are not specific to depression, but indicate dysphoria or general psychological distress (Kutcher & Marton, 1989).

Cutoff scores of 16 and 10 on the BDI maximize sensitivity and specificity of MDD and dysthymia diagnoses, respectively, in community samples (Barrera & Garrison-Jones, 1988); optimal cutoff scores for outpatient and inpatient adolescent samples generally are lower (e.g., Ambrosini et al., 1991). Additionally, sensitivity and specificity in treated samples are considerably lower than that in community samples (Barrerra & Garrison-Jones, 1988; Kashani, Sherman, Parker, & Reid, 1990). Other concerns include the lack of items relevant to school and the absence of parallel parent and teacher forms (Myers & Winters, 2002).

The BDI-II (Beck, Steer, & Brown, 1996), the most recent revision of the BDI, is updated to be consistent with DSM-IV criteria for MDD. According to the manual, the BDI-II is appropriate for adolescents as young as age 13; however, expert raters and inpatient adolescents identified some items that are less relevant to adolescent depression (e.g., "loss of interest in sex," "past failure") (Osman, Kopper, Barrios, Gutierrez, & Bagge, 2004). The BDI-II has high internal consistency (estimates $\geq .90$) in samples of adolescent inpatients (Krefetz, Steer, Gulab, & Beck, 2002; Kumar, Steer, Teitelman, & Villacis, 2002) and correlates with other depression rating scales, such as the RADS ($r = .84$; Krefetz et al., 2002), and suicide risk measures, such as suicidal ideation and feelings of hopelessness (Osman et al., 2004). BDI-II scores discriminate between adolescents who meet criteria for MDD and those who do not (Krefetz et al., 2002; Kumar et al.,

2002). In one study of adolescent inpatients (Kumar et al., 2002), a cutoff score of 21 demonstrated the highest positive predictive power of .85 (i.e., the proportion of adolescents scoring above the cutoff who meet diagnostic criteria for depression) and negative predictive power of .83 (i.e., the proportion of adolescents scoring below the cutoff who do *not* meet diagnostic criteria for depression).

Children's Depression Inventory

The Children's Depression Inventory (CDI; Kovacs, 1992) is a downward extension of the BDI, with language and format changes to accommodate youth age 7 and older. For each of 27 items, youth select one of three response alternatives that vary in severity. For approximately half of the items, alternatives are listed in order of increasing severity; the order is reversed for the remaining items. The CDI takes about 10–20 minutes to complete. An abbreviated version (Kovacs, 1992) and a parent version (Wierzbicki, 1987) are available. Correspondence of parent and teacher ratings with self-reports is low to moderate, with highest agreement about school functioning (Bennett, Pendley, & Bates, 1997; Ines & Sacco, 1992).

Internal consistency of the CDI exceeds .80 in most studies (e.g., Crowley, Worchel, & Ash, 1992; Smucker, Craighead, Craighead, & Green, 1986). Most studies report test–retest reliability coefficients close to .70, but coefficients range from as low as .38 (Saylor, Finch, Spirito, & Bennett, 1984) to as high as .88 (Finch, Saylor, Edwards, & McIntosh, 1987). The CDI correlates significantly with other depression self-report measures (e.g., Shain, Naylor, & Alessi, 1990). Evidence for discriminant validity is mixed. Some studies indicate that the CDI distinguishes between youth with depression and nondepressed youth (e.g., Timbremont, Braet, & Dreessen, 2004), but others suggest poor discriminant validity, sensitivity, and specificity (e.g., Ambrosini, 2000). For screening purposes, a cutoff score of 19 or 20 has been suggested for youth in the general population, where the prevalence of depression is low; cutoff scores of 12 or 13 have been recommended for clinic-referred samples (Kovacs, 1992). The CDI seems to be more sensitive to change in response to treatment than the Children's Depression Rating Scale—Revised and the Reynolds Child Depression Scale

(Stark, Reynolds, & Kaslow, 1987). However, some research documents significant reductions in CDI scores at a second assessment, when no treatment was provided (Meyer, Dyck, & Petrinack, 1989). Therefore, clinicians should use the CDI in combination with other information before concluding that there are positive treatment effects on depression.

Center for Epidemiologic Studies Depression Scale

The Center for Epidemiologic Studies Depression Scale (CES-D; Radloff, 1977), a 20-item measure, was originally developed for use with community samples of adults. Respondents indicate the frequency of depressive symptoms using a 3-point scale. Item content does not include all DSM criteria. Internal consistency of the CES-D with adolescent samples is high, with coefficients exceeding .85 (Garrison, Addy, Jackson, McKeown, & Waller, 1991; Roberts et al., 1991). The CES-D has only a moderate correlation with the Hamilton Depression Rating Scale (HDRS; $r = .48$; Roberts et al., 1991), but a high correlation with the RADS (r's > .74; Reynolds, 1987). Test–retest reliability in a community sample of adolescents was adequate ($r = .61$). The most frequently used cutoff score for the CES-D is 16, which indicates moderate depression, although several studies indicate that this cutoff yields false-positive diagnoses of depression in nondepressed youth (e.g., Roberts et al., 1991). Optimal cutoff scores for determining MDD in adolescents range from 12 to 22 for boys and 22 to 24 for girls (Garrison et al., 1991; Roberts et al., 1991). Convergence between CES-D scores indicating depression and K-SADS depression diagnoses is low (Roberts et al., 1991).

The child version of the CES-D, the CES-DC, does not correlate with the CDI in young children, but it has a moderate correlation ($r = .61$) in adolescents (Faulstich, Carey, Ruggiero, Enyart, & Gresham, 1986). Generally, the discriminant validity of the CES-DC is poor (Faulstich et al., 1986), because scores correlate moderately with conduct disorder (Andrews, Lewinsohn, Hops, & Roberts, 1993) and do not distinguish between depressed children and children with no diagnosis (Fendrich, Weissman, & Warner, 1990). Like the CES-D, the CES-DC has problems with sensitivity and specificity (Blatt, Hart, Quinlan, Leadbeater, &

Auerbach, 1993). Use of the CES-D or CES-DC to assess change in symptoms should be avoided given these problems.

Mood and Feelings Questionnaire

The Mood and Feelings Questionnaire (MFQ; Angold, Costello, et al., 1995), developed to assess symptoms of depression in youth ages 8–18, includes 30 or 35 items (depending on the version used) assessing DSM-III-R criteria for depressive disorders and other clinically significant symptoms. Respondents indicate the degree to which each statement applies to their experiences in the past 2 weeks using a 3-point Likert scale. A short form of the MFQ (SMFQ), composed of 13 items that showed optimal discriminative ability and internal consistency, is available. Parent versions of the full and short forms are available. The MFQ and SMFQ are strongly correlated (r's > .90) for both the child and parent versions (Angold, Costello, et al., 1995). The MFQ can be completed in about 10 minutes.

Stability estimates using the full MFQ exceed .70 (e.g., Costello, Benjamin, Angold, & Silver, 1991; Wood, Knoll, Moore, & Harrington, 1995). Concordance between child and parent reports is low (r's = .25 and .30, for the full and short forms, respectively). The full and short forms of the MFQ have moderate correlations with the CDI and the DISC-C, but the parent versions have low correlations with the CDI and DISC-P (Angold, Costello, et al., 1995). With a diagnosis of MDD on the K-SADS as the criterion, diagnostic accuracy of the MFQ child version is generally better than the MFQ parent version, and similar to the CDI and BDI (Wood et al., 1995). Scores on the MFQ child version discriminate between psychiatric inpatients with a DISC affective diagnosis and those with no affective diagnosis (Pellegrino et al., 1999).

Reynolds Adolescent Depression Scale and Reynolds Child Depression Scale

The Reynolds Adolescent Depression Scale (RADS; Reynolds, 1994) is a 30-item scale designed to assess depressive symptoms in youth ages 13 to 18. Seven items are uncharacteristic of depression to reduce the likelihood of response sets. Respondents indicate the frequency of each symptom on a 4-point scale;

possible scores range from 30 to 120. Content of the RADS does not include all symptoms of depression. Norms are based on an ethnically and geographically diverse sample of adolescents. The RADS takes about 10 minutes to complete (Reynolds, 1994).

Several studies report high internal consistency of the RADS in community and clinical samples, with estimates exceeding .90 (e.g., Dalley, Bolocofsky, Alcorn, & Baker, 1992; Reynolds, 1987, 1989). Test–retest reliability at 6 and 12 weeks is approximately .80 (Reynolds, 1987). The RADS has strong correlations with other depression measures, such as the CDI and CES-D, with correlations exceeding .70 (Reynolds, 1987). The RADS also is strongly correlated with the HDRS (r = .83; Reynolds, 1987) and the Children's Depression Rating Scale—Revised ([CDRS-R], r = .78; Shain et al., 1990). A cutoff score of 77 indicates clinically significant impairment in daily functioning. Using this cutoff score and diagnoses based on the HDRS, the RADS had high specificity (96%) but considerably lower sensitivity (62%) (Reynolds, 1987). The RADS can detect alleviation of adolescents' depressive symptoms but is less sensitive than the BDI in this regard (Reynolds & Coats, 1986). It is concerning that the recommended cutoff score misses one-third of depressed adolescents.

The Reynolds Child Depression Scale (RCDS; Reynolds, 1989), designed for use with children ages 8–13, consists of 30 items. Like the RADS, the normative sample for the RCDS is socioeconomically and ethnically diverse. Internal consistency of the RCDS in the normative sample (.90) is similar to that in other studies (e.g., Reynolds, 1989). Four-week test–retest reliability is .85 (Reynolds & Graves, 1989). The RCDS correlates strongly with the CDI (r's = .70–.79) (e.g., Bartell & Reynolds, 1986; Reynolds, 1989) and the CDRS-R (r = .76) (Reynolds, 1989). Additionally, several studies indicate that the RCDS is sensitive to change in depressive symptoms due to treatment (Crosbie-Burnett & Newcomer, 1990; Rawson & Tabb, 1993).

Review of Clinician Rating Scales

Hamilton Depression Rating Scale

The Hamilton Depression Rating Scale (HDRS; Hamilton, 1960; Warren, 1997) was designed to assess the severity of depressive symptoms in adults, but it is often used with adolescents (Myers & Winters, 2002). The HDRS includes 21 items, but Hamilton (1960) suggested that only the first 17 be used to compute the total score. Assessors rate both the presence or absence, and, if applicable, the severity of specified depressive symptoms during the past week. Objective criteria are available for some items; for others, the assessor uses judgment to decide whether symptoms are *mild*, *moderate*, or *severe*. There are no standardized interview questions; therefore, the quality of the data depends a great deal on the skill of the clinician or researcher. Administration time is 10–30 minutes.

There are limited data describing the psychometric properties of the HDRS in youth. One-week test–retest reliability in adolescents is high ($r = .90$) (Kutcher & Marton, 1989). In community samples, the HDRS has moderate correlations with the BDI ($r = .50$) and CES-D ($r = .48$) (Roberts et al., 1991) and a high correlation with the RADS ($r = .72$) (Reynolds, 1987). Among inpatient adolescents, the HDRS has high correlations with the CDRS ($r = .92$), BDI ($r = .72$), and CDI ($r = .73$) (Shain et al., 1990). The HDRS distinguishes between adolescent outpatients with major depression and nondepressed adolescents (Kutcher & Marton, 1989). Some studies indicate that the HDRS is sensitive to changes in response to pharmacotherapy (Ambrosini et al., 1999) and cognitive-behavioral therapy (Franklin et al., 1998). There is some concern that items assessing somatic complaints and anxiety minimize the ability of this measure to differentiate between depression and anxiety (Myers & Winters, 2002). In addition, differential weighting of items, overrepresentation of vegetative symptoms, and incomplete representation of DSM criteria make it difficult to interpret scores on the HDRS (Zimmerman, Posternak, & Chelminski, 2005).

Children's Depression Rating Scale—Revised

The Children's Depression Rating Scale—Revised (CDRS; Poznanski, Cook, & Carroll, 1979), a modification of the HDRS, is designed for use with children ages 6–12, but it is also used with adolescents (Myers & Winters, 2002). The current revised version, the CDRS-R (Poznanski & Mokros, 1999), includes 17 items. Fourteen items are rated on a 7-point severity scale, and the remaining items are rated on a 5-point severity scale. Assessors rate both the presence or absence, and, if applicable, the severity of each depressive symptom, and depressed facial affect, speech, and activity based on observations during the interview. It is recommended that the assessor interview youth and parents or other informants separately, then combine information from all sources. Possible scores for the child interview range from 17 to 113; possible scores for interviews with other informants range from 14 to 94. Administration time can exceed 30 minutes, depending on how many informants are interviewed (Overholser, Brinkman, Lehnert, & Ricciardi, 1995).

Two-week test–retest reliability of the CDRS is high ($r = .86$; Poznanski et al., 1984), and internal consistency is adequate (Myers & Winters, 2002). A number of studies show poor agreement between informants (e.g., Mokros, Poznanski, Grossman, & Freeman, 1987). The CDRS-R correlates significantly with the HDRS and with the CDI and RADS for females (r's = .89 and .86, respectively) but not for males (r's = .41 and .48, respectively). The CDRS-R has been used in treatment studies to assess change in severity of depression (e.g., Emslie et al., 1997). However, in preadolescent children, it might be less sensitive than the CDI (Stark et al., 1987). Given the inclusion of physiological symptoms, the CDRS might overpredict depression in children with medical or physical complaints (e.g., Aronen et al., 1996).

Review of Parent and Teacher Behavior Checklists and DSM-Referenced Scales

Achenbach Scales

The Achenbach System of Empirically Based Assessment (ASEBA) was designed to assess behavior problems and social competencies in preschool (ages 1½ to 5 years) and school-age (ages 6–18) youth. The Child Behavior Checklist (CBCL/6–18; Achenbach & Rescorla, 2001), one of the most widely used behavior rating scales, consists of 118 items, each rated on a 3-point scale. The CBCL yields information about a range of behavior syndromes, including anxious–depressed behavior, somatic complaints, withdrawn behavior, attention problems, social problems, and aggression–delinquency. These empirically derived scales can be combined to create overall internalizing, externalizing, and total problem scores. The CBCL has been normed in clinical and community samples by age and gender. A parallel Teacher Report Form (TRF/6–18; Achenbach & Rescorla, 2001) is available, with most items identical to the parent form. The CBCL and TRF can be completed in 8–10 minutes.

The reliability of CBCL depression items is low compared to the other scales (Clarizio, 1994), perhaps because these symptoms are less easily observed. The CBCL distinguishes between referred and nonreferred youth (Achenbach, 1991; Drotar, Stein, & Perrin, 1995), although it is less sensitive to variations in youth scoring in the normal range (Drotar et al., 1995) and less able to differentiate among specific dimensions of internalizing problems (Song, Singh, & Singer, 1994). For example, the Withdrawn scale predicts anxiety and depressive disorders (Kasius, Ferdinand, van den Berg, & Verhulst, 1997). Another concern is that the Anxious–Depressed subscale combines symptoms of anxiety and depression that have been shown to be distinct (e.g., Cantwell, 1988), and some items assessing depression (e.g., "unhappy, sad, depressed") are included on more than one scale. Consequently, the empirically derived scales of the CBCL have limited ability to predict depression. One study indicated that a subset of depression items from the CBCL discriminates between youth with MDD and those with no diagnosis (e.g., Rey & Morris-Yates, 1991); in another study, adolescents' scores on the Anxious–Depressed subscale predicted MDD analogue scores (Gerhardt, Compas, Connor, & Achenbach, 1999). Similarly, an empirically derived set of depression items showed greater sensitivity to MDD than did the Anxious–Depressed subscale (Lengua et al., 2001), suggesting that a subset of depression items might be useful for depression assessments.

Child Symptom Inventory

The Child Symptom Inventory (CSI) is a DSM-IV–referenced rating scale that screens for affective and behavioral symptoms of the major childhood disorders, including MDD and dysthymia (Gadow & Sprafkin, 2002). Items are rated on a 4-point scale. Parent and teacher versions are available. The 97-item parent version and the 77-item teacher version can be completed in 15–20 minutes. There are two options for scoring the CSI: a symptom severity score and a symptom count.

Internal consistency of the Major Depression and Dysthymia scales is moderate for the parent version (.59 and .68, respectively) and high for the teacher version (.75 and .73, respectively). Interrater reliability of the symptom severity scores for both depression scales is adequate ($r = .52$). The depression scales are significantly correlated with the Withdrawn, Somatic Complaints, and Anxious–Depressed subscales of the CBCL and TRF (Gadow & Sprafkin, 2002), providing evidence for good convergent validity but poor specificity (Mattison, Gadow, Sprafkin, Nolan, & Schneider, 2003). The teacher-rated CSI Depression scale distinguishes between youth classified as depressed and nondepressed according to DSM-IV criteria (Mattison et al., 2003).

Review of Peer Ratings

Many symptoms of depression (e.g., dysphoria, lack of involvement in activities) may be observed by peers during daily interactions. Peer ratings can be obtained in a number of settings, increasing their ecological validity. The best known peer-report method for assessing depression, the Peer Nomination Inventory for Depression (PNID; Lefkowitz & Tesiny, 1980), includes 20 items that assess four domains of functioning: affective, cognitive, motivational, and vegetative. Internal consistency is high ($r = .85$) (Lefkowitz & Tesiny, 1980), but there is limited information regarding the ability of the PNID to discriminate between youth with subclinical depressive symptoms and those with clinical depression. One study found that the PNID did not discriminate between major depression and dysthymic disorder (Ezpeleta, Polaino, Domenech, & Domenech, 1990). Use in clinical settings is limited by a variety of practical constraints, including time required to complete ratings and the absence of a stable peer group with sufficient familiarity to provide accurate ratings.

Review of Assessment Measures in Young Children

The only scale designed specifically to assess depressive symptoms in preschool age children is the Preschool Feelings Checklist (Luby,

Heffelfinger, Koenig-McNaught, Brown, & Spitznagel, 2004), a 16-item brief screening measure for parents. This measure has good internal consistency (alpha = .76) and discriminates between depressed and nondepressed preschool children. When used with a version of the DISC-IV modified for use with parents of preschool children, sensitivity and specificity are better than that found with the CBCL Internalizing scale (Luby et al., 2004).

The Berkeley Puppet Interview (BPI; Ablow et al., 1999), an interactive, semistructured interview, uses puppets to elicit ratings of psychiatric symptoms in young children. Test–retest reliability is moderately low in clinic and community samples (r's = .42 and .43, respectively). Internal consistency of the depression subscale is good in clinical samples (alpha = .75), but much lower in community samples (alpha = .36). The depression subscale of the BPI distinguishes between clinic-referred and community samples of children (Ablow et al., 1999).

The McArthur Health Behavior Questionnaire (HBQ; Essex et al., 2002) is designed to assess several aspects of young children's functioning, including depressive symptoms. Parent and teacher forms are available. Mother and teacher reports on the HBQ show adequate internal consistency and good test–retest reliability in clinic and community samples, and discriminate between clinic-referred and community samples of children (Ablow et al., 1999). In addition, mother report on the HBQ identifies more children with internalizing psychopathology than does the DISC-IV and is associated with teacher reports of impairment (Luby et al., 2002).

The CBCL and TRF have downward extensions that can be used with children as young as 18 months. These are the most widely used parent and teacher rating scales to assess psychopathology in young children (Achenbach & Rescorla, 2004), but the sensitivity of these measures to early MDD warrants further research (Luby et al., 2004). Diagnostic interviews also have been modified for use with young children. A downward extension of the CAPA, the Preschool Age Psychiatric Assessment (PAPA) (Egger & Angold, 2004), was developed for children ages 2 to 5. Interrater reliability is comparable to that of other semistructured diagnostic interviews. Similarly, a downward extension of the DISC-IV is being developed (Lucas, Fisher, & Luby, 1998).

ASSESSMENT OF CO-OCCURRING SYMPTOMS AND RELATED CONSTRUCTS

As noted earlier, a comprehensive assessment of depression includes the evaluation of co-occurring psychopathology and impairment across a variety of domains. Here we provide a brief summary of some relevant constructs of interest. Because many of the measures of related constructs have been used primarily in a research context, it is not always clear which of these would have utility in a clinical setting. Adapting these measures for application in practice and determining their clinical utility await further research.

Assessment of Co-Occurring Psychopathology

Both diagnostic interviews and rating scales may be used to assess co-occurring symptoms and disorders. However, self-report and other-informant rating scales often have limited discriminant validity. In particular, these measures tend not to distinguish adequately between depressive and anxiety disorders, due to their focus on symptoms of general distress (Joiner, Catanzaro, & Laurent, 1996). Consistent with contemporary theoretical conceptualizations of depression and anxiety, such as the tripartite model (Watson et al., 1995), it is becoming increasingly clear that assessment measures must differentiate between the shared (i.e., general distress) and unique components of depression (i.e., anhedonia and low positive affect), and anxiety (i.e., physiological arousal or somatic tension) (Lonigan, Carey, & Finch, 1994).

A few measures distinguish between components of depression and of anxiety. The Positive and Negative Affect Scale for Children (PANAS-C; Laurent et al., 1999) has high internal consistency, and good convergent and discriminant validity in community and inpatient samples (Laurent et al., 1999; Lonigan, Hooe, David, & Kistner, 1999). The PANAS-C includes 27 adjectives that reflect positive and negative affect. Youth rate the applicability of each adjective in the past few weeks, using a 5-point scale. Consistent with the tripartite model, the Negative Affect scale of the PANAS is associated with both anxiety and depression, whereas the Positive Affect scale is more strongly associated with depression than with anxiety (e.g., Lonigan, Phillips, & Hooe, 2003). The 18-item Physiological Hyperarousal Scale for Children (PH-C; Laurent,

Catanzaro, & Joiner, 2004), designed as a companion to the PANAS-C, has shown preliminary evidence of validity. The Affect and Arousal Scale for Children (AFARS; Chorpita et al., 2000) is a 27-item, self-report measure of positive and negative affect, and physiological hyperarousal. Respondents rate each item on a 4-point scale. The AFARS has high internal consistency and validity in a community sample (Chorpita et al., 2000; Daleiden, Chorpita, & Lu, 2000). In one study, both the PANAS-C and AFARS Negative Affect scales predicted self-reports of depression and anxiety. The PANAS-C Positive Affect scale discriminated between mood disorders and other disorders, but the AFARS Positive Affect scale did not (Chorpita & Daleiden, 2002), suggesting that the PANAS-C might be more useful for identifying depression. Although these measures include an assessment of (low) positive affect, they do not assess other aspects of anhedonia characteristic of depression (e.g., loss of pleasure, loss of interest in activities, boredom). Factor analyses of another recently developed measure, the Youth Mood and Anxiety Symptom Questionnaire (Y-MASQ; Rudolph et al., 2007), adapted from the adult version of this measure (MASQ; Watson et al., 1995), reveal that anhedonia emerges as a distinct factor from other dimensions of depression and anxiety in youth, suggesting that the specific assessment of anhedonia might be useful.

Assessment of Depression-Related Impairment

Biological Processes

Empirical examination of biological processes hypothesized to be associated with depression in youth has yielded mixed findings. Here we provide a brief overview of some methods to assess biological processes. If further research reveals evidence for the specificity of these methods to depression, their use in clinical practice to assess vulnerability to depression, to aid in diagnosis, or to evaluate treatment response should be considered.

Pharmacological challenge tests examine physiological responses to the administration of dexamethasone and growth hormone–releasing hormone (GHRH). Levels of hormones typically affected by these agents (cortisol for the former and growth hormone for the latter) are measured prior to and following the test. Atypical responses to these challenges (i.e., failure to suppress cortisol and blunted growth hormone responses) are characteristic of depressed and high-risk youth, but the specificity of these responses to depression is unclear (Dahl et al., 2000).

Possible sleep disturbances can be assessed using sleep polysomnography. This method typically requires an overnight stay in a sleep laboratory, where the individual is monitored while sleeping. Common forms of monitoring include electroencephalography (EEG; to record brain waves), electro-oculography (EOG; to record eye movement), and electrocardiography (ECG; to measure electrical activity in the heart). This procedure is minimally invasive. However, inconsistent findings regarding sleep abnormalities in depressed youth suggest that this method is not likely to be a useful approach for diagnosing depression (Bloch, 1997).

Identification of structural and functional brain abnormalities associated with depression requires the use of imaging techniques (e.g., magnetic resonance imaging [MRI] and computed tomography [CT]), and functional brain imaging techniques (e.g., single-photon emission computed tomography [SPECT] and positron emission tomography [PET]). The cost and equipment required for these methods limit their use in most settings, and minimal data recommend their use with depressed youth at this point. Other practical concerns also must be considered. For example, although MRI scanners do not use radiation, they might be noisy and are very sensitive to movement, which might make it difficult to obtain valid results in young children. Additionally, closed MRIs might cause discomfort in some youth. CT scans involve exposure to radiation in the form of X-rays, and the contrast dye used (often iodine) may cause an allergic reaction. Radioactive drugs also are used in PET (Rauch & Renshaw, 1995).

Thus, although emerging evidence points to some possible biological markers of depression in youth, many of the methods are not feasible in clinical settings due to the need for sophisticated equipment, invasive procedures, and appropriate training. Several of the methods are, of course, more feasible in hospital settings, in which access to equipment and training is more common. However, the inconsistency of evidence for particular types of biological dysfunction in depressed youth and the lack of specificity of many measures to depression limit their usefulness as diagnostic tools.

Social-Cognitive and Cognitive Processes

A large number of self-report measures have been developed to assess negative cognitions associated with depression, including constructs such as dysfunctional attitudes, pessimistic attributional style, low perceptions of competence and control, and hopelessness (for a review, see Winters, Myers, & Proud, 2002). These measures vary in their psychometric properties, and most lack sufficient normative information, which make recommendation of specific measures for use in clinical practice difficult.

Laboratory methods are less subject to the demand characteristics that might compromise the validity of self-report (Garber & Kaminski, 2000). Several information-processing tasks have demonstrated utility in distinguishing between youth with depressive symptoms or disorders and other youth. Incidental recall tasks present respondents with information of different valence and assess differential recall of positive versus negative information. It is hypothesized that depressed individuals recall information that is congruent with their depressive schemas regarding the self and others. Research generally supports this proposition (e.g., Cole & Jordan, 1995; Rudolph et al., 1997; Shirk et al., 1997), lending validity to these tasks as useful measures of depression-related memory biases. However, some aspects of memory biases might be age-dependent, not arising until adolescence (Cole & Jordan, 1995). Information-processing tasks (e.g., Stroop color-naming task) also have been used to assess attentional biases characteristic of depression, but research generally does not indicate an attentional bias for negative words among depressed youth (Neshat-Doost, Moradi, Taghavi, Yule, & Dalgleish, 2000). Because these studies employ methods developed for adults, additional research using developmentally based instruments is needed to examine attentional biases in depressed youth.

Depressed youth also may experience cognitive impairment, including deficits in intellectual functioning, speed of processing, and memory, although deficits may be more apparent in school performance than in cognitive abilities (Kovacs & Goldston, 1991). Empirical evidence is mixed, but some research indicates that, compared to nondepressed youth, depressed youth perform more poorly on complex reasoning and problem-solving tasks

(Kaslow, Tanenbaum, Abramson, Peterson, & Seligman, 1983), demonstrate larger Performance IQ deficits relative to their Verbal IQ (Brumback, Wilson, & Staton, 1984), and show a decreased posterior right-hemisphere bias in the processing of emotion (Flynn & Rudolph, 2007).

Selection of measures to assess social-cognitive processes depends on the construct(s) of interest and the purpose of the assessment (e.g., some measures show better discriminant validity for depression vs. anxiety). Developmental stage also is important to consider. Many of the measures were modified from those developed for adults, and adequate psychometric properties and clinical utility of these measures have not been established in youth, especially prior to adolescence. This is of particular concern given evidence that some aspects of cognitive vulnerability do not emerge until adolescence. Because assessment of these processes may inform possible targets for intervention or predictors of treatment outcome, further research aimed at standardization and validation for use in clinical settings would be helpful.

Interpersonal Processes

Impairment in social relationships may be assessed to a certain degree with depression rating scales and interviews, many of which assess certain aspects of interpersonal functioning (e.g., social withdrawal, feelings of loneliness). Structured behavioral observations of social interactions are another means of assessing the interpersonal aspect of depression. For these tasks, youth are observed participating in an interaction with another person in a controlled setting. For instance, specific tasks might focus on cooperation, problem solving, or conflict resolution (for a review, see Garber & Kaminski, 2000). Interactions typically are videotaped and coded for behaviors characteristic of depression. Behaviors of particular relevance include, for example, depressive affect or behaviors (e.g., dysphoria, withdrawal), aggression (e.g., irritability, argumentativeness), and deficits in problem solving. This method has demonstrated the ability to discriminate between depressed and nondepressed youth (e.g., Rudolph et al., 1994; Sanders et al., 1992). One advantage is that social interaction tasks provide information about sequences of behavior between depressed youth and others (e.g., how parents respond to youth depressive behaviors) that might prove useful for treatment planning. However, as discussed, questions remain about the extent to which these methods can be adequately and systematically transported for use in clinical practice. Other methods also have demonstrated utility for obtaining information about interpersonal functioning. These include assessments of youth responses to hypothetical social situations (e.g., Narrative Completion Task; Shirk, Boergers, Eason, Van Horn, 1998), semistructured interviews (e.g., Social Adjustment Inventory for Children and Adolescents; John, Gammon, Prusoff, & Warner, 1987), and self-report rating scales (e.g., Social Adjustment Scale—Self Report; Weissman, Orvaschel, & Padian, 1980). Once again, the lack of normative information and data about clinical utility for many of these measures limits their usefulness in clinical practice at this time.

Other Domains

Several other domains are reasonable candidates for inclusion in an assessment of depression given their relevance for prognosis, treatment planning, and evaluation of treatment outcome. Given the aggregation of depression in families, assessment of family history of psychopathology, especially affective disorders, is informative both for determining risk and predicting course. This information may be obtained from diagnostic interviews with family members or by asking informants about history of psychopathology in other family members. Several standardized and well-validated semistructured interviews to assess family history of psychopathology are available, such as the Family Informant Schedule and Criteria (Mannuzza & Fyer, 1990) and the Family History—Research Diagnostic Criteria (Andreasen, Endicott, Spitzer, & Winokur, 1977). The time required to complete these interviews can range from 10 to 50 minutes per family member. Screening measures, such as the Family History Screen (Weissman et al., 2000), are a useful alternative when interviews are not possible.

Because stressful life circumstances are associated with the onset and maintenance of depressive symptoms (Kessler, 1997), they may be a useful part of an assessment. Life stress can be assessed with self-report measures (e.g., Johnson & McCutcheon, 1980) or semistruc-

tured interviews (e.g., Rudolph et al., 2000; Williamson et al., 2003). Although interviews provide richer information about the context and timing of stress (Duggal et al., 2000), administration and coding of these interviews are quite time-consuming and may not always be practical in clinical settings.

Assessment of general psychosocial functioning is useful to determine severity of impairment. Some diagnostic interviews (e.g., CAPA) and rating scales (e.g., Achenbach scales) assess psychosocial functioning. Alternatively, psychosocial functioning can be assessed with measures specific to functional impairment, such as the clinician-rated Children's Global Assessment Scale (C-GAS; Shaffer et al., 1983), Child and Adolescent Functional Assessment Scale (Hodges, 1999), and the Psychosocial Schedule for School-Age Children—Revised (Puig-Antich, Lukens, & Brent, 1986). The Social Adjustment Scale—Self Report (Weissman et al., 1980), a self-report rating scale, has demonstrated greater sensitivity to treatment effects in adolescents with comorbid MDD and conduct disorder than the C-GAS (Rohde, Clarke, Mace, Jorgensen, & Seeley, 2004). Overall, a comprehensive assessment of depression should include evaluation of multiple domains of functioning to determine the severity of impairment, to inform prognosis and treatment planning, and to evaluate the effects of treatment and possible change processes.

SUMMARY AND RECOMMENDATIONS FOR ASSESSMENT OF YOUTH DEPRESSION

Research has established adequate psychometric properties and, to a more limited extent, clinical utility for a range of methods and measures designed to assess youth depression. A number of criteria must therefore be considered when determining the most appropriate assessment approach within both research and clinical settings.

1. *Select measures that are appropriate for the specific purpose and stage of assessment.* Selection of an appropriate assessment tool depends in part on the level of depression being assessed, which in turn reflects the taxonomic system of interest. Rating scales are appropriate if the goal is to assess symptom severity, whereas structured or semistructured inter-

views are required if the goal is to determine whether diagnostic criteria are met. The goal might depend in part on the stage of assessment. For example, in a "multiple-gating" approach (Reynold, 1994), ratings scales of depression and associated symptoms are used as screening tools, followed by more intensive interviews where indicated. Some ratings scales (e.g., CBCL/TRF, CDI) have extensive normative information and established cutoff scores that maximize their potential to select youth who will likely meet criteria for a diagnosis. However, these scales cannot be used as diagnostic instruments, because they have only moderate specificity for depression and do not provide information about the timing and duration of symptoms, history of disorder, associated impairment, or exclusionary criteria. Some rating scales demonstrate sensitivity to change in symptoms following treatment, suggesting that they may be useful at later stages of assessment to monitor treatment progress. Evaluating the psychometric adequacy of a measure also depends on the general purpose of the assessment. For example, the relative balance of desired sensitivity and specificity might be different for case formulation and prognosis versus treatment planning versus evaluation of treatment effectiveness. Different criteria for psychometric characteristics also are likely to be used in research versus clinical settings. Finally, the psychometric adequacy of measures must be considered for the particular population of interest (e.g., one with a low vs. a high base rate of depression; different ethnic and cultural groups).

2. *Select measures that are developmentally appropriate.* Another issue to consider is the developmental appropriateness of assessment tools. As discussed, the phenomenology of depression, the frequency of particular co-occurring symptoms and types of impairment, and the predictors of depression vary across development. These factors need to be considered both when selecting an assessment instrument and when interpreting results. For example, measures of adolescent depression that represent downward extensions of measures developed for adults might not fully assess the symptoms and domains of impairment most relevant to youth. Moreover, measures adapted from those used in adults tend not to have normative information on parallel parent and teacher versions, which are useful for assessing youth depression.

Additionally, the cognitive and language abilities of youth should guide the assessment strategy. Young children's reports of depressive symptoms are less reliable than those of adolescents (Edelbrock et al., 1985), because accurate reporting requires cognitive skills not present in preadolescents, such as the ability to gauge how often and how intensely they experience symptoms, and whether symptoms represent a change from prior functioning (Clarizio, 1994). Reading and language ability also should be considered in selection of measures and determination of how to administer self-report measures, particularly when measures originally designed for adults are used with youth. Self-report should be used with caution in children under 8 years of age, although the validity of self-report of depression has been shown in children as young as 5 (Ialongo, Edelsohn, & Kellam, 2001). Recently, methods for the assessment of depression in preschoolers have received more attention and show some promise. Given preliminary evidence that child- versus adolescent-onset depressive disorders might differ, more research on developmental changes in the nature of depression is needed to determine whether the best assessment methods vary across developmental stage.

3. *Carefully consider how to integrate information across informants and methods.* Regardless of the age of youth, multi-informant report typically is desirable. Unfortunately, few formal guidelines exist regarding how to integrate this information and to resolve discrepancies. Moreover, limited data are available on the incremental validity of particular measures when added to a comprehensive assessment battery, and no information is available on incremental validity for predicting clinically relevant outcomes (e.g., whether youth will benefit from certain types of treatment, optimal length of treatment). The recommended use of multiple measures, methods, and informants also must be balanced with the time and cost-effectiveness and the availability of trained personnel. One reasonable approach is the multiple-gating procedure described earlier, in which relatively low-cost screening methods are used at earlier stages of assessment, followed by more intensive methods as indicated. Continued research is needed to determine the incremental validity of measures and their ability to predict clinical outcomes.

4. *Select measures that are feasible and useful for the setting.* The choice of assessment

tools is clearly informed by pragmatic issues, such as the time and cost associated with training, administration, and scoring, and by their utility in a particular setting of interest. Because most measures of youth depression were developed for use in research, less attention has been devoted to establishing feasibility and utility of the measures, and their ecological validity in clinical settings. However, time-intensive measures might be modified for use in clinical settings. For example, if time and cost constraints prohibit the administration of a full semistructured interview, portions most relevant to youth (based on rating scales and family interviews) might be administered. Similarly, analogue behavioral observations developed for research may be modified for use in clinical settings. For example, instead of using highly trained, but uninvolved, observers to rate behaviors, therapists and clients can review target behaviors together as a part of treatment planning and evaluation (Mash & Foster, 2001).

5. *Assess co-occurring psychopathology.* Given high rates of comorbidity, a thorough assessment of depression should include an evaluation of other major disorders. This supplemental evaluation is needed to facilitate differential diagnosis, to determine whether depression is the primary diagnosis, and to provide information about concurrent symptoms that might influence the prognosis, selection of treatment, or treatment response. Diagnostic interviews and many rating scales include an assessment of other relevant psychopathology. Selection of other domains of assessment may be guided in part by knowledge about base rates of co-occurring problems. For example, although many ratings scales do not include an evaluation of eating disorders or substance abuse, the heightened rates of eating disorders in depressed female adolescents and of substance abuse in depressed male adolescents suggest the usefulness of screening for these symptoms within these particular groups. A comprehensive assessment also must include an evaluation of specific features of depression that might influence prognosis and treatment, such as suicidal ideation, symptoms of mania or hypomania, and psychosis.

6. *Assess related areas of impairment.* A thorough assessment involves examining several key areas of functioning that often are compromised in depressed youth, such as social-cognitive processes, academic perfor-

mance, and interpersonal relations. At a most basic level, this information can identify areas of dysfunction and distress that warrant attention. Moreover, this information may influence decisions about the setting (e.g., inpatient, outpatient) and the modality of treatment (e.g., family therapy, social skills training). An ongoing assessment of these areas throughout treatment also provides information about processes of change and clinically relevant outcomes (e.g., improvement in peer relations or academic performance). Although relatively little is known about the implications of impairment in various life domains for clinical outcomes, preliminary research identifies several factors that predict the course of depression. For example, a strong family history of depression, high levels of borderline personality disorder symptoms, and conflict with parents (in females) predict an increased likelihood of recurrence, whereas low levels of excessive emotional reliance, low levels of antisocial and borderline personality disorder symptoms, and a positive attributional style (in males) protect against recurrence (Lewinsohn et al., 2000; Rohde et al., 2005). More research is needed to examine the power of other characteristics of youth and their contexts to predict course and outcome, and to determine treatment-specific responsiveness. Based on this information, a better determination may be made about the utility of evaluating particular characteristics and experiences associated with depression.

Another challenge that arises in determining appropriate supplemental areas of assessment is that many of the measures for evaluating related constructs (e.g., life stress interviews, physiological assessments) were developed for use in research and are less practical in clinical settings. Moreover, these measures often lack normative information and are less standardized than measures of depression. Thus, recommendation of many of these measures in clinical settings is premature. More research is needed to standardize and adapt these measures for use in clinical settings and to determine their utility for predicting clinical outcomes.

7. *Consider the natural course of depression.* Data on the course of depression suggest that most disorders remit over time, but that ongoing subsyndromal symptoms and recurrence are common. Research points to some specific features that predict the likelihood of recurrence (see earlier sections). Assessment of

these aspects of personal and family history provides important supplemental information that may guide features of treatment such as involvement of family members and the need for periodic "booster" sessions after the completion of treatment. However, few scientific data are available on the utility of such features of treatment for decreasing the likelihood of recurrence. It also is important to consider that the course of depression is characterized by both disorder-specific and disorder-nonspecific continuity; that is, early onset of depression might predict not only future depression but also other disorders. Thus, even if depression is the primary initial diagnosis, ongoing evaluation for other disorders is necessary. Unfortunately, little research is available to guide prediction of whether depression will follow a disorder-specific or nonspecific course, with the exception that youth with a personal or family history of depression are more likely to show depression recurrence (Weissman, Wolk, Wickramaratne, et al., 1999) and those with co-occurring behavior disorders are more likely to show subsequent disorders other than depression (Harrington et al., 1990).

CONCLUSION

Given the prevalence of depressive symptoms and disorders in youth, particularly during adolescence, along with the accompanying impairment and risk for subsequent dysfunction, it is critical to develop guidelines for assessing depression that maximize the success of early identification, prevention, and intervention efforts for youth. Significant progress has been made in developing psychometrically sound methods for assessing depression and associated impairment in youth, but less attention has been paid to establishing the clinical utility and feasibility of these methods in applied settings. Future work should be directed toward facilitating the application of knowledge and methods developed in research to clinical settings.

REFERENCES

Abela, J. R. Z. (2001). The hopelessness theory of depression: A test of the diathesis–stress and causal mediation components in third and seventh grade children. *Journal of Abnormal Child Psychology, 29,* 241–254.

Ablow, J. C., Measelle, J., Kraemer, H., Harrington, R., Luby, J., & Smider, N. (1999). The MacArthur Three-City Outcome Study: Evaluating multiinformant measures of young children's symptomatology. *Journal of the American Academy of Child and Adolescent Psychiatry, 38,* 1580–1590.

Abramson, L. Y., Metalsky, G. I., & Alloy, L. B. (1989). Hopelessness depression: A theory-based subtype of depression. *Psychological Review, 96,* 358–372.

Achenbach, T. M. (1991). *Integrative guide for the 1991 CBCL/4–18, YSR, and TRF profiles.* Burlington: University of Vermont, Department of Psychiatry.

Achenbach, T. M., Conners, C. K., Quay, H. C., Verhulst, F. C., & Howell, C. T. (1989). Replication of empirically derived syndromes as a basis for taxonomy of child/adolescent psychopathology. *Journal of Abnormal Child Psychology, 17,* 299–323.

Achenbach, T. M., & Rescorla, L. A. (2001). *Manual for ASEBA school-age forms and profiles.* Burlington: University of Vermont, Research Center for Children, Youth, and Families.

Achenbach, T. M., & Rescorla, L. A. (2004). Empirically based assessment and taxonomy: Application to infants and toddlers. In R. DelCarmen-Wiggins & A. Carter (Eds.), *Handbook of infant, toddler, and preschool mental health assessment* (pp. 161–184). New York: Oxford University Press.

Ambrosini, P. J. (2000). Historical development and present status of the Schedule for Affective Disorders and Schizophrenia for School-Age Children (K-SADS). *Journal of the American Academy of Child and Adolescent Psychiatry, 39,* 49–58.

Ambrosini, P. J., Metz, C., Bianchi, M. D., Rabinovich, H., & Undie, A. (1991). Concurrent validity and psychometric properties of the Beck Depression Inventory in outpatient adolescents. *Journal of the American Academy of Child and Adolescent Psychiatry, 30,* 51–57.

Ambrosini, P. J., Wagner, K. D., Biederman, J., Glick, I., Tan, C., Elia, J., et al. (1999). Multicenter open-label sertraline study in adolescent outpatients with major depression. *Journal of the American Academy of Child and Adolescent Psychiatry, 38,* 566–572.

American Psychiatric Association. (2000). *Diagnostic and statistical manual of mental disorders* (4th ed., text rev.). Washington, DC: Author.

Andreasen, N. C., Endicott, J., Spitzer, R. L., & Winokur, G. (1977). The family history method using diagnostic criteria. *Archives of General Psychiatry, 34,* 1229–1235.

Andrews, J. A., Lewinsohn, P. M., Hops, H., & Roberts, R. E. (1993). Psychometric properties of scales for the measurement of psychosocial variables associated with depression in adolescence. *Psychological Reports, 73,* 1019–1046.

Angold, A. (2002). Diagnostic interviews with parents and children. In M. Rutter & E. Taylor (Eds.), *Child* and adolescent psychiatry: Modern approaches (4th ed., pp. 32–51). Oxford, UK: Blackwell Scientific.

Angold, A., & Costello, E. J. (1995). A test–retest reliability study of child-reported psychiatric symptoms and diagnoses using the Child and Adolescent Psychiatric Assessment (CAPA-C). Psychological Medicine, 25, 755–762.

Angold, A., & Costello, E. J. (2000). The Child and Adolescent Psychiatric Assessment (CAPA). Journal of the American Academy of Child and Adolescent Psychiatry, 39, 39–48.

Angold, A., Costello, E. J., & Erkanli, A. (1999). Comorbidity. Journal of Child Psychology and Psychiatry, 40, 57–87.

Angold, A., Costello, E. J., Messer, S. C., Pickles, A., Winder, F., & Silver, D. (1995). Development of a short questionnaire for use in epidemiological studies of depression in children and adolescents. International Journal of Methods in Psychiatric Research, 5, 237–250.

Angold, A., Costello, E. J., & Worthman, C. M. (1998). Puberty and depression: The roles of age, pubertal status, and pubertal timing. Psychological Medicine, 28, 51–61.

Angold, A., Prendergast, M., Cox, A., Harrington, R., Simonoff, E., & Rutter, M. (1995). The Child and Adolescent Psychiatric Assessment (CAPA). Psychological Medicine, 25, 39–753.

Angst, J., Sellaro, R., & Merikangas, K. R. (2000). Depressive spectrum diagnoses. Comprehensive Psychiatry, 41, 39–47.

Arnold, B. R., & Matus, Y. E. (2000). Test translation and cultural equivalence methodologies for use with diverse populations. In I. Cuellar & F. A. Paniagua (Eds.), Handbook of multicultural mental health (pp. 121–136). San Diego, CA: Academic Press.

Aronen, E. T., Teicher, M. H., Geenens, D., Curtin, S., Glod, C. A., & Pahlavan, K. (1996). Motor activity and severity of depression in hospitalized prepubertal children. Journal of the American Academy of Child and Adolescent Psychiatry, 35, 752–763.

Barrera, M., & Garrison-Jones, C. V. (1988). Properties of the Beck Depression Inventory as a screening instrument for adolescent depression. Journal of Abnormal Child Psychology, 16, 263–273.

Bartell, N. P., & Reynolds, W. M. (1986). Depression and self-esteem in academically gifted and nongifted children: A comparison study. Journal of School Psychology, 24, 55–61.

Beck, A. T. (1967). Depression: Clinical, experimental, and theoretical aspects. New York: Harper & Row.

Beck, A. T., Guth, D., Steer, R. A., & Ball, R. (1997). Screening for major depression disorders in medical inpatients with the Beck Depression Inventory for Primary Care. Behaviour Research and Therapy, 35, 785–791.

Beck, A. T., & Steer, R. (1993). Beck Depression Inventory. San Antonio, TX: Psychological Corporation.

Beck, A. T., Steer, R. A., & Brown, G. K. (1996). Manual for the Beck Depression Inventory–II. San Antonio, TX: Psychological Corporation.

Bell-Dolan, D. J., Reaven, N. M., & Peterson, L. (1993). Depression and social functioning: A multidimensional study of the linkages. Journal of Clinical Child Psychology, 22, 306–315.

Bennett, D. S., Ambrosini, P. J., Bianchi, M., Barnett, D., Metz, C., & Rabinovich, H. (1997). Relationship of Beck Depression Inventory factors to depression among adolescents. Journal of Affective Disorders, 45, 127–134.

Bennett, D. S., Pendley, J. S., & Bates, J. E. (1997). Daughter and mother report of individual symptoms on the Children's Depression Inventory. Journal of Adolescent Health, 20, 51–57.

Bird, H. R., Gould, M. S., & Staghezza, B. (1992). Aggregating data from multiple informants in child psychiatry epidemiological research. Journal of the American Academy of Child and Adolescent Psychiatry, 31, 78–85.

Birmaher, B., Arbelaez, C., & Brent, D. (2002). Course and outcome of child and adolescent major depressive disorder. Child and Adolescent Psychiatric Clinics of North America, 11, 619–638.

Birmaher, B., Dahl, R. E., Williamson, D. E., Perel, J. M., Brent, D. A., & Axelson, D. A. (2000). Growth hormone secretion in children and adolescents at high risk for major depressive disorder. Archives of General Psychiatry, 57, 867–872.

Birmaher, B., Kaufman, J., Brent, D. A., Dahl, R. E., Perel, J. M., Al-Shabbout, M., et al. (1997). Neuroendocrine response to 5-hydroxy-L-tryptophan in prepubertal children at high risk of major depressive disorder. Archives of General Psychiatry, 54, 1113–1119.

Birmaher, B., Ryan, N. D., Williamson, D. E., Brent, D. A., Kaufman, J., & Dahl, R. E. (1996). Childhood and adolescent depression: A review of the past 10 years: Part I. Journal of the American Academy of Child and Adolescent Psychiatry, 35, 1427–1439.

Blatt, S. J., Hart, B., Quinlan, D. M., Leadbeater, B., & Auerbach, J. (1993). Interpersonal and self-critical dysphoria and behavioral problems in adolescents. Journal of Youth and Adolescence, 22, 253–269.

Bloch, K. E. (1997). Polysomnography: A systematic review. Technology and Health Care, 5, 285–305.

Boyle, M. H., Offord, D. R., Racine, Y., Sanford, M., Szatmari, P., Feliming, J. E., et al. (1993). Evaluation of the Diagnostic Interview for Children and Adolescents for use in general population samples. Journal of Abnormal Child Psychology, 21, 663–681.

Boyle, M., & Pickles, A. (1997). Influence of maternal depressive symptoms on ratings of childhood behavior. Journal of Abnormal Child Psychology, 25, 399–412.

Brumback, R. A., Wilson, H., & Staton, R. D. (1984). Behavioural problems in children taking theophylline. Lancet, 1, 958.

Burke, K. C., Burke, J. D., Regier, D. A., & Rae, D. S. (1990). Age at onset of selected mental disorders in five community populations. *Archives of General Psychiatry, 47*, 511–518.

Cantwell, D. P. (1988). *DSM-III studies*. In M. Rutter, A. H. Tuma, & I. S. Lann (Eds.), *Assessment and diagnosis in child psychopathology* (pp. 3–36). New York: Guilford Press.

Carter, C. L., & Dacey, C. M. (1996). Validity of the Beck Depression Inventory, MMPI, and Rorschach in assessing adolescent depression. *Journal of Adolescence, 19*, 223–231.

Caspi, A., Sugden, K., Moffitt, T. E., Taylor, A., Craig, I. W., Harrington, H., et al. (2003). Influence of life stress on depression: Moderation by a polymorphism in the 5-HTT gene. *Science, 34*, 386–389.

Chang, D. F. (2002). Understanding the rates and distribution of mental disorders. In K. S. Kurasaki, S. Okazaki, & S. Sue (Eds.), *Asian American mental health: Assessment theories and methods* (pp. 9–27). New York: Kluwer Academic/Plenum Press.

Choi, H. (2002). Understanding adolescent depression in ethnocultural context. *Advances in Nursing Science, 25*, 71–85.

Chorpita, B. F., & Daleiden, E. L. (2002). Tripartite dimensions of emotion in a child clinical sample: Measurement strategies and implications for clinical utility. *Journal of Consulting and Clinical Psychology, 70*, 1150–1160.

Chorpita, B. F., Daleiden, E. L., Moffitt, C., Yim, L., & Umemoto, L. A. (2000). Assessment of tripartite factors of emotion in children and adolescents: I. Structural validity and normative data of an affect and arousal scale. *Journal of Psychopathology and Behavioral Assessment, 22*, 141–160.

Cicchetti, D., & Toth, S. L. (1998). The development of depression in children and adolescents. *American Psychologist, 53*, 221–241.

Clarizio, H. F. (1994). Assessment of depression in children and adolescents by parents, teachers, and peers. In W. M. Reynolds & H. F. Johnston (Eds.), *Handbook of depression in children and adolescents* (pp. 235–248). New York: Plenum Press.

Cole, D. A., & Jordan, A. E. (1995). Competence and memory: Integrating psychosocial and cognitive correlates of child depression. *Child Development, 66*, 459–473.

Cole, D. A., Martin, J. M., Peeke, L. G., Seroczynski, A. D., & Hoffman, K. (1998). Are cognitive errors of underestimation predictive or reflective of depressive symptoms in children?: A longitudinal study. *Journal of Abnormal Psychology, 107*, 481–496.

Cole, D. A., Martin, J. M., & Powers, B. (1997). A competency-based model of child depression: A longitudinal study of peer, parent, teacher, and self-evaluations. *Journal of Child Psychology and Psychiatry and Allied Disciplines, 38*, 505–514.

Compas, B. E. (1997). Depression in children and adolescents. In E. J. Mash & L. G. Terdal (Eds.), *Assessment of childhood disorders* (3rd ed., pp. 197–229). New York: Guilford Press.

Compas, B. E., Ey, S., & Grant, K. E. (1993). Taxonomy, assessment, and diagnosis of depression during adolescence. *Psychological Bulletin, 114*, 323–344.

Compas, B. E., Oppedisano, G., Connor, J. K., Gerhardt, C. A., Hinden, B. R., Achenbach, T. M., et al. (1997). Gender differences in depressive symptoms in adolescence: Comparison of national samples of clinically referred and nonreferred youths. *Journal of Consulting and Clinical Psychology, 65*, 617–626.

Costello, E. J., Angold, A., Burns, B. J., Stangl, D. K., Tweed, D. L., & Erkanli, A. (1996). The Great Smoky Mountains Study of youth: Goals, design, methods, and prevalence of DSM-III-R disorders. *Archives of General Psychiatry, 53*, 1129–1136.

Costello, E. J., Benjamin, R., Angold, A., & Silver, D. (1991). Mood variability in adolescents: A study of depressed, non-depressed and comorbid patients. *Journal of Affective Disorders, 23*, 199–212.

Crosbie-Burnett, M., & Newcomer, L. L. (1990). Group counseling children of divorce: The effects of a multimodal intervention. *Journal of Divorce, 13*, 69–78.

Crowley, S. L., Worchel, F. F., & Ash, M. J. (1992). Self-report, peer-report, and teacher-report measures of childhood depression: An analysis by item. *Journal of Personality Assessment, 59*, 189–203.

Dahl, R. E., Birmaher, B., Williamson, D. E., Dorn, L., Perel, J., Kaufman, J., et al. (2000). Low growth hormone response to growth hormone–releasing hormone in child depression. *Biological Psychiatry, 48*, 981–988.

Daleiden, E., Chorpita, B. F., & Lu, W. (2000). Assessment of tripartite factors of emotion in children and adolescents: II. Concurrent validity of the Affect and Arousal Scales for children. *Journal of Psychopathology and Behavioral Assessment, 22*, 161–182.

Dalley, M. B., Bolocofsky, D. N., Alcorn, M. B., & Baker, C. (1992). Depressive symptomatology, attributional style, dysfunctional attitude, and social competency in adolescents with and without learning disabilities. *School Psychology Review, 21*, 444–458.

Davidson, R. J., Pizzagalli, D., & Nitschke, J. (2002). The representation and regulation of emotion in depression: Perspectives from affective neuroscience. In I. H. Gotlib & C. L. Hammen (Eds.), *Handbook of depression* (pp. 219–244). New York: Guilford Press.

Dawson, G., Frey, K., Panagiotides, H., Osterling, J., & Hessl, D. (1997). Infants of depressed mothers exhibit atypical frontal brain activity: A replication and extension of previous findings. *Journal of Child Psychology and Psychiatry, 38*, 179–186.

Doi, Y., Roberts, R. E., Takeuchi, K., & Suzuki, S. (2001). Multiethnic comparison of adolescent major depression based on the DSM-IV criteria in a U.S.–Japan study. *Journal of the American Academy of Child and Adolescent Psychiatry, 40*, 1308–1315.

Dolan, B. M., Lacey, J. H., & Evans, C. (1990). Eating

behaviour and attitudes to weight and shape in British women from three ethnic groups. *British Journal of Psychiatry, 157*, 523–528.

Doss, A. J. (2005). Evidence-based diagnosis: Incorporating diagnostic instruments into clinical practice. *Journal of the American Academy of Child and Adolescent Psychiatry, 44*, 947–952.

Drotar, D., Stein, R. E. K., & Perrin, E. C. (1995). Methodological issues in using the Child Behavior Checklist and its related instruments in clinical child psychology research. *Journal of Clinical Child Psychology, 24*, 184–192.

Duggal, S., Malkoff-Schwartz, S., Birmaher, B., Anderson, B., Matty, M. K., Houck, P. R., et al. (2000). Assessment of life stress in adolescents: Self-report versus interview methods. *Journal of the American Academy of Child and Adolescent Psychiatry, 39*, 445–452.

Eaves, L. J., Silberg, J. L., Meyer, J. M., Maes, H. H., Simonoff, E., Pickles, A., et al. (1997). Genetics and developmental psychopathology: 2. The main effects of genes and environment on behavioral problems in the Virginia Twin Study of Adolescent Behavioral Development. *Journal of Child Psychology and Psychiatry and Allied Disciplines, 38*, 965–980.

Edelbrock, C., Costello, A. J., Dulcan, M. K., Kalas, R., & Conover, N. C. (1985). Age differences in the reliability of the psychiatric interview of the child. *Child Development, 56*, 265–275.

Egger, H. L., & Angold, A. (2004). The Preschool Age Psychiatric Assessment (PAPA): A structured parent interview for diagnosing psychiatric disorders in preschool children. In R. DelCarmen-Wiggins & A. Carter (Eds.), *Handbook of infant, toddler, and preschool mental health assessment* (pp. 223–243). New York: Oxford University Press.

Emslie, G. J., Rush, J., Weinberg, W. A., Kowatch, R. A., Hughes, C. W., Carmody, T., et al. (1997). A double–blind, randomized placebo-controlled trial of fluoxetine in children and adolescents with depression. *Archives of General Psychiatry, 54*, 1031–1037.

Emslie, G., Rush, J., Weinberg, W., Rintelmann, J., & Roffwarg, H. (1994). Sleep EEG features of adolescents with major depression. *Biological Psychiatry, 36*, 573–581.

Essex, M. J., Boyce, W. T., Goldstein, L. H., Armstrong, J. M., Kraemer, H. C., & Kupfer, D. J. (2002). The confluence of mental, physical, social, and academic difficulties in middle childhood: II. Developing the MacArthur Health and Behavior Questionnaire. *Journal of the American Academy of Child and Adolescent Psychiatry, 41*, 588–603.

Ezpeleta, L., de la Osa, N., Domenech, J. M., Navarro, J. D., Losilla, J. M., & Judez, J. (1997). Diagnostic agreement between clinicians and the Diagnostic Interview for Children and Adolescents—DICA-R—in an outpatient sample. *Journal of Child Psychology and Psychiatry and Allied Disciplines, 38*, 431–440.

Ezpeleta, L., Polaino, A., Domenech, E., & Domenech, J. M. (1990). Peer Nomination Inventory of Depression: Characteristics in a Spanish sample. *Journal of Abnormal Child Psychology, 18*, 373–391.

Faulstich, M. E., Carey, M. P., Ruggiero, L., Enyart, P., & Gresham, F. (1986). Assessment of depression in childhood and adolescence: An evaluation of the Center for Epidemiological Studies Depression Scale for Children (CES-DC). *American Journal of Psychiatry, 143*, 1024–1027.

Fendrich, M., Weissman, M. M., & Warner, V. (1990). Screening for depressive disorder in children and adolescents: Validating the Center for Epidemiologic Studies Depression Scale for Children. *American Journal of Epidemiology, 131*, 538–551.

Ferdinand, R. F., Hoogerheide, K. N., van der Ende, J., Heijmens V. J., Koot, H. M., Kasius, M. C., et al. (2003). The role of the clinician: Three-year predictive value of parents', teachers', and clinicians' judgment of childhood psychopathology. *Journal of Child Psychology and Psychiatry, 44*, 867–876.

Finch, A. J., Saylor, C. E., Edwards, G. L., & McIntosh, J. A. (1987). Children's Depression Inventory: Reliability over repeated administrations. *Journal of Clinical Child Psychology, 16*, 339–341.

Flannery, R. C. (1990). Methodological and psychometric considerations in child reports. In A. M. La Greca (Ed.), *Through the eyes of a child: Obtaining self-reports from children and adolescents* (pp. 57–82). Boston: Allyn & Bacon.

Flynn, M., & Rudolph, K. D. (2007). Perceptual asymmetry and youths' responses to stress: Understanding risk for depression. *Cognition and Emotion, 21*, 773–788.

Franklin, M. E., Kozak, M. J., Cashman, L. A., Coles, M. E., Rheingold, A. A., & Foa, E. B. (1998). Cognitive-behavioral treatment of pediatric obsessive–compulsive disorder: An open clinical trial. *Journal of the American Academy of Child and Adolescent Psychiatry, 37*, 412–419.

Gadow, K. D., & Sprafkin, J. (2002). *Child Symptom Inventory–4: Screening and norms manual.* Stony Brook, NY: Checkmate Plus.

Garber, J. (1984). Classification of childhood psychopathology: A developmental perspective. *Child Development, 55*, 30–48.

Garber, J., & Horowitz, J. L. (2002). Depression in children. In I. H. Gotlib & C. L. Hammen (Eds.), *Handbook of depression* (pp. 510–540). New York: Guilford Press.

Garber, J., & Kaminski, K. M. (2000). Laboratory and performance-based measures of depression in children and adolescents. *Journal of Clinical Child Psychology, 29*, 509–525.

Garber, J., Keiley, M. K., & Martin, N. C. (2002). Developmental trajectories of adolescents' depressive symptoms: Predictors of change. *Journal of Consulting and Clinical Psychology, 70*, 79–95.

Garrison, C. Z., Addy, C. L., Jackson, K. L., McKeown, R. E., & Waller, J. L. (1991). The CES-D as a screen for depression and other psychiatric disorders in adolescents. *Journal of the American Academy of Child and Adolescent Psychiatry, 30*, 636–641.

Gerhardt, C. A., Compas, B. E., Connor, J. K., & Achenbach, T. M. (1999). Association of a mixed anxiety–depression syndrome and symptoms of major depressive disorder during adolescence. *Journal of Youth and Adolescence, 28*, 305–323.

Goodman, S. H., & Gotlib, I. H. (1999). Risk for psychopathology in the children of depressed mothers: A developmental model for understanding mechanisms of transmission. *Psychological Review, 106*, 458–490.

Goodman, S. H., Schwab-Stone, M., Lahey, B., Shaffer, D., & Jensen, P. (2000). Major depression and dysthymia in children and adolescents: Discriminant validity and differential consequences in a community sample. *Journal of the American Academy of Child and Adolescent Psychiatry, 39*, 761–770.

Gotlib, I. H., & Hammen, C. (1992). *Psychological aspects of depression: Toward a cognitive-interpersonal integration*. London: Wiley.

Hamilton, M. (1960). A rating scale for depression. *Journal of Neurology, Neurosurgery, and Psychiatry, 23*, 56–61.

Hammack, P. L. (2003). Toward a unified theory of depression in urban African American youth: Integrating socioecologic, cognitive, family stress, and biopsychosocial perspectives. *Journal of Black Psychology, 29*, 187–209.

Hammen, C. (1992). Cognitive, life stress, and interpersonal approaches to a developmental psychopathology model of depression. *Development and Psychopathology, 4*, 191–208.

Hammen, C., & Rudolph, K. D. (2003). Childhood mood disorders. In E. J. Mash & R. A. Barkley (Eds.), *Child psychopathology* (2nd ed., pp. 233–278). New York: Guilford Press.

Hankin, B. L., & Abramson, L. Y. (2001). Development of gender differences in depression: An elaborated cognitive vulnerability–transactional stress theory. *Psychological Bulletin, 127*, 773–796.

Hankin, B. L., Abramson, L. Y., Moffitt, T. E., Silva, P. A., McGee, R., & Angell, K. E. (1998). Development of depression from preadolescence to young adulthood: Emerging gender differences in a 10-year longitudinal study. *Journal of Abnormal Psychology, 107*, 128–140.

Hankin, B. L., Fraley, R. C., Lahey, B. B., & Waldman, I. D. (2005). Is depression best viewed as a continuum or discrete category?: A taxometric analysis of childhood and adolescent depression in a population-based sample. *Journal of Abnormal Psychology, 114*, 96–110.

Harrington, R., Fudge, H., Rutter, M., Pickles, A., & Hill, J. (1990). Adult outcomes of childhood and adolescent depression: Psychiatric status. *Archives of General Psychiatry, 47*, 465–473.

Hayward, C., Gotlib, I. H., Schraedley, P. K., & Litt, I. F.

(1999). Ethnic differences in the association between pubertal status and symptoms of depression in adolescent girls. *Journal of Adolescent Health, 25*, 143–149.

Hodges, K. (1994). Evaluation of depression in children and adolescents using diagnostic clinical interviews. In W. M. Reynolds & H. F. Johnston (Eds.), *Handbook of depression in children and adolescents* (pp. 183–208). New York: Plenum Press.

Hodges, K. (1999). Child and Adolescent Functional Assessment Scale (CAFAS). In M. E. Maruish (Ed.), *The use of psychological testing for treatment planning and outcomes assessment* (2nd ed., pp. 631–664). Mahwah, NJ: Erlbaum.

Hope, T. L., Adams, C., Reynolds, L., Powers, D., Perez, R. A., & Kelley, M. L. (1999). Parent vs. self-report: Contributions toward diagnosis of adolescent psychopathology. *Journal of Psychopathology and Behavioral Assessment, 2*, 349–363.

Hovey, J. D., & King, C. A. (1996). Acculturative stress, depression, and suicidal ideation among immigrant and second-generation Latino adolescents. *Journal of the American Academy of Child and Adolescent Psychiatry, 35*, 1183–1192.

Ialongo, N., Edelsohn, G., & Kellam, S. G. (2001). A further look at the prognostic power of young children's reports of depressed mood and feelings. *Child Development, 72*, 736–747.

Ialongo, N., Edelsohn, G., Werthamer-Larsson, L., Crockett, L., & Kellam, S. G. (1993). Are self-reported depressive symptoms in first-grade children developmentally transient phenomena?: A further look. *Development and Psychopathology, 5*, 433–457.

Ines, T. M., & Sacco, W. P. (1992). Factors related to correspondence between teacher ratings of elmentary student depression and student self-ratings. *Journal of Consulting and Clinical Psychology, 60*, 140–142.

Jacques, H. A., & Mash, E. J. (2004). A test of the tripartite model of anxiety and depression in elementary and high school boys and girls. *Journal of Abnormal Child Psychology, 32*, 13–25.

Jensen, A. L., & Weisz, J. R. (2002). Assessing match and mismatch between practitioner-generated and standardized interview-generated diagnoses for clinic-referred children and adolescents. *Journal of Consulting and Clinical Psychology, 70*, 158–168.

Jensen, P. S., Rubio-Stipec, M., Canino, G., Bird, H. R., Dulcan, M. K., Schwab-Stone, M. E., et al. (1999). Parent and child contributions to diagnosis of mental disorder: Are both informants always necessary? *Journal of the American Academy of Child and Adolescent Psychiatry, 38*, 1569–1579.

John, K., Gammon, G. D., Prusoff, B. A., & Warner, V. (1987). The Social Adjustment Inventory for Children and Adolescents (SAICA): Testing of a new semistructured interview. *Journal of the American Academy of Child and Adolescent Psychiatry, 26*, 898–911.

Johnson, J. H., & McCutcheon, S. M. (1980). Assessing life stress in older children and adolescents: Preliminary findings with the Life Events Checklist. In I. G. Sarason & C. D. Spielberger (Eds.), *Stress and anxiety* (pp. 111–125). Washington, DC: Hemisphere.

Johnston, C., & Murray, C. (2003). Incremental validity in the psychological assessment of children and adolescents. *Psychological Assessment, 15,* 496–507.

Joiner, T. E., Catanzaro, S. J., & Laurent, J. (1996). Tripartite structure of positive and negative affect, depression, and anxiety in child and adolescent psychiatric inpatients. *Journal of Abnormal Psychology, 105,* 401–409.

Joiner, T. E., Coyne, J. C., & Blalock, J. (1999). On the interpersonal nature of depression: Overview and synthesis. In T. E. Joiner & J. C. Coyne (Eds.), *The interactional nature of depression* (pp. 3–19). Washington, DC: American Psychological Association.

Kandel, B., & Davies, M. (1982). Epidemiology of depressed mood in adolescents. *Archives of General Psychiatry, 39,* 1205–1212.

Kashani, J. H., Sherman, D. D., Parker, D. R., & Reid, J.C. (1990). Utility of the Beck Depression Inventory with clinic-referred adolescents. *Journal of the American Academy of Child and Adolescent Psychiatry, 29,* 278–282.

Kasius, M. C., Ferdinand, R. F., van den Berg, H., & Verhulst, F. C. (1997). Associations between different diagnostic approaches for child and adolescent psychopathology. *Journal of Child Psychology and Psychiatry and Allied Disciplines, 38,* 625–632.

Kaslow, N. J., Adamson, L. B., & Collins, M. H. (2000). A developmental psychopathology perspective on the cognitive components of child and adolescent depression. In A. J. Sameroff, M. Lewis, & S. M. Miller (Eds.), *Handbook of developmental psychopathology* (2nd ed., pp. 491–510). New York: Kluwer Academic/Plenum Press.

Kaslow, N. J., Tanenbaum, R. L., Abramson, L. Y., Peterson, C., & Seligman, M. E. (1983). Problem-solving deficits and depressive symptoms among children. *Journal of Abnormal Child Psychology, 11,* 497–501.

Kaufman, J., Birmaher, B., Brent, D., Rao, U., Flynn, C., Moreci, P., et al. (1997). Schedule for Affective Disorders and Schizophrenia for School-Age Children—Present and Lifetime Version (K-SADS-PL): Initial reliability and validity data. *Journal of the American Academy of Child and Adolescent Psychiatry, 36,* 980–988.

Kaufman, J., Martin, A., King, R. A., & Charney, D. (2001). Are child-, adolescent-, and adult-onset depression one and the same disorder? *Biological Psychiatry, 49,* 980–1001.

Kazdin, A. E. (1994). Informant variability in the assessment of childhood depression. In W. M. Reynolds & H. F. Johnston (Eds.), *Handbook of depression in children and adolescents* (pp. 249–271). New York: Plenum Press.

Kessler, R. C. (1997). The effects of stressful life events on depression. *Annual Review of Psychology, 48,* 191–214.

Kessler, R. C., Avenevoli, S., & Merikangas, K. R. (2001). Mood disorders in children and adolescents: An epidemiologic perspective. *Biological Psychiatry, 49,* 1002–1014.

Kessler, R. C., & Walters, E. E. (1998). Epidemiology of DSM-III-R major depression and minor depression among adolescents and young adults in the National Comorbidity Survey. *Depression and Anxiety, 7,* 3–14.

Klein, D. N., Dougherty, L. R., & Olino, T. M. (2005). Toward guidelines for evidence-based assessment of depression in children and adolescents. *Journal of Clinical Child and Adolescent Psychology, 34,* 412–432.

Klein, D. N., Lewinsohn, P. M., Rohde, P., Seeley, J. R., & Durbin, C. E. (2002). Clinical features of major depressive disorder in adolescents and their relatives: Impact on familial aggregation, implications for phenotype definition and specificity of transmission. *Journal of Abnormal Psychology, 111,* 98–106.

Klein, D. N., Ouimette, P. C., Kelly, H. S., Ferro, T., & Riso, L. P. (1994). Test–retest reliability of team consensus best-estimate diagnoses of Axis I and II disorders in a family study. *American Journal of Psychiatry, 151,* 1043–1047.

Kovacs, M. (1992). *Children's Depression Inventory manual.* North Tonawanda, NY: Multi-Health Systems.

Kovacs, M. (1996). Presentation and course of major depressive disorder during childhood and later years of the life span. *Journal of the American Academy of Child and Adolescent Psychiatry, 35,* 705–715.

Kovacs, M., & Goldston, D. (1991). Cognitive and social cognitive development of depressed children and adolescents. *Journal of the American Academy of Child and Adolescent Psychiatry, 30,* 388–392.

Krefetz, D. G., Steer, R. A., Gulab, N. A., & Beck, A. T. (2002). Convergent validity of the Beck Depression Inventory–II with the Reynolds Adolescent Depression Scale in psychiatric inpatients. *Journal of Personality Assessment, 78,* 451–460.

Kumar, G., Steer, R. A., Teitelman, K. B., & Villacis, L. (2002). Effectiveness of Beck Depression Inventory–II subscales in screening for major depressive disorders in adolescent psychiatric inpatients. *Assessment, 9,* 164–170.

Kutcher, S., Malkin, D., Silverberg, J., Marton, P., Williamson, P., Malkin, A., et al. (1991). Nocturnal cortisol, thyroid stimulating hormone, and growth hormone secretory profiles in depressed adolescents. *Journal of the American Academy of Child and Adolescent Psychiatry, 30,* 407–414.

Kutcher, S. P., & Marton, P. (1989). Utility of the Beck

Depression Inventory with psychiatrically disturbed adolescent outpatients. *Canadian Journal of Psychiatry*, *34*, 107–109.

Laurent, J., Catanzaro, S. J., & Joiner, T. E. (2004). Development and preliminary validation of the Physiological Hyperarousal Scale for Children. *Psychological Assessment*, *16*, 373–380.

Laurent, J., Catanzaro, S. J., Joiner, T. E., Rudolph, K. D., Potter, K. I., Lambert, S., et al. (1999). A measure of positive and negative affect for children: Scale development and preliminary validation. *Psychological Assessment*, *11*, 326–338.

Laurent, J., & Ettelson, R. (2001). An examination of the tripartite model of anxiety and depression and its application to youth. *Clinical Child and Family Psychology Review*, *4*, 209–230.

Lefkowitz, A., & Tesiny, E. (1980). Assessment of childhood depression. *Journal of Consulting and Clinical Psychology*, *48*, 43–50.

Lengua, L. J., Sadowski, C. A., Friedrich, W. N., & Fisher, J. (2001). Rationally and empirically derived dimensions of children's symptomatology: Expert ratings and confirmatory factor analyses of the CBCL. *Journal of Consulting and Clinical Psychology*, *69*, 683–698.

Lewinsohn, P. M., & Essau, C. A. (2002). Depression in adolescents. In I. H. Gotlib & C. L. Hammen (Eds.), *Handbook of depression* (pp. 541–559). New York: Guilford Press.

Lewinsohn, P. M., Hops, H., Roberts, R. E., Seeley, J. R., & Andrews, J. A. (1993). Adolescent psychopathology: I. Prevalence and incidence of depression and other DSM-III-R disorders in high school students. *Journal of Abnormal Psychology*, *102*, 133–144.

Lewinsohn, P. M., Rohde, P., Klein, D. M., & Seeley, J. R. (1999). Natural course of adolescent major depressive disorder: I. Continuity into young adulthood. *Journal of the American Academy of Child and Adolescent Psychiatry*, *38*, 56–63.

Lewinsohn, P., Rohde, P., & Seeley, J. (1994). Psychosocial risk factors for future adolescent suicide attempts. *Journal of Consulting and Clinical Psychology*, *62*, 297–305.

Lewinsohn, P. M., Rohde, P., Seeley, J. R., Klein, D. N., & Gotlib, I. H. (2000). Natural course of adolescent major depressive disorder in a community sample: Predictors of recurrence in young adults. *American Journal of Psychiatry*, *157*, 1584–1591.

Lewinsohn, P. M., Rohde, P., Seeley, J. R., Klein, D. N., & Gotlib, H. (2003). Psychosocial functioning of young adults who have experienced and recovered from major depressive disorder during adolescence. *Journal of Abnormal Psychology*, *112*, 353–363.

Lonigan, C. J., Carey, M. P., & Finch, A. J. (1994). Anxiety and depression in children and adolescents: Negative affectivity and the utility of self-reports. *Journal of Consulting and Clinical Psychology*, *62*, 1000–1008.

Lonigan, C. J., Hooe, E. S., David, C. F., & Kistner, J. A. (1999). Positive and negative affectivity in children: Confirmatory factor analysis of a two-factor model and its relation to symptoms of anxiety and depression. *Journal of Consulting and Clinical Psychology*, *67*, 374–386.

Lonigan, C. J., Phillips, B. M., & Hooe, E. S. (2003). Relations of positive and negative affectivity to anxiety and depression in children: Evidence from a latent variable longitudinal study. *Journal of Consulting and Clinical Psychology*, *71*, 465–481.

Luby, J. L., Heffelfinger, A., Koenig-McNaught, A. L., Brown, K., & Spitznagel, E. (2004). The Preschool Feelings Checklist: A brief and sensitive screening measure for depression in young children. *Journal of the American Academy of Child and Adolescent Psychiatry*, *43*, 708–717.

Luby, J. L., Heffelfinger, A., Measelle, J. R., Ablow, J. C., Essex, M. J., Dierker, L., et al. (2002). Differential performance of the MacArthur HBQ and DISC-IV in identifying DSM-IV internalizing psychopathology in young children. *Journal of the American Academy of Child and Adolescent Psychiatry*, *41*, 458–456.

Lucas, C., Fisher, P., & Luby, J. (1998). *Young-child DISC-IV research draft: Diagnostic Interview Schedule for Children*. New York: Columbia University.

Mannuzza, S., & Fyer, A. J. (1990). *Family Informant Schedule and Criteria (FISC), July 1990 revision*. New York: Anxiety Disorders Clinic, New York State Psychiatric Institute.

Manson, S. M., Ackerson, L. M., Dick, R. W., Baron, A. E., & Fleming, C. M. (1990). Depressive symptoms among American Indian adolescents: Psychometric characteristics of the Center for Epidemiologic Studies Depression Scale (CES-D). *Psychological Assessment*, *2*, 231–237.

Marmorstein, N. R., & Iacono, W. G. (2003). Major depression and conduct disorder in a twin sample: Gender, functioning, and risk for future psychopathology. *Journal of the American Academy of Child and Adolescent Psychiatry*, *42*, 225–233.

Mash, E. J., & Foster, S. L. (2001). Exporting analogue behavioral observation from research to clinical practice: Useful or cost-defective? *Psychological Assessment*, *13*, 86–98.

Mash, E. J., & Hunsley, J. (2005). Evidence-based assessment of child and adolescent disorders: Issues and challenges. *Journal of Clinical Child and Adolescent Psychology*, *34*, 362–379.

Mattison, R. E., Gadow, K. D., Sprafkin, J., Nolan, E., & Schneider, J. (2003). A DSM-IV-referenced Teacher Rating Scale for use in clinical management. *Journal of the American Academy of Child and Adolescent Psychiatry*, *42*, 442–449.

McCauley, E., Myers, K., Mitchell, J., Calderon, R., Schloredt, K., & Treder, R. (1993). Depression in young people: Initial presentation and clinical course. *Journal of the American Academy of Child and Adolescent Psychiatry*, *32*, 714–722.

McClure, E., Rogeness, G. A., & Thompson, N. M. (1997). Characteristics of adolescent girls with depressive symptoms in a so-called "normal" sample. *Journal of Affective Disorders, 42,* 187–197.

McGee, R., & Williams, S. (1988). A longitudinal study of depression in nine-year-old children. *Journal of the American Academy of Child and Adolescent Psychiatry, 27,* 342–348.

Meyer, N., Dyck, D., & Petrinack, R. (1989). Cognitive appraisal and attributional correlates of depressive symptoms in children. *Journal of Abnormal Child Psychology, 17,* 325–336.

Mitchell, J., McCauley, E., Burke, P. M., & Moss, S. J. (1988). Phenomenology of depression in children and adolescents. *Journal of the American Academy of Child and Adolescent Psychiatry, 27,* 12–20.

Mokros, H. B., Poznanski, E., Grossman, J. A., & Freeman, L. N. (1987). A comparison of child and parent ratings of depression for normal and clinically referred children. *Journal of Child Psychology and Psychiatry and Allied Disciplines, 28,* 613–627.

Myers, K., & Winters, N. C. (2002). Ten-year review of rating scales: II. Scales for internalizing disorders. *Journal of the American Academy of Child and Adolescent Psychiatry, 41,* 634–659.

Neshat-Doost, H. T., Moradi, A. R., Taghavi, M. R., Yule, W., & Dalgleish, T. (2000). Lack of attentional bias for emotional information in clinically depressed children and adolescents on the dot probe task. *Journal of Child Psychology and Psychiatry and Allied Disciplines, 41,* 363–368.

Nolen-Hoeksema, S. (2002). Gender differences in depression. In I. H. Gotlib & C. L. Hammen (Eds.), *Handbook of depression* (pp. 492–509). New York: Guilford Press.

Nyborg, V. M., & Curry, J. F. (2003). The impact of perceived racism: Psychological symptoms among African American boys. *Journal of Clinical Child and Adolescent Psychology, 32,* 258–266.

Okazaki, S. (2000). Asian American and white American differences on affective distress symptoms: Do symptom reports differ across reporting methods? *Journal of Cross-Cultural Psychology, 31,* 603–625.

Olsson, G., & von Knorring, A. L. (1997). Depression among Swedish adolescents measured by the self-rating scale Center for Epidemiology Studies—Depression Child (CES-DC). *European Child and Adolescent Psychiatry, 6,* 81–87.

Osman, A., Kopper, B. A., Barrios, F., Gutierrez, P. M., & Bagge, C. L. (2004). Reliability and validity of the Beck Depression Inventory–II with adolescent psychiatric inpatients. *Psychological Assessment, 16,* 120–132.

Overholser, J. C., Brinkman, D. C., Lehnert, K. L., & Ricciardi, A. M. (1995). Children's Depression Rating Scale—Revised: Development of a short form. *Journal of Clinical Child Psychology, 24,* 443–452.

Pellegrino, J. F., Singh, N., & Carmanico, S. J. (1999). Concordance among three diagnostic procedures for identifying depression in children and adolescents with EBD. *Journal of Emotional and Behavioral Disorders, 7,* 118–127.

Pine, D. S., Cohen, E., Cohen, P., & Brook, J. (1999). Adolescent depressive symptoms as predictors of adult depression: Moodiness or mood disorder? *American Journal of Psychiatry, 156,* 133–135.

Pine, D. S., Cohen, P., Gurley, D., Brook, J. S., & Ma, Y. (1998). The risk for early-adulthood anxiety and depressive disorders in adolescents with anxiety and depressive disorders. *Archives of General Psychiatry, 55,* 56–64.

Politano, P. M., Nelson, W. M., Evans, H. E., Sorenson, S. B., & Zeman, D. J. (1986). Factor analytic evaluation of differences between black and Caucasian emotionally disturbed children on the Children's Depression Inventory. *Journal of Psychopathology and Behavioral Assessment, 8,* 1–7.

Pomerantz, E. M., & Rudolph, K. D. (2003). What ensues from emotional distress?: Implications for competence estimation. *Child Development, 74,* 329–345.

Poznanski, E. O., Cook, S. C., & Carroll, B. J. (1979). A depression rating scale for children. *Pediatrics, 64,* 442–450.

Poznanski, E. O., Grossman, J. A., Buchsbaum, Y., Banegas, M., Freeman, L., & Gibbons, R. (1984). Preliminary studies of the reliability and validity of the Children's Depression Rating Scale. *Journal of the American Academy of Child Psychiatry, 23,* 191–197.

Poznanski, E. O., & Mokros, H. B. (1999). *Children's Depression Rating Scale—Revised (CDRS-R).* Los Angeles: Western Psychological Services.

Puig-Antich, J., & Chambers, W. (1978). *The Schedule for Affective Disorders and Schizophrenia for School-Age Children (Kiddie-SADS).* New York: New York State Psychiatric Institute.

Puig-Antich, J., Lukens, E., & Brent, D. (1986). *Psychosocial Schedule for School-Age Children—Revised.* Pittsburgh, PA: Western Psychiatric Institute and Clinic.

Puig-Antich, J., Lukens, E., Davies, M., Goetz, D., Brennan-Quattrock, J., & Todak, G. (1985). Psychosocial functioning in prepubertal major depressive disorders: II. Interpersonal relationships after sustained recovery from affective episode. *Archives of General Psychiatry, 42,* 511–517.

Puura, K., Almqvist, F., Tamminen, T., Piha, J., Kumpulainen, K., Rasanen, E., et al. (1998). Children with symptoms of depression—What do adults see? *Journal of Child Psychology and Psychiatry, 39,* 577–585.

Rao, U., Ryan, N. D., Birmaher, B., Dahl, R. E., Williamson, D. E., Kaufman, J., et al. (1995). Unipolar depression in adolescents: Clinical outcomes in adulthood. *Journal of the American Academy of Child and Adolescent Psychiatry, 34,* 566–578.

Radloff, L. S. (1977). A CES-D scale: A self-report depression scale for research in the general population. *Applied Psychological Measurement, 1,* 385–401.

Rauch, S. L., & Renshaw, P. F. (1995). Clinical neuroimaging in psychiatry. *Harvard Review of Psychiatry, 2,* 297–312.

Rawson, H. E., & Tabb, L. C. (1993). Effects of therapeutic intervention on childhood depression. *Child and Adolescent Social Work Journal, 10,* 39–51.

Reich, W. (2000). Diagnostic Interview for Children and Adolescents (DICA). *Journal of the American Academy of Child and Adolescent Psychiatry, 39,* 59–66.

Reich, W., Shayka, T., & Taibleson, C. (1991). *The Diagnostic Interview for Children and Adolescents—Revised.* St. Louis, MO: Washington University.

Rey, J. M., & Morris-Yates, A. (1991). Adolescent depression and the Child Behavior Checklist. *Journal of the American Academy of Child and Adolescent Psychiatry, 30,* 423–427.

Reynolds, W. M. (1987). *Reynolds Adolescent Depression Scale (RADS).* Odessa, FL: Psychological Assessment Resources.

Reynolds, W. M. (1989). *Reynolds Child Depression Scale (RCDS).* Odessa, FL: Psychological Assessment Resources.

Reynolds, W. M. (1994). Assessment of depression in children and adolescents by self-report questionnaires. In W. M. Reynolds & H. F. Johnston (Eds.), *Handbook of depression in children and adolescents* (pp. 209–234). New York: Plenum Press.

Reynolds, W. M., & Coats, K. I. (1986). A comparison of cognitive-behavioral therapy and relaxation training for the treatment of depression in adolescents. *Journal of Consulting and Clinical Psychology, 54,* 653–660.

Reynolds, W. M., & Graves, A. (1989). Reliability of children's reports of depressive symptomatology. *Journal of Abnormal Child Psychology, 17,* 647–655.

Rice, F., Harold, G. T., & Thapar, A. (2003). Negative life events as an account of age-related differences in the genetic aetiology of depression in childhood and adolescence. *Journal of Child Psychology and Psychiatry, 44,* 977–987.

Roberts, R. E., Lewinsohn, P. M., & Seeley, J. R. (1991). Screening for adolescent depression: A comparison of depression scales. *Journal of the American Academy of Child and Adolescent Psychiatry, 30,* 58–66.

Roberts, R. E., Phinney, J. S., Masse, L. C., Chen, Y. R., Roberts, C. R., & Romero, A. (1999). The structure of ethnic identity of young adolescents from diverse ethnocultural groups. *Journal of Early Adolescence, 19,* 301–322.

Roberts, R. E., Roberts, C. R., & Chen, Y. C. (1997). Ethnocultural differences in prevalence of adolescent depression. *American Journal of Community Psychology, 25,* 95–110.

Robins, L. N., Helzer, J. E., Croughan, J., & Ratcliff, K. S. (1981). National Institute of Mental Health Diagnostic Interview Schedule: Its history, characteristics, and validity. *Archives of General Psychiatry, 38,* 381–389.

Rogers, R. (2003). Standardizing DSM-IV diagnoses:

The clinical applications of structured interviews. *Journal of Personality Assessment, 81,* 220–225.

Rohde, P., Clarke, G. N., Mace, D. E., Jorgensen, J. S., & Seeley, J. R. (2004). An efficacy/effectiveness study of cognitive-behavioral treatment for adolescents with comorbid major depression and conduct disorder. *Journal of the American Academy of Child and Adolescent Psychiatry, 43,* 660–668.

Rohde, P., Lewinsohn, P. M., Klein, D. N., & Seeley, J. R. (2005). Association of parental depression with psychiatric course from adolescence to young adulthood among formerly depressed individuals. *Journal of Abnormal Psychology, 114,* 409–420.

Rubio-Stipec, M., Canino, G. J., Shrout, P., Dulcan, M., Freeman, D., & Bravo, M. (1994). Psychometric properties of parents and children as informants in child psychiatry epidemiology with the Spanish Diagnostic Interview Schedule for Children (DISC 2). *Journal of Abnormal Child Psychology, 22,* 703–720.

Rudolph, K. D. (2002). Gender differences in emotional responses to interpersonal stress during adolescence. *Journal of Adolescent Health, 30,* 3–13.

Rudolph, K. D., Flynn, M., & Abaied, J. L. (in press). A developmental perspective on interpersonal theories of youth depression. In J. R. Z. Abela & B. L. Hankin (Eds.), *Child and adolescent depression: Causes, treatment, and prevention.* New York: Guilford Press.

Rudolph, K. D., Hammen, C., & Burge, D. (1994). Interpersonal functioning and depressive symptoms in childhood: Addressing the issues of specificity and comorbidity. *Journal of Abnormal Child Psychology, 22,* 355–371.

Rudolph, K. D., Hammen, C., & Burge, D. (1997). A cognitive–interpersonal approach to depressive symptoms in preadolescent children. *Journal of Abnormal Child Psychology, 25,* 33–45.

Rudolph, K. D., Hammen, C., Burge, D., Lindberg, N., Herzberg, D. S., & Daley, S. E. (2000). Toward an interpersonal life-stress model of depression: The developmental context of stress generation. *Development and Psychopathology, 12,* 215–234.

Rudolph, K. D., Hammen, C., & Daley, S. E. (2006). Mood disorders. In D. A. Wolfe & E. J. Mash (Eds.), *Behavioral and emotional disorders in adolescents* (pp. 300–342). New York: Guilford Press.

Rudolph, K. D., Laurent, J. Joiner, T., Catanzaro, S., Lambert, S. M., Osborne, L., et al. (2007). *Development and validation of the Youth Mood and Anxiety Symptom Questionnaire (Y-MASQ).* Manuscript in preparation.

Rushton, J. L., Forcier, M., & Schectman, R. M. (2002). Epidemiology of depressive symptoms in the National Longitudinal Study of Adolescent Health. *Journal of the American Academy of Child and Adolescent Psychiatry, 41,* 199–205.

Ryan, N. D., Puig-Antich, J., Ambrosini, P., Rabinovich, H., Robinson, D., Nelson, B., et al.

(1987). The clinical picture of major depression in children and adolescents. *Archives of General Psychiatry, 44,* 66–74.

Sanders, M. R., Dadds, M. R., Johnston, B. M., & Cash, R. (1992). Childhood depression and conduct disorder: I. Behavioral, affective, and cognitive aspects of family problem-solving interactions. *Journal of Abnormal Psychology, 101,* 495–504.

Saylor, C. E., Finch, A. J., Spirito, A., & Bennett, B. (1984). The Children's Depression Inventory: A systematic evaluation of psychometric properties. *Journal of Consulting and Clinical Psychology, 52,* 955–967.

Shaffer, D., Fisher, P., Lucas, C. P., Dulcan, M. K., & Schwab-Stone, M. E. (2000). NIMH Diagnostic Interview Schedule for Children Version IV (NIMH DISC-IV): Description, differences from previous versions, and reliability of some common diagnoses. *Journal of the American Academy of Child and Adolescent Psychiatry, 39,* 28–38.

Shaffer, D., Gould, M. S., Brasic, J., Ambrosini, P., Fisher, P., Bird, H., et al. (1983). A Children's Global Assessment Scale (CGAS). *Archives of General Psychiatry, 40,* 1228–1231.

Shain, B. N., Naylor, M., & Alessi, N. (1990). Comparison of self-rated and clinician-rated measures of depression in adolescents. *American Journal of Psychiatry, 147,* 793–795.

Shirk, S. R., Boergers, J., Eason, A., & Van Horn, M. (1998). Dysphoric interpersonal schemata and preadolescents' sensitization to negative events. *Journal of Clinical Child Psychology, 27,* 54–68.

Shirk, S. R., Van Horn, M., & Leber, D. (1997). Dysphoria and children's processing of supportive interactions. *Journal of Abnormal Child Psychology, 25,* 239–249.

Siegel, J. M., Aneshensel, C. S., Taub, B., Cantwell, D. P., & Driscoll, A. K. (1998). Adolescent depressed mood in a multiethnic sample. *Journal of Youth and Adolescence, 27,* 413–427.

Smucker, M. R., Craighead, W. E., Craighead, L. W., & Green, B. J. (1986). Normative and reliability data for the Children's Depression Inventory. *Journal of Abnormal Child Psychology, 14,* 25–39.

Song, L., Singh, J., & Singer, M. (1994). The Youth Self-Report Inventory: A study of its measurement fidelity. *Psychological Assessment, 6,* 236–245.

Stark, K. D., Reynolds, W. M., & Kaslow, N. J. (1987). A comparison of the relative efficacy of self-control therapy and a behavioral problem-solving therapy for depression in children. *Journal of Abnormal Child Psychology, 15,* 91–113.

Sullivan, P. F., Neale, M. C., & Kendler, K. S. (2000). Genetic epidemiology of major depression: Review and meta-analysis. *American Journal of Psychiatry, 157,* 1552–1562.

Thapar, A., & McGuffin, P. (1998). Validity of the shortened Mood and Feelings Questionnaire in a community sample of children and adolescents: A preliminary research note. *Psychiatry Research, 81,* 259–268.

Thase, M. E., Jindal, R., & Howland, R. H. (2002). Biological aspects of depression. In I. H. Gotlib & C. L. Hammen (Eds.), *Handbook of depression* (pp. 192–218). New York: Guilford Press.

Timbremont, B., Braet, C., & Dreessen, L. (2004). Assessing depression in youth: Relation between the Children's Depression Inventory and a structured interview. *Journal of Clinical Child and Adolescent Psychology, 33,* 149–157.

Twenge, J. M., & Nolen-Hoeksema, S. (2002). Age, gender, race, socio-economic status, and birth cohort differences on the Children's Depression Inventory: A meta-analysis. *Journal of Abnormal Psychology, 111,* 578–588.

Verhulst, F. C., & van der Ende, J. (1992). Six-year developmental course of internalizing and externalizing problem behaviors. *Journal of the American Academy of Child and Adolescent Psychiatry, 31,* 924–931.

Wallace, J., Schnieder, T., & McGuffin, P. (2002). Genetics of depression. In I. H. Gotlib & C. L. Hammen (Eds.), *Handbook of depression* (pp. 169–191). New York: Guilford Press.

Warren, W. L. (1997). *Revised Hamilton Rating Scale for Depression (HRSD): Manual.* Los Angeles: Western Psychological Services.

Watson, D., Clark, L. A., Weber, K., Assenheimer, J. S., Strauss, M. E., & McCormick, R. A. (1995). Testing a tripartite model: II. Exploring the symptom structure of anxiety and depression in student, adult, and patient samples. *Journal of Abnormal Psychology, 104,* 15–25.

Weiss, B., & Garber, J. (2003). Developmental differences in the phenomenology of depression. *Development and Psychopathology, 15,* 403–430.

Weissman, M. M., Orvaschel, H., & Padian, N. (1980). Children's symptom and social functioning self-report scales: Comparisons of mothers' and children's reports. *Journal of Nervous and Mental Disease, 168,* 736–740.

Weissman, M. M., Wickramaratne, P., Adams, P., Wolk, S., Verdeli, H., & Olfson, M. (2000). Brief screening for family psychiatric history: The family history screen. *Archives of General Psychiatry, 57,* 675–682.

Weissman, M. M., Wolk, S., Goldstein, R. B., Moreau, D., Adams, P., Greenwald, S., et al. (1999). Depressed adolescents grown up. *Journal of the American Medical Association, 281,* 1707–1713.

Weissman, M. M., Wolk, S., Wickramaratne, P. J., Goldstein, R., Adams, P., Greenwald, S., et al. (1999). Children with prepubertal-onset major depressive disorder and anxiety grown up. *Archives of General Psychiatry, 56,* 794–801.

Weisz, J. R., Southam-Gerow, M. A., & McCarty, C. A. (2001). Control-related beliefs and depressive symptoms in clinic-referred children and adolescents: Developmental differences and model specificity. *Journal of Abnormal Psychology, 110,* 97–109.

Wichstrom, L. (1999). The emergence of gender difference in depressed mood during adolescence: The role of intensified gender socialization. *Developmental Psychology, 35,* 232–245.

Wierzbicki, M. (1987). A parent form of the Children's Depression Inventory: Reliability and validity in nonclinical populations. *Journal of Clinical Psychology, 43,* 390–397.

Williamson, D. E., Birmaher, B., Ryan, N. D., Shiffrin, T. P., Lusky, J. A., Protopapa, J., et al. (2003). The Stressful Life Events Schedule for children and adolescents: Development and validation. *Psychiatry Research, 119,* 225–241.

Winter, L. B., Steer, R. A., Jones-Hicks, L., & Beck, A. T. (1999). Screening for major depression disorders in adolescent medical outpatients with the Beck Depression Inventory for primary care. *Journal of Adolescent Health, 24,* 389–394.

Winters, N. C., Myers, K., & Proud, L. (2002). Ten-year review of rating scales. III: Scales assessing suicidality, cognitive style, and self-esteem. *Journal of the American Academy of Child and Adolescent Psychiatry, 41,* 1150–1181.

Wood, A., Knoll, L., Moore, A., & Harrington, R. (1995). Properties of the Mood and Feelings Questionnaire in adolescent psychiatric outpatients: A research note. *Journal of Child Psychology and Psychiatry and Allied Disciplines, 36,* 327–334.

World Health Organization. (1993). *The ICD-10 classification of mental and behavioural disorders: Diagnostic criteria for research.* Geneva: Author.

Yee, B. W., Huang, L. N., & Lew, A. (1998). Families: Life-span socialization in a cultural context. In L. C. Lee & N. W. S. Zane (Eds.), *Handbook of Asian American psychology* (pp. 83–135). Thousand Oaks, CA: Sage.

Yeh, M., & Yeh, J. W. (2002). The clinical assessment of Asian American children. In K. S. Kurasaki, S. Okazaki, & S. Sue (Eds.), *Asian American mental health: Assessment theories and methods* (pp. 233–249). New York: Kluwer Academic /Plenum Press.

Ying, Y. (2002). The conception of depression in Chinese Americans. In K. S. Kurasaki, S. Okazaki, & S. Sue (Eds.), *Asian American mental health: Assessment theories and methods* (pp. 173–183). New York: Kluwer Academic/Plenum Press.

Youngstrom, E., Izard, C., & Ackerman, B. (1999). Dysphoria-related bias in maternal ratings of children. *Journal of Consulting and Clinical Psychology, 67,* 905–916.

Zimmerman, M., Posternak, M. A., & Chelminski, I. (2005). Is it time to replace the Hamilton Depression Rating Scale as the primary outcome measure in treatment studies of depression? *Journal of Clinical Psychopharmacology, 25,* 105–110.

CHAPTER 6

Pediatric Bipolar Disorder

Eric Youngstrom

THE CONTROVERSY SURROUNDING PEDIATRIC BIPOLAR DISORDER

Pediatric bipolar disorder (PBD) is currently one of the most controversial diagnoses in child mental health (cf. Harrington & Myatt, 2003; Healy, 2006; Klein, Pine, & Klein, 1998; McClellan, 2005). Conventional wisdom has held that PBD is a relatively rare and serious mental illness, affecting about 1 in 100 adults in the general population. The age of onset also typically has been thought to be late adolescence or early adulthood (Klein et al., 1998). However, there has been an explosion of interest over the last decade in the diagnosis of "bipolar disorder" in children and adolescents. Bipolar diagnoses of preschoolers have been made by researchers (Tumuluru, Weller, Fristad, & Weller, 2003), and of toddlers by practicing clinicians (Papolos & Papolos, 2002). Parents sometimes describe their children as being bipolar "from birth," or even *in utero* (Papolos & Papolos, 2002).

Attention to the diagnosis also has dramatically increased. Whereas occasional case studies were published from the 1930s to the 1970s, the number of scholarly publications has risen geometrically since 1995 (Lofthouse & Fristad, 2004). There also has been a surge of attention in the popular media, ranging from special segments on news shows or Music Television (MTV™) to a cover article in *Time* mag-

azine (Kluger & Song, 2002), to nearly two dozen trade books aimed at parents and families, as well as health professionals (Lofthouse & Fristad, 2004).

Given this expansion of the age range and the surge of media attention, it is perhaps less surprising that the actual rates of diagnosis have increased. Even so, the magnitude of the change is remarkable. From virtually never being diagnosed prepubertally, PBD has become one of the more frequent diagnoses in many mental health settings. Rates of bipolar diagnoses in youth wards of the county in Illinois more than doubled, from 4 to 11% between 1994 and 2001 (Naylor, Anderson, Kruesi, & Stoewe, 2002), and similarly large increases have been documented in community mental health (Youngstrom, Youngstrom, & Starr, 2005) and other settings (Blader & Carlson, 2006). Marketing research estimated that nearly 100,000 youth were already taking medication for PBD in the United States in 2000, even prior to the wave of publicity around the diagnosis (Hellander, 2002).

Although there is speculation about both genetic and environmental changes that might lead to an increase in the rate of PBD (as discussed below), the acceleration in prevalence of the diagnosis is too rapid to be explained entirely by changes in risk factors. A major driver of the rise is changes in mental health practice. Changes in families' and practitioners' awareness of possible PBD, as well as changes in the conceptualization of what is considered "bipolar" disorder, play a huge role.

The surging diagnostic prevalence has provoked concern about "disease mongering": pathologizing behaviors that might be within normal limits, or promoting pharmacological interventions for problems that might be responsive to interpersonal interventions (Healy, 2006). PBD is much more rarely diagnosed in countries other than the United States (Soutullo et al., 2005). This is often attributed either to the "overdiagnosing" PBD (Harrington & Myatt, 2003), or possibly a greater incidence of PBD in the United States, perhaps as a result of the much more commonplace use of psychotropic medications (Reichart & Nolen, 2004).

Psychology as a profession has been much more skeptical than other health care professions about diagnosing bipolar disorder (BD) in children. Although critical thinking is certainly warranted, the skepticism has meant that there has been little in the way of development of rigorous assessment strategies. Similarly, relatively little effort has been invested in exploring psychosocial interventions: Only a few pioneering research groups have worked in this area, and without much extramural grant support until recently. As a consequence, the field of psychology has not been well prepared for the recent flood of referrals. Without proven assessment and psychosocial treatment techniques, there is a tremendous unmet need for helping families to make sense of their struggles and to address them constructively. Pediatricians, general practitioners, social workers, teachers, nurses, and parents have been trying to fill the gap, but psychological approaches clearly would be beneficial, too.

WHY BOTHER TO ASSESS FOR PBD?

In light of the justifiable reluctance to diagnose BD in children and adolescents, why should clinicians bother to assess for PBD? There are good reasons to be agnostic about PBD. "Agnosticism" in this context means being neither dogmatically certain that one will not encounter PBD in one's practice, nor suspending critical thought and labeling large numbers of cases with a trendy but probably relatively rare condition. The arguments for caution, which are described in detail below, include (1) the likely rarity of bipolar disorder in youth, (2) the diffi-

culty in disentangling mood symptoms from developmentally appropriate behavior or problems due to more common conditions (e.g., attention-deficit/hyperactivity disorder [ADHD] or unipolar depression), (3) frequent comorbidity that further obscures the clinical presentation, (4) lack of information about the developmental continuity of mood problems from youth into later life, and (5) a historical lack of proven assessment and therapeutic tools even if PBD were present.

On the other hand, BD has a large genetic contribution (Faraone, Tsuang, & Tsuang, 1999). The genes conveying risk are present from the moment of conception. Thus, the issue is determining how early adverse environmental experiences interact with genes to produce a pattern of behavior problems that we recognize as a mood disorder. Kraepelin (1921) diagnosed "manic depressive insanity" with some frequency in youth ages 13 and older, and more rarely in younger children. Case notes that paint a picture of mania in children extend back into the 17th century (Findling, Kowatch, & Post, 2003), and numerous other examples of published case presentations are scattered through the 20th century prior to 1990 (see Glovinsky, 2002, for a review). There is also no strong theoretical argument for why BD does not manifest until adulthood. Whereas some evidence suggests that changes in endocrine functioning associated with puberty might increase the hazard of developing BD, there are no models describing commonplace mechanisms that would later trigger a bipolar diathesis.

Perhaps the most compelling arguments in favor of careful assessment of possible PBD are pragmatic. In general, assessment should contribute to the clinical enterprise by *predicting* meaningful outcomes, by *prescribing* interventions (or contraindicating other approaches), or by measuring *processes* related to successful intervention. A case formulation involving PBD addresses all three of these domains. In terms of prediction, a bipolar diagnosis is associated with higher risk for many poor outcomes, including substance use, delinquency, and suicidality (Lewinsohn, Klein, & Seeley, 2000). Even when standard clinical care is available, PBD is associated with long periods of illness and high rates of relapse, and considerable functional impairment in terms of family conflict, educational failure, and poor peer relations (Birmaher et al., 2006; Geller, Tillman,

Craney, & Bolhofner, 2004; Lewinsohn et al., 2000).

With regard to prescription, a bipolar case formulation alerts a clinician to a set of potential concerns that extends beyond management of anger, impulse control, and internalizing problems, although these issues are likely also to be part of the presenting problem. In addition, a bipolar diagnosis should trigger a focus on sleep hygiene, activity scheduling, management of both positive and negative events, and evaluation of adherence to treatment (Danielson, Feeny, Findling, & Youngstrom, 2004). At present, there are no psychosocial or pharmacological treatments with enough demonstrated efficacy in youth samples to satisfy the highest standards for "empirically supported treatments" (Chambless & Hollon, 1998) or evidence-based practice (Guyatt & Rennie, 2002; Sackett, Straus, Richardson, Rosenberg, & Haynes, 2000). However, a growing body of evidence suggests that psychoeducational (Fristad, Gavazzi, & Mackinaw-Koons, 2003), family therapy (Miklowitz et al., 2004), cognitive behavioral therapy (Feeny, Danielson, Schwartz, Youngstrom, & Findling, 2006; Pavuluri et al., 2004), and other psychosocial interventions have value as adjunctive treatments. Practice parameters currently indicate that pharmacotherapy should be considered the first line of treatment for PBD, but they also make clear that psychosocial interventions are an essential component of the treatment package (Kowatch, Fristad, et al., 2005).

A bipolar diagnosis is also clinically helpful in terms of what approaches it contraindicates. At a pharmacological level, a bipolar diagnosis should probably rule out the use of stimulant medications as a way of managing hyperactivity and distractibility, at least without an additional mood-stabilizing agent already in use (Scheffer, Kowatch, Carmody, & Rush, 2005). Similarly, the U.S. Food and Drug Administration (FDA) has recommended that manufacturers of antidepressants voluntarily include language in packaging inserts alerting consumers and prescribers that thorough evaluation should rule out the possibility of bipolar illness before a person takes antidepressant medication to treat a depressive episode. There is widespread clinical concern that the well-intentioned use of stimulants or antidepressants is at best ineffective in managing bipolar illness and may even exacerbate the course of

illness instead (DelBello, Soutullo, et al., 2001; Geller, Fox, & Fletcher, 1993). Although it has proven difficult to demonstrate evidence of pharmacotoxicity in research studies (Carlson, 2003; Carlson & Mick, 2003), even the "best-case scenario" suggests that selection of inappropriate pharmacological interventions exposes patients to all of the potential risks, with little potential for benefit. Even though less work has targeted psychosocial interventions, it is also becoming evident that efficacious treatments for depression need some modification for work with BD, lest they accidentally trigger manic or mixed episodes (Fristad & Goldberg Arnold, 2004; Newman, Leahy, Beck, Reilly-Harrington, & Gyulai, 2002; Scott & Colom, 2005).

Additionally, a case formulation including a bipolar diagnosis generates a set of assessment goals and techniques geared toward supporting treatment. Besides routine evaluation of internalizing and externalizing symptoms, a bipolar formulation requires more systematic tracking of mood and energy levels. Unlike unipolar depression (see Rudolph & Lambert, Chapter 5, this volume), a bipolar diagnosis requires monitoring of highs, as well as lows and periods of irritability. Relapse prevention becomes an important formal component of treatment, so identification of "triggers" and early warning signs of mood destabilization ("roughening" of mood) (Sachs, Guille, & McMurrich, 2002) become paramount.

Finally, thorough assessment helps to reduce the rate of overdiagnosis of a trendy condition. Good evaluation not only leads to improved identification of those cases actually affected by PBD (i.e., raising the diagnostic "sensitivity") but also enhances correct recognition of cases without PBD (i.e., bettering the diagnostic "specificity"). Accurate identification of nonbipolar illnesses is of tremendous value to families. Correct diagnosis avoids unnecessarily exposing children to pharmacological agents that are less well investigated than stimulants or antidepressants in youth populations, yet clearly have risks of much more serious side effects (Findling, Feeny, Stansbrey, DelPorto-Bedoya, & Demeter, 2004). Besides lessening the risk of iatrogenic treatments, correctly labeling the nonbipolar condition connects to a much larger evidence base that can guide treatment. When we appropriately discern that the problems are due to ADHD, unipolar depression, or parent–child conflict, and not a bipolar illness, researchers and clinicians bring to bear much more experience and evidence.

For all of these reasons, it seems useful that cautious clinicians shift to an agnostic stance. Likewise, to avoid overdiagnosis, practitioners who have been diagnosing PBD would be prudent to adopt the most rigorous methods available. It behooves us to become familiar with the complexities of assessing BD in children and adolescents, as well as to learn about the tools and strategies that aid this high-stakes clinical decision.

DIAGNOSTIC CRITERIA

Diagnostic Categories

The challenges of assessing BD begin with the diagnostic criteria themselves. The fourth, text revised edition of the *Diagnostic and Statistical Manual of Mental Disorders* (DSM-IV-TR) currently delineates four different diagnoses that are clearly on the bipolar spectrum: bipolar I and bipolar II disorder, cyclothymia, and BD not otherwise specified (NOS) (American Psychiatric Association [APA], 2000). The In-

ternational Classification of Diseases (ICD-10) uses the same categories, but with slightly different criteria. However, diagnosing a mood disorder first requires gathering information about the lifetime history of mood *states*. Different *diagnoses* require different combinations of mood *states*, introducing a level of complexity not found in most other diagnoses. Adding more barriers to correct identification, people are unlikely to seek treatment for hypomania and rarely self-refer for treatment of mania. As a result, clinicians are much more likely to see patients during the depressed phase of a bipolar illness.

The mood states that must be assessed correctly to ascertain a DSM-IV-TR diagnosis of mood disorder include manic episode, mixed episode, major depressive episode, hypomanic episode, dysthymic episode, and dysthymia with superimposed hypomanic symptoms. Although the last mood state is not formally distinguished in DSM-IV-TR, it has been proven necessary to diagnose cyclothymia (which requires marked hypomanic *symptoms*, but not necessarily hypomanic *episodes* with duration of 4 or more days). Table 6.1 reviews the symp-

---

TABLE 6.1. Criteria for Manic or Hypomanic Episode

A. A distinct period of abnormally and persistently elevated, expansive, or irritable mood, clearly different from usual mood. *Duration*: At least 1 week (unless severe enough that hospitalization is necessary) for mania; at least 4 days for hypomanic episode.

B. During the mood episode, at least three of the following symptoms are also present to a significant degree (four or more if mood is mostly irritable):

    (1) inflated self-esteem or grandiosity
    (2) decreased need for sleep (such as feeling rested with only 3 hours of sleep)
    (3) pressured speech or more talkative than usual
    (4) flight of ideas or racing thoughts
    (5) distractibility
    (6) increased goal-directed activity or psychomotor agitation
    (7) excessive pleasurable activities with a high risk for painful or damaging consequences

C. If showing sufficient symptoms for both a manic episode and also major depressive episode for at least 1 week (or until hospitalized), then classify as "mixed episode"

D. *Mania*: Causes marked impairment in school, at home, or with peers; may also require hospitalization to prevent harm to self or others; may also have psychotic features.

    Hypomania: An unequivocal change in functioning from typical for person when not symptomatic, observable by others; but *not* severe enough to cause marked impairment, and with no psychotic features.

E. Rule out symptoms due to physiological effects of a substance (including stimulant or antidepressant medication), or symptoms due to a general medical condition.

Note. Adapted from American Psychiatric Association (2000). Copyright 2000 by the American Psychiatric Association. Adapted by permission.

toms and criteria for a DSM-IV-TR diagnosis of manic or hypomanic episodes. Rudolph and Lambert, Chapter 5, this volume, review the criteria for unipolar depression and dysthymia.

Some additional complexities are stipulated in the diagnosis of bipolar spectrum disorders. Bipolar II disorder requires both a major depressive episode and a hypomanic episode at some point in the person's life. Cyclothymia, on the other hand, involves depressive and hypomanic symptoms that are insufficient in severity to qualify for a full-blown major depressive or manic episode, at least during the first year of mood disturbance in children or adolescents, yet clearly mark a change from typical functioning or temperament. A bipolar I disorder diagnosis may be based on a single manic or mixed episode. One need never be depressed to be diagnosed with what used to be called "manic–depression"!

Little additional guidance is offered for assessment of mood disorders in children or adolescents. Besides noting that irritable mood may be more common than sad mood in depression for children, DSM-IV-TR does not make any developmental modifications of the symptom criteria for diagnosing any of the aforementioned mood states. The only developmental modification to the durational criteria is to accept a 1-year duration instead of a 2-year duration for dysthymic and cyclothymic episodes. Without good normative developmental data, it is difficult to tell whether these minimal adjustments are adequate. Research has concentrated on validating the extant diagnostic criteria in youth, then proposing incremental modifications for depression (Kovacs, 1989; Luby et al., 2003) and mania (Geller & Luby, 1997).

The following description of diagnoses is intended to provide an overview of the criteria, along with a discussion of the strengths and limitations of the current framework, especially as applied to children and adolescents.

Bipolar I

Considered the most serious form of bipolar illness, a bipolar I disorder diagnosis requires the presence of at least one manic or mixed episode during a person's lifetime. Once a manic or mixed episode has occurred, DSM and ICD nosologies consider the individual to have a lifetime diagnosis of bipolar I disorder. If the individual is currently functioning well, then the classification is bipolar I "in remission." If the person develops classic major depression, even years after the mania, then the correct diagnosis is "bipolar I, current episode: depressed." Both mania and mixed states require that the behavior be a change from typical functioning for the individual, and that the behavior causes impairment (even though it may not distress the person experiencing the mood disturbance). The mood disturbance must either occur much of the day for most days over a period of at least 1 week, or the mood disturbance must be so extreme as to result in psychiatric hospitalization, in which case the 1-week duration requirement is waived. Although a person need never be depressed to be diagnosed with bipolar I, depression is the more common phase of illness, at least in adults; and depression appears to impose a greater burden than does mania over the course of illness (Judd et al., 2005).

Bipolar II

Diagnosis of bipolar II disorder requires at least two lifetime mood states: both a major depressive episode and a hypomanic episode. Although generally considered less severe than bipolar I disorder, recent data indicate that bipolar II disorder may be associated with higher risk of suicide (Rihmer & Kiss, 2002). It is also much more difficult to diagnose than bipolar I, because hypomania is by definition more subtle and less impairing than mania. In addition, an affected individual is much more likely to seek treatment during the depressed phase of the illness, and neither the individual nor the interviewing clinician is likely to disclose or assess for the hypomanic episodes that distinguish between bipolar II illness and unipolar depression. Furthermore, bipolar II disorder has rarely been evaluated systematically in clinical or research settings with children (Youngstrom, Youngstrom, et al., 2005).

Put another way, clinicians are most likely to encounter bipolar II disorder during the depressed phase of the illness. There are no evidence-based indications that bipolar depression consistently presents differently than unipolar disorder at the symptom level. However, the bipolar–unipolar distinction is important in terms of suicide risk, substance use, choice of pharmacological agent, and possibly choice of strategies for psychotherapy. Unfortunately, available data also indicate that individuals affected with bipolar II disorder tend to first present clinically in the depressed phase of the illness, and early-onset depression may be a marker for BD (Birmaher, Arbelaez, & Brent, 2002; Kovacs, 1996). These findings suggest that many children and young adolescents afflicted with what appears to be depression might actually be experiencing the depressed phase of a bipolar illness.

Cyclothymia

The diagnosis of cyclothymic disorder requires that a period of mood disturbance last at least 1 year (2 years in adults), with no more than 2 months free of symptoms. The mood disturbance represents a clear change in the individual's typical pattern of behavior (distinguishing it from temperament) observable by others. The mood involves depressive or dysthymic symptoms, along with periods of hypomanic symptoms. During this index period, the depressive symptoms cannot become sufficiently severe to meet criteria for a major depressive episode (in which case the diagnosis changes to unipolar depression, or perhaps bipolar II disorder), nor can the hypomanic symptoms become too impairing (in which case the diagnosis changes to bipolar I disorder). It is possible to meet criteria for both cyclothymia and bipolar I disorder (much as it is possible to meet criteria for dysthymia and major depression over the course of lifetime—provided that the cyclothymic or dysthymic episode precedes the onset of the more severe mood state.

Cyclothymia is an especially slippery construct to assess on the bipolar spectrum. The long duration of the mood disturbance makes it hard to distinguish between temperamental traits and cyclothymic episodes, particularly for children: A year represents a much larger portion of a young child's life (blurring the boundary between an episode and a trait), and assessors need to rely more on collateral informants, such as parents or teachers, to identify changes in mood and energy. For this reason, in clinical practice, cyclothymia has rarely been diagnosed in youth even in the United States (Youngstrom, Youngstrom, et al., 2005). Some research groups are also reluctant to label youths with "cyclothymia," often lumping these clinical presentations into a "bipolar disorder not otherwise specified" category instead (Birmaher et al., 2006). However, it is worth noting that pediatric cyclothymia, when labeled as such, has been shown to be linked to high levels of impairment (Findling, Youngstrom, et al., 2005; Lewinsohn, Seeley, Buckley, & Klein, 2002), yet also often shows spontaneous remission or lack of progression to more severe forms of mood disorder (Kahana, Youngstrom, Calabrese, & Findling, under review; Lewinsohn et al., 2002).

Bipolar Disorder Not Otherwise Specified

Bipolar disorder not otherwise specified (BD NOS) is a residual category used to describe clinical presentations that appear to be on the bipolar spectrum but do not fit into any of the three aforementioned categories. DSM-IV-TR gives several examples of possible presentations for BD NOS, including repeated episodes of hypomania without lifetime history of manic, mixed, or depressive episodes—a presentation that is unlikely to come to clinical attention but has been described in studies of nonclinical adolescents and young adults (Depue, Krauss, Spoont, & Arbisi, 1989). Other presentations include manifesting an inadequate number of "B criteria" symptoms in the context of episodic mood disturbance, or showing sufficient symptoms, but for an insufficient duration to meet established criteria for a diagnosis. BD NOS, like cyclothymia, tends to be diagnosed only rarely in clinical practice (Youngstrom, Youngstrom, et al., 2005). In addition, different research groups tend to use different operational definitions of BD NOS (see Table 6.2). However, BD NOS is linked to substantial clinical impairment, including poor functioning academically and interpersonally, high rates of service utilization and suicide risk, and substantial mood disturbance, whether NOS is defined as insufficient number of symptoms (Lewinsohn, Seeley, & Klein, 2003), insufficient duration (Findling, Youngstrom, et al., 2005), or a combination of the two (Axelson et al., in press). BD NOS appears to show patterns of familial risk (Findling, Youngstrom, et al., 2005) and symptom severity (Axelson et al., 2006) that are consistent with it being on the bipolar spectrum; and more than one-fourth of youth with BD NOS progress to more fully syndromal bipolar presentations (i.e., meeting criteria for bipolar I or II disorder) within a few years of initially being diagnosed with BD NOS (Birmaher et al., 2006).

TABLE 6.2. Definitions of Bipolar Disorder, Bipolar Spectrum Disorder, and Research Definitions of Pediatric Bipolar Subtypes

Definition (source)	Comment
Bipolar I	• Requires lifetime presence of a manic or mixed-state episode, mood disturbance duration of 7 days or until hospitalization. • No requirement of depression—ever. • ICD-10 requires multiple episodes to be confident of diagnosis; only "provisional" with single episode, even in adults.
Bipolar II	• Requires lifetime combination of a major depressive episode and a hypomanic episode (of at least 4 days' duration).
Cyclothymia (DSM-IV-TR)	• Technically not considered a type of "bipolar NOS" in DSM. • Rarely diagnosed in children or adolescents in research or clinical settings (Youngstrom, Youngstrom, et al., 2005). • Many research groups lump cyclothymia with BD NOS (Birmaher et al., 2006). • Difficult to disentangle from normal development, temperament, and comorbid conditions due to the requirement that patient not meet criteria for full manic, mixed, or major depressive episode during initial year of illness. • Still possible to diagnose reliably, and associated with a significant amount of impairment (Findling, Youngstrom, et al., 2005).
Repeated hypomanias in the absence of lifetime mania or depression (DSM-IV-TR bipolar disorder not otherwise specified [BD NOS])	• Unlikely to be impairing enough to lead to treatment seeking; thus, not observed clinically. • Challenging to differentiate from behavior within developmental normal limits.
Insufficient duration of mood episodes (DSM-IV-TR). Leibenluft et al. (2003) further distinguish between cases with elated mood and/or grandiosity, and those with only irritability as mood disturbance; following Geller, Williams, et al. (1998).	• This appears to be a common presentation (Axelson et al., 2006; Findling, Youngstrom, et al., 2005). • It is associated with a high degree of impairment (Lewinsohn et al., 2000). • This definition may include cases with mood severity that would otherwise warrant a diagnosis of manic, mixed, or depressive state. • Also may include cases with mixed states that involve polarity shifts, if the diagnostician expects a week's worth of duration for either polarity. • Important to note that adult data are calling durations into question (Angst et al., 2003).
Insufficient number of manic symptoms. Leibenluft et al. (2003) included "irritable hypomania" and "irritable mania" as another "intermediate" phenotype, even if accompanied by four or more other manic symptoms.	• This also appears to be more prevalent than cases meeting strict DSM criteria for bipolar I or II disorder, both in adolescent data and in reanalyses of adult epidemiological data (Judd & Akiskal, 2003; Lewinsohn et al., 2000). • Captures a much more heterogeneous group, and it is possible to meet criteria for this category relying entirely on nonspecific symptoms (e.g., irritable mood plus distractibility, high motor activity, and rapid speech). • Research designs typically have not documented episodicity of symptoms (Judd & Akiskal, 2003; Lewinsohn et al., 2000). • In spite of these caveats, this definition of BD NOS is still associated with high rates of impairment and service utilization (Galanter et al., 2003; Hazell et al., 2003).
Severe mood dysregulation (previously referred to as a "broad phenotype") (Leibenluft et al., 2003, definition)	• Recommended criteria: Abnormal mood (anger or sadness) present at least half the day most days; accompanied by "hyperarousal" (insomnia*, agitation, distractibility, racing thoughts/flight of ideas; pressured speech, or social intrusiveness*); also shows increased reactivity to negative emotional stimuli compared to peers*; onset before age 12; duration at least 12 months, with no more than 2 months symptom free; symptoms severe in at least one setting.

(continued)

TABLE 6.2. *(continued)*

Definition (source)	Comment
	• Rule outs: elated mood, grandiosity, or episodically decreased need for sleep; distinct episodes of 4+ days' duration; meeting criteria for schizophreniform, schizophrenia, pervasive developmental disorder, or posttraumatic stress disorder; or meeting criteria for a substance use disorder in the past 3 months; or IQ < 80; or symptoms are attributable to a medication or general medical condition. • Comments: Not yet tested against data. The *exclusion* of episodicity and of several symptoms more specific to BD both are likely to select against bipolar spectrum cases. The inclusion of chronic presentations and sensitive but nonspecific symptoms are likely to include many individuals with presentations that are not on the bipolar spectrum. This category appears likely to include a blend of different etiologies and mechanisms as a result.
BD NOS—research criteria from "Course and Outcomes of Bipolar Youth" Study (NIMH Grant No. R01 MH059929) (Birmaher et al., 2006; Axelson et al., 2006)	• Requires "core positive"—presence of distinct period of abnormally elevated, expansive, or irritable mood. • Minimum of two other "B criteria" symptoms if mood is mostly elated; at least three "B criteria" if irritable. • Requires clear change from individual's typical functioning (consistent with DSM-IV and ICD guidelines for hypomania). • Requires 4+ hours of mood within a 24-hour period to be counted as an index "day" of disturbance. • Requires 4+ days at a minimum over the course of a lifetime to diagnose BD NOS; nonconsecutive days are acceptable. • Beginning to garner empirical support (Axelson et al., 2006). • Needs replication in other samples/research groups, but overlaps substantially with "insufficient duration" and "insufficient number of B criterion symptoms" definitions of BD NOS.
Child Behavior Checklist proxy diagnosis (after Mick et al., 2003). Often operationally defined as parent-reported *T*-scores of 70+ on Aggressive Behavior, Attention Problems, and Anxious–Depressed subscales.	• Convenient to use for large-sample studies. • Avoids problems of rater training and anchoring effects. • Prone to factors that might bias parent report. • Does not capture diagnostically specific symptoms; instead concentrates on sensitive symptoms that might also have high false-positive rate. • Focuses on symptoms that are likely to be "shared" with other disorders at a genetic level. • Concerns that agreement with clinical or research-interview-derived (K-SADS) diagnoses of bipolar spectrum might be modest.

Note. Expanded and adapted from Table 2 in Youngstrom, Birmaher, and Findling (under review).
*Symptom is not part of current DSM-IV nosology for mania.

Other Definitions of the Bipolar Spectrum

Several other definitions of "bipolar spectrum" diagnoses are sometimes used in the literature or clinically. One of the most important to consider clinically is "substance-induced mania." Manic-like symptoms may be induced not only by street drugs such as cocaine but also by prescription drugs, including corticosteroids (as happened with TV personality Jane Pauley). There also is concern that stimulant medications (Carlson & Mick, 2003; DelBello, Soutullo, et al., 2001), tricyclic antidepressants (Geller et al., 1993), or selective serotonin reuptake inhibitors (SSRIs) (Ghaemi, Hsu, Soldani, & Goodwin, 2003; Papolos, 2003; Reichart & Nolen, 2004) may induce manic symptoms. However, it is difficult to decide whether the appearance of manic symptoms in a person taking a medication represents (1) the spontaneous emergence of mania in someone already at risk, independent of the effects of the medication; (2) a side effect of the medication, irrelevant to the person's true status with regard to bipolar illness; (3) an "unmasking" of a previously undetected bipolar illness in someone already genetically at risk; or (4) an iatrogenic effect of medication that changes the nervous system in such a way that individuals not carrying genes of risk are still at risk of manifesting bipolar behaviors, even after medication is discontinued (a "scar hypothesis"). Recent research studies have failed to demonstrate clearly that medication use is associated with higher rates of mania (Carlson, 2003), and stimulants appear to be well tolerated when used in treatment for PBD in conjunction with mood-stabilizing compounds (Findling, McNamara, et al., 2005; Scheffer et al., 2005). For all these reasons, it is appropriate to follow the DSM recommendation to diagnose these cases as having "substance-induced mania" rather than "unmasked" bipolar I or bipolar II illness.

A second major category potential on the bipolar spectrum is represented by a subset of cases presenting with unipolar depression. People who have depression that onsets early, shows acute onset, is associated with atypical features (e.g., lethargy, hypersomnia, increased appetite or weight gain, and rejection sensitivity), recurrent depressive episodes, and in the context of a family history of BD are at higher risk of having depressed phases that ultimately prove to be bipolar illness (Birmaher et al., 2002; Kessler, Avenevoli, & Merikangas, 2001; Luby & Mrakotsky, 2003). Many researchers working with adults have tended to include these sorts of depressive presentations on the bipolar spectrum (Akiskal & Pinto, 1999; Ghaemi, Ko, & Goodwin, 2002; Sachs, 2004). Diagnosing depressed presentations in youth as bipolar spectrum illness is rare in clinical practice, and attempts to apply a "bipolar" label to depressed presentations in youth would be fraught with controversy. Yet epidemiological studies, longitudinal investigations of depression, and clinical referral patterns all indicate more than half of adults with bipolar illness likely sought help for depressive symptoms occurring in childhood or adolescence (Kessler, Berglund, Demler, Jin, & Walters, 2005; Perlis et al., 2004).

A third possible group on the bipolar spectrum includes those with "severe mood dysregulation," or what has sometimes been called the "broad phenotype" of bipolar illness (Leibenluft, Charney, Towbin, Bhangoo, & Pine, 2003). Key features of this presentation include chronic irritability and mood lability, along with a lack of distinct episodes with marked change in mood or energy. In some data, these presentations appear to be on a continuum with bipolar illnesses, albeit involving more rapid rates and briefer episodes of mood disturbance. Some have noted that this clinical presentation seems highly similar to borderline personality disorder (BPD) in adults, and may in fact be a juvenile precursor to BPD (MacKinnon & Pies, 2006). On the other hand, some investigators have found evidence that "chronic irritability," when precisely operationalized, may be more related to depression than to mania in terms of important correlates and associated features (Leibenluft, Cohen, Gorrindo, Brook, & Pine, 2006). This group must be considered potentially one of the most speculative categories on the bipolar spectrum. There are few data-based studies evaluating this presentation, and no significant longitudinal investigations, nor are treatment data informative about course and outcome. It is likely to be challenging to tease apart severe mood dysregulation from other, more common disorders of childhood, as well as from fluctuations of mood that fall within normal limits for child and adolescent behavior. Thus, it appears premature to begin applying the "severe mood dysregulation" label clinically, until sufficient data are available that the label predicts useful outcomes, prescribes intervention choices, or informs the process of treatment.

A fourth group sometimes considered on the bipolar spectrum is cases identified by means of a proxy measure rather than direct clinical interview. The two most common examples are the use of a profile of scores on the Child Behavior Checklist (CBCL; Achenbach, 1991a) or positive scores on a screener for BD, such as the Mood Disorder Questionnaire (Hirschfeld et al., 2000), as proxies for a bipolar diagnosis. These proxy definitions are typically used in research studies, especially in behavioral genetics work (Althoff, Rettew, Faraone, Boomsma, & Hudziak, 2006; Hudziak, Althoff, Derks, Faraone, & Boomsma, 2005) or in reanalyses of data initially gathered for purposes other than studying PBD (Galanter et al., 2003; Hazell, Carr, Lewin, & Sly, 2003; Reichart et al., 2004). As will become evident later in our discussion of the impact of illness base rates on the diagnostic efficiency of measures, the number of "proxy" cases that would actually be confirmed to have PBD in the event of a careful diagnostic interview can be wildly variable. The rate of "true" bipolar cases in a group of proxy-defined cases is likely to be low in most settings, especially in general population surveys. The low "positive predictive value" of a proxy diagnosis of PBD makes the interpretation of research relying on the proxy definition ambiguous at best. Furthermore, the substitution of a proxy definition for careful clinical diagnosis of PBD is clearly inappropriate in clinical practice.

RECOMMENDED CONSIDERATIONS FOR DIFFERENTIAL DIAGNOSIS IN CHILDREN

Comorbidity

BD has tremendously high rates of comorbidity with other mental disorders and substance use. In the first National Comorbidity Survey (NCS), 99% of adults meeting criteria for bipolar I illness met full criteria for at least one other lifetime Axis I diagnosis (Kessler, 1999). Rates of comorbidity appear similarly high in children and adolescents meeting criteria for BD (Geller et al., 2003; Kowatch, Youngstrom, Danielyan, & Findling, 2005). It is not straightforward to compare the rates of comorbid conditions between pediatric and adult samples, due to both developmental trends in the comorbid conditions and gaps in assessment batteries. For example, the high rates of substance use and antisocial behavior in adults with BD are likely much lower in youth by virtue of the generally later age of onset for these behaviors; youths show high rates of oppositional behavior and attention problems, but potential developmental continuity in these behaviors has been obscured by the lack of a clear adult analogue to oppositional defiant disorder (although it often is a precursor to antisocial behavior) (Moffit, Caspi, Dickson, Silva, & Stanton, 1996). Similarly, adult epidemiological studies or clinical investigations of adult BD until recently did not systematically evaluate ADHD, because conventional wisdom indicated that ADHD was a disorder of childhood and likely to remit spontaneously. However, newer studies evaluating ADHD in adults have found that BD is associated with a much higher lifetime rate of ADHD, as well as significantly more ADHD persisting into adulthood (Nierenberg et al., 2005).

The most common comorbidities identified in youths meeting criteria for BD are ADHD, oppositional defiant disorder, conduct disorder, and anxiety disorders (Kowatch, Youngstrom, et al., 2005); pediatric-onset BD may also be associated with higher risk of meeting criteria for other conditions, such as enuresis or eating disorders (Weckerly, 2002). The rate of comorbid ADHD was initially reported to be extremely high, in excess of 90% (Biederman et al., 1996; Geller et al., 2003). However, other investigations using different referral patterns or interview procedures have found that closer to 60% of youths with BD also meet criteria for ADHD. The lower rates are more similar to the rates of comorbid ADHD diagnosed clinically in youth treated for BD (Youngstrom, Youngstrom, et al., 2005). Even so, the rates for comorbid ADHD remain too remarkably high for these to be independent conditions. If ADHD were an unrelated illness that affects roughly 5% of the general population, then it should also manifest in roughly 5% of BD cases. The much higher rate of coincidence may be due to the pronounced overlap in diagnostic criteria. ADHD often involves distractibility, high motor activity, talkativeness, and impulsive behavior, all of which look like manic behaviors (Klein et al., 1998). Furthermore, youth with ADHD are often irritable and frequently meet criteria for comorbid oppositional or conduct disorders—potentially mimicking the irritable mood seen with mania. Conversely, a person who meets criteria for mania will also exhibit multiple symptoms that may appear consistent with ADHD. Thus, the high rate of comorbidity might be inflated by research interviewers or clinicians who do not sufficiently determine whether the symptom is most attributable to a mood disorder or another condition. However, other investigators argue that comorbid ADHD may represent a distinct subtype of BD, pointing to patterns of heritability and the fact that youth with comorbid ADHD and BD often show greater impairment and worse course (Biederman et al., 1996; Faraone, Biederman, Mennin, Wozniak, & Spencer, 1997).

Comorbid anxiety disorders are open to similar discussion: Rates of comorbidity vary too widely to be due merely to chance sampling differences (Kowatch, Youngstrom, et al., 2005). Higher comorbidity estimates may be due partially to diagnosis of anxiety disorders on the basis of anxious symptoms reported during the course of a mood episode. Again, "comorbid" anxiety is associated with greater impairment and worse course, but it is unclear whether this is due to the comorbidity, or whether the perceived "comorbidity" is another way to describe a person experiencing a greater number of total problems in the context of the illness.

Overall, it appears premature to report specific rates of comorbidity for different disorders, in light of both the potential methodological limitations and developmental changes in potential comorbid conditions. Clinically, one can expect to see "pure" bipolar presentations only rarely. It also makes sense to assess for attention problems and anxiety, as well as substance use and other antisocial behavior, when confronted with potential PBD. In terms of research, much more work is needed that looks for patterns of heterotypic continuity (e.g., oppositional behaviors in childhood persisting as more delinquent behaviors in adolescence, then as "antisocial personality" in adulthood). What are sometimes considered patterns of comorbidity may also prove to be useful endophenotypes, because they may reflect the activity of particular genes that are not uniformly present in all cases meeting DSM criteria for either disorder. For example, persons with BD and generalized anxiety disorder (GAD) may have behavioral inhibition system–related genes that are not present in other cases with PBD, and also mood-dysregulation genes not present in most individuals meeting criteria for GAD.

Rapid Cycling

BD, even in adults, is a recurrent illness. Few affected persons have only one episode of depression or mania over the course of their entire lifetime. However, many are able to go for periods of years, or even decades, between episodes of pathological mood disturbance (Goodwin & Jamison, 1990). Most people have more frequent relapses into mood states. "Rapid-cycling" mood disorder means that a person has at least four distinct mood episodes over the course of a year (APA, 2000; Dunner, Patrick, & Fieve, 1977). This pattern is vital to recognize: Rapid cycling prognosticates a more chronic course of illness, with greater comorbidity, less responsiveness to lithium, and higher risk of mortality (Coryell et al., 2003).

What defines a "cycle" or an "episode" is not universally agreed upon, and many adults with bipolar illness show a clear pattern of labile affective disturbance that does not fit into the strict DSM-IV definition of rapid cycling

(MacKinnon et al., 2003; Maj, Pirozzi, Formicola, & Tortorella, 1999). Some of the confusion is due to the lack of a precise definition for the end of a mood episode (Frank et al., 1991). A switch in polarity of mood (e.g., from mania to depression) may often occur within the course of a single episode (APA, 2000; Kraepelin, 1921). Some authors have described youth as having "ultradian" cycling, or polarity switches in the course of the same day (Geller et al., 1995). Sometimes these rates of daily polarity switches have been extrapolated to extend over the length of a year, or over the course of an even longer episode, then reported as the "rate of cycling" for youth, with estimates climbing up to the 10's of thousands (Geller, Williams, et al., 1998). These figures provoke understandable cynicism from those familiar with the adult presentation of BD, in which four distinct mood episodes within a single year portend a stormy course. The sheer quantitative discrepancy (four vs. thousands per year) may also raise concerns about whether we are confronting the same disorder in children and adults. Thus, it is crucial to realize that the described clinical presentations are actually quite similar, and the apparent discrepancies are due to slippage in the definition of terms. PBD is being described by multiple groups as involving rapid polarity switches, with brief durations at either extreme, yet each *episode* is a long period of dysregulated mood.

Mixed States

Mixed states involve symptoms of mania and of major depression during the same mood episode. According to DSM-IV-TR criteria, there must be an adequate number of symptoms present with sufficient intensity to meet criteria for both major depression and for mania. The duration of a mixed state is set at a week, unless symptoms are so severe as to require hospitalization, with the symptoms required to be present for "much of the day, nearly every day during at least a 1-week period (APA, 2000, p. 365). There are at least two ways that the requirement "much of the day" could be met. One would be for both manic and depressive symptoms to be present simultaneously in a single, homogeneous mood state. Kay Jamison (1995) has described this as a "black mania," combining the hopelessness, low self-esteem, pathological guilt, and despair of depression with the high energy, racing thoughts, and impulsivity of mania. Not surprisingly, such a mood state presents a high risk for suicide (Goodwin & Jamison, 1990).

In the other mixed presentation, mood oscillates rapidly between depressed and manic states over the course of the week, or even within the same day. Unstable and shifting moods were noted as a common presentation of mixed states by Kraepelin during his clinical observations (1921), and these have also been frequently documented in clinical observation of adults with BD (Kramlinger & Post, 1996), as well as prospective "life charting" of mood and energy (Denicoff et al., 1997) and objective markers of physical activity. This oscillating, labile form of "mixed state" is almost definitely what has been described by some as "ultradian cycling" in children (Geller & Cook, 2000).

Efforts to compare the adult and child phenomenology of BD have been hampered by terminology. Oscillating mixed states appear to be the most common presentation of BD in youth, consistent with age effects noted initially by Kraepelin (1921). At the same time, it is important to bear in mind that oscillating mixed states with pronounced mood lability are common in adults with mood disorder (MacKinnon & Pies, 2006). Conversely, the term "rapid cycling," as used in the adult literature, refers to the number of distinct mood *episodes* within a 1-year period rather than the number of *polarity shifts* of mood within a single episode. It appears relatively rare for children or adolescents to experience multiple remissions of their mixed state, then multiple relapses within the same year (Birmaher et al., 2006; Geller et al., 2004), particularly when "remission" is defined as a period of 2 months free of impairing symptoms (Findling et al., 2001; Frank et al., 1991). Thus, "rapid cycling" in the strictest sense appears to be uncommon in children, and there is instead a high rate of oscillating mixed states.

Major Symptom Dimensions and Associated Features

The two major dimensions involved in bipolar illness are depressive and manic symptoms. Counterintuitively, depression and mania do not appear to be opposite poles of a single dimension. Instead, they are two distinct sets of symptoms that can occur independently of each other or overlap. Mixed states involve high levels of both depressed and manic symptoms. A dimensional model resolves many of the problems noted with the current categorical classification system, including the large number of cases with "mixed hypomanias" or "anger attacks" in the context of depression, or agitated depressive presentations. Rather than requiring a proliferation of subcategories, these clinical presentations may be conceptualized as the coincidence of moderate levels of manic symptomatology during periods with higher levels of depressive symptoms. In fact, there is growing evidence that there might be different risk factors associated with triggering depressive versus hypomanic or manic symptoms (Johnson & Roberts, 1995). A major clinical implication is that assessment should include measures of both hypomanic/manic and depressed symptoms not only at intake but also as outcome measures, due to the potential for the emergence of new mood symptoms (including those of a different polarity than the presenting problem).

An alternative way of conceptualizing mania and depression is to link them to major motivational systems, such as Gray's behavioral inhibition system (BIS) and behavioral activation system (BAS; Fowles, 1994; Gray & McNaughton, 1996), or Depue's behavioral facilitation system (BFS; Depue & Iacono, 1989). These models put anxiety, depression, and mania within a larger evolutionary and neurobehavioral framework, where the clinical disorders are pathologically extreme or situationally inappropriate expressions of systems that otherwise serve important roles in the development of personality and healthy functioning. These models suggest linkages between mania and dopaminergic systems related to reward, extroversion, and approach-oriented behaviors (Depue & Collins, 1999). BIS–BAS models also predict a high degree of overlap between anxious and depressive symptoms, because both anxiety and depression involve high levels of BIS activation, also conceptualized as high levels of "negative affectivity" (Tellegen, Watson, & Clark, 1999). According to the "tripartite model" of depression and anxiety, negative affect, or high BIS activity, is a shared component of both anxiety and depression, whereas physiological hyperarousal is specific to anxiety, and low positive affect (or low BAS) is a specific marker for depression (Watson et al., 1995). The tripartite model's description of both depressed states and negative affect as a shared component of anxiety and depression has been replicated in multiple child and adolescent samples (Chorpita, 2002; Chorpita, Albano, & Barlow, 1998; Chorpita & Daleiden, 2002; Lonigan, Phillips, & Hooe, 2003). Although there are measures of BIS and BAS that include nonclinical behaviors (e.g., Carver & White, 1994), it is not clear that these instruments offer incremental value to clinical assessment. Instead, the clinical value of BIS and BAS models might lie primarily in the identification of "subsyndromal" or adaptive behaviors falling along the same dimension as mania or depression. Awareness of these behaviors might help to normalize and to depathologize some aspects, and also to monitor warning signs that presage the return of more severe mood disturbance. The BIS–BAS model also contributes a potential explanation for the frequent co-occurrence of anxious and depressive symptoms, which might otherwise be perceived as "comorbidity" of multiple disorders.

A third model of the dimensions of illness was first proposed by Kraepelin (1921). He described three clusters of symptoms involved in mood disorder: *cognitive or intellective*, including racing thoughts and heightened creativity at one extreme, and slowed thinking or dulled perceptions at the other; *vegetative*, including motor agitation and heightened energy at one extreme, and fatigue or psychomotor retardation at the other; and finally an *affective* component, ranging from manic excitement, expansiveness, and grandiosity to depressive hopelessness and despair. Kraepelin observed that these three clusters of symptoms were frequently out of phase with each other, giving rise to eight possible permutations of clinical presentation. Classic manic presentations entailed elevation of all three clusters, and classic depression reflected low levels of all three clusters. Agitated depression, in Kraepelin's model, involved high levels of the motor activity cluster of symptoms, whereas levels on the affective and cognitive dimensions remained low. Kraepelin provided an elegant and parsimonious way to describe clinically varied phenomena using a dimensional model. This framework also provided a means for integrating neuropsychological performance into a broader conceptual model of mood disorder. However, little recent work on neuropsychological performance in children or adolescents has included this historical model.

Several other features of PBD that deserve clinical attention include temperamental traits that are often associated with BD. Youth with PBD, compared to youth with ADHD or controls with no diagnosis, show higher novelty seeking and lower reward dependence behavior, lower persistence, and less self-direction and cooperativeness (Tillman et al., 2003). Youth at risk of developing BD because a biological parent has a bipolar history tend to show higher levels of trait negative affect, lower activity, and poorer sleep and rhythmicity (Chang, Blasey, Ketter, & Steiner, 2003). Rejection sensitivity also may be a prominent feature of bipolar illness, even when mood appears relatively stable (Benazzi, 2000; Fristad & Goldberg Arnold, 2004).These temperamental traits appear similar to many of the features seen in full-blown mood episodes, blurring the distinction between *character* and *mood episode*. However, BD appears to involve fluctuations or surges that noticeably amplify any temperamental qualities, suggesting that episodicity may be helpful in identifying youth at risk (Shaw, Egeland, Endicott, Allen, & Hostetter, 2005).

Epidemiology: Base Rates, Age of Onset, and Clinical Incidence

Epidemiological Data

A crucial question is how often PBD may be occurring both in the general population and in clinical settings. Epidemiological estimates convey a sense of the relative prevalence or rarity of different conditions, and the extent to which incidence varies by age or other demographic features. Epidemiological studies have found relatively low rates of mania in adolescents (Lewinsohn et al., 2002) and virtually no cases of mania in children (Costello et al., 1996; Shaffer et al., 1996). However, studies with adults reporting retrospectively about the onset of their mood symptoms indicate that more than 50% of adults with BD had their first mood symptoms before age 18 (Kessler, Rubinow, Holmes, Abelson, & Zhao, 1997), and often before the age of 16 (Perlis et al., 2004; Post et al., 2006). Surveys of adult consumers indicate median delays of 11–19 years between the beginning of mood symptoms and when treatment is sought and a correct diagnosis is made (Calabrese et al., 2001; Hirschfeld, Lewis, & Vornik, 2003;

Lish, Dime-Meenan, Whybrow, Price, & Hirschfeld, 1994).

There are several causes for caution in interpreting epidemiological results. First, most instruments used in epidemiological studies were written at a time when the prevailing wisdom was that mania did not occur in children, and only rarely in adolescents. As a result, there was little training for recognizing manic behavior and no attempts to modify descriptions or anchors to be developmentally appropriate. Subsequent experience indicates that some instruments, such as the Diagnostic Interview Schedule for Children (DISC; Shaffer et al., 1996), appear less sensitive to mania as a result. Second, epidemiological studies, with few exceptions, have not systematically assessed for hypomania. Without careful assessment of hypomania, only bipolar I illness can be diagnosed. As a result, most epidemiological studies have not tracked bipolar II illness, cyclothymia, or BD NOS. However, when assessed, these other bipolar spectrum diagnoses appear to be at least five times as common as bipolar I illness (Judd & Akiskal, 2003; Lewinsohn et al., 2002). Adding systematic assessment of just bipolar II disorder raises the estimated lifetime prevalence of BD in the adult U.S. population to 3.9% (Kessler et al., 2005). Although these other diagnoses have flown "under the radar" of most epidemiological studies, they are still associated with substantial burden and impairment. Third, some of the epidemiological studies have relied solely on self-report. It will become evident in later sections of this chapter that self-report often underestimates the occurrence and severity of manic and hypomanic symptoms. Due to these concerns, epidemiological studies should not yet be considered definitive. A balanced interpretation might be that the evidence suggests that BD is rare in children, somewhat more common in adolescents, and still more common in adults; at the same time, the "fuzzy" spectrum presentations outnumber clear cases of bipolar I illness at all ages.

Age of Onset

The age of onset of BD is also controversial. More recent epidemiological studies suggest that the median age of onset is currently around age 16 years (Kessler et al., 2005). However, data suggest a secular trend, with earlier ages of onset of mood disorder and

higher rates of mood disorder in each U.S. generation since World War II (Post, Leverich, Xing, & Weiss, 2001; Weissman et al., 1984). The youngest age cohort surveyed in the National Comorbidity Survey—Revised (NCS-R) had at least four times the lifetime hazard of developing BD (with an estimated prevalence of 6% by age 75) compared to the rate in the oldest age cohort (with a 1.5% lifetime prevalence). Onset in the United States also appears to be significantly earlier than that in Europe, based on both self-report measures and clinical interviews, and appears to be associated with higher rates of risk factors, including more familial history of mood disorder, higher familial rates of suicide, and greater exposure to childhood physical and sexual abuse (Post et al., 2006). Age of onset is an important prognostic variable: Earlier age of onset predicts higher rates of comorbidity with anxiety disorder and substance abuse, more rapid cycling, more chronic impairment, more days in poor mood state, greater risk of suicide or violence (Masi et al., 2006; Perlis et al., 2004), and possibly less responsiveness to lithium monotherapy (Duffy et al., 2002). "Take-home messages" for clinicians are that onset often occurs earlier than conventional wisdom has thought, and that early onset predicts a more challenging course of illness, requiring different forms of pharmacotherapy (and possibly other forms of psychosocial intervention).

Clinical Incidence

Information about clinical incidence is much more useful than general population epidemiological figures to practicing clinicians. Ideally, clinicians would have accurate statistics documenting the base rate of bipolar illness at their own setting. Failing that, it would be helpful to have estimates from similar clinical settings to use as benchmarks. Table 6.3 reports a broad sampling of published estimates from different clinical settings. There are important caveats to consider for any of these estimates. Referral patterns can vary dramatically between settings. Artifacts of the assessment process also generate highly discrepant estimates: Clinical diagnoses are more prone to the effects of heuristics than are semistructured diagnostic interviews, but interviews also involve varying degrees of clinical judgment (Garb, 1998). Differing conceptualizations of bipolar illness also influence the apparent rate. Estimates based on

TABLE 6.3. Base Rates of PBD in Different Clinical Settings

Setting (reference)	Base rate	Demography	Diagnostic method
High school epidemiological (Lewinsohn et al., 2000)	0.6%	Northwestern U.S. high school	K-SADS-PL[y]
Community mental health center (Youngstrom, Youngstrom, et al., 2005)	6%	Midwestern urban, 80% nonwhite, low-income area	Clinical interview and treatment [p,y]
General outpatient clinic; (Geller, Zimerman, et al., 2002)	6–8%	Urban academic research centers	WASH-UK-SADS[p,y]
County wards (DCFS) (Naylor et al., 2002)	11%	State of Illinois	Clinical interview and treatment[y]
Specialty outpatient service (Biederman et al., 1996)	15–17%	New England	K-SADS-E[p,y(only p young)]
Incarcerated adolescents (Teplin, Abram, McClelland, Dulcan, & Mericle, 2002)	2%	Midwestern urban area	DISC[y]
Incarcerated adolescents (Pliszka et al., 2000)	22%	Texas	DISC[y]
Acute psychiatric hospitalizations in 2002–2003—*adolescents* (Blader & Carlson, 2006)	21%	All of United States	Centers for Disease Control survey of discharge diagnoses
Inpatient service (Carlson & Youngstrom, 2003)	30% manic symptoms, < 2% strict BPI	New York City metropolitan region	DICA; K-SADS[p,y]
Acute psychiatric hospitalizations in 2002–2003—*children* (Blader & Carlson, 2006)	40%	All of United States	Centers for Disease Control survey of discharge diagnoses

Note. [p] Parent interviewed as component of diagnostic assessment; [y] youth interviewed as part of diagnostic assessment; K-SADS, Schedule for Affective Disorders and Schizophrenia for School-Age Children; PL, Present and Lifetime version; WASH-U, Washington University version; E, Epidemiological version of the K-SADS; DISC, Diagnostic Interview Schedule for Children; DICA, Diagnostic Interview for Children and Adolescents. From Youngstrom, Findling, et al. (2005, Table 1). Copyright 2005 by Erlbaum. Adapted with permission.

strict bipolar I illness are much lower than those including other diagnoses on the bipolar spectrum. Estimates that include parent report are more sensitive to PBD, but they may also increase the rate of false-positive diagnoses—both of which contribute to higher rates. All of these issues apply with equal force to estimates derived from one's own clinical practice. Thus, Table 6.3 offers an opportunity to compare the effects of different definitions and assessment methodologies, and to reflect on how one's own assessment methods might compare; it justifies three overarching conclusions: (1) Rates can be highly variable, even within the same setting, but (2) PBD occurs in clinical settings, and (3) rates are higher in clinical settings than in the general population, roughly corresponding to the intensity of services offered at the setting.

Domains of Impairment

BD is not simply associated with disturbances of mood and energy. The depressed phase of the illness brings with it all of the impairment and burden associated with unipolar depression (Judd et al., 2005). Manic episodes involve externalizing behaviors, along with the increased motor activity and poor concentration that are often typical of ADHD. Extreme mood states degrade executive function and cognitive performance, although these deficits do not appear to be specific to PBD (Henin, Mick, Nierenberg, & Biederman, 2006). Both depression and mania are associated with academic underachievement, poor educational attainment, peer rejection, and increased family conflict (Geller et al., 2000, 2004; Weckerly, 2002). PBD is also linked to increased use of alcohol and street drugs, and the combination of substance use and other impulsive behaviors greatly increases the risk of youth with PBD coming into contact with the justice system (Pliszka, Sherman, Barrow, & Irick, 2000). BD is a well-established risk factor for suicide (Brent et al., 1988), and earlier age of onset is related to elevated risk of suicide and of violent behavior in general (Perlis et al., 2004). Overall, PBD involves pervasive impairment across most social, emotional, cognitive, and vocational–educational areas of functioning. Without proper management, PBD puts an individual at higher risk of incarceration or suicide.

Demographic and Cultural Issues in Assessment

Sex Differences

Bipolar I disorder occurs equally often in men and women (Bebbington & Ramana, 1995; Kessler et al., 1997; Robb, Young, Cooke, & Joffe, 1998; Weissman et al., 1996). Pediatric data indicate no sex differences in the diagnosis of bipolar I disorder after adjusting for the fact that more young males present to clinics for externalizing problems in general (Biederman, Kwon, et al., 2004; Duax et al., 2005; Youngstrom, Youngstrom, et al., 2005). Bipolar II disorder may be more prevalent among adult women than among men (Berk & Dodd, 2005; cf. Kawa et al., 2005; Robb et al., 1998). The evidence on sex differences in the rate of juvenile bipolar II disorder is similarly mixed, with some data showing a possibly higher rate of bipolar II disorder in female than in male adolescents (Biederman, Kwon, et al., 2004; Birmaher et al., 2006; Faedda, Baldessarini, Glovinsky, & Austin, 2004). Developmental trends may account for adolescent girls' greater rates of depression, and perhaps for their greater rates of bipolar II disorder (Cyranowski, Frank, Young, & Shear, 2000). Alternatively, females may be more likely to acknowledge and/or seek treatment for depressive symptoms (Kessler, 1998), or there may be sex bias in sampling or diagnostic systems (Hartung & Widiger, 1998). Data for other bipolar spectrum diagnoses are scarce, but there is no evidence of sex difference in rates of cyclothymia or BD NOS. Although sex differences are an important consideration in PBD, sex has not proven to be predictive of length of illness or time until relapse (Geller et al., 2004).

Apparent sex differences in PBD are complicated by comorbid diagnoses such as ADHD, oppositional defiant disorder (ODD), and conduct disorder (CD) (Kowatch, Youngstrom, et al., 2005). In particular, ADHD has repeatedly shown higher rates of comorbidity in young males than in young females with BD (Biederman, Kwon, et al., 2004; Duax et al., 2005). Externalizing disorders are more common among boys than among girls (Costello et al., 1996), potentially leading to greater rates of boys also being diagnosed with PBD. It is still important for clinicians to recognize more subtle symptoms of PBD, so that children and adolescents seeking treatment for depressive symptoms, particularly females, do not go misdiagnosed or mistreated. Findings suggest that although separate sex norms or diagnostic criteria for PBD are probably unnecessary (Biederman, Kwon, et al., 2004), clinicians need to be more vigilant about PBD in females, whose presentation is less likely to show pure mania or hypomania.

Racial and Cultural Differences

Little is known about racial or cultural differences in the prevalence or phenomenology of PBD. However, minority youth with mood disorders are more likely to be misdiagnosed with CD or schizophrenia (DelBello, Lopez-Larson, Soutullo, & Strakowski, 2001), and more likely to be treated with older and/or depot antipsychotic medications (Arnold et al., 2004; DelBello, Soutullo, & Strakowski, 2000). Clinicians should assess systematically for mood disorder in ethnic/minority patients, particularly when the presenting problem involves aggressive behavior or psychosis. Clinicians should also be alert to the potential for racial bias in diagnosis when gathering family history data (Garb, 1998). Rather than taking family members' historical diagnoses at face value, it would be prudent to gather family history data at the symptom level whenever possible.

Young Adult Outcomes

Multiple longitudinal studies have published findings about stability, course, and outcome up to 4 years after the initial assessment identifying PBD. Youth initially diagnosed with BD typically experience at least partial remission of the illness: 37% having mania remit within the first year (Geller, Craney, et al., 2001), and 65% within the first 2 years, but 55% experience a relapse of mania within the same 2-year period (Geller, Craney, et al., 2002). Four-year follow-up of youth initially diagnosed with narrow phenotype PBD (requiring the presence of elated mood or grandiosity) indicated that they experienced hypomanic, manic, or mixed states for 57% of the follow-up period, and depressive states for 47% of follow-up (Geller et al., 2004). These findings have been cross-validated by a more recent, multisite study: 70% of patients recovered within an average follow-up period of 2 years, but 50% relapsed within the same time frame, and syndromal or subsyndromal mood symptoms were present during at least 60% of weeks during the follow-up period (Birmaher et al., 2006). Within the 2-year follow-up period, 25% of youth initially meeting criteria for cyclothymia or BD NOS had sufficiently worse mood states to meet strict criteria for bipolar II or bipolar I disorder. Youth with cyclothymia–BD NOS more often continued to have not only "subsyndromal" mood disturbance but also worse outcomes on most measures of functioning than did youth with more "classic, syndromal" presentations (Birmaher et al., 2006). In a much smaller follow-back study, in which 17 youth and parents were reinterviewed an average of 3 years after the initial diagnosis of cyclothymia or BD NOS, about one-third of youth developed more clearly syndromal bipolar presentations during subsequent years, compared to roughly one-third whose mood symptoms had remitted by the time of reevaluation (Kahana et al., under review).

These findings are similar to results from the follow-up waves of a longitudinal study of an epidemiological sample. Lewinsohn and colleagues (2000) found that adolescents meeting full criteria for BD (about 1% of the sample) showed significant risk of still meeting criteria for BD at follow-up. On the other hand, the 5% of the sample that met criteria for subsyndromal BD (the "core positive" definition provided in Table 6.2) did not show a significant rate of "conversion" into clear bipolar I or bipolar II disorder. However, the subsyndromal group continued to be highly impaired, showing increased risk for anxiety disorders, depression, antisocial behavior, suicidal ideation, and borderline personality traits (Lewinsohn et al., 2000). Taken together, findings suggest that

there are two subtypes—a more episodic version of mood disorder conforming to classic definitions and having a less chronic, although still highly impairing, course versus a more chronic pattern of mood dysregulation that does not meet full criteria for bipolar I or II disorder but tends to show developmental continuity and remain highly impairing.

Etiological Factors

A variety of risk factors are associated with BD (Tsuchiya, Byrne, & Mortensen, 2003). Genetic factors have received the most attention. BD and schizophrenia have similarly large genetic components, exceeding the heritability of all other major mental illnesses (Faraone et al., 1999; McGuffin et al., 2003). However, even monozygotic twins show roughly 80% concordance for BD, indicating that environmental factors play a role in the expression of illness even when genes are completely identical (Faraone et al., 1999). BD clearly involves multiple genes, which means that permutations or degrees of loading may be present in any given individual. There is also a genetic component to BD age of onset (Faraone, Glatt, Su, & Tsuang, 2004), suggesting that there may be a different, pediatric-onset subtype of BD with a distinct constellation of genetic factors (Biederman, Faraone, et al., 2004; Faraone, Glatt, & Tsuang, 2003). Retrospective data on adults with BD indicate that earlier age of onset is associated with more rapid cycling; more chronic course; and higher rates of comorbidity, suicidality, violent behavior, and substance use (Perlis et al., 2004)—similar to the phenomenology noted in child and adolescent samples (Kowatch, Youngstrom, et al., 2005).

Some of the work investigating the genetic architecture of PBD relies on the "bipolar profile" of scores on the CBCL described by Mick, Biederman, Pandina, and Faraone (2003). The profile has demonstrated a high degree of heritability (Althoff et al., 2006; Hudziak et al., 2005). However, in samples where PBD is rare, such as the general population, the majority of individuals with such a profile do not actually have a BD diagnosis (Volk, 2006). It is worth noting that this pattern of findings—a heritable behavior pattern that is not isolated to PBD—is entirely consistent with a polygenic model of illness. There may be a specific gene conferring risk for the "bipolar profile" of behaviors captured by the CBCL, and this gene might often be present in individuals with PBD. At the same time, the gene may also convey risk for aggressive behavior and occur in the context of other disorders, such as CD or ADHD.

Many other, more speculative mechanisms potentially contribute to risk for BD. One is genetic "anticipation," in which children inherit multiple copies of the same gene from a parent. For some conditions, there appears to be a dose–response relationship, in which receiving more copies of the same gene is associated with earlier onset of illness and more virulent course (Post, Weiss, & Leverich, 1994). This may contribute to the higher lifetime risk of BD in younger generations (e.g., Kessler et al., 2005). Another established risk factor for mood disorder is prenatal or perinatal trauma (Hack et al., 2004). It is possible that as medical technology saves more children who previously would have perished, some of the survivors may experience mood dysregulation as a result of subtle perinatal neural damage. It is possible that exposure to a virus or bacterium may trigger an autoimmune response that creates mood dysregulation similar to BD (Soto & Murphy, 2003).

Risk of bipolar illness might be influenced by diet, too. The popularity of omega-3 fatty acids as a remedy for BD stems from observations about epidemiological differences in fish intake, with populations with higher fish consumption showing lower rates of bipolar illness (Stoll, Locke, Marangell, & Severus, 1999). It also is noteworthy that the risk of BD increases with the onset of puberty (Nottelmann et al., 2001). Dietary changes in the United States have led to a dramatic rise in childhood obesity, along with puberty starting at a much younger age (Juul et al., 2006; Karlberg, 2002; Parent et al., 2003). Recent studies indicate that 14% of U.S. girls reach Tanner Stage 2 by age 8, and the national average for reaching Stage 2 of breast development is between 9.2 and 9.5 years (Lee, Guo, & Kulin, 2001). The endocrine changes associated with puberty are beginning at a younger age than previously, suggesting a mechanism for earlier onset of depression in girls (Cyranowski et al., 2000) and possibly increased aggression in boys (Rowe, Maughan, Worthman, Costello, & Angold, 2004). If these results prove robust, then diet-related findings suggest mechanisms for prevention models.

EVIDENCE-BASED APPROACHES TO DIAGNOSIS

Risk Assessment Model

The first piece of information to consider is the "base rate," or how common PBD is likely to be in a given setting. A practitioner in an inpatient unit is likely to see more individuals with PBD than would a school psychologist in a regular educational setting. The base rate provides an excellent foundation for the integration of additional information. Knowing that the base rate of PBD is around 5% in many outpatient clinics, for example, suggests that, on the one hand, BD is a diagnosis that should be considered and carefully assessed in some cases. On the other hand, a 5% prevalence reminds the practitioner that the diagnosis is likely to be rare, and other problems (including those with similar clinical presentations, such as ADHD or unipolar depression) are likely to be more common. This anchoring helps avoid over- or underdiagnosis due to availability heuristics that may be unduly influenced by the faddishness of a diagnosis (Davidow & Levinson, 1993). As I discussed in the earlier section "Clinical Incidence," clinicians can either rely on their own archival records to estimate the rate of PBD or use published estimates from similar clinical settings to provide a ballpark estimate. Table 6.3 provides some published estimates for calibration purposes, along with comments about the design of each study. If computerized, abstract databases are available, then it would be even better to search for newer benchmark estimates with key words such as "prevalence or incidence" and "bipolar disorder," along with terms describing the clinical context of interest (Youngstrom & Duax, 2005). Practitioners relying on local diagnoses should be aware that clinical diagnoses tend to underestimate the amount of comorbidity and may be particularly inaccurate in the case of PBD (Youngstrom, Youngstrom, et al., 2005).

Whether using local estimates or published values, the assessor should reflect on the procedures used to make the benchmark diagnoses, and consider the possible sources of bias and how they might influence initial estimates. A more thorough dissection of the validity of an estimate may be accomplished by comparing the design features to the 25 recommendations in the STAndardized Reporting of Diagnostic (STARD; Bossuyt et al., 2003) tests criteria, or by evaluating the applicability of the findings to the individual patient in question (Jaeschke, Guyatt, & Sackett, 1994b). Even when they are flawed, initial estimates of the base rate can lessen the impact of other factors that undermine the accuracy of the assessment process. Furthermore, if the practitioner follows other recommendations for evidence-based assessment, then periodically reevaluates the base rate of disorders, the process potentially becomes self-correcting. Reevaluation of base rates in one's own clinical setting is also good practice, because changes in public awareness and other external factors may also change the referral pattern over time.

Family History

Value of Gathering Family History

In a meta-analysis that reviewed over 100 articles discussing more than 30 different risk factors potentially associated with BD, only family history of BD was robust enough to merit clinical interpretation (Tsuchiya et al., 2003). Another meta-analysis found that, on average, 5% of children with a biological parent affected by BD already met criteria for a BD themselves at the time of the research assessment (Hodgins, Faucher, Zarac, & Ellenbogen, 2002). Conversely, no children in the "low risk" comparison groups developed bipolar spectrum illness in any of the studies reviewed. Having a bipolar parent also doubled the children's risk of developing psychopathology in general, and tripled the risk of developing mood disorders (not just bipolar spectrum illness). When interpreting the 5% rate of bipolar illness, one should remember that (1) family history of bipolar illness increases risk of psychopathology, and especially BD; (2) the vast majority of children with a parent diagnosed with BD still do not have PBD themselves; (3) they often show other, nonbipolar behavioral problems; and (4) youth participating in these studies were not followed into middle age, so it is impossible to know how many of them later developed full-blown bipolar illness.

Besides conveying information about the degree of risk of bipolarity for the youth, gathering family history also helps determine the family's strengths and challenges that may impinge upon therapy. Having a family member already in treatment for a mood disorder provides prior experience that shapes family attitudes toward intervention. If the prior treatment went well, then the family member offers a powerful role model and excellent potential social support for the youth. If prior experiences were negative, then it is crucial to find out family members' perceptions of what was suboptimal, so that one may pursue alternative recommendations or use other strategies to address the challenges and resistance. An adult's undiagnosed or poorly managed mood disorder often magnifies the chaos and conflict in a family, reducing the chances of good treatment adherence for the child. Family history may be informative about the likely course of illness for the youth, and may also have prescriptive value in shaping treatment selection. Children of parents with lithium-responsive BD tend to show better premorbid functioning, more distinct mood episodes, better interepisode functioning, and better response to lithium themselves (Duffy, Alda, Kutcher, Fusee, & Grof, 1998). Conversely, children whose parents had earlier onset, more rapid-cycling bipolar illness (which tends to be less lithium responsive) are themselves more likely to show a refractory and more chronically impaired course of illness (Duffy et al., 2002; Masi et al., 2006).

Challenges in Obtaining Family History

In spite of its proven clinical value, gathering a good family history may not always be possible. A common problem is that fathers often do not participate directly in the clinical evaluation process. In many families the biological father may have been absent from the child's life for years, or even since conception. When a parent is not directly evaluated, the clinician has to rely on information provided by the other available adult. Parents are often unfamiliar with the details of the other adult's mental health history, especially that in childhood. Indirect interviews are also prone to reporter bias. If the parents had an abusive relationship or an ugly divorce, then these circumstances may easily color the report about mental health history. If the child is placed in foster care or adopted, then there may be little or no information available about the biological parents. In school-based or forensic clinics, parents may not routinely be involved in clinical evaluations, and it may be difficult to include them.

Another consideration with BD is that historical diagnoses themselves may not have been accurate. A family-history diagnosis is almost always based on a prior clinical, not research, evaluation. Thus, a historical diagnosis is prone to all of the limitations of clinical diagnoses in general (Garb, 1998). On top of that is the fog added by imperfect awareness of other family members' diagnoses, as well as imperfect memory. Even worse are the factors related to race and ethnicity that might increase the likelihood of BD going undetected or misdiagnosed in African American or Latin American families (as discussed earlier). "Schizophrenia," "psychotic disorder," "antisocial personality," "drug and alcohol problems," or "conduct disorder" are all labels that could signify an undiagnosed bipolar illness, particularly in minority families. Finally, families typically do not have formal clinical training themselves, so their labels are more likely to be filtered through their own ethnographic lens. A relative with BD might be described as having "bad nerves," a "hot temper," or "anxiety attacks," for example.

Integrating Family History into a Risk Assessment Model

The more systematic and structured the interview, the more cost is added to the evaluation process, and the greater the burden imposed on families. For these reasons, clinicians need to see clear benefits before deciding to do more than a routine clinical assessment of family history. The differential diagnosis of PBD creates a situation in which the potential gains justify some increased time and burden. Accurate evaluation of familial history indicates the child's risk, and also informs case formulation and treatment strategies. Given how prone "historical" diagnoses are to error, simply asking whether anyone in the family has been diagnosed with BD is unlikely to be an adequate shortcut to evaluating family history.

One practical approach might be to ask the parents to fill out a brief screening measure, such as the Mood Disorder Questionnaire (MDQ; Hirschfeld et al., 2000), about themselves. The MDQ is a single page, with a low required reading level, yet it demonstrates high specificity to BD. The sensitivity of the MDQ appears to be moderate (often around .4 to .6), and it is poorer at detecting bipolar II and "bipolar spectrum" illnesses other than bipolar I illness (Miller, Klugman, Berv, Rosenquist, & Ghaemi, 2004), so it likely fails to identify the

relative who actually has a history of bipolar illness. It also is not known how well the MDQ would indirectly rate another adult relative (i.e., how accurately spouses' responses on the MDQ capture their partner's bipolar status). On the positive side, the MDQ has been validated in multiple languages, cultures, and settings, and shows fairly consistent performance (Isometsa et al., 2003); it also is free to use for private purposes, and very brief. The alternative might be to use the mood disorders module of a structured diagnostic interview, such as the Mini-International Neuropsychiatric Interview (MINI; Sheehan et al., 1998), to interview the parents. Completing the mood disorders module by itself generally takes only 5–15 minutes per relative. The MINI appears to be more structured than many instruments (improving the reliability and reducing the training demands) but less cumbersome than most other structured or semistructured interviews.

If a lifetime diagnosis of BD is found in a first-degree relative (e.g., biological mother, biological father, or a full biological sibling), then the child's risk of having BD increases by a factor of at least five (Youngstrom, Findling, Youngstrom, & Calabrese, 2005). This risk estimate is based on 5% of biologically at-risk youth manifesting BD (Hodgins et al., 2002), compared to a rough estimate of 1% of the general population of youth with any bipolar spectrum illness. Counterintuitively, it is more conservative to use a higher estimate of the prevalence in the general population; lower general prevalence estimates magnify the increase in risk associated with family history.

What if a second-degree relative, such as an aunt, uncle, grandparent, or half-sibling, has a bipolar illness? On average, these relatives share half as many genes with the youth in question compared to a first-degree relative. Therefore, the youth is half as likely to share the genes of risk, and the risk of BD increases by half as much, or a factor of 2.5.

Family history of mood disorder (including depression) also roughly doubles the risk of the child developing BD (Hodgins et al., 2002). "Fuzzy" presentations suggestive of possible BD, such as moodiness and alcoholism, or "schizophrenia" diagnosed in an ethnic/minority individual with a history of impulsivity and depression might also be treated as a "fuzzy" bipolar diagnosis, increasing the risk—but much less so than would a confirmed BD diagnosis (Youngstrom, Findling, et al., 2005).

Bayesian Approaches to Test Interpretation

How does a clinician incorporate information gleaned from family history into a case formulation? How best to combine findings during assessment is not intuitive. As an example, how worried would a clinician be that a child referred to an outpatient clinic had BD if the clinician learned that the child's biological father had been diagnosed with bipolar I disorder and responded well to lithium treatment? Clinicians typically interpret information informally and impressionistically, which avoids computation but is less accurate than actuarial approaches.

The other extreme is to take a strictly quantitative and actuarial approach to synthesizing the data gathered so far. An actuary would first establish the base rate of PBD at the outpatient clinic. At many outpatient settings, the rate of bipolar spectrum illness is likely to be around 5% (Youngstrom, Findling, et al., 2005; Youngstrom, Youngstrom, et al., 2005). An actuary would then combine the initial 5% risk with the five-fold increase in risk associated with having a first-degree relative diagnosed with BD. One method for calculating the revised risk estimate would be to use the Bayes Theorem to estimate the "posterior probability" of having BD, based on the new information about family history (Sackett et al., 2000). An algebraic way of accomplishing this would be to convert the prior probability (5%) into odds (5% divided by 95% = 1/19), then multiply the odds by the change in risk. The technical name for the change in risk is the "likelihood ratio," which is estimated by comparing the rate at which bipolar individuals versus nonbipolar individuals show the sign or symptom (resulting in a "false alarm" if the sign or symptom is treated as a positive indicator of BD) (Sackett et al., 2000). Multiplying the initial odds (1/19) by the likelihood ratio (5) yields the new odds that the child has BD (5/19). Odds are a familiar metric to those who engage in gambling or sports betting, but for most, probabilities are a more interpretable metric, so the new odds should be converted to a probability (using the formula probability = odds/[1 + odds]). In this particular instance, the actuary would estimate that the child had a 20.8% chance of having BD.

The 20.8% figure might be interpreted several different ways. One interpretation would be that out of a large group of patients at the clinic (where 5% have BD), roughly 21% of the subset of patients with a first-degree relative with BD will themselves have a bipolar spectrum illness. The other way of thinking about it is that each individual patient fitting that profile has a 21% risk of having BD. The technical name for the risk estimate is the "positive predictive power" or "positive predictive value" (PPV) of the assessment result (Kraemer, 1992). The PPV is loosely related to the diagnostic "sensitivity" of an assessment, but it is not the same thing. Sensitivity represents the rate at which a positive test result would occur in persons who truly have the disorder. PPV indicates the percentage of persons who have a positive score on the test and truly have the condition of interest. Because clinicians must make decisions about individual patients, and because they start with assessment results and need to infer the diagnosis (vs. already knowing the diagnoses for a group of patients, then comparing the test results in patients with and without the diagnosis, as would be done to estimate the sensitivity), the PPV is actually the more relevant statistic. The PPV is an estimate of how often a positive assessment result would be "right" as an indicator of the presence of illness.

Despite its greater clinical usefulness, the PPV is rarely reported, because it changes directly as a function of the disorder's base rate. The 21% risk of having BD when there is family history of BD is accurate in settings in which 5% of patients have BD. However, it would be an underestimate of a patient's risk in settings where BD is more common, and it would grossly overestimate the risk of BD in cases drawn from settings where BD is more rare. Based on the prevalence benchmarks from Table 6.3, for example, then, a positive family history would be associated with a 77% risk of BD in a child admitted to a psychiatric hospital (based on the 40% prevalence reported in clinical diagnoses reviewed by Blader & Carlson [2006]), but only a 2% risk in children seen in a public school setting. The degree of risk change associated with family history is the same in all three settings, but the degree of accuracy or decisiveness of the information changes dramatically depending on the base rate. Because base rates can change markedly across clinical settings (as in Table 6.3), it is impossible to establish PPV estimates that generalize across settings.

Introducing the Nomogram

Fortunately, there are alternatives to manual calculation of PPV with the Bayes Theorem. With the increasing popularity of "personal digital assistants" (PDAs) and other technology, it is possible to have software perform the necessary calculations. Another less technologically demanding approach is to use a "nomogram" to plot graphically the relationship between the initial risk estimate and the new information garnered by the assessment. Figure 6.1 presents a working nomogram, in which the first column marks the "prior probability," the second column indexes the likelihood ratio attached to the assessment result, and the third column yields the revised probability estimate. The nomogram approach is highly recommended, because (1) it requires no computation, (2) it is quick, (3) it is accurate, (4) it allows direct estimation of the PPV, and (5) it is highly flexible, allowing the inclusion of any

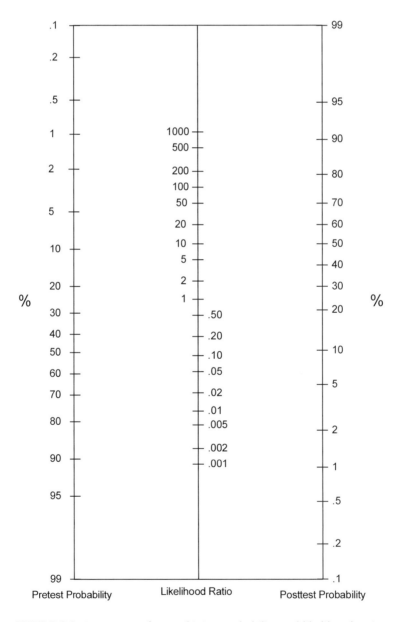

FIGURE 6.1. Nomogram for combining probability and likelihood ratios.

information that can be repackaged as a quantitative estimate of risk or of a likelihood ratio (Sackett et al., 2000). If one uses the nomogram in Figure 6.1 to interpret the change in risk associated with a positive family history, then one would start by finding the number corresponding to the base rate on the first line (5%, in the first example), then locating the likelihood ratio (5, for a first-degree relative) on the middle line. Connecting those two points and extending the line across the third line shows the revised probability. In this example, the line should cross the third, right-hand scale just above 20%. This corresponds quite closely to the calculated value of 20.8% if one uses the Bayes Theorem and a calculator instead. A nomogram is more flexible than a table of risk estimates, because it lets the clinician change the initial risk estimates, or change the likelihood ratio used (e.g., substituting 2.5 for the risk associated with family history, if an aunt or other second-degree relative has BD). This flexibility lends itself well to "sensitivity analysis," or seeing how changes in assumptions change the results (Sackett et al., 2000). Handbooks on evidence-based medicine provide much more detail about the likelihood ratio approach and provide examples of applying it to different medical conditions (Guyatt & Rennie, 2002; Sackett et al., 2000). Youngstrom and Duax (2005) provide a detailed case example using a nomogram to combine information about base rate and family history to evaluate potential PBD.

Behavior Checklists and Mood Rating Scales

There has been a surge in recent interest in the potential value of behavior checklists or mood rating scales as potential aids to improve the recognition of BD in both children and adults. Often these instruments are described as "screening tools," although, technically, screening is a relatively narrow role within the range of possible uses for tools to improve diagnosis. Screening, in the most precise sense, involves collecting inexpensive measures that are highly sensitive to a disorder, then referring patients with positive scores on the screening test for further evaluation. Screening tests need to be highly sensitive to avoid missing patients with the target condition. Negative results on a test with high sensitivity often decisively rule out the diagnosis (Sackett et al. [2000] suggest the mnemonic "SnNOut" [on a Sensitive test, a

Negative result helps rule Out a diagnosis]), whereas positive results tend to be more ambiguous, especially for rare disorders such as PBD. Although most patients with BD would score high on the test, nonbipolar patients may be so much more numerous that even fairly specific tests generate a large number of "false-positive" results.

For this reason, it is also valuable to have available tests that are more *specific* to BD. These tests set the bar higher, making false-positive results much less common. As a result, someone scoring high on a very specific test is much more likely to have BD (the SpPIn mnemonic [on a Specific test, a Positive result helps rule In a diagnosis]; Sackett et al., 2000). Ideally, clinicians would have multiple tests available, so that they could pick and choose more sensitive or specific tests based on which feature would be more helpful for a given situation, much as a golfer chooses among a variety of irons with different properties to use the tool most suited for the circumstances at hand. Almost as useful would be knowledge of the diagnostic value of multiple ranges of scores on the same test, so that the information offered by extremely low scores could be separated from indeterminate midrange or very high scores (Jaeschke et al., 1994b; Sackett et al., 2000).

Child Behavior Checklist and PBD

Systematic investigation of the diagnostic value of behavior checklists in children began with an article (Biederman et al., 1995) examining how well Achenbach's (1991a) Child Behavior Checklist (CBCL) distinguished between youth with research diagnoses of PBD and from youth with ADHD. More than eight different research groups on three different continents have replicated the result that youth with research diagnoses of BD score significantly higher than youth with ADHD or other comparison groups on multiple scales of the CBCL (Hazell, Lewin, & Carr, 1999; Kahana, Youngstrom, Findling, & Calabrese, 2003; Mick et al., 2003; Tramontina, Schmitz, Polanczyk, & Rohde, 2003; Youngstrom, Findling, Calabrese, et al., 2004). The profile of score elevations associated with PBD appears consistent across research groups (Mick et al., 2003) and correlates highly with the average pattern of problems in youth with clinical diagnoses of PBD (Youngstrom, Youngstrom, et al., 2005). Because of the extensive replication, some have suggested that the CBCL may be used to identify individuals with PBD, or that the CBCL profile may be used as a "proxy" definition of PBD in research or clinical settings in which detailed clinical interviews were not feasible (Mick et al., 2003). Indeed, the CBCL profile has been used as an operational definition of PBD in both behavioral genetics work (Hudziak et al., 2005) and reanalyses of treatment studies (Galanter et al., 2003).

Clinically, multiple analyses indicate that the Externalizing scale score on the CBCL is most powerfully associated with a bipolar diagnosis. Although PBD is linked with elevations on multiple syndrome scales, the Externalizing score does the best job of any CBCL scale at identifying BD, and no other scale, or combination of scales, provides incremental improvement in prediction after researchers control for Externalizing scores (Kahana et al., 2003; Youngstrom, Findling, Calabrese, et al., 2004). This simplifies test interpretation for the practitioner: If concerned about potential PBD, then the Externalizing score is the main CBCL score to consider in terms of changing diagnostic impression. The other scales do not add value in changing the diagnostic formulation, but provide information about domains of functioning and areas of impairment that may be important to address in treatment planning.

Studies that directly evaluate diagnostic efficiency tend to find that the CBCL is highly sensitive to PBD, but not very specific (Youngstrom, Findling, Calabrese, et al., 2004; Youngstrom, Youngstrom, et al., 2005). This makes sense, because the CBCL does not include a mania scale, nor do expert clinicians believe that a mania scale can be extracted from the CBCL item pool (Achenbach & Rescorla, 2001; Lengua, Sadowski, Friedrich, & Fisher, 2001). The CBCL mostly picks up the externalizing, disinhibited behavior component of manic and mixed states, and most youth with BD have episodes of these sorts of behavior. For this reason, low Externalizing levels on the CBCL lower the likelihood of a bipolar diagnosis a lot, ruling out the diagnosis in most settings (an example of the SnNOut rule described earlier). However, high CBCL scores are ambiguous, because they can be associated with a wide variety of diagnoses. The more diverse the range of diagnoses and comorbidities encountered at a clinical setting, the less specific are high scores on measures of general

pathology, such as the CBCL (Youngstrom, Meyers, Youngstrom, Calabrese, & Findling, 2006a).

Estimates of the likelihood ratios attached to different ranges of CBCL Externalizing scores have been published for two large samples of youth ages 5–10 and 11–17 years (Youngstrom, Findling, Calabrese, et al., 2004). These numbers make it possible for clinicians to use the nomogram and interpret CBCL scores directly for their individual patients. Table 6.4 reproduces the likelihood ratios for the extremely low and extremely high score intervals for various instruments. Table 6.5 presents the PPV estimates that would result from high CBCL scores when used in clinical settings with different prevalences. Readers interested in learning to use the nomogram may practice using the nomogram to connect different prevalences with the likelihood ratio associated with the CBCL score (4.3 for an Externalizing T-score of 85 or higher, per Table 6.4) and see how closely they duplicate PPV estimates in Table 6.5. Incorporation of CBCL scores into the evaluation of PBD has also been illustrated in detail in a published case example (Youngstrom & Youngstrom, 2005). An important implication of the PPV estimates in Table 6.5 is that treating a CBCL "test positive" as a proxy for PBD will be wrong in most cases drawn from most settings. Using CBCL Externalizing (or the "bipolar profile") as a proxy definition appears to be a reliable way to identify a group of youth with similar parent-reported behavior problems, but the majority of these youth will not meet strict criteria for a diagnosis of BD. Clinically, there is no substitute for thorough evaluation. Research based on proxy definitions cannot be interpreted as if it generalized to youth with strict diagnoses of BD (Volk, 2006).

Other Behavior Checklists

Various other measures are also in different stages of development and validation as diagnostic aids for PBD. Table 6.4 provides a listing of available measures as of April 2006, along with estimates of the area under the curve (AUC) and some comments about design features of studies that might affect clinical usage of the findings. When designs use comparable definitions of BD, as well as similar inclusion and exclusion criteria, the AUC provides a straightforward comparison of the overall di-

TABLE 6.4. Areas under the Curve (AUCs) and Likelihood Ratios for Potential Screening Measures for PBD

Screening measure (primary reference)	AUC	LR+ (score)	LR− (score)	Citation	Clinical generalizability
Adolescents (11–18 years)					
CBCL Externalizing T-score (Achenbach, 1991a)	.78 (*n* = 324)	4.3 (81+)	.04 (<54)	Youngstrom, Findling, Calabrese, et al. (2004)	High: Bipolar spectrum disorder (BPSD) versus all other diagnoses presenting to academic outpatient clinic, excluding pervasive developmental disorders and IQ < 80.
TRF Externalizing T-score (Achenbach, 1991b)	.70 (*n* = 324)	3.8 (77+)	.25 (<46)	Youngstrom, Findling, Calabrese, et al. (2004)	Same as above.
YSR Externalizing T-score (Achenbach, 1991c)	.71 (*n* = 324)	3.0 (77+)	.31 (<49)	Youngstrom, Findling, Calabrese, et al. (2004)	Same as above.
Parent-GBI—Hypomanic/Biphasic (Youngstrom, Findling, Danielson, & Calabrese, 2001)	.84 (*n* = 324)	9.2 (49+)	.06 (<9)	Youngstrom, Findling, Calabrese, et al. (2004)	Same as above. *Note*: Uses 0- to 3-point scale for scoring.
Parent-YMRS (Gracious et al., 2002)	.80 (*n* = 324) .70 (*n* = 124)	7.4 (28+)	.20 (<6)	Youngstrom, Findling, Calabrese, et al. (2004; Youngstrom, Meyers, et al. (2005)	Same as above. *Note*: Uses 0- to 4-point, 0- to 8-point scoring as per Young et al. (1978).
Adolescent-GBI—Hypomanic/Biphasic (Depue et al., 1981)	.62 (*n* = 324) .65 (*n* = 124)	3.9 (46+)	.33 (<10)	Youngstrom, Findling, Calabrese, et al. (2004); Youngstrom et al. (2005)	Same as above. *Note*. Uses 0- to 3-point scoring.
Parent-MDQ (Wagner et al., 2006)	~.84 (*n* < 150) .75 (*n* = 124)	3.9 (5+)	.32 (<5)	Wagner et al. (2006); Youngstrom et al. (2005)	High *Note*: Algorithm used by Wagner et al. (2006) requires co-occurring and at least moderate impairment.
Adolescent-MDQ (Hirschfeld et al., 2000)	~.59 (*n* < 150) .63 (*n* = 124)	1.5 (5+)	.84 (<5)	Wagner et al. (2006); Youngstrom, Meyers, et al. (2005)	*Note*: Hirschfeld's algorithm requires co-occurring and at least moderate impairment; Youngstrom, Meyers, et al. (2005) and Wagner et al. (2006) both found sensitivity improved by waiving these requirements.
Adolescent-YMRS (Youngstrom, Meyers, et al., 2005)	.50 (*n* = 124)	—	—	Youngstrom, Meyers, et al. (2005)	Very high: BPSD versus all others at community mental health center. *Note*: Do *not* use clinically!

(continued)

TABLE 6.4. *(continued)*

Screening measure (primary reference)	AUC	LR+ (score)	LR− (score)	Citation	Clinical generalizability
Children (5–10 years)					
CBCL Externalizing *T*-score (Achenbach, 1991a)	.82 (*n* = 318)	3.7 (73+)	.07 (<58)	Youngstrom, Findling, Calabrese, et al. (2004)	High: BPSD versus all other diagnoses presenting to academic outpatient clinic, excluding pervasive developmental disorders and IQ < 80.
TRF Externalizing *T*-score (Achenbach, 1991b)	.57 (*n* = 318)	1.4 (63+)	.78 (<57)	Youngstrom, Findling, Calabrese, et al. (2004)	Same as above. Do *not* use clinically!
Parent-GBI—Hypomanic/ Biphasic (Youngstrom et al., 2001)	.81 (*n* = 318)	6.3 (51+)	.10 (<11)	Youngstrom, Findling, Calabrese, et al. (2004)	Same as above. *Note*: Uses 0 to 3 scoring.
Parent-YMRS (Gracious et al., 2002)	.83 (*n* = 318) .66 (*n* = 141)	8.9 (35+)	.08 (<7)	Youngstrom, Findling, Calabrese, et al. (2004); Youngstrom, Meyers, et al. (2005)	Same as above. *Note*: Uses 0 to 4, 0 to 8 scoring as per Young et al. (1978).
Parent-MDQ (Wagner et al., 2006)	.72 (*n* = 141)	—	—	Youngstrom, Meyers, et al. (2005)	Very high: BPSD versus all others at community mental health center.
Combined samples (child and adolescent not reported separately)					
Parent-CMRS (Pavuluri et al., 2006)	.91 (*n* = 100)	13.7 (20+)	.19 (<20)	Pavuluri et al. (2006)	Limited: 50 BPSD versus 50 ADHD without mood disorder.
Two-Item Screen (Tillman & Geller, 2005)	.85 (*n* = 264) .70 (*n* = 500)	5.2* 1.6**	.31* .32**	Tillman & Geller (2005); Youngstrom, Meyers, et al. (2006); Papolos & Papolos (2002)	*Tillman and Geller recommend cutting at 9+ for ages 7–8 years, 8+ for 9–10 years, and 6+ for ages 11–17 years. **Threshold was chosen to be statistically optimal for entire sample.
Child Bipolar Questionnaire (Papolos & Papolos, 2002)	Not reported (*n* = 135)	7.1	N/A	Papolos, Hennen, Cockerham, Thode, & Youngstrom (2006)	Limited: K-SADS validation group comprised of bipolar spectrum, ADHD, or no diagnosis.
Child Symptom Inventory (Parent) (Gadow & Sprafkin, 1994)				No relevant data published yet	Adolescent version includes mania scale with DSM-IV items; mania items added to research version of child instrument (available from CSI authors upon request).
Adolescent Symptom Inventory (Gadow & Sprafkin, 1994)				No relevant data published yet	Includes mania scale with DSM-IV items.
Teacher Symptom Inventory (Gadow & Sprafkin, 1999)				No relevant data published yet	Includes mania scale with DSM-IV items.

Note. All studies used some version of K-SADS interview by a trained rater, combined with review by a clinician to establish consensus. LR+, change in likelihood ratio associated with a positive test score; LR−, likelihood ratio for a low score. LRs of 1 indicate that the test result did not change impressions at all. LRs larger than 10 or smaller than .10 are frequently clinically decisive; LRs of 5 or

TABLE 6.5. Examples of the Effects of Base Rate on the Positive Predictive Value (PPV) of High Scores on Two Screening Tests for Adolescent BD

Setting	Base rate	CBCL externalizing T-score (LR+)	PPV	P-GBI Hypomanic/ Biphasic score (LR+)	PPV
Public high school (Teplin et al., 2002)	0.6%	85 (4.3)	3%	54 (9.2)	5%
Juvenile detention (Youngstrom, Findling, et al., 2005)	2%	85 (4.3)	5%	54 (9.2)	16%
Outpatient clinic or community mental health (Naylor et al., 2002)	6%	85 (4.3)	21%	54 (9.2)	37%
County wards receiving mental health services (Pliszka et al., 2000)	11%	85 (4.3)	35%	54 (9.2)	53%
Juvenile detention (Blader & Carlson, 2006)	22%	85 (4.3)	55%	54 (9.2)	72%
Acute psychiatric hospitalization (based on Centers for Disease Control national data for discharge diagnoses in 2002–2003 (Thayer, 1996)	40%	85 (4.3)	74%	54 (9.2)	86%
Heavily enriched mood disorders study (many published analyses of diagnostic tests compare bipolar cases to an equal number of comparison cases)	50%	85 (4.3)	81%	54 (9.2)	90%

Note. The likelihood ratios associated with a positive test result (LR+) are from Table 4 of Youngstrom, Findling, Calabrese, et al. (2004).

agnostic efficiency of the tests. It also is possible to test whether the diagnostic performance of one test is significantly superior to another (Hanley & McNeil, 1983). These comparisons have more statistical power when the instruments are evaluated in the same sample, which also eliminates a wealth of other, potential confounds that might make it otherwise difficult to compare tests (Pepe, 2003).

Perusal of Table 6.4 indicates that more than 15 published measures include some endorsement that they might be helpful in assessing PBD. All except the CBCL have been published since 2001, in keeping with the rising interest in PBD. Few of the measures have published estimates of diagnostic efficiency available. A more subtle but crucial point is that the majority of the studies have design features that seriously limit the generalizability of findings into most clinical settings. The most common limitation involves filtering the sample in ways unlikely to be mirrored in clinical practice. This could include limiting the bipolar sample to bipolar I disorder cases, or to "narrow phenotype" cases (as described in Table 6.2). Focusing on bipolar I disorder would increase the severity of the manic or mixed symptoms sampled, thus increasing the apparent sensitivity of

the test. Including only narrow phenotype presentations might also enhance the sensitivity of measures that include the relevant symptoms (e.g., requiring periods of elated mood to satisfy inclusion criteria could make measures asking about elated mood appear more sensitive).

The inclusion and exclusion criteria also often change sample composition in ways that alter the diagnostic specificity. A common design in PBD research is use of two comparison groups: One with no Axis I diagnoses, and another with ADHD but no comorbid mood disorder (e.g., Geller, Warner, Williams, & Zimerman, 1998; Geller, Williams, et al., 1998; Pavuluri, Henry, Devineni, Carbray, & Birmaher, 2006; Tillman & Geller, 2005). This design was initially used to study the phenomenology of PBD, and to determine what behaviors indicated mania as opposed to normal childhood behaviors, or behaviors associated with ADHD—a disorder recognized as sharing many symptoms that could look like a manic presentation (Klein et al., 1998). Although the design makes good sense for phenomenological research, it distorts the performance of diagnostic tests markedly, unless practitioners employ the test in settings where children without uncomplicated ADHD or no diagnosis are systematically excluded. Including children with comorbid depression or other diagnoses produces much lower estimates of specificity (Youngstrom et al., 2006a). However, these humbler estimates are much more likely to generalize to clinical settings. These changes in performance offer concrete examples of why clinicians must pay attention to the design features of studies (Bossuyt et al., 2003) and weigh the appropriateness of applying findings to specific patients (Jaeschke, Guyatt, & Sackett, 1994a, 1994b; Sackett et al., 2000).

In spite of these limitations, several "take home" messages emerge from the studies reviewed in Table 6.4. First, there are promising diagnostic aids for PBD, at least under "efficacy" types of conditions. Second, measures that include more content pertaining to mania (e.g., the General Behavior Inventory [GBI], with 28 relevant items, or the MDQ, which asks about all DSM symptoms of mania) are much more specific to BD. As a consequence, high scores on these measures generate much larger likelihood ratios than do high scores on more general measures of psychopathology. Put another way, high scores on measures that systematically assess symptoms of mania are more powerful tools for helping to rule in PBD, whereas global measures of externalizing problems can be quite effective at ruling out PBD. Third, parent report measures appear to identify PBD better than do self- or teacher-reported measures. This holds true across studies, where parent reports produce AUCs in the .8–.9 range, compared to AUCs of .5–.7 for youth and teacher measures. The better performance of parent report has also been demonstrated in "head-to-head" comparisons between parent and youth report on the same instrument with the Achenbach scales (Youngstrom, Findling, Calabrese, et al., 2004), the GBI (Youngstrom, Findling, Calabrese, et al., 2004; Youngstrom, Meyers, et al., 2005), questionnaire versions of the Young Mania Rating Scale (Youngstrom, Meyers, et al., 2005), and the MDQ (Wagner, Findling, Emslie, Gracious, & Reed, 2006; Youngstrom, Meyers, et al., 2005). The better performance of the parent report is clearly not limited to a single instrument, or to a single research group's definition of PBD. It holds for both adolescents and younger children. This is an important finding, because it strongly contradicts the conventional clinical wisdom that self-report should be the preferred information source for evaluations of mood disorder (Loeber, Green, & Lahey, 1990).

Assessment and Treatment Thresholds

Are the combination of base-rate information, family history, and behavior checklists sufficient to do good case formulation and to begin treatment of BD? Most clinicians would say "no." Adopting these tools and the evidence-based framework described earlier would substantially improve the accuracy of clinical decision making about BD at a public health level, but it is not clear that these tools are powerful enough to justify making high-stakes decisions about individual cases.

Evidence-based medicine offers a helpful framework for answering the question, "How much is 'enough' confidence to have in a diagnosis to justify beginning treatment?" Certain diagnoses are so improbable that they are not worth the time and expense of clinical evaluation, even though they are theoretically possible. For example, the possibility of a heart attack in a 25-year-old is usually so low that it is not worth screening for it, let alone ordering an electrocardiogram for all 25-year-olds. However, for a specific case, other risk factors might raise the risk to a point that additional assessment makes good sense. If the 25-year-old has a family history with extensive early-onset heart disease or is taking a medication known to increase the risk of cardiac events, then the probability becomes high enough to merit additional assessment, even though the risk is still likely to be low. This exemplifies crossing a threshold of risk, below which the risk is so low that the expenditure of time, resources, and burden on the patient are not justified, and above which assessment would have utility. This has been called the "test/no-test threshold" (Guyatt & Rennie, 2002).

Similarly, there comes a point at which the diagnosis has been established with sufficient certainty that additional testing is unlikely to be helpful, and may actually become harmful due to the increased expense, burden, and risk involved for the patient, as well as the risk of potentially adding contradictory information that could lower the quality of the overall assessment (Kraemer, 1992). This has been called the "treatment threshold" (Guyatt & Rennie, 2002). The test and treatment thresholds carve the range of probability of a diagnosis into three segments: (1) below the test/no-test threshold, where risk is too low to justify the costs associated with assessment; (2) between the test and the treatment thresholds; or (3) above the treatment threshold, where confidence is high enough to discontinue diagnostic assessment and initiate intervention. If the probability falls in the midrange, then more assessment is required, until the new findings either decrease the probability back below the test threshold, or increase it beyond the treatment threshold.

Where should the test and treatment thresholds be set? Medical ethicists suggest that the thresholds should be set based on the costs and benefits associated with testing and with treatment (Guyatt & Rennie, 2002). There are situations in which the benefits of treatment are so high, and the costs and risks of treatment are so low, that it makes sense to skip assessment and treat everyone. This is true for many public health initiatives, such as iodizing table salt regardless of risk for thyroid dysfunction. In other scenarios, the risks of treatment are high enough that much greater diagnostic confidence is needed before starting the regimen. In light of the relative risks associated with atypical antipsychotic medications or mood stabilizers versus stimulant medication (Kowatch, Fristad, et al., 2005), the treatment threshold should be higher for a diagnosis of BD than for a diagnosis of ADHD. Although there are statistical models for determining the best places to set the threshold on a diagnostic test when

the costs and benefits (i.e., the "utilities") are known (Kraemer, 1992; Swets, Dawes, & Monahan, 2000), available data about the utilities relevant to PBD are not good. Thus it seems most appropriate for clinicians to talk individually with families and negotiate jointly the level of confidence required either to discontinue testing or to initiate treatment. Such discussions are empowering to the patient and family.

Table 6.5 presents the PPVs associated with high scores on the CBCL and the parent-completed GBI. Seen through the lens of the decision-making framework articulated here, PPVs for these tests probably fall in the "indeterminate" range. The PPVs are not high enough to justify starting high-risk interventions in most clinical settings, but they remain too high to effectively rule out a bipolar diagnosis. In other words, high scores on these tests are insufficiently accurate to be treated as a substitute for a diagnosis, but they should raise a "red flag" to trigger more thorough assessment. Table 6.6 lists other clinical features that should also provoke further assessment, even though quantitative risk estimates are not yet available.

Tests are much more helpful at ruling out PBD, reducing PBD probability below the test/no-test threshold. This is largely a function of the low base rate of PBD in most settings. If a disorder is already rare, then a test result that reduces risk is usually decisive. However, because many available tests are sensitive to PBD,

TABLE 6.6. Red Flags That Should Trigger Thorough Evaluation of Possible BD

Red flag	Description	References
Early-onset depression	Variously described as onset before age 25, or prepubertally	Kowatch, Youngstrom, et al. (2005)
Psychotic features	True delusions or hallucinations occurring in the context of mood	Kowatch, Youngstrom, et al. (2005)
Episodic aggressive behavior (including parent reports of extreme externalizing behavior)	Not specific to bipolar disorder, but most bipolar youth show this; more episodic should trigger evaluation to rule out	Hodgins et al. (2002)
Family history of BD	Five-fold increase in risk for first-degree relative; 2.5-fold for second-degree or "fuzzy" bipolar	Hodgins et al. (2002)
Atypical depression	Associated with hypersomnia (vs. insomnia), increased appetite and weight gain (vs. decrease), decreased energy, and interpersonal rejection sensitivity	Benazzi & Rihmer (2000); Birmaher et al. (1996)

low scores on them generate highly accurate negative predictive values (e.g., the SnNOut rule, or very small likelihood ratios).

Methods for Confirming Diagnosis

Diagnostic Interviews

One of the most powerful tools available for establishing a diagnosis is diagnostic interviews. These run the gamut from unstructured clinical interviews guided by the intuition and experience of the clinician, all the way to fully structured interviews that provide a rigid framework and clear scripting of the questions and probes. There are advantages and drawbacks to either extreme. Unstructured clinical interviews provide the greatest flexibility to maintain rapport, to be culturally competent, and to concentrate on issues that appear related to the presenting problem, but the price is lower reliability (i.e., results are unlikely to be duplicated by another clinician's interview) and greater susceptibility to heuristics that undermine the validity of decisions (Garb, 1998). Fully structured interviews offer the mirror image of strengths and weaknesses: Interviews can be structured to the point that they are delivered via computer. Questions are always asked and probed exactly the same way, maximizing interrater reliability (i.e., it does not matter which computer does the interview), but minimizing the flexibility, cultural competence, or other advantages offered by involving clinical judgment in the process.

At present, no fully structured diagnostic interview has demonstrated good validity for diagnosing PBD. Some instruments have failed to detect any cases of PBD in epidemiological studies (Costello et al., 1996; Shaffer et al., 1996), raising concerns about their sensitivity to bipolar diagnoses even when used in clinical settings where PBD might be reasonably common. Most published research on PBD has relied one of the several different versions of the Schedule for Affective Disorders and Schizophrenia for School-Age Children (K-SADS), including the Epidemiological version (K-SADS-E; Orvaschel, 1995), the Present and Lifetime version (K-SADS-PL; Kaufman et al., 1997), or the Washington University version (WASH-UK-SADS; Geller, Zimerman, et al., 2001). The K-SADS includes a mania module that has been validated down to at least age 5 (Nottelmann et al., 2001), and the WASH-U K-SADS includes extensive additional items potentially related to depression and mania in children beyond the core list of DSM symptoms. However, reliable K-SADS administration requires considerable training and supervision, and groups may differ in their conceptualization of symptoms and behaviors (cf. Geller, Zimerman, Williams, DelBello, Frazier et al., 2002; Wozniak et al., 1995). The K-SADS is also too cumbersome to use clinically. The core module of the PL version is nearly 200 pages long, with five additional supplements; and the WASH-U version is even more extensive. The complete KSADS interview with parent and child takes anywhere from 2 to 6 hours. Thus, training, expense, and burden on the family all mitigate against routine clinical use of the K-SADS.

The Children's Interview for Psychiatric Syndromes (ChIPS; Weller, Weller, Fristad, Rooney, & Schecter, 2000), a much briefer semistructured diagnostic interview, has shown promising validity for mood disorders (Fristad, Cummins, et al., 1998; Fristad, Glickman, et al., 1998). It is more likely to be viable for clinical use than the K-SADS due to lower training demands and briefer administration time. The ChIPS includes neither sufficient probes to capture cyclothymia nor some other variants of BD NOS; and its validity needs to be demonstrated in the hands of research groups other than its developers. Still, the combination of available validity data and the much more streamlined format makes ChIPS an attractive candidate, if a semistructured diagnostic interview is desired.

Concentrate on "Handle" Symptoms

Realistically, most practicing clinicians conduct unstructured diagnostic interviews rather than adopt one of the structured or semistructured interviews described earlier. To establish whether BD is present, it is essential to ask about all of the DSM symptoms of mania or hypomania. However, the symptoms are not equally useful indicators of potential BD (see Table 6.7). Many symptoms commonly seen in mania or hypomania (Kowatch, Youngstrom, et al., 2005) are frequently present in conditions other than BD (Carlson, 1998, 2002; Klein et al., 1998). Irritable mood, poor concentration, and high levels of motor activity are examples of symptoms that are highly sensitive but not specific to BD. Their high sensitivity means that the *absence* of the symptom may be helpful in ruling out a BD (SnNOut at the symptom level), but the presence of such symptoms is by itself ambiguous. Irritability is analogous to the "fever" or "pain" of child mental health: It indicates that something is wrong but does not provide much guidance in deciding what is wrong.

Other symptoms are more helpful in getting a "handle" on whether BD is present. Episodes of abnormally elated, expansive mood are one such symptom. Although elated mood is not the most impairing symptom associated with BD and is rarely high on the list of presenting problems, it is present in more than 80% of cases with PBD (Kowatch, Youngstrom, et al., 2005). Furthermore, elated mood that is noticeably more frequent, more intense, or longer in duration than would be developmentally appropriate rarely occurs in other child mental health syndromes (Kowatch, Fristad, et al., 2005). Grandiosity also appears fairly common in BD but less frequent in ADHD (Geller, Zimerman, Williams, DelBello, Bolhofner, et al., 2002). However, chronic grandiosity or an inflated but brittle sense of self-esteem is associated with CD (which was excluded from earlier studies of PBD), undermining the specificity of this symptom in settings in which antisocial behavior might occur.

Decreased need for sleep, which is not present in all cases, is highly specific to PBD and may be challenging to assess clinically for many reasons: Self-report is not very accurate about the onset and offset of sleep periods; parents may not know when the child is falling asleep or waking (especially if the parent is asleep at the time); and children often have televisions or computers in their room that contribute to poor sleep hygiene even when mood dysregulation is not a factor. In addition, sleep disturbance is more suggestive of BD when individuals are not sleeping because they have too much energy, or when they get less sleep than usual yet still feel energetic the following day. This should be distinguished from the insomnia often seen with unipolar depression, in which a person wants to sleep but has difficulty falling asleep despite low energy, due to stress and rumination about problems.

Hypersexuality is another symptom that deserves comment. Most children with PBD do not show hypersexuality (see Table 6.7). Indeed, hypersexuality is rarely present in prepubertal children outside of the context of either sexual abuse or mood disorder. Thus,

hypersexual behavior should trigger careful assessment of both possibilities.

Many other features that clinicians have noticed tend to occur with mood episodes. Table 6.7 (adapted from Youngstrom, Birmaher, & Findling, under review) lists the DSM-IV-TR and ICD-10 symptoms of mania, along with some clinically associated features. Where available, sensitivity estimates for the symptom or sign are provided. Quantitative estimates of specificity are more rare, and the few published estimates are unlikely to be clinically generalizable because of the inclusion and exclusion criteria used. Table 6.7 also offers brief comments about aspects of clinical presentation that would be more indicative of bipolar than of nonbipolar diagnoses.

For all of these symptoms, the case for BD is most compelling when the symptoms occur together in episodes that are a distinct shift from the person's typical functioning. Although not all authorities agree about the importance of distinct episodes, episodicity increases confidence in the diagnosis of mood disorders, particularly when mood episodes have recurred. The presence of episodes even when symptoms are prodromal or subthreshold also predicts later BD (Egeland, Hostetter, Pauls, & Sussex, 2000). Careful assessment of episodicity or fluctuations in symptom presentation also may help to clarify otherwise ambiguous symptoms. ADHD is associated with chronically high energy and poor concentration, for example. Hearing about a person suddenly having more energy than usual for periods of 1–2 weeks at a time and also difficulty staying focused on tasks sounds more like a mood disorder and less like ADHD. Careful evaluation of temperament and developmental history is vital to establish the backdrop against which these changes in functioning can be detected (Quinn & Fristad, 2004).

Mood and Energy Checkups

Prospectively gathering data about mood and energy over the course of treatment is a valuable tool for clarifying whether there are fluctuations suggestive of a mood disorder. This is a departure from the traditional model of bunching psychological assessment at the beginning of treatment. Instead, a more "dental model" of scheduling regular checkups to monitor mood and energy clarifies mood diagnosis in a way that a single panel of assessment can-

TABLE 6.7. Symptoms and Associated Features of BD

Symptom	Sensitivity to PBD[a]	Specificity to PBD	Features suggesting PBD	Features suggesting other diagnoses	Recommendation
Handle symptoms (high specificity)					
A.1. Elated, expansive, euphoric mood	70% (45–87%)	High	Extreme, causes impairment, situationally inappropriate, extreme duration	Transient, more responsive to redirection, more situationally driven; substance abuse, use of meds (e.g., corticosteroids)	Highly specific feature; its presence helps rule in diagnosis. Assess even though family may not consider it part of presenting problem.
A.2. Irritable mood	81% (55–94%)	Low	Irritability in context of other mood symptoms; high versus low energy irritability	Chronic oppositionality in absence of changes in mood or energy; it can be unipolar depression	Assess via collateral informant; self-report underestimates. If collaterals deny irritability, effectively rule out PBD because of high sensitivity. Embed in context of changes in mood and energy.
B.1. Grandiosity	78% (67–85%)	Moderately high; much lower if CD is included	Episodic quality, and should fluctuate with mood. Periods of grandiosity contrasted with low self-esteem, feeling worthless	More chronic, arrogant, not associated with mood is suggestive of CD/APD (antisocial personality disorder) or adolescent overconfidence; substance abuse	Worth emphasizing, but probably not specific enough to elevate to required feature. Fluctuations a key feature in discerning from CD/APD.
Increased energy	89% (76–96%); highest sensitivity in meta analysis	Low for "high energy," which is also common in ADHD; *episodic periods* of high energy would be more specific to mood disorder	Higher, if asked about fluctuation or change; lower, if asked about chronic (common feature in ADHD)	Chronic high motor activity	...eed to assess as change in functioning from youth's typical behavior. Episodic quality is more specific to bipolar disorder. Focus on *energy* versus motor activity for self-report; *change* in motor activity for collaterals.
Nonspecific symptoms (in descending order of sensitivity to BD)					
Pressured speech	82% (69–90%)	Unclear. Carlson (2002) raises issue of expressive language problems; but not evaluated yet in published samples	Episodic quality, change from typical for youth; set against slowed or impoverished speech during depression	Chronically "chatty" or talkative, more suggestive of ADHD	Emphasize changes from typical functioning embedded in shifts of mood or energy.
Racing thoughts	74% (51–88%)	Good, if embedded in mood context	Ask about imagery as well as words (Youngstrom et al., under review)	Distinguish from expressive language disorder and effects of substance abuse, medications	
Decreased need	72%	High, if framed as	High energy, actively	Decreased sleep due to	Emphasize decreased need for sleep, as

	Sensitivity				
for sleep	(53–86%)	decreased need, not insomnia; low, if just focus on trouble falling asleep	engaged in activities, does not miss sleep the next day	stimulant use (ADHD), use of substances or medications (e.g., asthma medications); difficulty falling asleep with unipolar depression (vs. decreased need for sleep). Depressed persons want to sleep but cannot	distinct from difficulty falling asleep (particularly due to stress or rumination). High energy, little diminution of energy despite decreased sleep.
Mood swings/lability	High	High, based on PGBI, CBCL, Conners items	Frequent, intense, with periods of long duration	May be induced by substance abuse, medications, medical/neurological illnesses, borderline personality traits, disruptive disorders	Parent report highly sensitive. PBD unlikely if parent denies. Specificity appears promising, based on multiple scales. Conceptualize as mixed state with volatile mood.
Hypersexuality	38% (31–45%)	High, typically either PBD or sexual abuse	Hypersexuality not characteristic, embedded in episodes of energy/mood; has pleasure-seeking quality	Sexual abuse linked to trauma, perhaps more seductive/reenacting quality than sensation-seeking; exposure to X-rated movies, actual sex	Insensitive to PBD, so absence not informative. Highly specific presence should trigger careful assessment of PBD and abuse (recognize that they could co-occur).
Distractibility	84% (71–92%)	Low, ADHD, unipolar, anxiety, PTSD, and low cognitive functioning all show this, too	Higher, if asked about change from typical; embedded in context of mood	Chronic problems much more suggestive of ADHD or neurological impairment	Probably important to assess via collateral instead of self-report. High sensitivity could make negative collateral report helpful in ruling out BD.
Poor judgment	69% (38–89%)	Moderate	Episodic, embedded in mood/energy, not a trait of youth	Impulsive or accident-prone, clumsy	Episodic, sensation seeking may be most specific presentation.
Flight of ideas	56% (46–66%)	Moderate		(Speech problems again) substance abuse, medication-induced effects	
Increased sense of well-being (ICD-10, p. 113)	Unknown	Unknown	Unknown, but theoretically likely to be low	Consistent with high positive affect model of mania	Needs investigation.
Increased sociability/people-seeking/overfamiliarity (ICD-10, p. 113); added to WASH-U K-SADS;	May be fairly sensitive	Unknown	Unknown		Needs investigation.

a Sensitivity estimates are from Kowatch, Youngstrom, et al. (2005) meta-analysis unless otherwise noted.

not. These checkups may be as basic as asking about changes in mood and energy at each appointment, or they could use brief checklists. Brevity is crucial to minimize burden and increase cooperation. Many instruments that would be good choices for an initial assessment battery are poor options for the repetitions needed to get prospective information.

At the opposite extreme, the "life-charting method" boils down questions to a bare minimum of two or three items (one rating energy, another rating mood and possibly distinguishing irritability from "up" or "down" moods), then has the patient or parent rate the items several times a day for several weeks or months (Denicoff et al., 1997). The life-charting method provides extremely detailed information about shifts in mood and energy, and it can be a powerful tool for identifying triggers that exacerbate mood disturbance. Several excellent examples of life charts are available at no charge on the Internet (Google searches on the term "bipolar life chart" provide multiple hits). Some families take readily to the life-charting methodology. Others find it too burdensome.

Methods Not Yet Diagnostically Informative

Many widely used procedures have not yet demonstrated validity for the assessment of PBD. Some have not been systematically investigated yet; others have some preliminary data available, but nothing that adequately draws inferences about the diagnostic validity of the tool applied in clinical settings. There have been no published evaluations of projective techniques such as the Rorschach Inkblot Test, the Thematic Apperception Test, or kinetic family drawing, despite a clinical lore that PBD might be associated with gory content (Popper, 1990). There also are no published studies with objective personality inventories yet. Without rigorous research, it is impossible to tell how helpful assessment results on any of these instruments might be in determining a bipolar diagnosis. Even face-valid results might occur frequently enough in nonbipolar cases to undermine the diagnostic value, much as the ubiquity of irritable mood offsets its high sensitivity to PBD. Other tests have shown statistically significant differences between bipolar and nonbipolar groups, including some neuropsychological and affective processing tasks (Dickstein et al., 2004, 2005; Henin et al., 2006; Rich, Bhangoo, et al., 2005; Rich,

Schmajuk, et al., 2005). However, these studies typically obtain effect sizes smaller than would be needed to classify individuals accurately based on test results, and they have used tight inclusion and exclusion criteria that increase internal validity (which is important for these novel investigations). Thus, clinicians attempting to use the same tools in clinical settings with fewer inclusion and exclusion criteria obtain even more modest results, further weakening the chances of a test contributing accurately to diagnostic formulation. Given the current evidence base:

1. There is no value added by administering any of these tests to aid in the differential diagnosis of PBD. Although many of these tools might demonstrate validity in future studies, at present they can only be considered unproven.
2. If these tests already have been given as part of an assessment battery, they should not be interpreted as changing the diagnostic formulation with regard to PBD.
3. These tests should only be added to an assessment battery in youth diagnosed with BD if the test serves some other, additional clinical purpose, such as ascertaining appropriate educational placement.

Cross-Informant Agreement and Implications for Impairment

A common issue in child assessment occurs when a parent (often the mother) reports lots of concerns about the child's behavior that do not appear to be corroborated by other perspectives, such as youth self-report or ratings provided by teachers. Clinicians are frequently worried that the parent might be hypervigilant or have unrealistic expectations about appropriate behavior, that ineffective parenting styles might be creating behavior problems that otherwise are well managed in the classroom and other settings, or that the parent's anxiety or depression might be biasing reports about the child's behavior (Richters, 1992). When parent and youth perceptions differ, clinicians tend to give more weight to youth report about internalizing problems, because youth have direct access to their own feelings (Loeber et al., 1990). Discrepancies between parent, teacher, and youth descriptions of behavior problems in PBD tend to be large (Hazell et al., 1999; Kahana et al., 2003; Youngstrom, Findling,

Calabrese, et al., 2004), raising concerns about both the accuracy of parent report and stability of behavior across settings (Thuppal, Carlson, Sprafkin, & Gadow, 2002).

Importantly, results have consistently demonstrated that parent appraisals of mood and behavior identify bipolar cases significantly better than do self- or teacher reports (Findling et al., 2002; Hazell et al., 1999; Kahana et al., 2003; Wagner et al., 2006; Youngstrom, Findling, Calabrese, et al., 2004; Youngstrom, Meyers, et al., 2005), even when predicting research diagnoses made on the basis of direct interviews of both the parent and child, as well as clinical observation. The greater validity of parent report persists in spite of high rates of mood disorder in the reporting parent in many of these samples, and in spite of the high levels of their own distress reported by parents (Youngstrom, Findling, & Calabrese, 2004).

The lower validity of teacher compared to parent reports appears to be due partly to the tendency of teachers to focus on increased motor activity and poor concentration, then to attribute these behaviors to ADHD (Abikoff, Courtney, Pelham, & Koplewicz, 1993). In fact, teachers do no better than chance at distinguishing between children with BD and those with ADHD (Youngstrom, Findling, Calabrese, et al., 2004) when using the Achenbach Teacher's Report Form (TRF; 1991b). Teachers might do better identifying bipolar cases using instruments that include item content more specific to mania, although some important behaviors, such as decreased need for sleep, are unlikely to be observed at school.

At least three factors undermine the validity of youth self-report: (1) Children and adolescents are often less cognitively capable of completing questionnaires, and less psychologically minded than adults; (2) social desirability effects might make youth minimize endorsement of irritable mood or hypersexuality; and (3) mania and hypomania tend to be more distressing to people around the affected person, rather than to the person him- or herself, and mood symptoms often are associated with a reduction in insight into one's own behavior (Dell'Osso et al., 2002; Pini, Dell'Osso, & Amador, 2001; Youngstrom, Findling, & Calabrese, 2004).

Agreement among informants about cases with PBD is actually higher than typically believed. According to both themselves and their teachers, affected youth experience more behavior problems than would be expected based on the level of problems described by the parent (Youngstrom, Meyers, Youngstrom, Calabrese, & Findling, 2006b). Interrater agreement appears to be even higher when focus is on mood symptoms in particular instead of behavior problems generally (Youngstrom, Findling, & Calabrese, 2004), so there is likely to be even more cross-situational consistency than current measures reveal. Even so, there appears to be a dose–response relationship, such that when manic symptoms are reported by more informants and in more settings, global functioning and objective measures of behavior on an inpatient unit all indicate progressively more severe impairment (Carlson & Youngstrom, 2003).

TREATMENT TARGETS: PROCESS AND OUTCOME MEASURES

Symptom Reduction

There are many rating instruments that measure symptoms during the course of treatment. Some are better suited for baseline and outcome evaluation; others are more suitable for monitoring progress during the course of treatment. It is worth bearing in mind that tools may play a valuable monitoring function without being top-tier outcome measures. The life-chart methodology or session-by-session checkups on mood and energy are cases in point. These are unlikely to be primary outcome measures, but they provide helpful weekly feedback about progress and setbacks in the course of treatment.

Clinician-Rated Measures of Symptom Severity

For clinical trials, the primary outcome measures are clinician-rated assessments of the severity of manic and depressive symptoms. The industry standards have been the Young Mania Rating Scale (YMRS; Young, Biggs, Ziegler, & Meyer, 1978) and the Child Depression Rating Scale—Revised (CDRS-R; Poznanski, Miller, Salguero, & Kelsh, 1984). The YMRS was originally designed for use with adults on an inpatient unit, with ratings completed by staff nurses based on direct observation of behavior over an 8-hour shift. With children and adolescents, YMRS ratings are typically based on clinician interviews with the child and the primary caregiver, and the reference period is usually extended to cover the past 2 weeks instead of 8 hours. Although the item anchors and weights were developed for use with inpatient adults, no adaptations have been made to make the anchors more developmentally appropriate for children or adolescents. The YMRS also includes some items covering behaviors that are not DSM symptoms of mania, and it omits other core symptoms (e.g., grandiosity or increased engagement in pleasurable but risky acts). In spite of these shortcomings, the YMRS has demonstrated considerable evidence of validity in youth (Fristad, Weller, & Weller, 1992, 1995; Youngstrom, Danielson, Findling, Gracious, & Calabrese, 2002). Even so, 2 of the 11 items on the YMRS are so weak as to lower the internal consistency of an already short scale. One of these is the "bizarre appearance" item, and the other is the item rating "lack of insight." Both items are also problematic in parent-report versions of the YMRS (Gracious, Youngstrom, Findling, & Calabrese, 2002; Youngstrom, Gracious, Danielson, Findling, & Calabrese, 2003). The calibration of YMRS scores across sites may also be different, such that similar clinical presentations earn widely divergent scores (Youngstrom, Findling, et al., 2003).

In contrast, the CDRS-R was developed specifically for use with children and adolescents, and the initial validation samples comprised youth (Poznanski et al., 1984).The CDRS-R includes 17 items rated on either a 1- to 5-point or 1- to 7-point scale, with higher scores signaling greater severity. Ratings are based on interviews with both the caregiver and the youth, with three items rated entirely on the basis of direct observation during the course of the youth interview. Strengths of the CDRS-R include its being designed specifically for youths, with developmentally appropriate anchors and validation samples; its high internal consistency (alphas often exceed .90); and its demonstrated sensitivity to treatment effects. Limitations of the CDRS-R are that it does not cover all DSM symptoms of depression, that it fails to distinguish between psychomotor agitation and retardation, that it does not assess both hypersomnia and insomnia (particularly problematic inasmuch as hypersomnia may denote bipolar depression), and that its scores also might depend substantially on the rater rather than on the severity of depression.

The degree to which clinician ratings are sus-

ceptible to variations in clinical judgment poses a major challenge not only for multisite trials but also for independent clinicians attempting to use the measures in their own practice. Without using standardized videotapes or training vignettes, a clinician has no means of knowing whether his or her perceived sense of mood severity corresponds with other clinicians' perceptions. In a recent study using videotapes, large differences were found between the scores assigned by American, Indian, and British psychiatrists (in descending order of average ratings) (Mackin, Targum, Kalali, Rom, & Young, 2006). The fact that so much variance in scores depends on the rater and not the diagnosis or the severity of illness obscures potential similarities across sites and studies. This state of affairs also means that we should not put great faith in commonly used rules of thumb, such as a YMRS score of 13 or higher to connote hypomania, or 16 or higher to designate moderate mania.

Newer measures of mania and depression, such as the K-SADS Mania Rating Scale and K-SADS Depression Rating Scale (Axelson et al., 2003), are designed to provide more thorough coverage of mood content, more consistent anchors and item score ranges, and other psychometric advantages. They represent a definite improvement over the prior generation of rating scales, but have not yet reached the tipping point at which their technical merits outweigh the inertia of the backlog of publications using the more familiar instruments. No clinician-rated instrument will resolve the problems associated with rater effects (e.g., different calibration across sites or raters) without requiring calibration against a standard set of training tapes, as is done with measures such as the Psychopathy Checklist—Revised (Hare, 1991).

Parent-Rated Measures of Severity and Outcome

Parent checklists are much easier to deploy in a standardized fashion across sites and clinics than are clinician-rated instruments. Training costs are lower, and susceptibility to idiosyncratic clinical interpretations of behaviors is also lessened. As yet there is no established front-runner for parent-reported symptom outcome measures. The CBCL often shows little improvement over the course of treatment, possibly because ratings cover a 6-month window, and acute clinical trials tend to be much shorter in length. The CBCL may also be hampered by the lack of scales with content specific to mood disorders. The MDQ focuses on symptoms of mania, but because it uses a simple present–absent format, it may not gather enough information about severity to be sensitive to treatment effects. The parent GBI has proven highly sensitive to treatment effects in open-label studies (Cooperberg, 2001; Youngstrom, Cooperberg, Findling, & Calabrese, 2003), showing large effects on both the manic–mixed and the depression scales. However, the reading level (roughly 12th grade) and the burden imposed by the GBI (10 pages of questions in 12-point font) hinder its utility as an outcome measure in clinical settings. Parent-rated YMRS scores appear less sensitive to treatment effects, in part due to the lower reliability of the instrument. Other parent-reported measures, such as the Child Bipolar Questionnaire (Papolos & Papolos, 2002) and the Child Mania Rating Scale (Pavuluri et al., 2006) (see Table 6.4) have not yet been evaluated as outcome measures.

Youth Self-Report Measures

As documented earlier, youth self-report, from a diagnostic perspective, does not efficiently identify BD. Youth might seek treatment for the depressed phase of illness, but they are very unlikely to self-refer for treatment during the manic, mixed, or hypomanic phases of illness. As a result, treatment referrals are often made by a concerned adult instead of the adolescent. It follows that the baseline levels of symptoms typically are lower when assessed via self-report than via collateral informants, because referrals are usually driven by the collateral perspective. The lack of initial insight and lower self-rated severity at baseline limit the room for improvement during therapy, ensuring that self-report will look like a relatively insensitive method for quantifying outcomes. Studies gathering both youth and parent report on the same measures have confirmed this expectation (Youngstrom, Cooperberg, et al., 2003).

Other Collateral Informants

Although there is a broad spectrum of possible informants about psychosocial functioning in youth, including siblings, peers, and teachers, among others, relatively little has been done to date in terms of collecting outcome data.

Outcome Benchmarks

"Social validation" provides an important set of methods for demonstrating meaningful clinical improvement (Kazdin, 1977). This involves confirming with parents, teachers, peers, or other significant individuals in the youth's life that they see observable improvement in the symptoms or functioning. Social validation also emphasizes the use of ecologically valid indicators of functioning. For PBD, these indicators might include improved school attendance, better grades, fewer disciplinary incidents, increases in the number of friends, or similar social, educational, or vocational gains.

A complementary system for measuring clinically significant change developed by Jacobson, Roberts, Berns, and McGlinchey (1999; Jacobson & Truax, 1991) has gained popularity among research-oriented clinicians. This approach to clinical significance involves using a relevant psychometric measure, then showing (1) that the scores change enough for clinicians to be confident that an individual patient really is improving given the precision of the instrument, and (2) that the scores have moved past a benchmark compared to clinical and nonclinical score distributions. The advantages of this approach to clinical significance include its feasibility, its strong psychometric underpinnings, and its reliance on empirically defined benchmarks (Jacobson et al., 1999). It also clearly focuses on whether treatment is helping each individual patient rather than on the way that effect sizes describe the average outcome for an aggregate of cases. The big drawback to the Jacobson and colleagues approach is that it requires psychometric information that is typically not reported in technical manuals or articles. Specifically, determination of "reliable change" requires knowledge of the standard error of the difference score for the measure. With regard to the three benchmarks, setting the threshold for getting the patient away from the clinical distribution requires having norms for a clinical population, or at least a mean and standard deviation for a representative clinical sample. Similarly, it is only possible to determine whether a patient has moved back into the nonclinical range of functioning (defined here as scoring within two standard deviations of the nonclinical mean) by having nonclinical norms available. The third threshold, crossing closer to the nonclinical than to the clinical mean, requires information about both the clinical and nonclinical distributions to calculate a weighted average.

To make it more practical for clinicians to apply the Jacobson and colleagues approach, Cooperberg (2001) meta-analyzed studies with relevant data on measures frequently used with PBD, generating pooled estimates of the mean and standard deviation for each measure in samples of youth with and without BD. The standard error of the difference was calculated with use of the standard error of the measure. Table 6.8 presents the standard error of the difference, allowing calculation of Jacobson's Reliable Change Index, but it also presents the number of change points needed to ensure 90 or 95% confidence (two-tailed) that the patient is improving. For most clinicians, the critical

scores are more useful, because they do not require computation. Table 6.8 also presents the benchmark values for moving away from the clinical distribution ("A"), back into the nonclinical range ("B"), or moving closer to the nonclinical than to the clinical average ("C").

In addition, Table 6.8 presents similar estimates for the CBCL and the Ohio Scales, based on the published standardization samples. These reference numbers are based on large and well-described samples. The "clinical" ranges for these measures are based on outpatient referrals, with or without a bipolar diagnosis, whereas the estimates for the mood-specific measures are based on an aggregate of multiple smaller samples with research diagnoses of mood disorder.

TABLE 6.8. Clinically Significant Change Benchmarks with Common Instruments and Mood Rating Scales

Measure	Cut scores[a]			Critical change (unstandardized scores)		
	A	B	C	95%	90%	$SE_{difference}$
Benchmarks based on published norms						
Beck Depression Inventory						
BDI Mixed Depression	4	22	15	9	8	4.8
CBCL *T*-scores (2001 norms)						
Total	49	70	58	5	4	2.4
Externalizing	49	70	58	7	6	3.4
Internalizing	n/a	70	56	9	7	4.5
Attention Problems	n/a	66	58	8	7	4.2
TRF *T*-scores (2001 norms)						
Total	n/a	70	57	5	4	2.3
Externalizing	n/a	70	56	6	5	3.0
Internalizing	n/a	70	55	9	7	4.4
Attention Problems	n/a	66	57	5	4	2.3
YSR *T*-scores (2001 norms)						
Total	n/a	70	54	7	6	3.3
Externalizing	n/a	70	54	9	8	4.6
Internalizing	n/a	70	54	9	8	4.8
Benchmarks based on bipolar spectrum samples (Cooperberg, 2002)						
Young Mania Rating Scale (Clinician-Rated)	6	2	2	12	10	6.2
Child Depression Rating Scale—Revised	n/a	40	29	8	7	4.0
Parent GBI, Hypomanic/Biphasic Scale	7	19	15	8	7	4.2
Parent GBI, Depression Scale	n/a	18	13	7	6	3.6
Adolescent GBI, Hypomanic/Biphasic Scale	n/a	32	19	8	7	4.4
Adolescent GBI, Depression Scale	n/a	47	27	10	9	5.2

[a] A, away from the clinical range; B, back into the nonclinical range; C, closer to the nonclinical than to the clinical mean.

Adherence

Nonadherence to treatment is a major issue when working with BD in children and adolescents, as well as adults. Patients frequently refuse to take medications, or they take them inconsistently due to attitudes about illness and treatment, concern about the side effects of the medications, or a lack of understanding about the recurrent nature of the illness. Consistent attendance at therapy appointments is also a difficulty, with the chaotic family environment often creating obstacles to compliance. It is crucial that practitioners monitor adherence to treatment recommendations. Psychoeducation about the nature of PBD, the potential benefits of medication and other treatment components, as well as potential side effects to monitor, has been demonstrated to improve adherence substantially, thus improving overall outcomes as well (Fristad, Gavazzi, et al., 2003; Fristad, Goldberg Arnold, & Gavazzi, 2003).

Quality of Life and Positive Aspects of Functioning

There is growing recognition that treatment should attend to improving quality of life and positive aspects of functioning versus focusing solely on symptom reduction. With children and adolescents, it is important to promote social and educational development, in addition to ameliorating problem behaviors. If a formal measure of quality of life is desired, then the two best-validated instruments currently available appear to be the KINDL (Ravens-Sieberer & Bullinger, 1998) and the Pediatric Quality of Life Scale (Varni, Seid, & Rode, 1999) based on a recent review (Harding, 2001). Whether or not a formal quality-of-life measure is used, clinicians should assess peer relationships, family functioning, and academic performance. Bipolar illness tends to have a detrimental effect on all of these areas of functioning, and interventions that address these deficits have a tremendous impact on both reducing the burden and improving the prognosis.

Differential Treatment Planning and Treatment Utility

Several factors deserve comment relative to how assessment may contribute to treatment planning. First, the distinction between unipolar and bipolar depression is important to make. Although the symptoms and presenting complaints of bipolar depression may appear similar to unipolar depression, the treatment response can be quite different. Antidepressant medications may be overactivating in BD, triggering mania or possibly increasing suicide risk (Carlson, 2003; Geller et al., 1993; Kowatch, Fristad, et al., 2005). Similarly, cognitive or social activation strategies need to be qualified to avoid the risk of not only lifting the person's depression but also triggering a mania episode (Newman et al., 2002). Besides avoiding unintended harmful effects, recognition of bipolar depression also suggests positive strategies that may be effective, including improved sleep hygiene and avoidance of self-medication of symptoms (Danielson et al., 2004).

Repeated assessment of mood and energy, whether by brief "checkups" at the beginning of each session, repetitions of a brief mood checklist, or via the life-charting method, is a powerful tool to discern whether there is an ebb and flow suggestive of a mood disorder or a more chronic condition. Once the case conceptualization includes a mood disorder, these repeated assessments become a valuable means of monitoring progress and identifying "triggers" that can worsen mood and functioning. Although there are many generic triggers, such as stress or sleep disruption, others will be more subtle or unique to the individual. These assessments are also valuable in learning the signs that indicate potential "roughening" or relapse (Sachs, 2004).

Clinicians also need to be alert to the frequent lack of insight into behavior, and the frequent differences in perspective, between the parent and the youth in bipolar illness. Many youth are not self-referred for treatment, and if their behaviors are driven by manic or mixed states, then they may perceive the problem as being other people's, not their own. What appears to be irritable mood to observers seems more like parents and teachers are "hassling," "nagging," or otherwise provoking the youth. Sometimes it may be possible to increase insight, but this is more often accomplished after the mood states are stabilized.

A final issue to consider in case formulation revolves around the "classic," or episodic, versus "chronic" presentation. Although this is not currently recognized as a formal distinction in DSM-IV-TR or ICD-10, the episodic versus chronic distinction is becoming a recurrent theme in the literature, both in youth and in adults. Youth with a more episodic presentation may have a better response to lithium and higher likelihood of a good prognosis (Ghaemi et al., 2002). Youth with the more chronic presentation, which may account for a large portion of youth diagnosed as "bipolar," show a poorer response to lithium, more comorbidity, and equal or higher levels of impairment. It is unclear whether this presentation is on the bipolar spectrum, or whether it represents a distinct syndrome. Most people with this presentation appear to continue to show chronic mood lability, suggesting that this might be the juvenile presentation of BPD (see Shiner, Chapter 17, this volume) in at least some cases. Interestingly, there is debate about whether BPD itself might be on the bipolar spectrum, representing the extreme of mood cycling or instability (MacKinnon & Pies, 2006). Besides indicating changes in pharmacotherapeutic approach, the episodic–chronic distinction may prove important for psychotherapy as well, perhaps suggesting that techniques drawn from dialectical behavioral therapy (Linehan, 1993) might be helpful in addressing the affective instability in the more chronic presentation.

OTHER ISSUES IN CASE FORMULATION

Developmental Factors

Developmental factors influence the assessment process in important ways. The younger the individual, the more conservative practitioners should be about applying a diagnosis of BD. On the one hand, genetic and environmental risk factors promoting development of BD may have been present since before birth, so it would be an error to assume dogmatically that BD cannot occur until after onset of puberty, and the hormonal cascade involved in puberty itself may be starting at unexpectedly young ages in some cases. However, the evidence also points to BD being more rare prepubertally, and other conditions that are much more common in children may also could account for mood lability. Normal development involves testing of limits, tantrums, and some aggression, and all these may interact powerfully with the family environment and parenting to produce coercive cycles of aggressive behavior (McMahon & Frick, 2005; Patterson, DeBaryshe, & Ramsey, 1989). Additionally, many

other childhood disorders, including anxiety disorders, pervasive developmental disorders, and unipolar depression, frequently have irritable mood and poor frustration tolerance as part of their presentation. The behavioral genetics literature sometimes described potential "phenocopies," or processes that produce a similar looking set of behaviors, but for different etiological reasons. These potential "phenocopies" may be more common than "true" PBD in most clinical settings.

Comorbidity is another challenge in case formulation. It is not parsimonious to diagnose a child with both anxiety and explosive, irritable mood as having both disorders, unless it can be shown that the two appear at separate times in at least some of the person's life (APA, 2000). Nor is it prudent from a risk management perspective to start simultaneously medications for both "comorbid" conditions; instead, the assessment process should clarify which problems are "primary"—in the sense of producing the biggest therapeutic gains and reductions in burden—and concentrate on alleviating them first. "Comorbidity" in the initial presentation might provide some useful distinctions about treatment selection in the future, but at present it seems to be more of a marker of severity. From a case formulation perspective, "comorbidity" may also provide a shorthand for a list of topics to revisit later in treatment, to "mop up" whatever has not resolved along with treatment of the primary problems.

Developmental stage changes the sources of information available for the assessment process, and also perhaps the weight that should be assigned to different perspectives. Younger children are able to fill out self-report questionnaires, and older youth may have difficulty depending on reading level. Youngsters also are less psychologically minded and often have difficulty both tolerating formal, semistructured diagnostic interviews and providing meaningful responses. Because referrals are usually driven by parental concerns, youth are frequently less motivated to cooperate in the interview. For all of these reasons, some groups and clinicians have not always interviewed youth under 12 years of age (e.g., Wozniak et al., 1995). Others have argued strongly that it is crucial to interview directly even young children, because they often provide different answers than their parents (Tillman et al., 2004). At a minimum, it seems like good practice to meet with children to understand their concerns, to assess their motivation for treatment, and also to make behavioral observations that can (1) corroborate or disconfirm parent report about mood and energy, (2) provide a sense of whether deficits in cognitive ability, a pervasive developmental disorder, or some other medical factor might be contributing to the mood dysregulation, and (3) gather some initial information about how the child responds interpersonally.

With adolescents, parent reports still remain valuable, but self-reports become more viable. Clinicians need to be sensitive to different mechanisms that might underlie apparent disagreements, including low insight and motivation contributing to adolescent underreporting or parent stress leading to overreporting. With adolescents, more thorough assessment of substance use should be a prominent feature of case formulation, and it should be revisited over the course of treatment, because mood disorders are linked to greatly increased risk of alcohol and drug use. Discussions about sexual activity may also be necessary; the impulsivity and fluctuating self-esteem associated with mood disorder contribute to risk of pregnancy, sexually transmitted infection, and poorer choices of partners.

Ethical and Legal Issues

The assessment and treatment of PBD raises multiple ethical and legal issues, three of which are especially salient:

1. Who is responsible for seeking and accepting treatment?
2. How do we proceed when a parent report does not appear to agree with other sources of information?
3. How do we ethically treat a potentially lethal condition that is difficult to recognize, in the absence of clear data about the long-term risks and benefits of different interventions? Does it make sense to try to treat prodromal BD?

First, the issue of responsibility for seeking and adhering to treatment is particularly complicated in PBD. In addition to the routine complexity of working with child patients in the legal custody of a parent or other caregiver (who ultimately is responsible for seeking and approving of treatment), BD often compromises patients' insight into their behavior. Fur-

thermore, many symptoms of mania are not distressing to the patient, whereas they are annoying or threatening to people around the patient. Hypomania and mania often feel pleasant, or at least not pathological, to the affected individual, yet these mood states can cause considerable social disruption. Behavior that feels "spontaneous" and "alive" to the youth can be perceived as obnoxious or threatening by others. The consequence is that youth with mania usually do not recognize their own mood disturbance, and instead project the blame for interpersonal conflict onto others. This lessens their motivation to participate in therapy, and it raises ethical concerns about continuing to treat them even when they are actively opposed to therapy. It also challenges conventional definitions of "impairment" emphasizing that the symptoms are causing distress (Wakefield, 1997).

Cross-informant agreement raises a second, related set of issues. Clinicians are often unimpressed by the level of agreement between parents and other informants. Given the heritable nature of BD, affected youth run a high risk of having affected parents as well. Clinicians are justifiably concerned about the possibility that a parent's own mood state might bias his or her description of the child's behavior. This undoubtedly occurs. However, countervailing trends need to be considered as well. As described earlier, these include the tendency for lack of insight to undermine the validity of self-report for mania, and the fact that most teacher-rated instruments do not include mania scales. Clinicians also need to bear in mind that most referrals are initiated by a parent, which means that the parent will on average be the most concerned party ("regression to the mean" produced by selecting cases based on one informant that is imperfectly correlated with other informants) (Campbell & Kenny, 1999). Many legitimate cases of PBD are referred by parents who themselves experience epochs of substantial mood disturbance. Clinicians need to balance recognition that adult mood can influence ratings of child behavior and the fact that parent report appears to be one of the most valid indicators of PBD, even when the adult also is affected by mood disorder (Youngstrom, Findling, & Calabrese, 2004).

Finally, there is the issue of how early in the course of illness to treat BD. Arguments for early intervention include the potential for better treatment response, possible neuroprotective effects that could lessen or avert the physiological and cognitive changes evident in recurrent illness, reduced risk of relapse, and the hope of better long-term functioning and quality of life (Chang, Steiner, et al., 2003). These potential benefits need to be weighed against the risks associated with early treatment, including the unknown long-term effects of medication, as well as the stigma of labeling people as having a mental illness and how this affects their relationships. Attempting to identify and treat BD at its earliest stages increases the challenge to differentiate between pathological mood states and typical functioning. Implicitly, arguments for early intervention lower the "treatment threshold" by accepting milder and fuzzier presentations as reasonable treatment targets. The case for prevention or early intervention is strengthened if there are low-cost or low-risk strategies that might help, such as changes in diet. Without more research about preventive techniques, as well as the long-term effects of more acute treatments, the best strategy might be "watchful waiting," with at-risk families documenting the emotional and behavioral functioning of children periodically as they grow up. With younger children, disruptive and aggressive behavior may demand treatment, but neither a PBD label nor pharmacological interventions should be used lightly.

CONCLUSION

BD in adolescence and childhood remains a controversial topic. Practitioners should be agnostic about the possibility of diagnosing it. Agnosticism implies being somewhat skeptical but open to the possibility, and looking for convincing data. Families are not well served by misdiagnosis in either direction.

Assessment of BD presents numerous challenges, such as a fluctuating presentation, complicated diagnostic criteria, and high rates of comorbidity. The hurdles to accurate recognition only grow higher with younger cases. At the same time, rapid progress has been made in demonstrating the validity of the diagnosis, understanding the associated burden, and learning about the prognosis over at least 4 years of follow-up. The field has also made gains in the number and quality of assessment tools available for diagnosis and for measuring progress and outcomes with children and adolescents.

The assessment model I have advocated in this chapter is heavily influenced by the recommendations of evidence-based medicine (Guyatt & Rennie, 2002; Sackett et al., 2000) and represents a different perspective than traditional approaches to psychological assessment. The information about the relative performance of tests and the clinical features associated with BD is valuable regardless of whether practitioners adopt other, more novel procedures, such as using the nomogram for estimating risk. There also are clear take-home messages, including some that counteract conventional wisdom about assessment, such as the importance of involving a parent or other familiar adult in the assessment of manic symptoms, compared to the relatively lower validity of self- or teacher-report. However, employing the rest of the evidence-based methods I have described here will help to make the best use of the assessment tools available, and to strike the balance between being open to the possibility of PBD yet avoiding overdiagnosis of a rare yet popularized condition.

ACKNOWLEDGMENT

This work was supported in part by National Institutes of Health Grant No. 5R01 MH066647 (Eric Youngstrom, Principal Investigator).

REFERENCES

Abikoff, H., Courtney, M., Pelham, W. E., & Koplewicz, H. S. (1993). Teachers' ratings of disruptive behaviors: The influence of halo effects. *Journal of Abnormal Child Psychology, 21,* 519–533.

Achenbach, T. M. (1991a). *Manual for the Child Behavior Checklist/4–18 and 1991 profile.* Burlington: University of Vermont, Department of Psychiatry.

Achenbach, T. M. (1991b). *Manual for the Teacher's Report Form and 1991 profile.* Burlington: University of Vermont, Department of Psychiatry.

Achenbach, T. M. (1991c). *Manual for the Youth Self-Report Form and 1991 profile.* Burlington: University of Vermont, Department of Psychiatry.

Achenbach, T. M., & Rescorla, L. A. (2001). *Manual for the ASEBA School-Age Forms and profiles.* Burlington: University of Vermont.

Akiskal, H. S., & Pinto, O. (1999). The evolving bipolar spectrum. Prototypes I, II, III, and IV. *Psychiatric Clinics of North America, 22,* 517–534, vii.

Althoff, R. R., Rettew, D. C., Faraone, S. V., Boomsma, D. I., & Hudziak, J. J. (2006). Latent class analysis shows strong heritability of the CBCL–juvenile bipolar phenotype. *Biological Psychiatry, 60,* 903–911.

American Psychiatric Association (APA). (2000). *Diagnostic and statistical manual of mental disorders* (4th ed., text rev.). Washington, DC: Author.

Angst, J., Gamma, A., Benazzi, F., Ajdacic, V., Eich, D., & Rossler, W. (2003). Toward a re-definition of subthreshold bipolarity: Epidemiology and proposed criteria for bipolar-II, minor bipolar disorders and hypomania. *Journal of Affective Disorders, 73,* 133–146.

Arnold, L. M., Strakowski, S. M., Schwiers, M. L., Amicone, J., Fleck, D. E., Corey, K. B., et al. (2004). Sex, ethnicity, and antipsychotic medication use in patients with psychosis. *Schizophrenia Research, 66,* 169–175.

Axelson, D. A., Birmaher, B., Strober, M., Gill, M. K., Valeri, S., Chiappetta, L., et al. (2006). Phenomenology of children and adolescents with bipolar spectrum disorders. *Archives of General Psychiatry, 63,* 1139–1148.

Axelson, D. A., Birmaher, B. J., Brent, D., Wassick, S., Hoover, C., Bridge, J., et al. (2003). A preliminary study of the Kiddie Schedule for Affective Disorders and Schizophrenia for School-Age Children mania rating scale for children and adolescents. *Journal of Child and Adolescent Psychopharmacology, 13,* 463–470.

Bebbington, P., & Ramana, R. (1995). The epidemiology of bipolar affective disorder. *Social Psychiatry and Psychiatric Epidemiology, 30,* 279–292.

Benazzi, F. (2000). Exploring aspects of DSM-IV interpersonal sensitivity in bipolar II. *Journal of Affective Disorders, 60,* 43–46.

Benazzi, F., & Rihmer, Z. (2000). Sensitivity and specificity of DSM-IV atypical features for bipolar II disorder diagnosis. *Psychiatry Research, 93,* 257–262.

Berk, M., & Dodd, S. (2005). Bipolar II disorder: A review. *Bipolar Disorders, 7,* 11–21.

Biederman, J., Faraone, S., Mick, E., Wozniak, J., Chen, L., Ouellette, C., et al. (1996). Attention-deficit hyperactivity disorder and juvenile mania: An overlooked comorbidity? *Journal of the American Academy of Child and Adolescent Psychiatry, 35,* 997–1008.

Biederman, J., Faraone, S. V., Wozniak, J., Mick, E., Kwon, A., & Aleardi, M. (2004). Further evidence of unique developmental phenotypic correlates of pediatric bipolar disorder: Findings from a large sample of clinically referred preadolescent children assessed over the last 7 years. *Journal of Affective Disorders, 82,* S45–S58.

Biederman, J., Kwon, A., Wozniak, J., Mick, E., Markowitz, S., Fazio, V., et al. (2004). Absence of gender differences in pediatric bipolar disorder: Findings from a large sample of referred youth. *Journal of Affective Disorders, 83,* 207–214.

Biederman, J., Wozniak, J., Kiely, K., Ablon, S., Faraone, S., Mick, E., et al. (1995). CBCL clinical scales discriminate prepubertal children with structured interview–derived diagnosis of mania from those with ADHD. *Journal of the American Academy of Child and Adolescent Psychiatry, 34,* 464–471.

Birmaher, B., Arbelaez, C., & Brent, D. (2002). Course and outcome of child and adolescent major depressive disorder. *Child and Adolescent Psychiatric Clinics of North America, 11,* 619–638.

Birmaher, B., Axelson, D., Strober, M., Gill, M. K., Valeri, S., Chiappetta, L., et al. (2006). Clinical course of children and adolescents with bipolar spectrum disorders. *Archives of General Psychiatry, 63,* 175–183.

Birmaher, B., Ryan, N. D., Williamson, D. E., Brent, D. A., Kaufman, J., Dahl, R. E., et al. (1996). Childhood and adolescent depression: A review of the past 10 years. Part I. *Journal of the American Academy of Child and Adolescent Psychiatry, 35,* 1427–1439.

Blader, J. C., & Carlson, G. (2006, April). *BPD diagnosis among child and adolescent U.S. psychiatric inpatients, 1996–2003.* Paper presented at the NIMH Pediatric Bipolar Disorder Conference, Chicago.

Bossuyt, P. M., Reitsma, J. B., Bruns, D. E., Gatsonis, C. A., Glasziou, P. P., Irwig, L. M., et al. (2003). Towards complete and accurate reporting of studies of diagnostic accuracy: The STARD initiative. *British Medical Journal, 326,* 41–44.

Brent, D. A., Perper, J. A., Goldstein, C. E., Kolko, D. J., Allen, J., Allman, C. J., et al. (1988). Risk factors for adolescent suicide: A comparison of adolescent suicide victims with suicidal inpatients. *Archives of General Psychiatry, 45,* 581–588.

Calabrese, J. R., Shelton, M. D., Bowden, C. L., Rapport, D. J., Suppes, T., Shirley, E. R., et al. (2001). Bipolar rapid cycling: Focus on depression as its hallmark. *Journal of Clinical Psychiatry, 62*(Suppl. 14), 34–41.

Campbell, D. T., & Kenny, D. A. (1999). *A primer on regression artifacts.* New York: Guilford Press.

Carlson, G. A. (1998). Mania and ADHD: Comorbidity or confusion. *Journal of Affective Disorders, 51,* 177–187.

Carlson, G. A. (2002). Bipolar disorder in children and adolescents: A critical review. In D. Shaffer & B. Waslick (Eds.), *The many faces of depression in children and adolescents* (Vol. 21, pp. 105–128). Washington, DC: American Psychiatric Association.

Carlson, G. A. (2003). The bottom line. *Journal of Child and Adolescent Psychopharmacology, 13,* 115–118.

Carlson, G. A., & Mick, E. (2003). Drug induced disinhibition in psychiatrically hospitalized children. *Journal of Child and Adolescent Psychopharmacology, 13,* 153–163.

Carlson, G. A., & Youngstrom, E. A. (2003). Clinical

implications of pervasive manic symptoms in children. *Biological Psychiatry, 53,* 1050–1058.

Carver, C. S., & White, T. L. (1994). Behavioral inhibition, behavioral activation, and affective responses to impending reward and punishment: The BIS/BAS Scales. *Journal of Personality and Social Psychology, 67,* 319–333.

Chambless, D. L., & Hollon, S. D. (1998). Defining empirically supported therapies. *Journal of Consulting and Clinical Psychology, 66,* 7–18.

Chang, K. D., Blasey, C. M., Ketter, T. A., & Steiner, H. (2003). Temperament characteristics of child and adolescent bipolar offspring. *Journal of Affective Disorders, 77,* 11–19.

Chang, K. D., Steiner, H., Dienes, K., Adleman, N., & Ketter, T. (2003). Bipolar offspring: A window into bipolar disorder evolution. *Biological Psychiatry, 53,* 945–951.

Chorpita, B. F. (2002). The tripartite model and dimensions of anxiety and depression: An examination of structure in a large school sample. *Journal of Abnormal Child Psychology, 30,* 177–190.

Chorpita, B. F., Albano, A. M., & Barlow, D. H. (1998). The structure of negative emotions in a clinical sample of children and adolescents. *Journal of Abnormal Psychology, 107,* 74–85.

Chorpita, B. F., & Daleiden, E. L. (2002). Tripartite dimensions of emotion in a child clinical sample: Measurement strategies and implications for clinical utility. *Journal of Consulting and Clinical Psychology, 70,* 1150–1160.

Cooperberg, M. (2001). *Clinically significant change for outcome measures used with pediatric bipolar disorders.* Unpublished doctoral dissertation, Case Western Reserve University, Cleveland, OH.

Coryell, W., Solomon, D., Turvey, C., Keller, M., Leon, A. C., Endicott, J., et al. (2003). The long-term course of rapid-cycling bipolar disorder. *Archives of General Psychiatry, 60,* 914–920.

Costello, E. J., Angold, A., Burns, B. J., Stangl, D. K., Tweed, D. L., Erkanli, A., et al. (1996). The Great Smoky Mountains Study of Youth: Goals, design, methods, and the prevalence of DSM-III-R disorders. *Archives of General Psychiatry, 53,* 1129–1136.

Cyranowski, J. M., Frank, E., Young, E., & Shear, K. (2000). Adolescent onset of the gender difference in lifetime rates of major depression. *Archives of General Psychiatry, 57,* 21–27.

Danielson, C. K., Feeny, N. C., Findling, R. L., & Youngstrom, E. A. (2004). Psychosocial treatment of bipolar disorders in adolescents: A proposed cognitive-behavioral intervention. *Cognitive and Behavioral Practice, 11,* 283–297.

Danielson, C. K., Youngstrom, E. A., Findling, R. L., & Calabrese, J. R. (2003). Discriminative validity of the General Behavior Inventory using youth report. *Journal of Abnormal Child Psychology, 31,* 29–39.

Davidow, J., & Levinson, E. M. (1993). Heuristic principles and cognitive bias in decision making: Implica-

tions for assessment in school psychology. *Psychology in the Schools, 30,* 351–361.

DelBello, M. P., Lopez-Larson, M. P., Soutullo, C. A., & Strakowski, S. M. (2001). Effects of race on psychiatric diagnosis of hospitalized adolescents: A retrospective chart review. *Journal of Child and Adolescent Psychopharmacology, 11,* 95–103.

DelBello, M. P., Soutullo, C. A., Hendricks, W., Niemeier, R. T., McElroy, S. L., & Strakowski, S. M. (2001). Prior stimulant treatment in adolescents with bipolar disorder: Association with age at onset. *Bipolar Disorders, 3,* 53–57.

DelBello, M. P., Soutullo, C. A., & Strakowski, S. M. (2000). Racial differences in treatment of adolescents with bipolar disorder. *American Journal of Psychiatry, 157,* 837–838.

Dell'Osso, L., Pini, S., Cassano, G. B., Mastrocinque, C., Seckinger, R. A., Saettoni, M., et al. (2002). Insight into illness in patients with mania, mixed mania, bipolar depression and major depression with psychotic features. *Bipolar Disorders, 4,* 315–322.

Denicoff, K. D., Smith-Jackson, E. E., Disney, E. R., Suddath, R. L., Leverich, G. S., & Post, R. M. (1997). Preliminary evidence of the reliability and validity of the prospective life-chart methodology (LCM-p). *Journal of Psychiatric Research, 31,* 593–603.

Depue, R. A., & Collins, P. F. (1999). Neurobiology of the structure of personality: Dopamine, facilitation of incentive motivation, and extraversion. *Behavioral and Brain Sciences, 22,* 491–569.

Depue, R. A., & Iacono, W. G. (1989). Neurobehavioral aspects of affective disorders. *Annual Review of Psychology, 40,* 457–492.

Depue, R. A., Krauss, S., Spoont, M. R., & Arbisi, P. (1989). General Behavior Inventory identification of unipolar and bipolar affective conditions in a nonclinical university population. *Journal of Abnormal Psychology, 98,* 117–126.

Depue, R. A., Slater, J. F., Wolfstetter-Kausch, H., Klein, D. N., Goplerud, E., & Farr, D. A. (1981). A behavioral paradigm for identifying persons at risk for bipolar depressive disorder: A conceptual framework and five validation studies. *Journal of Abnormal Psychology, 90,* 381–437.

Dickstein, D. P., Garvey, M., Pradella, A. G., Greenstein, D. K., Sharp, W. S., Castellanos, F. X., et al. (2005). Neurologic examination abnormalities in children with bipolar disorder or attention-deficit/hyperactivity disorder. *Biological Psychiatry, 58,* 517–524.

Dickstein, D. P., Treland, J., Snow, J., McClure, E. B., Mehta, M., Towbin, K. E., et al. (2004). Neuropsychological performance in pediatric bipolar disorder. *Biological Psychiatry, 55,* 32–39.

Duax, J., Scovil, K., Youngstrom, E. A., Bhatnagar, K. C., Williams, F., Calabrese, J. R., et al. (2005, June). *Effects of sex on rates of bipolar spectrum disorder and presenting mood state in youth ages 5–17.* Paper presented at the biennial meeting of the International Society for Bipolar Disorders, Pittsburgh, PA.

Duffy, A., Alda, M., Kutcher, S., Fusee, C., & Grof, P. (1998). Psychiatric symptoms and syndromes among adolescent children of parents with lithium-responsive or lithium-nonresponsive bipolar disorder. *American Journal of Psychiatry, 155,* 431–433.

Duffy, A., Alda, M., Kutcher, S., Cavazzoni, P., Robertson, C., Grof, E., et al. (2002). A prospective study of the offspring of bipolar parents responsive and nonresponsive to lithium treatment. *Journal of Clinical Psychiatry, 63,* 1171–1178.

Dunner, D. L., Patrick, V., & Fieve, R. R. (1977). Rapid cycling manic depressive patients. *Comprehensive Psychiatry, 18,* 561–566.

Egeland, J. A., Hostetter, A. M., Pauls, D. L., & Sussex, J. N. (2000). Prodromal symptoms before onset of manic–depressive disorder suggested by first hospital admission histories. *Journal of the American Academy of Child and Adolescent Psychiatry, 39,* 1245–1252.

Faedda, G. L., Baldessarini, R. J., Glovinsky, I. P., & Austin, N. B. (2004). Pediatric bipolar disorder: Phenomenology and course of illness. *Bipolar Disorders, 6,* 305–313.

Faraone, S. V., Biederman, J., Mennin, D., Wozniak, J., & Spencer, T. (1997). Attention-deficit hyperactivity disorder with bipolar disorder: A familial subtype? *Journal of the American Academy of Child and Adolescent Psychiatry, 36,* 1378–1387.

Faraone, S. V., Glatt, S. J., Su, J., & Tsuang, M. T. (2004). Three potential susceptibility loci shown by a genome-wide scan for regions influencing the age at onset of mania. *American Journal of Psychiatry, 161,* 625–630.

Faraone, S. V., Glatt, S. J., & Tsuang, M. T. (2003). The genetics of pediatric-onset bipolar disorder. *Biological Psychiatry, 53,* 970–977.

Faraone, S. V., Tsuang, M. T., & Tsuang, D. W. (1999). *Genetics of mental disorders: What practitioners and students need to know.* New York: Guilford Press.

Feeny, N. C., Danielson, C. K., Schwartz, L., Youngstrom, E. A., & Findling, R. L. (2006). CBT for bipolar disorders in adolescence: A pilot study. *Bipolar Disorders, 8,* 508–515.

Findling, R. L., Feeny, N. C., Stansbrey, R. J., DelPorto-Bedoya, D., & Demeter, C. (2004). Somatic treatment for depressive illnesses in children and adolescents. *Psychiatric Clinics of North America, 27,* 113–137.

Findling, R. L., Gracious, B. L., McNamara, N. K., Youngstrom, E. A., Demeter, C., & Calabrese, J. R. (2001). Rapid, continuous cycling and psychiatric co-morbidity in pediatric bipolar I disorder. *Bipolar Disorders, 3,* 202–210.

Findling, R. L., Kowatch, R. A., & Post, R. M. (2003). *Pediatric bipolar disorder: A handbook for clinicians.* London: Martin Dunitz.

Findling, R. L., McNamara, N. K., Youngstrom, E. A.,

Stansbrey, R., Gracious, B. L., Reed, M. D., et al. (2005). Double-blind 18-month trial of lithium versus divalproex maintenance treatment in pediatric bipolar disorder. *Journal of the American Academy of Child and Adolescent Psychiatry, 44,* 409–417.

Findling, R. L., Youngstrom, E. A., Danielson, C. K., DelPorto, D., Papish-David, R., Townsend, L., et al. (2002). Clinical decision-making using the General Behavior Inventory in juvenile bipolarity. *Bipolar Disorders, 4,* 34–42.

Findling, R. L., Youngstrom, E. A., McNamara, N. K., Stansbrey, R. J., Demeter, C. A., Bedoya, D., et al. (2005). Early symptoms of mania and the role of parental risk. *Bipolar Disorders, 7,* 623–634.

Fowles, D. C. (1994). A motivational theory of psychopathology. In W. D. Spaulding (Ed.), *Integrative views of motivation, cognition, and emotion* (Vol. 41, pp. 181–238). Lincoln: University of Nebraska Press.

Frank, E., Prien, R. F., Jarrett, R. B., Keller, M. B., Kupfer, D. J., Lavori, P. W., et al. (1991). Conceptualization and rationale for consensus definitions of terms in major depressive disorder. Remission, recovery, relapse, and recurrence. *Archives of General Psychiatry, 48,* 851–855.

Fristad, M. A., Cummins, J., Verducci, J. S., Teare, M., Weller, E., & Weller, R. A. (1998). Study IV: Concurrent validity of the DSM-IV revised Children's Interview for Psychiatric Syndromes (ChIPS). *Journal of Child and Adolescent Psychopharmacology, 8,* 227–236.

Fristad, M. A., Gavazzi, S. M., & Mackinaw-Koons, B. (2003). Family psychoeducation: An adjunctive intervention for children with bipolar disorder. *Biological Psychiatry, 53,* 1000–1008.

Fristad, M. A., Glickman, A. R., Verducci, J. S., Teare, M., Weller, E. B., & Weller, R. A. (1998). Study V: Children's Interview for Psychiatric Syndromes (ChIPS): Psychometrics in two community samples. *Journal of Child and Adolescent Psychopharmacology, 8,* 237–245.

Fristad, M. A., Goldberg Arnold, J. S., & Gavazzi, S. M. (2003). Multi-family psychoeducation groups in the treatment of children with mood disorders. *Journal of Marital and Family Therapy, 29,* 491–504.

Fristad, M. A., & Goldberg Arnold, J. S. (2004). *Raising a moody child: How to cope with depression and bipolar disorder.* New York: Guilford Press.

Fristad, M. A., Weller, E. B., & Weller, R. A. (1992). The Mania Rating Scale: Can it be used in children?: A preliminary report. *Journal of the American Academy of Child and Adolescent Psychiatry, 31,* 252–257.

Fristad, M. A., Weller, R. A., & Weller, E. B. (1995). The Mania Rating Scale (MRS): Further reliability and validity studies with children. *Annals of Clinical Psychiatry, 7,* 127–132.

Gadow, K. D., & Sprafkin, J. (1994). *Child Symptom Inventories manual.* Stony Brook, NY: Checkmate Plus.

Gadow, K. D., & Sprafkin, J. (1997). *Adolescent Symptom Inventory: Screening manual*. Stony Brook, NY: Checkmate Plus.

Gadow, K. D., & Sprafkin, J. (1999). *Youth's Inventory–4 manual*. Stony Brook, NY: Checkmate Plus.

Galanter, C., Carlson, G., Jensen, P., Greenhill, L., Davies, M., Li, W., et al. (2003). Response to methylphenidate in children with attention deficit hyperactivity disorder and manic symptoms in the Multimodal Treatment Study of Children with Attention Deficit Hyperactivity Disorder titration trial. *Journal of Child and Adolescent Psychopharmacology, 13*, 123–136.

Garb, H. N. (1998). *Studying the clinician: Judgment research and psychological assessment*. Washington, DC: American Psychological Association.

Geller, B., Bolhofner, K., Craney, J. L., Williams, M., DelBello, M. P., & Gundersen, K. (2000). Psychosocial functioning in a prepubertal and early adolescent bipolar disorder phenotype. *Journal of the American Academy of Child and Adolescent Psychiatry, 39*, 1543–1548.

Geller, B., & Cook, E. H., Jr. (2000). Ultradian rapid cycling in prepubertal and early adolescent bipolarity is not in transmission disequilibrium with val/met COMT alleles. *Biological Psychiatry, 47*, 605–609.

Geller, B., Craney, J. L., Bolhofner, K., DelBello, M. P., Axelson, D., Luby, J., et al. (2003). Phenomenology and longitudinal course of children with a prepubertal and early adolescent bipolar disorder phenotype. In B. Geller & M. P. DelBello (Eds.), *Bipolar disorder in childhood and early adolescence* (pp. 25–50). New York: Guilford Press.

Geller, B., Craney, J. L., Bolhofner, K., DelBello, M. P., Williams, M., & Zimerman, B. (2001). One-year recovery and relapse rates of children with a prepubertal and early adolescent bipolar disorder phenotype. *American Journal of Psychiatry, 158*, 303–305.

Geller, B., Craney, J. L., Bolhofner, K., Nickelsburg, M. J., Williams, M., & Zimerman, B. (2002). Two-year prospective follow-up of children with a prepubertal and early adolescent bipolar disorder phenotype. *American Journal of Psychiatry, 159*, 927–933.

Geller, B., Fox, L. W., & Fletcher, M. (1993). Effect of tricyclic antidepressants on switching to mania and on the onset of bipolarity in depressed 6- to 12-year-olds. *Journal of the American Academy of Child and Adolescent Psychiatry, 32*, 43–50.

Geller, B., & Luby, J. (1997). Child and adolescent bipolar disorder: A review of the past 10 years. *Journal of the American Academy of Child and Adolescent Psychiatry, 36*, 1168–1176.

Geller, B., Sun, K., Zimerman, B., Luby, J., Frazier, J., & Williams, M. (1995). Complex and rapid-cycling in bipolar children and adolescents: A preliminary study. *Journal of Affective Disorders, 34*, 259–268.

Geller, B., Tillman, R., Craney, J. L., & Bolhofner, K.

(2004). Four-year prospective outcome and natural history of mania in children with a prepubertal and early adolescent bipolar disorder phenotype. *Archives of General Psychiatry, 61*, 459–467.

Geller, B., Warner, K., Williams, M., & Zimerman, B. (1998). Prepubertal and young adolescent bipolarity versus ADHD: Assessment and validity using the WASH-U-KSADS, CBCL and TRF. *Journal of Affective Disorders, 51*, 93–100.

Geller, B., Williams, M., Zimerman, B., Frazier, J., Beringer, L., & Warner, K. L. (1998). Prepubertal and early adolescent bipolarity differentiate from ADHD by manic symptoms, grandiose delusions, ultra-rapid or ultradian cycling. *Journal of Affective Disorders, 51*, 81–91.

Geller, B., Zimerman, B., Williams, M., Bolhofner, K., Craney, J. L., DelBello, M. P., et al. (2001). Reliability of the Washington University in St. Louis Kiddie Schedule for Affective Disorders and Schizophrenia (WASH-U-KSADS) mania and rapid cycling sections. *Journal of the American Academy of Child and Adolescent Psychiatry, 40*, 450–455.

Geller, B., Zimerman, B., Williams, M., DelBello, M. P., Bolhofner, K., Craney, J. L., et al. (2002). DSM-IV mania symptoms in a prepubertal and early adolescent bipolar disorder phenotype compared to attention-deficit hyperactive and normal controls. *Journal of Child and Adolescent Psychopharmacology, 12*, 11–25.

Geller, B., Zimerman, B., Williams, M., DelBello, M. P., Frazier, J., & Beringer, L. (2002). Phenomenology of prepubertal and early adolescent bipolar disorder: Examples of elated mood, grandiose behaviors, decreased need for sleep, racing thoughts and hypersexuality. *Journal of Child and Adolescent Psychopharmacology, 12*, 3–9.

Ghaemi, S. N., Hsu, D. J., Soldani, F., & Goodwin, F. K. (2003). Antidepressants in bipolar disorder: The case for caution. *Bipolar Disorders, 5*, 421–433.

Ghaemi, S. N., Ko, J. Y., & Goodwin, F. K. (2002). "Cade's disease" and beyond: Misdiagnosis, antidepressant use, and a proposed definition for bipolar spectrum disorder. *Canadian Journal of Psychiatry, 47*, 125–134.

Glovinsky, I. (2002). A brief history of childhood-onset bipolar disorder through 1980. *Child and Adolescent Psychiatric Clinics of North America, 11*, 443–460.

Goodwin, F. K., & Jamison, K. R. (1990). *Manic–depressive illness*. New York: Oxford University Press.

Gracious, B. L., Youngstrom, E. A., Findling, R. L., & Calabrese, J. R. (2002). Discriminative validity of a parent version of the Young Mania Rating Scale. *Journal of the American Academy of Child and Adolescent Psychiatry, 41*, 1350–1359.

Gray, J. A., & McNaughton, N. (1996). The neuropsychology of anxiety: Reprise. In D. A. Hope (Ed.), *Perspectives in anxiety, panic and fear* (Vol. 43, pp. 61–134). Lincoln: University of Nebraska Press.

Guyatt, G. H., & Rennie, D. (Eds.). (2002). *Users'*

guides to the medical literature. Chicago: American Medical Association Press.

Hack, M., Youngstrom, E. A., Cartar, L., Schluchter, M., Gerry, T. H., Flannery, D., et al. (2004). Behavioral outcomes and evidence of psychopathology among very low birth weight infants at age 20 years. *Pediatrics, 114*, 932–940.

Hanley, J. A., & McNeil, B. J. (1983). A method of comparing the areas under receiver operating characteristic curves derived from the same cases. *Radiology, 148*, 839–843.

Harding, I.. (2001). Children's quality of life assessments: A review of generic and health related quality of life measures completed by children and adolescents. *Clinical Psychology and Psychotherapy, 8*, 79–96.

Hare, R. D. (1991). *Manual for the Psychopathy Checklist—Revised*. Toronto: Multi-Health Systems.

Harrington, R., & Myatt, T. (2003). Is preadolescent mania the same condition as adult mania?: A British perspective. *Biological Psychiatry, 53*, 961–969.

Hartung, C. M., & Widiger, T. A. (1998). Gender differences in the diagnosis of mental disorders: Conclusions and controversies of the DSM-IV. *Psychological Bulletin, 123*, 260–278.

Hazell, P. L., Carr, V., Lewin, T. J., & Sly, K. (2003). Manic symptoms in young males with ADHD predict functioning but not diagnosis after 6 years. *Journal of the American Academy of Child and Adolescent Psychiatry, 42*, 552–560.

Hazell, P. L., Lewin, T. J., & Carr, V. J. (1999). Confirmation that Child Behavior Checklist clinical scales discriminate juvenile mania from attention deficit hyperactivity disorder. *Journal of Paediatrics and Child Health, 35*, 199–203.

Healy, D. (2006). The latest mania: Selling bipolar disorder. *PLoS Medicine, 3*, e185.

Hellander, M. (2002). *Lithium testing in children: A public health necessity* [Testimony]. Washington, DC: U.S. Food and Drug Administration.

Henin, A., Mick, E., Nierenberg, A. A., & Biederman, J. (2006, April). *Neuropsychological performance in youths with bipolar disorder*. Paper presented at the NIMH Pediatric Bipolar Disorder Conference, Chicago.

Hirschfeld, R. M., Lewis, L., & Vornik, L. A. (2003). Perceptions and impact of bipolar disorder: How far have we really come?: Results of the National Depressive and Manic–Depressive Association 2000 survey of individuals with bipolar disorder. *Journal of Clinical Psychiatry, 64*, 161–174.

Hirschfeld, R. M., Williams, J. B., Spitzer, R. L., Calabrese, J. R., Flynn, L., Keck, P. E., Jr., et al. (2000). Development and validation of a screening instrument for bipolar spectrum disorder: The Mood Disorder Questionnaire. *American Journal of Psychiatry, 157*, 1873–1875.

Hodgins, S., Faucher, B., Zarac, A., & Ellenbogen, M. (2002). Children of parents with bipolar disorder. A population at high risk for major affective disorders.

Child and Adolescent Psychiatric Clinics of North America, 11, 533–553.

Hudziak, J. J., Althoff, R. R., Derks, E. M., Faraone, S. V., & Boomsma, D. I. (2005). Prevalence and genetic architecture of Child Behavior Checklist–juvenile bipolar disorder. *Biological Psychiatry, 58*, 562–568.

Isometsa, E., Suominen, K., Mantere, O., Valtonen, H., Leppamaki, S., Pippingskold, M., et al. (2003). The mood disorder questionnaire improves recognition of bipolar disorder in psychiatric care. *BMC Psychiatry 3*, 8.

Jacobson, N. S., Roberts, L. J., Berns, S. B., & McGlinchey, J. B. (1999). Methods for defining and determining the clinical significance of treatment effects: Description, application, and alternatives. *Journal of Consulting and Clinical Psychology, 67*, 300–307.

Jacobson, N. S., & Truax, P. (1991). Clinical significance: A statistical approach to defining meaningful change in psychotherapy research. *Journal of Consulting and Clinical Psychology, 59*, 12–19.

Jaeschke, R., Guyatt, G. H., & Sackett, D. L. (1994a). Users' guides to the medical literature: III. How to use an article about a diagnostic test: A. Are the results of the study valid? *Journal of the American Medical Association, 271*(5), 389–391.

Jaeschke, R., Guyatt, G. H., & Sackett, D. L. (1994b). Users' guides to the medical literature: III. How to use an article about a diagnostic test: B. What are the results and will they help me in caring for my patients? *Journal of the American Medical Association, 271*(9), 703–707.

Jamison, K. R. (1995). *An unquiet mind: A memoir of moods and madness*. New York: Vintage Books.

Johnson, S. L., & Roberts, J. E. (1995). Life events and bipolar disorder: Implications from biological theories. *Psychological Bulletin, 117*, 434–449.

Judd, L. L., & Akiskal, H. S. (2003). The prevalence and disability of bipolar spectrum disorders in the US population: Re-analysis of the ECA database taking into account subthreshold cases. *Journal of Affective Disorders, 73*, 123–131.

Judd, L. L., Akiskal, H. S., Schettler, P. J., Endicott, J., Leon, A. C., Solomon, D., et al. (2005). Psychosocial disability in the course of bipolar I and II disorders: A prospective, comparative, longitudinal study. *Archives of General Psychiatry, 62*, 1322–1330.

Juul, A., Teilmann, G., Scheike, T., Hertel, N. T., Holm, K., Laursen, E. M., et al. (2006). Pubertal development in Danish children: Comparison of recent European and US data. *International Journal of Andrology, 29*, 247–255; discussion, 286–290.

Kahana, S. Y., Youngstrom, E. A., Calabrese, J. R., & Findling, R. L. (under review). A three-year follow-up of youth initially diagnosed with subsyndromal bipolar disorder.

Kahana, S. Y., Youngstrom, E. A., Findling, R. L., & Calabrese, J. R. (2003). Employing parent, teacher, and youth self-report checklists in identifying pediatric bipolar spectrum disorders: An examination of diagnostic accuracy and clinical utility. *Journal of Child and Adolescent Psychopharmacology, 13,* 471–488.

Karlberg, J. (2002). Secular trends in pubertal development. *Hormone Research, 57*(Suppl. 2), 19–30.

Kaufman, J., Birmaher, B., Brent, D., Rao, U., Flynn, C., Moreci, P., et al. (1997). Schedule for Affective Disorders and Schizophrenia for School-Age Children—Present and Lifetime version (K-SADS-PL): Initial reliability and validity data. *Journal of the American Academy of Child and Adolescent Psychiatry, 36,* 980–988.

Kawa, I., Carter, J. D., Joyce, P. R., Doughty, C. J., Frampton, C. M., Wells, J. E., et al. (2005). Gender differences in bipolar disorder: Age of onset, course, comorbidity, and symptom presentation. *Bipolar Disorders, 7,* 119–125.

Kazdin, A. E. (1977). Assessing the clinical or applied importance of behavior change through social validation. *Behavior Modification, 1,* 427–452.

Kessler, R. C. (1998). Sex differences in DSM-III-R psychiatric disorders in the United States: Results from the National Comorbidity Survey. *Journal of American Medical Women's Association, 53,* 148–158.

Kessler, R. C. (1999). Comorbidity of unipolar and bipolar depression with other psychiatric disorders in a general population survey. In M. Tohen (Ed.), *Comorbidity in affective disorders* (pp. 1–25). New York: Marcel Dekker.

Kessler, R. C., Avenevoli, S., & Merikangas, K. R. (2001). Mood disorders in children and adolescents: An epidemiologic perspective. *Biological Psychiatry, 49,* 1002–1014.

Kessler, R. C., Berglund, P., Demler, O., Jin, R., & Walters, E. E. (2005). Lifetime prevalence and age-of-onset distributions of DSM-IV disorders in the National Comorbidity Survey Replication. *Archives of General Psychiatry, 62,* 593–602.

Kessler, R. C., Rubinow, D. R., Holmes, C., Abelson, J. M., & Zhao, S. (1997). The epidemiology of DSM-III-R bipolar I disorder in a general population survey. *Psychological Medicine, 27,* 1079–1089.

Klein, R. G., Pine, D. S., & Klein, D. F. (1998). Resolved: Mania is mistaken for ADHD in prepubertal children. *Journal of the American Academy of Child and Adolescent Psychiatry, 37,* 1093–1096.

Kluger, J., & Song, S. (2002, August 19). Young and bipolar. *Time,* pp. 39–47, 51.

Kovacs, M. (1989). Affective disorders in children and adolescents: Children and their development: Knowledge base, research agenda, and social policy application [Special issue]. *American Psychologist, 44,* 209–215.

Kovacs, M. (1996). Presentation and course of major depressive disorder during childhood and later years of the life span. *Journal of the American Academy of Child and Adolescent Psychiatry, 35,* 705–715.

Kowatch, R. A., Fristad, M. A., Birmaher, B., Wagner, K. D., Findling, R. L., & Hellander, M. (2005). Treatment guidelines for children and adolescents with bipolar disorder. *Journal of the American Academy of Child and Adolescent Psychiatry, 44,* 213–235.

Kowatch, R. A., Youngstrom, E. A., Danielyan, A., & Findling, R. L. (2005). Review and meta-analysis of the phenomenology and clinical characteristics of mania in children and adolescents. *Bipolar Disorders, 7,* 483–496.

Kraemer, H. C. (1992). *Evaluating medical tests: Objective and quantitative guidelines.* Newbury Park, CA: Sage.

Kraepelin, É. (1921). *Manic–depressive insanity and paranoia.* Edinburgh, UK: Livingstone.

Kramlinger, K. G., & Post, R. M. (1996). Ultra-rapid and ultradian cycling in bipolar affective illness. *British Journal of Psychiatry, 168,* 314–323.

Lee, P. A., Guo, S. S., & Kulin, H. E. (2001). Age of puberty: Data from the United States of America. *APMIS, 109,* 81–88.

Leibenluft, E., Charney, D. S., Towbin, K. E., Bhangoo, R. K., & Pine, D. S. (2003). Defining clinical phenotypes of juvenile mania. *American Journal of Psychiatry, 160,* 430–437.

Leibenluft, E., Cohen, P., Gorrindo, T., Brook, J. S., & Pine, D. S. (2006). Chronic versus episodic irritability in youth: A community-based, longitudinal study of clinical and diagnostic associations. *Journal of Child and Adolescent Psychopharmacology, 16,* 456–466.

Lengua, L. J., Sadowski, C. A., Friedrich, W. N., & Fisher, J. (2001). Rationally and empirically derived dimensions of children's symptomatology: Expert ratings and confirmatory factor analyses of the CBCL. *Journal of Consulting and Clinical Psychology, 69,* 683–698.

Lewinsohn, P. M., Klein, D. N., & Seeley, J. R. (1995). Bipolar disorders in a community sample of older adolescents: Prevalence, phenomenology, comorbidity, and course. *Journal of the American Academy of Child and Adolescent Psychiatry, 34,* 454–463.

Lewinsohn, P. M., Klein, D. N., & Seeley, J. (2000). Bipolar disorder during adolescence and young adulthood in a community sample. *Bipolar Disorders, 2,* 281–293.

Lewinsohn, P. M., Seeley, J. R., Buckley, M. E., & Klein, D. N. (2002). Bipolar disorder in adolescence and young adulthood. *Child and Adolescent Psychiatric Clinics of North America, 11,* 461–476.

Lewinsohn, P. M., Seeley, J. R., & Klein, D. N. (2003). Bipolar disorder in adolescents: Epidemiology and suicidal behavior. In B. Geller & M. P. DelBello (Eds.), *Bipolar disorder in childhood and early adolescence* (pp. 7–24). New York: Guilford Press.

Linehan, M. M. (1993). *Cognitive-behavioral treatment of borderline personality disorder.* New York: Guilford Press.

Lish, J. D., Dime-Meenan, S., Whybrow, P. C., Price, R. A., & Hirschfeld, R. M. (1994). The National Depressive and Manic–Depressive Association (DMDA) survey of bipolar members. *Journal of Affective Disorders, 31,* 281–294.

Loeber, R., Green, S. M., & Lahey, B. B. (1990). Mental health professionals' perception of the utility of children, mothers, and teachers as informants on childhood psychopathology. *Journal of Clinical Child Psychology, 19,* 136–143.

Lofthouse, N., & Fristad, M. (2004). Psychosocial interventions for children with early-onset bipolar spectrum disorder. *Clinical Child and Family Psychology Review, 21,* 71–89.

Lonigan, C. J., Phillips, B., & Hooe, E. (2003). Relations of positive and negative affectivity to anxiety and depression in children: Evidence from a latent variable longitudinal study. *Journal of Consulting and Clinical Psychology, 71,* 465–481.

Luby, J. L., & Mrakotsky, C. (2003). Depressed preschoolers with bipolar family history: A group at high risk for later switching to mania? *Journal of Child and Adolescent Psychopharmacology, 13,* 187–197.

Luby, J. L., Mrakotsky, C., Heffelfinger, A., Brown, K., Hessler, M., & Spitznagel, E. (2003). Modification of DSM-IV criteria for depressed preschool children. *American Journal of Psychiatry, 160,* 1169–1172.

Mackin, P., Targum, S. D., Kalali, A., Rom, D., & Young, A. H. (2006). Culture and assessment of manic symptoms. *British Journal of Psychiatry, 189,* 379–380.

MacKinnon, D. F., & Pies, R. (2006). Affective instability as rapid cycling: Theoretical and clinical implications for borderline personality and bipolar spectrum disorders. *Bipolar Disorders, 8,* 1–14.

MacKinnon, D. F., Zandi, P. P., Gershon, E., Nurnberger, J., Reich, T., & DePaulo, R. (2003). Rapid switching of mood in families with multiple cases of bipolar disorder. *Archives of General Psychiatry, 60,* 921–928.

Maj, M., Pirozzi, R., Formicola, A. M., & Tortorella, A. (1999). Reliability and validity of four alternative definitions of rapid-cycling bipolar disorder. *American Journal of Psychiatry, 156,* 1421–1424.

Masi, G., Perugi, G., Toni, C., Millepiedi, S., Mucci, M., Bertini, N., et al. (2006). The clinical phenotypes of juvenile bipolar disorder: Toward a validation of the episodic–chronic distinction. *Biological Psychiatry, 59,* 603–610.

McClellan, J. (2005). Commentary: Treatment guidelines for child and adolescent bipolar disorder. *Journal of the American Academy of Child and Adolescent Psychiatry, 44,* 236–239.

McGuffin, P., Rijsdijk, F., Andrew, M., Sham, P., Katz, R., & Cardno, A. (2003). The heritability of bipolar affective disorder and the genetic relationship to unipolar depression. *Archives of General Psychiatry, 60,* 497–502.

McMahon, R. J., & Frick, P. J. (2005). Evidence-based assessment of conduct problems in children and adolescents. *Journal of Clinical Child and Adolescent Psychiatry, 34,* 477–505.

Mick, E., Biederman, J., Pandina, G., & Faraone, S. V. (2003). A preliminary meta-analysis of the Child Behavior Checklist in pediatric bipolar disorder. *Biological Psychiatry, 53,* 1021–1027.

Miklowitz, D. J., George, E. L., Axelson, D. A., Kim, E. Y., Birmaher, B., Schneck, C., et al. (2004). Family-focused treatment for adolescents with bipolar disorder. *Journal of Affective Disorders, 82*(Suppl. 1), S113–S128.

Miller, C. J., Klugman, J., Berv, D. A., Rosenquist, K. J., & Ghaemi, S. N. (2004). Sensitivity and specificity of the Mood Disorder Questionnaire for detecting bipolar disorder. *Journal of Affective Disorders, 81,* 167–171.

Moffit, T. E., Caspi, A., Dickson, N., Silva, P., & Stanton, W. (1996). Childhood-onset versus adolescent-onset antisocial conduct problems in males: Natural history from ages 3 to 18 years. *Development and Psychopathology, 8,* 399–424.

Naylor, M. W., Anderson, T. R., Kruesi, M. J., & Stoewe, M. (2002, October). *Pharmacoepidemiology of bipolar disorder in abused and neglected state wards.* Poster presented at the National Meeting of the American Academy of Child and Adolescent Psychiatry, San Francisco.

Newman, C. F., Leahy, R. L., Beck, A. T., Reilly-Harrington, N. A., & Gyulai, L. (2002). *Bipolar disorder: A cognitive therapy approach.* Washington, DC: American Psychological Association.

Nierenberg, A. A., Miyahara, S., Spencer, T., Wisniewski, S. R., Otto, M. W., Simon, N., et al. (2005). Clinical and diagnostic implications of lifetime attention-deficit/hyperactivity disorder comorbidity in adults with bipolar disorder: Data from the first 1,000 STEP-BD participants. *Biological Psychiatry, 57,* 1467–1473.

Nottelmann, E., Biederman, J., Birmaher, B., Carlson, G. A., Chang, K. D., Fenton, W. S., et al. (2001). National Institute of Mental Health research roundtable on prepubertal bipolar disorder. *Journal of the American Academy of Child and Adolescent Psychiatry, 40,* 871–878.

Orvaschel, H. (1995). *Schizophrenia and Affective Disorders Schedule for Children—Epidemiological Version (KSADS-E).* Unpublished manuscript, Nova Southeastern University, Ft. Lauderdale, FL.

Papolos, D. F. (2003). Switching, cycling, and antidepressant-induced effects on cycle frequency and course of illness in adult bipolar disorder: A brief review and commentary. *Journal of Child and Adolescent Psychopharmacology, 13,* 165–171.

Papolos, D. F., Hennen, J., Cockerham, M. S., Thode, H. C., & Youngstrom, E. A. (2006). The Child Bipolar Questionnaire: A dimensional approach to screening for pediatric bipolar disorder. *Journal of Affective Disorders, 95,* 149–158.

Papolos, D. F., & Papolos, J. (2002). *The bipolar child: The definitive and reassuring guide to childhood's most misunderstood disorder* (2nd ed.). New York: Broadway Books.

Parent, A. S., Teilmann, G., Juul, A., Skakkebaek, N. E., Toppari, J., & Bourguignon, J. P. (2003). The timing of normal puberty and the age limits of sexual pre-cocity: Variations around the world, secular trends, and changes after migration. *Endocrine Reviews, 24,* 668–693.

Patterson, G. R., DeBaryshe, B. D., & Ramsey, E. (1989). A developmental perspective on antisocial behavior: Children and their development: Knowledge base, research agenda, and social policy application [Special Issue]. *American Psychologist, 44,* 329–335.

Pavuluri, M. N., Graczyk, P. A., Henry, D. B., Carbray, J. A., Heidenreich, J., & Miklowitz, D. J. (2004). Child- and family-focused cognitive-behavioral therapy for pediatric bipolar disorder: Development and preliminary results. *Journal of the American Academy of Child and Adolescent Psychiatry, 43,* 528–537.

Pavuluri, M. N., Henry, D. B., Devineni, B., Carbray, J. A., & Birmaher, B. (2006). Child Mania Rating Scale: Development, reliability, and validity. *Journal of the American Academy of Child and Adolescent Psychiatry, 45,* 550–560.

Pepe, M. S. (2003). *The statistical evaluation of medical tests for classification and prediction.* New York: Wiley.

Perlis, R., Miyahara, S., Marangell, L. B., Wisniewski, S. R., Ostacher, M., DelBello, M. P., et al. (2004). Long-term implications of early onset in bipolar disorder: Data from the first 1,000 participants in the Systematic Treatment Enhancement Program for Bipolar Disorder (STEP-BD). *Biological Psychiatry, 55,* 875–881.

Pini, S., Dell'Osso, L., & Amador, X. F. (2001). Insight into illness in schizophrenia, schizoaffective disorder, and mood disorders with psychotic features. *American Journal of Psychiatry, 158,* 122–125.

Pliszka, S. R., Sherman, J. O., Barrow, M. V., & Irick, S. (2000). Affective disorder in juvenile offenders: A preliminary study. *American Journal of Psychiatry, 157,* 130–132.

Popper, C. W. (1990). Diagnostic gore in children's nightmares. *American Academy of Child and Adolescent Psychiatry Newsletter, 17,* 3–4.

Post, R. M., Leverich, G., Luckenbaugh, D., Altshuler, L., Frye, M. A., Suppes, T., et al. (2006, April). *An excess of childhood-onset bipolar illness in the United States compared with Europe.* Paper presented at the NIMH Pediatric Bipolar Disorder Conference, Chicago.

Post, R. M., Leverich, G. S., Xing, G., & Weiss, S. R. B. (2001). Developmental vulnerabilities to the onset and course of bipolar disorder. *Development and Psychopathology, 13,* 581–598.

Post, R. M., Weiss, S. R. B., & Leverich, G. S. (1994). Recurrent affective disorder: Roots in developmental neurobiology and illness progression based on changes in gene expression: Neural plasticity, sensitive periods, and psychopathology [Special issue]. *Development and Psychopathology, 6,* 781–813.

Poznanski, E. O., Miller, E., Salguero, C., & Kelsh, R. C. (1984). Preliminary studies of the reliability and validity of the Children's Depression Rating Scale. *Journal of the American Academy of Child Psychiatry, 23,* 191–197.

Quinn, C. A., & Fristad, M. A. (2004). Defining and identifying early onset bipolar spectrum disorder. *Current Psychiatry Reports, 6,* 101–107.

Ravens-Sieberer, U., & Bullinger, M. (1998). Assessing health-related quality of life in chronically ill children with the German KINDL: First psychometric and content analytic results. *Quality of Life Research, 7,* 399–407.

Reichart, C. G., & Nolen, W. A. (2004). Earlier onset of bipolar disorder in children by antidepressants or stimulants?: An hypothesis. *Journal of Affective Disorders, 78,* 81–84.

Reichart, C. G., Wals, M., Hillegers, M. H., Ormel, J., Nolen, W. A., & Verhulst, F. C. (2004). Psychopathology in the adolescent offspring of bipolar parents. *Journal of Affective Disorders, 78,* 67–71.

Rich, B. A., Bhangoo, R. K., Vinton, D. T., Berghorst, L. H., Dickstein, D. P., Grillon, C., et al. (2005). Using affect-modulated startle to study phenotypes of pediatric bipolar disorder. *Bipolar Disorders, 7,* 536–545.

Rich, B. A., Schmajuk, M., Perez-Edgar, K. E., Pine, D. S., Fox, N. A., & Leibenluft, E. (2005). The impact of reward, punishment, and frustration on attention in pediatric bipolar disorder. *Biological Psychiatry, 58,* 532–539.

Richters, J. E. (1992). Depressed mothers as informants about their children: A critical review of the evidence for distortion. *Psychological Bulletin, 112,* 485–499.

Rihmer, Z., & Kiss, K. (2002). Bipolar disorders and suicidal behaviour. *Bipolar Disorders, 4,* 21–25.

Robb, J. C., Young, L. T., Cooke, R. G., & Joffe, R. T. (1998). Gender differences in patients with bipolar disorder influence outcome in the Medical Outcomes Survey (SF-20) subscale scores. *Journal of Affective Disorders, 49,* 189–193.

Rowe, R., Maughan, B., Worthman, C. M., Costello, E. J., & Angold, A. (2004). Testosterone, antisocial behavior, and social dominance in boys: Pubertal development and biosocial interaction. *Biological Psychiatry, 55,* 546–552.

Sachs, G. S. (2004). Strategies for improving treatment of bipolar disorder: Integration of measurement and management. *Acta Psychiatrica Scandinavica: Supplementum,* 7–17.

Sachs, G. S., Guille, C., & McMurrich, S. L. (2002). A clinical monitoring form for mood disorders. *Bipolar Disorders, 4,* 323–327.

Sackett, D. L., Straus, S. E., Richardson, W. S., Rosenberg, W., & Haynes, R. B. (2000). *Evidence-based medicine: How to practice and teach EBM* (2nd ed.). New York: Churchill Livingstone.

Scheffer, R. E., Kowatch, R. A., Carmody, T., & Rush, A. J. (2005). Randomized, placebo-controlled trial of mixed amphetamine salts for symptoms of comorbid ADHD in pediatric bipolar disorder after mood stabilization with divalproex sodium. *American Journal of Psychiatry, 162*, 58–64.

Scott, J., & Colom, F. (2005). Psychosocial treatments for bipolar disorders. *Psychiatric Clinics of North America, 28*, 371–384.

Shaffer, D., Fisher, P., Dulcan, M. K., Davies, M., Piacentini, J., Schwab-Stone, M. E., et al. (1996). The NIMH Diagnostic Interview Schedule for Children Version 2.3 (DISC-2.3): Description, acceptability, prevalence rates, and performance in the MECA study. *Journal of the American Academy of Child and Adolescent Psychiatry, 35*, 865–877.

Shaw, J. A., Egeland, J. A., Endicott, J., Allen, C. R., & Hostetter, A. M. (2005). A 10-year prospective study of prodromal patterns for bipolar disorder among Amish youth. *Journal of American Academy of Child and Adolescent Psychiatry, 44*, 1104–1111.

Sheehan, D. V., Lecrubier, Y., Sheehan, K. H., Amorim, P., Janavs, J., Weiller, E., et al. (1998). The Mini-International Neuropsychiatric Interview (M.I.N.I.): The development and validation of a structured diagnostic psychiatric interview for DSM-IV and ICD-10. *Journal of Clinical Psychiatry, 59*(Suppl. 20), 22–33; quiz, 34–57.

Soto, O., & Murphy, T. K. (2003). The immune system and bipolar affective disorder. In B. Geller & M. P. DelBello (Eds.), *Bipolar disorder in childhood and early adolescence* (pp. 193–214). New York: Guilford Press.

Soutullo, C. A., Chang, K. D., Diez-Suarez, A., Figueroa-Quintana, A., Escamilla-Canales, I., Rapado-Castro, M., et al. (2005). Bipolar disorder in children and adolescents: International perspective on epidemiology and phenomenology. *Bipolar Disorders, 7*, 497–506.

Stoll, A. L., Locke, C. A., Marangell, L. B., & Severus, W. E. (1999). Omega-3 fatty acids and bipolar disorder: A review. *Prostaglandins Leukotrines, and Essential Fatty Acids, 60*, 329–337.

Swets, J. A., Dawes, R. M., & Monahan, J. (2000). Psychological science can improve diagnostic decisions. *Psychological Science in the Public Interest, 1*, 1–26.

Tellegen, A., Watson, D., & Clark, L. A. (1999). On the dimensional and hierarchical structure of affect. *Psychological Science, 10*, 297–303.

Teplin, L. A., Abram, K. M., McClelland, G. M., Dulcan, M. K., & Mericle, A. A. (2002). Psychiatric disorders in youth in juvenile detention. *Archives of General Psychiatry, 59*, 1133–1143.

Thayer, R. E. (1996). *The origin of everyday moods: Managing energy, tension, and stress.* New York: Oxford University Press.

Thuppal, M., Carlson, G. A., Sprafkin, J., & Gadow, K. D. (2002). Correspondence between adolescent report, parent report, and teacher report of manic symptoms. *Journal of Child and Adolescent Psychopharmacology, 12*, 27–35.

Tillman, R., & Geller, B. (2005). A brief screening tool for a prepubertal and early adolescent bipolar disorder phenotype. *American Journal of Psychiatry, 162*, 1214–1216.

Tillman, R., Geller, B., Craney, J. L., Bolhofner, K., Williams, M., & Zimerman, B. (2004). Relationship of parent and child informants to prevalence of mania symptoms in children with a prepubertal and early adolescent bipolar disorder phenotype. *American Journal of Psychiatry, 161*, 1278–1284.

Tillman, R., Geller, B., Craney, J. L., Bolhofner, K., Williams, M., Zimerman, B., et al. (2003). Temperament and character factors in a prepubertal and early adolescent bipolar disorder phenotype compared to attention deficit hyperactive and normal controls. *Journal of Child and Adolescent Psychopharmacology, 13*, 531–543.

Tramontina, S., Schmitz, M., Polanczyk, G., & Rohde, L. A. (2003). Juvenile bipolar disorder in Brazil: Clinical and treatment findings. *Biological Psychiatry, 53*, 1043–1049.

Tsuchiya, K. J., Byrne, M., & Mortensen, P. B. (2003). Risk factors in relation to an emergence of bipolar disorder: A systematic review. *Bipolar Disorders, 5*, 231–242.

Tumuluru, R. V., Weller, E. B., Fristad, M. A., & Weller, R. A. (2003). Mania in six preschool children. *Journal of Child and Adolescent Psychopharmacology, 13*, 489–494.

Varni, J. W., Seid, M., & Rode, C. A. (1999). The PedsQL: Measurement model for the pediatric quality of life inventory. *Medical Care, 37*, 126–139.

Volk, H. (2006, April). *The CBCL bipolar profile is not looking bipolar.* Paper presented at the NIMH Pediatric Bipolar Disorder Conference, Chicago.

Wagner, K. D., Findling, R. L., Emslie, G. J., Gracious, B., & Reed, M. (2006). Validation of the Mood Disorder Questionnaire for bipolar disorders in adolescents. *Journal of Clinical Psychiatry, 67*, 827–830.

Wakefield, J. C. (1997). When is development disordered?: Developmental psychopathology and the harmful dysfunction analysis of mental disorder. *Development and Psychopathology, 9*, 269–290.

Watson, D., Clark, L. A., Weber, K., Assenheimer, J. S., Strauss, M. E., & McCormick, R. A. (1995). Testing a tripartite model: II. Exploring the symptom structure of anxiety and depression in student, adult, and patient samples. *Journal of Abnormal Psychology, 104*, 15–25.

Weckerly, J. (2002). Pediatric bipolar mood disorder. *Journal of Developmental and Behavioral Pediatrics, 23*, 42–56.

Weissman, M. M., Bland, R. C., Canino, G. J., Faravelli, C., Greenwald, S., Hwu, H.-G., et al. (1996). Cross-national epidemiology of major depression and bipolar disorder. *Journal of the American Medical Association, 276*(4), 293–299.

Weissman, M. M., Wickramaratne, P., Merikangas, K.

R., Leckman, J. F., Prusoff, B. A., Caruso, K. A., et al. (1984). Onset of major depression in early adulthood: Increased familial loading and specificity. *Archives of General Psychiatry, 41*, 1136–1143.

Weller, E. B., Weller, R. A., Fristad, M. A., Rooney, M. T., & Schecter, J. (2000). Children's Interview for Psychiatric Syndromes (ChIPS). *Journal of the American Academy of Child and Adolescent Psychiatry, 39*, 76–84.

Wozniak, J., Biederman, J., Kiely, K., Ablon, J. S., Faraone, S., Mundy, E., et al. (1995). Mania-like symptoms suggestive of childhood-onset bipolar disorder in clinically referred children. *Journal of the American Academy of Child and Adolescent Psychiatry, 34*, 867–876.

Young, R. C., Biggs, J. T., Ziegler, V. E., & Meyer, D. A. (1978). A rating scale for mania: Reliability, validity, and sensitivity. *British Journal of Psychiatry, 133*, 429–435.

Youngstrom, E. A., Birmaher, B., & Findling, R. L. (under review). Pediatric bipolar disorder: Validity, phenomenology, and recommendations for diagnosis. *Bipolar Disorders*.

Youngstrom, E. A., Cooperberg, M., Findling, R. L., & Calabrese, J. R. (2003, October). *Identifying the most sensitive outcome measure for pediatric bipolar disorder*. Paper presented at the annual meeting of the American Academy of Child and Adolescent Psychiatry, Miami Beach, FL.

Youngstrom, E. A., Danielson, C. K., Findling, R. L., Gracious, B. L., & Calabrese, J. R. (2002). Factor structure of the Young Mania Rating Scale for use with youths ages 5 to 17 years. *Journal of Clinical Child and Adolescent Psychology, 31*, 567–572.

Youngstrom, E. A., & Duax, J. (2005). Evidence based assessment of pediatric bipolar disorder: Part 1. Base rate and family history. *Journal of the American Academy of Child and Adolescent Psychiatry, 44*, 712–717.

Youngstrom, E. A., Findling, R. L., & Calabrese, J. R. (2004). Effects of adolescent manic symptoms on agreement between youth, parent, and teacher ratings of behavior problems. *Journal of Affective Disorders, 82*, S5–S16.

Youngstrom, E. A., Findling, R. L., Calabrese, J. R., Gracious, B. L., Demeter, C., DelPorto Bedoya, D., et al. (2004). Comparing the diagnostic accuracy of six potential screening instruments for bipolar disorder in youths aged 5 to 17 years. *Journal of the American Academy of Child and Adolescent Psychiatry, 43*, 847–858.

Youngstrom, E. A., Findling, R. L., Danielson, C. K., & Calabrese, J. R. (2001). Discriminative validity of parent report of hypomanic and depressive symptoms on the General Behavior Inventory. *Psychological Assessment, 13*, 267–276.

Youngstrom, E. A., Findling, R. L., Sachs, G., Carlson, G. A., Kafantaris, V., Wozniak, J., et al. (2003, March). *Manic symptoms in bipolar and nonbipolar youths across eleven research groups using the Young Mania Rating Scale*. Paper presented at the NIMH Conference on Pediatric Bipolar Disorder, Washington, DC.

Youngstrom, E. A., Findling, R. L., Youngstrom, J. K., & Calabrese, J. R. (2005). Toward an evidence-based assessment of pediatric bipolar disorder. *Journal of Clinical Child and Adolescent Psychology, 34*, 433–448.

Youngstrom, E. A., Gracious, B. L., Danielson, C. K., Findling, R. L., & Calabrese, J. R. (2003). Toward an integration of parent and clinician report on the Young Mania Rating Scale. *Journal of Affective Disorders, 77*, 179–190.

Youngstrom, E. A., & Youngstrom, J. K. (2005). Evidence based assessment of pediatric bipolar disorder: Part 2. Incorporating information from behavior checklists. *Journal of the American Academy of Child and Adolescent Psychiatry, 44*, 823–828.

Youngstrom, E. A., Meyers, O. I., Demeter, C., Youngstrom, J. K., Morello, L., Piiparinen, R., et al. (2005). Comparing diagnostic checklists for pediatric bipolar disorder in academic and community mental health settings. *Bipolar Disorders, 7*, 507–517.

Youngstrom, E. A., Meyers, O. I., Youngstrom, J. K., Calabrese, J. R., & Findling, R. L. (2006a). Comparing the effects of sampling designs on the diagnostic accuracy of eight promising screening instruments for pediatric bipolar disorder. *Biological Psychiatry, 60*, 1013–1019.

Youngstrom, E. A., Meyers, O. I., Youngstrom, J. K., Calabrese, J. R., & Findling, R. L. (2006b). Diagnostic and measurement issues in the assessment of pediatric bipolar disorder: Implications for understanding mood disorder across the life cycle. *Development and Psychopathology, 18*, 989–1021.

Youngstrom, E. A., Youngstrom, J. K., & Starr, M. (2005). Bipolar diagnoses in community mental health: Achenbach CBCL profiles and patterns of comorbidity. *Biological Psychiatry, 58*, 569–575.

CHAPTER 7

Adolescent Suicidal and Nonsuicidal Self-Harm Behaviors and Risk

David B. Goldston
Jill S. Compton

Suicidal and nonsuicidal self-harm behaviors are a serious public health problem among youth in the United States. Suicide is the third leading cause of death among 10- to 24-year-olds after accidents and homicide and accounts for a greater number of deaths than the next three leading causes of death (cancer, heart disease, congenital anomalies) combined within this age group (Centers for Disease Control and Prevention [CDC], 2006). Suicide also often leaves a traumatic toll on survivors (Jordan & McMenamy, 2004). In addition, about 1 in 12 high school students may be expected to attempt suicide yearly (Grunbaum et al., 2004). These nonlethal attempts result in a large proportion of adolescent psychiatric emergencies (Peterson, Zhang, Santa Lucia, King, & Lewis, 1996) and represent a significant burden on the health care system. Attempts are obviously associated with not only risk of physical injury, but also greater risk of repeat nonlethal suicidal behavior and eventual death by suicide (Goldston et al., 1999; Joiner et al., 2005; Leon, Friedman, Sweeney, Brown, & Mann, 1989; Lonnqvist & Ostamo, 1991). Although suicide deaths are often thought to be a permanent solution to the transient problems faced in youth, with proper identification and treatment, suicide should be preventable.

Nonetheless, despite increasing knowledge about the prevalence, course, and risk factors for suicidal behaviors, clinicians' ability to predict precisely who (on an individual level) is at risk for suicide, and when they are at risk, often is limited. Careful assessment of suicidal and nonsuicidal self-harm behaviors and risk can help clinicians better recognize and minimize the chances of future self-harm behaviors, and evaluate efforts to prevent or reduce suicidal behaviors.

Nonsuicidal self-harm behavior may be differentiated from suicidal behavior in that the former is not associated with intent to die. Nonsuicidal self-harm behavior, such as self-mutilation, has also become increasingly prevalent in adolescent populations (Laye-Gindhu & Schonert-Reichl, 2005). Nonsuicidal self-harm behavior is especially concerning in school settings, where such behavior sometimes occurs among groups of peers. Teachers and counselors recognize increased rates of these behaviors but often are ill-equipped to deal effectively with self-harming youth. There also appears to be an overlap between nonsuicidal self-harming behavior and suicidal behavior in adolescents (Laye-Gindhu & Schonert-Reichl, 2005). We hope that better assessment of nonsuicidal self-harm behavior and its functions (Nock & Prinstein, 2004, 2005) can improve our efforts at understanding the processes that are associated with and maintain this behavior, and ultimately help in prevention and treatment efforts.

PREVALENCE OF SUICIDAL AND NONSUICIDAL SELF-HARM

Prevalence estimates for suicide deaths across the lifespan, but especially in younger age groups, may be conservative given the likelihood that suicide deaths may be misclassified as accidental or undetermined causes of death (Mohler & Earls, 2001). The misclassification bias notwithstanding, the developmental trends in suicide rates are clear. Suicide deaths are very rare prior to age 15, increase between age 15 and 19, and are still more prevalent in young adulthood (CDC, 2007). For the year 2003, reported prevalence rates for suicide deaths in the United States were 1.3 per 100,000 for 10- to 14-year-olds, 8.2 per 100,000 for 15- to 19-year-olds, and 12.5 per 100,000 for 20- to 24-year-olds. Although the overall rates of youth suicide have decreased since 1995, contemporary rates of suicide among 15- to 24-year-olds continue to be considerably higher than estimates reported in the 1950s (National Center for Health Statistics [NCHS], 2002). Reports show that suicide among adolescents and young adults ages 15–24 declined substantially from 1995 to 2004 for young men (from 22.0 to 16.8 per 100,000) but not for young women (from 3.7 to 3.6 per 100,000) (CDC, 2006; NCHS, 2002). These trends for reduced suicide deaths among males have been viewed with cautious optimism, because the factors associated with decreasing suicide rates are not well understood. Hypotheses discussed in the literature include better recognition and treatment of depression in youth (especially in light of increased use of antidepressants, such as selective serotonin reuptake inhibitors), co-occurring decreases in substance use among younger cohorts, proportionately reduced use of firearms in suicide attempts, and a favorable socioeconomic climate in the United States during the period in question (Berman, 2003; Shaffer, Pfeffer, & the Workgroup on Quality Issues, 2001).

Prevalence rates of suicidal ideation, suicide attempts, and nonsuicidal self-harm vary as a function of assessment method (e.g., anonymous self-report questionnaires vs. face-to-face

psychiatric diagnostic interviews) and operational definitions of the terms (Meehan, Lamb, Saltzman, & O'Carroll, 1992). Nonetheless, it appears that suicide attempts are relatively uncommon before puberty, with rates of less than 1% for 5- to 11-year-olds (Lewinsohn, Rohde, Seeley, & Baldwin, 2001). Rates of suicide attempts increase rapidly with the onset of puberty, however. Anonymous self-report data from adolescents, collected as part of the Youth Risk Behavior Survey (YRBS) by the CDC, indicate that 8.4% of high school students in the United States endorsed having attempted suicide in the previous year, 2.3% reported making an attempt that required medical attention, 13.0% reported having made a specific plan to attempt suicide, and 16.9% reported seriously considering a suicide attempt in the same time frame (CDC, 2006).

Prevalence studies of nonsuicidal self-harm behavior among adolescents in the community are rare, and estimates vary considerably. For example, results from two studies with large representative samples of adolescents indicated nonsuicidal self-harm rates of 5.1 and 6.9% (Patton et al., 1997; Rodham, Hawton, & Evans, 2004). However, even these estimates are much lower than those in a recently published report showing that 15% of adolescents in a school-based sample of over 400 students reported engaging in self-harm behavior (Laye-Gindhu & Schonert-Reichl, 2005). Other research studies with slightly older samples of college undergraduates have yielded findings consistent with these higher figures and report prevalence estimates of 14 to 38% of students engaging in self-harm behavior (Favazza, 1992; Gratz, Conrad, & Roemer, 2002).

Adolescent and young adult males are more likely than females to die by suicide, whereas adolescent and young adult females report higher rates of nonsuicidal self-harm. According to data for the year 2004, there were 1.8 male suicide deaths for every female suicide death among children 10–14 years old, 3.6 male deaths for every female death in 15- to 19-year-olds, and 5.8 suicide deaths among males for every suicide death among females ages 20 to 24 (CDC, 2007). Moreover, the increase in suicide deaths among young people from the 1950s through the 1990s was also primarily attributable to increases in suicides among males. Specifically, the rate of suicide among 15- to 24-year-old males was 6.5/ 100,000 in 1950 and 18.4/100,000 in 1998 (NCHS, 2002). By contrast, the rate for females in the same age range was 2.6/100,000 in 1950 and 3.3/100,000 in 1998 (NCHS, 2002).

Gender differences emerge in the opposite direction when nonfatal suicide attempts and nonsuicidal self-harm behavior are examined among adolescents and young adults. In a longitudinal study of a community sample, Lewinsohn and colleagues (2001) found few gender differences in suicide attempters before age 12, but from age 12 through late adolescence, girls were more likely than boys to attempt suicide for the first time. At young adulthood, gender differences in incidence of suicide attempts dissipated, although females still tended to have higher rates than males (Lewinsohn et al., 2001). Higher rates of attempts among females also were found among high school students taking the YRBS (CDC, 2006) and in epidemiological studies with adults (Weissman et al., 1999). In a similar manner, data from a large study of high school students in Canada indicated that adolescent girls reported more nonsuicidal self-harm behavior than did adolescent boys (Laye-Gindu & Schonert-Reichl, 2005). Gender differences in adolescents' nonsuicidal self-harm behavior appear to be especially evident in clinical samples (Nixon, Cloutier, & Aggarwal, 2002).

Prevalence rates also differ among different ethnic and racial groups; such differences are presumed to reflect differences in culture and the socioenvironmental context of these behaviors (Goldston, Molock, et al., under review). For the years 1999 to 2004, the highest rates of suicide deaths for 10- to 24-year-olds were found among American Indian and Alaska Natives (19.3 and 5.5 per 100,000, for males and females, respectively; CDC, 2007). Among males, the lowest rate was found among Asian American and Pacific Islanders (6.5/100,000; CDC, 2007). Among females, the lowest rates were found among African Americans and Latinas (1.4 and 1.7 per 100,000, respectively; CDC, 2007).

Among nonlethal self-harm behaviors, YRBS data indicate that the highest rates of suicide attempts among females occur among American Indians, and Latinas (yearly rates of 21.8%[1] and 14.9%, respectively—Crosby, personal communication, January 2005; CDC, 2006). The highest rates of attempts for males were found for American Indians (13.9%;

Crosby, personal communication, January 2005). No comparable data regarding ethnic differences in nonsuicidal self-harm behavior were available.

METHODS AND MOTIVES OF SELF-HARM BEHAVIORS

The primary methods used for suicide for 10- to 24-year-olds in 2004 were firearms (47.0%), hanging or suffocation (37.4%), poisoning or overdose (8.2%), and falls or jumping (2.4%; CDC, 2007). Since 1990, there has been an increase in the proportion of suicides by hanging or suffocation (from 19.6%) and a decrease in the proportion of suicides by firearms (from 64.5%) among young people (CDC, 2007). Males accounted for 82% of the suicide deaths among people ages 10–24 in 2003, and compared to their female counterparts, used more firearms (51.3 vs. 27.4%) and less poisoning (6.1 vs. 18.0%; CDC, 2007).

Although the most common methods for attempting nonlethal suicide are ingestion and cutting, more than half of male adolescents' suicide attempts are by alternative means, such as guns, hanging, and other methods (Brent, 1987; Lewinsohn, Rohde, & Seeley, 1996; Spirito, Stark, Fristad, Hart, & Owens-Stively, 1987). By definition, suicide attempts are associated with at least some desire to die, but suicidal behavior often is associated with ambivalence and mixed motives. For many, suicide represents a way to get relief from difficult emotional states, to escape problems, to get back at others, or to make others feel sorry for their behavior (Boergers, Spirito, & Donaldson, 1998; Hawton, Cole, O'Grady, & Osborn, 1982; Kienhorst, DeWilde, Diekstra, & Wolters, 1995).

The most common method of nonsuicidal self-harm behavior is cutting with a sharp implement; other forms include burning, hitting, pinching, scratching, and biting (Ross & Heath, 2002). Teenagers engage in self-harm behavior for a variety of reasons: to cope with difficult feelings (e.g., depression and anxiety); to relieve unbearable tension, express frustration or anger, get revenge; to feel physical pain when other pain is unbearable; to distract attention away from unpleasant memories; to punish oneself, stop suicidal ideation, or avoid a suicide attempt; to stop feeling alone and empty; to gain control; and to stop feeling "numbed out" (Nixon et al., 2002). Additional

---

[1] Data for Native Americans were collected by the Bureau of Indian Affairs only for youth attending boarding schools.

findings suggest that nonsuicidal self-harm behavior among adolescents is typically an impulsive rather than well-planned act, and often occurs among adolescents whose friends engage in similar behavior patterns (Nock & Prinstein, 2005).

CO-OCCURRENCE WITH PSYCHIATRIC DISORDERS

Although there are rare instances in which suicide deaths occur without concurrent psychopathology, suicidal and nonsuicidal self-harm behaviors are thought to be so closely related to psychiatric illness that such behaviors are incorporated into the diagnostic criteria as symptoms of illness themselves (Brent, Perper, Moritz, & Allman, 1993). DSM-IV-TR (American Psychiatric Association [APA], 2000) criteria for major depressive disorder (MDD), for example, include recurring thoughts of death; suicidal ideation, with or without a plan; and suicide attempts as possible symptoms. Both suicidal and nonsuicidal self-harm behaviors are among the criteria accepted for borderline personality disorder (BPD; although the validity of diagnosing personality disorders in adolescents has been questioned; see Shiner, Chapter 17, this volume, for a discussion of personality disorders in adolescents). Despite the fact that suicidal and nonsuicidal self-harm behaviors often occur in the midst of mental health or substance use disorders, it is important to note that most adolescents with psychiatric disorders do not engage in suicidal or nonsuicidal self-harm behaviors.

Depressive and Anxiety Disorders

Studies in which the parents of adolescents who died by suicide (i.e., psychological autopsy studies) are interviewed have identified psychiatric disorders, especially depressive disorders, as primary risk factors for suicide (Shaffer, Gould, et al., 1996). These findings are consistent with data from longitudinal research with community-dwelling 9- to 16-year-olds in which depression with comorbid anxiety disorders or comorbid disruptive behavior disorders is strongly associated with suicidal thoughts and behavior (Foley, Goldston, Costello, & Angold, 2006). Similarly, in a longitudinal study of formerly psychiatrically hospitalized adolescents, Goldston, Daniel, and colleagues (under review) found that MDD and generalized anxiety disorder (GAD) are strongly related to suicide attempts, and that this relationship strengthens as individuals get older. When viewed prospectively, MDD is the psychiatric disorder that was most strongly predictive of repeat suicidal behaviors among hospitalized adolescents (Goldston et al., 1999). Finally, studies indicate that suicide risk is greater for adolescents with longer durations of illness (Brent, Kolko, Allan, & Brown, 1990) and shorter time to relapse compared to nonsuicidal adolescents (Lewinsohn, Clarke, Seeley, & Rhode, 1993).

Depression also appears to be related to nonsuicidal self-harm behaviors among adolescents (Garrison, Addy, McKeown, & Cuffe, 1993), and many teenagers report engaging in self-harm behaviors specifically to cope with their depression (Nixon et al., 2002). Adolescents with a history of both suicidal and nonsuicidal self-harm behavior have more depression than peers who have attempted suicide but have never engaged in nonsuicidal self-harm behavior (Guertin, Lloyd-Richardson, Spirito, Donaldson, & Boergers, 2001).

Substance Use Disorders

Among formerly psychiatrically hospitalized adolescents followed into young adulthood, the likelihood of suicide attempts was greater during episodes of substance use disorders, and the relationship between suicide attempts and substance use disorders strengthened as adolescents got older (Goldston, Daniel, et al., under review). Nonetheless, the relationship between substance abuse and suicidal self-harm behavior is complicated. The literature supports the notion that this relationship varies depending on age of onset, progression, severity or frequency, and level of substance use impairment, and that serious substance abuse is more likely to be associated with suicidal behavior (Goldston, 2004). For example, Esposito and Clum (2002) found that among high-risk youth in the schools, suicidal thoughts were related to the more severe drug and alcohol dependence disorders, but not significantly related to drug and alcohol abuse disorders. In addition, the relationship between substance abuse and suicidality is found more consistently in youth with more serious suicidal behaviors (Esposito-Smythers & Spirito, 2004; Goldston, 2004). For instance, Gould and colleagues (1998) found that suicide attempts, but not suicidal ideation, were associated with substance use disorders in an epidemiological sample. Both substance abuse and suicidal behaviors are associated with significant psychiatric comorbidity (e.g., Armstrong & Costello, 2002), prompting researchers to consider whether an independent relationship exists between adolescent self-harm behavior and substance abuse in the presence of co-occurring disorders such as depression (e.g., Esposito & Clum, 2002; Gould et al., 1998). In a case–control study, Brent and colleagues (1993) found that substance use disorders without mood disorders increased the risk of suicide three-fold, but in the presence of depression, the risk of suicide increased 17-fold.

The relationship between substance abuse and nonsuicidal self-harm behavior is less well studied. In a recent study, self-harm behavior among adolescents was most commonly an impulsive act that did not include the use of alcohol or drugs (Nock & Prinstein, 2005).

Disruptive Behavior Disorders

Disruptive behavior disorders also have been found to be associated with suicidal behaviors. For example, in a psychological autopsy case–control study, Shaffer, Gould, and colleagues (1996) found that disruptive behavior disorders were present among 50% of the adolescents who died by suicide. For adolescent males, but not females, the rates of conduct and oppositional disorders were greater than those observed in matched control subjects. However, disruptive behavior disorders were often comorbid with other disorders and did not appear to be independently related to suicide among adolescent males after the researchers controlled for the presence of past attempts and other diagnoses, such as mood and substance use disorders. In another psychological autopsy study, Brent and colleagues (1988) found no significant difference in the rates of disruptive behavior disorders of adolescent suicide victims and hospitalized suicidal adolescents. However, the adolescents who died by suicide did have higher rates of affective disorders with nonaffective comorbidity, including conduct disorder. In a review of the literature, James, Lai, and Dahl (2004) found that attention-deficit/hyperactivity disorder (ADHD) appeared to be modestly related to increased rates of suicide, especially among young males; this relationship appeared to be partially attrib-

utable to commonly associated comorbid conditions, including mood and conduct disorders.

In terms of nonlethal suicidal behavior, Goldston, Daniel, and colleagues (1999; under review) found that ADHD and conduct disorder were proximal risk factors for suicide attempts, but disruptive behavior disorders by themselves were not predictive of subsequent suicide attempts among formerly hospitalized adolescents. In addition, in a community sample, Gould and colleagues (1998) found that oppositional defiant disorder and conduct disorder were more common among youth who reported suicidal thoughts or attempts than among nonsuicidal adolescents. In another community study, Foley and colleagues (2006) found that disruptive behavior disorders were proximally related to suicidal thoughts and behaviors but primarily associated with risk when comorbid with depressive disorders.

In a follow-up study, Barkley and Fischer (2005) found that young adults diagnosed as hyperactive during childhood were more likely than comparison young adults to have considered suicide, to have made a suicide attempt, to have been hospitalized for suicidal behavior during their high school years, and to have considered suicide as an option after high school. Among the "grownup" hyperactive children, Barkley and Fischer found that the increased risk for suicide attempts was associated with lifetime histories of MDD, conduct disorder, and greater severity of ADHD.

RISK AND PROTECTIVE FACTORS

Aside from psychiatric and substance use disorders, a number of other factors have been found to be associated with risk for suicidal and nonsuicidal self-harm behaviors. Most of the research regarding risk and protective factors has been cross-sectional in nature. Although informative about associations with self-harm behavior, these studies do not necessarily shed light on the degree to which these factors are associated with risk for subsequent self-harm. Given the low base rate of suicide even among those at high risk, it is difficult to predict suicide accurately as an outcome. Moreover, risk and protective factors may differ in different risk or population groups because of different base rates of self-harm and risk factors. Risk and protective factors also may differ over time, or over the course of development, though research on these possibilities has been limited. Research on risk and protective factors also has often not differentiated between factors associated with short- and long-term risk for suicidal behavior (Hawton, 1987).

Both suicidal and nonsuicidal self-harm behaviors often occur in the context of immediate triggers or precipitants (proximal risk factors) and factors that may be associated with longer term risk (distal risk factors) (Moscicki, 1999). Although knowledge of proximal risk factors provides information about when individuals are at risk for suicidal or self-harm behavior, such knowledge does not necessarily provide information about who is at risk. Alternatively, distal risk factors may provide information about who is at risk for suicidal or nonsuicidal self-harm behavior, but not about when those individuals are at risk. In the following section, we review several groups of proximal and distal risk factors associated with suicidal and nonsuicidal self-harm behavior.

Previous Self-Harm Behavior

One obvious and pervasive concern for parents and providers of adolescents who engage in suicidal behavior is whether these acts will be repeated and ultimately lead to serious injury or death. Similar to other human behavior, a history of engaging in suicidal behavior is the best predictor of future suicide behavior, even after considering the effects of multiple risk factors (Joiner et al., 2005). Among adolescents, for instance, the number of prior suicide attempts has been found to be a strong predictor of future suicidal behavior (Goldston et al., 1999). Similarly, previous suicide attempts have been associated with significantly higher risk for repeated behavior among adults, with a suicide attempt increasing future risk by about 32% (Leon et al., 1989).

Some have argued that sensitization processes may account for increased risk associated with past suicidal behavior (Beck, 1996; Joiner, 2002). For example, previous experience with self-harm behavior may affect the capacity to participate in that behavior again in the future or sensitivity to cues associated with suicidal behavior. Alternatively, it is possible that the increased risk is associated with behavioral processes; for example, self-harm behavior may be associated with reinforcing consequences, such as reduction of painful affect,

that may increase the likelihood of its recurrence when in the presence of similar cues (Goldston, 2004; Goldston et al., 1999). Another possibility, which is not mutually exclusive, is that a subset of individuals is at risk for recurrent suicidal behaviors by virtue of historical, psychopathological, biological, environmental, or temperamental characteristics. Such individuals may simply be qualitatively different, or have different developmental trajectories, than individuals who engage in single attempts. In this regard, it is notable that outpatient children and adolescents with repeated suicide attempts had higher rates of sexual abuse, run-away behavior, and drug and alcohol use than first-time attempters (Mandell, Walrath, & Goldston, 2006; Walrath et al., 2001). In a similar manner, Esposito, Spirito, Boergers, and Donaldson (2003) found that adolescents presenting for emergency care after a repeat suicide attempt had more affective disorders, severe depressive symptoms, anger, disruptive behavior disorders, hopelessness, and self-mutilation than did adolescents with single attempts.

Although some researchers have noted that nonsuicidal self-harm behavior has addictive qualities (Nixon et al., 2002), the degree to which this behavior portends risk for future nonsuicidal self-harm or suicidal behaviors among adolescents has not been evaluated in prospective studies.

Impulsivity

Suicides among children and adolescents often are impulsive acts that correspond to recent stressors or crises (Hoberman & Garfinkel, 1988), and suicidal children have been found to have poorer impulse control than their nonsuicidal peers (Pfeffer, Hurt, Peskin, & Siefker, 1995). Impulsivity may be a relatively stable attribute of individuals, or it may reflect changes in cognitive or emotional states that result in a decreased ability to show restraint (Corruble, Damy, & Guelfi, 1999; Tice, Bratslavsky, & Baumeister, 2001; Weyrauch, Roy-Byrne, Katon, & Wilson, 2001). Nock and Prinstein (2005) have demonstrated that nonsuicidal self-mutilation among adolescents is typically an impulsive act. The degree to which impulsivity portends risk for future self-harm behavior is unclear.

Dougherty and colleagues (2004) have demonstrated that laboratory methods may be used to quantify different facets of impulsivity and their relationship to suicidality. For example, stop tasks may be used to assess aspects of impulsivity related to the ability to inhibit ongoing behavior. These tasks reveal increased impulsivity among adolescents with suicidal ideation (Dougherty, Mathias, Marsh, Moeller, & Swann, 2004; Mathias, Dougherty, Carrizal, & Marsh, 2003) and repeated suicide attempts (Prevette, Mathias, Marsh, & Dougherty, 2005). Continuous performance tasks may be used to assess aspects of impulsivity related to the accurate initiation of behavior. Adult suicide attempters show increased impulsivity on this task (Dougherty, Mathias, Marsh, Papageorgiou, et al., 2004; Horesh, 2001). Finally, delay-discounting procedures may be used to assess the ability to tolerate delay for a larger reward. On these tasks, adolescents with suicidal thoughts evidence increased impulsivity (Mathias et al., 2003).

Hopelessness

Hopelessness is a sense of extreme pessimism about the future. In his eloquent writings on the phenomenology of suicide, Shneidman (1996) has suggested that hopelessness is the common cognitive state among individuals who engage in suicidal behaviors. Hopelessness typically is associated with a sense of futility about life, or a viewpoint that problems will never be solved, or that life circumstances will never change. The negative view of the future is also a central tenet of the cognitive model of depression (Beck, Rush, Shaw, & Emery, 1979). Hopelessness has been found to predict repeat suicide attempts among adolescents following psychiatric hospitalization (Goldston et al., 2001), and it also appears to be associated with suicide intent (Nock & Kazdin, 2002; Spirito, Sterling, Donaldson, & Arrigan, 1996). Nonetheless, some researchers question the degree to which hopelessness is associated with suicidal ideation or behavior after controlling for depression (Asarnow & Guthrie, 1989; Goldston et al., 2001; Nock & Kazdin, 2002).

Adolescent suicide attempters with a history of nonsuicidal self-mutilation have been noted to have more hopelessness than adolescent attempters without self-mutilation (Guertin et al., 2001). In addition, hopelessness has been found to be associated with the negative reinforcement function of nonsuicidal self-mutilation (i.e., the degree to which such behavior is engaged in to relieve negative moods or affect) (Nock & Prinstein, 2005).

Reasons for Living

Clinicians working with suicidal patients often focus on helping patients recognize or develop new reasons for living. In one sense, it is intuitive that patients who have adequate reasons to continue living or have faith in their ability to cope generally do not take steps to end their lives. Indeed, there is evidence among previously hospitalized adolescents that individuals who endorse more reasons for living and, particularly, greater survival and coping beliefs, make fewer repeat suicide attempts over time (Goldston et al., 2001). Survival and coping beliefs also have been found to be negatively associated with hopelessness, dysfunctional attitudes, and suicidal thoughts, as well as estimates of future suicidal behavior (Cole, 1989b; Goldston et al., 2001). Jobes and Mann (1999) have suggested that the balance between reasons for living and reasons for dying is an important consideration in understanding risk for suicidality.

Problem-Solving Ability

Shneidman (1996) stated, "The common purpose of suicide is to seek a solution. Suicide is not a random act. It is never done without purpose. It is a way out of a problem, a dilemma, a bind, a difficulty, a crisis, an unbearable situation" (p. 130). This observation underscores the importance of problem-solving ability in the understanding of suicide and suicide risk. Shneidman also described the common perceptual state associated with suicide to be one of constriction, in which suicidal individuals often see suicide as their only option and are unable to identify other alternatives to this course of action. It is unclear whether the problem-solving deficits commonly observed among suicidal individuals are transient (state-like) or more stable over time (trait-like; Schotte, Cools, & Payvar, 1990). In addition, problem-solving difficulties may also be associated with hopelessness. For example, in the World Health Organization European (WHO/EURO) multicenter study on suicidal behavior, it was noted that passive–avoidant problem solving, characterized by "taking a gloomy view of the situation," a feeling of being "unable to do anything," and "the tendency to resign oneself to the situation," was associated with repetitive instances of self-harm behavior (McAuliffe et al., 2006). In a review of adolescent studies, Speckens and Hawton (2005) noted that in many studies, suicidal adolescents have more social problem-solving deficits than do nonsuicidal adolescents, but many of these differences appear to be accounted for (mediated) by depression and hopelessness.

Childhood Sexual Abuse

Childhood sexual abuse is a well-documented risk factor for many negative short- and long-term outcomes, and suicidal ideation and behavior are not exceptions. For example, in one study, adolescents and young adults who made medically serious suicide attempts were 6.5 times more likely to have histories of sexual abuse than case–control subjects in the community (Beautrais, Joyce, & Mulder, 1996). In a study of hospitalized youth, physical (nonsexual) and sexual abuse were associated with a higher number of past suicide attempts (Shaunesey, Cohen, Plummer, & Berman, 1993). In the National Comorbidity Study (NCS) sexual abuse was associated with histories of suicide attempts, even after considering other risk factors (Molnar, Berkman, & Buka, 2001). Moreover, concordance between parent and child in suicide attempts has been found to be more likely in the presence of parent and child sexual abuse (Brent et al., 2002).

There also is strong evidence of a relationship between childhood sexual abuse and nonsuicidal self-harm behavior (Briere & Gil, 1998; Santa Mina & Gallop, 1998; Zlotnick et al., 1996). In a study of adults, van der Kolk, Perry, and Herman (1991) found that earlier histories of trauma were associated with more cutting behavior. In a review focusing on self-injury among adults, Gratz (2003) suggested that there is much stronger evidence for an independent relationship between nonsuicidal self-harm behaviors and sexual abuse than for other forms of abuse.

Sexual Orientation

Young people who identify as gay, lesbian, or bisexual (GLB) appear to be at increased risk for suicidal behavior compared to heterosexual youth. Data from the YRBS indicated that GLB adolescents, or those unsure of their sexual ori-entation, were more likely than heterosexual youth to attempt suicide (Garofalo, Wolf, Wissow, Woods, & Goodman, 1999). Similarly, data from the National Longitudinal Study of Adolescent Health indicated that homosexual adolescents were at higher risk for suicidality, although this risk may have been mediated by common risk factors such as depression and hopelessness (Russell & Joyner, 2001). In a recent study, D'Augelli and colleagues (2005) found that in a sample of GLB adolescents, over half of the suicide attempts were related to sexual orientation. Factors associated with higher likelihood of attempts included parental psychological abuse, being considered gender-atypical in childhood by parents, and parental efforts to discourage GLB behaviors. Suicide attempts also were related to sexual victimization and loss of friends due to sexual orientation, and tended to occur after recognition of homosexual feelings but before disclosure to parents (D'Augelli, Hershberger, & Pilkington, 2001; Hershberger, Pilkington, & D'Augelli, 1997). Nonetheless, in one psychological autopsy study, adolescents who died by suicide did not appear to have increased minority sexual orientation (Shaffer, Fisher, Parides, & Gould, 1995), although it could be simply the case that informants were unaware of victims' sexual orientation or feelings.

Accessibility to Firearms

Presence of firearms in the home has been found to be more common among adolescents who die by suicide than by adolescents hospitalized for suicidality (Brent et al., 1988). In a recent case–control study, Grossman and colleagues (2005) found that the practices of locking up guns and ammunition, and storing guns unloaded, separately from ammunition, were associated with reduced firearm injuries and suicide attempts among children and adolescents. Parents, however, are often reluctant to remove guns from the homes to protect suicidal youth, even after counseling in this regard (Brent, Baugher, Birmaher, Kolko, & Bridge, 2000).

Family Psychiatric History

Suicidal behavior tends to run in families. Relatives of individuals who have engaged in suicidal behavior or died by suicide are themselves at higher risk for suicidal behavior (Brent, Bridge, Johnson, & Connolly, 1996), and there is greater concordance among monozygotic than among dizygotic twins for suicidal behavior (Roy & Segal, 2001; Roy, Segal, Centerwall, & Robinette, 1991). The children of adult suicide attempters are approximately six times more likely to engage in suicidal behavior than the children of adults who have not made suicide attempts (Brent et al., 2002). Although there is evidence that relatives of adolescents who have attempted or died by suicide have higher rates of psychiatric disorders than relatives of nonsuicidal adolescents (Wagner, 1997), the rates of family psychiatric disorders are comparable to those for similar-age peers in treatment settings. In contrast to what is known about familial risk of suicidal behavior, little research has documented associations between nonsuicidal self-harm behaviors and family psychiatric history.

Life Stress

Clearly, life stress is an obvious and overarching proximal risk factor for suicide. One study found that the great majority (80%) of adolescents who attempted suicide had experienced a major life stress in the prior 3 months (Heikkinen, Aro, & Lonnqvist, 1994). These findings have been replicated by research showing increased rates of stressful life events among adolescents and young adults in the 3 months prior to death by suicide, and more specifically, in the week prior to death (Cooper, Appleby, & Amos, 2002). Life events associated with increased risk for suicidal behaviors often include interpersonal difficulties, conflicts, or losses, and environmental consequences such as disciplinary action or legal problems (Adams, Overholser, & Spirito, 1994; Beautrais, Joyce, & Mulder, 1997; Gould, Fisher, Parides, Flory, & Shaffer, 1996). Some adolescents, however, do not report precipitants for their suicidal behavior (Beautrais et al., 1997), and the occurrence of life events may be related to young people's poor problem-solving skills or psychiatric difficulties.

The relationship between stressful life events and nonsuicidal self-harm behavior is less well documented. Garrison and colleagues (1993) found that nonsuicidal self-harm behaviors are also significantly correlated with the presence of undesirable life events. In clinical settings, interpersonal precipitants often appear to be associated with nonsuicidal self-harm behaviors.

Social Support

Shneidman (1996) has stated, "Suffering is half pain and half being alone with that pain. For some people, suicide is feeling entirely alone" (p. 119). In this regard, among high-risk adolescents in school, suicidal youth were found to have lower perceived social support from families, teachers, or friends than their nonsuicidal peers (Esposito & Clum, 2003). In particular, suicide attempters in one study were more likely than nonattempters to report that they would not go to a family member for assistance (O'Donnell, Stueve, Wardlaw, & O'Donnell, 2003). The relationship between social support and suicidality may differ by gender. For instance, peer support tends to increase as youth get older, and girls report more peer support than do boys. However, among girls in a hospitalized sample, perceived family support was related to hopelessness, depression, and suicidal thoughts, whereas among boys, peer support was most strongly related to depression and suicidal thoughts (Keer, Preuss, & King, 2006).

FUNCTIONAL IMPAIRMENT AND OUTCOMES

Suicidal adolescents evidence functional impairment in a variety of areas. For example, as assessed with the Child and Adolescent Functional Assessment Scale (CAFAS; Hodges & Wong, 1996), youth suicide attempters in outpatient settings showed greater impairment than their peers in home and school role performance, behavior toward others, and moods and emotions (Mandell et al., 2006). Repeat suicide attempters had the most impairment in moods and emotions, behavior toward others, and thinking.

Six months after entering treatment, suicidal youth continued to have difficulties in a number of areas of functioning (Mandell et al., 2006). For example, repeat suicide attempters were at higher risk than other youth for continuing to have problems in thinking and in behavior toward others, and first-time suicide attempters were at risk for continuing impairment in the home and substance use problems 6 months later. Repeat suicide attempters also were at increased risk for developing severe functional impairment in the areas of behavior toward others, moods and emotions, and self-harm. First-time attempters were primarily at risk for greater impairment in the area of self-harm 6 months later.

These varied areas of impairment dovetail with results from a review by Spirito, Boergers, and Donaldson (2002), indicating that youth often continue to have relational problems, difficulties with parents, and substance abuse, behavioral, and school problems following suicidal behavior. With particular reference to school impairment, youth who died by suicide were noted to have more school suspensions and failing grades than comparison youth in the community (Gould et al., 1996). Moreover, Daniel and colleagues (2006) found that suicidal ideation and attempts were related to reading disabilities and eventual dropout from school. In contrast to suicidal behavior, little is known about the various areas of impairment or of the prognosis for adolescents with nonsuicidal self-harm behaviors.

Summary

In this section, we have reviewed many factors associated with suicidal ideation and self-harm behavior among youth, including psychiatric factors (e.g., depressive disorders), cognitive factors (e.g., problem-solving ability, hopelessness), temperament (e.g., impulsivity), familial factors (e.g., family history of suicidal behavior), historical factors (e.g., history of suicide attempts, history of abuse), and facets of the environment (e.g., stressful life events, accessibility of firearms). We also have reviewed factors that may protect youth against suicidal behavior, such as perceived reasons for living. The large number of potential risk and protective factors may be daunting for clinicians working with multiproblem youth and trying to gauge or monitor both immediate and long-term risk. The large number of risk factors is partially a reflection of the current state of research in this area; most studies have focused on univariate relationships between risk or protective factors and self-harm behaviors. This univariate view of risk factors underscores that there are likely many interventions that prevent suicide and nonsuicidal self-harm behavior, but this approach provides limited information about which factor(s) are most important, for whom, and in what context. The factors often overlap; it is possible that some

may simply be correlates of others (e.g., hopelessness may be an indicator of depression), and some combinations of risk factors may be particularly important in portending later risk, or may portend risk for some, but not all, youth. Integrative models of risk and multivariate models regarding the evolution of risk over time are needed to help guide clinical practice, to help identify the most robust risk factors for particular individuals, and to guide assessment with more precision. In studies that have taken a multivariate approach, some of the strongest risk factors for future suicidal behavior across samples include diagnosis of depression (Goldston et al., 1999; Lewinsohn, Rohde, & Seeley, 1994) and past suicide attempts (Goldston et al., 1999; Joiner et al., 2005; Lewinsohn et al., 1994). Past suicidal behavior may also interact with other risk factors in contributing to risk. For example, in a clinically ascertained sample, Goldston and colleagues (1999, 2001) found that risk factors such as hopelessness and diagnosis of depression are more highly predictive of repeat than of first-time suicide attempts. As we describe in the next section, there are multiple approaches to assessment, and factors to be assessed depend in part on the intended purpose of an assessment.

PURPOSES OF ASSESSMENT OF SELF-HARM BEHAVIOR AND RISK

There are several purposes for assessing suicidal and nonsuicidal self-harm and risk, but the end goal is always the prevention of future suicidality and self-harm behavior. The first goal in suicide assessment is to identify imminent risk for self-harm behavior. Assessment of imminent risk helps to facilitate adequate monitoring and clinical intervention to diffuse crises and ensure immediate safety. Many suicidal crises are short-lived (Simon et al., 2001); hence, the importance of taking steps to diffuse such crises and ensure safety in the short run cannot be underestimated.

A second purpose of assessment is to predict future self-harm behaviors. Several approaches have been developed for estimating risk of future self-harm behavior. Unfortunately, however, despite cross-sectional correlations with histories of self-harm behaviors, it is still not clear that most assessments of "risk" actually predict (in a temporal or longitudinal sense) future self-harm behaviors. The prediction of self-harm behavior is an important part of many suicide prevention and treatment efforts with at-risk populations.

A third purpose of assessment related to suicidality and self-harm is that of treatment planning. In this regard, it is important to understand the functional context in which self-harm behavior occurs, including the precipitants or triggers for the behavior, the associated vulnerability and protective factors, the nature of the self-harm behavior itself, and the intrapersonal and environmental consequences of self-harm behavior. Functional analyses of suicidal and nonsuicidal self-harm behavior provide very useful information about possible targets for intervention. It is also important to identify whether the self-harm behavior occurs in the context of a psychiatric or substance use disorder, and to examine whether functional commonalities exist among self-harm and other problem behaviors, so that one can develop integrated treatment approaches. Furthermore, in recognition of the broader cultural context of self-harm behavior, it is important to assess the cultural nuances related to the specific precipitants, vulnerability and protective factors, expression, and consequences of suicidal and nonsuicidal self-harm behaviors for any given patient.

The last purpose of self-harm assessment is treatment monitoring. Ongoing assessment of suicidal and nonsuicidal self-harm ideation and behavior, and of risk and protective factors, provides information about the effectiveness of current interventions. Pharmacotherapy with antidepressant medications, for example, has been linked to small increases (about 2%) in self-harm adverse events for some youth (U.S. Food and Drug Administration [FDA], 2004; Treatment of Adolescent Depression Study [TADS] Team, 2004). Hence, it is particularly important to monitor self-harm behavior continuously when medications have been prescribed for emotional or behavioral problems.

USING A COMMON LANGUAGE

Professionals dealing with suicidal and nonsuicidal self-harm behavior have often used varied and inconsistent language to refer to key terms. As a result, it has been difficult for clinicians to compare findings across studies or even to communicate effectively (e.g., Garrison, Jackson, Addy, McKeown, & Waller, 1991; Goldston, 2003; Lewinsohn, Garrison, Langhinrichsen, & Marsteller, 1989). For example, many studies in the literature have focused only on suicidal behavior associated with medical consequences (e.g., Beautrais, 2003). Nonetheless, in the college sample of Meehan and colleagues (1992), 10% of students stated that they had attempted suicide sometime in their life, 5% said that they had experienced illness or injury because of a suicide attempt, and 3% stated that they had received medical attention because of suicidal behavior. Hence, studies that focus exclusively on suicidal behavior resulting in serious medical consequences may be very informative in their own right, but they may not adequately characterize the entire population of individuals engaging in suicidal behaviors. Additionally, most studies examining the predictive validity of clinical characteristics of suicidal behavior among adolescents have not found factors such as stated intent to be predictive of future suicidal behavior (Spirito, Lewander, Levy, Kurkjian, & Fritz, 1994).

In an article likening inconsistencies in the use of terms to describe suicidal behaviors to a "Tower of Babel," O'Carroll, Berman, Maris, and Moscicki (1996) summarized the findings of a workshop whose task it was to provide recommendations about the ways suicidal terms are operationally defined. In this recommended nomenclature, *suicide* was defined as "death from injury, poisoning or suffocation where there is evidence (either explicit or implicit) that the injury was self-inflicted and that the decedent intended to kill himself/herself" (pp. 246–247). A *suicide attempt* was operationally defined as "a potentially self-injurious behavior with a non-fatal outcome, for which there is evidence (either explicit or implicit) that the person intended at some (non-zero) level to kill himself/herself. A suicide attempt may or may not result in injuries" (O'Carroll et al., 1996, p. 247). The phrase "some (non-zero) level to kill himself/herself" is an implicit acknowledgment of the ambivalence that accompanies much suicidal behavior (Shneidman, 1996). *Suicidal ideation* was defined as "any self-reported thoughts of engaging in suicide-related behavior" (O'Carroll et al., 1996, p. 247).

Beyond this recommended nomenclature, several self-harm behaviors may be difficult to classify or characterize (Goldston, 2004). For example, adolescents sometimes make "aborted suicide attempts." The term "aborted suicide attempts" refers to occasions in which adolescents make preparations for suicide but decide not to follow through with their intentions (Barber, Marzuk, Leon, & Portera, 1998). For example, an adolescent may start to make an attempt by putting a noose around his neck and preparing to jump, but then at the last minute, decide that he is scared, or that the problem is not worth dying over. As described by Barber and colleagues (1998), "The essential characteristics of an aborted attempt are 1) intent to kill oneself, 2) a change of mind immediately before the actual attempt, and 3) absence of injury" (p. 385). Among adults, aborted suicide attempts appear to be more common among patients who have histories of actual suicide attempts than among patients without such histories (Barber et al., 1998).

Another example of suicidal behavior that does not fall neatly into the nomenclature of O'Carroll and colleagues (1996) is the "interrupted suicide attempt." In contrast to aborted suicide attempts, interrupted suicide attempts occur when an individual starts to attempt suicide, but the attempt is interrupted or prevented by others, or by external circumstances (Steer, Beck, Garrison, & Lester, 1988). For example, a suicidal adolescent may be getting ready to attempt suicide by holding a knife against her wrist, when a parent or friend arrives and takes the knife away. As noted previously (Goldston, 2004), interrupted suicide attempts may be particularly common among adolescents who still live in their parents' homes, where their suicide attempts have a high likelihood of being discovered. In adult patient samples, individuals whose suicide attempts have been interrupted are at increased risk for eventually dying by suicide compared to patients whose suicide attempts were not interrupted (Steer et al., 1988). It is not clear why individuals whose attempts are discovered should be at higher risk, but it may be that clinicians do not consider their behaviors to be as serious as those of individuals whose attempts are uninterrupted (Steer et al., 1988).

Passive suicide attempts represent another form of suicidal behavior. In passive suicidal behavior, adolescents may not take adequate precautions to save themselves when their lives are in danger, or necessary steps to prevent their demise. Adolescents with diabetes, for example, sometimes are persistently noncompliant with their medical regimen, despite health consequences. Although not all lack of adherence to the medical regimen is associated with

suicidality, Goldston, Kovacs, Ho, Parrone, and Stiffler (1994; Goldston et al., 1997) have noted an association between serious noncompliance and suicidal ideation and attempts.

Other suicidal youth may try to provoke peers, adversaries, or authorities to inflict harm upon them. Such behaviors, first described by Wolfgang (1959), are referred to as "victim-precipitated homicide." In contemporary society, such provocations may occur in the context of gang-related activity in urban areas or involve provocations of law enforcement officials. Such behaviors may be more common among groups in which suicide is associated with stigma.

Often confused with suicidal behaviors are nonsuicidal self-harm behaviors. There may be some similarities in the motives for nonsuicidal and suicidal self-harm behaviors, and certainly some youth engage in both forms of self-harm behaviors (Boergers et al., 1998; Nixon et al., 2002). Nonetheless, nonsuicidal self-harm behavior is not meant to end one's life. There have been suggestions, particularly by researchers studying adult clinical samples, that suicidal and nonsuicidal self-harm behaviors may sometimes be difficult to distinguish or classify (Isometsa & Lonnqvist, 1999). However, in most cases, nonsuicidal and suicidal self-harm behavior can be distinguished by asking respondents whether "any part of them" wanted to die when they engaged in this behavior.

WEIGHING DIFFERENT SOURCES OF INFORMATION

Given that suicidal behaviors are prevalent among adolescents and associated with a number of psychiatric disorders, it is important to inquire about the history of suicidal behavior, even when suicidal behavior is not the immediate referring problem. Likewise, in schools and other settings in which "gatekeepers" such as schoolteachers, coaches, or clergy may have contact with distressed youth, it is important for there to be recognition of the problem of suicide among young people. Gatekeepers who work with youth need to be comfortable asking about suicidality if they suspect that an individual is either considering or may already have attempted suicide. Direct inquiry (interviewing) is an appropriate method for asking about history of suicidal thoughts and behavior, and is the most commonly used approach. Nonetheless, it is striking that even trained mental health professionals are sometimes reluctant to ask a youth about suicidality. Professionals may not ask direct questions because of their own anxiety and apprehension about what they might need to do should they find out that someone is suicidal. Clinicians may also fear that by asking about suicide, they communicate an idea that the young person has not already had and may now consider and act upon. As a recent study pointed out, however, presenting suicidal adolescents with screening questions about suicidality does not increase rates of suicidal ideation or distress (Gould et al., 2005). In fact, the most vulnerable adolescents actually experienced some diminution in level of distress after being asked suicide-related questions (Gould et al., 2005). Moreover, as Fremouw, Perczel, and Ellis (1990) have pointed out, suicidal thoughts and behavior are common among individuals who are depressed, and queries about suicidality may communicate that clinicians recognize and understand the experience. Clinicians may actually run a greater risk when they do not ask about suicidal thoughts and behavior, because this omission may inadvertently reinforce adolescents' sense of alienation or the perception that no one really understands their experience.

For inquiries about suicidal behavior, adolescents should generally be relied upon more heavily than their parents or other adult informants. Suicidal behaviors, and certainly suicidal thoughts, are often not discussed with others, and several studies have found that youth tend to report suicidal behaviors that their parents know nothing about (Breton, Tousignant, Bergeron, & Berthiaume, 2002; Foley et al., 2006; Klimes-Dougan, 1998; Velez & Cohen, 1988; Walker, Moreau, & Weissman, 1990). For example, in a community survey, parents only correctly identified 6 of 59 adolescents who had reported suicidal thoughts, and 2 of the 36 adolescents who had attempted suicide (Breton et al., 2002). Similarly, in the Great Smoky Mountains epidemiological study (Foley et al., 2006), 69% of reports of suicidality consisted of positive reports by youths and negative reports by adults. It is sometimes the case that parents "miss" or misinterpret their child's suicidal behaviors either by not taking these behaviors seriously, believing that suicidal behaviors (or threats) are merely intended for instrumental purposes (e.g., to avoid punishment), failing to believe

that their child would want to kill him- or herself, or by simply being unaware of the behaviors (Goldston, 2003). Parental inaccuracies in perception of suicidal behavior also may be related to a lack of understanding of the fact that much adolescent suicidal behavior is associated with ambivalence and mixed motives. For example, it may be the case that adolescents simultaneously "want their way" in an argument with parents, want to avoid discipline, and also want to die because they feel so miserable.

Occasionally, reports of suicidality may not accurately reflect the level of distress experienced by an adolescent (Goldston, 2003). For example, an adolescent may deny feeling suicidal (and minimize other signs of distress) in an emergency room setting to avoid uncomfortable feelings or being hospitalized. Therefore, it is important for clinicians to consider alternative data sources, in addition to verbal reports, when evaluating suicide risk, particularly in an emergency setting. Similarly, adolescents may deny suicidality because they wish to be secretive about their intent or may desire to avoid unwanted attention or embarrassment. Thus, rapport with adolescents is especially important in eliciting accurate reports of suicidal behavior.

In contrast, sometimes there are occasions in which adolescents overreport suicidality. Communication of high suicide intent when it does not accurately reflect the feelings experienced by the adolescent may be associated with his or her desire to "mend" relationships (e.g., avoid breaking up), to be hospitalized, or to be taken out of a home environment that is experienced as intolerable (Goldston, 2003). Nonetheless, as pointed out by Goldston, Daniel, and Arnold (2006), "Child and adolescent report is certainly very important, but it should never preempt the judgment of a clinician. Clinicians should always err on the side of caution in making judgments about the risk of suicidal behavior; conversely, clinicians should be extraordinarily careful to not be dismissive of adolescent self-reports of suicidal ideation or behavior" (pp. 360–361).

STRATEGIES FOR ELICITING INFORMATION ABOUT SELF-HARM IN INTERVIEW

Shea (1999) has described several useful interviewing techniques that elicit information about suicidality. For example, individuals sometimes deny having a history of suicidality at first, but report suicidal behavior when asked follow-up questions about specific methods. In one example with adults, Barber, Marzuk, Leon, and Portera (2001) asked psychiatric inpatients about their past suicidal behavior, including aborted suicide attempts. When following up with the same patients after the initial assessment, Barber and colleagues found that 44% of adults who previously denied a history of aborted suicide attempts eventually reported such an attempt in response to specific queries.

In this regard, it also is very important to ask for concrete information or examples of suicidal behavior. For example, if a patient reports that he or she has attempted suicide "three or four times" in the past, it is useful to elicit as much information as possible about each suicide attempt, including approximate date, the method used, and the precipitants and consequences. This provides contextual information about the patterns of suicidal behavior that the clinician can use for treatment planning and understanding the current episode of suicidal behavior.

Normalization is another interviewing technique that is sometimes useful in the interview with suicidal patients (Shea, 1999). Although suicidality is often thought of as a difficult subject to discuss, framing questions about self-harm behavior in ways that minimize shame or embarrassment may help to "normalize" the topic. For example, the clinician may ask about suicidal behavior by prefacing the inquiry with a statement, such as "A lot of times when people are very upset, depressed, or feeling hopeless, they will think about wanting to attempt suicide. In the last week, how often have you had thoughts like that?"

Other useful techniques that elicit information about self-harm behavior include the gentle assumption and the amplification assumption (Shea, 1999). With the gentle assumption, the clinician implicitly makes an assumption that the patient has either thought about self-harm or has engaged in self-harm behavior (rather than asking the individual "whether" he or she has thought about or engaged in self-harm). For example, rather than asking a depressed adolescent, "Have you ever thought about suicide?", the clinician might ask, "When was the last time that you thought about killing yourself?" Similarly, rather than

asking an adolescent whether he or she has made a suicide attempt in the past, the clinician might ask how many suicide attempts he or she has made.

Using the amplification assumption, the clinician may try to make the adolescent feel more comfortable reporting self-harm behavior by assuming a degree of self-harm behavior that probably exceeds what the adolescent has experienced. For example, in assessing nonsuicidal self-harm, rather than asking the adolescent how often he or she cuts him- or herself, the clinician might ask, "In the last week, how many days have you cut on yourself at least five separate times?" Most self-harming adolescents do not engage in self-harm behavior at this frequency, so they may then feel more comfortable reporting rates that more closely resemble the actual frequency of their self-harm.

ASSESSMENT OF IMMINENT SUICIDALITY

One of the most important clinician tasks is to evaluate whether a patient is at imminent risk for suicidal behavior. Youth are generally considered to be at imminent risk when they state that they intend to kill themselves, feel that they can no longer keep themselves safe, or unable to say that they will refrain from attempting suicide, or cannot agree to a collaboratively developed safety plan.

Alternatively, the same conclusion may be reached by a clinician who thinks that despite what the adolescent says, his or her past behavior, history, and the nature of the current crisis suggest that the individual is at extraordinarily high risk of attempting suicide in the near future. When someone is thought to be at imminent risk for suicide, the clinician should first take immediate therapeutic steps to reduce this risk. However, if such efforts are not successful, the clinician may recommend hospitalization or another form of treatment that provides the monitoring necessary to ensure safety and prevent suicidal behavior.

Safety Plans as a Form of Assessment

Clinicians sometimes use various forms of nosuicide contracts in the hope that these will reduce immediate risk of self-harm behavior. Such contracts typically entail an explicit verbal or written statement that patients will not attempt to harm themselves within a specified period of time, or will tell someone if they feel that they cannot keep themselves safe. In theory, no-suicide contracts may have several advantages, including the fact that they represent a collaboration for safety between patient and clinician, encourage the patient to take responsibility for his or her own safety, entail a formal commitment not to engage in self-harm, and emphasize the clinician's concern about the patient's safety (Lee & Bartlett, 2005; Range et al., 2002). Nonetheless, the therapeutic value of no-suicide contracts has not been established. In fact, in the state of Minnesota, a " 'no-harm contract' was in place in almost every completed suicide occurring in an acute care facility" (Office of the Ombudsman for Mental Health and Mental Retardation, State of Minnesota, 2002). In addition, questions have been raised about whether no-suicide contracts may discourage patients from talking about suicidality, and encourage clinicians to become less vigilant in ongoing risk monitoring (Lee & Bartlett, 2005; Range et al., 2002). For these reasons, it is recommended that patients and therapists develop a collaborative safety plan in lieu of written or formal contracts. A safety plan differs from a no-suicide contract in that it outlines the steps agreed upon to ensure the safety of the patient in a suicidal crisis.

It is instructive that no-suicide contracts were originally developed as a method to assess suicide risk (Drye, Goulding, & Goulding, 1973). To the extent that patients cannot collaboratively develop a plan for safety and agree to refrain from efforts to kill themselves, they are by definition at imminent risk for suicidal behavior. Hence, regardless of whether clinicians use formal no-suicide contracts or develop safety plans, the fact that patients can or cannot agree to such terms provides important information about whether they are able to keep themselves safe.

Tasks for Assessing Imminent Suicidality

Bradley and Rotheram-Borus (1990) outlined five specific tasks (typically taking 20–30 minutes) to evaluate imminent danger of suicide among adolescents. The first task of the imminent danger assessment is to ascertain whether the adolescent is able to make positive statements about him- or herself; that is, adolescents should be able to recognize at least three positive attributes about themselves, their world, or at least about their interactions with

their therapist. Because most suicidal individuals tend to be entrenched in a negative and hopeless style of thinking, this task helps the clinician to evaluate the degree to which adolescents are in this negative mindset.

The second task in the assessment of imminent risk is to assess adolescents' capacity to assess their own feelings. In this regard, Rotheram (1987) suggests using a "feelings thermometer," wherein the adolescent can rate his or her feelings on a 0- to 100-point scale. The adolescent should be able to label both comfortable and uncomfortable feelings, and, specifically, should be able to label situations in which he or she has felt suicidal. To the degree that adolescents are able to recognize how they feel when they are becoming suicidal, they presumably will be better able to tell someone or take appropriate precautions to avoid acting on suicidal thoughts.

The third task used by Rotheram (1987) to assess current risk for suicide is to observe whether the adolescent is able to develop plans for coping with situations that have previously been (or might potentially be) associated with suicidal thoughts and feelings. This task is particularly useful in an emergency setting in which adolescents may state that they are no longer suicidal to avoid hospitalization or to stop further talk about the incident in front of family members. In their immediate desire to escape the situation, many adolescents may say that they are no longer suicidal, without having developed viable plans for dealing effectively with the situations that precipitated their suicidal behavior.

The fourth important task in the imminent danger assessment is the identification of three support individuals (Bradley & Rotheram-Borus, 1990). In this task, adolescents should be able to identify at least three individuals they can contact or speak with in the event that they are feeling suicidal or cannot keep themselves safe. The identification of support individuals is not only an assessment in and of itself (e.g., it is informative when individuals have so little perceived support that they cannot name three support people), but it also helps in the development of the therapeutic safety plan.

The fifth task in the evaluation of imminent danger is, of course, the solicitation of an agreement from the adolescent not to kill him- or herself, and an agreement to tell someone if he or she feels unable to stay safe. Rotheram (1987) suggests that "failure to perform these tasks is a behavioral indication of imminent danger; coping skills to ward off suicidal tendencies are not available" (p. 108).

Although these tasks are extremely useful in assessing risk, the clinician should consider other factors as well in evaluating whether someone is at imminent risk of self-harm. These factors include the youth's history, in particular, his or her history of suicidal behavior and adherence to safety agreements (e.g., reliability in letting others know when he or she feels suicidal), as well as parental history and capability of monitoring the adolescent and maintaining a safe environment in the home (e.g., making sure the adolescent does not have access to firearms when he or she is acutely suicidal). The final judgment of the clinician in assessing imminent danger to self should be made on the basis of all available information.

STANDARDIZED INSTRUMENTS FOR ASSESSING SELF-HARM BEHAVIORS AND RISK

There are a variety of instruments to screen and assess for suicidal or self-harm behavior among youths. Nonetheless, Prinstein, Nock, Spirito, and Grapentine (2001) have demonstrated that the agreement between different assessment instruments, methods, and sources of information in the assessment of suicidality is not always good. Hence, it behooves the clinician or researcher to obtain information from multiple sources, or to use multiple methods, basing final determination of clinical status on all available information.

One advantage to the use of standardized instruments is that they might help offset the unreliability of clinician judgment. For example, in a review of psychiatric assessments in an emergency setting, Way, Allen, Mumpower, Stewart, and Banks (1998) found that judgments about whether patients represented a "danger to themselves" were only modestly consistent among different clinicians (intraclass correlation coefficient = .44). Use of standardized instruments also may aid in the identification of suicidality that might otherwise not be detected (Malone, Szanto, Corbitt, & Mann, 1995). For example, hospital records of an adult sample indicated that clinicians failed to identify or document 12 of 50 instances in which patients were found to be depressed and to have histories of suicide attempts according to research assessments (Malone et al., 1995).

In considering instruments for assessing suicidality and risk among young people, Goldston (2003) recommended that four sets of question be asked. First, what is the level of precision in the definitions of suicidality? For example, are questions about suicidal thoughts separate from questions about thoughts of wanting to die or thoughts about death? Similarly, are there separate questions regarding suicidal and nonsuicidal self-harm behavior? Second, are items that assess whether the adolescent has engaged in suicidal behavior different or confounded by questions of degree of intent or the clinical characteristics of suicidal behavior? Instruments sometimes are designed to identify only suicidal behavior associated with "serious intent," despite the fact that findings regarding the relationship between intent and lethality among youth have not been consistent (DeMaso, Ross, & Beardslee, 1994; Lewinsohn et al., 1996; Nasser & Overholser, 1999; Plutchik, van Praag, Picard, Conte, & Korn, 1989). Third, is it clear from the queries that suicidal behavior is associated with "nonzero" intent to kill oneself? In this regard, queries assessing suicidality are sometimes worded so broadly (e.g., "Have you ever tried to hurt or harm yourself?") that they can elicit information about both suicidal and nonsuicidal self-harm. Finally, do questions about suicide attempt focus only on suicidal behavior that results in injury or requires medical attention? In the O'Carroll and colleagues (1996) recommended nomenclature, a suicide attempt by definition, does not have to result in injury; rather, it simply needs to be associated with the potential of injury. Restricting the focus to suicide attempts with injury excludes a subset of suicidal behavior, and the differences between suicide attempts that do and do not result in injury are not clear.

Detection Instruments

Detection instruments specifically assess current suicidality or self-harm behaviors, or one's history of such behavior. Some detection instruments focus on the assessment of suicidal behavior or thoughts but not on nonsuicidal self-harm or vice versa. In addition, some instruments focus on a continuum of severity of suicidality, whereas others focus on the presence or absence of self-harm behaviors or thoughts. Among the instruments used for detecting self-harm behaviors or thoughts are semistructured and structured psychiatric diagnostic instruments that have queries about self-harm, interviews developed specifically for assessing self-harm, self-report questionnaires or behavior checklists that include items assessing suicidality, or self-report questionnaires that focus solely on thoughts of self-harm or self-harm behaviors.

Although most psychiatric diagnostic interviews contain questions about suicidal ideation and attempts, two instruments in particular stand out because of the extent of their use and the amount of data available regarding their psychometric characteristics, the Schedule for Affective Disorders and Schizophrenia for School-Age Children—Epidemiological version (K-SADS-E) and the Diagnostic Interview Schedule for Children (DISC; see Goldston, 2003, for a comprehensive review of instruments for assessing suicidal behaviors and risk among children and adolescents).

The K-SADS-E (Orvaschel, 1994), a semistructured diagnostic interview for children and adolescents, provides interviewers the flexibility to clarify answers or ask questions beyond the required queries (Ambrosini, 2000). Interviewers for the K-SADS-E and other versions of the K-SADS are typically trained clinicians (Ambrosini, 2000). Because of the flexibility for additional questioning and clarification, and the use of clinicians as interviewers, the K-SADS-E can provide a systematic approach to assessment of psychiatric history in initial evaluations in clinical as well as research settings. The K-SADS-E typically takes between 2.5 and 3 hours to administer (Ambrosini, 2000) and has been used with youth in clinical (Brent et al., 1998), incarcerated (Rohde, Mace, & Seeley, 1997), and community (Lewinsohn et al., 1996) samples. The latest version of the K-SADS-E includes separate questions about recurrent thoughts of death, suicidal thoughts, suicide attempts, total number of past attempts, and nonsuicidal self-harm behavior. The query regarding suicide attempts ("Did you try to kill yourself?") is straightforward and implies a non-zero intent to kill oneself, without any reference to a requirement that the behavior results in injury. The question about suicidal ideation (thoughts about hurting or killing oneself) is so general that it likely elicits reports of thoughts of both suicidal and nonsuicidal self-harm.

The items regarding current thoughts of death and suicidal ideation, and past suicide attempt have high levels of interrater reliability (Lewinsohn, personal communication, September 1999). The suicidality items of the K-SADS-E have demonstrated concurrent validity, as reflected in associations with depression, poor coping skills, pessimism, and higher levels of suicidal ideation (Lewinsohn, Rohde, & Seeley, 1993; Rohde et al., 1997). In addition, these items have been found to be predictive of future suicidal behavior (Lewinsohn et al., 1994).

The DISC (Shaffer, Fisher, Lucas, Dulcan, & Schwab-Stone, 2000), a highly structured psychiatric diagnostic interview, has been used to evaluate suicidality in community- and school-based samples (Gould et al., 1998), clinical samples (Brent et al., 1986; Campbell, Milling, Laughlin, & Bush, 1993; King et al., 1997), and incarcerated samples (Kempton & Forehand, 1992) of youth. Although the structured format of the DISC makes possible its administration by individuals who do not necessarily have a clinical background, some training is required. The DISC takes approximately 1.5 to 2 hours for assessment of youth and approximately 1 hour for each informant (Shaffer et al., 2000).

The DISC has queries about thoughts of death, suicidal ideation, suicide plans, the association of suicidal thoughts with dysphoria, and lifetime number of suicide attempts. The DISC does not have queries about nonsuicidal self-harm behaviors, and the question asking the respondent whether he or she has "seriously" thought about suicide may yield conservative rates of suicidal thoughts. Although there is a separate question about suicide attempts requiring medical attention, the definition of "suicide attempts" is not confounded with a requisite degree of medical lethality or a requirement of injury. Moreover, the test–retest reliability of questions about suicide attempts is good to very good (Shaffer, personal communication, October 1999). In addition, DISC queries about suicidality have good concurrent validity, as evidenced by associations with "caseness" defined by cutoff scores on scales of suicidal ideation (King et al., 1997; Prinstein et al., 2001). Reports of current suicidal ideation and lifetime history of attempts were found to be related to subsequent suicidal behavior (Shaffer, personal communication, October 1999).

Interviews focused solely on assessment of suicidality or self-harm behaviors include the

Lifetime Parasuicide Count (LPC; Linehan & Comtois, 1997) and the Suicidal Behaviors Interview (SBI; Reynolds, 1989, 1990). The LPC was developed for adults and may be used to assess number of discrete episodes of both suicidal and nonsuicidal self-harm behaviors, although the instrument does not assess thoughts associated with self-harm. For most respondents, the LPC probably takes approximately 15 minutes or less (although administration time may vary with how well respondents remember the episodes and the number of self-harm episodes). Self-harm behaviors assessed with the LPC are classified as being associated with no intent to die (nonsuicidal self-harm), or with ambivalence and/or intent to die (both of the latter are considered to be suicide attempts). Relatively little psychometric information is available regarding the LPC, but it has been used in clinical settings, and adolescents with MDD, borderline personality disorder, and/or three or more Axis I psychiatric disorders were found to have more suicidal behaviors, as assessed with the LPC, than youth without these conditions (Velting & Miller, 1998).

The SBI, a 20-question semistructured interview, has been used with high-risk youth identified through screening evaluations in both school and clinical settings (Reynolds & Mazza, 1999). There are separate questions in the SBI about thoughts of wishing to be dead, thoughts of wanting to kill oneself, suicide attempts, and nonsuicidal self-harm behavior. The items regarding suicide attempts are consistent with the O'Carroll and colleagues (1996) nomenclature. The SBI has been found to have very high interrater reliability and internal consistency (Reynolds, 1990; Reynolds & Mazza, 1993), as well as considerable concurrent validity, as reflected in associations with number of past attempts, distress, and measures of depression (Champion, Carey, & Hodges, 1994; Reynolds, 1990; Reynolds & Mazza, 1999).

Depression questionnaires also often have items about suicidal thoughts that can be used as screens for the presence of suicidal ideation. For example, both the Beck Depression Inventory (BDI; Beck & Steer, 1987), which is appropriate for adolescents, and the Children's Depression Inventory (CDI), which is appropriate for children, have items assessing suicidal thoughts in the last 2 weeks. Both items assess severity of suicidal ideation, from no suicide ideation to thoughts of wanting to kill oneself (with no intent to do so), to a desire to kill oneself, if given the chance. These scales have been used in both community and clinical settings (Ivarsson, Gillbert, Arvidsson, & Broberg, 2002; Joiner, Rudd, Rouleau, & Wagner, 2000; Overholser, Adams, Lehnert, & Brinkman, 1995; Steer, Kumar, Ranieri, & Beck, 1998). Overholser and colleagues (1995) developed items that can be appended to the copyrighted version of the CDI to assess for previous suicidal behavior as well. This is particularly important, because suicidal thoughts may wax and wane over time, but past history of suicide attempts is one of the best predictors of future suicidal behavior (Joiner et al., 2005).

Several questionnaires of note have been developed specifically to assess severity of suicidal ideation or suicidal behaviors. The 14-item Suicidal Behaviors Questionnaire (SBQ-14) was developed to assess suicidal thoughts and behavior in adults (Linehan, 1996). A very brief, four-item version of the SBQ, the Suicidal Behaviors Questionnaire for Children (SBQ-C), was developed for use with children (Cotton & Range, 1993). Questions from the SBQ have been used with student (Cole, 1989a, 1989b; Osman et al., 1998), incarcerated (Cole, 1989b), and clinically ascertained samples (Kashden, Fremouw, Callahan, & Franzen, 1993; Osman et al., 1996). The SBQ-C has been used with children from both community and clinical settings (Payne & Billie, 1996). The SBQ-14 includes questions about frequency and intensity of suicidal ideation, suicide threats, suicide attempts and nonsuicidal self-harm behavior, and expectations about suicidal behavior. However, the initial question about suicidal ideation treats suicidal thoughts and suicide attempts as a continuum; one of the choices on this rating scale ("I attempted to kill myself, but I do not think I really meant to die") may be confusing in that suicide attempts are by definition considered to be associated with some intent to die. Items from the SBQ-14 have been shown to have concurrent validity, as reflected in correlations with rated reasons for living, depression, hopelessness, and impulsivity scales (Cole, 1989a, 1989b; Kashden et al., 1993; Osman et al., 1996, 1998). The four SBQ-C items are very similar to the items in the SBQ-14 that are used to assess suicidal thoughts and attempts, frequency of suicidal thoughts, telling others about suicidal thoughts, and expectations of suicide. However, the SBQ-C also includes the aforementioned potentially confusing query (from the SBQ-14) about suicide attempts without intent to die. The SBQ-C has been found to be internally consistent and scores on the SBQ-C have been found to be associated with depression and hopelessness scores (Payne & Billie, 1996).

The Beck Scale for Suicide Ideation (BSS; Beck & Steer, 1991), a questionnaire based on the interview-format Scale for Suicide Ideation (Beck, Kovacs, & Weissman, 1979), is one of the most widely used measures of suicidal ideation and includes items assessing passive suicidal ideation (when respondents state that they do not think they would take steps to save themselves if in harm's way). The scale also has one item assessing history of attempts. The BSS has been found to be internally consistent in clinical samples of adolescents (Kumar & Steer, 1995; Steer, Kumar, & Beck, 1993), but it is not clear whether it has been used with community samples. Severity scores on the BSS are predictably related to constructs such as depression, hopelessness, and another measure of suicidal thoughts (Kumar & Steer, 1995; Reinecke, DuBois, & Schultz, 2001; Steer et al., 1993).

The Suicidal Ideation Questionnaire (SIQ) was developed for use with high school youth, and the Suicidal Ideation Questionnaire—Junior (SIQ-JR), for use with junior high school (grades 7, 8, and 9) youth (Reynolds, 1988). Both scales assess a continuum of severity of thoughts of death to active suicidal ideation. Cutoffs on these scales denote clinically suicidal thoughts. One limitation of the scales when used as stand-alone screeners is that they do not include any items assessing suicidal or nonsuicidal self-harm behaviors. These reliable, highly internally consistent scales have been used in multiple clinical and nonclinical (primarily school) settings (Dick, Beals, Manson, & Bechtold, 1994; Hewitt, Newton, Flet, & Callander, 1997; Pinto, Whisman, & McCoy, 1997; Reynolds, 1988; Reynolds & Mazza, 1999). The scales have been well validated, as exemplified by correlations with depression, hopelessness, reasons for living, suicide attempts, and scores on other suicidality measures (Hewitt et al., 1997; King, Raskin, Gdowski, Butkus, & Opipari, 1990; Mazza, 2000; Pinto & Whisman, 1996; Pinto, Whisman, & Conwell, 1998; Reinecke et al., 2001; Reynolds, 1988). SIQ-JR scores also

have been found to predict later suicide attempts (King et al., 1995).

The Functional Assessment of Self-Harm (FASM; Lloyd, Kelley, & Hope, 1997) is a self-report instrument used to assess types and frequency of self-harm behavior (e.g., cutting and carving on oneself, pulling hair, biting self, "erasing skin," picking at wound, hitting self on purpose) during the past year. Questions on this instrument assess whether the self-harm behaviors are nonsuicidal or suicidal in nature, whether the respondent was using alcohol or drugs while engaging in self-harm, whether the self-harm was impulsive, and age of first self-harm. For treatment planning purposes, the scale additionally includes questions about the different anticipated functions of the self-harm behavior. The FASM has been used both with clinical and nonclinical samples of adolescents, and its scales have adequate internal consistency (Guertin et al., 2001; Lloyd et al., 1997; Nock & Prinstein, 2004, 2005).

Assessment in Prediction of Suicidality

Assessment of risk for future suicidality is also an important task for the practicing clinician. Risk assessment instruments are developed primarily to assess risk of future suicidality or to screen for individuals who may be at risk for suicidality. Despite the availability of a number of risk assessment instruments to assist clinicians in assessing risk, it is notable that many clinicians who work with suicidal clients do not routinely incorporate assessment instruments into their practice (Jobes, Eyman, & Yufit, 1995). Perhaps the most important function of a risk assessment instrument is the degree to which it is actually predictive of later suicidal behavior (i.e., has established predictive validity; Goldston, 2003). Many available risk assessment instruments have been shown to have only cross-sectional, rather than predictive, associations with suicidal behaviors. Nonetheless, not every factor associated with suicidal thoughts or behavior at a single point in time is related to later suicidal behavior.

Risk assessment instruments include several self-report questionnaires. Some of these focus on specific constructs associated with vulnerability and protective factors for suicidal behavior, whereas others include combinations of different risk and protective factors. With regard to self-report questionnaires, some of the most promising instruments focus on the assessment of cognitive states associated with suicidality. For example, the Beck Hopelessness Scale (BHS; Beck & Steer, 1988; Beck, Weissman, Lester, & Trexler, 1974; Steer & Beck, 1988), which was developed for adults, has also been used with adolescents in school and clinical settings for the assessment of pessimism or hopeless attitudes about the future (Brent et al., 1997, 1998; Goldston et al., 2001; Osman et al., 1998; Rotheram-Borus & Trautman, 1988). The BHS has been found to be internally consistent in samples of clinically ascertained suicidal adolescents (Steer et al., 1993), and to have a wealth of concurrent validity, as reflected in associations with assessments of depression, fewer reasons for living, and history of suicide attempts (Goldston et al., 2001; Osman et al., 1998; Reinecke et al., 2001). Most importantly, among outpatient adults, the BHS has been found to predict later suicide over a 20-year period of time (Brown, Beck, Steer, & Grisham, 2000), and in formerly hospitalized adolescents and adults in clinical settings, higher BHS scores have been found to predict repeat suicide attempts (Brittlebank et al., 1990; Goldston et al., 2001; Scott, House, Yates, & Harrington, 1997). Higher BHS scores also have been found to be associated with earlier discontinuation of treatment for depression among adolescents (Brent et al., 1997).

A child version of the BHS for youth as young as ages 6–13, the Hopelessness Scale for Children (HSC), has been developed (Kazdin, Rodgers, & Colbus, 1986) for assessments with children and adolescents in school and clinical settings (Asarnow & Guthrie, 1989; Cole, 1989a, 1989b; Hewitt et al., 1997; Kashani, Suarez, Allan, & Reid, 1997; Nock & Kazdin, 2002; Reifman & Windle, 1995). Particularly in clinical samples, the HSC has been found to be highly internally consistent (Kazdin et al., 1986; Spirito, Williams, Stark, & Hart, 1988). Similar to the BHS, a number of studies have documented the relationship between hopelessness assessed with the HSC and depression and fewer reasons for living (Asarnow & Guthrie, 1989; Cole, 1989a, 1989b; Pinto et al., 1998). However, findings are mixed pertaining to whether HSC scores are related to indices of suicidality cross-sectionally after controlling for depression (Asarnow & Guthrie, 1989; Cole, 1989a; Myers, McCauley, Calderon, Mitchell, et al., 1991; Nock & Kazdin, 2002). In one study of

hospitalized adolescents, HSC scores were found to predict suicide attempts within 18 months (Brinkman-Sull, Overholser, & Silverman, 2000). However, HSC scores were not related to subsequent suicidality in another study (Myers, McCauley, Calderon, & Treder, 1991).

As mentioned earlier, perceived reasons for living have been found to be a protective factor against suicide. The 48-item Reasons for Living Inventory (RFL-48), originally developed for assessing perceptions of reasons for not killing oneself in adult populations (Linehan, Goodstein, Nielsen, & Chiles, 1983), has also been used with adolescents (Goldston et al., 2001). Additional versions of this scale have been developed, including two versions specifically for use with adolescents: the Reasons for Living Inventory for Adolescents (RFL-A; Osman et al., 1998), and the Brief Reasons for Living Inventory for Adolescents (BRFL-A; Osman et al., 1996). Each version of the RFL has different subscales. However, on the RFL-48, the items on the Survival and Coping Beliefs subscale have the highest internal consistency (Pinto et al., 1998), and seem to be most highly related (in cross-sectional analyses) to suicidality, after controlling for severity of depression and hopelessness (Cole, 1989b). In a longitudinal study of formerly psychiatrically hospitalized adolescents, higher RFL-48 Survival and Coping Beliefs subscale scores were associated with fewer repeat suicide attempts over the course of the follow-up (Goldston et al., 2001). In cross-sectional studies, many of the subscales of the RFL-A and the BRFL-A were also predictably associated with constructs such as estimated suicide probability, suicidal ideation, and hopelessness (Gutierrez, Osman, Kopper, & Barrios, 2000; Osman et al., 1996, 1998). However, these latter RFL versions have not been demonstrated to be predictive of future suicidality (Goldston, 2003).

The BHS, HSC, and various versions of the RFL questionnaires are but a few of myriad risk assessment instruments available (Goldston, 2003). However, these questionnaires are among the very few that have demonstrated predictive validity, and, in at least some samples, scores on these questionnaires have been shown to predict later suicidal behavior. In addition, these questionnaires are brief and can be administered easily in school or clinical settings, typically taking 5–10 minutes for completion. Importantly, hopelessness and reasons for living in particular have the additional advantage of being easily targeted in treatments for suicidality. For example, a clinician may use cognitive therapy to help modify the maladaptive negative thoughts associated with hopelessness, and a variety of clinical approaches to strengthen existing reasons for living or develop new reasons for living.

A number of multistage screening procedures have been developed to assess suicide risk. Multistage approaches are advantageous insofar as screening with single instruments often results in unacceptable numbers of false positives (individuals identified as being "at risk" who are not at serious risk). Screening assessments are an integral part of suicide prevention efforts that focus on identifying individuals at risk in order to provide referrals to treatment or indicate selective prevention efforts. The first multistage suicide assessment system includes the Columbia Suicide Screen and the DISC (Shaffer & Craft, 1999; Shaffer, Wilcox, et al., 1996). The Columbia Suicide Screen is an 11-item self-report instrument that assesses suicide attempts and suicidal ideation, negative mood, substance abuse, and whether the respondent has a self-perceived need for treatment and is or is not receiving treatment (Shaffer et al., 2004). The algorithm for identifying risk on the Columbia Suicide Screen with the best balance between sensitivity and specificity yielded 75% sensitivity and 83% specificity (Shaffer et al., 2004). However, the 8-day test–retest reliability of this algorithm was only in the "fair" range (Altman, 1991), largely due to symptom attenuation (reduction of symptoms reporting at a second assessment). As noted by Shaffer and colleagues (2004), the significance of the drop-off in responding at a second assessment point is unclear, as is whether the initial or second assessment time points were more "valid." Because of these questions and the possibility for a large number of false positives when screening large groups of students (as is typically done with the Columbia Suicide Screen), it is recommended that the DISC be used as a second-stage screening to identify appropriate students (Shaffer et al., 2004). On the basis of these results, the clinician can meet individually with at-risk students to determine whether they need referrals for treatment. The Columbia Suicide Screen method is being increasingly disseminated and is capable of identifying many at-risk students in need of services. It is less clear whether referral to treatment actually reduces their risk for suicidal behavior, and studies are currently underway to examine this possibility. One practical concern that is sometimes voiced about large-scale screenings for suicide risk, such as the Columbia Suicide Screen, is that the number of students identified may potentially overwhelm school counselors' offices. Hence, it is important to ensure that resources are in place to meet the needs of newly identified at-risk students, and that referrals for treatment are available for students in need.

A second multistage screening assessment includes the Evaluation of Suicide Risk among Adolescents and the Imminent Danger Assessment (Bradley & Rotheram-Borus, 1990; Rotheram, 1987; Rotheram-Borus, 1989). The first-stage screening instrument may be used to help identify adolescents who are suicidal or at risk for suicidal behavior. This instrument includes a number of questions about both suicidality (e.g., lifetime suicide ideation and attempts, recent suicide attempts, exposure to suicidal behavior), and symptoms of depression and conduct disorder. Individuals who screen positive in the first-stage evaluation may then be evaluated with the Imminent Danger Assessment, described earlier in the section on assessing imminent risk of suicide. Interrater reliability for this set of assessment procedures was found to be very high (Rotheram-Borus & Bradley, 1991). These screening procedures have been used in settings with high-risk adolescents, including runaway teenagers, GLB teenagers, and teenagers who present for crisis services (Rotheram-Borus & Bradley, 1991; Rotheram-Borus, Hunter, & Rosario, 1994; Rotheram-Borus, Walker, & Ferns, 1996).

A third multistage screening assessment includes the High School Questionnaire (with the embedded Suicide Risk Screen [SRS]) and the Measure of Adolescent Potential for Suicide (MAPS) (Eggert, Thompson, & Herting, 1994; Eggert, Thompson, Herting, & Nicholas, 1995; Thompson & Eggert, 1999). In the first part of this assessment, adolescents are asked to complete the High School Questionnaire. Embedded within it are items assessing current suicidal thoughts and behavior, depression, and alcohol or substance use. Individuals who are considered at risk on the basis of the initial screen are then administered the MAPS via computer. The MAPS, a 2-hour assessment, covers "direct suicide risk factors" (e.g., suicidal thoughts, suicidal behaviors, exposure to suicide, preparation for suicide), "related risk factors" (e.g., depression, hopelessness, substance abuse, school dropout risk), and protective factors (e.g., self-esteem, support from others, sense of personal control). This screening system has been used to identify students thought to be at high risk for engaging in suicidal behavior in the schools (Eggert et al., 1994, 1995; Thompson & Eggert, 1999; Thompson, Eggert, & Herting, 2000; Thompson, Eggert, Randell, & Pike, 2001). Classifications of risk made with the SRS were found to be differentially and predictably related to both an independent measure of suicidal ideation and clinicians' judgments of risk (Thompson & Eggert, 1999). Ratings on the MAPS scales had correlations ranging from .52 to .79 with a scale of "suicide potential" (Eggert et al., 1994). Although this screening assessment is advantageous because of its assessment of multiple risk behaviors and its integration with a brief supportive intervention, difficulties may be encountered in its implementation or in sustaining its use in the school systems because of the large number of false positives associated with the first stage of screening (Hallfors et al., 2006).

The final multistage assessment combines the SIQ and the SBI (Reynolds, 1991). This multistage assessment differs from the others insofar as it focuses primarily on suicidal thoughts and suicidal behaviors rather than other risk and protective factors. Both of the instruments used in this multistage assessment have excellent psychometric properties and were described previously. However, Reynolds has suggested that screenings with the SIQ alone can result in an unacceptable number of false positives; for example, approximately 10% of screened adolescents tend to score above the cutoff (Reynolds, 1991). Hence, it is useful to follow up with more detailed assessment of suicidality and risk in individuals identified as suicidal in the initial screen. A potential difficulty with this approach is that the initial screen (the SIQ) assesses suicidal thoughts but not suicidal behavior (Goldston, 2003). Given that suicidal ideation may fluctuate over time, even among individuals with histories of suicidal behaviors, this screening approach may miss adolescents at high risk for subsequent suicidality by virtue of their past suicidal behaviors (Goldston, 2003).

Assessment of the Clinical Characteristics of Self-Harm Behaviors

The clinical characteristics of suicide attempts (e.g., stated intent, medical lethality) are often considered to be good indicators of risk for future suicidal behavior by treatment providers. For example, in a survey of psychologists, Peruzzi and Bongar (1999) found that "medical seriousness of past attempts" was rated the most important or critical factor by psychologists in estimating the degree of risk for suicidal behavior in a hypothetical patient with major depression. As described by Goldston (2003), a number of instruments assess clinical characteristics of suicidal behavior, such as intent or medical lethality. These instruments may be useful for descriptive purposes, in particular, for capturing the "topography" of suicidal behavior, such as methods, degree of planning, and so on—information that may be of use in treatment planning. In some cases, clinical characteristics have been found to be related to later suicidal behaviors in adult populations. However, the relationship between clinical characteristics of suicidal behavior and either the occurrence of future suicidal behavior among adolescents or the clinical characteristics of future suicidal behavior has not yet been demonstrated empirically (Goldston, 2003).

Examples of two instruments that assess clinical characteristics of suicidal behavior are the Beck Suicide Intent Scale (SIS; Beck, Schuyler, & Herman, 1974) and the Lethality of Suicide Attempt Rating Scale (Smith, Conroy, & Ehler, 1984). The SIS is administered as a semistructured interview and is considered by its authors to be appropriate for both adolescents and adults (Steer & Beck, 1988). The SIS comprises two parts—one assessing the objective intent associated with a suicide attempt, and the other assessing subjective intent. The part that assesses objective intent focuses on aspects of the suicidal behavior or context that can be observed, such as precautions taken against discovery, amount of planning, communications to others, and whether a suicide note was left. The section assessing subjective indications of intent includes the perceived seriousness of the suicide attempt and whether the respondent expected to die. The SIS has been used in clinical settings with adolescents who attempt suicide (Groholt, Ekeberg, & Haldorsen, 2000; Hawton, Kingsbury, Steinhardt,

James, & Fagg, 1999; Kingsbury, 1993; Nock & Kazdin, 2002; Spirito et al., 1994, 1996) and has been shown to have good interrater reliability (Brent et al., 1988). The subjective portion of the scale, in particular, was found to be internally consistent (Spirito et al., 1996). In one study, the two sections of the SIS were not strongly associated (Kingsbury, 1993), raising questions about the degree to which they are tapping into the same construct. SIS scores have concurrent validity, as evidenced by correlations with hopelessness, depression severity, and suicidal ideation constructs (DeMaso et al., 1994; Enns, Inayatulla, Cox, & Cheyne, 1997; Nock & Kazdin, 2002; Spirito et al., 1996). Among adults, suicide intent in previous suicide attempts, as assessed with the SIS, has been found to be related to eventual death by suicide (Harriss, Hawton, & Zahl, 2005; Suominen, Isometsa, Ostamo, & Lonnqvist, 2004), although the positive predictive value of intent as a predictor was low (Harriss et al., 2005). In adolescents, intent did not differentiate between single and repeat attempters in a 1-year follow-up (Hawton et al., 1999), nor was it related to repeat suicide attempts in a 3-month follow-up (Spirito et al., 1994).

The Lethality of Suicide Attempt Rating Scale (Smith et al., 1984), a clinician-rated scale of degree of medical lethality resulting from suicide attempts, has been used with adolescents in various settings (Lewinsohn, Rohde, & Seeley, 1993; Lewinsohn et al., 1994, 1996) and has demonstrated both good interrater reliability (Nasser & Overholser, 1999; Smith et al., 1984) and 6-month test–retest reliability (Nasser & Overholser, 1999). Higher ratings of medical lethality have been found to be related to more severe depression (Lewinsohn et al., 1996) and indications of higher suicide intent, such as taking precautions to prevent discovery, not communicating with others about the attempt, and higher expectations of death associated with attempts (Nasser & Overholser, 1999). Nonetheless, the predictive validity of the Lethality of Suicide Attempt Rating Scale with adolescents has yet to be examined.

ASSESSMENT FOR TREATMENT MONITORING

Several instruments may be used in clinical settings to monitor the process of treatment and clinical outcomes. For example, if the purpose of an intervention is to reduce the severity of an adolescent's suicidal thoughts, detection instruments may be used to monitor the course of suicidality or the effectiveness of the intervention. Additionally, it may be the case that an adolescent who is not suicidal at the beginning of an intervention needs to be monitored for the emergence of suicidality, because he or she is depressed or is receiving medications. Close monitoring is particularly important in conjunction with pharmacotherapy given recent findings of self-harm adverse events associated with antidepressant medications in youth (FDA, 2004; TADS Team, 2004). Finally, risk factors associated with suicidality are sometimes the target of treatment. For example, treatment may focus on the reduction of a factor, or set of factors, such as hopelessness. One of the most important considerations in choosing an instrument for treatment monitoring is sensitivity to changes in clinical status.

The two detection instruments that have been used most commonly for treatment monitoring are the BSS and the SIQ, both of which have been described previously (Beck & Steer, 1991; Reynolds, 1988). The BSS assesses suicidal ideation over the last week, whereas the SIQ assesses suicidal thoughts over the last month. With both the BSS and the SIQ, the clinician should also monitor suicide attempts since the last assessment. The SIQ does not include an item regarding self-harm behavior, and the single item regarding past attempts on the BSS may not be sensitive to recurrent suicidal behaviors.

The BSS was used successfully in a quasi-experimental study of dialectical behavior therapy (DBT) to demonstrate pre- to posttreatment reductions in suicidal ideation (Rathus & Miller, 2002). The SIQ was used to compare the effectiveness of DBT and treatment as usual (TAU) in an inpatient setting; both DBT and TAU resulted in significant reductions in suicidal ideation (Katz, Cox, Gunasekara, & Miller, 2004). No differences were found in SIQ suicidal ideation scores between adolescents randomized to routine care and those in routine care plus home visits and family intervention, although scores decreased in both groups over time (Harrington et al., 1998). However, in subgroup analyses, there were lower suicidal ideation scores in the experimental group condition relative to those in the routine care alone for youth without major depression; there were no treatment effects for youth with major depression (Harrington et al., 1998). In an open trial of fluoxetine for depression in adolescents, the medication resulted in significant reductions in SIQ-assessed suicidal thoughts for seven of the eight patients (Colle, Belair, DiFeo, Weiss, & LaRoche, 1994). In the TADS, 439 adolescents were randomized to four conditions: fluoxetine (and general support), placebo (and general support), cognitive-behavioral therapy, and combined fluoxetine and cognitive-behavioral therapy (TADS Team, 2004). Twelve weeks after the initiation of treatment, suicidal ideation, as assessed with the SIQ-JR, had been reduced in all four conditions. However, there were differences in the rates of reductions of suicidal ideation, with the combination treatment group evidencing greater rates of change than the placebo group, and the other two groups evidencing rates of change that did not differ significantly from placebo (TADS Team, 2004).

Hopelessness is a risk factor that has been targeted in different interventions, with the goal of reducing suicidality. A suicide prevention intervention in Israel resulted in reductions in hopelessness as assessed with the BHS for targeted students in some, but not all, schools in which the intervention was used (Orbach & Bar-Joseph, 1993). Formerly hospitalized suicidal teenagers receiving individual and family therapy evidenced reductions in BHS scores from initial assessments to 6-month follow-up later; similar changes in hopelessness were not evident for teenagers who declined treatment (Pillay & Wassenaar, 1995). Hopelessness as assessed with the HSC did not differ as an outcome between suicidal adolescents randomized to routine care and those randomized to routine care plus an in-home family intervention (Harrington et al., 1998).

ASSESSMENT FOR TREATMENT PLANNING PURPOSES: THE FUNCTIONAL ANALYSIS

There is much heterogeneity among youths who engage in self-harm behavior, and it is unlikely that a single intervention approach will be effective with every adolescent. Developing a functional analysis for an individual who is suicidal or self-harming is useful for understanding the context of self-harm behavior and may be helpful in developing an individualized, targeted treatment plan. One approach to

the development of a functional analysis is the S-O-R-C (stimulus–organism–response–consequences) model described by Goldfried and Sprafkin (1976). In the S-O-R-C model, the S refers to the discriminative stimuli or triggers thought to be associated with the behavior of interest (self-harm behavior). The O refers to vulnerability or protective factors that are specific to the organism or individual. These factors may moderate or mediate the relationship between the precipitants in the environment and the likelihood of a response of interest (suicidal or nonsuicidal self-harm behavior) occurring. For example, it may be the case that an adolescent attempts suicide in the aftermath of a breakup with a romantic partner. Clearly, not every adolescent attempts suicide when breaking off a relationship, so there must be factors that increase or decrease the likelihood of suicidal behavior occurring in the presence of those environmental events. The R in the S-O-R-C model represents the response of interest, in this case, suicidal or nonsuicidal self-harm behavior, and the topography of the responses (e.g., methods). The C in the model represents consequences that occur after an individuals engages in the self-harm behavior.

To illustrate how the functional analysis may be used in treatment planning, consider the S part of the model. The most common precipitants for suicidal behavior in adolescents are interpersonal loss or conflict and disciplinary or legal action (Adams et al., 1994; Beautrais et al., 1997; Gould et al., 1996). With information about the specific precipitants, the clinician can help the adolescent anticipate such situations and develop strategies for coping with or avoiding problematic situations. Alternatively, the clinician can help the adolescent ascertain whether the initial precipitating crisis has been resolved or is likely to recur, and plan steps to ensure that there is not a recurrence of these difficulties (e.g., family therapy to reduce the likelihood of arguments in the home).

With regard to the O part of the model, there are a number of risk and protective factors for suicidal behaviors, as described earlier in this chapter. With knowledge of these risk and protective factors on an individual basis, the clinician may focus on helping the adolescent to decrease risk and enhance protective factors. For example, an adolescent may evidence markedly poor problem-solving skills in the face of high levels or distress, and may fail to perceive that behavioral options other than continued misery or suicide exist. In such a case, the clinician can focus on problem-solving ability, working with the adolescent specifically to develop facility in generating and adopting alternative solutions to different problems. The clinician may try to reduce dysregulation of mood by focusing on associated cognitions with cognitive-behavioral approaches, or may focus on problematic patterns in relationships and role transitions that contribute to distress with interpersonal approaches. Alternatively, the clinician may help the adolescent to recognize or develop reasons for living, to plan for the future, or to participate in activities that may lead to increased positive social support.

Information about the response (self-harm behavior) itself can provide potentially useful information for treatment planning purposes. For example, with regard to information about the methods used, no research, to our knowledge, has demonstrated that individuals are more likely to choose the suicide method they used previously relative to other methods. However, the fact that the youth has used this method previously does let the clinician know that this method is in the youth's behavioral repertoire; there no longer is any doubt that the youth is capable of using this method to engage in self-harm. Similarly, suicidal thoughts and preparatory behaviors antecedent to actual suicide attempts may provide useful information about what the adolescent is considering, or how he or she goes about planning for suicide. The clinician may incorporate such information into safety planning, for example, restricting access to certain methods. For example, if an adolescent has thought about or tried to wreck a car as a way to attempt suicide, it makes sense to restrict access to the automobile and to driving, until the adolescent is no longer feeling suicidal.

Last, there are always consequences (the C in the functional analysis) following self-harm behavior. To the extent that the self-harm behavior results in a reduction in negative mood (e.g., relief or catharsis), the response will have been negatively reinforced. To the extent that self-harm behavior results in attention or support from peers or family that otherwise was not available, or to the extent that a difficult situation becomes resolved (because everyone realizes how "upset" the individual is), the response will be positively reinforced. In both cases, from a behavioral perspective, the response (self-harm) is more likely to occur when the individual is once again in the presence of the discriminative stimuli, because of the reinforcing consequences. To this end, the therapist may work to reduce sources of positive attention for self-harm behavior or to help the adolescent develop new behaviors that yield the same consequences of support or relief.

The Functional Analysis and Psychiatric Comorbidities

As described by Goldston (2004), when suicidal or self-harm behavior is comorbid with psychiatric disorders, for treatment planning purposes it often is useful to identify the functional similarities of the co-occurring problems. For example, to varying degrees, suicidal behavior may have antecedents, risk and protective factors, or consequences similar to the other problem behaviors. To the extent that such functional commonalities may be identified, chances of developing an integrated treatment approach increase and interventions may be selected to impact multiple problem areas.

An example of a functional analysis focusing on the similarities between suicidal behaviors and substance abuse is presented in Figure 7.1. The information presented in the boxes is the actual functional analysis (the precipitants, risk and protective factors, consequences, etc.). In the circles are examples of interventions that may be used to target different aspects of the functional analysis to reduce suicidal and substance use behaviors. The arrows from the circles to the boxes illustrate targeted aspects of the context of the problem behaviors.

As an illustration, for a particular teen, the antecedents of both suicidal behaviors and substance use may be chronic arguments with parents. Based on this analysis, the clinician can choose an intervention that focuses on reducing the pattern of conflict between the adolescent and parents. The adolescent may have poor problem-solving skills that make it difficult to choose alternative behaviors in stressful situations. The clinician may provide problem-solving training or help the adolescent to anticipate difficult situations, so that he or she can plan accordingly. To the extent that an adolescent engages in both substance use and self-harm behaviors to reduce negative affect (i.e., "self-medicates"), the clinician can focus on helping him or her to learn new coping strategies (e.g., relaxation techniques, meditation) to reduce or to help the adolescent "let go" of unpleasant feelings or increase positive feelings.

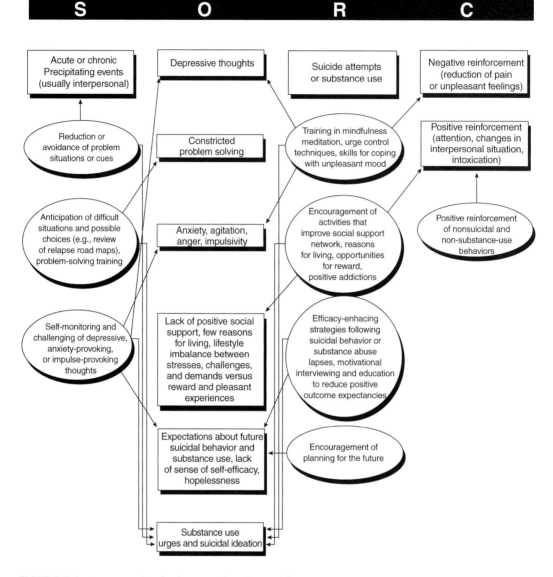

FIGURE 7.1. An example of a functional analysis of factors potentially affecting both suicidal behavior and substance use, and possible targets for intervention. From Goldston (2004). Copyright 2004 by Elsevier. Reprinted by permission.

The Functional Analysis and Cultural Considerations

A number of cultural differences and nuances in the context of suicidal behavior should be considered in assessment. These cultural differences in suicidal behavior and its context may also be described with the functional analytic model (Goldston et al., under review). For example, in terms of triggers, Asian Americans may experience "loss of face" when they do not meet expectations for their behavior or they "upset group harmony" (Zane & Mak, 2003). Loss of face in turn can be associated with depression and suicidal behavior. In another example, Zayas, Lester, Cabassa, and Fortuna (2005) noted that among Latinas, the precipitants for suicidal behavior often occur in the context of the family and may manifest as conflicts between the culture of origin and majority culture in areas such as role expectations and socialization (e.g., the centrality of the family, independence, dating).

In terms of vulnerability and protective factors, numerous examples of cultural nuances and differences should be considered in assessment related to suicidal risk. For example, among Native Americans, a sense of loss due to a history of forced relocations, suppression of traditional language and religion, and attempts at forced acculturation (e.g., boarding schools) is believed to be associated with hopelessness or demoralization (Brave Heart, 1998; 1999; Duran & Duran, 1995; O'Nell, 1993). Conversely, enculturation, or the degree to which an individual is involved in his or her traditional native activities or religion, or with tribal elders or extended family (Whitbeck, Adams, Hoyt, & Chen, 2004) may help to protect against mental health problems or suicidality (Goldston et al., under review). Similarly, among African Americans and other ethnic groups, perceived discrimination and racism may be associated with increased stress (Clark, Anderson, Clark, & Williams, 1999), and increased risk factors for suicidal behavior, such as hopelessness and increased substance use (Gibbons, Gerrard, Cleveland, Wills, & Brody, 2004; Nyborg & Curry, 2003; Wong, Eccles, & Sameroff, 2003). Nonetheless, the cultural cohesion of stable African American communities and extended family may help to impart a greater sense of ethnic identity, which in turn protects against various problem behaviors (Wong et al., 2003). Among both Latino and Asian American communities, acculturative stress may result in discrepancies in values, expectations for behaviors, and roles between the country of origin (or the parents' country of origin) and the majority culture. Such conflicts may increase distress and risk for suicidal behavior (e.g., Hovey, 2000a, 2000b).

The reactions to suicide and suicidal behavior in different cultures vary. For example, it has been noted that African American women sometimes "normalize" distress (Brown, Abe-Kin, & Barrio, 2003) and associated problems such as depression, considering such difficulties to be a "normal" part of day-to-day living that may be overcome through hard work and determination (Breland-Noble, 2004). Asian American families may be reluctant to talk about suicide because they fear the shame it will bring to the family (Morrison & Downey, 2000). Latino families may interpret suicidal behaviors as part of a cultural syndrome associated with distress, *ataques de nervios* (Zayas et al., 2005). In each of these cases, the cultural context tends to mitigate against seeking professional help for suicidal behaviors. Hence, careful assessment of the cultural context and reactions to suicidal behavior is critical to develop culturally relevant treatment plans to engage and retain individuals from diverse backgrounds.

ETHICAL CONSIDERATIONS IN ASSESSMENT AND MONITORING OF SUICIDAL PATIENTS

Careful assessment and monitoring of suicidal behaviors and risk are ethically mandated in clinical care. Berman, Jobes, and Silverman (2006) have pointed out that in general, two major issues are associated with liability in the care of suicidal patients. The first is *foreseeability*; that is, it is incumbent upon the health care provider to evaluate risk for suicidality by obtaining relevant history, current suicidal thoughts and intent, and information about risk factors for suicidal behaviors. This information should come from multiple sources, if possible, but particularly from direct interview and assessments with the adolescent patient and his or her parents or guardians. Foreseeability refers not only to the assessment of suicidal behaviors and risk at an initial assessment, but particularly for patients who are currently suicidal or thought to be at risk, also to an ongoing process of risk assessment.

In the second issue of liability, *reasonable care* (Berman, Jobes, & Silverman, 2006), the clinician should take appropriate and adequate steps to ensure development of a treatment plan to reduce the patient's suicidality and associated problems. This treatment plan should include steps by the clinician to assess safety issues and to develop an adequate safety plan that includes monitoring younger patients and removing means for attempting suicide. If the patient is not responding to treatment, the clinician should evaluate adequacy of the treatment approach. The instruments described in this chapter can help in the assessment of progress or adequacy of treatment over time. Reasonableness of care also refers to the ethical mandate not to abandon patients, particularly high-risk or suicidal patients.

As described earlier, one of the most important tasks for a clinician is the assessment of imminent risk for suicidal behaviors. In this regard, when an adolescent is imminently dangerous to him- or herself, confidentiality should be broken to ensure that parents or guardians are informed of the situation, and the patient is monitored adequately. The breaking of confidentiality when patients pose a danger to themselves is consistent with the ethical guidelines of the American Psychological Association and the American Psychiatric Association. In terms of reasonableness of care, clinicians should try to resolve crises or decrease distress without higher levels of care, but referral for evaluation of the need for hospitalization is sometimes necessary to ensure that the patient remains safe.

BEST-PRACTICES APPROACH TO EVALUATING SUICIDALITY IN CLINICAL PRACTICE

To summarize, there are multiple purposes and considerations in assessing suicidal and nonsuicidal self-harm behaviors and risk. Far too often, suicidal and nonsuicidal self-harm behaviors are simply not assessed, even in clinical settings, for a variety of reasons. This lack of assessment, particularly with youth known to have psychiatric, behavioral, or substance use difficulties, and especially with youth suspected of having depression or a high level of distress, is negligent and even dangerous. Hence, the first "best practice recommendation" is that self-harm behaviors and ideation about self-harm be routinely assessed in all youth in clinical settings, or known to have behavioral, emotional, or substance abuse problems, regardless of whether the "presenting problem" described by the youth or parents concerns suicidality. For youth with depression, a high degree of problem severity (e.g., as indicated by comorbidities or psychiatric hospitalization), a history of self-harm behavior (no matter how remote), or for youth receiving pharmacological treatment for depression, continued and ongoing monitoring of self-harm behavior and risk is recommended.

Youth often report considerably more self-harm behavior or thoughts of self-harm than adults in their lives report about them. Hence, a second best-practice recommendation is that assessment of suicidal behavior and risk should always include direct reports from youth themselves. Ideally, suicide assessments should include multiple methods (e.g., interview, observations, questionnaires) and multiple informants, but reports of the youth should always be considered. Granted, there may be occasions in which youth deny suicidal intent or provide "mixed signals" about their risk or suicidal intent; in such cases, the clinicians should always err on the side of safety and of being conservative, because the risks of not acting in such a matter (e.g., someone killing themselves) are simply too high.

In assessing imminent risk of self-harm, particularly in emergency settings, a third best-practice recommendation is that the clinician should consider youth reports not only about suicide intent (because he or she may be denying suicidality out of embarrassment or a desire to avoid hospitalization) but also about available support individuals, and whether the adolescent can articulate credible alternatives to suicidal behavior if crises continue or recur. Other factors that should be considered include youth history of self-harm, and parents' ability to monitor the youth and maintain a safe environment in the home.

A fourth best-practice recommendation is that when specific interviews, screens, or questionnaires are used to help in the detection of suicidality, clinicians use instruments that are known to be valid and to be reliable. Such detection instruments include diagnostic interviews such as the DISC and the K-SADS, interviews focused specifically on self-harm such as the SBI, and questionnaires such as the BSS and the SIQ. The latter two instruments have also proven to be useful in treatment monitoring.

A fifth best-practice recommendation is that when clinicians use "risk assessment" instruments to evaluate risk or self-harm behavior, the chosen instruments should be reliable and have predictive validity (which far too often is not the case). Available instruments that assess risk variables, such as hopelessness and severity of depression, and protective variables, such as perceived reasons for living, have demonstrated predictive validity with youth. In assessing risk, the clinician also should remember that many "detection instruments" have predictive validity insofar as past suicidal behavior is one the best predictors of future suicidal behavior. Information about clinical characteristics of past suicidal behavior, such as medical lethality or stated intent, should not be considered in risk assessments until such time that those clinical characteristics have actually been shown in prospective studies to portend higher risk among youth.

A sixth and final best-practice recommendation is that rather than a be-all and end-all, assessment of self-harm is part of a process that includes therapeutic action. For example, if a clinician determines that an adolescent is at imminent risk of suicidality, his or her obligation is to help ensure the safety of the adolescent, either by reducing risk or by referring the adolescent to a setting where he or she can be monitored more closely. If the clinician finds that a youth in treatment has thoughts about self-harm, he or she has an obligation to address these thoughts, to discuss safety considerations with both the adolescent and caretaker, and to develop a plan for reducing these thoughts and risk. If a youth continues to be suicidal, despite therapeutic efforts, the clinician has an ethical obligation to examine the adequacy of the treatment approach.

SUMMARY AND DIRECTIONS OF FUTURE ASSESSMENTS

For the reduction and prevention of adolescent self-harm behaviors, clinicians need to recognize and assess risk for self-harm and history of engaging in these behaviors. Careful clinical assessment is often useful in identifying youth at risk and in monitoring treatment progress. In this regard, it is notable that far fewer instruments are available for detecting the presence of nonsuicidal self-harm than for assessing the presence or severity of suicidal self-harm. It also is striking that against the backdrop of the large number of risk assessment instruments for suicidality, no instruments, to our knowledge, have been developed specifically to assess risk for nonsuicidal self-harm behaviors. To the extent that there is overlap between suicidal and nonsuicidal self-harm behaviors and their motivations (with the exception of wanting to die), it would be useful to evaluate whether risk assessment instruments developed for suicidal self-harm behaviors might also have utility in predicting nonsuicidal self-harm.

In addition, better understanding of the relationship between risk factors and suicidal behavior over time is needed. For example, many presumed risk factors may simply be covariates of increased distress, and it should be no surprise that distress is related to increased risk for self-harm behavior. Distress may wax and wane over time, and any predictive relationships between risk factors and

suicidality may similarly vary as a function of when those risk factors are assessed. To reduce long-term risk for self-harm behavior, it makes most sense for preventive and treatment interventions to target attributes associated with increased risk that are both modifiable and relatively stable over time. In this regard, a recent prospective study demonstrated that risk factors for adolescent and young adult suicide attempts include both trait and state variance, and the more stable trait variance in these measures is most strongly linked over time to suicide attempts (Goldston, Reboussin, & Daniel, 2006).

Research has increasingly focused on different facets of impulsivity assessed with laboratory measures and their relationship to different areas of brain functioning and suicidality (e.g., Dougherty, Mathias, et al., 2004; Mathias et al., 2003). Likewise, considerable research has focused on biological correlates and processes, particularly those related to serotonergic functioning, potentially associated with suicidal self-harm behaviors (e.g., Tyano et al., 2006). Nonetheless, despite a need for multimethod assessments, the utility of laboratory and biological measures in identifying individuals who may be at increased risk for subsequent suicidality has not been demonstrated and should be a focus of future research.

There is considerable heterogeneity among self-harming adolescents (e.g., Goldston et al., 1996, 1998; Mandell et al., 2006; Walrath et al., 2001). Different groups of self-harming adolescents are likely to have different characteristics and different developmental trajectories. Nonetheless, more research is needed to identify and characterize these different developmental trajectories and the varied courses of self-harming behaviors over time. Hand in hand with such efforts, we need to tailor assessment instruments more specifically toward identifying not only global risk for self-harm behaviors but also different groups of self-harming individuals with their own identifiable trajectories.

Finally, much research has been devoted to identifying who engages in self-harm, and the risk and protective factors for suicidal behavior. Recent research on adolescent nonsuicidal self-harm has taken this one step further by identifying the different behavioral functions of nonsuicidal self-harm behaviors. These functions, in turn, may be useful in developing individualized intervention plans for such adolescents. The utility of a functional analysis for understanding self-harm behaviors on an individual basis was described earlier in this chapter. As an adjunct to such efforts, the field would greatly benefit from assessment instruments that help to identify the functions associated with suicidal thoughts and behavior, in a way that leads to a clearer understanding of the context of these behaviors and needed directions for treatment efforts.

REFERENCES

Adams, J., Overholser, J., & Spirito, A. (1994). Stressful life events associated with adolescent suicide attempts. *Canadian Journal of Psychiatry, 39*, 43–48.

Altman, D. (1991). *Practical statistics for medical research.* London: Chapman & Hall.

Ambrosini, P. (2000). The historical development and present status of the Schedule for Affective Disorders and Schizophrenia for School-Aged Children (K-SADS). *Journal of the American Academy of Child and Adolescent Psychiatry, 39*, 49–58.

American Psychiatric Association (APA). (2000). *Diagnostic and statistical manual of mental disorders* (4th ed., text rev.). Washington, DC: Author.

Armstrong, T., & Costello, E. (2002). Community studies on adolescent substance use, abuse, or dependence and psychiatric comorbidity. *Journal of Consulting and Clinical Psychology, 70*, 1224–1239.

Asarnow, J., & Guthrie, D. (1989). Suicidal behavior, depression, and hopelessness in child psychiatric inpatients: A replication and extension. *Journal of Clinical Child Psychology, 18*, 129–136.

Barber, M., Marzuk, P., Leon, A., & Portera, L. (1998). Aborted suicide attempts: A new classification of suicidal behavior. *American Journal of Psychiatry, 155*, 385–389.

Barber, M., Marzuk, P., Leon, A., & Portera, L. (2001). Gate questions in psychiatric interviewing: The case of suicide assessment. *Journal of Psychiatric Research, 35*, 67–69.

Barkley, R., & Fischer, M. (2005). Suicidality in children with ADHD. *ADHD Report, 13*, 1–4.

Beautrais, A. (2003). Suicide and serious suicide attempts in youth: A multiple group comparison study. *American Journal of Psychiatry, 160*, 1093–1099.

Beautrais, A., Joyce, P., & Mulder, R. (1996). Risk factors for serious suicide attempts among youth aged 13 through 24 years. *Journal of the American Academy of Child and Adolescent Psychiatry, 35*, 1174–1182.

Beautrais, A., Joyce, P., & Mulder, R. (1997). Precipitating factors and life events in serious suicide attempts among youth aged 13 through 24 years. *Journal of the American Academy of Child and Adolescent Psychiatry, 36*, 1543–1551.

Beck, A. T. (1996). Beyond belief: A theory of modes, personality, and psychopathology. In P. M. Salkovskis (Ed.), *Frontiers of cognitive therapy* (pp. 1–25). New York: Guilford Press.

Beck, A. T., Kovacs, M., & Weissman, A. (1979). Assessment of suicidal intention: The Scale for Suicidal Ideation. *Journal of Consulting and Clinical Psychology, 47*, 343–352.

Beck, A. T., Rush, A. J., Shaw, B. F., & Emery, G. (1979). *Cognitive therapy of depression.* New York: Guilford Press.

Beck, A. T., Schuyler, D., & Herman, I. (1974). Development of suicidal intent scales. In A. Beck, H. Resnik, & D. Lettieri (Eds.), *The prediction of suicide.* Bowie, MD: Charles Press.

Beck, A. T., & Steer, R. (1987). *Manual for the Beck Depression Inventory.* San Antonio, TX: Psychological Corporation.

Beck, A. T., & Steer, R. (1988). *Beck Hopelessness Scale manual.* San Antonio, TX: Psychological Corporation.

Beck, A. T., & Steer, R. (1991). *Manual for the Beck Scale for Suicidal Ideation.* San Antonio, TX: Psychological Corporation.

Beck, A. T., Weissman, A., Lester, D., & Trexler, L. (1974). The measurement of pessimism: The Hopelessness Scale. *Journal of Consulting and Clinical Psychology, 42*, 861–865.

Berman, A. (2003, April). *Why are suicide rates declining? A panel discussion.* Paper presented at the annual meeting of the American Association of Suicidology, Santa Fe, NM.

Berman, A., Jobes, D., & Silverman, M. (2006). *Adolescent suicide: Assessment and intervention.* Washington, DC: American Psychological Association Press.

Boergers, J., Spirito, A., & Donaldson, D. (1998). Reasons for adolescent suicide attempts: Associations with psychological functioning. *Journal of the American Academy of Child and Adolescent Psychiatry, 37*, 1287–1293.

Bradley, J., & Rotheram-Borus, M. (1990). *Evaluation of imminent danger for suicide: A training manual.* Tulsa, OK: National Resource Center for Youth Services.

Brave Heart, M. (1998). The return to the Sacred Path: Healing the historical trauma and historical unresolved grief response among the Lakota through a psychoeducational group intervention. *Smith College Studies in Social Work, 68*, 287–305.

Brave Heart, M. (1999). Gender differences in the historical grief response among the Lakota. *Journal of Health and Social Policy, 10*, 1–21.

Breland-Noble, A. (2004). Mental healthcare disparities affect treatment of black adolescents. *Psychiatric Annals, 34*, 534–538.

Brent, D. (1987). Correlates of the medical lethality of suicide attempts in children and adolescents. *Journal of the American Academy of Child and Adolescent Psychiatry, 26*, 87–91.

Brent, D., Baugher, M., Birmaher, B., Kolko, D., & Bridge, J. (2000). Compliance with recommendations to remove firearms in families participating in a clinical trial for adolescent depression. *Journal of the American Academy of Child and Adolescent Psychiatry, 39,* 1220–1226.

Brent, D., Bridge, J., Johnson, B., & Connolly, J. (1996). Suicidal behavior runs in families: A controlled family study of adolescent suicide victims. *Archives of General Psychiatry, 53,* 1145–1152.

Brent, D., Holder, D., Kolko, D., Birmaher, B., Baugher, M., Roth, C., et al. (1997). A clinical psychotherapy trial for adolescent depression comparing cognitive, family, and supportive therapy. *Archives of General Psychiatry, 54,* 877–885.

Brent, D., Kalas, R., Edelbrock, C., Costello, A., Dulcan, M., & Conover, N. (1986). Psychopathology and its relationship to suicidal ideation in childhood and adolescence. *Journal of the American Academy of Child and Adolescent Psychiatry, 25,* 666–673.

Brent, D., Kolko, D., Allan, M., & Brown, R. (1990). Suicidality in affectively disordered inpatients. *Journal of the American Academy of Child and Adolescent Psychiatry, 29,* 586–593.

Brent, D., Kolko, D., Birmaher, B., Baugher, M., Bridge, J., Roth, C., et al. (1998). Predictors of treatment efficacy in a clinical trial of three psychosocial treatments for adolescent depression. *Journal of the American Academy of Child and Adolescent Psychiatry, 37,* 906–914.

Brent, D., Oquendo, M., Birmaher, B., Greenhill, L., Kolko, D., Stanley, B., et al. (2002). Familial pathways to early-onset suicide attempt: Risk for suicidal behavior in offspring of mood-disordered suicide attempters. *Archives of General Psychiatry, 59,* 801–807.

Brent, D., Perper, J., Goldstein, C., Kolko, D., Allan, M., Allman, C., et al. (1988). Risk factors for adolescent suicide: A comparison of adolescent suicide victims with suicidal inpatients. *Archives of General Psychiatry, 45,* 581–588.

Brent, D., Perper, J., Moritz, G., & Allman, C. (1993). Psychiatric risk factors for adolescent suicide: A case–control study. *Journal of the American Academy of Child and AdolescentPsychiatry, 32,* 521–529.

Breton, J., Tousignant, M., Bergeron, L., & Berthiaume, C. (2002). Informant-specific correlates of suicidal behavior in a community survey of 12- to 14-year-olds. *Journal of the American Academy of Child and Adolescent Psychiatry, 41,* 723–730.

Briere, J., & Gil, E. (1998). Self-mutilation in clinical and general population samples: Prevalence, correlates, and functions. *American Journal of Orthopsychiatry, 68,* 609–620.

Brinkman-Sull, D., Overholser, J., & Silverman, E. (2000). Risk of future suicide attempts in adolescent psychiatric inpatients at 18-month follow-up. *Suicide and Life-Threatening Behavior, 30,* 327–340.

Brittlebank, A., Cole, A., Hassanyeah, F., Kenny, M., Simpson, D., & Scott, J. (1990). Hostility, hopelessness and deliberate self-harm: A prospective follow-up study. *Acta Psychiatrica Scandinavica, 81,* 280–283.

Brown, C., Abe-Kim, J., & Barrio, C. (2003). Commentary: "Treatment is not enough: We must prevent depression in women," by Le, Munoz, Ippen, & Stoddard (20030. *Prevention and Treatment, 6,* 18.

Brown, G., Beck, A., Steer, R., & Grisham, J. (2000). Risk factors for suicide in psychiatric outpatients: A 20-year prospective study. *Journal of Consulting and Clinical Psychology, 68,* 371–377.

Campbell, N., Milling, L., Laughlin, A., & Bush, E. (1993). The psychosocial climate of families with suicidal pre-adolescent children. *American Journal of Orthopsychiatry, 63,* 142–145.

Centers for Disease Control and Prevention (CDC). (2006). Youth risk behavior surveillance—United States, 2005. *MMWR Surveillance Summary, 55*(No. SS-51).

Centers for Disease Control and Prevention (CDC). (2007). *National Center for Injury Prevention and Control: Web-based Injury Statistics Query and Reporting System(WISQARS).* Available at *www.cdc.gov/ncipc/wisqars*

Champion, K., Carey, M., & Hodges, K. (1994). *Hopelessness, depression, recklessness and suicidal behavior in hospitalized adolescents.* Unpublished manuscript.

Clark, R., Anderson, N., Clark, V., & Williams, D. (1999). Racism as a stressor for African Americans: A biopsychosocial model. *American Psychologist, 54,* 805–816.

Cole, D. (1989a). Psychopathology of adolescent suicide: Hopelessness, coping beliefs, and depression. *Journal of Abnormal Psychology, 9,* 248–255.

Cole, D. (1989b). Validation of the Reasons for Living Inventory in general and delinquent adolescent samples. *Journal of Abnormal Child Psychology, 17,* 13–27.

Colle, L., Belair, J., DiFeo, M., Weiss, J., & La Roche, C. (1994). Extended open-label fluoxetine treatment of adolescents with major depression. *Journal of Child and Adolescent Psychopharmacology, 4,* 225–232.

Cooper, J., Appleby, L., & Amos, T. (2002). Life events preceding suicide by young people. *Social Psychiatry and Epidemiology, 37,* 271–275.

Corruble, E., Damy, C., & Guelfi, J. (1999). Impulsivity: A relevant dimension in depression regarding suicide attempts? *Journal of Affective Disorders, 53,* 211–215.

Cotton, C., & Range, L. (1993). Suicidality, hopelessness, and attitudes toward life and death in children. *Death Studies, 17,* 185–191.

Daniel, S., Walsh, A., Goldston, D., Arnold, E., Reboussin, B., & Wood, F. (in press). Suicidality, school drop-out, and reading problems among adolescents. *Journal of Learning Disabilities, 39,* 507–514.

D'Augelli, A., Grossman, A., Salter, N., Vasey, J., Starks, M., & Sinclair, K. (2005). Predicting the suicide attempts of lesbian, gay, and bisexual youth. *Suicide and Life-Threatening Behavior, 35,* 646–660.

D'Augelli, A., Hershberger, S., & Pilkington, N. (2001). Suicidality patterns and sexual orientation-related factors among lesbian, gay, and bisexual youths. *Suicide and Life-Threatening Behavior, 31*, 250–264.

DeMaso, D., Ross, L., & Beardslee, W. (1994). Depressive disorders and suicidal intent in adolescent suicide attempters. *Developmental and Behavioral Pediatrics, 15*, 74–77.

Dick, R., Beals, J., Manson, S., & Bechtold, D. (1994). *Psychometric properties of the suicidal ideation questionnaire in American Indian adolescents.* Unpublished manuscript, University of Colorado Health Sciences Center, Denver.

Dougherty, D., Mathias, C., Marsh, D., Moeller, F., & Swann, A. (2004). Suicidal behaviors and drug abuse: Impulsivity and its assessment. *Drug and Alcohol Dependence, 76*(Suppl.), 93–105.

Dougherty, D., Mathias, C., Marsh, D., Papageorgiou, T., Swann, A., & Moeller, F. (2004). Laboratory measured behavioral impulsivity relates to suicide attempt history. *Suicide and Life-Threatening Behavior, 34*, 374–385.

Drye, R., Goulding, R., & Goulding, M. (1973). No-suicide decisions: Patient monitoring of suicidal risk. *American Journal of Psychiatry, 130*, 171–174.

Duran, E., & Duran, B. (1995). *Native American postcolonial psychology.* Albany: State University of New York Press.

Eggert, L., Thompson, E., & Herting, J. (1994). A Measure of Adolescent Potential for Suicide (MAPS): Development and preliminary findings. *Suicide and Life-Threatening Behavior, 24*, 359–381.

Eggert, L, Thompson, E., Herting, J., & Nicholas, L. (1995). Reducing suicide potential among high-risk youth: Tests of a school-based prevention program. *Suicide and Life-Threatening Behavior, 25*, 276–296.

Enns, M., Inayatulla, M., Cox, B., & Cheyne, L. (1997). Prediction of suicide intent in Aboriginal and non-Aboriginal adolescent inpatients: A research note. *Suicide and Life-Threatening Behavior, 27*, 218–224.

Esposito, C., & Clum, G. (2002). Psychiatric symptoms and their relationship to suicidal ideation in a high-risk adolescent community sample. *Journal of American Academy of Child and Adolescent Psychiatry, 41*, 44–51.

Esposito, C., & Clum, G. (2003). The relative contribution of diagnostic and psychosocial factors in the prediction of adolescent suicidal ideation. *Journal of Clinical Child and Adolescent Psychology, 32*, 386–395.

Esposito, C., Spirito, A., Boergers, J., & Donaldson, D. (2003). Affective, behavioral, and cognitive functioning in adolescents with multiple suicide attempts. *Suicide and Life-Threatening Behavior, 33*, 389–399.

Esposito-Smythers, C., & Spirito, A. (2004). Adolescent substance use and suicidal behavior: A review with implications for treatment research. *Alcoholism, Clinical and Experimental Research, 28*, 77S–88S.

Favazza, A. (1992). Repetitive self-mutilation. *Psychiatric Annals, 22*, 60–63.

Foley, D., Goldston, D., Costello, E., & Angold, A. (2006). Proximal psychiatric risk factors for suicidality in youth: The Great Smoky Mountains Study. *Archives of General Psychiatry, 63*, 1017–1024.

Fremouw, W., Perczel, M., & Ellis, T. (1990). *Suicide risk: Assessment and response guidelines.* New York: Pergamon Press.

Garofalo, R., Wolf, R., Wissow, L., Woods, E., & Goodman, E. (1999). Sexual orientation and risk of suicide attempts among a representative sample of youth. *Archives of Pediatrics and Adolescent Medicine, 153*, 487–493.

Garrison, C., Addy, C., McKeown, R., & Cuffe, S. (1993). Nonsuicidal physically self-damaging acts in adolescents. *Journal of Child and Family Studies, 2*, 339–352.

Garrison, C., Jackson, K., Addy, C., McKeown, R., & Waller, J. (1991). Suicidal behaviors in young adolescents. *American Journal of Epidemiology, 133*, 1005–1014.

Gibbons, F., Gerrard, M., Cleveland, M., Wills, T., & Brody, G. (2004). Perceived discrimination and substance use in African American parents and their children: A panel study. *Journal of Personality and Social Psychology, 86*, 517–529.

Goldfried, M., & Sprafkin, J. (1976). Behavioral personality assessment. In J. Spence, R. Carson, & J. Thibaut (Eds.), *Behavioral approaches to therapy.* Morristown, NJ: General Learning Press.

Goldston, D. (2003). *Measuring suicidal behaviors and risk among children and adolescents.* Washington, DC: American Psychological Press.

Goldston, D. (2004). Conceptual issues in understanding the relationship between suicidal behavior and substance abuse during adolescence. *Drug and Alcohol Dependence, 76*(Suppl.), S79–S91.

Goldston, D. B., Daniel, S. S., & Arnold, E. M. (2006). Suicidal and nonsuicidal self-harm behaviors. In D. A. Wolfe & E. J. Mash (Eds.), *Behavioral and emotional disorders in adolescents: Nature, assessment, and treatment* (pp. 343–380). New York: Guilford Press.

Goldston, D., Daniel, S., Melton, B., Reboussin, D., Kelley, A., & Frazier, P. (1998). Psychiatric disorders among previous suicide attempters, first-time, and repeat attempters on an adolescent inpatient psychiatry unit. *Journal of the American Academy of Child and Adolescent Psychiatry, 37*, 924–932.

Goldston, D., Daniel, S., Reboussin, B., Frazier, P., Treadway, L., & Mayfield, A. (under review). *Proximal psychiatric diagnoses and suicide attempts among adolescents and young adults: A longitudinal study.*

Goldston, D., Daniel, S., Reboussin, D., Kelley, A., Ievers, C., & Brunstetter, R. (1996). First-time suicide attempters, repeat attempters, and previous attempters on an adolescent inpatient psychiatry unit. *Journal of the American Academy of Child and Adolescent Psychiatry, 35*, 631–639.

Goldston, D., Daniel, S., Reboussin, B., Reboussin, D., Frazier, P., & Harris, A. (2001). Cognitive risk factors and suicide attempts among formerly hospitalized adolescents: A prospective naturalistic study. *Journal of the American Academy of Child and Adolescent Psychiatry, 40,* 91–99.

Goldston, D., Daniel, S., Reboussin, D., Reboussin, B., Frazier, P., & Kelley, A. (1999). Suicide attempts among formerly hospitalized adolescents: A prospective naturalistic study or risk during the first 5 years after discharge. *Journal of the American Academy of Child and Adolescent Psychiatry, 38,* 660–671.

Goldston, D., Kelley, A., Reboussin, D., Daniel, S., Smith, J., Schwartz, R., et al. (1997). Suicidal ideation and behavior and noncompliance with the medical regimen among diabetic adolescents. *Journal of the American Academy of Child and Adolescent Psychiatry, 36,* 1528–1536.

Goldston, D., Kovacs, M., Ho, V., Parrone, P., & Stiffler, L. (1994). Suicidal ideation and suicide attempts among youth with insulin-dependent diabetes mellitus. *Journal of the American Academy of Child and Adolescent Psychiatry, 33,* 240–246.

Goldston, D., Molock, S., Whitbeck, L., Murikami, J., Zayas, L., & Hall, G. (under review). *Cultural considerations in adolescent suicide prevention and psychosocial treatment.*

Goldston, D., Reboussin, B., & Daniel, S. (2006). Predictors of suicide attempts: State and trait components. *Journal of Abnormal Psychology, 115,* 842–849.

Gould, M., Fisher, P., Parides, M., Flory, M., & Shaffer, D. (1996). Psychosocial risk factors of child and adolescent completed suicide. *Archives of General Psychiatry, 53,* 1155–1162.

Gould, M., King, R., Greenwald, S., Fisher, P., Schwab-Stone, M., Kramer, R., et al. (1998). Psychopathology associated with suicidal ideation and attempts among children and adolescents. *Journal of the American Academy of Child and Adolescent Psychiatry, 37,* 915–923.

Gould, M., Marrocco, F., Kleinman, M., Thomas, J., Mostkoff, K., Cote, J., et al. (2005). Evaluating iatrogenic risk of youth suicide screening programs: A randomized controlled trial. *Journal of the American Medical Association, 293,* 1635–1643.

Gratz, K. (2003). Risk factors for and functions of deliberate self-harm: An empirical and conceptual review. *Clinical Psychology: Science and Practice, 10,* 192–205.

Gratz, K., Conrad, S., & Roemer, L. (2002). Risk factors for deliberate self-harm among college students. *American Journal of Orthopsychiatry, 72,* 128–140.

Groholt, B., Ekeberg, O., & Haldorsen, T. (2000). Adolescents hospitalised with deliberate self-harm: The significance of an intention to die. *European Child and Adolescent Psychiatry, 9,* 244–255.

Grossman, D., Mueller, B., Riedy, C., Dowd, M., Villaveces, A., Prodzinski, J., et al. (2005). Gun storage practices and risk of youth suicide and unintentional firearm injuries. *Journal of the American Medical Association, 293,* 707–714.

Guertin, T., Lloyd-Richardson, E., Spirito, A., Donaldson, D., & Boergers, J. (2001). Self-mutilative behavior in adolescents who attempt suicide by overdose. *Journal of the American Academy of Child and Adolescent Psychiatry, 40,* 1062–1069.

Gutierrez, P., Osman, A., Kopper, B., & Barrios, F. (2000). Why young people do not kill themselves: The Reasons for Living Inventory for Adolescents. *Journal of Clinical Child Psychology, 29,* 177–187.

Hallfors, D., Brodish, P., Khatapoush, S., Sanchez, V., Cho, H., & Steckler, A. (2006). Feasibility of screening adolescents for suicide risk in "real world" high school settings. *American Journal of Public Health, 96,* 282–287.

Harrington, R., Kerfoot, M., Dyer, E., McNiven, F., Gill, J., Harrington, V., et al. (1998). Randomized trial of a home-based family intervention for children who have deliberately poisoned themselves. *Journal of the American Academy of Child and Adolescent Psychiatry, 37,* 512–518.

Harriss, L., Hawton, K., & Zahl, D. (2005). Value of measuring suicidal intent in the assessment of people attending hospital following self-poisoning or self-injury. *British Journal of Psychiatry, 186,* 60–66.

Hawton, K. (1987). Assessment of suicide risk. *British Journal of Psychiatry, 150,* 145–153.

Hawton, K., Cole, D., O'Grady, J., & Osborn, M. (1982). Motivational aspects of deliberate self-poisoning in adolescents. *British Journal of Psychiatry, 141,* 286–291.

Hawton, K., Kingsbury, S., Steinhardt, K., James, A., & Fagg, J. (1999). Repetition of deliberate self-harm by adolescents: The role of psychological factors. *Journal of Adolescence, 22,* 369–378.

Heikkinen, M., Aro, H., & Lonnqvist, J. (1994). Recent life events, social support and suicide. *Acta Psychiatrica Scandinavica, 377*(Suppl.), 65–72.

Hershberger, S., Pilkington, N., & D'Augelli, A. (1997). Predictors of suicide attempts among gay, lesbian, and bisexual youth. *Journal of Adolescent Research, 12,* 477–497.

Hewitt, P., Newton, J., Flett, G., & Callander, L. (1997). Perfectionism and suicide ideation in adolescent psychiatric patients. *Journal of Abnormal Child Psychology, 25,* 95–101.

Hoberman, H., & Garfinkel, B. (1988). Completed suicide in children and adolescents. *Journal of the American Academy of Child and Adolescent Psychiatry, 27,* 689–695.

Hodges, K., & Wong, M. (1996). Psychometric characteristics of a multidimensional measure to assess impairment: The Child and Adolescent Functional Assessment Scale. *Journal of Child and Family Studies, 5*(4), 445–467.

Horesh, N. (2001). Self-report vs. computerized measures of impulsivity as a correlate of suicidal behavior. *Crisis, 22,* 27–31.

Hovey, J. (2000a). Acculturative stress, depression, and

suicidal ideation among Central American immigrants. *Suicide and Life-Threatening Behavior, 30,* 125–139.

Hovey, J. (2000b). Acculturative stress, depression, and suicidal ideation in Mexican immigrants. *Cultural Diversity and Ethnic Minority Psychology, 6,* 134–151.

Isometsa, E., & Lonnqvist, J. (1999). Suicide attempts v. deliberate self-harm: A reply. *British Journal of Psychiatry, 175,* 90.

Ivarsson, T., Gillberg, C., Arvidsson, T., & Broberg, A. (2002). The Youth Self-Report (YSR) and the Depression Self-Rating Scale (DSRS) as measures of depression and suicidality among adolescents. *European Child and Adolescent Psychiatry, 11,* 31–37.

James, A., Lai, F., & Dahl, C. (2004). Attention deficit hyperactivity disorder and suicide: A review of possible associations. *Acta Psychiatrica Scandinavica, 110,* 408–415.

Jobes, D., Eyman, J., & Yufit, R. (1995). How clinicians assess suicide risk in adolescents and adults. *Crisis Intervention and Time-Limited Treatment, 2,* 1–12.

Jobes, D., & Mann, R. (1999). Reasons for living versus reasons for dying: Examining the internal debate of suicide. *Suicide and Life-Threatening Behavior, 29,* 97–104.

Joiner, T. (2002). The trajectory of suicidal behavior over time. *Suicide and Life-Threatening Behavior, 32,* 33–41.

Joiner, T., Conwell, Y., Fitzpatrick, K., Witte, T., Schmidt, N., Berlim, N., et al. (2005). Four studies on how current and past suicidality relate even when "everything but the kitchen sink" is covaried. *Journal of Abnormal Psychology, 114,* 291–303.

Joiner, T., Rudd, D., Rouleau, M., & Wagner, K. (2000). Parameters of suicidal crises vary as a function of previous suicide attempts in young inpatients. *Journal of the American Academy of Child and Adolescent Psychiatry, 39,* 876–880.

Jordan, J., & McMenamy, J. (2004). Interventions for suicide survivors: A review of the literature. *Suicide and Life-Threatening Behavior, 34,* 337–349.

Kashani, J., Suarez, L., Allan, W., & Reid, J. (1997). Hopelessness in inpatient youths: A closer look at behavior, emotional expression, and social support. *Journal of the American Academy of Child and Adolescent Psychiatry, 36,* 1625–1631.

Kashden, J., Fremouw, W., Callahan, T., & Franzen, M. (1993). Impulsivity in suicidal and nonsuicidal adolescents. *Journal of Abnormal Child Psychology, 21,* 339–353.

Katz, L., Cox, B., Gunasekara, S., & Miller, A. (2004). Feasibility of dialectical behavior therapy for suicidal adolescent inpatients. *Journal of the American Academy of Child and Adolescent Psychiatry, 43,* 276–282.

Kazdin, A., Rodgers, A., & Colbus, D. (1986). The Hopelessness Scale for Children: Psychometric characteristics and concurrent validity. *Journal of Consulting and Clinical Psychology, 54,* 241–245.

Keer, D., Preuss, L., & King, C. (2006). Suicidal adolescents' social support from family and peers: Gender-specific associations with psychopathology. *Journal of Abnormal Child Psychology, 34* (electronic publication ahead of print).

Kempton, T., & Forehand, R. (1992). Suicide attempts among juvenile delinquents: The contribution of mental health factors. *Behaviour Research and Therapy, 30,* 537–541.

Kienhorst, I., DeWilde, E., Diekstra, R., & Wolters, W. (1995). Adolescents' image of their suicide attempt. *Journal of the American Academy of Child and Adolescent Psychiatry, 34,* 623–628.

King, C., Katz, S., Ghaziuddin, N., Brand, E., Hill, E., & McGovern, L. (1997). Diagnosis and assessment of depression and suicidality using the NIMH Diagnostic Interview Schedule for Children (DISC-2.3). *Journal of Abnormal Child Psychology, 25,* 173–181.

King, C., Raskin, A., Gdowski, C., Butkus, M., & Opipari, L. (1990). Psychosocial factors associated with urban adolescent female suicide attempts. *Journal of the American Academy of Child and Adolescent Psychiatry, 29,* 289–294.

King, C., Segal, H., Kaminski, K., Naylor, M., Ghaziuddin, N., & Radpour, L. (1995). A prospective study of adolescent suicidal behavior following hospitalization. *Suicide and Life-Threatening Behavior, 25,* 327–338.

Kingsbury, S. (1993). Clinical components of suicidal intent in adolescent overdose. *Journal of the American Academy of Child and Adolescent Psychiatry, 32,* 518–520.

Klimes-Dougan, B. (1998). Screening for suicidal ideation in children and adolescents: Methodological considerations. *Journal of Adolescence, 21,* 435–444.

Kumar, G., & Steer, R. (1995). Psychosocial correlates of suicidal ideation in adolescent psychiatric inpatients. *Suicide and Life-Threatening Behavior, 25,* 339–346.

Laye-Gindhu, A., & Schonert-Reichl, K. (2005). Nonsuicidal self-harm among community adolescents: Understanding the "whats" and "whys" of self-harm. *Journal of Youth and Adolescence, 34,* 447–457.

Lee, J., & Bartlett, M. (2005). Suicide prevention: Critical elements for managing suicidal clients and counselor liability without the use of a no-suicide contract. *Death Studies, 29,* 847–865.

Leon, A., Friedman, R., Sweeney, J., Brown, R., & Mann, J. (1989). Statistical issues in the identification of risk factors for suicidal behavior: The application of survival analysis. *Psychiatry Research, 31,* 99–108.

Lewinsohn, P., Clarke, G., Seeley, J., & Rohde, P. (1994). Major depression in community adolescents: Age at onset, episode duration, and time to recurrence. *Journal of the American Academy of Child and Adolescent Psychiatry, 33,* 809–818.

Lewinsohn, P., Garrison, C., Langhinrichsen, J., & Marsteller, F. (1989). *The assessment of suicidal behavior in adolescents: A review of scales suitable for epidemiologic and clinical research.* Washington, DC: U.S. Government Printing Office.

Lewinsohn, P., Rohde, P., & Seeley, J. (1993). Psychosocial characteristics of adolescents with a history of suicide attempt. *Journal of the American Academy of Child and Adolescent Psychiatry, 32,* 60–68.

Lewinsohn, P., Rohde, P., & Seeley, J. (1994). Psychosocial risk factors for future adolescent suicide attempts. *Journal of Consulting and Clinical Psychology, 62,* 297–305.

Lewinsohn, P., Rohde, P., & Seeley, J. (1996). Adolescent suicidal ideation and attempts: Prevalence, risk factors, and clinical implications. *Clinical Psychology: Science and Practice, 3,* 25–46.

Lewinsohn, P., Rohde, P., Seeley, J., & Baldwin, C. (2001). Gender differences in suicide attempts from adolescence to young adulthood. *Journal of the American Academy of Child and Adolescent Psychiatry, 40,* 427–434.

Linehan, M. (1996). *Suicidal Behaviors Questionnaire (SBQ).* Unpublished instrument, University of Washington, Seattle.

Linehan, M., & Comtois, K. (1997). *Lifetime Parasuicide Count.* Unpublished instrument, University of Washington, Seattle.

Linehan, M., Goodstein, J., Nielsen, S., & Chiles, J. (1983). Reasons for staying alive when you are thinking of killing yourself: The Reasons for Living Inventory. *Journal of Consulting and Clinical Psychology, 51,* 276–286.

Lloyd, E., Kelley, M., & Hope, T. (1997, April). *Self-mutilation in a community sample of adolescents: Descriptive characteristics and provisional prevalence rates.* Paper presented at the annual meeting of the Society for Behavioral Medicine, New Orleans, LA.

Lonnqvist, J., & Ostamo, A. (1991). Suicide following the first suicide attempt: A five-year follow-up using a survival analysis. *Psychiatria Fennica, 22,* 171–179.

Malone, K., Szanto, K., Corbitt, E., & Mann, J. (1995). Clinical assessment versus research methods in the assessment of suicidal behavior. *American Journal of Psychiatry, 152,* 1601–1607.

Mandell, D., Walrath, C., & Goldston, D. (2006). Variation in functioning, psychosocial characteristics, and six month outcomes among suicidal youth in comprehensive community Mental Health Services. *Suicide and Life-Threatening Behavior, 36,* 349–362.

Mathias, C., Dougherty, D., Carrizal, M., & Marsh, D. (2003, April). *Impulsivity in adolescents with suicidal ideation.* Poster session presented at the 36th annual meeting of the American Association of Suicidology, Santa Fe, NM.

Mazza, J. (2000). The relationship between posttraumatic stress symptomatology and suicidal behavior in school-based adolescents. *Suicide and Life-Threatening Behavior, 30,* 91–103.

McAuliffe, C., Corcoran, P., Keeley, H., Arensman, A., Bille-Brahe, U., DeLeo, D., et al. (2006). Problem-solving ability and repetition of self-harm: A multicentre study. *Psychological Medicine, 36,* 45–55.

Meehan, P., Lamb, J., Saltzman, L., & O'Carroll, P. (1992). Attempted suicide among young adults: Progress toward a meaningful estimate of prevalence. *American Journal of Psychiatry, 149,* 41–44.

Mohler, B., & Earls, F. (2001). Trends in adolescent suicide: Misclassification bias? *American Journal of Public Health, 91,* 150–153.

Molnar, B., Berkman, L., & Buka, S. (2001). Psychopathology, childhood sexual abuse, and other childhood adversities: Relative links to subsequent suicidal behaviour in the US. *Psychological Medicine, 31,* 965–977.

Morrison, L., & Downey, D. (2000). Racial differences in self-disclosure of suicidal ideation and reasons for living: Implications for training. *Cultural Diversity and Ethnic Minority Psychology, 6,* 374–386.

Moscicki, E. (1999). Epidemiology of suicide. In D. Jacobs (Ed.), *The Harvard Medical School guide to suicide assessment and intervention* (pp. 40–51). San Francisco: Jossey-Bass/Pfeiffer.

Myers, K., McCauley, E., Calderon, R., Mitchell, J., Burke, P., & Schloredt, K. (1991). Risks for suicidality in major depressive disorder. *Journal of the American Academy of Child and Adolescent Psychiatry, 30,* 86–94.

Myers, K., McCauley, E., Calderon, R., & Treder, R. (1991). The 3-year longitudinal course of suicidality and predictive factors for subsequent suicidality in youths with major depressive disorder. *Journal of the American Academy of Child and Adolescent Psychiatry, 30,* 804–810.

Nasser, E., & Overholser, J. (1999). Assessing varying degrees of lethality in depressed adolescent suicide attempters. *Acta Psychiatrica Scandinavica, 99,* 423–431.

National Center for Health Statistics (NCHS). (2002). *Health, United States, 2002: With Chartbook on Trends in the Health of Americans.* Hyattsville, MD: Author.

Nixon, M., Cloutier, P., & Aggarwal, S. (2002). Affect regulation and addictive aspects of repetitive self-injury in hospitalized adolescents. *Journal of the American Academy of Child and Adolescent Psychiatry, 41,* 1333–1341.

Nock, M., & Kazdin, A. (2002). Examination of affective, cognitive, and behavioral factors and suicide-related outcomes in children and young adolescents. *Journal of Clinical Child and Adolescent Psychology, 31,* 48–58.

Nock, M., & Prinstein, M. (2004). A functional approach to the assessment of self-mutilative behavior. *Journal of Consulting and Clinical Psychology, 72,* 885–890.

Nock, M., & Prinstein, M. (2005). Contextual features

and behavioral functions of self-mutilation among adolescents. *Journal of Abnormal Psychology, 114,* 140–146.

Nyborg, V., & Curry, J. (2003). The impact of perceived racism: Psychological symptoms among African American boys. *Journal of Clinical Child and Adolescent Psychology, 32,* 258–266.

O'Carroll, P., Berman, A., Maris, R., & Moscicki, E. (1996). Beyond the Tower of Babel: A nomenclature for suicidology. *Suicide and Life-Threatening Behavior, 26,* 237–252.

O'Donnell, L., Stueve, A., Wardlaw, D., & O'Donnell, C. (2003). Adolescent suicidality and adult support: The Reach For Health study of urban youth. *American Journal of Health Behavior, 27,* 633–644.

Office of the Ombudsman for Mental Health and Mental Retardation, State of Minnesota. (2002). *Suicide prevention alert.* Available at *www.ombudmhmr. state.mn.us/alerts/suicidepreventionalert.htm*

O'Nell, T. (1993). "Feeling worthless": An ethnographic investigation of depression and problem drinking at the Flathead reservation. *Culture, Medicine and Psychiatry, 16,* 447–469.

Orbach, I., & Bar-Joseph, H. (1993). The impact of a suicide prevention program for adolescents on suicidal tendencies, hopelessness, ego identity, and coping. *Suicide and Life-Threatening Behavior, 23,* 120–129.

Orvaschel, H. (1994). *Schedule for Affective Disorders and Schizophrenia for School-Aged Children—Epidemiologic Version 5 (K-SADS-E).* Unpublished instrument, Nova Southeastern University, Ft. Lauderdale, FL.

Osman, A., Downs, W., Kopper, B., Barrios, F., Baker, M., Osman, J., et al. (1998). The Reasons for Living Inventory for Adolescents (RFL-A): Development and psychometric properties. *Journal of Clinical Psychology, 54,* 1063–1078.

Osman, A., Kopper, B., Barrios, F., Osman, J., Besett, T., & Linehan, M. (1996). The Brief Reasons for Living Inventory for Adolescents (BRFL-A). *Journal of Abnormal Child Psychology, 24,* 433–443.

Overholser, J., Adams, D., Lehnert, K., & Brinkman, D. (1995). Self-esteem deficits and suicidal tendencies among adolescents. *Journal of the American Academy of Child and Adolescent Psychiatry, 34,* 919–928.

Patton, G., Harris, R., Carlin, J., Hibbert, M., Coffey, C., Schwartz, M., et al. (1997). Adolescent suicidal behavior: A population-based study of risk. *Psychological Medicine, 27,* 715–724.

Payne, B., & Billie, S. (1996, March). *Reliability and validity of the Suicidal Behaviors Questionnaire for Children.* Paper presented at the annual meeting of the Southeastern Psychological Association, Norfolk, VA.

Peruzzi, N., & Bongar, B. (1999). Assessing risk for completed suicide in patients with major depression: Psychologists' view of critical factors. *Professional Psychology: Research and Practice, 30,* 576–580.

Peterson, B., Zhang, H., Santa Lucia, R., King, R., & Lewis, M. (1996). Risk factors for presenting problems in child psychiatric emergencies. *Journal of the American Academy of Child and Adolescent Psychiatry, 35,* 1162–1173.

Pfeffer, C., Hurt, S., Peskin, J., & Siefker, C. (1995). Suicidal children grow up: Ego functions associated with suicide attempts. *Journal of the American Academy of Child and Adolescent Psychiatry, 34,* 1318–1325.

Pillay, A., & Wassenaar, D. (1995). Psychological intervention, spontaneous remission, hopelessness, and psychiatric disturbance in adolescent parasuicides. *Suicide and Life-Threatening Behavior, 25,* 386–392.

Pinto, A., & Whisman, M. (1996). Negative affect and cognitive biases in suicidal and nonsuicidal hospitalized adolescents. *Journal of the American Academy of Child and Adolescent Psychiatry, 35,* 158–165.

Pinto, A., Whisman, M., & Conwell, Y. (1998). Reasons for living in a clinical sample of adolescents. *Journal of Adolescence, 21,* 397–405.

Pinto, A., Whisman, M., & McCoy, K. (1997). Suicidal ideation in adolescents: Psychometric properties of the Suicidal Ideation Questionnaire in a clinical sample. *Psychological Assessment, 9,* 63–66.

Plutchik, R., van Praag, H., Picard, S., Conte, H., & Korn, M. (1989). Is there a relationship between the seriousness of suicidal intent and the lethality of the suicide attempt? *Psychiatry Research, 27,* 71–79.

Prevette, K., Mathias, C., Marsh, D., & Dougherty, D. (2005, November). *Impulsivity in suicidal adolescent inpatients.* Poster presented at the annual meeting of the International Society for Research on Impulsivity, Washington, DC.

Prinstein, M., Nock, M., Spirito, A., & Grapentine, W. (2001). Multimethod assessment of suicidality in adolescent psychiatric inpatients: Preliminary results. *Journal of the American Academy of Child and Adolescent Psychiatry, 40,* 1053–1061.

Range, L., Campbell, C., Kovac, S., Marion-Jones, M., Aldridge, H., Kogos, S., et al. (2002). No-suicide contracts: An overview and recommendations. *Death Studies, 26,* 51–74.

Rathus, J., & Miller, A. (2002). Dialectical behavioral therapy adapted for suicidal adolescents. *Suicide and Life-Threatening Behavior, 32,* 146–157.

Reifman, A., & Windle, M. (1995). Adolescent suicidal behaviors as a function of depression, hopelessness, alcohol use, and social support: A longitudinal investigation. *American Journal of Community Psychology, 23,* 329–354.

Reinecke, M., DuBois, D., & Schultz, T. (2001). Social problem solving, mood, and suicidality among inpatient adolescents. *Cognitive Therapy and Research, 25,* 743–756.

Reynolds, W. (1988). *Suicidal Ideation Questionnaire: Professional manual.* Odessa, FL: Psychological Assessment Resources.

Reynolds, W. (1989). *Suicidal Behaviors Inventory (SBI).* Unpublished instrument, University of Wisconsin, Madison.

Reynolds, W. (1990). Development of a semistructured clinical interview for suicidal behaviors in adolescents. *Psychological Assessment, 2,* 382–393.

Reynolds, W. (1991). A school-based procedure for the identification of adolescents at risk for suicidal behaviors. *Family and Community Health, 14,* 64–75.

Reynolds, W., & Mazza, J. (1993). *Evaluation of suicidal behavior in adolescents: Reliability of the Suicidal Behaviors Interview.* Unpublished manuscript, University of British Columbia, Vancouver, Canada.

Reynolds, W., & Mazza, J. (1999). Assessment of suicidal ideation in inner-city children and young adolescents: Reliability and validity of the Suicidal Ideation Questionnaire–JR. *School Psychology Review, 28,* 17–30.

Rodham, K., Hawton, K., & Evans, E. (2004). Reasons for deliberate self-harm: Comparison of self-poisoners and self-cutters in a community sample of adolescents. *Journal of American Academy of Child and Adolescent Psychiatry, 43,* 80–87.

Rohde, P., Mace, D., & Seeley, J. (1997). The association of psychiatric disorders with suicide attempts in a juvenile delinquent sample. *Criminal Behaviour and Mental Health, 7,* 187–200.

Ross, S., & Heath, N. (2002). A study of the frequency of self-mutilation in a community sample of adolescents. *Journal of Youth and Adolescence, 31,* 67–77.

Rotheram, M. (1987). Evaluation of imminent danger for suicide among youth. *American Journal of Orthopsychiatry, 57,* 102–110.

Rotheram-Borus, M. (1989). Evaluation of suicide risk among youths in community settings. *Suicide and Life-Threatening Behavior, 19,* 108–119.

Rotheram-Borus, M., & Bradley, J. (1991). Triage model for suicidal runaways. *American Journal of Orthopsychiatry, 61,* 122–127.

Rotheram-Borus, M., Hunter, J., & Rosario, M. (1994). Suicidal behavior and gay-related stress among gay and bisexual male adolescents. *Journal of Adolescent Research, 9,* 498–508.

Rotheram-Borus, M., & Trautman, P. (1988). Hopelessness, depression, and suicidal intent among adolescent suicide attempters. *Journal of the American Academy of Child and Adolescent Psychiatry, 27,* 700–704.

Rotheram-Borus, M., Walker, J., & Ferns, W. (1996). Suicidal behavior among middle-class adolescents who seek crisis services. *Journal of Clinical Psychology, 52,* 137–143.

Roy, A., & Segal, N. (2001). Suicidal behavior in twins: A replication. *Journal of Affective Disorders, 66,* 71–74.

Roy, A., Segal, N., Centerwall, B., & Robinette, D. (1991). Suicide in twins. *Archives of General Psychiatry, 48,* 29–32.

Russell, S., & Joyner, K. (2001). Adolescent sexual orientation and suicide risk: Evidence from a national study. *American Journal of Public Health, 91,* 1276–1281.

Santa Mina, E., & Gallop, R. (1998). Childhood sexual and physical abuse and adult self-harm and suicidal behaviour: A literature review. *Canadian Journal of Psychiatry, 43,* 793–800.

Schotte, D., Cools, J., & Payvar, S. (1990). Problem-solving deficits in suicidal patients: Trait vulnerability or state phenomenon? *Journal of Consulting and Clinical Psychology, 58,* 562–564.

Scott, J., House, R., Yates, M., & Harrington, J. (1997). Individual risk factors for early repetition of deliberate self-harm. *British Journal of Medical Psychology, 70,* 387–393.

Shaffer, D., & Craft, L. (1999). Methods of adolescent suicide prevention. *Journal of Clinical Psychiatry, 60,* 70–74.

Shaffer, D., Fisher, P., Lucas, C., Dulcan, M., & Schwab-Stone, M. (2000). NIMH Diagnostic Interview Schedule for Children, Version IV (NIMH DISC-IV): Description, differences from previous versions, and reliability of some common diagnoses. *Journal of the American Academy of Child and Adolescent Psychiatry, 39,* 28–38.

Shaffer, D., Fisher, P., Parides, M., & Gould, M. (1995). Sexual orientation in adolescents who commit suicide. *Suicide and Life-Threatening Behavior, 25*(Suppl.), 64–71.

Shaffer, D., Gould, M., Fisher, P., Trautman, P., Moreau, D., Kleinman, M., et al. (1996). Psychiatric diagnoses in child and adolescent suicide. *Archives of General Psychiatry, 53,* 339–348.

Shaffer, D., Pfeffer, C., & the Workgroup on Quality Issues. (2001). Practice parameters for the assessment and treatment of children and adolescents with suicidal behavior. *Journal of the American Academy of Child and Adolescent Psychiatry, 40,* 24S–51S.

Shaffer, D., Scott, M., Wilcox, H., Maslow, C., Hicks, R., Lucas, C., et al. (2004). The Columbia Suicide Screen: Validity and reliability of a screen for youth suicide and depression. *Journal of the American Academy of Child and Adolescent Psychiatry, 43,* 71–79.

Shaffer, D., Wilcox, H., Lucas, C., Hicks, R., Busner, C., & Parides, M. (1996, October). *The development of a screening instrument for teens at risk for suicide.* Poster presented at the annual meeting of the Academy of Child and Adolescent Psychiatry, New York.

Shaunesey, K., Cohen, J., Plummer, B., & Berman, A. (1993). Suicidality in hospitalized adolescents: Relationship to prior abuse. *American Journal of Psychiatry, 63,* 113–119.

Shea, S. (1999). *The practical art of suicide assessment: A guide for mental health professionals and substance abuse counselors.* Hoboken, NJ: Wiley.

Shneidman, E. (1996). *The suicidal mind.* New York: Oxford University Press.

Simon, T., Swann, A., Powell, K., Potter, L., Kresnow, M., & O'Carroll, P. (2001). Characteristics of impulsive suicide attempts and attempters. *Suicide and Life-Threatening Behavior, 32*(Suppl.), 49–59.

Smith, K., Conroy, R., & Ehler, B. (1984). Lethality of

Suicide Attempt Rating Scale. *Suicide and Life-Threatening Behavior, 14,* 215–242.

Speckens, A., & Hawton, K. (2005). Social problem-solving in adolescents with suicidal behavior: A systematic review. *Suicide and Life-Threatening Behavior, 35,* 365–387.

Spirito, A., Boergers, J., & Donaldson, D. (2002). Adolescent suicide attempters: Post-attempt course and implications for treatment. *Clinical Psychology and Psychotherapy, 7(3),* 161–173.

Spirito, A., Lewander, W., Levy, S., Kurkjian, J., & Fritz, G. (1994). Emergency department assessment of adolescent suicide attempters: Factors related to short-term follow-up outcome. *Pediatric Emergency Care, 10,* 6–12.

Spirito, A., Stark, L., Fristad, M., Hart, K., & Owens-Stively, J. (1987). Adolescent suicide attempters hospitalized on a pediatric unit. *Journal of Pediatric Psychology, 12,* 171–189.

Spirito, A., Sterling, C., Donaldson, D., & Arrigan, M. (1996). Factor analysis of the Suicide Intent Scale with adolescent suicide attempters. *Journal of Personality Assessment, 67,* 90–101.

Spirito, A., Williams, C., Stark, L., & Hart, K. (1988). The Hopelessness Scale for Children: Psychometric properties with normal and emotionally disturbed adolescents. *Journal of Abnormal Child Psychology, 16,* 445–458.

Steer, R., & Beck, A. (1988). Use of the Beck Depression Inventory, Hopelessness Scale, Scale for Suicidal Ideation, and Suicidal Intent Scale with adolescents. *Advances in Adolescent Mental Health, 3,* 219–231.

Steer, R., Beck, A., Garrison, B., & Lester, D. (1988). Eventual suicide in interrupted and uninterrupted attempters: A challenge to the cry-for-help hypothesis. *Suicide and Life-Threatening Behavior, 18,* 119–128.

Steer, R., Kumar, G., & Beck, A. (1993). Self-reported suicidal ideation in adolescent psychiatric inpatients. *Journal of Consulting and Clinical Psychology, 61,* 1096–1099.

Steer, R., Kumar, G., Ranieri, W., & Beck, A. (1998). Use of the Beck Depression Inventory–II with adolescent psychiatric outpatients. *Journal of Psychopathology and Behavioral Assessment, 20,* 127–137.

Suominen, K., Isometsa, E., Ostamo, A., & Lonnqvist, J. (2004). Level of suicide intent predicts overall mortality and suicide after attempted suicide: A 12-year follow-up study. *BMC Psychiatry, 4,* 11.

Thompson, E., & Eggert, E. (1999). Using the Suicide Risk Screen to identify suicidal adolescents among potential high school dropouts. *Journal of the American Academy of Child and Adolescent Psychiatry, 36,* 1506–1514.

Thompson, E., Eggert, L., & Herting, J. (2000). Mediating effects of an indicated prevention program for reducing youth depression and suicide risk behaviors. *Suicide and Life-Threatening Behaviors, 30,* 252–271.

Thompson, E., Eggert, E., Randell, B., & Pike, K.

(2001). Evaluation of indicated suicide risk prevention approaches for potential high school dropouts. *American Journal of Public Health, 91,* 742–752.

Tice, D., Bratslavsky, E., & Baumeister, R. (2001). Emotional distress regulation takes precedence over impulse control: If you feel bad, do it! *Journal of Personality and Social Psychology, 80,* 53–67.

Treatment of Adolescent Depression Study Team (TADS). (2004). Fluoxetine, cognitive-behavioral therapy, and their combination for adolescents with depression. *Journal of the American Medical Association, 292,* 807–820.

Tyano, S., Zalsman, G., Ofek, H., Blum, I., Apter, A., Wolovik, L., et al. (2006). Plasma serotonin levels and suicidal behavior in adolescents. *European Neuropsychopharmacology, 16,* 49–57.

U.S. Food and Drug Administration (FDA). (2004). *FDA Public Health Advisory: Suicidality in children and adolescents being treated with antidepressant medications.* Available at *www.fda.gov/cder/drug/antidepressantss/SSRIPHA200410.htm*

van der Kolk, B., Perry, J., & Herman, L. (1991). Childhood origins of self-destructive behavior. *American Journal of Psychiatry, 146,* 490–494.

Velez, C., & Cohen, P. (1988). Suicidal behavior and ideation in a community sample of children: Maternal and youth reports. *Journal of the American Academy of Child and Adolescent Psychiatry, 27,* 349–356.

Velting, D., & Miller, A. (1998, November). Diagnostic risk factors for adolescent parasuicidal behavior. In J. Pearson (Chair), *Suicidality in youth: Developing the knowledge base for youth at risk.* Presentation at the NIMH Workshop, Bethesda, MD.

Wagner, B. (1997). Family risk factors for child and adolescent suicidal behavior. *Psychological Bulletin, 121,* 246–298.

Walker, M., Moreau, D., & Weissman, M. (1990). Parents' awareness of children's suicide attempts. *American Journal of Psychiatry, 147,* 1364–1366.

Walrath, C., Mandell, D., Liao, Q., Holden, E. W., DeCarolis, G., Santiago, R., et al. (2001). Suicidal behaviors among children in the Comprehensive Community Mental Health Services for Children and Their Families program. *Journal of the American Academy of Child and Adolescent Psychiatry, 40,* 1197–1205.

Way, B., Allen, M., Mumpower, J., Stewart, T., & Banks, S. (1998). Interrater agreement among psychiatrists in psychiatric emergency assessments. *American Journal of Psychiatry, 155,* 1423–1428.

Weissman, M., Bland, R., Canino, G., Greenwald, S., Hwu, H., Joyce, P., et al. (1999). Prevalence of suicide ideation and suicide attempts in nine countries. *Psychological Medicine, 29,* 9–17.

Weyrauch, K., Roy-Byrne, P., Katon, W., & Wilson, L. (2001). Stressful life events and impulsiveness in failed suicide attempt. *Suicide and Life-Threatening Behavior, 31,* 311–319.

Whitbeck, L., Adams, G., Hoyt, D., & Chen, X. (2004). Conceptualizing and measuring historical trauma among American Indian people. *American Journal of Community Psychology, 33,* 119–130.

Wolfgang, M. (1959). Suicide by means of victim-precipitated homicide. *Journal of Clinical and Experimental Psychopathology, 20,* 335–349.

Wong, C., Eccles, J., & Sameroff, A. (2003). The influence of ethnic discrimination and ethnic identification on African American adolescents' school and socioemotional adjustment. *Journal of Personality, 71,* 1197–1232.

Zane, N., & Mak, W. (2003). Major approaches to the measurement of acculturation among ethnic minority populations: A content analysis and an alternative empirical strategy. In K. Chun, P. Organista, & G. Marin (Eds.), *Acculturation: Advances in theory, measurement, and applied research* (pp. 39–60). Washington, DC: American Psychological Association.

Zayas, L., Lester, R., Cabassa, L., & Fortuna, L. (2005). "Why do so many Latina teens attempt suicide?": A conceptual model for research. *American Journal of Orthopsychiatry, 75*(2), 275–287.

Zlotnick, C., Shea, T., Pearlstein, T., Simpson, E., Costello, E., & Begin, A. (1996). The relationship between dissociative symptoms, alexithymia, impulsivity, sexual abuse, and self-mutilation. *Comprehensive Psychiatry, 37,* 12–16.

PART IV

Anxiety Disorders

CHAPTER 8

Anxiety in Children and Adolescents

Michael A. Southam-Gerow
Bruce F. Chorpita

Problems related to fears and anxiety in youth are relatively common, with lifetime prevalence rates of clinical disorders ranging from 6 to 15% in epidemiological studies (e.g., Silverman & Ginsburg, 1998; U.S. Public Health Service, 2000). Youth with anxiety problems experience significant and often lasting psychosocial impairment, such as poor school performance, social problems, and familial conflict (e.g., Langley, Bergman, McCracken, & Piacentini, 2004; Silverman & Ginsburg, 1998). The co-occurrence of these problems with disruptive behavior problems, depression, or additional anxiety disorders is also quite high, with rates of co-occurrence ranging up to 65% in epidemiological samples (Fergusson, Horwood, & Lynskey, 1993; Zoccolillo, 1992) and up to 84% in clinic samples (e.g., Albano, Chorpita, & Barlow, 2003; Kendall et al., 1997). Thus, the problems found in these youth are substantial (e.g., Costello, Angold, & Keeler, 1999; Pine, Cohen, Gurley, Brook, & Ma, 1998).

Accumulating evidence also supports the notion that such problems have an early onset in childhood and adolescence. Among the anxiety disorders, separation anxiety disorder and specific phobia have the earliest average onset (approximately age 7), whereas generalized anxiety disorder and obsessive–compulsive disorder typically have their onset in middle childhood (age 9–10); onset of social phobia is typically in early adolescence, and onset of panic disorder comes latest, around the age of 15 (e.g., Morris & March, 2004). Anxiety also appears to run a chronic course into adulthood (Albano et al., 2003; Pine et al., 1998). Thus, the impairment associated with anxiety in youth has important long-term implications for adult functioning (Pine et al., 1998), with most research suggesting that anxiety symptoms actually worsen over time (Kendall, 1994) and possibly lead to depression (e.g., Chorpita & Barlow, 1998) or substance use disorders (e.g., Compton, Burns, Egger, & Robertson, 2002; Grant et al., 2004). Survey data from public schools using a conjunction of various measures of impaired functioning indicate that 45.8% of children diagnosed with anxiety disorders are also classified as seriously emotionally disturbed (Costello, Angold, & Burns, 1996).

Given the heightened prevalence of problematic fears and anxiety among children and adolescents, the long-term and broad implications of not addressing these problems (Albano et al., 2003; Ollendick, King, & Chorpita, 2005; Pine et al., 1998), and the significant degree of distress and impairment experienced by anxious and fearful youth across a range of activities and situations, research on which treatments are most effective and useful has grown substantially (Chorpita & Southam-Gerow, 2006). Most treatments, however, depend heavily on the clinician's ability to assess a child's anxiety and evaluate his or her need for treatment. Fortunately, developments in the area of assessment have made similar strides in helping professionals to identify youth with anxiety-related problems, so that treatment may be provided when necessary (Chorpita & Southam-Gerow, 2006; see also Compton et al., 2004; Ollendick et al., 2005).

This chapter examines the research literature on assessment of anxiety in children and adolescents. We begin with a discussion of the various anxiety disorders common among children and adolescents. Next, we discuss conceptual issues relevant to assessment, including the importance of multimethod assessment approaches and the distinction between content and process in assessment. Next, we describe the purposes of assessment and provide a brief overview of common assessment methods. We then present a comprehensive review of instruments used in the assessment of anxiety in children; in this review, we offer specific assessment approach recommendations. Finally, we offer some suggestions for future research. Our focus throughout the chapter is on the real-world applicability of assessment. As clinical researchers move toward understanding factors essential to dissemination of research-based interventions, many have encouraged the need for a similar direction for clinical assessment (e.g., Mash & Hunsley, 2005; Silverman & Ollendick, 2005). We hope that this chapter serves as a basis for clinicians and administrators in selecting assessment tools for use in applied settings.

CHILDHOOD ANXIETY DISORDERS

In the fourth, text revised version of the *Diagnostic and Statistical Manual of Mental Disorders* (DSM-IV-TR; American Psychiatric Association [APA], 2000), children may be diagnosed with any of nine anxiety disorders: separation anxiety disorder (SAD), panic disorder (PD), agoraphobia, generalized anxiety disorder (GAD, formerly overanxious disorder), social phobia/social anxiety disorder, specific (simple) phobia, obsessive–compulsive disorder (OCD), posttraumatic stress disorder (PTSD), and acute stress disorder. These disor-

ders share the emotion of anxiety as the predominant feature, expressed through specific and discrete cognitive, physiological, and behavioral reactions. What distinguishes one anxiety disorder from the next is often the focus of the child's anxiety. In this section we define the core and associated features of specific anxiety disorders affecting children and adolescents. A listing of DSM-IV-TR criteria is provided in Table 8.1 for each disorder. The reader interested in the assessment of PTSD and acute stress disorder is referred to Fletcher (Chapter 9, this volume) for a comprehensive review (see also Chorpita & Southam-Gerow, 2006, for discussion of the treatment of PTSD). This review of childhood anxiety disorders and their features is designed to be brief and illustrative. Interested readers are referred to more in-depth discussion of these topics elsewhere (e.g., Albano et al., 2003; Beidel & Turner, 2005; Morris & March, 2004).

Separation Anxiety Disorder

SAD is the only true *childhood* anxiety disorder that remained when DSM-IV (APA, 1994) was published. The essential feature of SAD is excessive anxiety and fear concerning separation from home or from those to whom the child is attached (e.g., parents or caretakers). Such anxiety must be inappropriate for the child's age and expected developmental level given that separation anxiety is a normal developmental phenomenon from approximately age 7 months to 6 years (Beidel & Turner, 2005; Silverman & Dick-Niederhauser, 2004). Children must evidence at least three of the eight symptoms for at least 4 weeks to qualify for a diagnosis of SAD. Moreover, the disturbance must be accompanied by clinically significant distress or impairment in social, academic, or other important areas of functioning. Table 8.1 highlights the DSM-IV criteria for SAD.

Children diagnosed with SAD are more likely to report somatic complaints than children diagnosed with phobic disorders (e.g., Beidel & Turner, 2005; Last, 1991). Children with SAD may also drop out of activities such as clubs or sports, if their parents are not actively involved, but not for lack of interest in the activity. Friendships may wane due to the child's repeated refusal to attend activities away from home, although children with SAD in general are socially skilled and well liked by

TABLE 8.1. Brief Diagnostic Criteria for anxiety Disorders from DSM-IV-TR

Separation anxiety disorder (SAD)	• Developmentally inappropriate and excessive anxiety concerning separation from home or from those to whom the individual is attached • Duration: at least 4 weeks
Generalized anxiety disorder (GAD)	• Excessive worry about multiple situations • Perception that worry is uncontrollable • At least three physiological/cognitive symptoms • Duration: at least 6 months
Social phobia	• Excessive and disabling fear of social or evaluative situations. • Avoidance of situations or endurance with extreme distress • Duration: at least 6 months
Obsessive–compulsive disorder (OCD)	• Obsessions (recurrent intrusive unwanted thoughts) and/or compulsions (repetitive behavior or mental act that person is driven to do, usually to reduce distress caused by obsession)
Specific phobia	• Excessive and disabling fear of specific stimuli • Avoidance of situations or endurance with extreme distress • Duration: at least 6 months
Panic disorder	• 1+ panic attacks for no discernible reason • Persistent concern about having additional attacks or worry about the implications of the attack or its consequences (e.g., losing control, having a heart attack, "going crazy") or a significant change in behavior related to the attacks • Duration: at least 1 month.

Note. All disorders have as one criterion that the symptoms must cause significant distress and/or functional impairment. From American Psychiatric Association (2000). Copyright 2000 by the American Psychiatric Association. Adapted by permission.

peers (Last, 1989). Academic performance may be compromised by the child's repeated requests to leave class, and distress and preoccupation with separation concerns. In extreme form, children with SAD who refuse to attend school miss important social and academic experiences available only in the school setting (Kearney, 2001). At times, efforts are made to provide these children with tutoring and assignments to complete at home; however, repeated absences place a child at risk for failure to meet the standards for attendance set forth in state regulations. Consequently, some children are then required to repeat the academic year and, in extreme cases, are remanded to the legal system for compliance with school attendance.

Epidemiological studies have suggested the prevalence of SAD ranges from 2.0 to 12.9%, with higher prevalence rates for studies involving younger children (e.g., Silverman & Dick-Niederhauser, 2004). However, more recent studies have reported somewhat lower prevalence rates, under 5% (e.g., Bolton et al., 2005;

Ford, Goodman, & Meltzer, 2003; Shaffer, Fisher, Dulcan, & Davies, 1996). Gender discrepancies have been reported, with more females than males having the disorder, but the finding is not consistent across all studies (e.g., Beidel & Turner, 2005; Silverman & Dick-Niederhauser, 2004). SAD is the least stable of the anxiety disorders, with some studies suggesting up to 80% natural remission (e.g., Foley, Pickles, Maes, Silberg, & Eaves, 2004). However, in studies of youth with SAD who later do not meet SAD criteria often meet criteria for another anxiety disorder diagnosis (Beidel & Turner, 2005).

Generalized Anxiety Disorder

The core symptoms of GAD in DSM-IV-TR are listed in Table 8.1. The disorder is characterized by excessive and uncontrollable worry about multiple topics that lasts at least 6 months. Because there is a high rate of comorbidity among anxiety disorders (see below), an important diagnostic consideration relates to the focus of the youth's worries. If restricted solely to (1) separation from an attachment figure (SAD), (2) social situations (social phobia), or (3) a specific event, stimulus, or situation (specific phobia), GAD is not the appropriate diagnosis. It is worth noting that until the release of DSM-IV (APA, 1994, 2000), overanxious disorder (OAD; DSM-III, APA [1980] and DSM-III-R, APA [1987]), was considered the diagnosis for youth who worried excessively. As a result, research on GAD in youth has only been amassed in the past 12 years.

Vasey's (1993) developmental theory of worry contends (1) that GAD should be more prevalent in older compared to younger children; (2) that older youth worry about a greater diversity of topics; and that (3) with age, a youth's ability to elaborate cognitively on worries increases. Evidence has generally supported these propositions. For example, although worry is common across childhood, it is more prevalent in older children (e.g., Vasey, 1993). Worry topics shift across development, too. Younger children worry more about their *physical* well-being, whereas older children worry more about their behavioral competence, social evaluation, and *psychological* well-being. Evidence also suggested that as age increases, children's ability to elaborate the potential negative consequences of worries increases. Different comorbidity patterns are also present in youth with GAD, depending on age, with younger children (ages 5–11) more likely presenting with separation concerns and - attention-deficit/hyperactivity disorder (ADHD), and older children showing more comorbid major depression and specific phobias (Masi, Favilla, Mucci, & Millipiedi, 2000; Strauss, Lease, Last, & Francis, 1988). In addition to the aforementioned symptoms, disturbing dreams have been associated with GAD in adolescents, especially girls (Nielsen et al., 2000). Finally, because headaches, stomachaches, muscle tension, sweating, and trembling are commonly reported physical complaints of children with GAD, many children are referred for treatment by their pediatricians or by gastrointestinal specialists (e.g., Bell-Dolan & Brazeal, 1993).

As a result of the shift from OAD to GAD, epidemiological studies of GAD in youth are relatively few. We also examined studies of OAD because, in general, research has suggested that youth diagnosed with OAD have tended to be diagnosed with GAD when DSM-IV criteria were applied (Kendall & Warman, 1996; Tracey, Chorpita, Douban, & Barlow, 1997). Community studies have reported prevalence rates for OAD ranging from less than 2 to 19%. Rates of GAD appear lower, ranging from 0.4 to 4.2%. Childhood anxiety disorder clinic studies have reported the prevalence of disorders in their samples, with prevalence of OAD and GAD being quite high, from about 20% to over 70% depending on the clinic (see Chorpita & Southam-Gerow, 2006, for review). In clinics serving a general clinical population, rates of OAD and GAD are considerably lower, in the 5–10% range (e.g., Southam-Gerow, Weisz, & Kendall, 2003).

Social Phobia

In DSM-IV, the essential feature of social phobia is a marked and persistent fear of one or more social or performance situations in which the person fears that embarrassment may occur. Upon exposure to the social or performance situation, the person almost invariably experiences an immediate anxiety response that may take the form of a panic attack. Individuals with social phobia may either avoid these situations or endure them with extreme distress. DSM-IV-TR criteria for social phobia are highlighted in Table 8.1. If the fear includes most social situations, a specifier of "generalized" is added.

Children with social phobia present with significantly higher levels of depressed mood than do normal children (Beidel, Turner, & Morris, 1999; La Greca & Lopez, 1998). Moreover, compared to their nonanxious peers, these children generally endorse significantly lower perceptions of cognitive competence and higher trait anxiety (Beidel & Turner, 2005; Beidel et al., 1999), with higher self-reported state anxiety during an evaluative task (Beidel, 1991). Furthermore, many youth with social phobia appear to have impaired social skills, as assessed in observational studies (Beidel et al., 1999; Spence, Donovan, & Brechman-Toussaint, 1999). Youth with social phobia may also become oppositional about going to school (Kearney, 2001).

Community epidemiological studies suggest that between 0.5 and 2.8% of youth meet criteria for social phobia (Beidel & Turner, 2005; Beidel, Turner, & Morris, 1995; Canino et al., 2004; Ford et al., 2003; Shaffer et al., 1996). Rates are generally higher for older youth and females; also, rates in studies in the United States and Puerto Rico were higher than those in studies in Britain. The vast majority of youth with social phobia, up to 92% in some studies, meet criteria for the "generalized" type (e.g., Beidel, Morris, & Turner, 2004; Hofmann et al., 1999). In addition, adolescents with generalized social phobia are distinguished from those with the nongeneralized form by (1) earlier age of onset, (2) greater impairment in functioning, (3) higher risk for the development of comorbid conditions, and (4) greater likelihood of earlier inhibited temperament or familial adversities (see Velting & Albano, 2001, for a review). Onset for social phobia is typically in early adolescence (age 11–12 years; Beidel et al., 2004; Beidel & Turner, 2005). In specialty anxiety clinic samples, rates of social phobia are in the 15–25% range (e.g., Kendall, Brady, & Verduin, 2001; Silverman et al., 1999).

Obsessive–Compulsive Disorder

OCD is characterized by recurrent and intrusive obsessions and compulsions that are time-consuming (greater than 1 hour per day) and cause marked distress for the child or significant functional impairment (APA, 2000). Table 8.1 provides a summary of the DSM-IV-TR criteria for OCD. In contrast to the adult criteria, the DSM does not require the child to realize that his or her obsessions or compulsions are excessive or unreasonable. Typical obsessions in youth include contamination fears, sexual or religious themes, or aggressive/violent images, and typical compulsions include washing, checking, ordering, and arranging (March, Franklin, Leonard, & Foa, 2004; Piacentini & Langley, 2004).

Comorbid anxiety and depression are among the most common associated features of OCD (March et al., 2004; Piacentini & Langley, 2004; Wewetzer et al., 2001), though concurrent mood disorders are typically more prevalent in older children (Geller et al., 2001). Earlier age of onset has been associated with an increased risk of ADHD and other anxiety disorders, including specific phobia, GAD, and separation anxiety (Geller et al., 2001; March et al., 2004). There is a higher incidence of OCD in children and adults with Tourette's disorder (35 to 50%); the incidence of Tourette's disorder in children and adults with OCD is lower, with estimates ranging between 5 and 7% (e.g., Geller et al., 2001).

Epidemiological studies suggest that between 1 and 2% of children meet DSM criteria for OCD (Geller et al., 1998; Piacentini & Langley, 2004), with studies that obtained higher rates relying on self-report checklists rather than clinical interviews. In childhood and early adolescence, there are slightly more males than females with OCD; with age, this gender discrepancy disappears (Beidel & Turner, 2005; March et al., 2004). Age of onset has ranged from 7 to 10 years according to the literature (e.g., Geller et al., 1998).

Specific Phobias

Specific phobia is diagnosed in youth who have a marked and persistent fear of certain objects or situations; the feared stimuli cannot include social situations, fear of having a panic attack, or separation concerns. As with social phobia, exposure to the stimulus is met with a severe fear response and is either avoided or endured with distress. Unlike adults, children may not recognize that the fear is excessive or unreasonable. Table 8.1 outlines the DSM-IV-TR symptoms for specific phobia. Common subtypes of specific phobia include fear of animals, blood, injection/injury, and natural environment.

Oppositional behavior is common in youth with a specific phobia insofar as they oppose adult efforts to expose them to the feared stimulus. As discussed below, specific phobia often co-occurs with other anxiety disorders, particularly GAD. A key to diagnosing specific phobia lies in differentiating between normal fears that are common throughout childhood, and the severe and impairing fears associated with specific phobia.

Reported rates of specific phobia are typically between 3 and 10%, with lower rates in studies relying on clinical interviews and rigorously adhering to the DSM impairment criteria (Essau, Conradt, & Petermann, 2000; Ollendick, King, & Muris, 2002; Verhulst, van der Ende, Ferdinand, & Kasius, 1997). Animal and natural environment phobias were the most common subtypes, with high levels of psychosocial impairment reported during the worst episode of the disorder. Despite such impairment, few adolescents receive any help for their phobia. Not surprisingly, phobias are especially common in childhood anxiety clinics. Ollendick and colleagues (2002) report that 15% of youth in such clinics meet criteria for a phobia diagnosis, though rates as high as 48% have been reported in the literature (Kendall et al., 1997). The disorder is more common among girls and younger children than among boys and older children (e.g., King, Muris, & Ollendick, 2004; Muris, Schmidt, & Merckelbach, 1999).

Panic Disorder

Until recently, many in the clinical and research communities debated whether children and adolescents can have panic disorder, believing that youth were not capable of having the catastrophic cognitions that typify panic disorder (see Kearney & Silverman, 1992; Moreau & Weissman, 1992; Nelles & Barlow, 1988). However, it is now generally accepted that panic attacks and panic disorder can occur in youth (e.g., Hayward, Killen, Kraemer, & Taylor, 2000; Kearney, Albano, Eisen, Allan, & Barlow, 1997; Ollendick, Mattis, & King, 1994). Panic disorder is defined by the occurrence of at least one *unexpected* panic attack, followed by at least 1 month of any one (or more) of the following: persistent fear of experiencing future attacks, worry about the implications of the attack or its consequences, or a significant change in behavior related to the attacks (APA, 2000). Table 8.1 outlines the diagnostic criteria for panic disorder.

In addition to panic symptoms, children and adolescents with panic disorder may display concomitant "agoraphobia," defined as the fear of being in situations from which escape may be difficult or embarrassing, or in which help is not readily available in the event of a panic attack (Kearney et al., 1997; Masi et al., 2000). A child with panic disorder may also avoid school situations, such as riding the bus and going to gym class, or refuse to attend school. Youth with panic disorder may also present with comorbid GAD, specific phobias, SAD, and depression (Kearney et al., 1997; Masi et al., 2000).

Rates of panic disorder in children and adolescents are not very well known given how recently the diagnosis in this age range has been given serious attention. Nevertheless, available estimates range from 0.5 to 5.3% for panic disorder, with rates of panic attacks being much higher—as high 63% in some reports (Lewinsohn, Hops, Roberts, Seeley, & Andrews, 1993; Masi et al., 2000; Ollendick, Birmaher, & Mattis, 2004; Verhulst et al., 1997). Panic disorder rates as high as 10% have been reported in mental health service settings (e.g., Kearney et al., 1997). Evidence suggests that rates are higher for females and increase with age across childhood and adoles-

cence (Ollendick et al., 2004). Peak age of onset occurs in late adolescence, though 10–20% of youth with panic disorder report that their first panic attack occurred before age 10 (Ollendick et al., 2004).

Other Descriptive Issues

In the following three sections, we discuss a few additional issues related to childhood anxiety disorders. First, we briefly describe common psychiatric comorbidities associated with anxiety disorders. Then we provide a concise review of the sparse research on childhood anxiety in diverse samples. We conclude with a short précis of research and theory concerning the etiology of anxiety.

Common Comorbidities

The issue of comorbidity in the childhood anxiety disorders plays a critical role in the understanding of childhood anxiety more generally (e.g., Caron & Rutter, 1991; Doss & Weisz, 2006). The focus of our chapter precludes a more than cursory review of the important data on common comorbidities. For more, the reader is referred to recent texts that focus more on childhood psychopathology (e.g., Albano et al., 2003). Evidence is clear that youth with anxiety disorders are likely to have at least one comorbid disorder (Brady & Kendall, 1992; Russo & Beidel, 1994), with rates in excess of 65% in epidemiological (Angold, Costello, & Erkanli, 1999; Bird, Gould, & Staghezza, 1993) and clinically referred samples (Kendall et al., 1997; Silverman & Ginsburg, 1998) commonly reported. In particular, comorbidity among the anxiety disorders is common, with GAD, SAD, and social phobia frequently co-occurring. Among the anxiety disorder diagnoses, OCD is the least likely to be associated with a comorbid anxiety disorder diagnosis, though comorbidity is still relatively common (e.g., Beidel & Turner, 2005). Aside from other anxiety disorders, depressive disorders are another common comorbidity (Brady & Kendall, 1992). As we discuss later, there are some theoretical reasons that this overlap makes sense (see "Conceptual Issues in Assessment"). Finally, there is also frequent comorbidity with disruptive behavior disorders, such as oppositional defiant disorder (ODD) and ADHD (e.g., Russo & Beidel, 1994).

A primary implication of comorbidity in the assessment of anxiety is that an assessor needs expertise in more than anxiety assessment tools. Conducting a differential diagnosis becomes an essential task. As an example, endorsement of the symptom "difficulty concentrating" might reflect at least three different diagnostic considerations within the mental health domain: an anxiety disorder diagnosis (e.g., GAD), a depressive disorder diagnosis, or ADHD. Thus, although we believe this chapter provides a comprehensive overview of the tools needed for anxiety assessment, we strongly advise mental health professionals to read the remaining chapters of this book and apply the lessons from them, before assessing a child suspected of having an anxiety disorder.

Anxiety in Diverse Samples

Despite calls for work with diverse samples, research with such samples has been lacking. In this brief section, we provide an overview of the literature focused on anxiety in youth, with regard to gender, ethnicity, and family income; our discussion is illustrative. The presence of gender differences in anxiety disorders among adults has been a robust finding (Yonkers & Gurguis, 1995). In youth, gender differences are also present, though they appear to emerge for many anxiety disorders in late childhood or early adolescence, in a manner similar to that found in the depression literature (e.g., Albano & Krain, 2005; Muris, Mayer, et al., 1998). As noted earlier, male cases predominate in samples of children with OCD until adolescence, at which point the male:female ratio becomes equivalent (e.g., March et al., 2004; Piacentini & Langley, 2004).

In general, very little research has focused on childhood anxiety in low-income samples. Some evidence does suggest that lower socioeconomic status and lower parental education level are associated with a greater prevalence and risk of anxiety disorders (Bird, Gould, Yager, Staghezza, & Canino, 1989; Last, Hersen, Kazdin, Finkelstein, & Strauss, 1987; Valez, Johnson, & Cohen, 1989). Recent work by Southam-Gerow and colleagues (Southam-Gerow, Chorpita, Miller, & Taylor, 2007; Southam-Gerow, Weisz, et al., 2003) has suggested that youth with anxiety disorders who present in clinics serving low-income families are more likely to have multiple disorders and increased family difficulty. The lack of research on childhood anxiety in low-income families is particularly problematic given the link between income and child psychopathology, particularly externalizing disorders (e.g., Atkins, Graczyk, & Frazier, 2003; Attar, Guerra, & Tolan, 1994; Costello, Compton, Keeler, & Angold, 2003; Kim-Cohen, Moffitt, & Caspi, 2004). Thus, future research should include more low-income families.

There are relatively more studies that include participants from diverse ethnic backgrounds, although, overall, this literature, too, is greatly lacking (e.g., Austin & Chorpita, 2004; Safren et al., 2000). Some studies have found differing levels of anxiety symptoms in African American versus European American youth, though the direction of the difference has not been consistent across studies (e.g., Compton, Nelson, & March, 2000; Last & Perrin, 1993). Issues of culture and ethnicity are important to consider in the assessment of childhood anxiety, because they play an important role in determining how child behaviors are perceived within a cultural group. For example, one behavior may generate a clinical referral in one cultural group, whereas in another, it may not. Relatedly, cultural and ethnic variables impact emotional development, and not all cultures share the same views on emotion expression and regulation (e.g., Fredrickson, 1998; Friedlmeier & Trommsdorff, 1999; Matsumoto, 1990).

In summary, although a growing body of research has focused directly on the demographic composition of anxiety disorders in children and adolescents, the available data are still too limited to allow for broad inferences. Studies vary on selection and recruitment procedures, geographical boundaries, incentives for participation, and opportunities for treatment. Cultural or racial biases may influence whether children from specific minority groups are referred for treatment of internalizing disorders such as anxiety. Moreover, the majority of studies in the literature with clinic-referred youth stem from specialty clinics for anxiety disorders in youth, whose samples have the potential for recruitment bias. Families who seek mental health services may be in a better position to be referred or to afford such services, and the clinical assessment literature is best interpreted with these caveats in mind.

Major Etiological Perspectives

A complete review of the major etiological perspectives of anxiety disorders is beyond the scope of this chapter, and the interested reader is referred elsewhere (e.g., Albano et al., 2003;

Beidel & Turner, 2005; Morris & March, 2004). Albano and colleagues (2003) summarized the "triple vulnerability" model of anxiety development (Barlow, 2000, 2002) as involving the interaction of a heritable biological diathesis, a psychological vulnerability related to "feeling" an uncontrollable/unpredictable threat or danger, and early learning experiences.

In terms of the first vulnerability, considerable evidence supports the notion that anxiety has a heritable component (Eaves et al., 1997; Eley et al., 2003). Many have suggested that this vulnerability for the development of anxiety manifests as an "inhibited" temperamental style, defined as the tendency to withdraw from novel or social experiences (e.g., Biederman et al., 1993; Kagan, Reznick, & Snidman, 1988). Other models of temperament and anxiety have focused more directly on the organization of biological systems that underlie motivation and emotion (e.g., Gray & McNaughton, 1996). For example, Gray's (1982) model of inhibition, independent of Kagan's work, has inspired rich theorizing regarding the relation of biological and temperamental factors to anxiety and anxiety disorders (e.g., Barlow, Chorpita, & Turovsky, 1996; Lonigan & Philips, 2001). Yet another area of temperament research has focused on the relation of anxiety disorders and depression to broader personality and affective variables, such as those represented in the Big Five model (i.e., Surgency/Extraversion, Agreeableness, Conscientiousness, Emotional Stability/Neuroticism, and Openness).

One of the most well researched of these models is Clark and Watson's (1991) tripartite model of emotion and its relation to anxiety and depression in children, a perspective suggesting that factors of positive affectivity (PA), negative affectivity (NA), and physiological hyperarousal (PH) account for the relation of anxiety and depression (Mineka, Watson, & Clark, 1998). This model has found empirical support in childhood anxiety research (e.g., Chorpita, Albano, & Barlow, 1998; Lonigan, Hooe, David, & Kistner, 1999) and has led to new assessment developments, as we discuss in some detail below.

Complementing these genetic and temperament models, several psychosocial factors associated with the development of anxiety disorders include coping strategies (Kendall, 1994), social–familial transmission (Chorpita, Albano, & Barlow, 1996), information processing (Vasey, Daleiden, Williams, & Brown, 1995), and complex forms of conditioning (Bouton, Mineka, & Barlow, 2001). One organizing theme involves the role of perceptions of control in both the expression and the development of negative emotions (Barlow, 2000, 2002; Chorpita, 2001). Many treatment approaches have focused on information-processing and learning histories as the key correlates, as evidenced by the prominence of cognitive-behavioral treatments in the child anxiety area (e.g., Chorpita & Southam-Gerow, 2006). Still, relational factors represent another important risk factor. For example, insecure early attachment is related to the development of anxiety disorders (Manassis, 2001; Warren, Huston, & Egeland, 1997), and problem-solving styles appear to be consistent within families of youth with anxiety disorders, such that avoidant strategies are emphasized (Chorpita et al., 1996).

The third area of vulnerability, as articulated by Barlow (2001), involves specific learning experiences that may precipitate specific disorders. For example, youth with existing inhibited temperament in conjunction with psychosocial risk factors of uncontrollability or poor problem solving are thought to be at increased risk to develop an anxiety disorder upon experiencing a specific fearful conditioning event. In general, early theories of how such conditioning occurs are quite diverse, including notions of associative and instrumental learning (Delprato & McGlynn, 1984; Mowrer, 1960), observational learning (Bandura, 1977), and verbal instruction (e.g., Rachman, 1977). Such concepts have now been incorporated in more contemporary, integrative developmental models (Albano et al., 2003; Chorpita, 2001; Vasey & Dadds, 2001) that emphasize core developmental psychopathology concepts such as temperament–environment fit, multifinality, equifinality, and multiple and reciprocal determinism (cf. Kazdin & Kagan, 1994; Sroufe, 1990).

CONCEPTUAL ISSUES IN ASSESSMENT

Proper assessment rests upon assumptions about a clearly articulated theory, and the child anxiety literature has faced some historical challenges in this area. Cronbach and Meehl (1955) offered the term *nomological network* to describe "the interlocking system of laws which constitute a theory" (p. 290) and argued that to understand the meaning of any chosen construct (e.g., childhood fear or anxiety), we must have certain ideas about how it will relate to other constructs.

Presumably, "anxiety" is a central construct in the relevant theoretical network, but to what degree is "anxiety" related to constructs such as "fear," "panic," "dread," "sadness," "inhibition," and so forth? Because many of the most widely used measures of childhood anxiety were originally developed prior to the contemporary theoretical positions regarding negative emotions (e.g., Barlow, 1988; Clark & Watson, 1991, Gray & McNaughton, 1996), a number of measures represent constructs in a network that has since been refined or strongly challenged by the accumulation of new evidence.

For example, the behavioral and emotional outputs of brain systems underlying fear and anxiety are consistent with a number of constructs related to vulnerability for anxiety disorders and depressive disorders from other literatures (Brown, Chorpita, & Barlow, 1998; Clark & Watson, 1991; Gray & McNaughton, 1996). Clark, Watson, and Mineka (1994) described NA as a "stable, highly heritable general trait dimension with a multiplicity of aspects ranging from mood to behavior" (p. 104). Thus, NA may be of considerable value in predicting the future emergence of anxious pathology. Furthermore, the model allows for improved understanding of the comorbidity among disorders of emotion. Perhaps most importantly, tests of the model in the context of dimensions of anxiety and depression have revealed the benefit of a hierarchical assessment framework (e.g., Chorpita, 2002; Zinbarg & Barlow, 1996); that is, it appears important to assess not only the symptoms of particular disorders or syndromes but also the higher-order affective and arousal dimensions related to those syndromes.

Research has provided at least an initial outline of the relation between the constructs of NA and PH, and has resolved the issues of terminology to some degree as well (Brown et al., 1998; Chorpita, 2001; Chorpita et al., 1996; Chorpita, Plummer, & Moffitt, 2000; Joiner, Catanzaro, & Laurent, 1996; Lonigan et al., 1999). Figure 8.1 shows the basic relations identified in children among dimensions outlined in the DSM-IV and the broader constructs of NA and PH. This general model has been confirmed in four studies in children and adolescents in both clinical and nonclinical

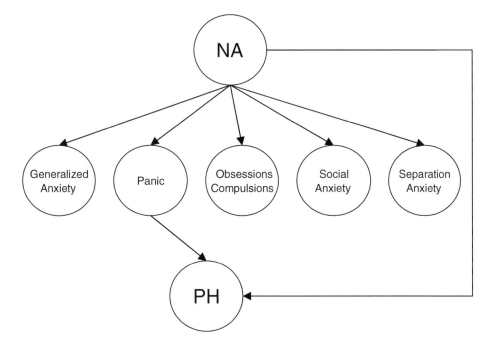

FIGURE 8.1. Model of relations among affective dimensions.

samples, and suggests that NA serves as a risk factor for all of the anxiety syndromes, whereas PH is related only to particular dimensions (Brown et al., 1998). Similar results from an adult clinical sample warranted the reformulation of the tripartite model (Mineka et al., 1998): Rather than being uniformly associated with anxiety, PH is associated with only particular anxiety syndromes (e.g., panic; Brown et al., 1998).

This integration of the literature on PH and NA with diagnostic syndromes also serves to explain the historical divergence of the child assessment literature and the diagnostic classification system. It seems likely that most of the traditional measures of anxiety in children were designed to assess broad trait dimensions; hence, they converged with broader constructs such as NA. More recent strategies keyed to diagnostic symptoms yielded confirmation of those respective syndromes. Taken together, these results illustrate two conceptual levels by which to consider clinical manifestations of fear and anxiety in youth. Given the current state of the literature, it appears that an understanding of both general factors (i.e., negative affect and arousal) and specific syndromes (e.g., clinical disorders) are important in terms of informing the treatment of anxious psychopathology.

Because accumulating evidence suggests that the broad term "anxiety" may be multifactorial, traditional measures of "anxiety" may be conceptually overinclusive. Not surprisingly, early measures of childhood anxiety had demonstrated problems with discriminant validity. For example, Perrin and Last (1992) found that the Revised Children's Manifest Anxiety Scale [RCMAS], the Fear Survey Schedule for Children—Revised [FSSC-R], and a modified version of the State–Trait Anxiety Inventory for Children—Trait [STAIC-T] (Fox & Houston, 1983) failed to discriminate between boys with anxiety disorders and those with ADHD, and that the FSSC-R failed to discriminate between boys with anxiety disorders and those with no history of psychiatric illness. The laws of the nomological network, however preliminary, suggest that children with anxiety disorders should score higher on anxiety measures than children with other disorders or no disorders. Similar results have been found with the related construct of anxiety sensitivity, a measure of which failed to discriminate between children with ADHD and those with

anxiety disorders (e.g., Rabian, Peterson, Richters, & Jensen, 1993). Given these issues, Stark and Laurent (2001) have considered whether "it is time to move to [the] next generation of measures" in assessing childhood anxiety (and depression). Fortunately, some new measures (reviewed later in the chapter) are consistent with the multidimensional and hierarchical nature of the nomological network.

QUESTIONS RELEVANT TO ASSESSMENT

In this section, we cover two topics: the purposes of assessment, as we see it, and assessment methods typically employed.

Purposes of Assessment

Essentially, assessment is an activity performed to inform a plan. That plan may include educational placement, a psychosocial treatment plan, the decision to start day care, the use of medication, and so forth. Assessment approaches for childhood fears and anxieties (see below) are extremely diverse. However, given issues related to stigmatization and test error, assessors should generally employ incremental approaches, and use increasingly more tests only as dictated by a lack of clarity for impending clinical or caregiver decisions.

Assessment generally informs three major decisions: (1) identification–screening, (2) triage–treatment planning, and (3) outcome assessment. The first decision involves determining whether the child has a fear or anxiety disorder that warrants treatment; that is, one must identify (1) whether the condition is developmentally inappropriate in the observed context, and (2) whether the condition causes sufficient distress or interference to merit being addressed formally in some way. We refer to this as the identification and screening phase. The first part of this decision is often guided by measures of anxiety or related constructs, to determine whether intensity or severity is outside of the developmentally normative range. The second part of that decision, however, must typically be informed by a measure related not to fear or anxiety per se, but to its functional consequences. For example, failure to attend school, lack of friends, feelings of extreme distress, and academic impairment—all indicators of possible need for treatment—are not always assessed solely by anxiety measures.

A related screening purpose that is becoming more common, universal screening for identification of at-risk youth (e.g., for prevention programs), may also be called prescreening, because the goal is not so much to determine need for treatment as to determine need for further screening. We differentiate this *prescreening* from the screening that might happen at the time of a mental health referral, because the latter also represents the beginning of the second purpose of assessment, treatment planning.

Once sufficient information is available to suggest the need for treatment, the second decision involves determining the nature of the fear or anxiety, so that appropriate treatments can be tailored to the condition. We refer to this phase as triage and treatment planning. Traditions for informing this decision vary widely, from diagnosis to functional analysis, to various case conceptualization approaches; these methods are reviewed in some detail below.

Finally, the third assessment decision typically involves measuring the ongoing effects of a plan or intervention (i.e., outcome measurement). Such measurement strategies typically involve brief, focused measures that provide regular feedback about the effects of treatment and its components. For example, weekly observation of the frequency of speaking in class might indicate whether particular aspects of a social anxiety intervention are working as intended. These repeated assessments are typically briefer and more focused than the earlier comprehensive assessments, although they often share common measurement tools.

Sometimes, all three assessment goals—identification–screening, triage–treatment planning, and outcome measurement—may be served by the same assessment tool; however, this is not often the case. A measurement tool designed to differentiate between normal and abnormal levels of anxiety may not inform treatment planning well, except to indicate that treatment is indicated. For example, a high score on the Screen for Child Anxiety Related Emotional Disorders (SCARED; Birmaher et al., 1997) informs the assessor about broad diagnostic areas of concern (e.g., separation anxiety) but does not identify the proximal influences on those concerns (i.e., the related antecedents, behaviors, and consequences that need to be addressed to remedy the problem). As another example, relevant outcomes may shift throughout treatment as the client improves, or as new treatment goals emerge. As such, outcome measurement needs to shift and may often be different than the initial assessment tools used to screen or identify treatment foci. Throughout our review of the available assessment tools, we clarify the use(s) of each tool for these three purposes.

Assessment Methods

In this section, we briefly describe the primary methods used to assess child anxiety. The primary assessment methods in the child anxiety literature are similar to those in other areas and consistent with the multifaceted nature of anxiety in youth. These methods include questionnaires, structured diagnostic interviews, direct observation, and physiological assessment. Our discussion of questionnaires and interviews here is brief and restricted to providing an overview of the method; the subsequent measures review provides specific examples of measures, along with psychometric data. Our discussion of observational and physiological methods is more extended, because we do not provide a review of specific methods in the review section later. We conclude the section with a description of case conceptualization, a method frequently used in practice, but one for which it is difficult to gather traditional psychometric data.

Questionnaires

Questionnaires possess tremendous efficiency, especially in clinical practice. Most questionnaires do not require expertise for administration; thus, they are easily implemented in a busy clinical practice by an assistant. In some instances, computer-aided administration is possible, allowing the client to complete the questionnaire at home in between sessions. Questionnaires also permit a high degree of respondent confidentiality/privacy, in the sense that the respondent is permitted to reveal personal feelings without having to speak them to another person. Questionnaires also have the advantage of being the most thoroughly researched assessment methods. As such, there is a relative plethora of data on the performance of many of questionnaires. Furthermore, questionnaires have the advantage of multiple versions to include multiple reporters, a key issue in assessing children. Disadvantages to the use of questionnaires include the lack of a systematic way to follow up on responses to clarify meaning or to ensure validity. As an example, a respondent who may not fully understand the meaning of a question might respond in a less than valid manner. Another problem with questionnaires is that the information gleaned is limited to what is asked. Finally, questionnaires require literacy. This issue complicates their use with younger children, youth (and parents) with limited literacy, and youth for whom a questionnaire is not available in his or her primary language.

Structured Diagnostic Interviews

The current state of the art for clinical diagnosis involves the structured diagnostic interview (Shaffer, Lucas, & Richters, 1999). Compared with unstructured clinical interviews, structured diagnostic interviews (1) yield more objective and quantifiable data, (2) facilitate comprehensive assessment of a range of disorders, and (3) increase the specificity of the information gathered (Costello, Egger, & Angold, 2005; Shaffer et al., 1999). One of the main limitations of these interviews is the lengthy administration time. Assessment of a child and parent with a typical interview may take up to 4–5 hours, not including scoring and interpretation. Although the data obtained are often quite rich, such procedures are likely not feasible in many service settings. As a compromise, it may be preferable to administer the portions of a structured interview that seem relevant based on some screening work (via phone, etc.). In an investigation of such an approach, Chorpita, Yim, and Tracey (2002) report that preliminary evidence suggests similar accuracy can be obtained in less time, when screens are performed with carefully selected instruments.

In general, two types of structured interviews are available: (1) respondent-based and (2) interviewer-based (e.g., Shaffer et al., 1999). The former interview has as its prime advantage the ability to use lay interviewers. With respondent-based approaches, the format of the interview is tightly controlled, requiring mostly yes–no responses. The questions are also worded such that no special knowledge of the DSM is needed to administer the interview. Interviewer reliability, then, is rarely an issue so long as the interviewers are well trained to follow the protocol. However, such interviews have the possible disadvantage of respondent unreliability given that an interviewer is allowed to clarify only conceptual issues (e.g.,

the meaning of "obsessions") within certain limits. Furthermore, an interviewer is not permitted to probe yes–no answers, even when he or she suspects that the respondent misunderstood a question. Interviewer-based approaches, on the other hand, require a clinically trained interviewer who is familiar with the DSM. Such interviews allow the interviewer to ask multiple questions to gather a thorough understanding of responses.

Observational Methods

Because relying on child and parent report alone limits what one can learn, it is often advisable to use assessment procedures other than questionnaires and interviews. The most common observational procedure for anxiety assessment, the behavioral avoidance test (BAT), can be administered in either laboratory or naturalistic settings. These procedures have been used to assess fears of heights (Van Hasselt, Hersen, Bellack, Rosenblum, & Lamparski, 1979), social interaction (Eisen & Silverman, 1991), blood (Van Hasselt et al., 1979), animals (Evans & Harmon, 1981), and darkness (Kelly, 1976). For the most part, these measures were designed for specific, idiographic purposes, and not for nomothetic standardization. In other words, these measures were created and adapted to specific uses within a particular study, or for the treatment of a specific child. As a result, they do not possess the same evidence base as the interviews and questionnaires we describe shortly. However, because of the utility of BATs in clinical practice, we recommend their use as a means of assessing treatment progress and outcome. The BAT has numerous advantages, including (1) a straightforward procedure, (2) a direct relevance to desired outcomes, and (3) concurrent monitoring of different types of responses (e.g., physiological responses and motor behavior).

That said, there are also several limitations of the BAT. First, as we noted, the absence of a standardized BAT procedure makes cross-study comparisons difficult. This can also complicate interpretation of BAT results. For example, criteria used to determine clinical severity (e.g., the need for formal intervention) of a particular response may be rather subjective, with some judges, but not others, interpreting a given response as abnormal. Second, as typically used, a BAT affords the subject a high level of control, a factor that is not likely to occur in natural settings. Although the BAT may track a specific outcome of interest, it is not clear how well BAT results generalize to new situations and contexts. Thus, clinicians may choose to design BATs that include less control for clients, and that are implemented in natural or varied settings.

As an illustration, we routinely use questionnaire data both to conduct initial assessment and to track progress and outcome. Questionnaires are generally designed to capture broad patterns of symptoms or functioning. Often, however, treatment for a youth with an anxiety disorder may have a few specific outcomes in mind, such as a return to school or an increase in social interaction. The use of a BAT to track these specific outcomes is often more sensitive and outcome-relevant than questionnaire or interview data. In the case of Frank, an 11-year-old youth with school refusal behavior stemming from social and separation anxiety, we used multiple questionnaires throughout treatment. However, a key index was observing and tracking his approach and avoidance behaviors regarding school. We implemented a naturalistic, "moving-target" BAT with school attendance as the goal, so that as Frank was successful in lower level approach behaviors, we continually updated the goal criterion. At first, this meant that time he spent in the parking lot of the school was tracked. However, as treatment progressed, we tracked the time spent in the classroom. In parallel fashion, we also measured Frank's specific avoidance behaviors, such as covering his head with his coat. In the end, although other, more general outcome indices showed improvement as well, these specific areas tapped by a customized BAT very likely assessed the most important outcome from the perspective of the consumers.

There are some measurement issues that all observational methods have in common (Barrios & Hartmann, 1997). One such issue is accuracy, which is the ability to obtain data that reflect without distortion the domain under investigation (Foster, Bell-Dolan, & Burge, 1988). To ensure accuracy, observational methods must be compared with an objective criterion; however, oftentimes such a criterion does not exist, so the accuracy of observational methods cannot be ensured (Foster & Cone, 1980). Another issue is reactivity, which means that the mere presence of observers can influence the behavior being observed (Tyron, 1998), leading subjects to act differently than they would otherwise act. There is some evidence, however, that children are not as prone as adults to reactivity

(Foster & Cone, 1980). Some methods for minimizing reactivity include using participant observers, and video cameras or tape recorders; minimizing subject–observer interaction; and allowing enough time for reactivity to lessen (Haynes & Horn, 1982). Yet another issue is factors that may bias the reports of observers, such as expectancies and observer drift. For example, knowing the experimenter's expectations might influence observers. "Observer drift" describes tendency of trained observers to rate the same events differently over time (Tyron, 1998). Regular agreement checks and effective observer training are important to minimize observer bias (Harris & Lahey, 1982). A final problem is that direct observation methods often lack feasibility in applied settings. They are not only more challenging to administer but also the chances that such methods in clinical settings have the same scope of dissemination and penetration as standardized questionnaires and checklists—now often available on the Internet—seem relatively low.

In summary, observation methods clearly have a place in assessment of anxiety. However, given the lack of standardization and norms, they likely work best when supplemented with other methods, such as structured interviews, self-report measures, and psychophysiological measurement to obtain a full picture of the phenomenon of anxiety. Furthermore, observational methods are most useful as measures of treatment planning and outcome rather than for screening purposes. Indeed, repeated BATs in some ways are difficult to distinguish from treatment itself. Finally, although observational measures have been used for many years, their psychometric standing is relatively unknown in clinical populations of children. As our review indicates, only a handful of studies have examined the properties of these assessment methods. In the end, though observational measures are important tools in the assessment armamentarium, they no longer play the central role they played in the past (Mash & Foster, 2001).

Physiological Assessment

Another assessment method that eliminates the reliance on potentially subjective reporting is using physiological indices, such as heart rate, blood pressure, cortisol levels, or galvanic skin response (Beidel, 1988, 1991). Although measurement of anxiety with physiological methods makes theoretical sense, because anxiety (and stress) have clear physiological manifestations and underpinnings (Barlow, 2002), anxiety-focused research on such measures with children is rare (e.g., Beidel & Turner, 2005; see also Wilhelm & Roth, 2001, for discussion of the rarity of such measures in adult anxiety research). Thinking broadly, physiological measurement of reactivity to stress typically focuses on two systems: the hypothalamic–pituitary–adrenal (HPA) and the sympathetic–adrenal–medullary (SAM) systems (e.g., Bauer, Quas, & Boyce, 2002). In the child anxiety literature, most measures have focused on the SAM system, relying on indices such as heart rate (HR) or blood pressure (BP). Some studies have also used galvanic skin response (GSR). To date, the number of such studies that has examined psychometric properties of these methods is quite small; hence, we do not review them in the section below.

As noted, HR and BP (and, to a lesser extent, GSR) are used as indices of SAM activity. Recent psychophysiological research has suggested that better measures for SAM activity may exist, so that it is possible to disentangle sympathetic and parasympathetic arousal (e.g., Brenner, Beauchaine, & Sylvers, 2005; deGeus & van Doornen, 1996). Both HR and BP gauge the combined activity of the two systems (Bauer et al., 2002). Two indices, heart rate variability (HRV; essentially, variance in observed HR) and respiratory sinus arrhythmia (RSA; HR fluctuation as it relates to respiration), are thought to tap parasympathetic arousal. There is some controversy as to the optimal way to gauge RSA and HRV, discussion of which is beyond the scope of this chapter (de Geus & van Doornen, 1996). A third index, the preejection period (PEP; time between two cardiac events—the depolarization of left ventricle and ejection of blood into the aorta), is thought to index sympathetic arousal. Together, RSA or HRV and PEP afford a good way to gauge the complexity of SAM activity (de Geus & van Doornen, 1996). However, the utility of these indices for anxiety assessment is less clear for at least two reasons. First, we could not identify any studies that specifically link any of these measures to anxiety in a child population. Thus, there is too little research in the area to judge the value of these measures. Second, because all three measures are likely to gauge constructs broader than anxiety alone (e.g., Beauchaine, 2001; Thayer & Lane, 2000), their use in assessment of anxiety (e.g., vs. negative temperament, depression) is not clear. Still, there has been increasing interest in these measures to gauge several anxiety-related constructs, including children's stress reactivity, child temperament, and child emotion regulation (e.g., Alkon et al., 2003; Boyce et al., 2001; Calkins & Dedmon, 2001; Granger, Weisz, & Kauneckis, 1994; Kagan et al., 1988). Thus, future researchers should consider including measures such as RSA, HRV, or PEP in their child anxiety studies to inform the field as to their helpfulness.

Studies concerning markers of the HPA system in the child anxiety literature are even rarer than those that focus on the SAM system, perhaps because such measurement entails collection of blood, urine, or saliva, adding both complexity to the study design and implementation, and a potentially unpleasant demand on participants. HPA activity is usually assessed through measurement of cortisol levels (in blood, urine, or saliva) or, less often, measurement of adrenocorticotropic hormone (Bauer et al., 2002). Some have advocated measuring HPA activity via other means (e.g., dehydroepiandrosterone [DHEA] and its sulfated ester [DHEAS]; Granger & Kivlighan, 2003). Research on HPA activity has been somewhat more common in youth with depressive or conduct disorders (e.g., Goodyer, Park, & Herbert, 2001; Pajer, Gardner, Rubin, Perel, & Neal, 2001; van Goozen, Matthys, Cohen-Kettenis, Thijssen, & van Engeland, 1998). Similar to our conclusions about the newer indices of the SAM system, research is needed to determine the utility of biochemical markers of the HPA system for assessing anxiety.

In summary, physiological measures represent an exciting yet understudied area in the assessment of anxiety in children. Because of scant available data about the performance of these measures in assessing anxiety in children, we cannot yet recommend them for any of the three primary purposes of clinical assessment: (1) screening, (2) treatment planning, or (3) outcome measurement. However, we do see a potential for growth in the role of these measures in the coming years, especially as they are better studied and their methods become less intrusive. Indeed, there may be a time when physiological measurement becomes a key part of screening for anxiety or anxiety risk, as well as an important outcome measure. It is even conceivable that should methods become more accessible, treatment planning might be aided by physiological measurement.

Case Conceptualization

We conclude our review of assessment methods with a brief description of a method that is an important component of any assessment, yet is not itself subject to scientific study: *case conceptualization*. Although case conceptualization takes many forms, we focus here on functional assessment (FA). The basic premise behind case conceptualization is that in addition to nomothetically oriented assessment tools, an idiographic formulation is needed for each client/patient to individualize treatment (e.g., Freeman & Miller, 2002). A case conceptualization is essentially a "story" that describes the client's problems and strengths, posits hypotheses for why they have come to be, and offers possible remedies for the problems (e.g., Freeman & Miller, 2002). In this way, case conceptualizations must be rooted in theoretical assumptions about the variables that cause and influence behavior. Two recent treatment programs, multisystemic therapy (MST; Henggeler, Schoenwald, Rowland, & Cunningham, 2002) and primary and secondary control enhancement training (PASCET; Weisz, Southam-Gerow, Gordis, & Connor-Smith, 2003), include aspects of case conceptualization. In the case of MST, there is explicit and ongoing use of the specific case conceptualization method FA throughout treatment.

In FA, a number of steps are followed. The problem(s) is defined as behaviorally as possible. Then, a number of factors relevant to the problem are identified, including (1) background/historical variables assessed, (2) antecedent events, (3) established operations (i.e., events or conditions that alter the effect of other events or conditions), and (4) consequences. Once the relevant factors are identified, hypotheses are developed that connect the factors to the problem, then tested in the treatment process, and the new data that emerge are used to modify the case conceptualization. In this way, case conceptualization that uses FA is an ongoing and iterative process: The case formulation is fluid and not static.

INSTRUMENT REVIEW

Review Parameters and Procedures

Our intention in this chapter is to identify the most commonly used instruments for child anxiety and to review their psychometric prop-

erties to help guide assessors in selecting the best instruments for the assessment task. To do that, we have used several strategies. First, we conducted a PsycINFO search using the following parameters: [anxiety or fear or worry or panic or avoidance or phobia or obsession or compulsion or stress] and [measure or instrument or scale or questionnaire or assessment] and [child or children or youth or adolescent]. We included only articles from 1970 to the present. The PsycINFO search netted 6,052 articles. In addition, we searched through the reference lists of anxiety measurement review articles (e.g., Barrios & Hartmann, 1997; Myers & Winters, 2002), related chapters on treatment (e.g., Chorpita & Southam-Gerow, 2006), and the reference lists of articles we retrieved from the initial search. With additional articles added from reference list searches, we identified a pool of 7,218 articles. We then screened this pool using the criteria listed in Table 8.2.

From our initial sample of over 7,200 articles, 188 met the criteria in Table 8.2. A team of coders examined these studies using a detailed coding manual (available upon request). The coding process involved extracting data from the articles in the categories listed in Table 8.3, consistent with criteria proposed by Stallings and March (1995; see also Greco & Morris, 2004). Coding meetings were held at least biweekly during the coding, and all coders were in regular contact. Of the 188 articles, 15% (30) were double-coded to ensure consistency. Interrater kappa coefficients were over .90 for all codes.

Results and Discussion of Review

As noted earlier, there are different procedures and methods that can be used to assess anxiety, including questionnaires, interviews, observations, and physiological measures. The two former methods have received the most research attention by far, at least according to the criteria we used to establish our sample. With regard to questionnaires, we found 150 articles that met our criteria, whereas for interviews, we found 33 articles meeting those same criteria.

The number of articles meeting our criteria that focused on physiological or observational measures was considerably smaller. This outcome was not surprising for physiological measures given their expense and concerns raised

TABLE 8.2. Screening Criteria for Article Coding

1. The article evaluated a measure that purports to assess an *anxiety-related* construct, including *but not limited to*:

   - Anxiety
   - Fear
   - Worry
   - Panic
   - Avoidance
   - Any DSM anxiety disorder (e.g., phobia, OCD, GAD)
   - But *not* including the following
     - Traumatic stress or PTSD
     - Anxiety-relevant temperamental characteristics
     - Test anxiety
     - Medical- or dental-related anxiety

   To meet this criterion, the evaluated measure must have at least one anxiety-specific scale. Measures that included broad anxiety/depression scales only (e.g., Child Behavior Checklist) were not included.

2. The study had a minimum sample size of 25 child/adolescent (i.e., ages 5–18) cases. Studies of infants, toddlers, and preschoolers were not included.

3. The primary or secondary focus of the article was an examination of a measure's psychometric properties (reliability and/or validity and/or factor analysis). In other words, the study must have as one of its purposes the examination of the psychometric properties of a measure of an anxiety-related construct.

about their reliable use with children (e.g., Beidel, 1991). Because we were able to identify only a handful of studies that examined physiological measures and met our inclusion criteria, we chose not to discuss specific physiological measures in this chapter.

It was surprising that our search identified so few psychometric studies of observational measures, in contrast to earlier chapters on fears and anxieties (e.g., Barrios & Hartmann, 1997). Our review suggests that questionnaires and interviews are now the prominent methods of assessment. Furthermore, inspection of the studies on observational measures in earlier chapters reveals that most of the cited studies had very small samples, many with an *n* of 1. Our criterion requiring a minimum sample size

TABLE 8.3. Coding Categories

- Article information
- Study parameters (e.g., number of participants, sociodemographic characteristics)
- Measure parameters (e.g., number of items, number of scales)
- Reliability data (e.g., internal consistency, retest reliability)
- Validity data (e.g., convergent, divergent, and discriminant validity)
- Factor-analytic findings

of 25 excluded many of these studies. Even studies with sample sizes above 25 were primarily treatment studies, whose focus was evaluation of a treatment and not the psychometric properties of any particular measure. As a result, available psychometric data of the observational measure were inadequate. Furthermore, as described earlier, the measures were typically designed for a specific study and were often idiographic (i.e., designed for a specific child's clinical presentation). Thus, we do not discuss observational measures further.

Questionnaires

We identified 151 articles examining the psychometric properties of 48 different questionnaires. Among the 48 questionnaires were multiple variants of certain questionnaires; for example, the FSSC has multiple revisions and has been translated into several languages. Almost one-third of the articles we identified were published in 2000 or later, indicating an accelerating trend in anxiety assessment research. Questionnaires studied ranged in size from 10 items to over 400. Overall, the large majority of questionnaires had child report versions (38 of the 48 questionnaires). We identified 13 different measures in our review that had parent report versions, 6 that had a teacher report version, and 2 that had a clinician report version. From a purely quantitative view, the RCMAS (Reynolds & Richmond, 1978), the STAIC (Spielberger, 1973), and the FSSC-R (Ollendick, 1983) were the most studied measures, with more than 15 articles on each of the measures. However, since 2000, the most frequently studied measures were the SCARED (Birmaher et al., 1997), the STAIC, and the Childhood Anxiety Sensitivity Inventory (CASI; Silverman, Fleisig, Rabian, & Peterson, 1991). Descriptive data on the 14 most studied questionnaires are listed in Table 8.4.

The discussion of our findings is divided into two sections. First, we provide a brief description of the 14 instruments that received the most empirical attention (see Table 8.4). After a brief description of each measure, we discuss the psychometric characteristics of each. Because of the great number of questionnaires studied, we focus our discussion here on the 14 most frequently studied measures.

OVERVIEW OF QUESTIONNAIRES

We identified three basic types of questionnaires in our review. First, there were two "trait" measures referred to by Muris, Merckelbach, and colleagues (2002) as "traditional" anxiety measures: the RCMAS (Reynolds & Richmond, 1978) and the STAIC (Spielberger, 1973). Second, there were several "multidimensional" anxiety questionnaires, most of which focus on DSM-IV categories, including the Revised Child Anxiety and Depression Scale (RCADS; Chorpita, Yim, Moffitt, Umemoto, & Francis, 2000), the SCARED (Birmaher et al., 1997), and the Spence Child Anxiety Scale (SCAS; Spence, 1998). The Multidimensional Anxiety Scale for Children (MASC; March, Conners, et al., 1999), another multidimensional instrument, does not follow DSM criteria as closely in its construction. Finally, several questionnaires assessed more specific problem areas or *syndromes* within the anxiety spectrum, including social anxiety, OCD, worry, phobias/fears, and school refusal. In this section, we briefly describe each of these 14 measures to provide an overview before presenting the psychometric characteristics of each.

We begin with the two trait measures of anxiety, the STAIC and the RCMAS. Explicitly based on the state–trait distinction (Gaudry, Vagg, & Spielberger, 1975), the STAIC includes

two separate 20-item scales (i.e., state and trait anxiety) that may be administered separately or together.[1] The measure consists of statements (e.g., "I worry too much," "I get jittery") for which a respondent is rated on a 3-point scale (*Hardly ever, Sometimes, Often*). The STAIC has been translated in to multiple languages, including Chinese (e.g., Li, Cheung, & Lopez, 2004a, 2004b), Dutch (Muris, Gadet, Moulaert, & Merckelbach, 1998), and Thai (Chaiyawat & Brown, 2000). Another traditional trait measure, the RCMAS, is a 37-item instrument that possesses a "total" scale, three anxiety-related subscales (i.e., worry/oversensitivity, concentration, and physiological anxiety), and a "lie" scale. The RCMAS comprises a series of yes–no questions (e.g., "Often I have trouble getting my breath," "I often worry about something bad happening to me").

Alternatively, the multidimensional measures of anxiety include three DSM-IV–based scales and one additional multidimensional scale (see Table 8.5). The RCADS, a 47-item DSM-IV–based instrument, includes a total anxiety and depression scale and a total anxiety scale. In addition, there are five anxiety disorder–related scales and a major depressive disorder scale (see Table 8.5). RCADS items are designed to index DSM-IV syndromes; a respondent uses a 4-point scale (*Never, Sometimes, Often, Always*). Another DSM-IV–based instrument, the SCARED, has two different versions: the original SCARED and a revised version (SCARED-R). The former has 41 items (e.g., "I am nervous," "When I get frightened, my heart beats fast") and possesses a "total" scale and five DSM-IV subscales (see Table 8.5). The SCARED-R has 66 items, with a "total" scale and nine DSM subscales (see Table 8.5). The SCARED and SCARED-R both employ a 3-point scale (i.e., *Almost Never, Sometimes, Often*). The SCAS, the final DSM-IV–based scale, has 44 items (e.g., "I worry about being away from my parents," "I feel afraid if I have to talk in front of my class") and includes a "total" scale and six DSM-IV subscales (see Table 8.5). The SCAS uses a 4-point scale (i.e., *Never, Sometimes, Often, Always*). Although all three of these instruments are DSM-IV–

---

[1] Although data exist with regard to the State version, our discussion here is focused on the Trait version of the measure.

TABLE 8.4. Descriptive Information for Selected Questionnaires

Measure name	Abbrev.	Type	Construct	No. of subscales	No. of items	Time to complete (min)	Cost (company)?
Revised Children's Manifest Anxiety Scale	RCMAS	Trait	Anxiety	3	37	9	Yes (Pro-Ed)
State–Trait Anxiety Inventory for Children	STAIC	Trait	Trait (and State) anxiety	2	20 or 40	5 or 10	Yes (Mind Garden)
Multidimensional Anxiety Scale for Children	MASC	Multidimensional	Non-DSM anxiety	4	39	10	Yes (Harcourt)
Revised Child Anxiety and Depression Scale	RCADS	Multidimensional	DSM anxiety disorders	6	47	12	No
Screen for Child Anxiety Related Emotional Disorders	SCARED	Multidimensional	DSM anxiety disorders	5 or 9	38 or 66	9 or 16	No
Spence Children's Anxiety Scale	SCAS	Multidimensional	DSM anxiety disorders	6	44	11	Maybe (Permission needed for commercial use)
Childhood Anxiety Sensitivity Index	CASI	Syndrome	"Panic" and anxiety sensitivity	1 or 2	18 or 44	5 or 11	No
Children's Yale–Brown Obsessive–Compulsive Scale	CY-BOCS	Syndrome	OCD	4	10 or 79	3 or 20	No
Fear Survey Schedule for Children	FSSC	Syndrome	"Phobias"	5	80 or 78	20 or 19	No
Leyton Obsessional Inventory—Child Version	LOI-C	Syndrome	OCD	4	20	5	No
Penn State Worry Questionnaire for Children	PSWQ-C	Syndrome	GAD	1	14	4	No
School Refusal Assessment Scale	SRAS	Syndrome	School refusal	4	16 or 24	4 or 6	No
Social Anxiety Scale	SAS	Syndrome	Social phobia	3	22	6	No
Social Phobia and Anxiety Inventory	SPAI	Syndrome	Social phobia	2	26	7	Yes (Harcourt)

Informants	No. of papers since 1970	No. of papers since 2000	Countries tested in	Age range	No. of studies with >20% minorities?	Studies include boys and girls?	Variants	Languages/cultural adaptations
Child, Parent	29	4	USA, Australia, Belgium, Canada, Netherlands, Uruguay, Zimbabwe	5–19	9	Yes		English, Dutch, French, Spanish
Child, Parent	20	7	USA, Australia, Belgium, Canada, China, Netherlands, Thailand	6–18	4	Yes	Original, Adolescent	English, Chinese, Thai, Dutch
Child	6	3	USA, Belgium	8–18	3	Yes		English, Dutch
Child	2	2	USA	6–18	2	Yes		English
Child, Parent	15	8	USA, Belgium, Germany, Netherlands, South Africa	8–19	1	Yes	Original, Revised	English, Dutch, German, Afrikaans
Child, Parent	8	6	Australia, Belgium, Germany, Netherlands, South Africa	7–19	0	Yes		English, Dutch, German, Afrikaans
Child	12	7	USA, Netherlands, Spain	8–18	3	Yes	Original, Revised	English, Catalan, Dutch
Child	3	3	USA	5–19	0	Yes	Interview, Checklist	English
Child, Parent	17	3	USA, Australia, Belgium, China, Greece, Netherlands	3–19	2	Yes	Revised, II	English, Chinese, Greek, Hawaiian, Dutch
Cild	2	2	USA	8–17	0	Yes		English
Child	3	1	USA, Netherlands	6–18	0	Yes		English, Dutch
Child, Parent	3	2	USA	6–17	1	Yes	Original, Revised	English
Child	12	6	USA, Spain		4	Yes	Child, Child–Revised, Adolescent	English, Spanish
Child	10	5	USA, Spain	8–18	1	Yes		English, Spanish

TABLE 8.5. DSM Disorder Coverage for Multidimensional Anxiety Measures

	RCADS	SCARED	SCARED-R	SCAS
GAD	✓	✓	✓	✓
SAD	✓	✓	✓	✓
Social phobia	✓	✓	✓	✓
Panic disorder	✓	✓	✓	✓
OCD	✓		✓	✓
PTSD			✓	
Specific phobia			✓	
School phobia		✓		
Other anxiety problems				✓
Major depression	✓			

based, they do not cover the same disorders (see Table 8.5 for details).

The final multidimensional measure of anxiety, the MASC, does not draw solely on a DSM conceptualization of anxiety. The MASC is a 39-item (e.g., "I feel tense or uptight," "I get scared when my parents go away") measure that indexes a single personality dimension, as well as physiological arousal and two clinical syndromes. The MASC possesses a "total" scale and four subscales: (1) Harm Avoidance, (2) Physical Symptoms, (3) Separation Anxiety, and (4) Social Anxiety. In addition, two other subscales have been developed for the MASC, an Anxiety Disorder Index and a 10-item "Short" version of the total instrument. The MASC uses a 4-point scale (i.e., *Never true, Rarely true, Sometimes true, Often true*).

In addition to the trait and multidimensional measures, we also identified several measures that trade off bandwidth for fidelity (e.g., Cronbach, 1970) by focusing exclusively on narrow, anxiety-related syndromes (e.g., social anxiety, phobias/fears). For example, two measures of social anxiety received a lot of empirical attention: the Social Anxiety Scale and variants (SAS; e.g., La Greca, Dandes, Wick, & Shaw, 1988) and the Social Phobia and Anxiety Inventory and variants (SPAI; Beidel et al., 1995). The SAS, a 22-item (e.g., "I worry about what others think of me," "I get nervous when I talk to peers I don't know very well") measure, has been studied in its child (SASC), revised child (SASC-R), and adolescent (SAS-A) versions. Across all versions, there has been a "total" scale and three subscales: (1) Fear of Negative Evaluation, (2) Social Avoidance and

Distress–New Situations, and (3) Social Avoidance and Distress–General Situations. The SAS uses a 5-point scale (i.e., from *Definitely not true* to *Definitely true*). The child version of the SPAI, the SPAI-C, is a 26-item (e.g., "I avoid social situations," "I feel afraid if have to ask questions in class") measure with a "total" scale and three subscales: (1) Fear of Adults, (2) Fear of Familiar Peers, and (3) Fear of Unfamiliar Peers. However, these scales have not been consistently confirmed across all studies; some researchers have posited other scales based on factor analysis (e.g., Storch, Masia-Warner, Dent, Roberti, & Fisher, 2004). The SPAI-C uses a 3-point scale (i.e., *Never, Sometimes, Most of the time/Always*).

Of the several measures of OCD receiving empirical attention, only the Child Yale–Brown Obsessive–Compulsive Scale (CY-BOCS; e.g., Scahill, Riddle, & McSwiggin-Hardin, 1997) and the Leyton Obsessional Inventory—Child version (LOI-C; e.g., Berg, Rapoport, & Flament, 1986) have been studied psychometrically. The CY-BOCS, based on an OCD measure for adults, was originally developed as a clinical interview, later adapted into a clinician-administered questionnaire, and has recently been adapted into a checklist. There is a 10-item clinician-administered version of the measure comprises a "total" scale and three (or four) subscales (depending on the study): (1) Obsessions, (2) Compulsions, (3) Severity, and (4) Disturbance. There is also a 79-item checklist of the measure that can be self-administered; this version possesses a "total" scale and the four subscales listed earlier. The CY-BOCS uses a 5-point scale (i.e., higher ratings indicate greater severity). The LOI-C has 20- and 44-item versions (e.g., "Do you hate dirt and dirty things?"; "Do thoughts or words ever keep going over and over in your mind?"). Across several studies, different factor structures have been reported, from a total score plus two-factor (i.e., Total Obsessive and Total Interference scales) version to a total score plus four-factor (i.e., General Obsessive, Numbers/ Luck, Dirt/Contamination, School) version. The LOI-C employs a yes–no response format.

Although several measures that were studied tapped worries, only one measure was the focus of more than one study: the Penn State Worry Questionnaire for Children (PSWQ-C; Chorpita, Tracey, Brown, Collica, & Barlow, 1997). This 14-item (e.g., "My worries really bother me," "I am always worrying about something") measure has a single total scale. The PSWQ-C employs a 4-point scale (i.e., *Never true, Sometimes true, Most times true, Always true*).

Another "syndrome" measure, the School Refusal Assessment Scale (SRAS; Kearney & Silverman, 1993), is a 24-item (e.g., "How often do you have bad feelings about going to school because you are afraid?"; "How often do you feel you would rather be with your parents than go to school?") instrument designed to assess the function of the school refusal. The measure has four "scales," essentially the four "functions" of school refusal: (1) Attention Getting, (2) Avoidance/Negative, (3) Escape/ Negative Affect, and (4) Tangible Rewards. The SRAS employs a 0- to 6-point scale (*Never* to *Always*).

The FSSC measure and its variants are designed to tap the severity of fears in childhood and as such represent a gauge of the DSM category specific phobia. For our review, we included studies of the FSSC-R and the second version of the FSSC. The FSSC-R has 80 items (e.g., "Being killed or murdered," "My parents criticizing me") and the FSSC-II, 78 items. The FSSC-R uses a 3-point scale (*None, Some, A lot*). It has a "total" scale and five subscales reflecting specific domains of fear: (1) Fear of Animals/Minor Injuries, (2) Fear of Death/ Danger, (3) Fear of Failure and Criticism, (4) Fear of the Unknown, and (5) Medical Fears. However, not all studies have identified the same factor structure. Finally, we note that there are psychometric data for Chinese (e.g., Dong, Xia, Lin, Yang, & Ollendick, 1995), Greek (e.g., Mellon, Koliadis, & Paraskevo-

poulos, 2004), and Hawaiian (e.g., Shore & Rapport, 1998) versions of the FSSC and variants.

Both the CASI (Silverman et al., 1991) and its revised version (CASI-R; Muris, 2002) are 18-item (e.g., "It scares me when I feel shaky," "When my stomach hurts, I worry I might be really sick") measures, although a 44-item version has also been studied. As described earlier, the CASI "fits" into either the syndrome or response domain category and is often used in studies of panic as an outcome measure and as a marker of sensitivity to the physiological component of anxiety. The CASI employs a 1- to 3-point scale (i.e., *None* to *A lot*). The measure is generally thought to possess a single "total" scale, though factor-analytic work, described later, has suggested up to five scales.

RELIABILITY

Overall, the literature has no lack of studies examining the reliability of the measures; internal consistency (tapped by Cronbach's alpha) is by far the most frequently examined psychometric characteristic. Many studies also examined retest reliability using the Pearson *r* or, more recently, the intraclass correlation coefficient (ICC). Interpretation of the reliability of tests measuring psychological constructs is not a straightforward endeavor; hence, a few prefatory remarks are in order. First, our discussion focuses on measures that tap "trait" (vs. state) experiences (Gaudry et al., 1975). As a result, retest reliability in particular becomes an important indicator. Furthermore, recent emphasis on the multidimensionality of anxiety, discussed throughout this chapter, implies that both total scales and subscales should possess strong reliability. Finally, although the literature has relied almost exclusively on Cronbach's alpha as an estimate of internal reliability, we do note the current controversy concerning the use of that estimate; the interested reader is referred to this literature (e.g., Becker, 2000; Schmidt, Le, & Ilies, 2003; Zinbarg, Revelle, Yovel, & Li, 2005).

INTERNAL CONSISTENCY

Classic test theory suggests that internal consistency statistics above .80 represent high reliability; estimates between .70 and .80, moderate to low reliability; and scores below .70 represent low reliability (e.g., Murphy &

Davidshofer, 1998). Internal consistency coefficients below .70 raise obvious concern about the reliability of a measure; less obvious are the concerns raised by coefficients that are "too" high. For example, Streiner and Norman (2003) have noted that internal consistency scores exceeding .90 suggest significant item redundancy, a problem that impacts the efficiency of the measure, especially for use in busy clinical settings. Thus, we examined our data for measures scoring "too high" or "too low." We follow our framework of discussing measures in the following order: (1) trait measures, (2) multidimensional measures, and (3) syndrome measures.

Most studies, and most scales, were found to have strong internal consistency. Table 8.6 summarizes data for the 14 instruments. In particular, the "total" scores for all measures had at least moderate reliability, with the exception of one estimate for the STAIC, which scored .69 (Papay & Hedl, 1978). This is not surprising, because "total" scores represent a reliability estimate with the greatest number of items for each scale; Cronbach's alpha increases as the number of items increases (Anastasi, 1988). Examining the performance of the subscales of the various measures, we found that most also met the criterion of .80 or higher.

Examining the extreme ends of the spectrum, however, we did find "problems" at both the high and low ends of reliability. Several instruments were found to have reliability estimates exceeding .90. Of the instruments with "high" internal consistency coefficients, the two scales measuring social anxiety (SPAI-C, and SASC and SAS-A) demonstrated potential item redundancy. Concern about the performance of the FSSC-R is also warranted because of the high cost of that measure with regard to item number. Although the SCARED and the SCAS exhibited "excessive" internal consistency coefficients, both screening measures are designed to cover a lot of conceptual ground. As such, the high number of items seems justified. Still, the SCAS appears to be the more efficient measure, if judged solely by internal consistency standards.

Examining the low end of the internal consistency spectrum, none of the "total" scales for any instrument had an internal consistency coefficient below .70. However, several of the instruments' subscales did yield "low" internal consistency estimates, including scales from the RCMAS, SCARED, SCAS, MASC, SASC-R, and FSSC-R.

Taken together, these various internal consistency findings yield a few conclusions. First, as would be expected, the "total" scale for each measure performs better than the various subscales. Thus, in general, confidence in the reliability of a measure is greatest for the "total" score. A few instruments were notable for their strong reliability results, including the CASI, RCADS, PSWQ-C, SRAS, and STAIC. Furthermore, many of the subscales from the MASC, SCAS, and SCARED also merit mention. However, as noted, some of the scales were "poor performers"—and some were consistently so. For example, the Concentration and Physiological Anxiety subscales of the RCMAS performed consistently poorly, whereas the Worry subscale of that measure showed more mixed findings.

RETEST RELIABILITY

Given their long history, it was surprising to see a relatively small number of studies examining the retest reliability of the RCMAS and STAIC. Comparably more studies were identified for newer measures such as the SCARED, SCAS, and MASC. In general, most of the statistics were positive: More than 80% of the findings reported a retest correlation above .50. Table 8.6 summarizes the findings from our review. As would be expected, most of the highest coefficients were for relatively brief time periods, 1 to 3 weeks. However, several measures had retest correlations above .70 for time periods of 3 months or longer, including the RCMAS (parent and child report), the CASI, and the SCARED. There was a clear pattern, with longer retest intervals associated with lower reliability estimates.

In short, retest reliability estimates of these various child anxiety measures were strong. However, retest reliability was relatively infrequently assessed. Thus, the strength of our conclusions is limited by the relative paucity of studies, especially in comparison to the much larger number of studies examining internal consistency. Given that the test–retest paradigm measures a different test property than does internal consistency, and is arguably a more robust index of reliability, more research on the reliability of common measures seems warranted.

TABLE 8.6. Aggregated Ranges of Several Types of Reliability Estimates for Questionnaires

Instrument	Citation(s)	Internal consistency (α)	Test–retest (r)	Test–retest (ICC)
Childhood Anxiety Sensitivity Index	Chorpita, Albano, & Barlow (1996); Chorpita & Daleiden (2000); Fullana, Servera, Weems, Totella-Feliu, & Caseras (2003); Lambert, Cooley, Campbell, Benoit, & Stansbury (2004); Muris (2002); Muris & Meesters (2004); Rabian, Embry, & MacIntyre (1999); Rabian, Peterson, Richters, & Jensen (1993); Silverman et al. (1991); van Widenfelt, Siebelink, Goedhart, & Treffers (2002); Walsh, Stewart, McLaughlin, & Comeau (2004); Weems, Hammond-Laurence, Silverman, & Ginsburg (1998)	.81 to .93	.52 to .66	
Children's Yale–Brown Obsessive–Compulsive Scale	McKay et al. (2003, 2005); Storch et al. (2005)	.47 to .95		
Fear Survey Schedule for Children (multiple versions)	Bouldin & Pratt (1998); Burnham & Gullone (1997); Dong et al. (1995); Gullone, King, & Cummins (1996); Gullone & King (1992); King & Ollendick (1992); Mellon, Koliadis, & Paraskevopoulos (2004); Muris & Ollendick (2002); Muris, Merckelbach, Ollendick, King, & Bogie (2002); Muris, Merckelbach, Mayer, et al. (1998); Ollendick, King, & Frary (1989); Ollendick (1983); Perrin & Last (1992); Sarphare & Aman (1996); Shore & Rapport (1998); Weems, Silverman, Saavedra, Pina, & Lumpkin (1999)	.57 to .97	.37 to .90	
Multidimensional Anxiety Scale for Children	March, Sullivan, & Parker (1999); March, Parker, Sullivan, Stallings, & Conners (1997); Muris, Merckelbach, Ollendick, King, & Bogie (2002); Muris, Gadet, Moulaert, & Merckelbach (1998); Olason, Sighvatsson, & Smami (2004); Rynn et al. (2006)	.62 to .90		.34 to .93
Negative Affectivity Self-Statement Questionnaire	Lerner et al. (1999); Muris, Mayer, Snieder, & Merckelbach (1998); Ronan, Kendall, & Rowe (1994)	.79 to .84	.96	
Positive and Negative Affect Schedule for Children	Crook, Beaver, & Bell (1998); Laurent et al. (1999)	.86	.66 to .74	
Penn State Worry Questionnaire for Children	Chorpita, Tracey, Brown, Collica, & Barlow (1997); Muris, Meesters, & Gobel (2001); Muris, Merckelbach, Wessel, & van de Ven (1999)	.82 to .89	.92	
Revised Child Anxiety and Depression Scale	Chorpita, Moffitt, & Gray (2005); Chorpita, Yim, Moffitt, Umemoto, & Francis (2000); deRoss, Gullone, & Chorpita (2002)	.61 to .85	.64 to .80	
Revised Children's Manifest Anxiety Scale	Epkins (1993); Joiner, Schmidt, & Schmidt (1996); Lee, Piersel, Friedlander, & Collamer (1988); Mattison, Bagnato, & Brubaker (1988); Merritt, Thompson, Keith, & Gustafson (1995); Muris, Merckelbach, Ollendick, King, & Bogie (2002); Muris, Merckelbach, Mayer, et al. (1998); Paget & Reynolds (1984); Perrin & Last (1992); Reynolds (1980, 1981, 1985); Reynolds & Paget (1981); Reynolds & Richmond (1978, 1979); Richmond, Rodrigo, & de Rodrigo (1988); Ryngala, Shields, & Caruso (2005); Tannenbaum, Forehand, &	.49 to .92	.68 to .75	

(continued)

TABLE 8.6. *(continued)*

Instrument	Citation(s)	Internal consistency (α)	Test–retest (r)	Test–retest (ICC)
Revised Children's Manifest Anxiety Scale *(cont.)*	Thomas (1992); Turgeon & Chartrand (2003); Wilson, Chibaiwa, Majoni, Masukume, & Nkoma (1990); Wolfe, Finch, Saylor, & Blount (1987)			
Social Anxiety Scale for Children/ Adolescents (original and revised)	Epkins (2002); Ginsburg, La Greca, & Silverman (1998); Inderbitzen & Hope (1995); Inderbitzen-Nolan & Walters (2000); Inderbitzen-Nolan, Davies, & McKeon (2004); La Greca, Dandes, Wick, Shaw, & Stone (1988); La Greca & Lopez (1998); La Greca & Stone (1993); Olivares et al. (2005); Sarphare & Aman (1996); Storch, Eisenberg, Roberti, & Barlas (2003); Storch, Masia-Warner, Dent, Roberti, & Fisher (2004)	.70 to .89	.46 to .71	
Screen for Child Anxiety Related Disorders (original and revised)	Birmaher et al. (1997); Boyd, Ginsburg, Lambert, Cooley, & Campbell (2003); Essau, Muris, & Ederer (2002); Hale, Raaijmakers, Muris, & Meeus (2005); Muris, Gadet, Moulaert, & Merckelbach (1998); Muris, Merckelbach, Mayer, et al. (1998); Muris, Merckelbach, Moulaert, & Gadet (2000); Muris, Merckelbach, Ollendick, King, & Bogie (2002); Muris, Merckelbach, Schmidt, & Mayer (1999); Muris, Merckelbach, van Brakel, & Mayer (1999); Muris, Merckelbach, van Brakel, Mayer, & van Dongen (1998); Muris, Merckelbach, Wessel, & van de Ven (1999); Muris, Schmidt, & Merckelbach (2000); Muris, Schmidt, Engelbrecht, & Perold (2002); Muris & Steerneman (2001)	.66 to .96		.86
Spence Children's Anxiety Scale	Essau, Muris, & Ederer (2002); Muris, Merckelbach, Ollendick, King, & Bogie (2002); Muris, Schmidt, & Merckelbach (2000); Muris, Schmidt, Engelbrecht, & Perold (2002); Nauta et al. (2004); Spence, Barrett, & Turner (2003); Spence (1997, 1998)	.57 to .92	.45 to .75	
Social Phobia and Anxiety Inventory for Children	Beidel, Turner, & Fink (1996); Beidel, Turner, & Morris (1995); Beidel, Turner, Hamlin, & Morris (2000); Clark, Turner, & Beidel (1994); Epkins (2002); Inderbitzen-Nolan, Davies, & McKeon (2004); Morris & Masia (1998); Olivares, García-López, Hidalgo, Turner, & Beidel (1999); Storch, Masia-Warner, Dent, Roberti, & Fisher (2004)		.63 to .91	
State–Trait Anxiety Inventory for Children	Chaiyawat & Brown (2000); Cross & Huberty (1993); Gaudry & Poole (1975); Kirisci, Clark, & Moss (1996); Li, Cheung, & Lopez (2004a, 2004b); Muris & Meesters (2004); Muris, Merckelbach, Ollendick, King, & Bogie (2002); Muris, Merckelbach, van Brakel, Mayer, & van Dongen (1998); Nelson, Finch, Kendall, & Gordon (1977); Papay & Hedl (1978); Papay & Spielberger (1986); Perrin & Last (1992); Psychountaki, Zervas, Karteroliotis, & Spielberger (2003); Reynolds (1980); Schisler, Lander, & Fowler-Kerry (1998); Southam-Gerow, Flannery-Schroeder, & Kendall (2003); Steele, Phipps, & Srivastava (1999); Turgeon & Chartrand (2003); Wolfe, Finch, Saylor, & Blount (1987)	.82 to .89		.68 to .79

Note. Measures for which reliability coefficients could not be coded are not included in the table. α, Cronbach's alpha; *r*, Pearson correlation; ICC, intraclass correlation coefficient.

RELIABILITY: SUMMARY

Overall, there is a reasonable level of confidence in the reliability of many of the questionnaires developed to gauge child anxiety. In particular, the "total" scale of all of the measures performed well. Although this same point also holds for many of the subscales of the measures, there were notable exceptions, especially with respect to scales tapping fears and phobias. We also noted that despite this relatively high level of reliability, the efficiency of some measures must be considered. Measures with potential redundancy generally provide more detailed item-level information; thus, they may be best suited for screening/identification and treatment planning, but not outcome measurement. Finally, data on retest reliability, though somewhat sparse, suggest good support for the measures studied.

VALIDITY

We coded articles for four validity-related measurements: convergent validity (concurrent and predictive), divergent validity, and discriminant validity. In general, the validity evidence amassed for anxiety questionnaires was less impressive than the reliability evidence. Table 8.7 summarizes validity data for the 14 instruments.

The most common pattern in the studies we reviewed was to examine concurrent convergent validity and to do so within informant (e.g., positive correlations of two self-report measures of the same or similar constructs). In these cases, most studies had modestly supportive results. Such a procedure may inflate validity estimates, because some of the shared variance between scores represents informant and method variance (Campbell & Fiske, 1959; Cronbach & Meehl, 1955). When validity was assessed across reporters, correlations were typically not as impressive—an unsurprising finding. Cross-informant discrepancies in reporting on psychopathology are the rule in the literature (Meyer et al., 2001). Thus, it is not clear that poor cross-informant correlations suggest poor validity (Achenbach, McConaughy, & Howell, 1987). Nevertheless, our review suggests that evidence for the validity of many measures of childhood anxiety is still relatively tenuous.

Throughout our discussion of the validity findings for the 14 measures, we focus on the validity of the "total" scales. We only examine validity evidence of the subclass for the multidimensional measures and the SRAS (by design, the SRAS does not have a "total" scale).

A variety of studies speak to the validity of the "Total Anxiety" subscales of two trait anxiety measures: RCMAS and STAIC. In a particularly informative study evaluating the RCMAS and STAIC, Muris, Merckelbach, and colleagues (2002) reported correlations among these two and four other anxiety measures: FSSC-R, MASC, SCAS, and SCARED. Intercorrelations among these six scales were quite high, exceeding .50 in all cases for the "total" scales of each.

Evidence for the RCMAS is also moderately strong with regard to convergent validity, with correlations with other anxiety measures in appropriate ranges (i.e., above .50). However, correlations with the Children's Depression Inventory (CDI) were quite high (above .65) across several studies, suggesting the measure may lack divergent validity. Discriminative validity evidence was mixed with some, but not other, studies reporting positive results (e.g., Perrin & Last, 1992). The RCMAS did consistently distinguish between anxious and nonclinical youth groups, but evidence for distinctions among multiple clinical groups was less positive. For example, Chorpita, Moffitt, and Gray (2005) showed that the RCMAS did not significantly discriminate between children with anxiety disorders and children with other disorders (alpha = .01), and that the effect size for this discrimination was approximately one-third that for the RCADS in making the same discrimination.

Finally, regarding the STAIC, there were many more studies examining the validity of the Trait than the State scale. Correlations with contemporary anxiety scales suggested good validity for the STAIC–Trait, with some coefficients exceeding .80 (e.g., RCMAS, SCARED). Evidence was also relatively supportive of the distinction between the Trait and State scales, with correlations falling below .45 across multiple studies. The only study that measured divergent validity for STAIC examined the parent report version (Southam-Gerow, Flannery-Schroeder, & Kendall, 2003); findings suggest moderate divergent validity support, with the STAIC-Trait correlating below .35 with measures of child aggression and externalizing behavior problems. Evidence of discriminative validity was similar to that found for the

TABLE 8.7. Aggregated Ranges of Convergent Validity Estimates for Questionnaires

Instrument	Citation(s)	Pearson r
Childhood Anxiety Sensitivity Index	Chorpita, Albano, & Barlow (1996); Chorpita & Daleiden (2000); Fullana, Servera, Weems, Totella-Feliu, & Caseras (2003); Lambert, Cooley, Campbell, Benoit, & Stansbury (2004); Muris (2002); Muris & Meesters (2004); Rabian, Embry, & MacIntyre (1999); Rabian, Peterson, Richters, & Jensen (1993); Silverman et al. (1991); van Widenfelt, Siebelink, Goedhart, & Treffers (2002); Walsh, Stewart, McLaughlin, & Comeau (2004); Weems, Hammond-Laurence, Silverman, & Ginsburg (1998)	−.08 to .93
Children's Yale–Brown Obsessive–Compulsive Scale	McKay et al. (2003, 2005); Storch et al. (2005)	−.19 to .76
Fear Survey Schedule for Children (multiple versions)	Bouldin & Pratt (1998); Burnham & Gullone (1997); Dong et al. (1995); Gullone, King, & Cummins (1996); Gullone & King (1992); King & Ollendick (1992); Mellon, Koliadis, & Paraskevopoulos (2004); Muris & Ollendick (2002); Muris, Merckelbach, Ollendick, King, & Bogie (2002); Muris, Merckelbach, Mayer, et al. (1998); Ollendick, King, & Frary (1989); Ollendick (1983); Perrin & Last (1992); Sarphare & Aman (1996); Shore & Rapport (1998); Weems, Silverman, Saavedra, Pina, & Lumpkin (1999)	.01 to .85
Multidimensional Anxiety Scale for Children	March, Sullivan, & Parker (1999); March, Parker, Sullivan, Stallings, & Conners (1997); Muris, Merckelbach, Ollendick, King, & Bogie (2002); Muris, Gadet, Moulaert, & Merckelbach (1998); Olason, Sighvatsson, & Smami (2004); Rynn et al. (2006)	−.11 to .79
Negative Affectivity Self-Statement Questionnaire	Lerner et al. (1999); Muris, Mayer, Snieder, & Merckelbach (1998); Ronan, Kendall, & Rowe (1994)	.07 to .79
Penn State Worry Questionnaire for Children	Chorpita, Tracey, Brown, Collica, & Barlow (1997); Muris, Meesters, & Gobel (2001); Muris, Merckelbach, Wessel, & van de Ven (1999)	.23 to .73
Revised Child Anxiety and Depression Scale	Chorpita, Moffitt, & Gray (2005); Chorpita, Yim, Moffitt, Umemoto, & Francis (2000); deRoss, Chorpita, & Gullone (2002)	.34 to .72
Revised Children's Manifest Anxiety Scale	Epkins (1993); Joiner, Schmidt, & Schmidt (1996); Lee, Piersel, Friedlander, & Collamer (1988); Mattison, Bagnato, & Brubaker (1988); Merritt, Thompson, Keith, & Gustafson (1995); Muris, Merckelbach, Ollendick, King, & Bogie (2002); Muris, Merckelbach, Mayer, et al. (1998); Paget & Reynolds (1984); Perrin & Last (1992); Reynolds (1980, 1981, 1985); Reynolds & Paget (1981); Reynolds & Richmond (1978, 1979); Richmond, Rodrigo, & de Rodrigo (1988); Ryngala, Shields, & Caruso (2005); Tannenbaum, Forehand, & Thomas (1992); Turgeon & Chartrand (2003); Wilson, Chibaiwa, Majoni, Masukume, & Nkoma (1990); Wolfe, Finch, Saylor, & Blount (1987)	−.58* to .93
Social Anxiety Scale for Children/Adolescents (Original and Revised)	Epkins (2002); Ginsburg, La Greca, & Silverman (1998); Inderbitzen & Hope (1995); Inderbitzen-Nolan & Walters (2000); Inderbitzen-Nolan, Davies, & McKeon (2004); La Greca, Dandes, Wick, Shaw, & Stone (1988); La Greca & Lopez (1998); La Greca & Stone (1993); Olivares et al. (2005); Sarphare & Aman (1996); Storch, Eisenberg, Roberti, & Barlas (2003); Storch, Masia-Warner, Dent, Roberti, & Fisher (2004)	.06 to .79

(continued)

TABLE 8.7. *(continued)*

Instrument	Citation(s)	Pearson *r*
Screen for Child Anxiety Related Disorders (Original and Revised)	Birmaher et al. (1997); Boyd, Ginsburg, Lambert, Cooley, & Campbell (2003); Essau, Muris, & Ederer (2002); Hale, Raaijmakers, Muris, & Meeus (2005); Muris, Gadet, Moulaert, & Merckelbach (1998); Muris, Merckelbach, Mayer, et al. (1998); Muris, Merckelbach, Moulaert, & Gadet (2000); Muris, Merckelbach, Ollendick, King, & Bogie (2002); Muris, Merckelbach, Schmidt, & Mayer (1999); Muris, Merckelbach, van Brakel, & Mayer (1999); Muris, Merckelbach, van Brakel, Mayer, & van Dongen (1998); Muris, Merckelbach, Wessel, & van de Ven (1999); Muris, Schmidt, & Merckelbach (2000); Muris, Schmidt, Engelbrecht, & Perold (2002); Muris & Steerneman (2001)	−.25* to .89
Spence Children's Anxiety Scale	Essau, Muris, & Ederer (2002); Muris, Merckelbach, Ollendick, King, & Bogie (2002); Muris, Schmidt, & Merckelbach (2000); Muris, Schmidt, Engelbrecht, & Perold (2002); Nauta et al. (2004); Spence, Barrett, & Turner (2003); Spence (1997, 1998)	.08 to .86
Social Phobia and Anxiety Inventory for Children	Beidel, Turner, & Fink (1996); Beidel, Turner, & Morris (1995); Beidel, Turner, Hamlin, & Morris (2000); Clark et al. (1994); Epkins (2002); Inderbitzen-Nolan, Davies, & McKeon (2004); Morris & Masia (1998); Olivares et al. (1999); Storch, Masia-Warner, Dent, Roberti, & Fisher (2004)	−.45 to .79
School Refusal Assessment Scale	Higa, Daleiden, & Chorpita (2002); Kearney (2002); Kearney & Silverman (1993)	
State–Trait Anxiety Inventory for Children	Chaiyawat & Brown (2000); Cross & Huberty (1993); Gaudry & Poole (1975); Kirisci, Clark, & Moss (1996); Li, Cheung, & Lopez (2004); Muris & Meesters (2004); Muris, Merckelbach, Ollendick, King, & Bogie (2002); Muris, Merckelbach, van Brakel, Mayer, & van Dongen (1998); Nelson, Finch, Kendall, & Gordon (1977); Papay & Hedl (1978); Papay & Spielberger (1986); Perrin & Last (1992); Psychountaki, Zervas, Karteroliotis, & Spielberger (2003); Reynolds (1980); Schisler, Lander, & Fowler-Kerry (1998); Southam-Gerow, Flannery-Schroeder, & Kendall (2003); Steele, Phipps, & Srivastava (1999); Turgeon & Chartrand (2003); Wolfe, Finch, Saylor, & Blount (1987)	−.15 to .88

Note. Measures for which convergent validity coefficients could not be coded are not included in the table.
* Negative association was predicted (i.e., criterion should be negatively correlated with scale).

RCMAS and the FSSC-R; the STAIC-Trait distinguishes between anxious and nonclinical youth groups, but does not distinguish between anxious and other clinical groups (Perrin & Last, 1992).

Among the multidimensional measures, validity evidence was relatively strong for the "total" scales. For example, the SCARED total scale correlated very highly with the SCAS, RCMAS, MASC, and STAIC total scales (*r* > .80) and nearly at that level with the Youth Self-Report Internalizing Scale (.77), a broad self-report measure of anxiety, depression, withdrawal, and other internalizing dimensions (Achenbach & Rescorla, 2001). Another notable fact about the SCARED is that compared to any other questionnaire, more studies examined its validity. In comparison, the validity coefficients for the SCAS were also high but not consistently above .80 as were those of the SCARED. Still, most correlations reported for the "total" scale were above .70, suggesting rather strong relationships among these measures of anxiety. Another DSM-based scale, the RCADS, showed similarly high correlations with the RCMAS. However, there were relatively fewer data on the RCADS compared to the SCARED.

The MASC is another measure designed to index multiple dimensions of anxiety, but it does not rely solely on a DSM conceptualization. Validity evidence for this measure is comparable to that of the SCAS and RCADS, in that correlations were above .60 and often exceeded .70 for relevant child report anxiety measures (e.g., RCMAS, STAIC, SCAS, SCARED).

Overall, the "total" scales for the MASC, RCADS, SCAS, and SCARED all performed quite well with regard to within-reporter correlations. Evidence for cross-reporter correlations is sparse for these measures, and existing data are not highly positive. As an example, the MASC "total" scale correlated .14 with parent report STAIC, despite correlating .60 with the child report STAIC.

Validity data concerning the subscales of the multidimensional scales are best for the SCARED, SCAS, and RCADS. Much of the relevant data concerning the SCARED and SCAS come from a Muris, Merckelbach, and colleagues (2002) study comparing the two instruments (along with four others). On the positive side, the SCARED GAD subscale correlated highly with the PSWQ-C, the RCMAS Worry subscale, and the SCAS GAD subscale. Furthermore, two articles indicated good discriminative validity for the SCARED (Birmaher et al., 1997; Muris & Steerneman, 2001). The SCARED OCD subscale has not been examined in a study including another OCD subscale (e.g., LOI-C, CY-BOCS) except the SCAS OCD subscale; correlations between the two scales were above .65 across two articles. No relevant discriminative validity evidence exists. Similarly, the SCARED Panic Disorder subscale correlates well with the SCAS Panic Disorder subscale (above .73 across two articles). However, the scale correlation is also nearly as high with more general scales, such as the RCMAS (.73) and the STAIC–Trait (.71).

The SCARED SAD scale correlated highly with the SCAS SAD subscale (above .78) across two articles; correlation with the MASC Separation Anxiety subscale was also consistent with expectation (above .60). However, the correlations with the STAIC–Trait and RCMAS total scale were quite high (above .65), reducing the strength of confidence in the distinctness of the scale. The discriminative validity evidence for the scale is positive, however, showing good discrimination even in youth with anxiety disorder diagnoses. The SCARED Social Anxiety subscale did not perform as well. Although correlations with broader measures were lower than the other subscales reviewed, correlations with the SCAS Social Phobia subscale was lower than expected, around .40, and lower at times than other correlations with other, less relevant scales (e.g., the SCAS OCD subscale). Furthermore, discriminative validity was modest: The scale discriminated between anxious and non-anxious and youth with disruptive behavior disorders, but no within-anxiety specificity was demonstrated. Finally, the evidence for the Phobia subscales of the SCARED was less impressive, mirroring the reliability evidence reported earlier. As an example, the Animal Phobia subscale did not correlate particularly highly with the Animal Fears subscale of the FSSC-R. Because the majority of evidence for the SCARED scales was from studies also examining the SCAS, similar conclusions may be drawn about the subscales of that measure. The SCAS GAD subscale was correlated with the SCARED GAD subscale, though it was as highly correlated with the STAIC–Trait and RCMAS, as well as the SCARED Panic Disorder subscale. Discriminative validity evidence was not strong for the measure. A somewhat better result was found for the SCAS OCD subscale, which correlated highly with the SCARED OCD subscale but less so with more general scales (e.g., RCMAS, STAIC–total), though these correlations were still above .55. The SCAS Panic Disorder subscale was highly (.80) correlated with its corresponding SCARED scale, with other scales correlating moderately to highly (r's ≤ .71). A similar pattern was found for the SCAS SAD subscale, though correlations were in general lower across the various measures. Finally, as noted earlier, the SCAS Social Phobia subscale did not correlate as highly as would be expected with the SCARED Social Phobia subscale (below .60).

Recent tests of the validity of the RCADS in a clinical sample lend relatively strong support to its validity. For example, the subscales all correlated positively with the RCMAS (r's = .59 to .72), with interview-derived ratings of corresponding clinical syndromes (r's = .34 to .54), and with similar clinician ratings derived from parent interviews (r's = .22 to .31). As a point of comparison, the RCMAS validity coefficients with these same parent interview–derived ratings ranged from −.01 to .16 (all nonsignificant). In a stringent test of divergent validity, four of the five RCADS anxiety scales (all but panic) failed to correlate significantly with depression scores controlled for variance, as measured by the RCMAS. Thus, although there are few studies on this measure, its psychometric support is so far quite strong.

Next we turn to the validity evidence for the syndrome measures, starting with the social anxiety questionnaires: the SPAI-C and the SASC and SAS-A. Relative to the SPAI-C, a much greater number of studies have focused on the SAS and its variants. Correlations between the two "total" scales have been greater than .60. A positive finding is that both measures correlate more highly with each other than with anxiety measures with more bandwidth, though correlations with these broadband measures are generally above .40. The "total" scale of the SAS and its variants also had modest relationships with a variety of measures of social competence (e.g., number of friends), with Pearson r's in the range of .15 to .30. Correlations were typically higher for girls than for boys, although examinations of difference were not always reported. Similarly, the SPAI-C "total" scale was modestly related to observed social behavior, again in the .15 to .30 range, though some relationships approached .40 (e.g., speech latency).

Although the SPAI-C has several subscales, we deemed the evidence too preliminary to evaluate their validity, particularly given the notion that the measure itself may possess greater validity for subdimensions than the criteria to which it might be compared (Cronbach & Meehl, 1955). The subscales of the SAS and variants have received somewhat more empirical attention. The SAS has three subscales: (a) Fear of Negative Evaluation (FNE), (2) Social Avoidance/Distress–General (SA/D-Gen), and (3) Social Avoidance/Distress–New Situations (SA/D-New). In general, these scores had intercorrelations in the .50–.60 range, suggesting that though they do have considerable overlap, there is also support for their distinctness. For convergent validity, studies compared the subscales with the RCMAS or measures of social and relational functioning. The FNE subscale correlated above .50 with the RCMAS across three articles, whereas the magnitude of the correlations for the other two subscales (SA/D-Gen and SA/D-New) was somewhat lower across these studies, with correlations around .40. All three scales also correlated with the Social Acceptance subscale of the Harter Social Competence Measure; these correlations were

higher for girls than boys. For the FNE and SA/D-New subscales, correlations with other measures of social competence (e.g., number of friends, social skills) were modest (.20 and below); somewhat stronger (r = .30) relationships emerged between these same indices and the SA/D-Gen. In general, the subscales did not perform as well as the "total" scale. In general, both the SAS and the SPAI subscales face the challenge of validation in an area in which suitable validity criteria are difficult to identify. Although evidence does not appear to favor either instrument, data to date are more plentiful for the SAS (and variants).

As noted earlier, the FSSC and variants (e.g., revised version, non-English versions, FSSC-II) tap fears and phobia. The measure has demonstrated moderately strong convergent validity evidence, with correlations above .50 with the RCMAS, STAIC, MASC, SCAS, and SCARED. However, some studies have reported correlations as low as .31. The two articles reporting discriminative validity evidence were mixed: One (Ollendick, 1983) found that the measure distinguished between phobic and normal youth, whereas the other (Perrin & Last, 1992) found that the measure did not distinguish between anxious and normal youth or those with ADHD.

Turning now to measures of OCD, we note preliminarily that the CY-BOCS was sometimes administered as a questionnaire and sometimes as an interview. For this discussion, we include data on both versions. Between the LOI-C and CY-BOCS, the latter has the best validity profile, with relevant validity correlations exceeding .60 for the total scale. Furthermore, correlations with general anxiety measures (e.g., RCMAS, MASC total) were appropriately lower (below .40), suggesting that the CY-BOCS is not simply a measure of general anxiety. We discuss the factor-analytic results of the measure shortly. However, there is little discriminant validity evidence for the measure. Evidence for the LOI-C is much weaker. In fact, of the two articles we identified that examined the validity of the measure, neither was particularly supportive. None of its scales correlated significantly with relevant measures in one article (Berg et al., 1986). Although some discriminant validity evidence was reported insofar as the measure distinguished between youth with OCD and nonclinical controls, the measure did not consistently distinguish between youth with OCD and those with other psychiatric diagnoses (Berg et al., 1986). It is notable, too, that the validity of the measure has not been examined in almost two decades.

As noted earlier, only one measure of worry in children has been examined by more than one study—the PSWQ-C. Extant data are promising for the measure; correlations were above .60 for other measures of worry or GAD, such as the RCMAS Worry subscale and the SCARED GAD subscale. Furthermore, although correlations with other anxiety measures were also high, the correlation for the most relevant scale was always highest (e.g., correlation with SCARED GAD was higher than any other SCARED subscale). In the Chorpita et al. (1997) study, other indices of validity were positive: the PSWQ-C correlated highly with the number and intensity of worries, as well as symptom reports on the Anxiety Disorders Interview Schedule—Child version (ADIS-C) of uncontrollable worry. Correlations with excessive worry were more modest, suggesting the measure may not capture either the "excessive worry" or the "uncontrollable" aspects of GAD.

Validity of the SRAS was examined across three articles, with one focusing primarily on factor analysis (discussed below). In general, results are supportive of the four subscales. In the original development paper, Kearney and Silverman (1993) confirmed their hypotheses that the Escape, Avoidance, and Attention Getting subscales correlated above .30 with anxiety measures, whereas the Tangible Rewards subscale correlated below .10. Similarly, the Tangible Rewards and Attention Getting subscales were correlated more highly with the Child Behavior Checklist (CBCL) Externalizing subscale. A similar pattern emerged in the Higa, Daleiden, and Chorpita (2002) study of the measure; for example, the patterns of youth meeting criteria for internalizing versus externalizing disorders mapped as expected onto the four SRAS subscales. In short, the validity evidence for the SRAS is promising, though limited by a small number of studies.

Finally, overall validity evidence for the CASI is rather modest. The measure correlates rather highly with a variety of other anxiety measures, such as FSSC-R, RCMAS, STAIC, and MASC, with validity coefficients ranging from .50 to .74. Arguably, the measure should have as its highest correlates measures related to the physiology of anxiety. Although the measure did correlate highest with the SCAS Panic Disorder subscale (among the various SCAS subscales), correlations with other physiology-related measures were less consistent. Furthermore, one discriminative validity study (Rabian et al., 1993) suggested that although the measure did discriminate between anxious and nonanxious youth, it was not able to discriminate between anxious youth and those with externalizing behavior problems. Furthermore, the effect size for the CASI in discriminating children with panic disorder from those with other anxiety disorders was found to be lower than that of the STAIC (Chorpita & Lilienfeld, 1999), casting some doubts about the relevance of the CASI to panic disorder in youth.

Interviews

Our review identified 33 articles examining the psychometric properties of structured diagnostic interviews, representing 11 instruments. As noted earlier, there are two basic types of structured interview: (1) respondent-based and (2) interviewer-based (Shaffer et al., 1999). Respondent-based interviews attempt to maximize reliability through standardization of the interview, such that most responses to questions can be "yes" or "no" and do not require the interviewer to know much about DSM criteria. As such, with adequate training, these interviews may be employed by lay interviewers. They are typically viewed as ideal for epidemiological settings, but not in clinical settings. On the other hand, interviewer-based interviews require a high level of professional knowledge given that the interview is only semistructured, such that probe and follow-up questions are at the discretion of the interviewer. Therefore, a clinician is required to conduct the interview. Furthermore, their reliability, particularly interrater reliability, requires close scrutiny. We summarize the reliability findings for the interviews in Table 8.8.

In the study of anxiety disorders in youth, only one respondent-based interview has been examined in a study reporting psychometric data, the Diagnostic Interview Schedule for Children (DISC; Shaffer, Fisher, Dulcan, & Davies, 1996). Several interviewer-based interviews have reported psychometric data, including the Anxiety Disorders Interview Schedule, Child and Parent versions (ADIS-C/P; Silverman & Albano, 1996; Silverman &

TABLE 8.8. Aggregated Ranges of Reliability Estimates for Interviews

Instrument	Citation(s)	Internal consistency (α)	Test–retest	Interrater
Anxiety Disorders Interview Schedule for Children and Parents	Lyneham & Rapee (2005); Silverman & Eisen (1992); Silverman & Nelles (1988); Silverman & Rabian (1995); Silverman, Saavedra, & Pina (2001)	—	–.06 to .86 (r) .15 to 1.0 (κ)	.35 to 1.0 (κ) .90 to 1.0 (r)
Anxiety Rating for Children—Revised	Bernstein, Crosby, Perwien, & Borchardt, (1996)	.69 to .80	—	—
Child Assessment Schedule	Hodges, Cools, & McKnew (1989); Hodges, McKnew, Burbach, & Roebuck (1987); Hodges, McKnew, Cytryn, Stern, & Kline (1982); Hodges, Saunders, Kashani, & Hamlett, (1990)	.57 to .88	.66 to .88 (r) .38 to .88 (κ)	—
Children's Anxiety Evaluation Form	Hoehn-Saric, Maisami, & Wiegand (1987)	—	—	—
Children's Yale–Brown Obsessive Compulsive Scale	Scahill et al. (1997); Storch et al. (2004)	.80 to .90	.70 to .76 (ICC)	.66 to .91 (ICC)
Diagnostic Interview for Children, Adolescents	Boyle, Offord, Racine, Szatmari, Sanford, & Fleming, (1997); Sylvester, Hyde, & Reichler (1987); Welner, Reich, Herjanic, Jung, & Amado (1987)	—	.61 to .64 (ICC) .30 to .57 (κ)	—
Diagnostic Interview Schedule for Children	Ribera et al. (1996); Roberts, Solovitz, Chen, & Casat (1996); Schwab-Stone, Shaffer, Dulcan, & Jensen (1996); Shaffer, Fisher, Dulcan, & Davies (1996)	—	–.05 to .73 (ICC) –.27 to .75 (κ)	–.27 to 1.0 (κ)
Dominic—Revised	Murphy, Marelich, & Hoffman (2000); Valla, Bergeron, & Smolla (2000)	.66 to .78	.71 to .77 (ICC) .70 to .76 (κ)	.73 to .81 (κ)
Pictorial Diagnostic Instrument	Ernst, Godfrey, Silva, Pouget, & Welkowitz (1994)	.85	—	—
Pictorial Instrument for Children, Adolescents	Ernst, Cookus, & Moravec (2000)	.54	—	—
Schedule for Affective Disorders and Schizophrenia for School-Age Children	Chambers (1985); Hodges, McKnew, Burbach, & Roebuck (1987); Kaufman, Birmaher, Brent, & Rao (1997); Kolaitis, Korpa, Kolvin, & Tsiantis (2003)	.44	.10 to .53 (ICC) .60 to .78 (κ)	.80 (κ)
Terry	Bidaut-Russell, Valla, Thomas, Begeron, & Lawson (1998); Valla et al. (2000)	.65 to .90	.72 (ICC) .70 to .76 (κ)	—

Note. α, Cronbach's alpha; ICC, intraclass correlation coefficient; κ, Cohen's kappa; r, Pearson correlation.

Nells, 1988), the Child and Adolescent Psychiatric Assessment (CAPA; Angold & Costello, 2000), the Children's Assessment Schedule (Hodges, McKnew, Cytryn, Stern, & Kline, 1982), the Diagnostic Interview for Children and Adolescents (DICA; Welner, Reich, Herjanic, Jung, & Amado, 1987), and the Schedule for Affective Disorders and Schizophrenia for School-Age Children (K-SADS; Kaufman, Birmaher, Brent, & Rao, 1997). A unique aspect of the ADIS-C/P compared to the other interviews is its use of dimensional ratings concerning severity, intensity, interference, avoidance, and uncontrollability at the symptom and syndrome levels. In addition, three separate picture-based interviews identified in our review are discussed separately. Our review and discussion are by instrument, starting with the respondent-based interview. Although we identified 11 separate instruments in our review, our discussion is limited to those with the most data.

As noted, the DISC is a respondent-based interview that, among other advantages, is designed for lay interviewers. We identified six articles on the psychometrics of the DISC that specifically included at least one childhood anxiety disorder diagnosis. Studies of retest and interrater reliability have been reported (see Table 8.8). Retest reliability coefficients, with retest periods of 1–3 weeks, varied by diagnosis. With such small time frames, these coefficients represent a reasonable gauge of the measure's reliability. Coefficients (kappa or ICC were typically reported) for specific/simple phobia, SAD, GAD/OAD, and social phobia were highest, with mean coefficient values above .50. Panic disorder and agoraphobia mean coefficients were both below .50, and those for panic disorder, .22.

Interrater reliability has also been reported for the DISC. An interesting artifact of the development of the DISC is the use of lay and professional (i.e., MD or PhD) interviewers. As a result, interrater reliability has been studied within and across these categories of interviewer, something that occurs rarely in studies of the other interviews. These data have been reported for agoraphobia, GAD/OAD, SAD, simple/specific phobia, and social phobia. Across the two articles examining interrater reliability, coefficients were highest when parent and combined reports were considered, with mean kappas for all diagnoses around .50 for each, whereas the kappa for interrater reliabil-

ity for child reports was .25. For the combined and parent report kappas, social and simple/specific phobia had the best overall coefficients (.55–.60), with GAD/OAD in the middle (about .50), and SAD the lowest (below .45). Comparing lay versus lay and lay versus psychiatrist interrater reliability did not suggest notable differences in the magnitude of kappa, suggesting that lay interviewers agreed with each other about as well as lay interviewers agreed with psychiatrists using the DISC. In general, these interrater reliability coefficients are not promising, especially given the design of the DISC as a highly standardized instrument, a point to which we return in our conclusion to this section on interviews.

Turning to the interviewer-based interviews, we start with the ADIS-C/P, which, not surprisingly, was the most commonly studied interview for childhood anxiety disorders. Retest reliability data, reported in the 1- to 3-week range, are largely positive, with coefficients above .70 for most diagnoses. A few general findings emerge. First, concerning age differences, older group tended to have *lower* retest reliability. A good example of this phenomenon is found for GAD, reported in a study by Silverman, Saavedra, and Pina (2001). Child, parent, and combined report diagnoses were examined across a 10-day period. The retest coefficient for the younger (ages 7–11) children was above .70 for GAD in all three reports (i.e., child report, parent report, and combined report) whereas for older (ages 12–16) children, only one of the three was at .70 (combined), with the other two below .60. A second general finding is that the "combined" report yielded the best retest coefficients, followed by parent report.

Although fewer interrater than retest reliability data are reported for the ADIS-C/P, there is still a reasonable database on this property of the interview. Again, the data are largely positive. As noted earlier, kappa coefficients above .74 (e.g., Landis & Koch, 1977) are typically considered adequate for diagnostic interviews. Studies have demonstrated the ADIS-C/P meets this standard often, though not always. For example, the kappa for OAD was below criterion for parent and combined reports in the Silverman and Eisen (1992) article. Similarly low coefficients for social phobia were reported in the same study by combined and child reports. However, the general trend was for acceptable kappas for the ADIS-C/P. Buttressing this conclusion is the finding by Lyne-ham and Rapee (2005) that kappas were acceptable for in-person compared to phone interviews across multiple diagnoses (i.e., specific phobia, social phobia, SAD, and GAD). Despite these rather positive data, there is a notable lack of data for the OCD diagnosis, though, most likely a result of its rarity.

Four other interviewer-based interviews have psychometric data available concerning anxiety disorders: CAPA, CAS, DICA, and K-SADS. For all four, however, data are rather limited. Taking the CAS as an example, data for the instrument are only available for two diagnoses (OAD and SAD). Retest data are modestly supportive for SAD (.56) and less so for OAD (.38). Interrater reliability data are even sparser, with a pre–DSM-III-R study by Hodges, McKnew, and colleagues (1982) noting that such reliability was above .70. Data on the K-SADS, though more recent, are equally meager. Retest data are available for the DICA in one study across 17 days for two diagnoses (OAD and SAD), and coefficients are moderate to weak (.57 and .32, respectively). Kaufman and colleagues (1997) reported better results for the K-SADS, with kappa at or above .70, but only for GAD and "any anxiety diagnosis." No interrater reliability data were available for either DICA or K-SADS. Unlike the other interviews, however, CAS, DICA, and K-SADS have some reported validity evidence. For example, in a rare study comparing two structured diagnostic interviews, Hodges, McKnew, Burbach, and Roebuck (1987) found moderate to low agreement between CAS and K-SADS for "any anxiety disorder" diagnosis, with kappas ranging from .37 to .54. Boyle and colleagues (1997) compared the diagnoses achieved using the DICA compared to the Ontario Child Health Study (OCHS), a behavior problem checklist; kappas were poor for SAD and OAD (below .40). Overall, data for these three interviews is spare. Although data for the K-SADS and CAPA are relatively stronger than those for the other two interviews, there is overall very little known about these four interviews concerning childhood anxiety disorders.

The most important point to make about interviews is that despite the promise for improved reliability afforded by the DSM, surprisingly little evidence supports the use of DSM-based interviews for anxiety disorders, with one important exception, the ADIS-C/P. Given that the ADIS-C/P was developed specif-

ically for anxiety disorders in children, it is not surprising that this interview stood out in our review. Still, it is worth noting that the ADIS-C/P is the only structured interview with reliability data for all of the anxiety disorder diagnoses. Although the DISC is a well-studied instrument, reliability estimates for the anxiety disorders are not particularly strong, especially in comparison to the ADIS-C/P. The other structured interviews have fewer studies, making any conclusions about their use premature.

We conclude our discussion of interviews by noting the emergence of a small number of *picture-based* diagnostic interviews that decrease reliance on verbal report as a means of interviewing children about symptoms related to DSM diagnoses. Two interviews, the Dominic and the Terry, have received attention across multiple studies. In both interviews, a child is shown a series of pictures in which a child exhibits DSM symptoms, and is asked, "Have you ever felt sad (for example), like Terry/Dominic?" Terry and Dominic are the same except that the Terry contains drawings of a black youth and the Dominic depicts a white youth. Psychometric data for the three anxiety disorder diagnoses (OAD, SAD, phobia) covered by the instrument are positive. Retest reliability coefficients exceeded .70 over 10 days. Interrater reliability estimates also exceeded .70. Limited validity evidence has been reported, however. These interviews represent a promising effort to expand the reach of diagnostic interviews.

Before we move to the more general conclusion of our review, we reiterate a point we made earlier concerning the types of interviews. In clinical circumstances, interviewer-based interviews appear to be the preferred choice when design alone is considered. Also, we were somewhat surprised to discover that respondent-based interviews, despite their high degree of structure, did not yield better reliability estimates. As a result, use of an interviewer-based interview such as the ADIS-C/P makes both clinical and empirical sense.

General Summary and Conclusions

Our review revealed a rich literature on the assessment of child anxiety. Since 1970, more than 180 articles have been published, representing more than 700 studies conducted on over 75 measures. Using our search parameters, the literatures on questionnaires and interviews are the best developed. Research on observational measures, once considered to have the best psychometric evidence (e.g., Barrios & Hartmann, 1997), has shown a decline over time in psychometric studies. On the other hand, physiological measures, once considered too unreliable with children (e.g., Beidel, 1991), are beginning to receive more attention, though, thus far, mainly in literatures beyond the scope of our review.

We conclude our review with a set of general recommendations. Before doing so, we offer a brief discussion of the clinical feasibility of measurement. Thus far, our focus has been on the traditional psychometric topics of reliability and validity. Although both are necessary properties of a useful instrument, neither dimension speaks directly to *clinical feasibility and utility*. Recently, increasing emphasis on real-world applicability has increased the importance of the feasibility of measures in clinical practice (Mash & Hunsley, 2005; Silverman & Ollendick, 2005). From our perspective, feasibility involves calculation of the *relative economy* of a given measure (compared to its psychometrically equivalent alternatives). A first property to consider here is *time required*, gauged by the number of items or the time needed to complete a given assessment (e.g., interview, observation). Table 8.4 provides the total number of items for each of the questionnaires we have described in detail, along with an estimate of the time required to administer the instrument. Time estimates for interviews are harder to gauge; although some articles indicated the estimated time to conduct the interviews, the estimates varied considerably. Thus, we do not provide any specific estimates except to say that diagnostic interviews typically take at least 60 minutes per reporter (i.e., 120 minutes for a child and a parent); the duration is also typically longer if the child is more symptomatic. Hence, interview times in epidemiological studies are briefer than those in clinical studies. Time required represents one component of the instrument's "cost." As time increases, child and/or parent fatigue has the potential to degrade the *yield* (i.e., decrease validity) and to impact the satisfaction of the client (thus, increasing chance that he or she will stop treatment or seek it elsewhere). Furthermore, in most clinical settings, financial considerations limit the time dedicated to assessment (Sanchez & Turner, 2003). Thus, a clinician

must carefully consider how much time to spend using assessment tools.

Another cost associated with some measures is an actual financial cost. Some of the measures are copyrighted and have a cost associated with their use (see Table 8.4). The ADIS-C/P and the DISC are also copyrighted instruments with cost associated with their use. Obviously, financial cost has implications for feasibility. As an example, within the health care system, consumers are increasingly seeing coinsurance fees for medical tests (e.g., strep test, cholesterol test). It is conceivable that such issues will arise in mental health practice, particularly if the number of "free" measures decreases.

Economizing on *time required* and reducing actual *financial cost* are components of feasibility. However, another important consideration concerns the ultimate *yield* of the measure. In other words, how much information does a measure generate considering its cost (e.g., in time, financial cost)? Although our field has not elaborated a method for determining this ratio, we offer the following preliminary framework to guide our discussion.

Considering the purposes of assessment we discussed earlier (identification/screening, triage/treatment planning, and treatment evaluation), a yield for a measure varies depending on which purpose it is meant to serve. We posit that the overall *yield* curve is likely to have a bell shape. Specifically, at the identification phase, keeping *time required* low is likely to be critical, because relatively few youth who complete the screen will need any follow-up. Thus, engaging in extensive measurement does not appear necessary or feasible. However, in the triage/treatment planning phase, greater tolerance for cost is likely. During this phase, an assessor seeks to identify *caseness*, to triage the client into the appropriate treatment(s), and to identify key treatment goals. Thus, a wider net is preferred. Furthermore, at the outset of treatment, extended time for assessment may be expected and "billable" within mental health systems. Overall, the need for sensitivity may make the relative cost of the time spent lower during screening and treatment planning.

Note, however, that the yield of a measure for triage/treatment planning purposes is likely maximized as the ratio between the number of relevant constructs measured (e.g., DSM disorders) and the time spent increases; lower ratios are associated with higher "cost" insofar as the measure does not provide much information despite the time spent. Thus, despite greater tolerance for higher cost, economic concerns remain in the triage/treatment planning stage.

As one moves to outcome measurement, efficiency remains a prime concern, because of the limited time available during and after treatment for lengthy assessments. Furthermore, the focus of treatment is likely to be narrow; thus, measurement of those specific goals may be most critical in gauging the effects of treatment.

We pause briefly to point out that this focused measurement stands in contrast to a typical, randomized, controlled trial posttreatment battery, which often contains multiple measures of similar constructs. Although such measurement represents a state-of-the-art approach to clinical assessment in a research trial, the context of that assessment must be considered. In the absence of real-world financial and time pressures, such an extensive battery of measurements may indeed be the best choice. As valuable as such assessments are to the science of outcome assessment, however, the practice of outcome assessment must by necessity be more parsimonious.

In addition to the notion of feasibility, another dimension relevant to applied use of these instruments involves optimal conditions of use. A close read of our discussion thus far suggests that some measures are better suited for a certain purpose, whereas others are better suited for other purposes. Table 8.9 summarizes our recommendations.

For the purpose of identification, questionnaires represent the best choice. Because parsimony is of the essence, a measure such as the STAIC–Trait is a strong choice, with only 20 items. We also recommend the Positive and Negative Affect Scale for Children (PANAS-C), because it has stronger conceptual ties to notions of temperament, although is not an anxiety measure per se. Although the DSM-based scales are lengthier, several offer norms that allow for the determination of percentile or T-scores, which can help in determining whether or not treatment is warranted. Of these, RCADS is the briefest and covers several anxiety diagnoses, as well as depression.

For triage and treatment planning, working with one of the DSM-based scales makes best sense in terms of locating the type of anxiety and degree of comorbid elevations. Despite their length, such measures may be worthwhile because of their superior precision in identifying areas for treatment focus. Indeed, as we and others have discussed elsewhere (e.g., Chorpita & Nakamura, 2004), use of DSM-based questionnaires may also represent a way to plan for the efficient use of an accompanying structured diagnostic interview. The choice among the three anxiety-related DSM questionnaires is not simple, because of the lack of uniform coverage of the DSM disorders (see Table 8.5). The SCARED-R has the broadest scope, screening for all seven of the DSM-IV anxiety disorders; the first version of the SCARED only included four diagnoses (plus school phobia). The RCADS affords the advantage of screening for depression and anxiety

TABLE 8.9. Recommendations by Assessment Purpose

Purpose	Identification	Triage/treatment planning	Outcome during treatment	Outcome posttreatment
Questionnaire	STAIC[a]	RCADS	Syndrome questionnaire	Syndrome questionnaire
Questionnaire	PANAS-C	SCARED		RCADS
Questionnaire	RCADS	SCAS		SCARED
Interview		ADIS-C/P		ADIS-C/P
Interview		K-SADS		K-SADS
Other		Process measures (e.g., SRAS, functional assessment)	Idiographic measures (e.g., number of panic attacks)	Idiographic measures (e.g., number of panic attacks)
Other		Idiographic measures (e.g., number of panic attacks)		

[a] Although there are data on the State version, our focus here is the Trait version of the STAIC.

but does not screen for PTSD and specific phobia. The SCAS screens for the same anxiety disorders as the RCADS (with the addition of physical injury fears) but does not screen for depression. Considering coverage, the RCADS would appear to be a reasonable choice. However, psychometric evidence for the measure, although uniformly positive, is not as extensively documented as that for the SCARED and SCAS. Furthermore, if full coverage of the anxiety disorders is desired, especially PTSD (though see Fletcher, Chapter 9, this volume), the SCARED-R may be preferable. Use of the trait measures is not recommended at the treatment planning stage.

The use of a structured diagnostic interview is clearly an important tool for treatment planning. The data clearly identify the ADIS-C/P as the superior interview for anxiety disorders. If cost is an issue, the K-SADS may be a viable option, though data are sparse. However, because all structured interviews are costly with regard to time and training required, we recommend using one of the DSM-based multidimensional questionnaires in clinical practice as a way to identify components of diagnostic interviews most worth administering (cf. Chorpita & Nakamura, in press).

A notable gap in the assessment literature is the paucity of process- or function-oriented measures that offer data on the mechanisms causing or maintaining the problem behaviors. This is a critical gap, because an important goal of treatment planning involves hypothesizing the causal or maintaining factors of the anxiety. However, almost all of the measures we identified gauge only symptom severity, frequency, or interference, not their presumed causes. In most clinical situations, data on functions of the problem behaviors are obtained with loosely structured, clinical interviewing techniques. As discussed earlier, we prefer the use of functional assessment (FA) as a guide to identifying the "process" of the problem(s) identified. Our recommendation comes from the accumulation of related data reported by those using FA and similar approaches (e.g., Francis & Chorpita, 2004; Henggeler et al., 2002; Persons, 1989). Although some of the gap in measuring causal variables may be due to the relatively poor understanding of etiology and mechanisms of treatment action in general (Kazdin, 2001), this understanding cannot be advanced without strategies to measure potential mediators and moderators of treatment.

A small number of questionnaires appear potentially useful in the regard, specifically, the SRAS and CASI. In cases of school refusal, the SRAS is a tool to gauge the reasons for the school refusal and to plan treatment. Least clear is the role of the CASI in developing a treatment plan. Although anxiety sensitivity is related to several anxiety disorders, no studies have demonstrated any added benefit of using the CASI along with other questionnaires in treatment planning.

Regarding outcome measurement, there are two types of outcome one may be interested in assessing: (1) ongoing, during-treatment assessment and (2) posttreatment assessment. One way to address the first of these is to use the instruments recommended for triage/treatment planning questionnaires: RCADS, SCARED, or SCAS. However their use may not warranted in many cases, because the focus of treatment is generally more limited. Thus, there may be more parsimonious ways to assess outcome, and more focused assessment methods are typically recommended. Specifically, ongoing assessment of outcome can be measured efficiently by an instrument specific to the syndrome in question. For example, one could choose between SPAI-C or the SAS and variants to measure social anxiety. Our review recommends the latter, because there are relatively more data on the measure, and it has four fewer items.

A problem with this plan emerges for problem areas without a specific measure. For example, panic disorder and SAD do not have stand-alone questionnaires specifically designed for them. Furthermore, although the FSSC-R taps fear severity, it is not likely to serve as a particularly useful outcome tool for treatment of specific phobia, because treatment will likely focus on a finite number of specific fears; thus, their declining severity and reduced avoidance is of more of interest than an inventory of a child's fear of a wide array of stimuli. In short, then, use of syndrome-specific questionnaires for outcome measurement is limited to GAD, OCD, and social phobia.

An alternative may be to extract individual scales from the DSM-based multidimensional questionnaires. A problem with this procedure concerns the lack of psychometric data for the scales as stand-alone measures. Furthermore, as noted earlier, available psychometric data on some of the scales are not particularly strong. For example, doubts concerning the reliability of the OCD and phobia scales make their use questionable. Still, use of these scales individually merits consideration and may prove to be a fruitful future research direction. Furthermore, the CY-BOCS represents a strong choice for OCD, so the only diagnoses that are not well covered may be phobias. And, as we discuss shortly, idiographic measurement may represent the best choice in this instance anyway.

Observational measures may also serve as good, idiographic ways to track ongoing treatment progress. Homework assignments, though not usually conceptualized as such, are often assessments of treatment progress. In exposure-based treatments, administration of a BAT may be used to determine treatment progress. This may be the optimal method for tracking progress in treating phobias. Less formal observational measures, such as client self-monitoring, also may provide insight into treatment effects. However, as noted, psychometric study of these methods is challenging, and little research has documented the reliability or validity of these methods.

To this point, we have suggested tracking treatment progress for discrete syndromes or problems. However, in cases with multiple diagnoses identified at the initial assessment, for which treatment has been multiply focused, such an approach may be less helpful. Furthermore, because estimates of comorbidity are high across epidemiological and clinical studies, this situation is likely to be quite common. In these instances, the broader DSM screening instruments may be needed to track ongoing treatment progress.

At posttreatment, if there is interest in identifying response generalization effects of treatment (i.e., reductions in other problems areas), broader instruments or a structured diagnostic interview may be the best route. Such methods allow the clinician to confirm that no (additional) problems remain (or have emerged). Considering economy, on the other hand, a clinician may again choose to use a specific questionnaire, perhaps paired with areas selected from a follow-up structured diagnostic interview. In addition, in some cases, the use of a BAT may also be a useful way to conclude treatment, allowing the client to demonstrate gains made in treatment in a more obvious way than might be achieved with a questionnaire or interview.

As summarized in Table 8.9, our recommendations with regard to assessment tools depend on the purpose of assessment. Furthermore, some of our recommendations are more tentative than others, because important gaps that remain in the literature preclude stronger recommendations. Finally, we remind the reader of our overall caveat for the chapter. Our focus has been on measures of child anxiety. As such, we have not discussed measures of other problem areas (e.g., disruptive behavior disorders, general child functioning measures). Thus, our recommendations are limited to anxiety-related measures. If we were recommending measures for broad clinical assessment, we would change our list. Overall, our review and the related recommendations are meant as a guide for clinicians to make evidence-based decisions for the assessment of child anxiety.

FUTURE DIRECTIONS

A review of nearly 40 years of research on assessment of anxiety in children points to several issues in the literature that call for additional research. First, there appears to be a need for additional evidence on parent report questionnaires. It is well documented that parents and youth often disagree about the psychological symptoms the youth is experiencing (e.g., DiBartolo, Albano, Barlow, & Heimberg, 1998; Frick, Silverthorn, & Evans, 1994). As a result, considerable debate exists regarding the preferred reporter of children's anxious symptomatology—parent or child. Some researchers have suggested that children may be better reporters of their own distress (e.g., Edelbrock, Costello, Dulcan, Conover, & Kala, 1985; Jensen, Traylor, Xenakis, & Davis, 1988), whereas others have found that parents may more reliably report their children's anxious distress (e.g., DiBartolo, Albano, Barlow, & Heimberg, 1998; Rapee, Barrett, Dadds, & Evans, 1994; Schniering, Hudson, & Rapee, 2000).

The controversy over whose report is preferable notwithstanding, few disagree that the use of parent reports in conjunction with child reports confers significant advantages over an exclusive reliance on youth self-report. It is unclear how reliable the reports of younger children (before age 10) are in discriminating subtle emotional states such as worry, anxiety, and depression (e.g., Edelbrock, Costello, Dulcan, Conover, & Kala, 1985; Harris, 1993; Silverman & Eisen, 1992; but see Silverman &

Rabian, 1995). Schniering and colleagues (2000) reported a trend in which children have more difficulty reporting on complex details, such as the duration and onset of symptoms. Similarly, Perez, Ascaso, Massons, and de la Osa Chaparro (1998) found that children demonstrate difficulties in thinking retrospectively and in answering questions that require the most metacognition (e.g., questions about internal thoughts or feeling states). Because children almost never refer themselves for clinical treatment, ignoring the parent's view seems clinically contraindicated. Finally, with only one reporter, assessment or diagnostic inferences cannot be corroborated as easily. Thus, we urge measure designers to continue to develop and investigate parent report versions of questionnaires.

Second, it appears more generally that the field would benefit simply from more measurement research. The child anxiety measurement literature is replete with "single-study" instruments (i.e., measures developed and tested in one [or a few] studies, only to be replaced or eclipsed by another, similar "single-study" instrument). Given that establishing the validity of an instrument and articulating its boundaries conditions (e.g., clinical, school samples) are highly complex endeavors (Cronbach & Meehl, 1955), it seems advisable that there be at a minimum some additional research on the field's most commonly used measures.

Loevinger (1957) outlined three components of construct validity that are worth considering here: substantive validity, structural validity, and external validity (for more recent expositions of construct validity, see Embretson, 1983; Hogan & Nicholson, 1988; Messick, 1995). In short, these components respectively imply that (1) the content of the items on a test should be consistent with the investigator's theory regarding the trait being assessed, (2) the structural relations among the items of a measure should correspond to theoretical expectations (e.g., internal consistency or factor structure), and (3) the measure's relations with extratest correlates should accord with theoretical prediction. Few of the instruments reviewed here have demonstrated strong findings in all of these areas.

Most lacking across the board is the evidence for substantive validity (cf. content validity; Haynes, Richard, & Kubany, 1995); that is, many measures appear to have been designed with an initially underdeveloped item pool,

such that factor-analytic findings often yield two- or three-item factors, or scales are otherwise underrepresented or unclearly related to theoretical domains (e.g., Chorpita & Daleiden, 2000). This observation suggests that future test development and revision should seek to be quite clear about the theory of the constructs in question, and should be explicitly overinclusive with initial item pools (Loevinger, 1957) to clearly demarcate an instrument's construct boundaries.

With respect to screening/identification, we agree with the now not-so-recent sentiment of Stark and Laurent (2001) regarding the need for a new generation of measures. On the one hand, multidimensional scales, particularly those that index DSM syndromes, appear to have high utility for identifying areas of concern. For the purpose of measuring treatment progress and outcome, on the other hand, it would be helpful to continue to develop and refine the more focused measures, obviating the need for the use of extended measures at repeated intervals (unless, of course, comorbidity is an issue, in which case multidimensional approach remains a strong choice). That said, the vast majority of research on the assessment of child anxiety involves single-instrument evaluation. Although important, single-instrument approaches to assessment are rarely appropriate in clinical circumstances. More studies on how various measures may be used in conjunctive accord and on empirical tests of combinatorial algorithms would be highly useful for the field. There has been little or no research on the use of data combination strategies other than rule-based interviews and linear sums of questionnaire items. More sophisticated approaches such as item–response theory (Reise, Ainsworth, & Haviland, 2005), associative network theory (Peng & Reggia, 1996), and Bayesian logic models (e.g., Chorpita et al., 2000) may ultimately point the way to the optimal inference strategies that draw from an efficient yet comprehensive battery of instruments. The promise of these new approaches is not well known in this context; we hope, therefore, that they will be frequent subjects of study as assessment approaches continue to be developed and improved for youth with anxiety.

Finally, that despite increasing calls for research with diverse sample, our review indicates that most of the evidence to date involves samples of mostly white youth. Given sociodemographic trends in the United States and other countries, the evidence base needs major work in this area if we are to maintain confidence in its external validity. In the area of child anxiety assessment, the work needed is both practical and conceptual. On the practical end, we simply need more studies with diverse samples. Although diversity of ethnic groups is one important direction (Austin & Chorpita, 2004; Safren et al., 2000), we also need work that examines measurement with poor and rural youth (e.g., Atkins et al., 2003; Costello et al., 2003). On the conceptual end, we also may need to rethink assumptions about anxiety measurement, because cross-cultural research has identified different manifestations of anxiety symptomatology in different cultural groups. For nations with increasing multicultural populations, sensitivity to such differences becomes a critical public health issue.

ACKNOWLEDGMENTS

Preparation of this chapter was supported in part through a grant from the Hawaii Department of Health, through the Research Network on Youth Mental Health, sponsored by the John D. and Catherine T. MacArthur Foundation, and by National Institute of Mental Health Grant No. K23 MH69421. We would like to thank Lauren Akselrod, Lauren Brown, Joella Newgen, Kathryn Taylor, and Katie Burns for their assistance with materials for this chapter.

REFERENCES

Achenbach, T. M., McConaughy, S. H., & Howell, C. T. (1987). Child/adolescent behavioral and emotional problems: Implications of cross-informant correlations for situational specificity. *Psychological Bulletin, 101,* 213–232.

Achenbach, T. M., & Rescorla, L. A. (2001). *Manual for the ASEBA School-Age Forms & Profiles.* Burlington: University of Vermont, Research Center for Children, Youth, and Families.

Albano, A. M., Chorpita, B. F., & Barlow, D. H. (2003). Childhood anxiety disorders. In E. J. Mash & R. A. Barkley (Eds.), *Child psychopathology* (2nd ed., pp. 279–329). New York: Guilford Press.

Albano, A. M., & Krain, A. L. (2005). Anxiety and anxiety disorders in girls. In D. J. Bell, S. L Foster, & E. J. Mash (Eds.), *Handbook of behavioral and emotional problems in girls* (pp. 79–116). New York: Kluwer Academic/Plenum Press.

Alkon, A., Goldstein, L. H., Smider, N., Essex, M. J., Kupfer, D. J., Boyce, W. T., et al. (2003). Developmental and contextual influences on autonomic reactivity in young children. *Developmental Psychobiology, 42,* 64–78.

American Psychiatric Association (APA). (1980). *Diagnostic and statistical manual of mental disorders* (3rd ed.). Washington, DC: Author.

American Psychiatric Association (APA). (1987). *Diagnostic and statistical manual of mental disorders* (3rd ed., rev.). Washington, DC: Author.

American Psychiatric Association (APA). (1994). *Diagnostic and statistical manual of mental disorders* (4th ed.). Washington, DC: Author.

American Psychiatric Association (APA). (2001). *Diagnostic and statistical manual of mental disorders* (4h ed., rev.). Washington, DC: Author.

Anastasi, A. (1988). *Psychological testing* (6th ed.). New York: Macmillan.

Angold, A., & Costello, E. J. (2000). The Child and Adolescent Psychiatric Assessment (CAPA). *Journal of the American Academy of Child and Adolescent Psychiatry, 39,* 39–48.

Angold, A., Costello, E. J., & Erkanli, A. (1999). Comorbidity. *Journal of Child Psychology and Psychiatry, 40,* 57–87.

Atkins, M. S., Graczyk, P. A., & Frazier, S. L. (2003). Toward a new model for promoting urban children's mental health: Accessible, effective, and sustainable school-based mental health services. *School Psychology Review, 32,* 503–514.

Attar, B. K., Guerra, N. G., & Tolan, P. H. (1994). Neighborhood disadvantage, stressful life events, and adjustment in urban elementary school children. *Journal of Clinical Child Psychology, 23,* 391–400.

Austin, A. A., & Chorpita, B. F. (2004). Temperament, anxiety, and depression: Comparisons across five ethnic groups of children. *Journal of Clinical Child and Adolescent Psychology, 33,* 216–226.

Bandura, A. (1977). *Social learning theory.* New York: General Learning Press.

Barlow, D. H. (1988). *Anxiety and its disorders: The nature and treatment of anxiety and panic.* New York: Guilford Press.

Barlow, D. H. (2000). Unraveling the mysteries of anxiety and its disorders from the perspective of emotion theory. *American Psychologist, 55,* 1245–1263.

Barlow, D. H. (2002). *Anxiety and its disorders: The nature and treatment of anxiety and panic* (2nd ed.). New York: Guilford Press.

Barlow, D. H., Chorpita, B. F., & Turovsky, J. (1996). Fear, panic, anxiety, and the disorders of emotion. In D. A. Hope (Ed.), *Nebraska Symposium on Motivation: Integrated views of motivation and emotion* (Vol. 43, pp. 251–328). Lincoln: University of Nebraska Press.

Barrios, B. A., & Hartmann, D. P. (1997). Fears and anxieties. In E. J. Mash & L. G. Terdal (Eds.), *Assessment of childhood disorders* (2nd ed., pp. 196–262). New York: Guilford Press.

Bauer, A. M., Quas, J. A., & Boyce, W. T. (2002). Associations between physiological reactivity and children's behavior: Advantages of a multisystem approach. *Journal of Developmental and Behavioral Pediatrics, 23,* 102–113.

Beauchaine, T. P. (2001). Vagal tone, development, and Gray's motivational theory: Toward an integrated model of autonomic nervous system functioning in psychopathology. *Development and Psychopathology 13*, 183–214.

Becker, G. (2000). How important is transient error in estimating reliability?: Going beyond simulation studies. *Psychological Methods, 5*, 370–379.

Beidel, D. C. (1988). Psychophysiological assessment of anxious emotional states in children. *Journal of Abnormal Child Psychology, 97*, 80–82.

Beidel, D. C. (1991). Determining the reliability of psychophysiological assessment in childhood anxiety. *Journal of Anxiety Disorders, 5*, 139–150.

Beidel, D. C., Morris, T. L., & Turner, M. W. (2004). Social phobia. In T. L. Morris & J. S. March (Eds.), *Anxiety disorders in children and adolescents* (2nd ed., pp. 141–163). New York: Guilford Press.

Beidel, D. C., & Turner, S. M. (2005). *Childhood anxiety disorders: A guide to research and treatment.* New York: Routledge.

Beidel, D. C., Turner, S. M., & Fink, C. M. (1996). Assessment of childhood social phobia: Construct, convergent, and discriminative validity of the Social Phobia and Anxiety Inventory for Children (SPAI-C). *Psychological Assessment, 8*, 235–240.

Beidel, D. C., Turner, S. M., Hamlin, K., & Morris, T. L. (2000). The Social Phobia and Anxiety Inventory for Children (SPAI-C): External and discriminative validity. *Behavior Therapy, 31*, 75–87.

Beidel, D. C., Turner, S. M., & Morris, T. L. (1995). A new inventory to assess childhood social anxiety and phobia: The Social Phobia and Anxiety Inventory for Children. *Psychological Assessment, 7*, 73–79.

Beidel, D. C., Turner, S. M., & Morris, T. L. (1999). Psychopathology of childhood social phobia. *Journal of the American Academy of Child and Adolescent Psychiatry, 38*, 643–650.

Bell-Dolan, D., & Brazeal, T. J. (1993). Separation anxiety disorder, overanxious disorder, and school refusal. *Child and Adolescent Psychiatric Clinics of North America, 2*, 563–580.

Berg, C. J., Rapoport, J. L., & Flament, M. (1986). The Leyton Obsessional Inventory—Child Version. *Journal of the American Academy of Child and Adolescent Psychiatry, 25*, 84–91.

Bernstein, G. A., Crosby, R. D., Perwien, A. R., & Borchardt, C. M. (1996). Anxiety rating for children-revised: Reliability and validity. *Journal of Anxiety Disorders, 10*, 97–114.

Bidaut-Russell, M., Valla, J., Thomas, J. M., Begeron, L., & Lawson, E. (1998). Reliability of the Terry: A mental health cartoon-like screener for African-American children. *Child Psychiatry and Human Development, 28*, 249–263.

Biederman, J., Rosenbaum, J. F., Bolduc-Murphy, E. A., Faraone, S., Chaloff, J., Hirshfeld, D. R., et al. (1993). Behavioral inhibition as a temperamental risk factor for anxiety disorders. *Child and Adolescent Psychiatric Clinics of North America, 2*, 667–684.

Bird, H. R., Gould, M. S., & Staghezza, B. M. (1993). Patterns of diagnostic comorbidity in a community sample of children aged 9 through 16 years. *Journal of the American Academy of Child and Adolescent Psychiatry, 32*, 361–368.

Bird, H. R., Gould, M. S., Yager, T., Staghezza, B., & Canino, G. (1989). Risk factors for maladjustment in Puerto Rican children. *Journal of the American Academy of Child and Adolescent Psychiatry, 28*, 847–850.

Birmaher, B., Khetarpal, S., Brent, D., Cully, M., Balach, L., Kaufman, J., et al. (1997). The Screen for Child Anxiety Related Emotional Disorders (SCARED): Scale construction and psychometric characteristics. *Journal of the American Academy of Child and Adolescent Psychiatry, 36*, 545–553.

Bolton, D., Eley, T. C., O'Connor, T. G., Perrin, S., Rabe-Hesketh, S., Rijsdijk, F., et al. (2006). Prevalence and genetic and environmental influences on anxiety disorders in 6-year-old twins. *Psychological Medicine, 36*, 335–344.

Bouldin, P., & Pratt, C. (1998). Utilizing parent report to investigate young children's fears: A modification of the Fear Survey Schedule for Children–II: A research note. *Journal of Child Psychology and Psychiatry, 39*, 271–277.

Bouton, M. E., Mineka, S., & Barlow, D. H. (2001). A modern learning-theory perspective on the etiology of panic disorder. *Psychological Review, 108*, 4–32.

Boyce, W. T., Quas, J., Alkon, A., Smider, N. A., Essex, M. J., Kupfer, D. J., et al. (2001). Autonomic reactivity and psychopathology in middle childhood. *British Journal of Psychiatry, 179*, 144–150.

Boyd, R. C., Ginsburg, G. S., Lambert, S. F., Cooley, M. R., & Campbell, K. D. M. (2003). Screen for child anxiety related emotional disorders (SCARED): Psychometric properties in an African-American parochial high school sample. *Journal of the American Academy of Child and Adolescent Psychiatry, 42*, 1188–1196.

Boyle, M. H., Offord, D. R., Racine, Y. A., Szatmari, P., Sanford, M., & Fleming, J. E. (1997). Adequacy of interviews vs. checklists for classifying childhood psychiatric disorder based on parent reports. *Archives of General Psychiatry, 54*, 793–799.

Brady, E., & Kendall, P. C. (1992). Comorbidity of anxiety and depression in children and adolescents. *Psychological Bulletin, 111*, 244–255.

Brenner, S. L., Beauchaine, T. P., & Sylvers, P. D. (2005). A comparison of psychophysiological and self-report measures of BAS and BIS activation. *Psychophysiology, 42*, 108–115.

Brown, T. A., Chorpita, B. F., & Barlow, D. H. (1998). Structural relationships among dimensions of the DSM-IV anxiety and mood disorders and dimensions of negative affect, positive affect, and autonomic arousal. *Journal of Abnormal Psychology 107*, 179–192.

Burnham, J. J., & Gullone, E. (1997). The Fear Survey Schedule for Children–II: A psychometric investigation with American data. *Behaviour Research and Therapy, 35,* 165–173.

Calkins, S. D., & Dedmon, S. E. (2000). Physiological and behavioral regulation in two-year-old children with aggressive/destructive behavior problems. *Journal of Abnormal Child Psychology, 28,* 103–118.

Campbell, D. P., & Fiske, D. W. (1959). Convergent and discriminant validity by the multi-trait–multi-method matrix. *Psychological Bulletin, 56,* 81–105.

Canino, G., Shrout, P. E., Rubio-Stipec, M., Bird, H. R., Bravo, M., Ramirez, R., et al. (2004). The DSM-IV rates of child and adolescent disorders in Puerto Rico. *Archives of General Psychiatry, 61,* 85–93

Caron, C., & Rutter, M. (1991). Comorbidity in child psychopathology: Concepts, issues and research strategies. *Journal of Child Psychology and Psychiatry, 32,* 1063–1080.

Chaiyawat, W., & Brown, J. K. (2000). Psychometric properties of the Thai versions of State–Trait Anxiety Inventory for Children and Child Medical Fear Scale. *Research in Nursing and Health, 23,* 406–414.

Chambers, W. J. (1985). The assessment of affective disorders in children and adolescents by semistructured interview: Test-retest reliability of the Schedule for Affective Disorders and Schizophrenia for School-Age Children, Present Episode Version. *Archives of General Psychiatry, 42,* 696–702.

Chorpita, B. F. (2001). Control and the development of negative emotions. In M. W. Vasey & M. R. Dadds (Eds.), *The developmental psychopathology of anxiety* (pp. 112–142). New York: Oxford University Press.

Chorpita, B. F. (2002). The tripartite model and dimensions of anxiety and depression: An examination of structure in a large school sample. *Journal of Abnormal Child Psychology, 30,* 177–190.

Chorpita, B. F., Albano, A. M., & Barlow, D. H. (1996). Child Anxiety Sensitivity Index: Considerations for children with anxiety disorders. *Journal of Clinical Child Psychology, 25,* 77–82.

Chorpita, B. F., Albano, A. M., & Barlow, D. H. (1998). The structure of negative emotions in a clinical sample of children and adolescents. *Journal of Abnormal Psychology, 107,* 74–85.

Chorpita, B. F., & Barlow, D. H. (1998). The development of anxiety: The role of control in the early environment. *Psychological Bulletin, 117,* 3–19.

Chorpita, B. F., & Daleiden, E. L. (2000). Properties of the childhood Anxiety Sensitivity Index in Children with anxiety disorders: Autonomic and nonautonomic factors. *Behavior Therapy, 31,* 327–349.

Chorpita, B. F., & Lilienfeld, S. O. (1999). Clinical assessment of anxiety sensitivity in children: Where do we go from here? *Psychological Assessment, 11,* 212–224.

Chorpita, B. F., Moffitt, C. E., & Gray, J. (2005). Psychometric properties of the Revised Child Anxiety and Depression Scale in a clinical sample. *Behaviour Research and Therapy, 43,* 309–322.

Chorpita, B. F., & Nakamura, B. J. (in press). Dynamic

structure in diagnostic structured interviewing: A comparative test of accuracy and efficiency. *Journal of Psychopathology and Behavioral Assessment.*

Chorpita, B. F., Plummer, C., & Moffitt, C. E. (2000). Relations of tripartite dimensions of emotion to childhood anxiety and mood disorders. *Journal of Abnormal Child Psychology, 28,* 299–310.

Chorpita, B. F., & Southam-Gerow, M. A. (2006). Fears and anxieties. In E. J. Mash & R. A. Barkley (Eds.), *Treatment of childhood disorders* (3rd ed., pp. 271–335). New York: Guilford Press.

Chorpita, B. F., Tracey, S. A., Brown, T. A., Collica, T. J., & Barlow, D. H. (1997). Assessment of worry in children and adolescents: An Adaptation of the Penn State Worry Questionnaire. *Behaviour Research and Therapy, 35,* 569–581.

Chorpita, B. F., Yim, L., Moffitt, C., Umemoto, L. A., & Francis, S. E. (2000). Assessment of symptoms of DSM-IV anxiety and depression in children: A Revised Child Anxiety and Depression Scale. *Behaviour Research and Therapy, 38,* 835–855.

Chorpita, B. F., Yim, L. M., & Tracey, S. A. (2000). Feasibility of a simplified and dynamic Bayesian system for use in structured diagnostic interviews. *Journal of Psychopathology and Behavioral Assessment, 24,* 13–23.

Clark, D. B., Turner, S. M., & Beidel, D. C. (1994). Reliability and validity of the Social Phobia and Anxiety Inventory for adolescents. *Psychological Assessment, 6,* 135–140.

Clark, L. A., & Watson, D. (1991). A tripartite model of anxiety and depression: Psychometric evidence and taxonomic implications. *Journal of Abnormal Psychology, 100,* 316–336.

Clark, L. A., Watson, D., & Mineka, S. (1994). Temperament, personality, and the mood and anxiety disorders. *Journal of Abnormal Psychology 103,* 103–116.

Compton, S. N., Burns, B. J., Egger, H. L., & Robertson, E. (2002). Review of the evidence base for treatment of childhood psychopathology: Internalizing disorders. *Journal of Consulting and Clinical Psychology, 70,* 1240–1266.

Compton, S. N., March, J. S., Brent, D., Albano, A. M., Weersing, V. R., & Curry, J. (2004). Cognitive-behavioral psychotherapy for anxiety and depressive disorders in children and adolescents: An evidence-based medicine review. *Journal of the American Academy of Child and Adolescent Psychiatry, 43,* 930–959.

Compton, S. N., Nelson, A. H., & March, J. S. (2000). Social phobia and separation anxiety symptoms in community and clinical samples of children and adolescents. *Journal of the American Academy of Child and Adolescent Psychiatry, 39,* 1040–1046.

Costello, E. J., Angold, A., & Burns, B. J. (1996). The Great Smoky Mountains Study of Youth: Functional impairment and serious emotional disturbance. *Archives of General Psychiatry, 53,* 1137–1143.

Costello, E. J., Angold, A., & Keeler, A. (1999). Adolescent outcomes of childhood disorders: The consequences of severity and impairment. *Journal of the American Academy of Child and Adolescent Psychiatry, 38,* 121–128.

Costello, E. J., Compton, S. N., Keeler, G., & Angold, A. (2003). Relationships between poverty and psychopathology: A natural experiment. *Journal of the American Medical Association, 290,* 2023–202.

Costello, E. J., Egger, H., & Angold, A. (2005). 10-Year research update review: The epidemiology of child and adolescent psychiatric disorders: I. Methods and public health burden. *Journal of the American Academy of Child and Adolescent Psychiatry, 44,* 972–986.

Cronbach, L. J. (1970). *Essentials of psychological testing* (3rd ed.). New York: Harper.

Cronbach, L. J., & Meehl, P. E. (1955). Construct validity in psychological tests. *Psychological Bulletin, 52,* 281–302.

Crook, K., Beaver, B. R., & Bell, M. (1998). Anxiety and depression in children: A preliminary examination of the utility of the PANAS-C. *Journal of Psychopathology and Behavioral Assessment, 20,* 333–350.

Cross, R. W., & Huberty, T. J. (1993). Factor analysis of the State–Trait Anxiety Inventory for children with a sample of seventh- and eighth-grade students. *Journal of Psychoeducational Assessment, 11,* 232–241.

de Geus, E. J. C., & van Doornen, L. J. C. (1996). Ambulatory assessment of parasympathetic/sympathetic balance by impedance cardiography. In J. Fahrenberg & M. Myrtek (Eds.), *Ambulatory assessment: Computer-assisted psychological and psychophysiological methods in monitoring and field studies* (pp. 141–163). Ashland, OH: Hogrefe & Huber.

Delprato, D. J., & McGlynn, F. D. (1984). Behavioral theories of anxiety disorders. In S. M. Turner (Ed.), *Behavioral theories and treatment of anxiety* (pp. 1–49). New York: Plenum Press.

deRoss, R., Chorpita, B. F., & Gullone, E. (2005). The Revised Child Anxiety and Depression Scale: A psychometric investigation with Australian youth. *Behaviour Change, 19,* 90–101.

DiBartolo, P. M., Albano, A. M., Barlow, D. H., & Heimberg, R. G. (1998). Cross-informant agreement in the assessment of social phobia in youth. *Journal of Abnormal Child Psychology, 26,* 213–220.

Dong, Q., Xia, Y., Lin, L., Yang, B., & Ollendick, T. H. (1995). The stability and prediction of fears in Chinese children and adolescents: A one-year follow-up. *Journal of Child Psychology and Psychiatry and Allied Disciplines, 36,* 819–831.

Doss, A. J., & Weisz, J. R. (2006). Syndrome co-occurrence and treatment outcomes in youth mental health clinics. *Journal of Consulting and Clinical Psychology, 74,* 416–425.

Eaves, L. J., Silberg, J. L., Maes, H. H., Simonoff, E., Pickles, A., Rutter, M., et al. (1997). Genetics and developmental psychopathology: 2. The main effects of genes and environment on behavioral problems in the Virginia Twin Study of Adolescent Behavioral Development. *Journal of Child Psychology and Psychiatry and Allied Disciplines, 38,* 965–980.

Edelbrock, C., Costello, A. J., Dulcan, M. K., Conover, N. C., & Kala, R. (1986). Age differences in the reliability of the psychiatric interview of the child. *Child Development, 56,* 265–275.

Eisen, A. R., & Silverman, W. K. (1991). Treatment of an adolescent with bowel movement phobia using self-control therapy. *Journal of Behavior Therapy and Experimental Psychiatry 22,* 45–51.

Eley, T. C., Bolton, D., O'Connor, T., Perrin, S., Smith, P., & Plomin, R. (2003). A twin study of anxiety-related behaviours in young children. *Journal of Child Psychology and Psychiatry and Allied Disciplines, 44,* 945–960.

Embretson, S. (1983). Construct validity: Construct representation versus nomothetic span. *Psychological Bulletin, 93,* 179–197.

Epkins, C. C. (1993). A preliminary comparison of teacher ratings and child self-report of depression, anxiety, and aggression in inpatient and elementary school samples. *Journal of Abnormal Child Psychology, 21,* 649–661.

Epkins, C. C. (2002). A comparison of two self-report measures of children's social anxiety in clinic and community samples. *Journal of Clinical Child and Adolescent Psychology, 31,* 69–79.

Ernst, M., Cookus, B. A., & Moravec, B. C. (2000). Pictorial Instrument for Children and Adolescents (PICA-III-R). *Journal of the American Academy of Child and Adolescent Psychiatry, 39,* 94–99.

Ernst, M., Godfrey, K. A., Silva, R. R., Pouget, E. R., & Welkowitz, J. (1994). A new pictorial instrument for child and adolescent psychiatry: A pilot study. *Psychiatry Research, 51,* 87–104.

Essau, C. A., Conradt, J., & Petermann, F. (2000). Frequency, comorbidity, and psychosocial impairment of specific phobia in adolescents. *Journal of Clinical Child Psychology, 29,* 221–231.

Essau, C. A., Muris, P., & Ederer, E. M. (2002). Reliability and validity of the Spence Children's Anxiety Scale and the Screen for Child Anxiety Related Emotional Disorders in German children. *Journal of Behavior Therapy and Experimental Psychiatry, 33,* 1–18.

Evans, P. D., & Harmon, G. (1981). Children's self-initiated approach to spiders. *Behaviour Research and Therapy 19,* 543–546.

Fergusson, D. M., Horwood, L. J., & Lynskey, M. T. (1993). Prevalence and comorbidity of DSM-III—R diagnoses in a birth cohort of 15 year olds. *Journal of the American Academy of Child and Adolescent Psychiatry, 32,* 1127–1134.

Foley, D. L., Pickles, A., Maes, H. M., Silberg, J. L., & Eaves, L. J. (2004). Course and short-term outcomes of separation anxiety disorder in a community sample of twins. *Journal of the American Academy of Child and Adolescent Psychiatry, 43,* 1107–1114.

Ford, T., Goodman, R., & Meltzer, H. (2003). The British Child and Adolescent Mental Health Survey 1999: The prevalence of DSM-IV disorders. *Journal of the American Academy of Child and Adolescent Psychiatry, 42,* 1203–1211.

Foster, S. L., Bell-Dolan, D. J., & Burge, D. A. (1988). Behavioral observation. In A. S. Bellack & M. Hersen (Eds.), *Behavioral assessment: A practical handbook* (3rd ed., pp. 199–160). Elmsford, NY: Pergamon Press.

Foster, S. L., & Cone, J. D. (1980). Current issues in direct observation. *Behavioral Assessment 2,* 313–338.

Fox, J. E., & Houston, B. K. (1983). Distinguishing between cognitive and somatic trait and state anxiety in children. *Journal of Personality and Social Psychology, 45,* 862–870.

Francis, S. E., & Chorpita, B. F. (2004). Behavioral assessment of children in outpatient settings. In M. Hersen (Series Ed.) & S. N. Haynes & E. M. Heiby (Vol. Eds.), *Comprehensive handbook of psychological assessment: Vol. 3. Behavioral assessment* (pp. 291–319). Hoboken, NJ: Wiley.

Fredrickson, B. L. (1998). Cultivated emotions: Parental socialization of positive emotions and self-conscious emotions. *Psychological Inquiry, 9,* 279–281.

Freeman, K. A., & Miller, C. A. (2002). Behavioral case conceptualization for children and adolescents. In M. Hersen (Ed.), *Clinical behavior therapy: Adults and children* (pp. 239–255). New York: Wiley.

Frick, P. J., Silverthorn, P., & Evans, C. (1994). Assessment of childhood anxiety using structured interviews: Patterns of agreement among informants and association with maternal anxiety. *Psychological Assessment, 6,* 372–379.

Friedlmeier, W., & Trommsdorff, G. (1999). Emotion regulation in early childhood: A cross-cultural comparison between German and Japanese toddlers. *Journal of Cross-Cultural Psychology, 30,* 684–711.

Fullana, M. A., Servera, M., Weems, C. F., Tortella-Feliu, M., & Caseras, X. (2003). Psychometric properties of the Childhood Anxiety Sensitivity Index in a sample of Catalan school children. *Anxiety, Stress, and Coping, 16,* 99–107.

Gaudry, E., & Poole, C. (1975). A further validation of the state–trait distinction in anxiety research. *Australian Journal of Psychology, 2,* 119–125.

Gaudry, E., Vagg, P., & Spielberger, C. D. (1975). Validation of the state–trait distinction in anxiety research. *Multivariate Behavioral Research, 3,* 331–341.

Geller, D. A., Biederman, J., Faraone, S. V., Bellordre, C. A., Kim, G. S., Hagermoser, L., et al. (2001). Disentangling chronological age from age of onset in children and adolescents with obsessive–compulsive disorder. *International Journal of Neuropsychopharmacology, 4,* 169–178.

Geller, D. A., Biederman, J., Jones, J., Shapiro, S., Schwartz, S., & Park, K. S. (1998). Obsessive–compulsive disorder in children and adolescents: A review. *Harvard Review of Psychiatry, 5,* 260–273.

Ginsburg, G. S., La Greca, A. M., & Silverman, W. K.

(1998). Social anxiety in children with anxiety disorders: Relation with social and emotional functioning. *Journal of Abnormal Child Psychology, 26,* 175–185.

Goodyer, I. M., Park, R. J., & Herbert, J. (2001). Psychosocial and endocrine features of chronic first-episode major depression in 8–16 year olds. *Biological Psychiatry, 50,* 351–357.

Granger, D. A., & Kivlighan, K. T. (2003). Integrating biological, behavioral, and social levels of analysis in early child development: Progress, problems and prospects. *Child Development, 74,* 1058–1063.

Granger, D. A., Weisz, J. R., & Kauneckis, D. (1994). Neuroendocrine reactivity, internalizing behavior problems, and control-related cognitions in clinic-referred children and adolescents. *Journal of Abnormal Psychology, 103,* 267–276.

Grant, B. F., Stinson, F. S., Dawson, D. A., Chou, P., Dufour, M. C., Compton, W., et al. (2004). Prevalence and co-occurrence of substance use disorders and independent mood and anxiety disorders: Results from the National Epidemiologic Survey on Alcohol and Related Conditions. *Archives of General Psychiatry, 61,* 807–816.

Gray, J. A., & McNaughton, N. (1996). The neuropsychology of anxiety: A reprise. In D. A. Hope (Ed.), *Nebraska Symposium on Motivation: Perspectives on anxiety, panic, and fear* (Vol. 43, pp. 61–134). Lincoln: University of Nebraska Press.

Greco, L. A., & Morris, T. L. (2004). Assessment. In T. L. Morris & J. S. March (Eds.), *Anxiety disorders in children and adolescents* (2nd ed., pp. 99–121). New York: Guilford Press.

Gullone, E., & King, N. J. (1992). Psychometric evaluation of a revised fear survey schedule for children and adolescents. *Journal of Child Psychology and Psychiatry, 33,* 987–998.

Gullone, E., King, N. J., & Cummins, R. A. (1996). Fears in youth with mental retardation: Psychometric evaluation of the Fear Survey Schedule for Children–II (FSSC-II). *Research in Developmental Disabilities, 17,* 269–284.

Hale, W. W., Raaijmakers, Q., Muris, P., & Meeus, W. (2005). Psychometric properties of the Screen for Child Anxiety Related Emotional Disorders (SCARED) in the general adolescent population. *Journal of the American Academy of Child and Adolescent Psychiatry, 44,* 283–290.

Harris, F. C., & Lahey, B. B. (1982). Recording system bias in direct observational methodology: A review and critical analysis of factors causing inaccurate coding behavior. *Clinical Psychology Review, 2,* 539–556.

Harris, P. L. (1993). Understanding emotion. In M. Lewis & J. M. Haviland (Eds.), *Handbook of emotions* (pp. 237–246). New York: Guilford Press.

Haynes, S. N., & Horn, W. F. (1982). Reactivity in behavioral observation: A review. *Behavioral Assessment, 4,* 369–385.

Haynes, S. N., Richard, D. C., & Kubany, E. S. (1995).

Content validity in psychological assessment: A functional approach to concepts and methods. *Psychological Assessment, 7*, 238–247.

Hayward, C., Killen, J. D., Kraemer, H. C., & Taylor, C. B. (2000). Predictors of panic attacks in adolescents. *Journal of the American Academy of Child and Adolescent Psychiatry 39*, 207–214.

Henggeler, S. W., Schoenwald, S. K., Rowland, M. D., & Cunningham, P. B. (2002). *Serious emotional disturbance in children and adolescents: Multisystemic therapy.* New York: Guilford Press.

Higa, C. K., Daleiden, E. L., & Chorpita, B. F. (2002). Psychometric properties and clinical utility of the School Refusal Assessment Scale in a multiethnic sample. *Journal of Psychopathology and Behavioral Assessment, 24*, 247–258.

Hodges, K., Cools, J., & McKnew, D. (1989). Test–retest reliability of a clinical research interview for children: The Child Assessment Schedule. *Psychological Assessment, 1*, 317–322.

Hodges, K., Kline, J., Stern, L., Cytryn, L., & McKnew, D. (1982). The development of a child assessment interview for research and clinical use. *Journal of Abnormal Child Psychology, 10*, 173–189.

Hodges, K., McKnew, D., Burbach, D. J., & Roebuck, L. (1987). Diagnostic concordance between the Child Assessment Schedule (CAS) and the Schedule for Affective Disorders and Schizophrenia for School-Age Children (K-SADS) in an outpatient sample using lay interviewers. *Journal of the American Academy of Child and Adolescent Psychiatry, 26*, 654–661.

Hodges, K., McKnew, D., Cytryn, L., Stern, L., & Kline, J. (1982). The Child Assessment Schedule (CAS) diagnostic interview: A report on reliability and validity. *Journal of the American Academy of Child and Adolescent Psychiatry, 21*, 468–473.

Hodges, K., Saunders, W. B., Kashani, J., & Hamlett, K. (1990). Internal consistency of DSM-III diagnoses using the symptom scales of the Child Assessment Schedule. *Journal of the American Academy of Child and Adolescent Psychiatry, 29*, 635–641.

Hoehn-Saric, E., Maisami, M., & Wiegand, D. (1987). Measurement of anxiety in children and adolescents using semistructured interviews. *Journal of the American Academy of Child and Adolescent Psychiatry, 26*, 541–545.

Hofmann, S., Albano, A. M., Heimberg, R. G., Tracey, S., Chorpita, B. F., & Barlow, D. H. (1999). Subtypes of social phobia in adolescents. *Depression and Anxiety, 9*, 8–15.

Hogan, R., & Nicholson, R. A. (1988). The meaning of personality test scores. *American Psychologist, 43*, 621–626.

Inderbitzen, H. M., & Hope, D. A. (1995). Relationship among adolescent reports of social anxiety, anxiety, and depressive symptoms. *Journal of Anxiety Disorders, 9*, 385–396.

Inderbitzen-Nolan, H., Davies, C. A., & McKeon, N. D. (2004). Investigating the construct validity of the SPAI-C: Comparing the sensitivity and specificity of the SPAI-C and the SAS-A. *Journal of Anxiety Disorders, 18*, 547–560.

Inderbitzen-Nolan, H. M., & Walters, K. S. (2000). Social Anxiety Scale for Adolescents: Normative data and further evidence of construct validity. *Journal of Clinical Child Psychology, 29*, 360–371.

Jensen, P. S., Traylor, J., Xenakis, S. N., & Davis, H. (1988). Child psychopathology rating scales and interrater agreement: I. Parents' gender and psychiatric symptoms. *Journal of the American Academy of Child and Adolescent Psychiatry, 27*, 442–450.

Joiner, T. E., Jr., Catanzaro, S. J., & Laurent, J. (1996). Tripartite structure of positive and negative affect, depression, and anxiety in child and adolescent psychiatric inpatients. *Journal of Abnormal Psychology, 105*, 401–409.

Joiner, T. E., Schmidt, K. L., & Schmidt, N. B. (1996). Low-end specificity of childhood measures of emotional distress: Differential effects for depression and anxiety. *Journal of Personality Assessment, 67*, 258–271.

Kagan, J., Reznick, J. S., & Snidman, N. (1988). Biological bases of childhood shyness. *Science, 240*, 167–171.

Kaufman, J., Birmaher, B., Brent, D., & Rao, U. (1997). Schedule for Affective Disorders and Schizophrenia for School-Age Children—Present and Lifetime version (K-SADS-PL): Initial reliability and validity data. *Journal of the American Academy of Child and Adolescent Psychiatry, 36*, 980–988.

Kazdin, A. E. (2001). Bridging the enormous gaps of theory with therapy research and practice. *Journal of Clinical Child Psychology, 30*, 59–66.

Kazdin, A. E., & Kagan, J. (1994). Models of dysfunction in developmental psychopathology. *Clinical Psychology: Science and Practice, 1*, 35–52.

Kearney, C. A. (2001). *School refusal behavior in youth: A functional approach to assessment and treatment.* Washington, DC: American Psychological Association.

Kearney, C. A. (2002). Identifying the function of school refusal behavior: A revision of the School Refusal Assessment Scale. *Journal of Psychopathology and Behavioral Assessment, 24*, 235–245.

Kearney, C. A., Albano, A. M., Eisen, A. R., Allan, W. D., & Barlow, D. H. (1997). The phenomenology of panic disorder in youngsters: An empirical study of a clinical sample. *Journal of Anxiety Disorders, 11*, 49–62.

Kearney, C. A., & Silverman, W. K. (1992). Let's not push the "panic" button: A critical analysis of panic and panic disorder in adolescents. *Clinical Psychology Review, 12*, 293–305.

Kearney, C. A., & Silverman, W. K. (1993). Measuring the function of school refusal behavior: The school assessment scale. *Journal of Clinical Child Psychology, 22*, 85–96.

Kelley, C. K. (1976). Case histories and shorter communications: Play desensitization of fear of darkness in playschool children. *Behavior Research and Therapy 14*, 79–81.

Kendall, P. C. (1994). Treating anxiety disorders in children: Results of a randomized clinical trial. *Journal of Consulting and Clinical Psychology, 62*, 100–110.

Kendall, P. C., Brady, E. U., & Verduin, T. L. (2001). Comorbidity in childhood anxiety disorders and treatment outcome. *Journal of the American Academy of Child and Adolescent Psychiatry, 40*, 787–794.

Kendall, P. C., Flannery-Schroeder, E. C., Panichelli-Mindel, S. P., Southam-Gerow, M. A., Henin, A., & Warman, M. J. (1997). Therapy for youths with anxiety disorders: A second randomized clinical trial. *Journal of Consulting and Clinical Psychology, 65*, 366–380.

Kendall, P. C., & Warman, M. J. (1996). Anxiety disorders in youth: Diagnostic consistency across DSM-III-R and DSM-IV. *Journal of Anxiety Disorders, 10*, 453–463.

Kim-Cohen, J., Moffitt, T. E., & Caspi, A. (2004). Genetic and environmental processes in young children's resilience and vulnerability to socioeconomic deprivation. *Child Development, 75*, 651–668.

King, N. J., Muris, P., & Ollendick, T. H. (2004). Specific phobia. In T. L. Morris & J. S. March (Eds.), *Anxiety disorders in children and adolescents* (2nd ed., pp. 263–279). New York: Guilford Press.

King, N. J., & Ollendick, T. H. (1992). Reliability of the Fear Survey Schedule for Children—Revised. *Australian Educational and Developmental Psychologist, 9*, 55–57.

Kirisci, L., Clark, D. B., & Moss, H. B. (1996). Reliability and validity of the State–Trait Anxiety Inventory for Children in adolescent substance abusers: Confirmatory factor analysis and item response theory. *Journal of Child and Adolescent Substance Abuse, 5*, 57–69.

Kolaitis, G., Korpa, T., Kolvin, I., & Tsiantis, J. (2003). Schedule for Affective Disorders and Schizophrenia for school-age children—present episode (K-SADS-P): A pilot inter-rater reliability study for Greek children and adolescents. *European Psychiatry, 18*, 374–375.

La Greca, A. M., Dandes, S. K., Wick, P., Shaw, K., & Stone, W. L. (1988). Development of the Social Anxiety Scale for Children: Reliability and concurrent validity. *Journal of Clinical Child Psychology, 17*, 84–91.

La Greca, A. M., & Lopez, N. (1998). Social anxiety among adolescents: Linkages with peer relations and friendships. *Journal of Abnormal Child Psychology, 26*, 83–94.

La Greca, A. M., & Stone, W. L. (1993). Social Anxiety Scale for Children—Revised: Factor structure and concurrent validity. *Journal of Clinical Child Psychology, 22*, 17–27.

Lambert, S. F., Cooley, M. R., Campbell, K. D. M., Benoit, M. Z., & Stansbury, R. (2004). Assessing anxiety sensitivity in inner-city African American children: Psychometric properties of the Childhood

Anxiety Sensitivity Index. *Journal of Clinical Child and Adolescent Psychology, 33*, 248–259.

Landis, J. R., & Koch, G. G. (1977). The measurement of observer agreement for categorical data. *Biometrics, 33*, 159–174.

Langley, A. K., Bergman, L., McCracken, J., & Piacentini, J. C. (2004). Impairment in childhood anxiety disorders: Preliminary examination of the Child Anxiety Impact Scale—Parent Version. *Journal of Child and Adolescent Psychopharmacology, 14*, 105–114.

Last, C. G. (1989). Anxiety disorders. In T. H. Ollendick & M. Hersen (Eds.), *Handbook of child psychopathology* (2nd ed., pp. 219–227). New York: Plenum Press.

Last, C. G. (1991). Somatic complaints in anxiety disordered children. *Journal of Anxiety Disorders, 5*, 125–138.

Last, C. G., Hersen, M., Kazdin, A., Finkelstein, R., & Strauss, C. C. (1987). Comparison of DSM-III separation anxiety and overanxious disorders: Demographic characteristics and patterns of comorbidity. *Journal of the American Academy of Child and Adolescent Psychiatry 26*, 527–531.

Last, C. G., & Perrin, S. (1993). Anxiety disorders in African-American and white children. *Journal of Abnormal Child Psychology, 21*, 153–164.

Laurent, J., Catanzaro, S. J., Joiner, T. E. J., Rudolph, K. D., Potter, K. I., & Lambert, S., et al. (1999). A measure of positive and negative affect for children: Scale development and preliminary validation. *Psychological Assessment, 11*, 326–338.

Lee, S., W., Piersel, W. C., Friedlander, R., & Collamer, W. (1988). Concurrent validity of the Revised Children's Manifest Anxiety Scale (RCMAS) for adolescents. *Educational and Psychological Measurement, 48*, 429–433.

Lerner, J., Safren, S. A., Henin, A., Warman, M., Heimberg, R. G., & Kendall, P. C. (1999). Differentiating anxious and depressive self-statements in youth: Factor structure of the Negative Affect Self-Statement Questionnaire among youth referred to an anxiety disorders clinic. *Journal of Clinical Child Psychology, 28*, 82–93.

Lewinsohn, P. M., Hops, H., Roberts, R. E., Seeley, J. R., & Andrews, J. A. (1993). Adolescent psychopathology: I. Prevalence and incidence of depression and other DSM-III-R disorders in high school students. *Journal of Abnormal Psychology, 102*, 133–144.

Li, H., Cheung, W., & Lopez, V. (2004a). Psychometric evaluation of the Chinese version of the State Anxiety Scale for Children. *Research in Nursing and Health, 27*, 198–207.

Li, H., Cheung, W., & Lopez, V. (2004b). The reliability and validity of the Chinese version of the Trait Anxiety Scale for Children. *Research in Nursing and Health, 27*, 426–434.

Loevinger, J. (1957). Objective tests as instruments of psychological theory. *Psychological Reports, 3*, 635–694.

Lonigan, C. J., Hooe, E. S., David, C. F., & Kistner, J. A. (1999). Positive and negative affectivity in children: Confirmatory factor analysis of a two-factor model and its relation to symptoms of anxiety and depression. *Journal of Consulting and Clinical Psychology*, 67, 374–386.

Lonigan, C. J., & Phillips, B. M. (2001). Temperamental influences on the development of anxiety disorders. In M. W. Vasey & M. R. Dadds (Eds.), *The developmental psychopathology of anxiety* (pp. 60–91). New York: Oxford University Press.

Lyneham, H. J., & Rapee, R. M. (2005). Agreement between telephone and in-person delivery of a structured interview for anxiety disorders in children. *Journal of the American Academy of Child and Adolescent Psychiatry*, 44, 274–282.

Manassis, K. (2001). Child–parent relations: Attachment and anxiety disorders. In W. K. Silverman & P. D. Treffers (Eds.), *Anxiety disorders in children and adolescents: Research, assessment and intervention* (pp. 255–272). New York: Cambridge University Press.

March, J. S., Conners, C., Arnold, G., Epstein, J., Parker, J., & Hinshaw, S., et al. (1999). The Multidimensional Anxiety Scale for Children (MASC): Confirmatory factor analysis in a pediatric ADHD sample. *Journal of Attention Disorders*, 3, 85–89.

March, J. S., Franklin, M. E., Leonard, H. L., & Foa, E. B. (2004). Obsessive–compulsive disorder. In T. L. Morris & J. S. March (Eds.), *Anxiety disorders in children and adolescents* (2nd ed., pp. 212–240). New York: Guilford Press.

March, J. S., Parker, D. A., Sullivan, K., Stallings, P., & Connors, C. K. (1997). The Multidimensional Anxiety Scale for Children (MASC): Factor structure, reliability, and validity. *Journal of the American Academy of Child and Adolescent Psychiatry*, 36, 554–565.

March, J. S., Sullivan, K., & Parker, J. D. (1999). Test–retest reliability of the Multidimensional Anxiety Scale for Children. *Journal of Anxiety Disorders*, 13, 349–358.

Mash, E. J., & Foster, S. L. (2001). Exporting analogue behavioral observation from research to clinical practice: Useful or cost-defective? *Psychological Assessment*, 13, 86–98.

Mash, E. J., & Hunsley, J. (2005). Evidence-based assessment of child and adolescent disorders: Issues and challenges. *Journal of Clinical Child and Adolescent Psychology*, 34, 362–379

Masi, G., Favilla, L., Mucci, M., & Millepiedi, S. (2000). Depressive comorbidity in children and adolescents with generalized anxiety disorder. *Child Psychiatry and Human Development*, 30, 205–215.

Matsumoto, D. (1990). Cultural similarities and differences in display rules. *Motivation and Emotion*, 14, 195–214.

Mattison, R. E., Bagnato, S. J., & Brubaker, B. H. (1988). Diagnostic utility of the Revised Children's Manifest Anxiety Scale in children with DSM-III

anxiety disorders. *Journal of Anxiety Disorders*, 2, 147–155.

McKay, D., Piacentini, J., Greisberg, S., Graae, F., Jaffer, M., & Miller, J. (2005). The structure of childhood obsessions and compulsions: Dimensions in an outpatient sample. *Behaviour Research and Therapy*, 44, 137–146.

McKay, D., Piacentini, J., Greisberg, S., Graae, F., Jaffer, M., & Miller, J., et al. (2003). The children's Yale–Brown Obsessive–Compulsive Scale: Item structure in an outpatient setting. *Psychological Assessment*, 15, 578–581.

Mellon, R., Koliadis, E. A., & Paraskevopoulos, T. D. (2004). Normative development of fears in Greece: Self-reports on the Hellenic Fear Survey Schedule for Children. *Journal of Anxiety Disorders*, 18, 233–254.

Merritt, K. A., Thompson, R. J., Keith, B. R., & Gustafson, K. E. (1995). Screening for child-reported behavioral and emotional problems in primary care pediatrics. *Perceptual and Motor Skills*, 80, 323–329.

Messick, S. (1995). Validity of psychological assessment: Validation of inferences from person's responses and performances as scientific inquiry into score meaning. *American Psychologist*, 50, 741–749.

Meyer, G. J., Finn, S. E., Eyde, L. D., Kay, G. G., Moreland, K. L., Dies, R. R., et al. (2001). Psychological testing and psychological assessment: A review of evidence and issues. *American Psychologist*, 56, 128–165.

Mineka, S., Watson, D. W., & Clark, L. A. (1998). Psychopathology: Comorbidity of anxiety and unipolar mood disorders. *Annual Review of Psychology*, 49, 377–412.

Moreau, D., & Weissman, M. M. (1992). Panic disorder in children and adolescents: A review. *American Journal of Psychiatry*, 149, 1306–1314.

Morris, T. L., & March, J. S. (Eds.). (2004). *Anxiety disorders in children and adolescents* (2nd ed.). New York: Guilford Press.

Morris, T. L., & Masia, C. (1998). Psychometric evaluation of the Social Phobia and Anxiety Inventory for Children: Concurrent validity and normative data. *Journal of Clinical Child Psychology*, 27, 452–458.

Mowrer, O. H. (1960). *Learning theory and behavior.* New York: Wiley.

Muris, P. (2002). An expanded Childhood Anxiety Sensitivity Index: Its factor structure, reliability, and validity in a non-clinical adolescent sample. *Behaviour Research and Therapy*, 40, 299–311.

Muris, P., Gadet, B., Moulaert, V., & Merckelbach, H. (1998). Correlations between two multidimensional anxiety scales for children. *Perceptual and Motor Skills*, 87, 269–270.

Muris, P., Mayer, B., Snieder, N., & Merckelbach, H. (1998). The relationship between anxiety disorder symptoms and negative self-statements in normal children. *Social Behavior and Personality*, 26, 307–316.

Muris, P., & Meesters, C. (2004). Children's somatization symptoms: Correlations with trait anxiety, anxiety sensitivity, and learning experiences. *Psychological Reports, 94,* 1269–1275.

Muris, P., Meesters, C., & Gobel, M. (2001). Reliability, validity, and normative data of the Penn State Worry Questionnaire in 8–12-yr-old children. *Journal of Behavior Therapy and Experimental Psychiatry, 32,* 63–72.

Muris, P., Merckelbach, H., Mayer, B., van Brakel, A., Thissen, S., & Moulaert, V., et al. (1998). The Screen for Child Anxiety Related Emotional Disorders (SCARED) and traditional childhood anxiety measures. *Journal of Behavior Therapy and Experimental Psychiatry, 29,* 327–339.

Muris, P., Merckelbach, H., Moulaert, V., & Gadet, B. (2000). Associations of symptoms of anxiety disorders and self-reported behavior problems in normal children. *Psychological Reports, 86,* 157–162.

Muris, P., Merckelbach, H., Ollendick, T., King, N., & Bogie, N. (2002). Three traditional and three new childhood anxiety questionnaires: Their reliability and validity in a normal adolescent sample. *Behaviour Research and Therapy, 40,* 753–772.

Muris, P., Merckelbach, H., Schmidt, H., & Mayer, B. (1999). The revised version of the Screen for Child Anxiety Related Emotional Disorders (SCARED-R): Factor structure in normal children. *Personality and Individual Differences, 26,* 99–112.

Muris, P., Merckelbach, H., van Brakel, A., & Mayer, B. (1999). The revised version of the Screen for Child Anxiety Related Emotional Disorders (SCARED-R): Further evidence for its reliability and validity. *Anxiety, Stress, and Coping, 12,* 411–425.

Muris, P., Merckelbach, H., van Brakel, A., Mayer, B., & van Dongen, L. (1998). The Screen for Child Anxiety Related Emotional Disorders (SCARED): Relationship with anxiety and depression in normal children. *Personality and Individual Differences, 24,* 451–456.

Muris, P., Merckelbach, H., Wessel, I., & van de Ven, M. (1999). Psychopathological correlates of self-reported behavioural inhibition in normal children. *Behaviour Research and Therapy, 37,* 575–584.

Muris, P., & Ollendick, T. H. (2002). The assessment of contemporary fears in adolescents using a modified version of the Fear Survey Schedule for Children—Revised. *Journal of Anxiety Disorders, 16,* 567–584.

Muris, P., Schmidt, H., Engelbrecht, P., & Perold, M. (2002). DSM-IV-defined anxiety disorder symptoms in South African children. *Journal of the American Academy of Child and Adolescent Psychiatry, 41,* 1360–1368.

Muris, P., Schmidt, H., & Merckelbach, H. (1999). The structure of specific phobia symptoms among children and adolescents. *Behaviour Research and Therapy, 37,* 863–868.

Muris, P., Schmidt, H., & Merckelbach, H. (2000). Correlations among two self-report questionnaires for measuring DSM-defined anxiety disorder symptoms

in children: The Screen for Child Anxiety Related Emotional Disorders and the Spence Children's Anxiety Scale. *Personality and Individual Differences, 28,* 333–346.

Muris, P., & Steerneman, P. (2001). The Revised version of the Screen for Child Anxiety Related Emotional Disorders (SCARED-R): First evidence for its reliability and validity in a clinical sample. *British Journal of Clinical Psychology, 40,* 35–44.

Murphy, D. A., Marelich, W. D., & Hoffman, D. (2000). Assessment of anxiety and depression in young children: Support for two separate constructs. *Journal of Clinical Child Psychology, 29,* 383–391.

Murphy, K. R., & Davidshofer, C. O. (1998). *Psychological testing: Principles and applications* (4th ed.). Upper Saddle River, NJ: Prentice-Hall.

Myers, K., & Winters, N. C. (2002). Ten-year review of rating scales II: Scales for internalizing disorders. *Journal of the American Academy of Child and Adolescent Psychiatry, 41,* 634–659.

Nauta, M. H., Scholing, A., Rapee, R. M., Abbott, M., Spence, S. H., & Waters, A. (2004). A parent-report measure of children's anxiety: Psychometric properties and comparison with child-report in a clinic and normal sample. *Behaviour Research and Therapy, 42,* 813–839.

Nelles, W. B., & Barlow, D. H. (1988). Do children panic? *Clinical Psychology Review, 8,* 359–372.

Nelson, W. M., Finch, A. J., Kendall, P. C., & Gordon, R. H. (1977). Anxiety and locus of conflict in normal children. *Psychological Reports, 41,* 375–378.

Nielsen, T. A., Laberge, L., Paquet, J., Tremblay, R. E., Vitaro, F., & Montplaisir, J. (2000). Development of disturbing dreams during adolescence and their relation to anxiety symptoms. *Sleep, 23,* 727–736.

Olason, D. T., Sighvatsson, M. B., & Smari, J. (2004). Psychometric properties of the Multidimensional Anxiety Scale for Children (MASC) among Icelandic schoolchildren. *Scandinavian Journal of Psychology, 45,* 429–436.

Olivares, J., García-López, L. J., Hidalgo, M. D., Turner, S. M., & Beidel, D. C. (1999). The Social Phobia and Anxiety Inventory: Reliability and validity in an adolescent Spanish population. *Journal of Psychopathology and Behavioral Assessment, 21,* 67–78.

Olivares, J., Ruiz, J., Hidalgo, M. D., Joaquín, L., García-López, L. J., & Rosa, A. I., et al. (2005). Social Anxiety Scale for Adolescents (SAS-A): Psychometric properties in a Spanish-speaking population. *International Journal of Clinical and Health Psychology, 5,* 85–97.

Ollendick, T. H. (1983). Reliability and validity of the Revised Fear Survey Schedule for Children (FSSC-R). *Behaviour Research and Therapy, 21,* 685–692.

Ollendick, T. H., Birmaher, B., & Mattis, S. G. (2004). Panic disorder. In T. L. Morris & J. S March (Eds.), *Anxiety disorders in children and adolescents* (2nd ed., pp. 189–211). New York: Guilford Press.

Ollendick, T. H., King, N. J., & Chorpita, B. F. (2005).

Empirically supported treatments for children and adolescents: The movement to evidence-based practice. In P. C. Kendall (Ed.), *Child and adolescent therapy: Cognitive-behavioral procedures* (3rd ed., pp. 492–520). New York: Guilford Press.

Ollendick, T. H., King, N. J., & Frary, R. B. (1989). Fears in children and adolescents: Reliability and generalizability across gender, age, and nationality. *Behaviour Research and Therapy, 27*, 19–26.

Ollendick, T. H., King, N. J., & Muris, P. (2002). Fears and phobias in children: Phenomenology, epidemiology and aetiology. *Child and Adolescent Mental Health, 7*, 98–106.

Ollendick, T. H., Mattis, S. G., & King, N. J. (1994). Panic in children and adolescents: A review. *Journal of Child Psychology and Psychiatry, 35*, 113–134.

Paget, K. D., & Reynolds, C. R. (1984). Dimensions, levels and reliabilities on the Revised Children's Manifest Anxiety Scale with learning disabled children. *Journal of Learning Disabilities, 17*, 137–141.

Pajer, K., Gardner, W., Rubin, R. T., Perel, J., & Neal, S. (2001). Decreased cortisol levels in adolescent girls with conduct disorder. *Archives of General Psychiatry 58*, 297–302.

Papay, J. P., & Hedl, J. J. (1978). Psychometric characteristics and norms for disadvantaged third and fourth grade children on the State–Trait Anxiety Inventory for Children. *Journal of Abnormal Child Psychology, 6*, 115–120.

Papay, J. P., & Spielberger, C. D. (1986). Assessment of anxiety and achievement in kindergarten and first- and second-grade children. *Journal of Abnormal Child Psychology, 14*, 279–286.

Peng, Y., & Reggia, J. A. (1989). A connectionist model for diagnostic problem solving. *IEEE Transactions on Systems, Man, and Cybernetics, 19*, 285–298.

Perez, R. G., Ascaso, L. E., Massons, J. M. D., & de la Osa Chaparro, N. (1998). Characteristics of the subject and interview influencing the test-retest reliability of the Diagnostic Interview for Children and Adolescents—Revised. *Journal of Child Psychology and Psychiatry, 39*, 963–972.

Perrin, S., & Last, C. G. (1992). Do childhood anxiety measures measure anxiety? *Journal of Abnormal Child Psychology, 20*, 567–578.

Persons, J. B. (1989). *Cognitive therapy in practice: A case formulation approach.* New York: Norton.

Piacentini, J., & Langley, A. K. (2004). Cognitive-behavioral therapy for children who have obsessive–compulsive disorder. *Journal of Clinical Psychology, 60*, 1181–1194.

Pine, D. S., Cohen, P., Gurley, D., Brook, J., & Ma, Y. (1998). The risk for early-adulthood anxiety and depressive disorders in adolescents with anxiety and depressive disorders. *Archives of General Psychiatry, 55*, 56–64.

Psychountaki, M., Zervas, Y., Karteroliotis, K., & Spielberger, C. (2003). Reliability and validity of the Greek version of the STAIC. *European Journal of Psychological Assessment, 19*, 124–130.

Rabian, B., Embry, L., & MacIntyre, D. (1999). Behavioral validation of the Childhood Anxiety Sensitivity Index in children. *Journal of Clinical Child Psychology, 28*, 105–112.

Rabian, B., Peterson, R. A., Richters, J., & Jensen, P. S. (1993). Anxiety sensitivity among anxious children. *Journal of Clinical Child Psychology, 22*, 441–446.

Rachman, S. (1977). The conditioning theory of fear-acquisition: A critical examination. *Behaviour Research and Therapy, 15*, 375–387.

Rapee, R. M., Barrett, P. M., Dadds, M. R., & Evans, L. (1994). Reliability of the DSM-III—R childhood anxiety disorders using structured interview: Interrater and parent–child agreement. *Journal of the American Academy of Child and Adolescent Psychiatry, 33*, 984–992.

Reise, S. P., Ainsworth, A. T., & Haviland, M. G. (2005). Item response theory: Fundamentals, applications, and promise in psychological research. *Current Directions in Psychological Science, 14*, 95–101.

Reynolds, C. R. (1980). Concurrent validity of What I Think and Feel: The Revised Children's Manifest Anxiety Scale. *Journal of Consulting and Clinical Psychology, 48*, 774–775.

Reynolds, C. R. (1981). Long-term stability of scores on the Revised Children's Manifest Anxiety Scale. *Perceptual and Motor Skills, 53*, 702.

Reynolds, C. R. (1985). Multitrait validation of the Revised Children's Manifest Anxiety Scale for children of high intelligence. *Psychological Reports, 56*, 402.

Reynolds, C. R., & Paget, K. D. (1981). Factor analysis of the Revised Children's Manifest Anxiety Scale for blacks, whites, males, and females with a national normative sample. *Journal of Consulting and Clinical Psychology, 49*, 352–359.

Reynolds, C. R., & Richmond, B. O. (1978). What I Think and Feel: A revised measure of children's manifest anxiety. *Journal of Abnormal Child Psychology, 6*, 271–280.

Reynolds, C. R., & Richmond, B. O. (1979). Factor structure and construct validity of "What I Think and Feel": The Revised Children's Manifest Anxiety Scale. *Journal of Personality Assessment, 43*, 281–283.

Ribera, J., Canino, G., Rubio-Stipec, M., Bravo, M., Bauermeister, J. J., Alegria, M., et al. (1996). The Diagnostic Interview Schedule for Children (DISC-2.1) in Spanish: Reliability in a Hispanic population. *Journal of Child Psychology and Psychiatry, 37*, 195–204.

Richmond, B. O., Rodrigo, G., & de Rodrigo, M. (1988). Factor structure of a Spanish version of the Revised Children's Manifest Anxiety Scale in Uruguay. *Journal of Personality Assessment, 52*, 165–170.

Roberts, R. E., Solovitz, B. L., Chen, Y., & Casat, C. (1996). Retest stability of DSM-III-R diagnoses among adolescents using the Diagnostic Interview Schedule for Children (DISC-2.1C). *Journal of Abnormal Child Psychology, 24*, 349–362.

Ronan, K. R., Kendall, P. C., & Rowe, M. (1994). Negative affectivity in children: Development and validation of a self-statement questionnaire. *Cognitive Therapy and Research*, 18, 509–528.

Russo, M. F., & Beidel, D. C. (1994). Comorbidity of childhood anxiety and externalizing disorders: Prevalence, associated characteristics, and validation issues. *Clinical Psychology Review*, 14, 199–221.

Ryngala, D. J., Shields, A. L., & Caruso, J. C. (2005). Reliability generalization of the Revised Children's Manifest Anxiety Scale. *Educational and Psychological Measurement*, 65, 259–271.

Rynn, M. A., Barber, J. P., Khalid-Khan, S., Siqueland, L., Dembiski, M., McCarthy K. S., et al. (2006). The psychometric properties of the MASC in a pediatric psychiatric sample. *Journal of Anxiety Disorders*, 200, 139–157.

Safren, S. A., Heimberg, R. G., Lerner, J., Henin, A., Warman, M., & Kendall, P. C. (2000). Differentiating anxious and depressive self-statements: Combined factor structure of the Anxious Self-Statements Questionnaire and the Automatic Thoughts Questionnaire—Revised. *Cognitive Therapy and Research*, 24, 327–344.

Sanchez, L. M., & Turner, S. M. (2003). Practicing psychology in the era of managed care: Implications for practice and training. *American Psychologist*, 58, 116–129.

Sarphare, G., & Aman, M. G. (1996). Parent- and self-ratings of anxiety in children with mental retardation: Agreement levels and test–retest reliability. *Research in Developmental Disabilities*, 17, 27–39.

Scahill, L., Riddle, M. A., & McSwiggin-Hardin, M. (1997). Children's Yale–Brown Obsessive Compulsive Scale: Reliability and validity. *Journal of the American Academy of Child and Adolescent Psychiatry* 36, 844–852.

Schisler, T., Lander, J., & Fowler-Kerry, S. (1998). Assessing children's state anxiety. *Journal of Pain and Symptom Management*, 16, 80–87.

Schmidt, F. L., Le, H., & Ilies, R. (2003). Beyond alpha: An empirical examination of the effects of different sources of measurement error on reliability estimates for measures of individual differences constructs. *Psychological Methods*, 8, 206–224.

Schniering, C. A., Hudson, J. L., & Rapee, R. M. (2000). Issues in the diagnosis and assessment of anxiety disorders in children and adolescents. *Clinical Psychology Review* 20, 453–478.

Schwab-Stone, M. E., Shaffer, D., Dulcan, M. K., & Jensen, P. S. (1996). Criterion validity of the NIMH Diagnostic Interview Schedule for Children Version 2.3 (DISC-2.3). *Journal of the American Academy of Child and Adolescent Psychiatry*, 35, 878–888.

Shaffer, D., Fisher, P., Dulcan, M. K., & Davies, M. (1996). The NIMH Diagnostic Interview Schedule for Children Version 2.3 (DISC-2.3): Description, acceptability, prevalence rates, and performance in the MECA study. *Journal of the American Academy of Child and Adolescent Psychiatry*, 35, 865–877.

Shaffer, D., Lucas, C. P., & Richters, J. E. (Eds.). (1999). *Diagnostic assessment in child and adolescent psychopathology*. New York: Guilford Press.

Shore, G. N., & Rapport, M. D. (1998). The Fear Survey Schedule for Children—Revised (FSSC-HI): Ethnocultural variations in children's fearfulness. *Journal of Anxiety Disorders*, 12, 437–461.

Silverman, W. K., & Albano, A. M. (1996). *The Anxiety Disorders Interview Schedule for DSM-IV—Child and Parent Versions*. San Antonio, TX: Graywind.

Silverman, W. K., & Dick-Niederhauser, A. (2004). Separation anxiety disorder. In T. L. Morris & J. S. March (Eds.), *Anxiety disorders in children and adolescents* (2nd ed., pp. 164–188). New York: Guilford Press.

Silverman, W. K., & Eisen, A. R. (1992). Age differences in the reliability of parent and child reports of child anxious symptomatology using a structured interview. *Journal of the American Academy of Child and Adolescent Psychiatry*, 31, 117–124.

Silverman, W. K., Fleisig, W., Rabian, B., & Peterson, R. A. (1991). Child Anxiety Sensitivity Index. *Journal of Clinical Child Psychology*, 20, 162–168.

Silverman, W. K., & Ginsburg, G. S. (1998). Anxiety disorders. In T. H. Ollendick & M. Hersen (Eds.), *Handbook of child psychopathology* (3rd ed., pp. 239–268). New York: Plenum Press.

Silverman, W. K., Kurtines, W. M., Ginsburg, G. S., Weems, C. F., Lumpkin, P. W., & Carmichael, D. H. (1999). Treating anxiety disorders in children with group cognitive-behavioral therapy: A randomized clinical trial. *Journal of Consulting and Clinical Psychology*, 67(6), 995–1003.

Silverman, W. K., & Nelles, W. B. (1988). The Anxiety Disorders Interview Schedule for Children. *Journal of the American Academy of Child and Adolescent Psychiatry*, 27, 772–778.

Silverman, W. K., & Ollendick, T. H. (2005). Evidence-based assessment of anxiety and its disorders in children and adolescents. *Journal of Clinical Child and Adolescent Psychology*, 34, 380–411.

Silverman, W. K., & Rabian, B. (1995). Test–retest reliability of the DSM-III-R childhood anxiety disorders symptoms using the Anxiety Disorders Interview Schedule for Children. *Journal of Anxiety Disorders*, 9, 139–150.

Silverman, W. K., Saavedra, L. M., & Pina, A. A. (2001). Test–retest reliability of anxiety symptoms and diagnoses with anxiety disorders interview schedule for DSM-IV: Child and parent versions. *Journal of the American Academy of Child and Adolescent Psychiatry* 40, 937–944.

Southam-Gerow, M. A., Chorpita, B. F., Miller, L. M., & Taylor, A. (2007). *Are children with anxiety disorders self-referred to a university clinic like those from the public mental health system?* Manuscript under review.

Southam-Gerow, M. A., Flannery-Schroeder, E. C., &

Kendall, P. C. (2003). A psychometric evaluation of the parent report form the State–Trait Anxiety Inventory for Children—Trait Version. *Journal of Anxiety Disorders, 17,* 427–446.

Southam-Gerow, M. A., Weisz, J. R., & Kendall, P. C. (2003). Youth with anxiety disorders in research and service clinics: Examining client differences and similarities. *Journal of Clinical Child and Adolescent Psychology, 32,* 375–385.

Spence, S. H. (1997). Structure of anxiety symptoms among children: A confirmatory factor-analytic study. *Journal of Abnormal Psychology, 106,* 280–297.

Spence, S. H. (1998). A measure of anxiety symptoms among children. *Behaviour Research and Therapy, 36,* 545–566.

Spence, S. H., Barrett, P. M., & Turner, C. M. (2003). Psychometric properties of the Spence Children's Anxiety Scale with young adolescents. *Journal of Anxiety Disorders, 17,* 605–625.

Spence, S. H., Donovan, C., & Brechman-Toussaint, M. (1999). Social skills, social outcomes, and cognitive features of childhood social phobia. *Journal of Abnormal Psychology, 108,* 211–221.

Spielberger, C. D. (1973). *Preliminary test manual for the State–Trait Anxiety Inventory for Children.* Palo Alto, CA: Consulting Psychologists Press.

Sroufe, L. A. (1990). Considering the normal and abnormal together: The essence of developmental psychopathology. *Development and Psychopathology, 2,* 335–347.

Stallings, P., & March, J. S. (1995). Assessment. In J. S. March (Ed.), *Anxiety disorders in children and adolescents* (pp. 125–147). New York: Guilford Press.

Stark, K. D., & Laurent, J. (2001). Joint factor analysis of the Children's Depression Inventory and the Revised Children's Manifest Anxiety Scale. *Journal of Clinical Child Psychology, 30,* 552–567.

Steele, R. G., Phipps, S., & Srivastava, D. K. (1999). Low-end specificity of childhood measures of emotional distress: Consistent effects for anxiety and depressive symptoms in a nonclinical population. *Journal of Personality Assessment, 73,* 276–289.

Storch, E. A., Eisenberg, P. S., Roberti, J. W., & Barlas, M. E. (2003). Reliability and validity of the Social Anxiety Scale for Children—Revised for Hispanic children. *Hispanic Journal of Behavioral Sciences, 25,* 410–422.

Storch, E. A., Masia-Warner, C., Dent, H. C., Roberti, J. W., & Fisher, P. H. (2004). Psychometric evaluation of the Social Anxiety Scale for Adolescents and the Social Phobia and Anxiety Inventory for Children: Construct validity and normative data. *Journal of Anxiety Disorders, 18,* 665–679.

Storch, E. A., Murphy, T. K., Geffken, G. R., Bagner, D. M., Soto, O., & Sajid, M., et al. (2005). Factor analytic study of the Children's Yale–Brown Obsessive–Compulsive Scale. *Journal of Clinical Child and Adolescent Psychology, 34,* 312–319.

Storch, E. A., Murphy, T. K., Geffken, G. R., Soto, O., Sajid, M., Allen, P., et al. (2004). Psychometric evaluation of the Children's Yale–Brown Obsessive–Compulsive Scale. *Psychiatry Research, 129,* 91–98.

Strauss, C. C., Lease, C. A., Last, C. G., & Francis, G. (1988). Overanxious disorder: An examination of developmental differences. *Journal of Abnormal Child Psychology, 16,* 433–443.

Streiner, D. L., & Norman, G. R. (2003). *Health measurement scales: A practical guide to their development and use* (3rd ed.). New York: Oxford University Press.

Sylvester, C. E., Hyde, T. S., & Reichler, R. J. (1987). The Diagnostic Interview for Children and Personality Inventory for Children in studies of children at risk for anxiety disorders or depression. *Journal of the American Academy of Child and Adolescent Psychiatry, 26,* 668–675.

Tannenbaum, L. E., Forehand, R., & Thomas, A. M. (1992). Adolescent self-reported anxiety and depression: Separate constructs or a single entity. *Child Study Journal, 22,* 61–72.

Thayer, J. F., & Lane, R. D. (2000). A model of neurovisceral integration in emotion regulation and dysregulation. *Journal of Affective Disorders 61,* 201–216.

Tracey, S. A., Chorpita, B. F., Douban, J., & Barlow, D. H. (1997). Empirical evaluation of DSM-IV generalized anxiety disorder criteria for children and adolescents. *Journal of Clinical Child Psychology, 26,* 404–414.

Turgeon, L., & Chartrand, É. (2003). Psychometric properties of the French Canadian version of the State–Trait Anxiety Inventory for Children. *Educational and Psychological Measurement, 63,* 174–185.

Turgeon, L., & Chartrand, É. (2003). Reliability and validity of the Revised Children's Manifest Anxiety Scale in a French-Canadian sample. *Psychological Assessment, 15,* 378–383.

Tyron, W. W. (1998). The inscrutable null hypothesis. *American Psychologist, 53,* 796.

U.S. Public Health Service. (2000). *Report of the Surgeon General's Conference on Children's Mental Health: A national action agenda.* Washington, DC: Department of Health and Human Services.

Valez, C. N., Johnson, J., & Cohen, P. (1989). A longitudinal analysis of selected risk factors for childhood psychopathology. *Journal of the American Academy of Child and Adolescent Psychiatry, 28,* 861–864.

Valla, J., Bergeron, L., & Smolla, N. (2000). The Dominic-R: A pictorial interview for 6- to 11-year-old children. *Journal of the American Academy of Child and Adolescent Psychiatry, 39,* 85–93.

van Goozen, S. H., Matthys, W., Cohen-Kettenis, P. T., Thijssen, J. H., & van Engeland, H. (1998). Adrenal androgens and aggression in conduct disorder prepubertal boys and normal controls. *Biological Psychiatry 43,* 156–158.

Van Hasselt, V. B., Hersen, M., Bellack, A. S.,

Rosenblum, N., & Lamparski, D. (1979). Tripartite assessment of the effects of systematic desensitization in a multiphobic child: An experimental analysis. *Journal of Behavior Therapy and Experimental Psychiatry, 10,* 51–56.

van Widenfelt, B. M., Siebelink, B. M., Goedhart, A. W., & Treffers, P. D. A. (2002). The Dutch Childhood Anxiety Sensitivity Index: Psychometric properties and factor structure. *Journal of Clinical Child and Adolescent Psychology, 31,* 90–100.

Vasey, M. W. (1993). Development and cognition in childhood anxiety: The example of worry. *Advances in Clinical Child Psychology, 15,* 1–39.

Vasey, M. W., & Dadds, M. R. (2001). *The developmental psychopathology of anxiety.* London: Oxford University Press.

Vasey, M. W., Daleiden, E. L., Williams, L. L., & Brown, L. M. (1995). Biased attention I childhood anxiety disorders: A preliminary study. *Journal of Abnormal Child Psychology, 23,* 267–279.

Velting, O. N., & Albano, A. M. (2001). Current trends in the understanding and treatment of social phobia in youth. *Journal of Child Psychology and Psychiatry and Allied Disciplines, 42,* 127–140.

Verhulst, F. C., van der Ende, J., Ferdinand, R. F., & Kasius, M. C. (1997). The prevalence of DSM-III-R diagnoses in a national sample of Dutch adolescents. *Archives of General Psychiatry, 54,* 329–336.

Walsh, T. M., Stewart, S. H., McLaughlin, E., & Comeau, N. (2004). Gender differences in Childhood Anxiety Sensitivity Index (CASI) dimensions. *Journal of Anxiety Disorders, 18,* 695–706.

Warren, S. L., Huston, L., & Egeland, B. (1997). Child and adolescent anxiety disorders and early attachment. *Journal of the American Academy of Child and Adolescent Psychiatry, 36,* 637–644.

Weems, C. F., Hammond-Laurence, K., Silverman, W. K., & Ginsburg, G. S. (1998). Testing the utility of the anxiety sensitivity construct in children and adolescents referred for anxiety disorders. *Journal of Clinical Child Psychology, 27,* 69–77.

Weems, C. F., Silverman, W. K., Saavedra, L. M., Pina, A. A., & Lumpkin, P. W. (1999). The discrimination of children's phobias using the Revised Fear Survey Schedule for Children. *Journal of Child Psychology and Psychiatry and Allied Disciplines, 40,* 941–952.

Weisz, J. R., Southam-Gerow, M. A., Gordis, E. B., & Connor-Smith, J. K. (2003). Primary and secondary control enhancement training for youth depression: Applying the Deployment-Focused Model of treatment development and testing. In A. E. Kazdin & J. R. Weisz (Eds.), *Evidence-based treatments for children and adolescents* (pp. 165–183). New York: Guilford Press.

Welner, Z., Reich, W., Herjanic, B., Jung, K. G., & Amado, H. (1987). Reliability, validity, and parent–child agreement studies of the Diagnostic Interview for Children and Adolescents (DICA). *Journal of the American Academy of Child and Adolescent Psychiatry, 26,* 649–653.

Wewetzer, C., Jans, T., Muller, B., Neudorfl, A., Bucherl, U., Remschmidt, H., et al. (2001). Long-term outcome and prognosis of obsessive-compulsive disorder with onset in childhood or adolescence. *European Child and Adolescent Psychiatry, 10,* 37–46.

Wilhelm, F. H., & Roth, W. T. (2001). The somatic symptom paradox in DSM-IV anxiety disorders: Suggestions for a clinical focus in psychophysiology. *Biological Psychology, 57,* 105–140.

Wilson, D. J., Chibaiwa, D., Majoni, C., Masukume, C., & Nkoma, E. (1990). Reliability and factorial validity of the Revised Children's Manifest Anxiety Scale in Zimbabwe. *Personality and Individual Differences, 11,* 365–369.

Wolfe, V. V., Finch, A. J., Saylor, C. F., & Blount, R. L. (1987). Negative affectivity in children: A multitrait-multimethod investigation. *Journal of Consulting and Clinical Psychology, 55,* 245–250.

Yonkers, K., & Gurguis, G. (1995). Gender differences in the prevalence and expression of anxiety disorders. In M. V. Seeman (Ed.), *Gender and psychopathology* (pp. 113–130). Washington, DC: American Psychiatric Association.

Zinbarg, R. E., & Barlow, D. H. (1996). Structure of anxiety and the anxiety disorders: A hierarchical model. *Journal of Abnormal Psychology, 105,* 181–193.

Zinbarg, R. E., Revelle, W., Yovel, I., & Li, W. (2005). Cronbach's alpha, Revelle's beta, and McDonald's omega$_H$: Their relations with each other and two alternative conceptualizations of reliability. *Psychometrika, 70,* 123–133.

Zoccolillo, M. (1992). Co-occurrence of conduct disorder and its adult outcomes with depressive and anxiety disorders: A review. *Journal of the American Academy of Child and Adolescent Psychiatry, 31,* 547–556.

CHAPTER 9

Posttraumatic Stress Disorder

Kenneth E. Fletcher

The evaluation of posttraumatic stress reactions in children, adolescents, and young adults is not as straightforward a process as it might first appear. Whereas the assessment process shares similar challenges with any assessment of behavioral and emotional problems in children, it faces additional challenges of its own, some of which may not be readily apparent to clinicians who are less familiar with the research on childhood posttraumatic stress disorder (PTSD). PTSD, for example, is one of the few mental disorders that requires exposure to a high-magnitude stressor that has the potential for producing traumatic reactions. Some of the challenges clinicians face in this regard are to establish whether the child under consideration was exposed to a stressor, whether that stressor qualifies as a potentially traumatic stressor, whether the child experienced it as such, and finally whether the child's behaviors that appear to be symptomatic of PTSD actually began as a consequence of exposure to the stressor under consideration. The first section of this chapter describes these and other factors that need to be taken into account in the process of evaluating traumatic responses. The second section suggests which of the currently available assessment tools might allow the clinician to evaluate children for PTSD most effectively.

The need to assess the possible presence of traumatic reactions in an infant, child, adolescent, or young adult may arise in a variety of circumstances. An informed caregiver or other adult in the child's life may be concerned for the child after a particularly difficult crisis disrupts the child's life. This is most likely to happen after a major disaster that affects entire communities, such as hurricanes or tsunamis often do, or the disaster may have more personal repercussions for the child, such as the loss of a home to fire. Increasingly, children are being referred for assessment after they are discovered in homes embroiled in domestic violence. Victims of physical or sexual abuse (see Crooks & Wolfe, Chapter 14, and Wolfe, Chapter 15, this volume), and sometimes of emotional abuse or neglect, are likely to be referred for evaluation as well.

At other times, children may be referred for reasons seemingly unrelated to posttraumatic stress, but someone, perhaps even the clinician, recognizes the need to examine them for possible posttraumatic reactions, if only for purposes of differential diagnosis. Children's traumatic reactions are frequently not recognized as such, in part, due to adults in their lives minimizing the possibility of traumatic reactions in their children. It may also be due to lack of recognition of the potential stress an event might pose for the child. In other instances, adults in the child's life may simply be unaware of the kinds of stressful experiences to which a child is exposed. Some children, for example, live with daily bullying on the way to school and again on the way home, but never reveal these experiences to an adult. On the other hand, a conspiracy of silence may surround a child who is the victim of maltreatment.

In this sense, posttraumatic stress can be a silent referral. Therefore, clinicians need to be particularly alert to the possibility that a good many symptomatic behaviors that at first suggest other problems may actually be symptoms of reactions to traumatic experiences. Referrals for problems related to apparent hyperactivity, aggressiveness, social withdrawal, depression, anxiety, separation anxiety, dissociative experiences, substance abuse, runaway behavior, excessive risk-taking behavior, and sexual acting out all may provide clues to the possible presence of traumatic reactions in infants, children, adolescents, and young adults. In addition, many difficult or inexplicable physical complaints, such as gastrointestinal problems, chronic pain of any kind, or fibromyalgia, among others, also may point to traumatic experiences.

The likelihood that children referred for reasons other than trauma reactions have been exposed to one or more potentially traumatic events is surprisingly high. In one large, longitudinal study (Costello, Erkanli, Fairbank, & Angold, 2002), one in every four children reported experiencing at least one event of high-magnitude stress by the time he or she reached the age of 16. High-magnitude stressor events in this study encompassed the extreme stressors referred to in the fourth edition of the *Diagnostic and Statistical Manual of Mental Disorders* (DSM-IV; American Psychiatric Association [APA], 1994), including serious accidents, serious illnesses, natural disasters, fires, war, terrorism, violence within or outside the family, sexual abuse, rape, coercion, death of a loved one, witnessing such an event, or learning about such an event, among others. Of the children who had been exposed to high-magnitude stressors in this study, 18% reported exposure to two such events, and 10% reported experiencing three or more. Moreover, 6% of all of the children in the study reported exposure to a high-magnitude stressor within the past 3 months.

With these results in mind, clinicians might do well to consider first taking a history of any possible high-magnitude stressors children have experienced over their lifetime, then inquiring about current stressors in children's lives on a regular basis thereafter, regardless of the reasons for the child's referral. This is not to say that clinicians should screen all children for PTSD. However, taking a history of lifetime and current stressors in each child's life might prove informative in several ways. Most obviously, it would assist in identifying circumstances in the child's life that might warrant further assessment for possible traumatic reactions to those circumstances. Cohen and colleagues (1998) pointed out that "routine screening for exposure to domestic or community violence, child abuse, and other common stressors is essential in making [the] determination" (p. 9S) that symptoms of avoidance, numbing, and overarousal were not present prior to exposure to the high-magnitude stressor for which a child is being assessed. Less obviously perhaps, routine screening for exposure to high-magnitude stressors may provide information about life experiences that might be relevant for other problems in the child's life. In fact, given the association between chronic traumatization and major somatic complaints (as described later in this chapter in the discussion of complex PTSD), family physicians and pediatricians would be well advised to screen for such occurrences among their infant, child, adolescent, and young adult patients on a regular basis as well.

THE FULL SPECTRUM OF POSTTRAUMATIC STRESS RESPONSES

Anyone, from infant to older adult, regardless of age, can react adversely when high-magnitude stressors intrude on his or her life (Fletcher, 2003). Reactions to extreme adversity need not necessarily develop into PTSD, however. Other possible reactions include grief, depression, anxiety, fear, and dissociative states, among others. This chapter is concerned with those reactions to high-magnitude stressors that form the cluster of symptoms associated with PTSD.

High-magnitude stressors play an important role in the diagnosis of PTSD. Prior to DSM-IV, PTSD was the only DSM disorder that for diagnosis required exposure to a high-magnitude stressor. A second disorder that depends on such exposure, acute stress disorder (ASD), was added in DSM-IV. The etiology and symptomatology of PTSD and ASD and are closely related, to the point that they may represent different points on a spectrum of posttraumatic stress reactions. If, as its name suggests, ASD can be considered to represent *acute* reactions to high-magnitude stressors, it has been proposed that many of the symptoms listed in DSM-IV as "associated or descriptive features" of PTSD might represent the other end of the spectrum of *chronic* reactions. In fact, these so-called "associated" symptoms were derived from a proposed syndrome for DSM-IV that has been referred to by various names, such as disorders of extreme stress not otherwise specified (DES NOS) or, more recently, complex PTSD (Kilpatrick et al., 1998). Evidence is accumulating that the proposed syndrome complex PTSD provides a reliable and valid clustering of symptoms that should be considered in particular circumstances (van der Kolk, Roth, Pelcovitz, Sunday, & Spinazzola, 2005), which I describe briefly later in the chapter. Moreover, there is evidence that treating the distinctive symptoms of complex PTSD as "associated" or comorbid conditions rather than as an integral part of the posttraumatic response leads to markedly reduced response to treatment (van der Kolk & Courtois, 2005; van der Kolk et al., 2005). All three of these "syndromes"—ASD, PTSD, and complex PTSD—share several characteristics, as I describe later in the chapter. All three syndromes can be distinguished from adjustment disorder based on the criterion that they all represent traumatic reactions to high-magnitude stressors. In fact, DSM-IV specifies that a diagnosis of adjustment disorder should be made when nonextreme stressors are involved, such as moving to a new neighborhood, starting a new school, or the birth of a sibling. This chapter is concerned only with those disorders that develop as a reaction to high-magnitude stressors, including the two DSM-IV disorders, ASD and PTSD, as well as the proposed disorder currently not recognized by DSM-IV, complex PTSD. For the sake of simplicity, complex PTSD is referred to as a syndrome or disorder in the rest of this chapter, despite its lack of recognition in DSM-IV.

The view I take in this chapter is that these three syndromes represent a continuum of posttraumatic stress responses. Someone who has experienced a catastrophic event can only be classified as reacting with symptoms of ASD within 1 month of the event. A victim of traumatic events cannot be classified as having PTSD, until more than 1 month has passed since the traumatic event. Symptoms that typify complex PTSD tend to appear after exposure to the most extreme kinds of interpersonal trauma, such as sexual, physical, or emotional maltreatment, or after being held captive and tortured. Moreover, these traumatic events tend to be of extended duration and/or to be repetitive in nature, and the responses tend to be of longer duration and more likely to effect substantial changes in the victim's personality.

Etiology of Posttraumatic Stress Responses

The majority (approximately two-thirds according to one meta-analysis; Fletcher, 2003) of children exposed to high-magnitude stressors do *not* develop enough posttraumatic stress symptoms to qualify for a diagnosis of PTSD. The etiology of posttraumatic stress response syndromes such as ASD, PTSD, and complex PTSD appears to depend on a complex interaction of characteristics of the event itself (e.g., its nature, cause, severity, duration, and the child's exposure to or dosage of particularly distressing aspects of the event); the child's cognitive, emotional, psychobiological, and behavioral responses to the event; personal characteristics of the child (including biological vulnerabilities, previous exposure to and reaction to other stressors, developmental stage, age, gender, ethnicity, coping skills, etc.); and characteristics of the social environment (e.g., socioeconomic status, support received from the family and community, the caregivers' own responses to the child's experiences, etc.). Several models have been suggested to depict the possible interactions of all of these influences on the child's ultimate reaction to potentially traumatic events (Fletcher, 2003; Green, Wilson, & Lindy, 1985; La Greca, Silverman, Vernberg, & Prinstein, 1996; Ursano, Fullerton, & McCaughey, 1994). Detailed consideration is given later in the chapter to many of these issues, such as the importance of the characteristics of the stressor, age and developmental stage, gender and ethnic differences, and important beliefs affected by traumatic experience. There is not space to give full coverage to the other factors mentioned here. However, clinicians should always keep in mind the multiple possible pathways to dysfunctional responses to high-magnitude stressors, so the potential influence of the remaining factors is touched upon here. For a more detailed discussion of all of these factors, the reader is referred to Fletcher (2003).

Emotional Reactions

DSM-IV criterion A2 (see Table 9.1) requires an emotional reaction of horror, fear, or helplessness to the high-magnitude stressor, which may also be expressed as disorganized or agitated behavior in young children. Research gives substance to this requirement. Children who lived through Hurricane Hugo and reported feelings of sadness, worry, fear, loneliness, or anger during the hurricane were more likely to respond with symptoms of PTSD afterwards (Shannon, Lonigan, Finch, & Taylor, 1994). Their emotional responses were more strongly associated with symptomatology than with the amount of hurricane damage to their households. Other studies have also indicated that the more fear children experience during a high-magnitude stressor (their emotional peritraumatic response), the more likely they are to develop symptoms of PTSD in the aftermath, whether they are very young children (e.g., ages 4–9) (Rossman, Bingham, & Emde, 1997), adolescents (Udwin, Boyle, Yule, Bolton, & O'Ryan, 2000), or young adults in college (Bernat, Ronfeldt, Calhoun, & Arias, 1998). Clearly, assessing the child's emotional reactions during the course of the stressor can provide important information about the likely course of his or her reactions once the experience concludes.

Appraisals and Attributions

APPRAISALS

Cognitive appraisals are evaluations that people make concerning the importance and meaning of events in terms of their own personal health and safety (Lazarus & Folkman, 1984). Peterson and Seligman (1983) attempted to apply their theory of learned helplessness to traumatic experience, suggesting that an aversive situation must be appraised as inescapable and unpredictable, if a sense of helplessness is to be felt. Foa, Steketee, and Rothbaum (1989) proposed that exposure to high-magnitude stressors can cause "fear structures" to develop. These "programs for escape or avoidance behavior" (p. 166) include at least three kinds of information: characteristics of the stressful situation, personal interpretations of the meaning of the situation, and procedures for responding to the threat of the situation.

ATTRIBUTIONS

When people attempt to make sense of their unpredictable, uncontrollable, aversive experiences, they tend to attribute them to either internal or external causes, to stable or unstable conditions over time, and to specific or more global conditions (Abramson, Seligman, & Teasdale, 1978). Self-blame or guilt has been found to be associated with children's posttraumatic stress symptomatology (Realmuto et al., 1992; Udwin et al., 2000). A "foreshortened" or pessimistic view of the future, in which survivors of high-magnitude stressors do not believe they will live a long and productive life, is an example of an attribution of stable (prolonged) insecurity and lack of safety into the future. Global attributions of causality ("all adults are untrustworthy" vs. "just the adult who abused is untrustworthy") have been found to be associated with abuse among children (Wolfe, Gentile, Michienzi, Sas, & Wolfe, 1991).

Neurobiological Changes Due to Stressful Experiences

Physiological arousal among individuals with PTSD can manifest as increased heart rate, respiration rate, and skin conductivity (Jones & Barlow, 1990). Evidence is accumulating that exposure to high-magnitude stressors can lead to changes in brain structure and functioning, particularly in the hypothalmic–pituitary–adrenal (HPA) axis, a part of the neuroendocrine system that controls reactions to stress (Bremner, Southwick, & Charney, 1999; Golier & Yehuda, 1998). When exposed to a stressor, neurons in the hypothalamus release a chemical called CRF (corticotrophin-releasing factor), which in turn causes the pituitary gland to release another chemical, ACTH (adrenocorticotropic hormone), which then stimulates the adrenal cortex to release cortisol, a chemical that influences the body's response to stress (e.g., it causes the heart to beat faster) (Graham, Heim, Goodman, Miller, & Nemeroff, 1999). Early exposure to chronic abuse and neglect activates the HPA axis, which, because the infant's neural circuitries are still developing, may lead to permanent changes in the HPA axis and re-

TABLE 9.1. DSM-IV-TR Diagnostic Criteria for Posttraumatic Stress Disorder

A. The person has been exposed to a traumatic event in which both of the following were present:

   (1) the person experienced, witnessed, or was confronted with an event or events that involved actual or threatened death or serious injury, or a threat to the physical integrity of self or others

   (2) the person's response involved intense fear, helplessness, or horror. Note: In children, this may be expressed instead by disorganized or agitated behavior.

B. The traumatic event is persistently reexperienced in one (or more) of the following ways:

   (1) recurrent and intrusive distressing recollections of the event, including images, thoughts, or perceptions. Note: In young children, repetitive play may occur in which themes or aspects of the trauma are expressed.

   (2) recurrent distressing dreams of the event. Note: In children, there may be frightening dreams without recognizable content.

   (3) acting or feeling as if the traumatic event were recurring (includes a sense of reliving the experience, illusions, hallucinations, and dissociative flashback episodes, including those that occur on awakening or when intoxicated). Note: In young children, trauma-specific reenactment may occur.

   (4) intense psychological distress at exposure to internal or external cues that symbolize or resemble an aspect of the traumatic event

   (5) physiological reactivity on exposure to internal or external cues that symbolize or resemble an aspect of the traumatic event.

C. Persistent avoidance of stimuli associated with the trauma and numbing of general responsiveness (not present before the trauma), as indicated by three (or more) of the following:

   (1) efforts to avoid thoughts, feelings, or conversations associated with the trauma

   (2) efforts to avoid activities, places, or people that arouse recollections of the trauma

   (3) inability to recall an important aspect of the trauma

   (4) markedly diminished interest or participation in significant activities

   (5) feeling of detachment or estrangement from others

   (6) restricted range of affect (e.g., unable to have loving feelings)

   (7) sense of a foreshortened future (e.g., does not expect to have a career, marriage, children, or a normal life span).

D. Persistent symptoms of increased arousal (not present before the trauma), as indicated by two (or more) of the following:

   (1) difficulty falling or staying asleep

   (2) irritability or outbursts of anger

   (3) difficulty concentrating

   (4) hypervigilance

   (5) exaggerated startle response

E. Duration of the disturbance (symptoms in Criteria B, C, and D) is more than 1 month.

F. The disturbance causes clinically significant distress or impairment in social, occupational, or other important areas of functioning.

Specify if:
   Acute: if duration of symptoms is less than 3 months
   Chronic: if duration of symptoms is 3 months or more

Specify if:
   With Delayed Onset: if onset of symptoms is at least 6 months after the stressor.

(continued)

TABLE 9.1. *(continued)*

Associated descriptive features and mental disorders. Individuals with Posttraumatic Stress Disorder may describe painful guilt feelings about surviving when others did not survive or about the things they had to do to survive. Avoidance patterns may interfere with interpersonal relationships. . . . The following associated constellation of symptoms may occur and are more commonly seen in association with an interpersonal stressor (e.g., childhood sexual or physical abuse, domestic battering): impaired affect modulation; self-destructive and impulsive behavior; dissociative symptoms; somatic complaints; feelings of ineffectiveness, shame, despair, or hopelessness; feeling permanently damaged; a loss of previously sustained beliefs; hostility; social withdrawal; feeling constantly threatened; impaired relationships with others; or a change from the individual's previous personality characteristics.

Posttraumatic Stress Disorder is associated with increased rates of Major Depressive Disorder, Substance-Related Disoders, Panic Disorder, Agoraphobia, Obsessive–Compulsive Disorder, Generalized Anxiety Disorder, Social Phobia, Specific Phobia, and Bipolar Disorder. These disorders can either precede, follow, or emerge concurrently with the onset of Posttraumatic Stress Disorder.

Note. From American Psychiatric Association (2000). Copyright 2000 by the American Psychiatric Association. Reprinted by permission.

sponse to stress. High levels of cortisol can also accelerate death of neurons, predisposing the child to cognitive and memory impairments, and perhaps affective disorders in adulthood (Graham et al., 1999).

Individual Characteristics

BIOLOGICAL VULNERABILITY

Some researchers are investigating the possibility of familial predispositions to posttraumatic responses, although little conclusive evidence has yet been found (Koenen, 2003). It appears that

> there is likely no "PTSD gene" that is necessary and sufficient for the development of the disorder. Instead, there are probably many different genes, each of which contributes interchangeably and additively, in a probabilistic fashion, to the inherited liability for PTSD. (Koenen, 2003, p. 1)

Temperament, however, may play a role in posttraumatic response. Research on resilience suggests that resilient children tend to be more outgoing, positive in mood, and adaptable to change as infants (Werner & Smith, 1982). Higher intelligence also may mitigate some of the effects of traumatic experiences (Silva et al., 2000; Werner & Smith, 1982).

PSYCHOLOGICAL STRENGTHS AND VULNERABILITIES

Because traumatic experiences tend to be experienced as uncontrollable, it has been suggested that a sense of self-efficacy or control in stressful situations can attenuate the traumatic ef-

fects of such experiences (Bandura, Taylor, Williams, Mefford, & Barchas, 1985; Foa, Zinbarg, & Rothbaum, 1992). Maltreated adolescent girls with low self-esteem, who consider themselves at the mercy of the environment (demonstrating an external locus of control), have reported higher levels of depression than maltreated girls with high self-esteem, who believe they are in control over their environment (an internal locus of control; Moran & Eckenrode, 1992).

There is good evidence that past experience with high stressors can incline a child to react with symptoms of posttraumatic stress to the current stressful circumstances (Fletcher, 2003). This is particularly true if the child has reacted with posttraumatic symptomatology to past high-magnitude stressors (Daviss, Mooney, et al., 2000; Fremont, 2004; Kassam-Adams & Winston, 2004; Stoddard & Saxe, 2001). A history of stressful life events prior to the high-magnitude stressor has repeatedly been associated with higher levels of PTSD in children after exposure to high-magnitude stressors (Mannarino, Cohen, & Berman, 1994; Seifer, Sameroff, Baldwin, & Baldwin, 1992).

Early stressful experience may not always sensitize a child to later stress, however. The impact of earlier stressful experience may depend more on how the child reacted to that experience than on the fact of exposure itself (Rutter, 1983). Past experience of mastering threatening experiences may help the child deal with later stressful experiences (Rutter, 1983). This suggests that choice of coping strategies can affect posttraumatic stress response. In one study (Stallard, Velleman, Langsford, & Baldwin, 2001), children and adolescents diagnosed with PTSD after motor vehicle accidents did not differ from those not diagnosed with PTSD in their use of active coping strategies of seeking social support, problem solving, and cognitive restructuring. However, children with PTSD were more likely to report the use of avoidant, emotional coping strategies of social withdrawal, distraction, emotional regulation, and blaming others.

Social Characteristics

Children's reactions to high-magnitude stressors are often closely related to the reactions of their caregivers, especially the mother (Ajdukovic, 1998; Milgram & Toubiana, 1996; Winje & Ulvik, 1998), especially for younger children (Pynoos & Eth, 1985). Social support of any kind is associated with lower levels of PTSD symptomatology (Ajdukovic, 1998; Kendall-Tackett, Williams, & Finkelhor, 1993; La Greca et al., 1996; Udwin et al., 2000). Caregiver parenting style can affect children's ability to cope with extremely stressful experience. A flexible (Baumrind, 1971), warm, caring, and attentive parenting style (Maccoby & Martin, 1983) appears to encourage the development of a sense of competence and self-reliance in children. On the other hand, rigid, coercive parenting appears to reduce children's sense of self-esteem and self-competence (Slater & Power, 1987). The quality of the parental relationship may also have an important impact on children's ability to deal with traumatic experiences. Family conflict prior to, during, and after the traumatic experience has been found to be associated with more severe PTSD symptomatology in children (Green et al., 1991; Pelcovitz et al., 1998; Wasserstein & La Greca, 1998).

Shared Characteristics of the Three Posttraumatic Stress Syndromes

By definition, all three posttraumatic stress syndromes consist of physiological and psychological responses to events "that the person experienced, witnessed, or was confronted with . . . that involved actual or threatened death or serious injury, or a threat to the physical integrity of self or others" and "the person's response involved intense fear, helplessness, or horror," which is the description of criterion A

for both PTSD and ASD in the fourth, text revised edition of DSM-IV-TR (APA, 2000; see Tables 9.1 and 9.2). As noted earlier, ASD is diagnosable if symptoms occur within the first month after exposure to a traumatic event and have endured for at least 2 days. Symptoms of PTSD can be diagnosed only after 1 month has passed since the traumatic experience. Complex PTSD is considered to be a consequence of exposure to "early onset, multiple, extended, and sometimes highly invasive traumatic events, frequently of an interpersonal nature, often involving a significant amount of stigma or shame" (Briere & Spinazzola, 2005, p. 401).

Posttraumatic Stress Disorder

PTSD, ASD, and complex PTSD have many symptoms in common, as well. Someone who appears to manifest the complex PTSD symptom constellation nearly always also meets criteria for PTSD (van der Kolk et al., 2005). The "core symptoms" of PTSD, according to DSM-IV, are symptoms of reexperiencing, avoidance of reminders, and overarousal due to reminders of the stressful event(s). These symptoms are common to all three of the posttraumatic stress syndromes: ASD, complex PTSD, and PTSD. Survivors of traumatic experiences who develop any or all of these disorders tend to be subjected to unbidden thoughts, feelings, or memories (frequently of physical sensations, as well as visual images or sounds) that they associate with the traumatic experience. These memories make survivors feel as though they are reexperiencing or reliving the traumatic event or events (criterion B). Because recall of the memories is involuntary, survivors' sense of helplessness is intensified. In an attempt to regain control over an environment that survivors feel is increasingly out of control, they begin to anticipate danger, and become overaroused and easily startled (criterion D). In an attempt to moderate their overwhelming feelings of fear and anxiety, survivors often try to avoid anything that might remind them of their traumatic experience; in some cases this can lead to social withdrawal, flat affect, and an emotional "shutting down" or numbing (criterion C).

In school-age and younger children, upsetting dreams about the stressful experience can change over time into nightmares of monsters or other fearful and threatening experiences. Reliving of the event(s) may also take the form of "traumatic play," wherein aspects of the experience are recreated in play. British children, for instance, played airplane games during the bombing of London in World War II (Freud & Burlingham, 1943), and children held hostage on a school bus played school bus games (Terr, 1981). There have been some reports of a sense of "foreshortened future" among traumatized children, wherein they report feeling as though they will not live to be very old. Anxiety also may be expressed in traumatized children as physical symptoms, such as stomachaches and headaches.

For a diagnosis of PTSD to be made, the child must have been exposed to an event or events wherein death or serious injury was involved or threatened, and the child or adolescent must have reacted with feelings of intense fear, horror, or helplessness (criterion A; see Table 9.1). *The child or adolescent need not have been directly involved in the event or even in direct danger. He or she may have* witnessed *the event happening to others, or he or she may only have* heard about *such an event from others, as when told by others* (Saigh, 1985, 1991) *or they may have only viewed such events on television* (Pfefferbaum et al., 2000). The division of traumatic events into two broad types has proved to have heuristic utility (Fletcher, 2003). Type I traumatic events may be considered acute high-magnitude stressors, because they tend to occur once and are of relatively short duration. Natural disasters, such as hurricanes, and man-made calamities, such as fires, are examples of Type I high-magnitude stressors. Type II traumatic events tend to be of prolonged duration, with multiple repetitions. They also tend to be interpersonal and violent. Sexual abuse and physical abuse are examples of Type II high-magnitude stressors, as are violent political kidnappings, witnessing parental torture, and possibly domestic violence between caretakers and their partners. ASD tends to result from Type I traumatic events, and complex PTSD symptoms typically arise from exposure to extremely traumatizing Type II events. PTSD can result from both types of traumatic events, although symptomatic reactions may differ depending on the type of event (Fletcher, 2003).

DSM-IV requires one symptom of reexperiencing of the event after exposure occurs (criterion B). Also required are three symptoms of denial, avoidance, withdrawal, or numbing (criterion C). Requiring three symptoms of de-

nial or avoidance may be too restrictive (Green, 1993), because it is difficult to identify such symptoms, whether the identification is made by the survivor, an observer, or the person making the assessment. This may be difficult when assessing the reactions of children (Scheeringa & Zeanah, 2003; Schwarz & Kowalski, 1991) and particularly when assessing reactions of infants (Scheeringa & Zeanah, 1995).

Criterion D of DSM-IV requires two reactions symptomatic of overarousal to make a diagnosis of PTSD. Criterion E requires that symptoms have endured for at least 1 month. Criterion F requires that these symptoms cause clinically significant distress or disrupt important activities in the child's or adolescent's life. Criterion F needs serious consideration by the clinician. It is likely that disruption in more than one sphere of the child's or adolescent's life is associated with greater severity of the disorder. Restoring a sense of safety and meaningfulness to these important activities should be an essential and concrete goal in therapy.

Some clinicians and therapists have argued that symptom lists for PTSD included in DSM-IV and in the 10th revision of the *International Classification of Diseases* (ICD-10; World Health Organization, 1992) may not be inclusive enough (Keane, 1993), especially when the reactions of children or infants (Scheeringa, Zeanah, Drell, & Larrieu, 1995) are involved (Armsworth & Holaday, 1993). Still others question the reliance on diagnostic criteria, arguing that a dimensional approach to the assessment of posttraumatic stress responses, rather than the dichotomous diagnostic method of DSM-IV and ICD-10, might prove more fruitful in the long run for both the researcher and the clinician (Keane, 1993; Putnam, 1998).

These points may be illustrated with the results of a study of the aftereffects on first- and third-grade children exposed to a hostage-taking incident in Paris (Vila, Porsche, & Mouren-Simeoni, 1999). The researchers reported the number of children who not only met DSM-IV diagnostic criteria for PTSD, but also those who did not meet full PTSD criteria but did meet all criteria except one of criterion C (avoidance) and one of criterion D (overarousal). Children who met this reduced set of criteria were said to have subclinical posttraumatic stress. They found that 7 (26.9%) of 26 children met the full DSM criteria for PTSD at some time during the 18-month follow-up period, whereas 13 (50%) met criteria for subclinical posttraumatic stress, while never meeting the full DSM-IV criteria for PTSD diagnosis. Moreover, of the seven children who met the full criteria at some point during the follow-up period, three children originally only met criteria for subclinical posttraumatic stress when they were first assessed.

Prevalence and Incidence

The prevalence of PTSD among children in the community has been estimated to be between 1 and 14% (APA, 1994). However, these figures apply to children and adolescents regardless of whether they have ever been exposed to a high-magnitude stressor. Incidence rates among those who have actually experienced trauma provide more meaningful information for clinical and research purposes. Even then the picture is complicated by the need to take into account the kinds of stressful events involved, the ages and developmental stages of the children or adolescents exposed to the events, their gender and ethnicity, how their reactions were assessed, how soon after their exposure their reactions were assessed, and other potential mediators and moderators of the impact of the stressful events on the survivors (Fletcher, 2003).

After Hurricane Hugo, 5,687 youths between the ages of 9 and 19 were surveyed for their reactions (Lonigan, Shannon, Finch, Daugherty, & Taylor, 1991; Shannon et al., 1994). The overall incidence of those who met criteria A–D of DSM-III-R (APA, 1987) was 5.4%. Girls were more likely (6.9%) than boys (3.8%) to meet all of these criteria. There were no significant differences observed among the ethnic groups, with an incidence of 6.3% among African Americans (who represented 25.8% of the sample), whereas it was 5.1% among all of the other ethnic groups. The incidence was 9.2% among school-age children (ages 9–12), which was higher than the 4.2% rate for those ages 13–15, and the 3.1% rate for those ages 16–19.

The estimated incidence rates of this study are likely to be conservative and perhaps not as accurate as they might have been if a different assessment tool had been employed. The researchers in this particular instance used one of the first assessment tools developed to measure childhood PTSD, the Child Posttraumatic Stress Reaction Index (CPTS-RI; Frederick, 1985b; Frederick, Pynoos, & Nader, 1992; Pynoos et al., 1987; see Appendix 9.5). The CPTS-RI was not designed to be used to determine PTSD diagnosis using DSM-IV criteria. To do so, researchers are forced to modify the way the measure is scored (Nader, 1993, 1999). Estimates of incidence rates depend on the manner in which researchers choose to dichotomize the 5-point scale response categories for each item. Two choices are possible: (1) to consider a symptom as present if the relevant item is rated with one of the two highest responses, or (2) to use the three highest responses as indicative of the presence of a symptom. The first approach obviously produces lower estimates (as demonstrated by Schwarz & Kowalski, 1991). Shannon and colleagues (1994) and Lonigan and colleagues (1991) used the first, more conservative approach, which may have underestimated incidence rates of PTSD among the children of Hurricane Hugo.

Other studies have found higher incidence rates. Of 1,019 fourth- to eighth-grade students in North Carolina surveyed after a major fire in a chicken-processing plant in the community, 11.9% met DSM-III-R criteria for PTSD (March, Amaya-Jackson, Terry, & Costanzo, 1997). In another study of urban youth exposed to community violence, 24% met PTSD criteria (Breslau, Davis, Andeski, & Peterson, 1991), whereas in a similar study, 34.5% of youth met full PTSD criteria (Berman, Kurtines, Silverman, & Serafini, 1996). A meta-analysis of the empirical literature (Fletcher, 2003) found incidence rates similar to those in the two preceding studies, with estimated rates of 39% for preschool children (≤ 7 years old), 33% for school-age children (6–12 years old), and 27% for adolescents (12 years and older).

Gender Differences

Whether or not gender differences are found among children and adolescent survivors of extremely stressful events depends on several factors. Boys and girls tend to be exposed to different kinds of interpersonal violence. Girls, for instance, are more likely than boys to report having experienced sexual abuse or rape, whereas boys are more likely to report having been a victim of community violence (Bergen, Martin, Richardson, Allison, & Roeger, 2004; Garland et al., 2001; Helzer, Robins, & McEvoy, 1987).

Girls and boys may also react differently to the same traumatic events. Girls may be more likely to react with internalizing behavior problems, such as clinging, worrying, sullenness; whereas, boys may be more likely to react with both internalizing and externalizing behavior problems, such as argument, hot temper, impulsivity, or hyperactivity (Bolton, O'Ryan, Udwin, Boyle, & Yule, 2000; Jaffe, Wolfe, Wilson, & Zak, 1986; Winje & Ulvik, 1998). Sexually abused girls between the ages of 2 and 6 years in one study (Kiser et al., 1988) tended to feel sad and depressed, whereas boys the same age who had been sexually abused tended to act with rage and aggression. Girls reported significantly more feelings of fear, horror, and helplessness in response to a hurricane than did boys (Goenjian et al., 2001). Moreover, although significant bivariate associations indicated that girls reported more symptoms of PTSD than did boys, gender differences disappeared in multivariate analyses when subjective reactions were considered as well. This suggests the possibility that girls may report higher levels of PTSD symptomatology than boys, because girls are liable to experience more fear, horror, and helplessness in the face of traumatic events. Some support for this possibility was found in assessments of reactions of children and adolescents to Hurricane Hugo (Lonigan et al., 1991; Shannon et al., 1994). There, too, girls reported more PTSD symptoms than did boys; in addition, they were more likely to report being distressed by the hurricane, feeling upset by thoughts of it, fearing its recurrence, avoiding reminders of the hurricane, avoiding feelings about it, and experiencing affective numbing, somatic complaints, guilt feelings, and increased startle response.

On the other hand, the coping strategies of girls may be more adaptive than those of boys. Girls may be more likely to seek social support, whether from a caregiver or from peers, after experiencing a severe trauma, and they may be more likely to receive social support from important others once they seek it (Milgram & Toubiana, 1996; Rossman, 1992). Moreover, girls' use of anger seems to decline with age; although its use by boys appears to decline between ages 8 and 9 years, it seems to increase again between ages 10 and 12 (Rossman, 1992).

Even the time of assessment relevant to the potentially traumatic experience may make a difference in gender-reported symptomatology.

The sexually abused preschool boys observed by Kiser and colleagues (1988) were more likely than sexually abused girls to be withdrawn immediately after their abuse was discovered; whereas, a year later, girls were more likely to be withdrawn. Posttraumatic stress symptomatology among boys after a nuclear waste disaster decreased over time, whereas it increased among girls (Korol, Green, & Gleser, 1999). Similarly, displaced boys in wartime Bosnia showed more symptoms of anxiety, overarousal, and intrusive thoughts than girls at first assessment, but 8 months later, girls were more symptomatic in these areas than boys (Stein, Comer, Gardner, & Kelleher, 1999).

Ethnic and Cultural Variations

There is ample evidence that PTSD occurs among children of different cultural and ethnic backgrounds (Ahmad & Mohamad, 1996; Beals et al., 1997; DeJong, Emmett, & Hervada, 1982; Diehl, Zea, & Espino, 1994; DiNicola, 1996; Jones, Dauphinais, Sack, & Somervell, 1997; Lindholm & Willey, 1986; Pierce & Pierce, 1984). On the whole, when exposed to Type I, acute, nonabusive stressors of high magnitude, children of non-European descent may present with more severe levels of posttraumatic symptomatology than children of other ethnic backgrounds. Of the 5,587 youth ages 9–19 whose reactions to Hurricane Hugo were assessed (Shannon et al., 1994), the majority were of European American descent (67.3%), whereas 25.8% were African American, 3.6% were Asian American, 1.4% were Hispanic American, and 1.9% were from "other minority" groups. Even after controlling for the severity of the traumatic experience and for levels of trait anxiety, African American children and adolescents reported more symptoms of criteria A through D of DSM-III-R PTSD than did the European American or other, non–African American minority children and adolescents. At the same time, the proportion of African Americans (6.3%) who met the core criteria, A through D for PTSD, did not differ significantly from the proportion of other children and adolescents (5.1%) who met the same criteria.

On the other hand, ethnic group differences were observed in a prospective study of the reactions to Hurricane Andrew of 442 fifth, sixth, and seventh graders (La Greca et al.,

1996). European American children constituted 45.7% of the sample, whereas Hispanic American and African American children each comprised 23.5% of the sample, and Asian Americans, 3.4%. The Hispanic American and African American children reported similar levels of posttraumatic symptomatology, at levels that were approximately one-half a standard deviation higher than those reported by the European American children. Moreover, the African American and Hispanic American children were less likely to demonstrate improved PTSD symptomatology over time. As the authors remarked, "These ethnic differences in PTSD reporting may be related to other variables associated with minority status, such as the limited availability of financial resources" (p. 721), but the reasons for the differences remain unclear.

Cultural and ethnic differences become more complex when Type II chronic or abusive stressors of high magnitude are considered. Upon review of the medical records of four groups of American children—80 of African, 69 of Asian, 89 of European, and 80 of Hispanic origin—referred to a clinic for sexual abuse, several differences among the groups emerged (Rao, DiClemente, & Ponton, 1992). Sexual acting out was least likely to be observed among Asian American children (1.4% vs. 15.0% among African Americans, 17.5% among European Americans, and 12.8% among Hispanic Americans). Asian American children were also the least likely to display anger (8.7% vs. 21.3% among African Americans, 22.5% among European Americans, and 20.0% among Hispanic Americans). Urinary problems were least frequently found among Asian American children (2.9%) and most frequently among European Americans (17.5%), with the frequency among African Americans (10.0%) and Hispanic Americans (6.3%) in between the two extremes. On the other hand, suicide attempts or ideation occurred most frequently among Asian American children (21.7% vs. 11.3% among African Americans, 15.0% among European Americans, and 10.0% among Hispanic Americans).

Cultural background may affect how PTSD symptomatology is manifested (Cohen et al., 1998). DSM-IV (APA, 1994) notes that children of Hispanic or Latin American origins, for example, may manifest symptoms as the culture-bound syndrome of *susto*, also known as "fright sickness," literally meaning a loss of the soul from the body (Rubel, O'Nell, &

Collado-Ardon, 1984). The cause is a sudden frightening experience such as an accident, a fall, witnessing a relative's sudden death, or any other potentially dangerous event. Symptoms include nervousness, anorexia, insomnia, listlessness, despondence, involuntary muscle tics, and diarrhea. A diagnosis is based on the symptom complex and the associated history of a traumatic event. Unfortunately, research on the impact of culture and ethnicity among non-American cultures, especially immigrants and refugees, is in its early stages at best (Jaycox et al., 2002; Sattler et al., 2002).

The many issues surrounding cross-cultural and multiethnic assessment of trauma are far too complex to consider here in depth (Manson, 1997; Marsella, Friedman, Gerrity, & Scurfield, 1996; Stamm & Friedman, 2000). However, it was considered of such importance that Appendix I of DSM-IV is devoted to an "Outline for Cultural Formulation and Glossary of Culture-Bound Syndromes." Manson (1997), a member of the NIMH-sponsored Culture and Diagnosis Group that wrote that appendix for DSM-IV (Mezzich, 1995), provides a discussion and example of how to conduct a cultural formulation when taking a client's history. Every clinician should be able to conduct a cultural formulation, not only because immigrants, and in particular refugees from war torn third-world countries, are increasingly likely to settle in areas other than their traditional ports of entry, but because even within the United States there are ethnic and cultural differences that should be considered when assessing and treating trauma with Native Americans, Hispanics who themselves are not a homogeneous culture, and black Americans born in this country. The National Child Traumatic Stress Network (Ko, 2005, p. 1) notes the extent of the problem in the United States:

> Research indicates that children and adolescents from minority backgrounds are at increased risk for trauma exposure and development of Posttraumatic Stress Disorder [PTSD; Jaycox et al., 2002; Norris, Byrne, Diaz, & Kaniasty, 2002]. For example, African American, American Indian, and Latin American children are overrepresented in reported cases of child maltreatment, and in foster care [U.S. Department of Health and Human Services, Administration for Children and Families, 2002]. Further, research indicates that disasters pose particular burdens in mental health for ethnic minority and developing country popu-

lations, especially for children, due to social, economic, and political marginalization, deprivation, and powerlessness [Sattler et al., 2002]. Consequently, minority children fare worse in the aftermath of trauma, often experiencing more severe symptomatology for longer periods of time, than their majority group counterparts [Cohen, Deblinger, Mannarino, & de Arellano, 2001; Jones, Hadder, Carvajal, Chapman, & Alexander, 2006; Norris & Alegria, 2005].

Acute Stress Disorder

If posttraumatic reactions are restricted to 1 month after traumatic exposure, PTSD may not be diagnosed. ASD, however, can be, if symptomatology meets DSM-IV criteria. Whereas some of the symptomatology of ASD (see Table 9.2) parallels that of PTSD, the pri-

mary distinction, besides timing of responses, is dissociative symptomatology. Although this includes the absence of emotional responsiveness, a general sense of detachment or emotional numbing, which is included as a symptom of avoidance or withdrawal in PTSD, it includes additional symptoms not considered essential for PTSD diagnosis. Survivors might experience a reduction of awareness of the surroundings, of "being in a daze," for example, and may find it difficult to recall some or all aspects of their experience. A feeling that their experience cannot have been real (derealization) is also possible. Their sense of detachment from their experience may become so extreme that they begin to feel that what they are living is not happening to them, that it is all a dream (depersonalization). To meet criteria for diag-

---

TABLE 9.2. DSM-IV-TR Diagnostic Criteria for Acute Stress Disorder

A. The person has been exposed to a traumatic event in which both of the following were present:

(1) the person experienced, witnessed, or was confronted with an event or events that involved actual or threatened death or serious injury, or a threat to the physical integrity of self or others
(2) the person's response involved intense fear, helplessness, or horror

B. Either while experiencing or after experiencing the distressing event, the individual has three (or more) of the following dissociative symptoms:

(1) a subjective sense of numbing, detachment, or absence of emotional responsiveness
(2) a reduction in awareness of his or her surroundings (e.g., "being in a daze")
(3) derealization
(4) depersonalization
(5) dissociative amnesia (i.e., inability to recall an important aspect of the trauma)

C. The traumatic event is persistently reexperienced in one (or more) of the following ways: recurrent images, thoughts, dreams, illusions, flashback episodes, or a sense of reliving the experience or perceptions; or distress on exposure to reminders of the traumatic event.

D. Marked avoidance of stimuli that arouse recollections of the trauma (e.g., thoughts, feelings, conversations, activities, places, people).

E. Marked symptoms of anxiety or increased arousal (e.g., difficulty sleeping, irritability, poor concentration, hypervigilance, exaggerated startle response, motor restlessness).

F. The disturbance causes clinically significant distress or impairment in social, occupational, or other important areas of functioning or impairs the individual's ability to pursue some necessary task, such as obtaining necessary assistance or mobilizing personal resources by telling family members about the traumatic experience.

G. The disturbance lasts for a minimum of 2 days and a maximum of 4 weeks and occurs within 4 weeks of the traumatic event.

H. The disturbance is not due ot the direct physiological effects of a substance (e.g., a drug of abuse, a medication) or a general medical condition, is not better accounted for by Brief Psychotic Disorder, and is not merely an exacerbation of a preexisting Axis I or Axis II disorder.

Note. From American Psychiatric Association (2000). Copyright 2000 by the American Psychiatric Association. Reprinted by permission.

nosis, survivors must manifest three or more of these symptoms. On the other hand, they are not required to have more than one symptom of each of the "core" PTSD symptoms: re-experiencing, avoidance of stimuli associated with the traumatic event(s), and increased arousal. Note that symptoms of *both* avoidance and numbing or dissociation are required to meet the criteria for diagnosis of ASD, unlike the criteria for PTSD, which require three symptoms of avoidance, withdrawal, *or* numbing (but not dissociation). Moreover, the symptoms of dissociation can manifest *during* the traumatic event(s), as well as immediately after.

The definition of ASD has been controversial since its inception in DSM-IV (Davidson et al., 1996; Marshall, Spitzer, & Liebowitz, 1999; Rothbaum & Foa, 1993). The objective was to allow identification of clinically important responses to high-magnitude stressors in the immediate aftermath of the experience, during the 4-week period in which PTSD could not be diagnosed, while avoiding the possibility of assigning a diagnosis to survivors who would eventually recover on their own (Davidson et al., 1996; Marshall et al., 1999). At that time, several studies found that dissociative responses during or immediately after traumatic experiences were predictive of eventual diagnosis of PTSD (see Cardeña, Lewis-Fernández, Bear, Pakianathan, & Spiegel, 1996, for a review). Information on the incidence of ASD after exposure to high-magnitude stressors has yet to be explored adequately. Nor is there currently much generally agreed-upon information about the risk factors for developing ASD after exposure to extreme stressors, the association of its occurrence with the development of PTSD, or other factors that might influence its etiology and prognosis. What little evidence exists regarding ASD among children and adolescents suggests that the incidence of dissociative symptoms after high-magnitude stressors, key criteria for diagnosis of ASD, is considerably less than that found among adults (Daviss, Mooney, Racusin, Fleischer, et al., 2000; Daviss, Mooney, Racusin, Ford, et al., 2000; Kassam-Adams & Winston, 2004) and does not predict later incidence of PTSD. The requirement for symptoms of dissociation has thus far led to lower incident rates for diagnosis of ASD than for subsyndromal ASD. Rates of ASD among children and adolescents after hospitalization for injuries were 7.4%, whereas rates for subsyndromal ASD were 22% (Daviss, Mooney,

Racusin, Ford, et al., 2000). Similarly, rates for full versus subsyndromal ASD were 8% versus 14% among traffic accident survivors (Kassam-Adams & Winston, 2004), and 19.4% versus 24.7% among children and adolescents involved in assaults or motor vehicle accidents (Stedman, Yule, Smith, Glucksman, & Dalgleish, 2005). In all of these studies, however, although diagnosis of ASD was a good predictor of later PTSD, dissociation did not play a significant role in the prediction. The number of ASD symptoms (which does not depend on endorsement of dissociative symptoms) is what predicts later PTSD rather than the diagnosis of ASD (which does depend on endorsement of dissociative symptoms). Much more research is clearly needed regarding the incidence of ASD among children, with special attention to the predictability of later PTSD from ASD severity versus diagnosis. The development of good measures of ASD symptomatology is required for such research. Fortunately, work has begun in this area, as described in a later section of this chapter.

Complex PTSD

The DSM-IV-TR (APA, 2000) definition of PTSD implicitly acknowledges the development of more severe symptoms as the duration of the condition increases, noting that duration of symptoms for less than 3 months is indicative of acute PTSD, whereas longer duration indicates chronic PTSD (see Table 9.1). The literature has increasingly noted the greater likelihood of comorbid conditions developing the longer PTSD persists (Keane & Kaloupek, 1997; van der Kolk et al., 2005). Foa, Friedman, and Keane (2000) note that more than 80% of patients with PTSD suffer from comorbid conditions. Many PTSD researchers and clinicians have proposed that most of the symptoms that DSM-IV lists as associated symptoms actually provide a description of complex PTSD, and that this syndrome "provides a clear delineation of the enduring developmental effects of trauma" and "is helpful in conceptualizing the complex adaptations to trauma over the lifespan" (van der Kolk & Courtois, 2005, p. 386).

Pain (2002) has suggested that this conceptualization of complex PTSD fits Kardiner's original (1941) conceptualization of the developmental course of traumatic reactions. She noted that he postulated a two-stage response to trauma that also takes into account how the disorder changes as it becomes long-standing. He described the core response to trauma and first stage as expressed in the symptoms of PTSD. Stage two—the change from simple PTSD to PTSD with comorbidity, or what we are calling complex PTSD or DESNOS—represents the personality's adaptation and reorganization in response to the compromised function caused by failure to recover from the original trauma(s). This concept is salient in the case of individuals who suffered repeated and prolonged psychological trauma during childhood, which disturbed the normal developmental trajectory. (p. 13)

Because complex PTSD is not a recognized disorder in DSM-IV, there is no formal definition of the syndrome. However, criteria for complex PTSD were created for the DSM-IV field trial for PTSD, which also explored the viability and utility of a separate diagnostic category for complex PTSD (Kilpatrick et al., 1998; van der Kolk et al., 1996). Since that time various listings of symptom categories have been suggested, but most include the following seven categories: (1) difficulties regulating affect and impulses, (2) alterations in attention or consciousness, (3) somatization, (4) distorted self-perception, (5) distorted perceptions of the perpetrator, (6) difficult relations with others, and (7) alterations in systems of meaning. Descriptions of the kinds of symptoms in each of the seven categories may be found in Table 9.3, in which categories and symptoms are based on similar listings in Herman (1992), Pelcovitz and colleagues (1997), and van der Kolk and colleagues (2005).

Very little is known about the manifestation of complex PTSD symptoms among children and adolescents. However, the DSM-IV field trial for PTSD included adolescents age 15 years and older who were identified as meeting criteria for complex PTSD (van der Kolk et al., 1996, 2005). Moreover, research has shown that traumatized children have problems with unmodulated impulse control and aggression (Cole & Putnam, 1992; Steiner, Garcia, & Matthews, 1997), may be prone to dissociation and to problems maintaining attention (Perry, 2001; Perry, Pollard, Blakley, Baker, & Vigilante, 1995; Teicher et al., 2003), and have difficulties forming trusting relationships with both caregivers and peers (Schneider-Rosen & Cicchetti, 1984). Thus, growing evidence indi-

cates that children, adolescents, and young adults can and do develop clusters of symptoms that bear a strong resemblance to the proposed syndrome of complex PTSD. Even if this cluster of symptoms is not accepted as an official syndrome, clinicians should be alert to the possibility of such associated and related symptoms of PTSD developing among children exposed to abuse and neglect of any kind, especially if the abuse started when they were young and continued over a prolonged period of time.

Other Comorbid Disorders

As noted earlier, survivors of traumatic experiences who react with symptoms of PTSD are more likely than not to show signs of other disorders as well. For children and adolescents these include substance abuse (Kilpatrick et al., 2000), adjustment, panic, depressive (Kilpatrick et al., 2003), anxious, dissociative, attention deficit (Saigh, Yasik, Sack, & Koplewicz, 1999), and eating disorders (Breslau, Davis, Andreski, Peterson, & Schultz, 1991; Cloitre, Chase Stovall-McClough, Miranda, & Chemtob, 2004; Finkelhor & Kendall-Tackett, 1997; Zlotnick et al., 1996). There is increasing evidence that adults who suffered childhood abuse may have long-term medical problems as well, including cardiovascular, immunological, metabolic, and sexual problems (Briere & Elliott, 2003; Dube et al., 2001; Felitti et al., 1997; Hulme, 2000; van der Kolk et al., 2005). Clinicians need to be aware of the possible existence of such comorbid disorders, both when assessing and treating children clearly identified as survivors of high-magnitude stressors and when seeing children with these conditions who have not been identified as survivors of potentially traumatic events.

ASSESSMENT OF PTSD IN CHILDREN

Practice parameters for the assessment and treatment of children and adolescents with PTSD have been published by the American Academy of Child and Adolescent Psychiatry (AACAP; Cohen et al., 1998). This article includes a review of several measures of childhood PTSD, as does another review (Ohan, Myers, & Collett, 2002) by the same journal. The AACAP practice parameters appear to be directed primarily toward the clinician situated in the clini-

TABLE 9.3. Complex PTSD Symptom Constellation Arranged into Categories

I. Difficulty regulating affect and impulses

A. Affect regulation
  • Easily upset. Difficulty calming down once upset.
  • Persistent dysphoria.
B. Modulation of anger
  • Persistent feelings of anger.
  • Difficulty controlling anger.
C. Self-destructive
  • Either deliberate hurting of self or involvement in an unusual number of serious "accidents."

D. Suicidal preoccupation
E. Difficulty modulating sexual involvement
  • Sexual preoccupation, from fantasy to situations that put self at risk or in danger.
F. Excessive risk taking

II. Alteration in attention or consciousness

A. Amnesia
  • Unable to remember important parts of life history, or confusion or uncertainty about whether certain events did or did not take place.
B. Transient dissociative episodes
  • Difficulty keeping track of time in daily life.
  • "Spacing out" when feeling frightened or under stress.

C. Depersonalization or derealization
  • Feeling unreal or as if living in a dream. Events do not seem real.
D. Reliving the traumatic experiences
  • Through intrusive memories, etc., as in PTSD, or through ruminative preoccupation with the events or similar kinds of events.

III. Somatization

A. Digestive system
  • Unexplained nausea, abdominal pain, intolerance of food, vomiting, diarrhea.
B. Chronic pain
  • Recurrent, unexplained pain in arms, legs, back, joints, genitals, while urinating, headaches.
C. Cardiopulmonary symptoms
  • Shortness of breath, dizziness, heart palpitations, chest pain.

D. Conversion symptoms
  • Unexplained difficulties remembering things, difficulties swallowing, losing one's voice, blurred vision, actual blindness, fainting and losing consciousness, seizures and convulsions, difficulties walking, muscle weakness or paralysis, difficulties urinating.
E. Sexual symptoms
  • Unexplained burning sensations in sexual organs or rectum (not during intercourse); impotence for males; irregular menstrual periods, excessive premenstrual tension, excessive menstrual bleeding for females.

IV. Distorted self-perception

A. Ineffectiveness
  • Feelings of having no control over what happens to self.
  • Can manifest as paralysis of initiative.
B. Permanent damage
  • Feelings of having something wrong with self that can never be fixed.
C. Guilt and self-blame
  • Persistent and recurring feelings of guilt about many things.
  • A readiness to assume guilt in new situations.

D. Shame
  • Feelings of deep shame.
  • Poor self-esteem.
E. Nobody can understand
  • Feelings of being different and set apart from others.
F. Minimizing
  • Minimizing one's own victimization and the victimization of others.

V. Distorted perceptions of the perpetrator

A. Adopting distorted beliefs
  • Believing that one deserved to be hurt or "punished."
B. Idealization of the perpetrator
  • Unrealistic attribution of total power to perpetrator.
  • Paradoxical gratitude.

C. Preoccupation with relationship with the perpetrator, including preoccupation with revenge
  • Sense of special or supernatural relationship.
D. Identification with the perpetrator
  • Acceptance of beliefs or rationalizations of the perpetrator.

(continued)

TABLE 9.3. *(continued)*

VI. Difficult relations with others

A. Inability to trust
  - Difficulties forming and keeping intimate relationships.
B. Isolation and withdrawal
  - May alternate with repeated search for rescuer.

C. Revictimization
  - Vulnerability to being victimized in a manner similar to the original trauma and in new kinds of traumas.
D. Victimizing others
  - Victimizing others in a manner similar to the original trauma.

VII. Alterations in systems of meaning

A. Despair and hopelessness

B. Loss of previously sustaining beliefs
  - Loss of belief in the meaningfulness of life. Loss of religious beliefs or other previous sustaining beliefs.

---

cal setting. As such, they do not address the particular needs of assessment outside the clinical setting. Assessment needs in the field during and immediately after the occurrence of a high-magnitude stressor, such as Hurricane Katrina, call for a different approach to assessment—a two-stage process: a quick screening, followed by a more intensive assessment for individuals who screen positive for posttraumatic stress reactions. Because clinicians may be asked to assist in crisis situations, the unique assessment needs associated with the initial screening for the possible presence of ASD or PTSD are considered here as well. Since the AACAP Workgroup on Quality Issues made its recommendations (Cohen et al., 1998), and since Ohan and colleagues made their recommendations in 2002, much more has been learned about the assessment of children's reactions to high-magnitude stressors, and many more assessment tools have been created and tested. As such, measures recommended in this chapter frequently differ from the AACAP and Ohan and colleagues recommendations.

Factors to Consider When Choosing Assessment Tools

As noted earlier, simply being exposed to a potentially traumatic event does not necessarily mean a child will develop ASD, PTSD, complex PTSD, or any other adverse reaction. Children's and adolescents' responses to high-magnitude stressors may be affected by quite a few factors, many of which need to be considered during the assessment process (for more detailed consideration of these factors, see Fletcher, 2003; Nader, 1997; and, in particular, Nader, in press). Some of the more salient factors were discussed briefly earlier. Additional factors that need to be considered in assessment include the age and developmental stage of the youth, the youth's reading level and verbal comprehension, the purpose of the assessment, the type of stressor to which the youth was exposed, how close the youth was to the central aspects of the stressor, how long the exposure lasted, and how the youth's parents reacted to his or her experience. It is particularly important to be mindful of the psychometric properties of the measures.

Clinical Utility

One criterion for choosing a clinical measure that is more often assumed than explicitly considered, both by clinicians and by those who develop such measures, is clinical utility. Of course, no one would create or choose to use a clinical measure unless it was thought to have some sort of clinical utility. Just what that utility might be, however, is not always considered beyond accurate assessment and diagnosis, and perhaps as a measure of success or failure of clinical interventions (a use that unfortunately is found more often in research than in clinical practice). Part of the reason for the lack of clarity on the clinical utility of such measures may be the lack of a formal definition for the term, especially as it relates to clinical measures. One notable attempt to define "clinical utility" has been made as it relates to the clinical utility of psychiatric diagnoses. First and colleagues (2004) define clinical utility in this regard as the extent to which DSM assists clinical decision makers in fulfilling the various clinical functions of a psychiatric classification system. These functions include assisting clinicians and other users with the following:

1. Conceptualizing diagnostic entities
2. Communicating clinical information to practitioners, patients and their families, and health care systems administrators
3. Using diagnostic categories and criteria sets in clinical practice (including for diagnostic interviewing and differential diagnosis)
4. Choosing effective interventions to improve clinical outcomes
5. Predicting future clinical management needs (p. 947)

With minimal revision this could be applied to a definition of the clinical utility of a clinical assessment tool. Measures of ASD, PTSD, and complex PTSD should be able to guide the clinician's conceptualization of each of these diagnostic entities. Inasmuch as a measure includes assessment of all suggested symptoms and rules for determining whether requirements are met for each criterion associated with these syndromes, it can be said to meet the first requirement of clinical utility set forth by Fast et al. Many measures of childhood PTSD do not explicitly address criterion E (the duration of symptoms must be more than 1 month posttrauma) or criterion F (the symptoms must lead to clinically significant distress and substantial social dysfunction). The clinician needs to consider whether associated symptoms should also be measured, in addition to the required symptoms, such as criteria A–F for PTSD. In some cases, for example, among the very young, some relevant symptoms may not even be considered by most of the child PTSD assessment tools currently available, as noted in the later discussion of developmental issues related the assessment of childhood PTSD.

Communicating clinical information to the child and family, as well as to other practitioners and administrators, not to mention health insurance agencies—the second point in the First and colleagues (2004) definition of clinical utility—can be facilitated by an assessment tool that allows the clinician to determine the child's precise responses to his or her traumatic experience during the event, immediately after it, and over time. Information obtained using a reliable and valid instrument can provide insight to clinician, child, and family, as well as detailed and documented support for the clinician's diagnosis. Copies of the responses to standardized interviews or surveys placed in the child's medical record can help to ensure that other clinicians and therapeutic caregivers have an adequate understanding of the child's reactions as well.

The third part of the definition of clinical utility is perhaps the most salient reason for creating and using diagnostic assessment tools: diagnostic interviewing and differential diagnosis. It is important to remember that differential diagnosis is a necessary part of the assessment, however. It is also important to remember that PTSD is frequently comorbid with other disorders that also are responses to the same traumatic circumstances. Grief or depression, for example, may also be posttraumatic responses, not just ASD, PTSD, or complex PTSD. Most current PTSD measures (other than the general diagnostic measures described in Appendix 9.3) do not provide screening for other responses so clinicians need to supplement PTSD-specific measures with assessment tools for other possible responses. This is especially the case for children referred for violent, interpersonal stressors of long duration, such as abuse, in which case symptoms of complex PTSD should be assessed, as well as the DSM-IV symptoms of PTSD.

The last two points of the definition of clinical utility—choosing effective interventions and predicting future clinical needs—are clearly related. The results of the first assessment should provide guidelines for how the clinician may best proceed with the initial stages of any intervention. An overemphasis on symptoms of avoidance, numbing, and overarousal may suggest to the clinician that the child is not ready to be asked to focus attention on the details of the traumatic experience at this point. Perhaps issues of trust, therapeutic bonding, and reassurance of security would be good places to start with this particular child. At the same time, the clinician should be alert to the fact that such heightened attention to defending against reminders may indicate the intensity with which such reminders are likely to return once the child does gain a minimum sense of safety and reassurance, and be prepared for the fear that such intense reminders are likely to inspire in the child.

The anticipation of dynamic changes over time in presenting symptomatology when treating individuals with posttraumatic stress suggests another aspect of the clinical utility of measures of PTSD that is not explicitly considered in First and colleagues' (2004) definition: the ability to monitor a child's changing symptomatology. For the most part, of course, clinicians monitor the progress of their client's symptomatology on a regular but unstructured basis as they discuss their progress. However, an occasional formal assessment of current symptomatology can ensure that no possible symptoms are being overlooked. Such assessments also provide an opportunity to examine the child's progress by comparing the child's current and previous responses. This can be particularly productive in the group setting, where some children may tend to participate in group discussion less than others. Formal assessment also assists in the evaluation of different types of intervention. In fact, only in this context has the ability of a measure to monitor children's progress been assessed to any degree thus far. For a measure to serve as a useful monitoring tool, it needs to be able to reflect actual changes accurately in children's posttraumatic stress symptomatology; that is, it needs to be responsive to true change in symptomatology. There are formal methods of assessing a measure's responsiveness to change, but these methods have yet to be used to test the responsivity of any of the currently available measures of childhood ASD, PTSD, or complex PTSD.

The Clinical Assessment

In what follows, the terms "child" and "children" include infants, children, adolescents, and young adults unless otherwise noted. A clinician attempting to determine a child's reactions to high-magnitude stressors ideally should collect information from as many sources as possible, including not only the child and one or more caregivers, but also others who knew the child prior to, during, and after the event(s). Additional reporters might include relatives other than the primary caregivers, siblings, teachers, peers, and others who were affected by the event(s), especially those who lived through it with the child. When the stressor involves abuse or domestic violence, any alleged offending caregiver need not be interviewed, although a report from sources involved with eliciting the offender's report of the event(s) can be helpful.

OBTAIN A HISTORY

The article "*Practice Parameters for the Assessment and Treatment of Children and Adolescents with Posttraumatic Stress Disorder*" (Cohen et al., 1998) recommends the same course of assessment for the parent and the child. The first step is to obtain a thorough history of the child. Whenever possible, information should be sought regarding the child's psychiatric history, including any partial or inpatient hospitalizations, medications (especially psychotropic), and outpatient psychotherapy. This would include any history of mood disorders, anxiety disorders, PTSD symptomatology, and substance abuse, as well as medical conditions that may present as anxiety or mood disorders, such as thyroid disease. An understanding of the medical and psychiatric history of other members of the family may also be very helpful.

The clinician is encouraged to assess the extent to which other stressors have played a part in the child's life, both in the distant past and more recently. As noted earlier, previous exposure to other stressors may have an important impact on the child's reaction to the event(s) under consideration. The clinician should inquire not only into the child's history of exposure to high-magnitude stressors such as abuse or neglect, and exposure to domestic or community violence, but also into the occurrence of and reaction to other, lesser stressors, such as family illnesses, deaths, conflict, separation, or divorce, as well as frequent moves, school changes, or problems in the school or with peers.

Any parental history of exposure to potentially traumatic events also should be considered, whether or not the child might be aware of this history. Any familial history of PTSD is particularly important to determine, because this can have repercussions on the child's outlook on life and ability to cope with stressful events. It also can affect the caregiver's reactions to the child's potentially traumatic experience, especially if that experience mirrors the caregiver's own traumatic experience. The reactions of mothers to their children's abuse experience may be greatly complicated if the mothers themselves have a history of childhood abuse, for example. The clinician should ascertain whether the caregiver was exposed to the same event(s) as the child and if so, the nature of the caregiver's own reactions during and after experiencing the event(s), and the extent to which the caregiver may have reacted to the experience with symptoms of posttraumatic stress. The parents' own reactions to the *child's* traumatic experiences also should be explored, because children, especially younger children, often use their parents' reactions to the experience to determine how they themselves should be reacting (Fletcher, 2003).

DEVELOPMENTAL CONSIDERATIONS

During the assessment process, the clinician must make an effort to pay attention to developmental variations in the child's reactions. This is particularly important when assessing preschool-age children. Scheeringa, Peebles, Cook, and Zeanah (2001; Scheeringa & Zeanah, 1995; Scheeringa, Zeanah, Myers, & Putnam, 2003) devised and examined the predictive ability of a revised set of particularly interesting criteria for this age group. Their criteria are dependent more on behavioral observations than on verbal descriptions of symptoms (Scheeringa et al., 2003):

> Some symptoms had to be developmentally modified because they were derivative functions of memory, abstract thought, emotional processing, or language, which are all in a state of emerging development in young children. Several symptoms could not be used because they were inappropriate for the developmental capacities of young children (e.g., sense of a foreshortened future). The A(2) criterion (the person's immediate response must show extreme emotional or behavioral reactions) was not required, because if the child is perverbal, and an adult is not present to witness the child's reaction, then this symptom is undetectable. One completely new symptom—loss of previously acquired developmental skills such as toileting or speech—was added to cluster C. It was a common symptom in prior studies and fit conceptually with the avoidance/numbing symptoms. An entirely new cluster was added that contained three symptoms that had also been frequently observed: new separation anxiety, new aggression, and new fears that seemed unrelated to trauma reminders. These symptoms did not fit conceptually into the existing cluster so they were placed in a new cluster for further research. Finally, the algorithm threshold was changed so that only one avoidance/numbing symptom (cluster C) was needed instead of three. Only one hyperarousal symptom (cluster D) was needed instead of two. One symptom from the new cluster was needed. (pp. 561–562)

Among 62 children exposed to high-magnitude stressors, none met DSM-IV criteria for PTSD, though 67.9% had at least one symptom of criterion B, reexperiencing (Scheeringa et al., 2003). After examining several alternatives, the researchers concluded that the optimal algorithm was one symptom of both criteria B and C and two of criterion D. Scheeringa and colleagues used this algorithm to diagnose 26% of the young children with PTSD. Children diagnosed with PTSD using this method (Scheering, Zeanah, Myers, & Putnam, 2005) were significantly more likely than those not diagnosed with PTSD to show functional impairment 1 and 2 years later, and were more likely 2 years later to be diagnosed with PTSD using DSM-IV criteria per the National Institute of Mental Health (NIMH) Diagnostic Interview Schedule for Children, Version IV (DISC—Shaffer, Fisher, & Lucas, 2000; see Appendix 9.3). Importantly, other research has replicated these findings (Ippen, Briscoe-Smith, & Lieberman, 2004; Ohmi et al., 2002). Much of the criteria used in Scheeringa and Zeanah's measure (see Posttraumatic Stress Disorder Semistructured Interview and Observational Record for Infants and Young Children in Appendix 9.4 for the current version of the measure used) has been adopted for use in the Diagnostic Classification of Mental Health and Developmental Disorders of Infancy and Early Childhood: Revised Edition (DC:0–3R; Zero to Three, 2005) diagnosis of PTSD in this age group.

UNDERSTANDABILITY OF QUESTIONS

It also is important to determine the extent to which all informants, child and adult, are able to understand the meaning of each question asked of them. Too many assessment tools for children and adolescents have been based on adult measures, with no attempt to rewrite questions to make them more child-friendly. One of the original and most widely used measures of childhood PTSD, the Child Posttraumatic Stress Reaction Index (CPTS-RI—Frederick et al., 1992; see Appendix 9.5), is an unfortunate example of this problem. The clinician should carefully read and assess each measurement tool prior to administering it to caregiver or child and be ready to provide clarifying prompts or explanations, if respondents do not appear to understand any question.

ASSESS THE FULL RANGE OF RESPONSES

The assessment of posttraumatic symptomatology should include the full range of possible reactions. Thus, it should ideally include an assessment of ASD symptomatology, especially if the event occurred less than 1 month prior to the assessment. The dissociative symptoms of ASD are rarely assessed in measures of the core DSM-IV criteria of PTSD, even though the presence of such symptoms more than 1 month after the occurrence of the event(s) may be indicative of more severe reactions to the traumatic event(s). Moreover, if the event(s) to which the child's reactions are being assessed might qualify as "early onset, multiple, extended, and sometimes highly invasive traumatic events, frequently of an interpersonal nature, often involving a significant amount of stigma or shame" (Briere & Spinazzola, 2005, p. 401), then the clinician should attempt to assess possible symptoms of complex PTSD as well. This is particularly important because, as noted earlier, there is evidence that treating the distinctive symptoms of complex PTSD as comorbid conditions rather than as an integral part of the posttraumatic response can lead to markedly reduced response to treatment (van der Kolk & Courtois, 2005; van der Kolk et al., 2005).

Approximate onset dates of traumatic symptoms should be ascertained as often as possible. Only those symptoms with onset after exposure can be considered diagnostic of ASD or PTSD. Duration of symptoms can provide evidence regarding the severity of the traumatic response as well. Some assessment tools ascertain whether symptoms have occurred within the past week or past month. Others specifically determine dates of onset for symptoms that children endorse. Clinicians should be mindful that children younger than 8 years vary in their ability to answer reliably time-related questions about date of onset and duration, or even whether symptoms have occurred within a specific time frame, such as 1 month ago. Certainly children younger than 6 years have great difficulty with such concepts, and caregivers must be relied upon for such information. Caregivers, too, however, are often limited in their ability to answer such questions, particularly if the symptoms refer to internal states. Even their dating of externalizing behaviors may be inaccurate, if onset occurred outside their purview, such as during recess time at school or afterschool play. Therefore, assessments of onset and duration of symptoms should be considered approximations rather than definitive responses.

When responses from different sources conflict, the child's responses should be considered the most compelling, particularly if the questions concern internal processes, unless there are reasons to question the veracity of the child's statements or his or her ability to recall or articulate the experiences. Generally, the older the child, the more weight his or her responses should be accorded. Responses of primary caregivers, whether parent, grandparent, stepparent, or other, should generally carry nearly as much weight as the child's responses, perhaps even more in some cases, such as those regarding externalizing behaviors. When considering the responses of others who have some knowledge of the child, keep in mind the circumstances under which the respondent and the child normally interact. Teachers, for example, tend to interact with their students in a much narrower set of situations than do primary caregivers, even though the teachers spend several hours a day, 5 days a week with their students. Fathers, or the family's primary source of income, too, may spend less time with the child than do mothers, or the family's primary caregiver, in general. In the final analysis, children who are age 8 and older might be considered to know more about their own experiences, especially their own internal processes, than any adult who knows or cares for them.

Caregiver Assessment

When possible, it is often helpful to obtain as much information as possible from adults in the child's life regarding the stressor(s) to which the child has been exposed, and the child's reactions to the stressor(s), before interviewing the child in any depth concerning his or her experience. In addition to providing valuable information regarding specific details of the traumatic event or stressor(s), caregivers also can supply information about the child's level of functioning. Primary caregivers provide the most detailed and accurate reports about the child's experiences, behavior, and emotional and social life prior to and after the occurrence of the stressful event(s). If the child is of school age, a report on the child's performance at school, including academic performance, social behavior at school, activity level, and interactions with teachers and other authority figures, may provide information complementary to that of the caregiver regarding the child's posttraumatic functioning outside the home, in situations where the caregiver is rarely present.

Child Assessment

After interviewing the child's caregiver, the clinician should then interview the child, and starts by eliciting the child's understanding of the reason for the referral. The clinician encourages the child to describe the experience(s) from his or her own point of view. Asking for some description of the stressful experience(s) is useful in many ways, because it allows the clinician to develop a picture of the child's subjective experience during and immediately after the traumatic event, and provides an indication of the detail and accuracy of the child's memories of the event(s). It is primarily the child's *perception* of the experience and its consequences, rather than the "objective" description of the event(s) or the caregiver's perceptions of the event, that affects the child's reactions: what he or she saw and experienced, what those experiences meant to the child during the event and afterwards, and, in particular, what thoughts and feelings the experience evoked in the child. At the same time, the child should be allowed to give as much, or as little, information as he or she is willing to divulge during the first interview. More information may be forthcoming as the child becomes more comfortable with the interviewer and the interview process itself.

The clinician tries to discover who or what the child considers responsible for the event(s), whether the child feels responsible to any degree, and whether the child feels that he or she reacted inappropriately to the event(s), or could or should have reacted differently. It is important to determine the extent to which the child *perceives* caregivers and important others to have been distressed by the experience themselves. The younger the child, the more likely his or her reactions are a reflection of the reactions of caregivers and important others (Fletcher, 2003). The interviewer should also attempt to evaluate the level of support the child feels he or she has received from caregivers and important others. In addition, an

understanding of the extent to which the child feels the experience has resulted, or will result, in stigmatization or ostracism by family or peers may be helpful during both the assessment process and treatment. In a similar vein, the interviewer should attempt to determine the child's perceptions concerning his or her reactions to the stressful event(s), in particular, whether the child feels that his or her reactions are "normal." Reassuring children regarding misattributions of self-responsibility for the event(s) and the "normality" of any reactions to it may encourage children to describe their experiences and reactions more openly and honestly, as well as relieve some of their distress.

Assessing the Stressor

Prior to assessing the child's reactions to exposure to a potentially traumatic event or events, the clinician must first develop an understanding of the stressful experience itself. When possible, a detailed description of the events leading up to, during, and following the stressor is important when assessing the child's reactions to the stressful event(s). Discrepancies between the child's description and the "actual" event may provide useful diagnostic information. If a primary caregiver was not present, reports from other sources, including police reports, news reports, and reports of emergency response teams, may be useful in developing a description of the stressor prior to hearing the child's own description.

Assessing Exposure to High-Magnitude Stressors

In some cases, the clinician may not know whether the child has ever been exposed to a high-magnitude stressor. This is often the case when a child is being administered a general psychiatric examination, for example. In those situations, it may be necessary to ask whether or not the child has ever experienced any of a list of potential high-magnitude stressors. Such lists are included in the PTSD module of nearly all of the general child psychiatric interviews listed in Appendix 9.3. There are also standalone measures of exposure to stressful experiences available. These are described in Appendix 9.1. Some of these measures assess only exposure to high-magnitude stressors. Other measures assess a wide array of stressors, including not only potentially high-magnitude stressors, such as abuse, kidnapping, torture, or natural disasters, but also stressors of generally lesser magnitude (e.g., overnight stay in a hospital prior to routine surgery to remove the child's tonsils, the death of a pet, or extended periods of separation from the caregiver, especially at earlier ages), to which past exposure might contribute to the child's reactions to a more current high-magnitude stressor.

Few of the measures that assess only exposure to high-magnitude stressors described in Appendix 9.1 have been examined for their psychometric properties, and none have had both their reliability and validity assessed. Of those with some evidence of acceptable to good test–retest and interrater reliability, the Traumatic Events Screening Inventory (TESI; Ford et al., 2002) seems to show the most promise. Available in both child and parent forms, the TESI is an interview that comprises 16 questions regarding high-magnitude stressors, arranged so that questions about exposure to the lowest magnitude stressors are first and those regarding sexual abuse are last, to help the child and parent tolerate the potentially stressful nature of the questions. Probes assist the interviewer to determine whether or not any endorsed event met both parts of criterion A of DSM-IV PTSD diagnosis. If criterion A is met for a particular type of stressor, the interviewer asks for more specifics about the event(s), the age of the child when it occurred, who else was involved, and whether anyone was hurt and needed medical attention. The TESI is designed to assess exposure to high magnitude stressors among children aged 8 to 18. The parent form (TESI-P—Ghosh Ippen et al., 2002; see Appendix 9.1) was designed to assess children ages 0–18 years. The interviewer should be a qualified mental health professional, or an advanced trainee supervised by a qualified mental health professional.

Assessing Exposure to a Range of Stressors

The AACAP practice parameters for the assessment and treatment of children and adolescents with PTSD (Cohen et al., 1998) emphasize that to develop a full understanding of the child's reactions to any particular high-magnitude stressor, the clinician must understand the child's history of and reactions to a wide range of possible stressors, such as significant family conflict, separation or divorce, frequency of moves, school changes, family deaths, illnesses,

and exposure to domestic and community violence. To accomplish this, it is recommended that some measure of exposure to lifetime stressors be administered to the parent and/or child—preferably both, whenever possible—to help determine the extent to which the child has been exposed to a range of stressors, *in addition to* high-magnitude stressors.

Several instruments are available to assess both high-magnitude stressors and those of a generally lesser magnitude. The appropriateness of the measures described in Appendix 9.1 depends on the developmental level of the child, adolescent, or young adult who is being assessed.

ASSESSING STRESSORS IN PRESCHOOL AND SCHOOL-AGE CHILDREN

There are currently no measures that assess a full range of high-, moderate-, and low-magnitude stressors among preschool or school-age children. Only some of the interviews and self-report measures with good psychometric properties that assess a child's exposure to community violence also assess sexual abuse, physical abuse, and neglect, and none assesses stressors of lesser magnitude. The Juvenile Victimization Questionnaire (JVQ—Finkelhor, Hamby, Ormrod, & Turner, 2005; see Appendix 9.1), a very promising new measure with good psychometric properties, assesses exposure to (1) conventional crime, (2) child maltreatment, (3) peer and sibling victimization, (4) sexual victimization, and (5) witnessing and indirect victimization. Exposure is assessed for the previous year and over the lifetime of the child. As an interview, the JVQ can be used with children 8 years and older. It can be administered in a self-report format with juveniles 12 years and older, including young adults. A parent version of the JVQ can be used to assess the exposure history of children age 2 years and older.

The Preschool Age Psychiatric Assessment (PAPA) Life Events Scale (Egger & Angold, 2004; Appendix 9.1) is part of the full PAPA psychiatric assessment interview (see Appendix 9.3). The Life Events Scale assesses a particularly good selection of high- and lesser-magnitude stressors in the lives of the very youngest children, ages 3–6 years, such as a reduction in the family's standard of living, attending unsafe day care, a detailed history of accidents and hospitalization, separation from significant attachment figures for more than 1 week, and becoming homeless. These potentially stressful experiences for very young children are rarely assessed by other stressor scales and interviews. Related interviews include life events scales for older children and adolescents ages 9–17 (Child and Adolescent Psychiatric Assessment [CAPA] Life Events Scale; Angold & Costello, 2000, Tables 5 and 6) and for young adults 18 years or older (Young Adult Psychiatric Assessment [YAPA] Life Events Scale; Angold & Costello, 2000, Tables 5 and 6).

The Tough Times Checklist (Fletcher, 1996f; Appendix 9.1) is a self-report measure for children with a third-grade or higher reading level (approximately age 7 years and older), that assesses the child's lifetime exposure to stressors of both high and moderate magnitude. It does not assess any type of sexual abuse or neglect, although the child is asked whether any peers, adult strangers, or known adults ever made him or her do "something horrible." Assessors are then required to inquire as to the nature of that event, if the child endorses it. Children indicate whether they have ever experienced each of the stressors. A version for adolescents, the Teen Tough Times Checklist (Fletcher, 1996f; Appendix 9.1) assesses exposure in the previous year and over the lifetime to the same stressors included in the Tough Times Checklist. Rather than a simple checklist, respondents rate each stressor on a 4-point scale: *Never happened* (0); *Happened, but the worst time was not upsetting* (1); *Happened, and the worst time was somewhat upsetting* (2); and *Happened, and the worst time was very upsetting* (3). A caregiver version for children of any age, the Child's Upsetting Times Checklist (Fletcher, 1996f; Appendix 9.1) asks the caregiver to rate the child's exposure to the same stressors, using the same response format as the Teen Tough Times Checklist. Of these three related measures, the Child's Upsetting Times Checklist is the only one that has any psychometric information. It has been shown to correlate significantly with both the child's own report and the parent's report of the child's PTSD symptomatology (Fletcher, 1996b).

ASSESSING STRESSORS IN ADOLESCENTS AND YOUNG ADULTS

The Young Adults Upsetting Times Checklist, a paper-and-pencil self-report measure (Fletcher, 1996f; Fletcher & Skidmore, 1997), is currently the only available measure of stressor exposure for adolescents and young adults that assesses both moderate- and high-magnitude stressors, including a variety of sexual abuse experiences, both prior to and after age 18 years. It has accumulated good evidence for its reliability and validity. The measure is suitable for adolescents, young adults, and older adults. Depending on the maturity of the child, it might be suitable for children as young as 11 or 12 years. Respondents rate each item as *Never happened* (0); *Happened, but the worst time was not upsetting* (1); *Happened, and the worst time was somewhat upsetting* (2); *Happened, and the worst time was very upsetting* (3); and *Happened, and the worst time was extremely upsetting* (4). Two additional items ask respondents to rate (1) the worst thing that happened to them in the past year and (2) the worst thing that ever happened to them prior to the last year. Total scores can be computed for the previous year, for any time before the past year, and for any time over the lifetime, including the past year. Each of these totals correlates significantly with measures of posttraumatic stress (see Appendix 9.1 for more details).

Assessing the Traumatic Characteristics of Stressful Events

Simple assessment of the kinds and number of potentially stressful events to which children have been exposed can provide useful information, but it is unlikely to tell the whole story regarding the child's peritraumatic experience. No two events are exactly alike. Even stressful events of the same type are likely to differ substantially from each other. Moreover, the same event is never experienced either subjectively or objectively in exactly the same way by people who live through it together. Each stressful event is a unique phenomenological experience for everyone who lives through it. The fact that not everyone who lives through the same high-magnitude stressor develops PTSD illustrates this point. Despite this, the literature does suggest that specific characteristics or dimensions of high-magnitude stressors increase the likelihood that anyone exposed to events that manifest these dimensions will react with symptoms of PTSD (Fletcher, 2003).

The Dimensions of Stressful Events (DOSE) scale (Fletcher, 1996d) was designed to assess the characteristics or dimensions of high-magnitude stressor events suggested by the literature to increase the likelihood of a child or adolescent responding with PTSD symptomatology. The measure is divided into two sections. The first section contains 25 items that assess such things as the child's proximity to the event; viewing of blood; whether anyone was injured or killed; whether the child was separated from caretakers; the child's relationship to any perpetrator and other victims; the perception of stigmatization associated with the experience(s); the suddenness and unexpectedness of the event(s); the perceived uncontrollability of the event(s); the duration and frequency of exposure to the event(s); whether the event was caused by humans rather than nature; whether the adverse consequences of the event(s) are long lasting, irreversible, and liable to recur; whether the event(s) involved moral conflicts for the child; whether the child perceived the event(s) as a threat to family or friends; and whether the event(s) originated within the family. The second DOSE section contains 24 items that assess the frequency and degree of child abuse experiences, as well as experiences that may mitigate the child's responses, such as the extent to which the parents support the child's claim. The psychometric properties of the first section (none are yet available for the second section) are very good. Scores on the DOSE appear to provide better prediction of adverse outcomes than do counts of the number of lifetime stressors to which a child has been exposed (Fletcher, 1996b; Fletcher, Cox, Skidmore, Janssens, & Render, 1997; Fletcher, Spilsbury, Creedan, & Friedman, 2006). These results suggest that the DOSE might provide a means of screening for posttraumatic stress responses without asking about any DSM-IV symptomatic responses. See Appendix 9.2 for more details on psychometric properties of the measure.

ASSESSING EMOTIONAL RESPONSES TO HIGH-MAGNITUDE STRESSORS

Interviews. Determining that the child has been exposed to high-magnitude stressors with characteristics that increase the likelihood of traumatic responses meets only the first half of DSM-IV criterion A. The clinician also must determine that the child's "response involved intense fear, helplessness, or horror" or "disorganized or agitated behavior" (see Table 9.1). Most of the general psychiatric interviews that

have PTSD modules (see Appendix 9.3) include questions designed to assess the child's response to their potentially traumatic experience, although some interviews are more thorough than others in that they ask about several specific kinds of possible responses, while others try to make do with one or two very general questions. It is generally best to be more specific when asking questions of children and adolescents. Few interviews that ask about specific responses sacrifice much time to do so; therefore, when choosing from among general psychiatric interviews, the Child and Adolescent Psychiatric Assessment (CAPA) Scale (Angold & Costello, 2000) and its associated versions for preschool children (the PAPA) and for young adults (the YAPA), would seem the best choice, because each explores the child's responses in more detail than do others, while not sacrificing too much time in the process. If one prefers to focus only on the assessment of PTSD and does not wish to conduct a full-scale diagnostic interview but would still like to conduct an interview, the Children's PTSD Inventory (CPTSDI; Saigh, 1998a, 1998b) is a good choice. It asks preliminary questions about four types of high-magnitude stressors to which children might be exposed, followed by four questions on their reactions to any stressor.

Self-Report Questionnaires. If an interview is not possible, or if a self-report assessment tool is required to examine children's responses to high-magnitude stressors, perhaps as part of a screening process, then the choices currently are limited. For exposure to high-magnitude stressors that do not involve abuse, the Exposure Questionnaire (EQ—Nader, 1993, 1999; see Appendix 9.2) might be a good choice. Similar to the DOSE, the EQ assesses aspects of the event(s) associated with increased PTSD symptomatology—such as whether there was threat to life, threat of injury, subjective proximity to the events, relationship to victims, worries about others, property damage, and helping efforts. In addition, it assesses the child or adolescent's emotional reactions during the event, such as helplessness, fear, horror, panic, and guilt, both during and after the traumatic experience. It inquires about the frequency and intensity of the reactions. Two versions are available, one for Postwar Questions and one for Postdisaster or Violence Questions. Scores on the *EQ* have been shown to be associated with exposure and severity levels for children in war zones (Nader & Fairbanks, 1994; Nader, Pynoos, Fairbanks, Al-Ajeel, & Al-Asfour, 1993), providing some preliminary evidence of the validity of the measure. Another, shorter scale that might be considered, the Peritraumatic Response Scale (Pfefferbaum et al., 2002), consists of just 12 questions that address the child's peritraumatic responses of fear, arousal, and dissociation at the time of the incident. Unfortunately, no information about its psychometric properties is currently available.

When assessing the peritraumatic responses of children who have been abused, the Children's Peritraumatic Experiences Questionnaire (CPEQ—Wolfe & Birt, 1993; see Appendix 9.2) is an appropriate choice. The CPEQ is a 33-item scale designed to assess children's emotional reactions during their sexual abuse experiences, or for nonabused children, their most negative life experience. The CPEQ assesses feelings and thoughts of helplessness, fear, terror, sadness, and anger related to DSM-IV criterion A2. Items are divided into five subscales, derived from a principal components analysis: Extreme Reactions (e.g., thoughts of being killed or killing the perpetrator, fear of death and injury, becoming ill, wanting to throw something, terror, or fainting), Fear/Anxiety, Negative Affect, Dissociation, and Guilt. The measure appears to have good psychometric properties (Wolfe & Birt, 2002b; see Appendix 9.2). The CPEQ is now included with the Children's Impact of Traumatic Events Scale–II (CITES-II—Wolfe et al., 1991; see Appendix 9.5).

Assessing the Full Range of Posttraumatic Stress Reactions

Assessing ASD

ASSESSING ASD WITH A GENERAL PSYCHIATRIC INTERVIEW

There are currently very few measures of ASD available for children ages 6–18 (see Appendix 9.3). An exception is the Children's Interview for Psychiatric Syndromes (ChIPS—Rooney, Fristad, Weller, & Weller, 1999; Weller, Weller, Fristad, Rooney, & Schecter, 2000; Weller, Weller, Rooney, & Fristad, 1999), a highly structured interview that screens for 20 DSM-IV Axis I disorders, as well as psychosocial stressors such as emotional, physical, or sexual abuse and neglect. In doing so, it assesses both ASD and PTSD. If the stressor occurred within

4 weeks of the interview, children are asked six questions to assess whether they reacted with symptoms of dissociation or derealization, such as whether they have felt as if they were not themselves and as if they were no longer real (depersonalization), and whether they have trouble remembering things about the event(s). Then seven questions are asked that assess reexperiencing symptoms, two that assess feeling "upset" by reminders of the experience(s), and one that assesses physical reactions to reminders, such as stomachaches or trouble breathing. If none of these symptoms is endorsed, the rest of the Stress Disorder questions are skipped. Otherwise, 10 questions are asked that assess symptoms of avoidance and withdrawal. If at least one of these is answered in the affirmative, one question is asked about changes in moods or emotions since the event(s), one about feelings of numbness since the event(s), and two about anticipating a foreshortened future (feeling as if one will not live a long life). Then six questions are asked about symptoms of overarousal, anger, and difficulty concentrating. If none of these questions is endorsed, one question is asked about a tendency to startle easily.

The interviewer is provided with two algorithms to determine whether the child meets criteria for ASD or PTSD, or neither. Next the child is asked when the symptoms began, then whether he or she is still troubled by the symptoms; if not, an attempt is made to determine when the symptoms stopped. Children who meet criteria for ASD are asked whether the symptoms began within 4 weeks of the event(s), lasted more than 2 days, and lasted for less than 4 weeks. Children who meet criteria for PTSD are asked whether the symptoms have lasted longer than 1 month. Finally, children are asked whether "these problems cause you trouble" at home, at school, and with other kids. If the duration of symptoms can be determined, the interviewer can indicate whether the PTSD can be classified as acute or chronic in duration, and whether or not symptoms had a regular onset (within 6 months of the event[s]) or a delayed onset (more than 6 months after the event[s]). ChIPS is designed to be administered by people with at least a bachelor's degree in a field associated with mental health. It is recommended that a clinician familiar with DSM-IV who has undergone similar training on ChIPS train lay interviewers. Unfortunately, the psychometric properties of the ChIPS have yet to be established satisfactorily (see Appendix 9.3).

ASSESSING ASD WITH A CARETAKER REPORT OF ASD AND PTSD

The Child Stress Disorders Checklist (CSDC; Saxe, 2004) is a 42-item, paper-and-pencil scale that asks parents, guardians, or other observers to report on the child's reaction to high-magnitude stressors. Unlike most other child PTSD measures to date, the CSDC allows assessment of symptoms of both DSM-IV PTSD and ASD. The respondent is first asked to indicate whether the child has been exposed to any of eight kinds of high-magnitude stressors, including an "other" category. Age of exposure is requested for all endorsed stressors. Next, five questions are asked regarding the child's emotional reactions to the experience(s), then seven items assess symptoms of reexperiencing, five assess avoidance, eight assess numbing and dissociation, six assess increased arousal, and four assess functional impairment. Responses to each question can be either *Not true* (as far as you know), *Somewhat true*, or *Very true*. Psychometric properties for the measure are currently sparse but encouraging (see Appendix 9.5).

ASD SELF-REPORT

There is currently only one self-report measure devoted to the assessment of ASD in children. Fortunately, it appears to have very good psychometric properties (see Appendix 9.7 for details). The Acute Stress Checklist for Children (ASC-Kids; Kassam-Adams, 2006), a 29-item self-report measure, comprises 25 items assessing ASD according to DSM-IV criteria: 4 items assessing whether the experience was horrible, frightening, beyond the child or adolescent's control, or whether the child feared for his or her life; 4 items assessing emotional numbing, derealization, and dissociation; 15 items assessing the remaining DSM-IV criteria; 1 item assessing the degree to which the child or adolescent was emotionally upset by the experience; 1 item assessing disruptions to social interaction with meaningful others; 2 items assessing social functioning at school and with the immediate family; 1 item assessing social support; and 1 item assessing self-perceived coping skill. Most response categories are *Never/Not true* (0), *Sometimes/Somewhat* (1) and *Often/Very true* (2). Items rated a score of 2 indicate that

a DSM-IV symptom is present. Symptom category subscales include Dissociation, Reexperiencing, Avoidance, and Overarousal/Anxiety. The ASC-Kids is appropriate for children ages 8–17, although the author suggests that the items should be read to children age 9 and younger, as well as to any 10- or 11-year-old who appears to require assistance.

Assessing PTSD

ASSESSING PTSD WITH A GENERAL PSYCHIATRIC INTERVIEW

Several general psychiatric interviews for children that include PTSD modules are available (see Appendix 9.3). Of these, the Diagnostic Interview for Children and Adolescents—Revised (DICA-R; Kaplan & Reich, 1991) was among the first to include a PTSD module. A semistructured interview, the DICA-R is a modification of the Diagnostic Interview for Children and Adolescents (DICA; Herjanic & Reich, 1983a, 1983b), developed to allow the assessment of diagnoses in children 6–17 years old. The DICA-R, a modified form of the DICA, allows assessment of DSM-III-R criteria. Questions were rephrased in a more conversational manner, and questions related to DSM-III-R diagnoses were added (Kaplan & Reich, 1991), including a PTSD module. The DICA-R was then itself revised to allow assessment of DSM-IV diagnoses. There are versions for younger children, ages 6–12 years, for adolescents, and for parents. The time required for administration of the full DICA-R is approximately 1.5 hours. With training, the interview may be administered by research assistants with no more than a bachelor's degree.

Unfortunately, psychometric information on the DICA-R is questionable. Some 7-year-olds have been reported to have difficulty understanding some of the DICA-R questions, supposedly written for interviewing 6- to 12-year-olds (reported in Nader, 1997). The PTSD module was unable to distinguish between adolescents who were exposed to wildfires and those who were not (Jones, Ribbe, & Cunningham, 1994). To add to the confusion, the DICA-R has been replaced by the Missouri Assessment of Genetics Interview for Children (MAGIC—Reich & Todd, 2002; see Appendix 9.3), for which full psychometric information is still unavailable.

The Child and Adolescent Psychiatric Assessment Scale (CAPA; Angold & Costello,

2000) appears to be one of the few general child psychiatric interviews containing a PTSD module for which there is specific information regarding its reliability and validity. However, psychometric properties for the PTSD module are still sketchy at this point. The CAPA was designed to be administered to children between the ages of 9 and 17 years. A version for young adults, the Young Adults Psychiatric Assessment (YAPA; see Appendix 9.6) is also available, although there is not yet any psychometric information for the interview. The Preschool Age Psychiatric Assessment (PAPA—Egger & Angold, 2004; Egger, Ascher, & Angold, 1999; Egger et al., 2004; see Appendix 9.3) is a substantial rewrite of the CAPA for preschool children ages 3–6 years. Changes include DSM-IV and ICD-10 criteria that better reflect experiences of younger children. Symptoms and diagnoses included in the Diagnostic Classification of Mental Health and Developmental Disorders of Infancy and Early Childhood, Revised Edition (DC:0–3R; Zero to Three, 2005) were added to the PAPA as well. Relevant items from other preschool measures not covered by the CAPA also were included. Changes appropriate for preschool children were made to the family functioning and relationships sections. Alternate PTSD and reactive attachment disorder diagnostic criteria were based on criteria suggested by Zeanah, Boris, and Scheeringa (Boris, Zeanah, Larrieu, Scheeringa, & Heller, 1998; Scheeringa et al., 1995, 2001; Scheeringa & Zeanah, 1995). Detailed information is gathered by the PAPA regarding 21 changes in the child's behaviors, emotions, or relationships that might have occurred as a result of exposure to the potentially traumatizing event(s), such as new fears or anxieties, increased crying, increased aggression, regression of toileting skills or language, and changes in the child's interactions with others (Egger & Angold, 2004). Each symptom is rated for frequency, intensity, duration, and date of onset. If the caregiver indicates that at least one high-magnitude stressor has occurred in the child's life, and if the caregiver believes that experience is related to at least one symptom (new fears, separation anxiety, etc.), then the interviewer asks the questions in the PTSD section. PAPA requires the same type and duration of training as is required for the CAPA and YAPA. Certification by a qualified PAPA trainer is required before using the PAPA in the field. Unfortunately, very little psycho-

metric information is yet available for the PAPA.

Another promising general psychiatric interview for children, the ChIPS (Rooney et al., 1999; Weller et al., 1999, 2000) was discussed earlier in the section that describes measures of ASD, because it assesses both ASD and PTSD.

PTSD-SPECIFIC CHILD INTERVIEWS

PTSD Interviews for Preschool Children. Levonn: A Cartoon-Based Structured Interview for Assessing Young Children's Distress Symptoms (Martinez & Richters, 1993; Richters, Martinez, & Valla, 1990) was written for young, school-age children. Shahinfar, Fox, and Leavitt (2000) devised a version for preschool children. Levonn, a 39-item, cartoon-based, structured interview of children's distress symptoms, is based on an earlier cartoon-based interview of general psychiatric symptoms, Dominique (Valla, 1989). The Dominique interview was revised, so that the main character Levonn represents an urban child. The Levonn includes cartoons of symptoms associated with PTSD, with two- or three-sentence scripts included for each cartoon. The response format comprises three thermometers filled with varying degrees of mercury, indicating increasing levels of frequency. Thermometers are labeled *Never, Some of the time*, and *A lot of the time*. Before administration of the PTSD interview, children are taught how to use the thermometer response format correctly.

After each cartoon is described by the interviewer, children draw a circle around a thermometer to indicate how often they have felt like Levonn. On one page, for example, the three thermometers take up the top one-third of the page. On the right, lower half of the page are three cartoons, laid out vertically, one over the other. In the top cartoon, a frowning young boy with a white face is shown in his pajamas walking somewhat slouched over away from a bed, with his head slightly bent down. The middle cartoon shows the boy, now dressed for school, walking, again slouched over, head bent, and frowning, dragging a book bag along the ground. In the bottom cartoon, Levonn, again in pajamas, stands facing his bed, frowning, with his head bent. In the middle of the left bottom portion of the page is the following script, which the interviewer reads to the child being interviewed: "Here is Levonn feeling very sad for a whole day. He gets up in the morning feeling sad, he feels sad all day, and he still feels sad at bedtime. How many times have you felt like Levonn?" (Martinez & Richters, 1993, p. 26). The scale comprises four subscales measuring Depression, Anxiety/Recurring Thoughts, Sleep Problems, and Impulsiveness.

In the revised version for preschoolers (Shahinfar et al., 2000), the symptoms assessed include sadness, lack of appetite, fear of going outside because of possible violence, intrusive traumatic memories, and nightmares. Thus, a DSM-IV diagnosis is not possible with Levonn. In a study of 155 primarily (98.8%) African American children between the ages of 3.5 and 4.5, the authors carefully debriefed children after administering the revised Levonn. Shahinfar and colleagues reported that very few of the children indicated either verbally or behaviorally that they had been upset by the interview. Unfortunately, most of the available psychometric data are based on the original Levonn for school-age children.

PTSD Interviews for School-Age Children and Older. The Clinician-Administered PTSD Scale for Children and Adolescents (CAPS-CA—Newman et al., 2004; see Appendix 9.5) is an interview based on the Clinician-Administered PTSD Scale for adults (CAPS; Weathers et al., 2004). The CAPS-CA is currently considered the "gold standard" interview for childhood PTSD. Comprising approximately 53 items that assess things such as the intensity of the experience and its duration, it is an extremely complete, detailed, well-thought-out interview. The PTSD-specific items inquire about the occurrence, intensity, and frequency of endorsed symptoms both for the past month and over the lifetime. The interview begins with a script to establish the meaning of a month's time for those younger children who might have trouble with the concept. To establish criterion A, 17 different types of high-magnitude stressors are described one by one, and the child or adolescent is asked to indicate whether each event actually happened to him or her, or whether he or she *Saw it, Learned about it,* is *Not sure,* or it *Never happened* to him or her. If none of the 17 events is endorsed, four additional prompts are provided to attempt to elicit an experience of a high-magnitude stressor. If three or more events are endorsed, the interviewer tries to determine whether the experiences evoked fear or terror, a sense of helplessness, horror, or disorganized agitation. Various optional prompts for eliciting this information are provided the interviewer, using wording appropriate for children and adolescents. The interviewer rates whether each event was a life threat, a serious injury or threat to physical integrity, and whether each of the four emotional reactions just listed occurred when the exposure occurred.

When a child's responses meet DSM-IV criterion A, questions related to each symptom listed in DSM-IV are administered. First, a practice question teaches the child or adolescent how to respond to the questions about frequency and intensity of events. After questions that assess DSM-IV criteria B–D, two questions related to the duration of symptoms (criterion E) are then asked, followed by four questions regarding subjective distress and social, scholastic, and developmental (loss of acquired skill) functioning (criterion F). Three global rating scales are available: (1) overall validity of the responses, (2) overall severity of PTSD symptoms, and (3) improvement for instances of repeated administration of the interview over time. Six items examine the presence of seven associated features: guilt over acts of commission or omission, survivor guilt when there were multiple victims, shame, reduction of awareness of surroundings, derealization, depersonalization, and changes in attachment. Three open-ended questions determine how the child or adolescent thinks the event has affected his or her life, what has helped him or her feel better since the event, and what coping strategies he or she uses.

The interviewer's guide and summary scoring sheet for the CAPS-CA (Newman et al., 2004) includes scoring for ASD, although no algorithms are provided for actually deriving a diagnosis of ASD. There is a lot to like about the CAPS-CA but, unfortunately, despite the general conception that the CAPS-CA represents the "gold standard" for the assessment of childhood PTSD, the psychometric properties of the interview have yet to be thoroughly explored. Moreover, although no information is available on the average administration time required by the interview for children who have PTSD symptoms, the level of detail required by the full interview is likely to take a considerable amount of time. However, the authors do indicate that "it is possible to customize the interview by eliminating less relevant components or changing the time frames" (p.

4). Still, the dearth of psychometric information for the CAPS-CA (see Appendix 9.5 for details) means it cannot yet be recommended for clinical use.

The Children's PTSD Inventory (CPTSDI; Saigh, 1998a, 1998b), an interview for children ages 7 years and older, has excellent psychometric data (see Appendix 9.5). In fact, the procedures followed by Saigh and his colleagues (2000) for developing and assessing the psychometric properties of their interview could serve as a model for anyone who wishes to examine the psychometric characteristics of a new measure. The CPTSDI is a 47-question interview designed to provide a DSM-IV diagnosis of childhood PTSD. The child is first read a sample list of traumatic events, then is asked four questions to examine exposure to high-magnitude stressors, and four questions to assess possible traumatic reactivity to the exposure, per both parts of criterion A of DSM-IV. If this criterion is not met, the interview terminates. Eleven questions examine the presence or absence of symptoms of intrusion (criterion B of DSM-IV). Sixteen questions address criterion C, avoidance and numbing symptoms. Seven questions address criterion D symptoms of overarousal. Five questions assess the duration of symptoms (criterion E) and significant impairment in functioning (criterion F). Each item measures a symptom or criterion and is scored as present or absent. The interview requires 15–20 minutes when administered to youth with a trauma history, and only 5 minutes to administer to youth with no trauma history (Saigh et al., 2000). The psychometric properties of the CPTSDI make it the best choice for a PTSD-specific interview for children age 7 years and older.

PTSD-SPECIFIC CHILD PAPER-AND-PENCIL SELF-REPORTS

Self-reports for preschool children are rare, and the few that are available tend to be cartoon based (e.g., Levonn, described above; see Appendix 9.4), and tend to assess symptoms that are not directly associated with DSM-IV PTSD criteria. The Posttraumatic Symptom Inventory for Children (PT-SIC; Eisen, 1997), a promising self-report measure for children ages 4–8 that does attempt to assess the DSM-IV PTSD criteria, is a 30-item questionnaire that assesses PTSD symptoms based on DSM-IV criteria. Questions are read to the child by the clinician or administrator and are addressed in two stages. A child is first asked if a symptom ever happens. If the child answers affirmatively, he or she is asked to indicate the frequency of such occurrences: *A real lot—like everyday* (scored 2) or *Just sometimes* (scored 1). The PT-SIC includes a checklist to screen for 11 high-magnitude stressors (e.g., car crashes, sexual abuse, witnessing or being a victim of community violence). The PT-SIC is a newer scale and cannot yet be considered to have established psychometric properties, but its use with children ages 4–8 years might provide useful insight into the young child's personal reactions to exposure to high-magnitude stressors.

Although several child paper-and-pencil self-report measures are currently available, few assess all of the core DSM-IV criteria A–F symptoms or have amassed enough evidence of reliability and validity to make them good candidates for clinical use. The Child Posttraumatic Stress Reaction Index (CPTS-RI—Frederick et al., 1992; also known as the PTSD-RI and the CPTSD-RI) was one of the first measures written to assess childhood PTSD. It has become the most frequently used outcome measure in research on childhood PTSD. Based on Frederick's (1985a, 1985b) measure of PTSD in adults, the CPTS-RI does not appear to have ever been assessed for readability or reading level among children, which is troubling, because some of the language might be considered confusing for adults. Originally intended to be used as an interview, the CPTS-RI has frequently been used as a self-report measure in research, with little or no evidence that it is suitable for such use. Information on the psychometric properties was nonexistent for quite some time, and that currently available is minimal (see Appendix 9.5). Moreover, the measure was never intended to be used to make PTSD diagnosis, nor is it possible to do so in its current form. It does not assess the full range of DSM-IV symptomatology. Items are assessed with a 5-point Likert-like scale, which makes it difficult to decide what kind of response indicates the presence of a symptom. Estimates of diagnosis obviously vary depending on whether one decides to use the middle, or the second highest response or higher as the indicator of symptom endorsement, as demonstrated by Schwarz and Kowalski (1991).

A revised version of the CPTS-RI has been created: the UCLA PTSD Reaction Index for DSM-IV (UPRID—Pynoos, Rodriquez, Steinberg, Stuber, & Frederick, 1998; see Appendix 9.5). The UPRID has been selected to be the primary PTSD screening measure for the National Child Traumatic Stress Network. It is a 49-item scale derived from the CPTS-RI, but with much better written questions. A parent version is available. An original adolescent version (Rodriguez, Steinberg, Saltzman, & Pynoos, 2001a) was eventually merged with the child version (Steinberg, Brymer, Decker, & Pynoos, 2004). Two shorter versions, one with seven items and the other with nine, are available for screening. The measure is designed to be administered three different ways: (1) as a self-report; (2) as one-on-one "interview," wherein the items are read to the child; and (3) for group administration.

The first 13 items of the UPRID assess exposure to different high-magnitude stressors for children. Stressors assessed include community violence, natural disaster, medical trauma, and abuse. These are followed by an item that asks children to select the experience that bothers them the most and rate how bothersome it was for them, using a 3-point scale: *A little* (1), *Somewhat* (2), or *A lot* (3). The next 13 items assess different responses to the experience that children might have had at the time. These items are intended to establish whether children responded with fear, helplessness, or horror, per DSM-IV criterion A2, but one item is about reactions of confusion, another is about upset or disorganized behavior, and still another is about feelings of unreality. These are rated as either yes or no. Of the final 22 questions, 20 assess the presence of symptoms related to DSM-IV criteria B–D, and, in addition, fear of recurrence of the trauma and trauma-related guilt are assessed by one item each. These items are rated from *None of the time* (0) to *Most of the time* (5). The questionnaire is accompanied by a frequency rating sheet that visually assists children in providing accurate responses about how often the reaction has occurred over the past month. Although the instrument was not created to be a diagnostic tool, there also is a score sheet that allows one to make a preliminary DSM-IV diagnosis. It is recommended that the instructions and questions be read aloud to children under the age of 12 or to youth with reading comprehension problems. When children meet criterion A, and when they sufficiently endorse each of the B–D criteria categories at the top two rating categories (*Much of the time* or *Most of the time*), a likely diagnosis of PTSD is made. When chil-

dren meet criterion A and only two of symptom criteria B–D, they are scored as "partial" PTSD. A cutoff of 38 or greater has the greatest sensitivity and specificity for detecting PTSD (Rodriguez et al., 2001a, 2001b).

It is difficult to evaluate the psychometric properties of the UPRID, because the authors appear to report results of CPTS-RI psychometric testing as if they were representative of the psychometrics of the UPRID (Steinberg et al., 2004). To further complicate the matter, both the CPTS-RI and the UPRID have undergone several revisions, and the reported psychometric properties of the UPRID as reported by Steinberg and colleagues (2004) appear to be based on tests of different iterations of both scales. Needless to say, this is confusing at best, as well as misleading. The two measures are not the same: Their structures differ; the questions are worded very differently; the response categories differ; and each measure contains questions that are not included on the other measure. The psychometrics of one measure cannot be substituted for the psychometrics of the other. On the other hand, some of the earlier reports regarding the measure (Rodriguez, 2001; Rodriguez et al., 2001a, 2001b), as well as the latest (Rodriguez, in press), do seem to report solely on the psychometric properties of the UPRID. Thus, although it is currently difficult to determine with certainty the reliability and validity of the UPRID, its psychometric properties as reported by Rodriguez (2001, in press) do suggest that it is a promising PTSD-specific measure for use with children age 7 years and older. It is certainly to be preferred as an alternative to the CPTS-RI.

The Child PTSD Symptom Scale (CPSS—Foa, Johnson, Feeny, & Treadwell, 2001; see Appendix 9.5) is one of the best of the currently available self-report measures of childhood PTSD that may be used to make a tentative clinical diagnosis of PTSD in children 8 years or older. It is based on a psychometrically sound measure of PTSD in adults, the Posttraumatic Diagnostic Scale (Foa, Cashman, Jaycox, & Perry, 1997). The language of the adult scale was modified to be more appropriate for children. The 26-item CPSS includes 2 items assessing exposure to a high-magnitude stressor (DSM-IV criterion A); 17 items assessing symptoms of reexperiencing, avoidance, and overarousal (criteria B–D); and 7 items assessing impaired functioning (criterion F). Children and adolescents are asked to indicate how often the 17 PTSD symptoms bothered them in the past month, with responses of *Not at all* (0), *Once a week or less* (1), *2 to 4 times a week* (2), and *5 or more times a week* (3). The 17 PTSD symptoms yield a total symptom severity score ranging from 0 to 51, as well as symptom severity scores for each of the three core DSM-IV criteria B–D. These items can also be scored dichotomously, presumably scoring ratings of 2 or 3 as symptom present; thus, a tentative DSM-IV diagnosis can be made based on responses to the 2 criterion A items, the 17 criteria B–D items, and the 7 criterion F items. Children indicate whether or not their symptoms cause them difficulty in each of the following seven areas of functioning: prayers, chores and duties, relationships with friends, fun and hobbies, schoolwork, relationships with family, and general happiness with life. These responses are scored as either *Absent* (0) or *Present* (1).

The psychometrics of the CPSS are impressive, although they may be considered preliminary in some respects, because they are based on a study wherein the measure was administered by examiners who read the questions aloud to children. Also assessed were reactions to a high-magnitude stressor that had occurred over 2 years prior to the administration; the primary measure of convergent validity, the CPTS-RI (Frederick et al., 1992; see Appendix 9.5), as described earlier, may not represent a "gold standard" against which to measure, especially because it neither assesses the full spectrum of DSM-IV symptoms of PTSD nor does it allow diagnosis of PTSD according to DSM-IV standards (as the authors themselves note; Foa et al., 2001, p. 377). Nonetheless, the psychometric studies are relatively thorough compared to those conducted for other paper-and-pencil, child self-report measures, and the results suggest that the CPSS is an excellent self-report measure of PTSD among school-age children, adolescents, and young adults.

ASSESSING CHILDREN'S PTSD WITH CAREGIVER REPORTS

Most parent or caregiver versions of children's PTSD assessment measures are versions of child self-report measures. Of the interviews that include PTSD as part of a broader assessment of several psychiatric disorders, those associated with the CAPA are among the best and most useful, especially if the child is to be interviewed with the CAPA (see Appendix 9.3) or

one of its variants, the PAPA (see Appendix 9.3) or the YAPA (see Appendix 9.6). Two of the PTSD-specific measures, one an interview and the other a parent self-report on the child's reactions, that currently appear to have the best psychometrics are the Childhood PTSD Interview—Parent Form (Fletcher, 1996b, 1996c) and the Parent Report of the Child's Reaction to Stress (PRCRS; Fletcher, 1996b, 1996e). These measures are from the same author and ask similar but not entirely parallel questions.

The Childhood PTSD Interview—Parent Form (Fletcher, 1996b, 1996c; see Appendix 9.5) is a semistructured interview of the caretaker regarding the child's reactions to the stressor(s). It allows DSM-IV criteria to be assessed and diagnosis to be made. It contains one item that allows the interviewer to rate how well the caregiver's description of the event(s) matches that of the child. Sixty-two questions assess DSM-IV PTSD criteria A–D. Unlike most other measures of childhood PTSD, all symptoms are assessed by at least two different questions to increase the reliability of the measure. Four questions assess criterion A. Nineteen questions assess the five symptoms of criterion B. The seven symptoms of criterion C are assessed by 24 questions. The five criterion D symptoms are assessed by 15 questions (see Appendix 9.5 for details).

An optional, additional 26 questions on the interview assess associated symptoms. Interviewers may choose to ask some, all, or none of these questions. Five questions assess symptoms of anxiety; three assess symptoms of depression; two assess indications of whether the child perceives certain prestressor events as omens; two assess symptoms of survivor guilt; and two assess symptoms of guilt or self-blame, at which point the interviewer is asked to indicate to what extent the child might actually be considered to have some responsibility for events. Two questions assess indications of fantasy denial; three assess possible self-destructive or suicidal thoughts and behaviors; four assess symptoms of dissociation; three assess antisocial behavior; two assess risk-taking behavior; and a final two assess changed eating habits. Answers to these questions can provide indications of whether the child should be assessed for ASD or complex PTSD.

The PRCRS (Fletcher, 1996b, 1996e; see Appendix 9.5) is a 78-item, paper-and-pencil report by the parent about the child's reaction to exposure to a high-magnitude stressor. The first 51 questions allow the assessment of DSM-IV PTSD criteria A–D. The first 4 questions assess criterion A; 20 questions assess the five symptoms of criterion B; 21 assess the seven symptoms of criterion C; and 12 assess criterion D's five symptoms. Associated symptoms are assessed by an additional 27 questions on the PRCRS (see Appendix 9.5 for details). Most items are answered using 6-point, Likert-like response categories, ranging from *Never* to *Always*, and many include a seventh *Don't know* category. Children's positive responses to some of the items are followed by a request that they explain or describe the reason for the response. Scorers of the responses are cautioned to consider these explanations carefully before rating the response. For example, parent or guardians are asked to explain what makes them believe their child behaves in new and unusual ways since the event(s).

Psychometrics for these two parent reports are promising, but they are based on a small sample of only 30 caregivers (Fletcher, 1996b). Of particular interest is the degree to which each of these parent measures demonstrated good agreement with child reports. The Parent Interview correlated .69 with the Childhood PTSD Interview—Child Form (Fletcher, 1996c; see Appendix 9.5) and .59 with the When Bad Things Happen scale (WBTH—Fletcher, 1996g; see Appendix 9.5) self-report. The PRCRS correlated .60 with the Parent Interview and .54 with the WBTH self-report.

Assessing Complex PTSD

SELF-REPORT ASSESSMENT OF COMPLEX PTSD AMONG PRESCHOOL CHILDREN

The Angie/Andy Cartoon Trauma Scales (Praver & Pelcovitz, 1996; Praver, Pelcovitz, & DiGiuseppe, 1998; see Appendix 9.7) were created specifically to assess complex PTSD in children ages 3–4 years and older. Modeled on the cartoon-based child interview, Levonn: A Cartoon-Based Structured Interview for Assessing Young Children's Distress Symptoms (Richters et al., 1990; see Appendix 9.4), this interview is a child version of the Structured Interview for Disorders of Extreme Stress Not Otherwise Specified (SIDES; see Appendix 9.7 and description below). It contains 44 full-page cartoons illustrating DSM-IV symptomatic responses to high-magnitude stressors plus the

additional symptoms associated with complex PTSD (see Table 9.3). As such, it is primarily a measure of reactions to prolonged, repeated abuse; thus, it is probably more appropriate for assessing complex PTSD among young children. However, it does allow posttraumatic stress symptomatology to be assessed. The Angie/Andy Cartoon Trauma Scales include scales of Attention and Consciousness, Dysregulation of Affect and Impulses, Relations with Others, Self-Perception, Somatization, and Systems of Meaning. Symptoms such as despair, hopelessness, and loss of previously sustained beliefs are included. Two summary scores are computed: one for Posttraumatic Stress symptoms and one for Total Associated symptoms. The associated items are relevant for the assessment of complex PTSD. The child rates how often he or she feels like the child in the drawing, using four separate thermometers that are filled to levels corresponding to a response of *Never, Just a few times, Some of the time*, and *A lot of the time*. There are parallel Angie/Andy Parent Rating Scales available, which ask the parent to assess the same symptoms in the child, minus the cartoons.

The Structured Interview for Disorders of Extreme Stress Not Otherwise Specified (SIDES; Pelcovitz et al., 1997), a 48-item interview, can also be administered as a paper-and-pencil self-report measure. It was designed to assess the suggested criteria for complex PTSD (also known as disorder of extreme stress not otherwise specified, or DES NOS). The SIDES was used to investigate the viability of a separate diagnostic category for complex PTSD during the DSM-IV field trials (Kilpatrick et al., 1998; van der Kolk et al., 1996). Questions on the SIDES assess specific symptoms of the domains of complex PTSD. In the domain of alteration in regulation of affect and impulses, three questions assess problems with affect regulation in general; four assess problems modulating anger; three assess self-destructive behaviors; one assesses suicidal preoccupation; seven assess difficulty modulating preoccupation with sexual involvement; and one assesses excessive risk-taking behavior. In the domain of alterations in attention or consciousness, one item assesses amnesia, four assess transient dissociative episodes and depersonalization, and one assesses a sense of ineffectiveness. The domains alteration in self-perception, sense of ineffectiveness; sense of permanent damage to the self; guilt and responsibility; shame; feeling that nobody can understand; and minimizing the traumatic experience(s) are all assessed with one question each. In the domain of alterations in perception of the perpetrator, the adoption of distorted beliefs about the perpetrator; idealization of the perpetrator; and preoccupation with hurting the perpetrator are assessed with one question each. In the domain of alterations in relations with others, three items assess the inability to trust others, one assesses the occurrence of revictimization experiences, and one assesses the tendency to victimize others. In the domain of somatization, problems with the digestive system and chronic pain are assessed by one question each, whereas cardiopulmonary symptoms are assessed with one item, wherein the respondent can indicate whether any of four different symptoms have been experienced; conversion symptoms are assessed with one item, wherein the respondent can indicate whether any of nine different symptoms have been experienced; and sexual symptoms are assessed with one item, wherein up to four symptoms can be endorsed. In the domain of alterations in systems of meaning, three items assess a pessimistic attitude toward the future (also known as foreshortened future), and two items assess a loss of previously sustaining beliefs. Endorsement of complex PTSD is met when criteria for all scales except that assessing alterations in perceptions of the perpetrator are met (Pelcovitz et al., 1997).

FUTURE DIRECTIONS

Measures written specifically to assess PTSD in children did not exist 15 years ago. As this chapter demonstrates, there is now a large but potentially confusing array from which to select. Which measure or measures the clinician chooses depend on the purposes of the assessment, the respondents, time constraints, and other logistical and procedural considerations. However, a great deal of the choice also should depend on the psychometric properties of the measure(s) to be used. Instruments that are without empirical support and that do not measure what they purport to measure are of little use. Similarly, important decisions about the state of mind and emotions of a child who has been exposed to a potentially traumatic experience should not rely on unreliable measures that cannot be assumed to reflect the true state of affairs from one day to the next. I hope that

the information in this chapter helps readers make better informed choices of the most empirically supported and clinically practical assessment tools for assessing childhood PTSD in the full range of its manifestation.

At the same time, it must be admitted that very few of the many measures of childhood PTSD now available have sufficient data on their psychometric properties. Fortunately, clinicians and researchers alike are becoming increasingly aware of the necessity for testing the reliability, validity, and clinical utility of measures that may ultimately help determine the welfare of traumatized children, adolescents, and young adults. One of the developments we are most likely to see in the near future are more reports regarding the assessment of the psychometric properties of many of the measures described in this chapter. Important information regarding certain psychometric properties is still lacking on nearly all of the measures discussed in this chapter. Few have had their factor structure examined, for example. Fewer still have been assessed using Item Response Theory, which can provide more precise information regarding the contribution of each item to the overall score. Nearly all of the measures of childhood PTSD currently available lack information regarding how well their scores are able to reflect progress shown in treatment. Knowledge of a measure's responsivity to intervention can help guide clinicians in their choice of measures to use when monitoring a child's response to treatment. To date no measures of childhood PTSD have been formally assessed for their ability to detect treatment response. However, a few have demonstrated an ability to detect effective interventions for posttraumatic stress. These include the Child and Adolescent Trauma Survey (CATS; March, Amaya-Jackson, et al., 1997; March, Amaya-Jackson, Murray, & Schulte, 1998), the CPTS-RI (Frederick et al., 1992; Goenjian et al., 2001), the CAPS-CA (March et al., 1998; Newman et al., 2004), and the Kauai Recovery Index (KRI—Hamada, Kameoka, & Yanagida, 1996; Hamada, Kameoka, Yanadiga, & Chemtob, 2003) (see Appendix 9.5 for all of these measures).

Another current shortcoming in the field is the fragmentation or compartmentalization of measures that assess the full range of posttraumatic stress symptomatology. Newer measures do seem to be developing in the direction of integrating assessment of the related symptomatology of ASD and PTSD. This is particularly true of general psychiatric interviews for children, such as the CAPA, PAPA, YAPA, and ChIPS. However, far too many measures still tend to focus only on PTSD symptomatology, and, in fact, the majority do not evaluate all DSM-IV A (both parts) through F criteria, assessing only the 17 symptoms listed in DSM-IV for the core criteria B, C, and D instead. This may be adequate for screening purposes. However, by not evaluating the full range of possible reactions to high-magnitude stressors, these measures make it all too easy to misdiagnose children and to miss additional and "associated" symptomatology that may in fact be more relevant for treatment of dysfunctional children. This is particularly likely to occur among children exposed to the most horrendous experiences over extended periods of time: sexual, physical, and emotional abuse and neglect. Any clinician who evaluates maltreated children but does not examine the possibility that the children are experiencing symptoms associated with such traumatic experiences, symptoms that go far beyond the 17 core symptoms of PTSD listed in DSM-IV, places those children at risk for a lifetime of increasingly disabling behavioral and medical problems, ranging from chronic, unexplainable medical problems to substance abuse, social and sexual problems, and borderline personality disorder. The few currently available measures that include questions about at least some of the additional and associated symptoms included in DSM-IV can sometimes provide important insight into symptoms associated with more extreme traumatization. However, none of today's measures, not even the interviews, allows for assessment of the full range of symptoms associated with complex PTSD, with the possible exception of the Angie/Andy Cartoon Trauma Scales (Praver & Pelcovitz, 1996; Praver, Pelcovitz, & DiGiuseppe, 1998) and its associated measure for parents (see Appendix 9.7).

Measures that provide assessment of the full spectrum of posttraumatic stress responses should be able to evaluate whether a child has ever been exposed to a stressor with the qualities most likely to lead the child to respond with symptoms of posttraumatic stress. The clinician, in addition to probing for exposure to known high-magnitude stressors, would consider other experiences that the child him- or herself experienced as extremely stressful. Assessment of the experience should go beyond

simply noting whether exposure to a potentially traumatic event has taken place. It should include the child's emotional reactions to the event as it took place and immediately afterward, with questions that help elucidate the extent to which the child's emotional reactions meet criterion A2 of DSM-IV. It would also mean attempting to come to a more detailed understanding of the actual circumstances surrounding the child's experience of the event. Particularly important is the extent to which the event involved those characteristics that, according to the literature, increase the likelihood of children responding with posttraumatic stress symptomatology, measured in a standardized manner similar to that employed by the DOSE scale.

Once a clinician develops an understanding of the child's experience, he or she can assess the child's initial and continuing responses. This involves assessment of a full complement of the possible reactions, including those associated with ASD, PTSD, and complex PTSD, as well as other important possibilities, such as grief reactions or changes in cognitive processing. Elaboration of the assessment of disruptions in the child's functioning as a result of the traumatic experience (criterion F of DSM-IV diagnostic criteria for PTSD) is useful as part of both the assessment process and treatment planning and monitoring.

Beyond refining and integrating assessment tools for the full spectrum of a potentially traumatic event and the child's reactions to it, both during the event and afterward, the field is ready to move into areas of assessment that go beyond the mere determination of symptomatology and diagnosis. It is time to make tools available to examine further ramifications of the traumatic experience and its aftermath. This already is starting to happen. A good example of a new measure that assesses important, possibly long-term reactions to traumatic experiences not captured by DSM-IV symptomatology is the World View Survey (Fletcher, 1996h; Skidmore & Fletcher, 1997; see Appendix 9.7), which assesses important beliefs about the self and others that appear to be the result of traumatic experience. Several theorists have suggested that posttraumatic stress responses represent a survivor's attempt to accommodate to and assimilate experiences that challenge the victim's whole worldview (e.g., Chemtob, Roitblat, Hamada, Carlson, & Twentyman, 1988; Foa et al., 1989; Horowitz,

1976a, 1976b). Some theorists (Epstein, 1990; Janoff-Bulman, 1989; McCann & Pearlman, 1990a, 1990b; Norris & Kaniasty, 1991) contend that stressful events become traumatic when they shatter certain basic beliefs that people normally assume about themselves and the world in which they live. Alteration in meaning is one of the symptoms of complex PTSD (see Table 9.3), but beliefs related to meaning are not the only beliefs that can be affected by traumatic experiences. High-magnitude stressors can pose overwhelming threats to beliefs about the safety and security of the world—its certainty, orderliness, predictability, and controllability—and to beliefs in one's competence and general self-esteem, not to mention the trustworthiness of important others (Fletcher, 1988; Janoff-Bulman, 1989, 1992; Norris & Kaniasty, 1991).

The World View Survey (Skidmore & Fletcher, 1997) assesses 50 beliefs that reflect the basic assumptions thought to be affected by traumatic experience (Epstein, 1990; Janoff-Bulman, 1989). The measure also includes potentially positive beliefs (e.g., that it is good to be alive, or that having lived through traumatic experiences, one now feels capable of handling anything). The authors determined the psychometric properties of the measure using responses of undergraduate college students, but the measure has been used successfully with adolescent psychiatric inpatients as well, most of whom had a diagnosis of PTSD (Skidmore & Fletcher, 1997). Factor analysis produced nine factors, and a second-order factor analysis suggested that the nine factors fell under two superordinate factors.

The first higher-order factor comprised six of the original factors, all of which were related to the basic assumptions put forth by Epstein (1990) and Janoff-Bulman (1989): (1) Anxious Uncertainty (exemplified by beliefs such as "Life does not seem to make much sense anymore"); (2) Inadequacy (e.g., "I am a jinx"); (3) Dangerous World (e.g., "The world is a dangerous place to live"); (4) Self-Abnegation (e.g., "Sometimes I think I am not a very good person"); (5) Lack of Control (e.g., "I feel like I have control over my life"—if disagreed with); and (6) Poor Attachment (e.g., "It is easy for me to make friends"—if disagreed with). The second higher-order factor comprised four of the original factors, most of which were originally intended to indicate positive beliefs, but which correlations with PTSD symptoms indi-

cated should be scored in a negative direction: (1) Poor Ego-Strength (e.g., "Since I have lived through some bad times, I have a better idea of what is important to me and what is not"—if disagreed with); (2) Poor Attachment (e.g., "It is easy for me to make friends"—if disagreed with); (3) Lack of Personal Empowerment (e.g., "I feel like nothing can keep me from getting what I want out of life anymore"—if disagreed with); and (4) Negative Outlook (e.g., "Nowadays I feel like every new day I am alive is a gift"—if disagreed with). Poor Attachment loaded on both higher-order factors.

Examination of the ramifications of a traumatic experience for the adolescent's or young adult's belief system with a measure such as the World View Survey can provide guidance relative to the goals and progress of treatment for these youth. This is an example of the possibilities for assessment that go beyond determining the degree to which a child meets DSM-IV criteria for PTSD.

In summary, this chapter has emphasized the need to consider much more than just DSM-IV's 17 core symptoms of PTSD when attempting to assess the reactions of infants, children, adolescents, and young adults to high-magnitude stressors. During the process of making such an assessment, the clinician will do well to keep in mind several key ideas. First, exposure to even the most extreme stressor does not automatically lead to reactions symptomatic of posttraumatic stress in anyone of any age. Second, whenever possible, the child should be allowed to give an account of his or her experience of, and reactions to, the stressor, although accounts of important others, especially caregivers, should also be given due consideration. Third, children should be interviewed in a manner appropriate to their developmental stage and in language suitable to their ability to comprehend. A corollary to this is that when children are asked to respond to standardized measures, the interview should endeavor to ensure that they have an adequate grasp of the possible response categories. It is not good practice to assume that the questions and response categories will be clearly understandable to a child just because the measure has been published and/or used by others to assess PTSD in children. Fourth, possible responses to traumatic events are not limited to PTSD. Some children who exhibit few or no symptoms of PTSD possibly exhibit other symptoms that seem to be related to the traumatic experience (e.g., depression, fear, or panic attacks), and others who clearly have PTSD symptoms also may exhibit additional symptoms that need more immediate attention than the core symptoms of PTSD (e.g., self-cutting or suicidal behavior). In short, the child's experience is uniquely her or his own and should be examined as such, rather than as something that one assumes it *should* be or is *supposed* to be. The best assessment tools help the clinician, child, and caregiver to come to a collaborative understanding of the child's experience. This collaborative understanding then provides a sound basis for a treatment plan that will help the child respond more adaptively to the earth-shattering experience and move beyond it to more positive growth experiences.

REFERENCES

Abramson, L. Y., Seligman, M. E. P., & Teasdale, J. D. (1978). Learned helplessness in humans: Critique and reformulation. *Journal of Abnormal Psychology*, 87, 49–94.

Achenbach, T. (1991a). *Child Behavior Checklist/4–18*. Burlington: University of Vermont, Department of Psychiatry.

Achenbach, T. (1991b). *Youth Self-Report*. Burlington: University of Vermont, Department of Psychiatry.

Achenbach, T. M., & Edelbrock, C. (1983). *Manual for the Child Behavior Checklist and the Revised Child Behavior Profile*. Burlington: University of Vermont.

Administration for Children and Families. (Accessed April 9, 2006). In National Survey of Child and Adolescent Well-Being (NSCAW): CPS sample component wave 1 data analysis. Appendix B: Reliability of NSCAW measures. Available at *www.acf.hhs.gov/ programs/opre/abuse_neglect/nscaw/reports/cps_sample/cps_appb_tab1.html*

Ahmad, A., & Muhamad, K. (1996). The socioemotional development of orphans in orphanages and traditional foster care in Iraqi Kurdistan. *Child Abuse and Neglect*, 20, 1161–1173.

Ajdukovic, M. (1998). Displaced adolescents in Croatia: Sources of stress and posttraumatic stress reaction. *Adolescence*, 33, 209–217.

Amaya-Jackson, L., McCarthy, C., Newman, E., & Cherney, M. (1995). *Child PTSD checklist*. Unpublished manuscript, Duke University, Durham, NC.

Ambrosini, P. J., & Dixon, J. F. (2000). *Schedule for Affective Disorders and Schizophrenia for School Age Children (6–18 yrs.), KIDDIE-SADS (K-SADS) (Present State and Lifetime Version), K-SADS-IVR (Revision of K-SADS-IIIR)*. Unpublished instrument, Medical College of Pennsylvania, Eastern Pennsylvania Psychiatric Institute, Philadelphia.

American Psychiatric Association (APA). (1987). *Diagnostic and statistical manual of mental disorders* (3rd ed., rev.). Washington, DC: Author.

American Psychiatric Association (APA). (1994). *Diagnostic and statistical manual of mental disorders* (4th ed.). Washington, DC: Author.

American Psychiatric Association (APA). (2000). *Diagnostic and statistical manual of mental disorders* (4th ed., text rev.). Washington, DC: Author.

Amorim, P., Lecrubier, Y., Weiller, E., Hergueta, T., & Sheehan D. (1998). DSM-III-R psychotic disorders: Procedural validity of the Mini-International Neuropsychiatric Interview (M.I.N.I.): Concordance and causes for discordance with the CIDI. *European Psychiatry*, 13, 26–34.

Angold, A., & Costello, E. J. (1995). A test–retest reliability study of child-reported psychiatric symptoms and diagnoses using the Child and Adolescent Psychiatric Assessment (CAPA-C). *Psychological Medicine*, 25, 755–762.

Angold, A., & Costello, E. (2000). The Child and Adolescent Psychiatric Assessment (CAPA). *Journal of the American Academy of Child and Adolescent Psychiatry*, 39, 39–48.

Armstrong, J., Putnam, F., & Carlson, E. (1993, October). *The Adolescent Dissociative Experiences Scale (A-DES; Version 1.0)*. Paper presented at the Ninth Annual Meeting of the International Society for Traumatic Studies. San Antonio, TX.

Armsworth, M. W., & Holaday, M. (1993). The effects of psychological trauma on children and adolescents. *Journal of Counseling and Development*, 72, 49–56.

Bandura, A., Taylor, C. B., Williams, S. L., Mefford, I. N., & Barchas, J. D. (1985). Catecholamine secretion as a function of perceived coping self-efficacy. *Journal of Consulting and Clinical Psychology*, 53, 406–415.

Baumrind, D. (1971). Current patterns of parental authority. *Developmental Psychology Monographs*, 4, 1–101.

Beals, J., Piasecki, J., Nelson, S., Jones, M., Keane, E., Dauphnais, P., et al. (1997). Psychiatric disorder among American Indian adolescents: Prevalence in Northern American Plains youth. *Journal of the American Academy of Child and Adolescent Psychiatry*, 36, 1252–1259.

Bean, T., Derluyn, I., Eurelings-Bontekoe, Broekaert, E., & Spinhover, P. (2006). Validation of the multiple language versions of the Reactions of Adolescents to Traumatic Stress Questionnaire. *Journal of Traumatic Stress*, 19, 241–255.

Bean, T., Eurelings-Bontekoe, E. H. M., Derluyn, I., & Spinhover, P. (2004a). *HSCL-37A user's manual*. Retrieved May 15, 2005, from *www.centrum45.nl/research/amaenggz/ukamtool.php*.

Bean, T. Eurelings-Bontekoe, E. H. M., Derluyn, I., & Spinhover, P. (2004b). *RATS user's manual*. Retrieved May 15, 2005, from *www.centrum45.nl/research/amaenggz/ukamtool.php*.

Bean, T. Eurelings-Bontekoe, E. H. M., Derluyn, I., &

Spinhover, P. (2004c). *SLE user's manual.* Retrieved May 15, 2005, from *www.centrum45.nl/research/amaenggz/ukamtool.php.*

Bergen, H. A., Martin, G., Richardson, A. S., Allison, S., & Roeger, L. (2004). Sexual abuse, antisocial behaviour and substance use: Gender differences in young community adolescents. *Australian and New Zealand Journal of Psychiatry, 38,* 34–41.

Berman, S. L., Kurtines, W. M., Silverman, W. K., & Serafini, L. T. (1996). The impact of exposure to crime and violence on urban youth. *American Journal of Orthopsychiatry, 66,* 329–336.

Bernat, J. A., Ronfeldt, H. M., Calhoun, K. S., & Arias, I. (1998). Prevalence of traumatic events and peritraumatic predictors of posttraumatic stress symptoms in a non-clinical sample of college students. *Journal of Traumatic Stress, 11,* 645–664.

Birleson, P. (1981). The validity of depressive disorder in childhood and the development of a self-rating scale: A research report. *Journal of Child Psychology and Psychiatry and Allied Disciplines, 22,* 73–88.

Bolton, D., O'Ryan, D., Udwin, O., Boyle, S., & Yule, W. (2000). The long-term psychological effects of a disaster experienced in adolescence: II. General psychopathology. *Journal of Child Psychology and Psychiatry, and Allied Disciplines, 41,* 513–523.

Boris, N. W., Zeanah, C. H., Larrieu, J. A., Scheeringa, M. S., & Heller, S. S. (1998). Attachment disorders in infancy and early childhood: A preliminary investigation of diagnostic criteria. *American Journal of Psychiatry, 155,* 295–297.

Bremner, J. D., Southwick, S. M., & Charney, D. S. (1999). The neurobiology of posttraumatic stress disorder: An integration of animal and human research. In P. Saigh & D. Bremner (Eds.), *Post-traumatic stress disorder* (pp. 103–143). Washington, DC: American Psychological Press.

Breslau, N., Davis, G. C., Andreski, P., & Peterson, E. (1991). Traumatic events and posttraumatic stress disorder in an urban population of young adults. *Archives of General Psychiatry, 48,* 216–222.

Briere, J. (1996a). *Psychometric review of Trauma Symptom Checklist for Children (TSCC).* In B. H. Stamm (Ed.), *Measurement of stress, trauma, and adaptation* (pp. 378–380). Lutherville, MD: Sidran Press.

Briere, J. (1996b). *Trauma Symptom Checklist for Children (TSCC) professional manual.* Odessa, FL: Psychological Assessment Resources.

Briere, J. (2000). *Trauma Symptom Checklist for Young Children (TSCYC) professional manual.* Odessa, FL: Psychological Assessment Resources.

Briere, J., & Elliott, D. M. (2003). Prevalence and psychological sequelae of self-reported childhood physical and sexual abuse in a general population sample of men and women. *Child Abuse and Neglect, 27,* 1205–1222.

Briere, J., Johnson, K., Bissada, A., Damon, L., Crouch, J., Gil, E., et al. (2001). Trauma Symptom Checklist for Young Children (TSCYC): Reliability and association with abuse exposure in a multi-site study. *Child Abuse and Neglect, 25,* 1001–1014.

Briere, J., & Lanktree, C. B. (1995). *The Trauma Symptom Checklist for Children (TSCC): Preliminary psychometric characteristics.* Unpublished manuscript, Department of Psychiatry, University of Southern California School of Medicine, Los Angeles, CA.

Briere, J., & Spinazzola, J. (2005). Phenomenology and psychological assessment of complex posttraumatic states. *Journal of Traumatic Stress, 18,* 401–412.

Buka, S., Selner-O'Hagan, M., Kindlon, D., & Earls, F. (1996). *My Exposure to violence and my child's exposure to violence.* Unpublished manual, Harvard School of Publis Health, Boston.

Cardeña, E., Lewis-Fernández, R., Bear, D., Pakianathan, I., & Spiegel, D. (1996). Dissociative disorders. In T. A. Widiger, A. J. Frances, H. A. Pincus, R. Ross, M. B. First, & W. W. Davis (Eds.), *DSM-IV sourcebook* (Vol. 2, pp. 973–1005). Washington, DC: American Psychiatric Press.

Carrion, V. G., Weems, C. F., Ray, R. D., & Reiss, A. L. (2002). Toward an empirical definition of pediatric PTSD: The phenomenology of PTSD symptoms in youth. *Journal of the American Academy of Child and Adolescent Psychiatry, 41,* 166–173.

Chaffin, M., & Schultz, S. (2001). Psychometric evaluation of the Children's Impact of Traumatic Events Scale—Revised. *Child Abuse and Neglect, 25,* 401–411.

Chaffin, M., Wherry, J., Newlin, C., Crutchfield, A., & Dykman, R. (1997). The Abuse Dimensions Inventory: Initial data on a research measure of abuse severity. *Journal of Interpersonal Violence, 12,* 569–589.

Chemtob, C. M., Nakashima, J., Hamada, R. S., & Carlson, J. G. (2002). Brief-treatment for elementary school children with disaster-related posttraumatic stress disorder: A field study. *Journal of Clinical Psychology, 59,* 99–112.

Chemtob, C., Roitblat, H. C., Hamada, R. S., Carlson, J. G., & Twentyman, C. T. (1988). A cognitive action theory of post-traumatic stress disorder. *Journal of Anxiety Disorders, 2,* 253–275.

Children and War Foundation. (1998). *The Children's Impact of Events Scale (13) (CRIES-13).* Available online at *www.childrenandwar.org*

Cloitre, M., Chase Stovall-McClough, K., Miranda, R., & Chemtob, C. (2004). Therapeutic alliance, negative mood regulation, and treatment outcome in child abuse-related posttraumatic stress disorder. *Journal of Consulting and Clinical Psychology, 72,* 411–416.

Cohen, J., Bernet, W., Dunne, J. E., Adair, M., Arnold, V., Benson, S., Bukstein, O., et al. (1998). Practice parameters for the assessment and treatment of children and adolescents with posttraumatic stress disorder. *Journal of the American Academy of Child and Adolescent Psychiatry, 37*(Suppl.), 4S—26S.

Cohen, J. A., Deblinger, E., Mannarino, A. P., & de

Arellano, M. A. (2001). The importance of culture in treating abused and neglected children: An empirical review. *Child Maltreatment, 6*, 148–157.

Cole, P., & Putnam, F. W. (1992). Effect of incest on self and social functioning: A developmental psychopathology perspective. *Journal of Consulting and Clinical Psychology, 60*, 174–184.

Cooley, M. R., Turner, S. M., & Beidel, D. C. (1995). Assessing community violence: The children's report of exposure to violence. *Journal of the American Academy of Child and Adolescent Psychiatry, 34*, 201–208.

Cooley-Quille, M. R., Turner, S. M., & Beidel, D. C. (1995). Emotional impact of children's exposure to community violence: A preliminary study. *Journal of the American Academy of Child and Adolescent Psychiatry, 34*, 1362–1368.

Costello, E. J., Angold, A., March, J., & Fairbank, J. (1998). Life events and posttraumatic stress: The development of a new measure for children and adolescents. *Psychological Medicine, 28*, 1275–1288.

Costello, J., Erkanli, A., Fairbank, J. A., & Angold, A. (2002). The prevalence of potentially traumatic events in childhood and adolescence. *Journal of Traumatic Stress, 15*, 99–112.

Crouch, J. L., Smith, D. W., Ezzell, C. E., & Saunders, B. E. (1999). Measuring reactions to sexual trauma among children: Comparing the Children's Impact of Traumatic Events Scale and the Trauma Symptom Checklist for Children. *Child Maltreatment, 4*, 255–263.

Cunningham, P. B., Jones, R. T., & Yang, B. (1994). *Impact of community violence on African American children and adolescents in high violent crime neighborhoods: Preliminary findings.* Poster presented at the seventh annual research conference, A System of Care for Children's Mental Health: Expanding the Research Base, Tampa, FL.

Davidson, J. R. T., Foa, E. B., Blank, A. S., Brett, E. A., Fairbank, J., Green, B. L., et al. (1996). Posttraumatic stress disorder. In T. A. Widiger, A. J. Frances, H. A. Pincus, R. Ross, M. B. First, & W. W. Davis (Eds.), *DSM-IV sourcebook* (Vol. 2, pp. 577–606). Washington, DC: American Psychiatric Press.

Daviss, W. B., Mooney, D., Racusin, R., Fleischer, A., Mooney, D., Ford, J. D., et al. (2000). Acute stress disorder symptomatology during hospitalization for pediatric injury. *Journal of the American Academy of Child and Adolescent Psychiatry, 39*, 569–575.

Daviss, W. B., Mooney, D., Racusin, R., Ford, J. D., Fleischer, A., & McHugo, C. J. (2000). Predicting posttraumatic stress after hospitalization for pediatric injury. *Journal of the American Academy of Child and Adolescent Psychiatry, 39*, 576–583.

DeJong, A. R., Emmett, G. A., & Hervada, A. R. (1982). Sexual abuse of children: Sex-, race-, and age-dependent variations. *American Journal of Diseases of Children, 136*, 129–134.

Derogatis, L. R. (1977). *SCL-90: Administration, scoring and Procedure Manual-I for the R (Revised) version.* Baltimore: Johns Hopkins University School of Medicine.

Derogatis, L. R., & Melisaratos, N. (1983). The Brief Symptom Inventory: An introductory report. *Psychological Medicine, 13*, 595–605.

Diaz, J. (1994). *The impact of sexual abuse on adolescent females: Factors influencing subsequent psychological adjustment and sexual behaviour.* Unpublished doctoral dissertation. Columbia University, New York, NY.

Diehl, V. A., Zea, M. C., & Espino, C. M. (1994). Exposure to war violence, separation from parents, posttraumatic stress and cognitive functioning in Hispanic children. *Interamerican Journal of Psychology, 28*, 25–41.

DiNicola, V. F. (1996). Ethnocentric aspects of posttraumatic stress disorder and related disorders among children and adolescents. In A. J. Marsella, M. J. Friedman, E. T. Gerrity, & R. M. Scurfield (Eds.), *Ethnocultural aspects of posttraumatic stress disorder: Issues, research and clinical applications* (pp. 389–414). Washington, DC: American Psychological Press.

Dise-Lewis, J. E. (1988). The Life Events and Coping Inventory: An assessment of stress in children. *Psychosomatic Medicine, 50*, 484–499.

Dube, S. R., Anda, R. F., Felitti, V. J., Chapman, D. P., Williamson, D. F., & Giles, W. H. (2001). Childhood abuse, household dysfunction, and the risk of attempted suicide through the life span: Findings from the Adverse Childhood Experiences Study. *Journal of the American Medical Association, 286*, 3089–3096.

Dunn, L. M., & Dunn, L. M. (1981). *Peabody Picture Vocabulary Test—Revised.* Circle Pines, MN: American Guidance Service.

Dyregrov, A., Kuterovac, G., & Barath, A. (1996). Factor analysis of the Impact of Event Scale with children in war. *Scandinavian Journal of Psychology, 36*, 339–350.

Egger, H. L., & Angold, A. (2004). The Preschool Age Psychiatric Assessment (PAPA): A structured parent interview for diagnosing psychiatric disorders in preschool children. In R. Delcarmen-Wiggens & A. Carter (Eds.), *A handbook of infant, toddler, and preschool mental health assessment* (pp. 224–243) New York: Oxford University Press.

Egger, H., Ascher, B., & Angold, A. (1999). *Preschool Age Psychiatric Assessment—Parent Interview.* Unpublished manuscript, Center for Developmental Epidemiology, Department of Psychiatry and Behavioral Sciences, Duke University Medical Center, Durham, NC.

Egger, H., Erkanli, A., Keeler, G., Potts, E., Walter, B. K., & Angold, A. (2004). *Test–retest reliability for the Preschool Age Psychiatric Assessment (PAPA).* Unpublished manuscript, Duke University Medical Center, Durham, NC.

Eisen, M. L. (1997). *The development and validation of

a new measure of PTSD for young children. Unpublished manuscript, California State University, Los Angeles.

Elliot, D. M., & Briere, J. (1994). Forensic sexual abuse evaluations in older children: Disclosures and symptomatology. *Behavioural Sciences and the Law, 12,* 261–277.

Epstein, S. (1990). The self-concept, the traumatic neurosis, and the structure of personality. In D. Ozer, J. M. Healey, Jr., & A. J. Stewart (Eds.), *Perspectives on personality* (Vol. 3, pp. 63–98). Greenwich, CT: JAI Press.

Evans, J. J., & Briere, J., Boggiano, A. K., & Barrett, M. (1994). *Reliability and validity of the Trauma Symptom Checklist for Children in a normative sample.* Paper presented at the Conference on Responding to Child Maltreatment, San Diego, CA.

Eyberg, S. M., & Ross, A. W. (1978). Assessment of child behavior problems: The validation of a new inventory. *Journal of Clinical Child Psychology, 7,* 113–116.

Felitti, V. J., Anda, R. F., Nordenberg, D., Williamson, D. F., Spitz, A. M., Edwards, V., et al. (1997). Relationship of childhood abuse and household dysfunction to many of the leading causes of death in adults: The Adverse Childhood Experiences (ACE) study. *American Journal of Preventive Medicine, 14,* 245–258.

Finkelhor, D., Hamby, S. L., Ormrod, R., & Turner, H. (2005). The Juvenile Victimization Questionnaire: Reliability, validity, and national norms. *Child Abuse and Neglect, 29,* 383–412.

Finkelhor, D., & Kendall-Tackett, K. (1997). A developmental perspective on the childhood impact of crime, abuse and violent victimization. In D. Cicchetti & S. Toth (Eds.), *Rochester Symposium on Developmental Psychopathology and Developmental Perspectives on Trauma* (pp. 1–32). Rochester, NY: University of Rochester Press.

First, M., Gibbon, M., Williams, J. B., & Spitzer, R. L. (1996). *Structured Clinical Interview for the DSM-IV (SCID).* Biometrics Research Department, New York State Psychiatric Institute, New York, NY.

First, M. B., Pincus, H. A., Levine, J. B., Williams, J. B. W., Ustun, B., & Peele, R. (2004). Clinical utility as a criterion for revising psychiatric diagnoses. *American Journal of Psychiatry, 161,* 946–954.

Fisher, P., Hoven, C. W., Moore, R. E., Bird, H., Chiang, P., Lichtman, J., et al. (1993, October). *Evaluation of a method to assess PTSD in children and adolescents.* Poster presented at the American Public Health Association meeting, San Francisco.

Fletcher, K. E. (1988). Belief systems, exposure to stress, and post-traumatic stress disorder in Vietnam veterans (Doctoral dissertation, University of Massachusetts at Amherst, 1988). *Dissertation Abstracts International, 49,* 1981B.

Fletcher, K. E. (1996a). Childhood posttraumatic stress disorder. In E. J. Mash & R. A. Barkley (Eds.), *Child psychopathology* (1st ed., pp. 242–275). New York: Guilford Press.

Fletcher, K. E. (1996b, November). *Measuring school-aged children's PTSD: Preliminary psychometrics of four new measures.* Paper presented at the 12th Annual Meeting of the International Society for Traumatic Stress Studies, San Francisco.

Fletcher, K. E. (1996c). Psychometric review of Childhood PTSD Interview. In B.H. Stamm (Ed.), *Measurement of stress, trauma, and adaptation* (pp. 87–89). Lutherville, MD: Sidran Press.

Fletcher, K. E. (1996d). Psychometric review of Dimensions of Stressful Events (DOSE) rating scale. In B. H. Stamm (Ed.), *Measurement of stress, trauma, and adaptation* (pp. 144–150). Lutherville, MD: Sidran Press.

Fletcher, K. E. (1996e). Psychometric review of the Parent Report of the Child's Reaction to Stress. In B. H. Stamm (Ed.), *Measurement of stress, trauma, and adaptation* (pp. 225–227). Lutherville, MD: Sidran Press.

Fletcher, K. E. (1996f). Psychometric review of Tough Times Checklist, Teen Tough Times Checklist, Child's Upsetting Times Checklist, and Young Adult's Upsetting Times Checklist. In B. H. Stamm (Ed.), *Measurement of stress, trauma, and adaptation* (pp. 358–361). Lutherville, MD: Sidran Press.

Fletcher, K. E. (1996g). Psychometric review of the When Bad Things Happen scale. In B. H. Stamm (Ed.), *Measurement of stress, trauma, and adaptation* (pp. 435–437). Lutherville, MD: Sidran Press.

Fletcher, K. E. (1996h). Psychometric review of the World View Survey. In B. H. Stamm (Ed.), *Measurement of stress, trauma, and adaptation* (pp. 443–445). Lutherville, MD: Sidran Press.

Fletcher, K. E. (2003). Childhood posttraumatic stress disorder. In E. J. Mash & R. A. Barkley (Eds.), *Child psychopathology* (2nd ed., pp. 330–371). New York: Guilford Press.

Fletcher, K. E., Cox, W. D., Skidmore, G. L., Janssens, D., & Render, T. (1997, November). *Multimethod assessment of traumatization and PTSD among adolescent psychiatric inpatients.* Paper presented at the 13th Annual Meeting of the International Society for Traumatic Stress Studies, Montreal, Canada.

Fletcher, K. E., & Skidmore, G. L. (1997, November). *The impact of lifetime exposure to stress among college students.* Paper presented at the 13th Annual Meeting of the International Society for Traumatic Stress Studies, Montreal, Canada.

Fletcher, K. E., Spilsbury, J. C., Creeden, R., & Friedman, S. (2006, November). *Psychometric properties of the Dimensions of Stressful Events (DOSE) scale.* Paper presented at the 22nd Annual Meeting of the International Society for Traumatic Stress Studies, Hollywood, CA.

Flowers, A., Lanclos, N. F., & Kelley, M. L. (2002). Validation of a screening instrument for exposure to violence in African American children. *Journal of Pediatric Psychology, 27*, 351–361.

Flowers, A. L., Hastings, T. L., & Kelley, M. L. (2000). Development of a screening instrument for exposure to violence in children: The KID-SAVE. *Journal of Psychopathology and Behavioral Assessment, 22*, 91–104.

Foa, E. B., Cashman, L., Jaycox, L., & Perry, K. (1997). The validation of a self-report measure of posttraumatic stress disorder: The Posttraumatic Diagnostic Scale. *Psychological Assessment, 9*, 445–451.

Foa, E. B., Johnson, K. M., Feeny, N. C., & Treadwell, K. R. H. (2001). The Child PTSD Symptom Scale: A preliminary examination of its psychometric properties. *Journal of Clinical Child Psychology, 30*, 376–384.

Foa, E., Keane, T. M., & Friedman, M. J. (2000). *Effective treatments for PTSD: Guidelines from the International Society of Traumatic Stress Studies.* New York: Guilford Press.

Foa, E. B., Steketee, G., & Rothbaum, B. O. (1989). Behavioral/cognitive conceptualizations of posttraumatic stress disorder. *Behavior Therapy, 20*, 155–176.

Foa, E. B., Zinbarg, R., & Rothbaum, B. O. (1992). Uncontrollability and unpredictability in post-traumatic stress disorder: An animal model. *Psychological Bulletin, 112*, 218–238.

Ford, J. D., Racusin, R., Rogers, K., Ellis, C., Schiffman, J., Ribbe, D., et al. (2002). *Traumatic Events Screening Inventory for Children (TESI-C) Version 8.4.* National Center for PTSD and Dartmouth Child Psychiatry Research Group, White River Junction, UT.

Ford, J. D., & Rogers, K. (1997, November). *Empirically-based assessment and relatedness in trauma and disorganized attachment.* Paper presented at the Annual Convention of the International Society for Traumatic Stress Studies, Montreal, Canada.

Fox, N. A., & Leavitt, L. A. (1995). *The Violence Exposure Scale for Children—VEX (Preschool Version).* College Park: Department of Human Development, University of Maryland.

Frederick, C. J. (1985a). Children traumatized by catastrophic situations. In S. Eth & R. S. Pynoos (Eds.), *Post-traumatic stress disorder in children* (pp. 73–99). Washington, DC: American Psychiatric Press.

Frederick, C. J. (1985b). Selected foci in the spectrum of posttraumatic stress disorders. In J. Laube & S. A. Murphy (Eds.), *Perspectives on disaster recovery* (pp. 110–130). East Norwalk, CT: Appleton–Century–Crofts.

Frederick, C. J., Pynoos, R. S., & Nader, K. O. (1992). *Childhood Posttraumatic Stress Reaction Index (CPTS-RI).* Los Angeles: Authors.

Fremont, W. P. (2004). Childhood reactions to terrorism-induced trauma: A review of the past 10 years. *Journal of the American Academy of Child and Adolescent Psychiatry, 43*, 381–392.

Freud, A., & Burlingham, D. T. (1943). *War and children.* Westport, CT: Greenwood Press.

Friedrich, W. N. (1991). Sexual behaviour in sexually abused children. In J. Briere (Ed.), *Treating victims of child abuse* (pp. 15–28). San Francisco: Jossey-Bass.

Friedrich, W. N. (1998). *The Child Sexual Behavior Inventory professional manual.* Odessa, FL: Psychological Assessment Resources.

Freidrich, W. N., & Jaworski, T. M. (1995). *Measuring dissociation and sexual behaviours in adolescents and children.* Unpublished manuscript, Mayo Clinic, Rochester, MN.

Fristad, M. A., Cummins, J., Verducci, J. S., Teare, M., Weller, E. B., & Weller, R. A. (1998). Study IV: Concurrent validity of the DSM-IV revised Children's Interview for Psychiatric Syndromes (ChIPS). *Journal of Child and Adolescent Psychopharmacology, 8*, 227–236.

Fristad, M. A., Glickman, A. R., Verducci, J. S., Teare, M., Weller, E. B., & Weller, R. A. (1998). Study V: Children's Interview for Psychiatric Syndromes (ChIPS): Psychometrics in two community samples. *Journal of Child and Adolescent Psychopharmacology, 8*, 237–245.

Garland, A. F., Hough, R. L., McCabe, K. M., Yeh, M., Wood, P. A., & Aarons, G. A. (2001). Prevalence of psychiatric disorders in youths across five sectors of care. *Journal of the American Academy of Child and Adolescent Psychiatry, 40*, 409–418.

Ghosh Ippen, C., Ford, J., Racusin, R., Acker, M., Bosquet, M., Rogers, K., et al. (2002). *Traumatic Events Screening Inventory—Parent Report Revised.* VT: National Center for PTSD Dartmouth Child Trauma Research Group, White River Junction, VT.

Gilbert, A. M. (2004). Psychometric properties of the Trauma Symptom Checklist for Young Children (TSCYC). *Dissertation Abstracts International, 65*(1-B), 478.

Goenjian, A. K., Molina, L., Steinberg, A. M., Fairbanks, L. A., Alvarez, M. L., Goenjian, H. A., et al. (2001). Posttraumatic stress and depressive reactions among Nicaraguan adolescents after Hurricane Mitch. *American Journal of Psychiatry, 158*, 788–794.

Golier, J., & Yehuda, R. (1998). Neuroendocrine activity and memory-related impairments in posttraumatic stress disorder. *Development and Psychopathology, 10*, 857–869.

Graham, Y. P., Heim, C., Goodman, S. H., Miller, A. H., & Nemeroff, C. B. (1999). The effects of neonatal stress on brain development: Implications for psychopathology. *Development and Psychopathology, 11*, 545–565.

Green, B. L. (1993). Disasters and posttraumatic stress disorder. In J. R. T. Davidson & E. B. Foa (Eds.), *Posttraumatic stress disorder: DSM-IV and beyond* (pp. 75–97). Washington, DC: American Psychiatric Association.

Green, B. L., Korol, M., Grace, M. C., Vary, M. G.,

Leonard, A. C., Gleser, G. C., et al. (1991). Children and disaster: Age, gender, and parental effects on PTSD symptoms. *Journal of the American Academy of Child and Adolescent Psychiatry, 30,* 945–951.

Green, B. L., Wilson, J. P., & Lindy, J. D. (1985). Conceptualizing post-traumatic stress disorder: A psychosocial framework. In C. R. Figely (Ed.), *Trauma and its wake* (Vol. 1, pp. 53–69). New York: Brunner/Mazel.

Greenwald, R. (1997). *Child and Parent Reports of Post-Traumatic Symptoms (CROPS & PROPS): Copyrighted instruments.* Towson, MD: Sidran Institute.

Greenwald, R., & Rubin, A. (1999). Brief assessment of children's post-traumatic symptoms: Development and preliminary validation of parent and child scales. *Research on Social Work Practice, 9,* 61–75.

Greenwald, R., Satin, M. S., Azubuike, A. A., Borgen, R., & Rubin, A. (2001, December). *Trauma-informed multi-component treatment for juvenile delinquents: Preliminary findings.* Poster session presented at the annual meeting for the International Society for Traumatic Stress Studies, New Orleans, LA.

Hamada, R. S., Kameoka, V., & Yanagida, E. (1996, November). *The Kauai Recovery Index (KRI): Screening for post-disaster adjustment problems in elementary-aged populations.* Paper presented at the 12th Annual Meeting of the International Society for Traumatic Stress Studies, San Francisco.

Hamada, R. S., Kameoka, V., Yanagida, E., & Chemtob, C. M. (2003). Assessment of elementary school children for disaster-related posttraumatic stress disorder symptoms: The Kauai Recovery Index. *Journal of Nervous and Mental Disorders, 191,* 268–272.

Hastings, T., & Kelley, M. (1997a). Development of a screening instrument for exposure to violence in children: The KID-SAVE. *Journal of Psychopathology and Behavioral Assessment, 22,* 91–104.

Hastings, T., & Kelley, M. (1997b). Development and validation of the Screen for Adolescent Violence Exposure (SAVE). *Journal of Abnormal Child Psychology, 25,* 511–520.

Helzer, J. E., Robins, L. N., & McEvoy, L. (1987). Posttraumatic stress disorder in the general population. *New England Journal of Medicine, 317,* 1630–1634.

Herjanic, B., & Reich, W. (1983a). *Diagnostic Interview for Children and Adolescents (DICA-C): Child version.* St. Louis, MO: Washington University School of Medicine.

Herjanic, B., & Reich, W. (1983b). *Diagnostic Interview for Children and Adolescents (DICA-P): Parent version.* St. Louis, MO: Washington University School of Medicine.

Herman, J. L. (1992). Complex PTSD: A syndrome in survivors of prolonged and repeated trauma. *Journal of Traumatic Stress, 5,* 377–391.

Horowitz, M. J. (1976a). Psychological response to serious life events. In V. Hamilton & D. M. Warburton (Eds.), *Human stress and cognition* (pp. 235–263). New York: Wiley.

Horowitz, M. (1976b). *Stress response syndromes.* New York: Aronson.

Horowitz, M., Wilner, N., & Alvarez, W. (1979). Impact of Events Scale: A measure of subjective stress. *Psychosomatic Medicine, 41,* 209–218.

Hulme, P. A. (2000). Symptomatology and health care utilization of women primary care patients who experienced childhood sexual abuse. *Child Abuse and Neglect, 24,* 1471–1484.

Hyman, I., Snook, P., Lurkis, L., Phan, C., & Britton, G. (2001, August). *Student Alienation and Trauma Scale: Assessment, research and practice.* Paper presented at the 109th Annual Convention of the American Psychological Association, San Francisco.

Hyman, I., Zelikoff, W., & Clarke, J. (1988). *School Trauma Survey—Student Form.* Philadelphia: National Center for Study of Corporal Punishment and Alternatives in Schools (NCSCPAS), Temple University.

Ippen, C., Briscoe-Smith, A., & Lieberman, A. (2004, November). *PTSD symptomatology in young children.* Presented at the 20th Annual Meeting of the International Society for Traumatic Stress Studies, New Orleans, LA.

Jaffe, P., Wolfe, D., Wilson, S. K., & Zak, L. (1986). Family violence and child adjustment: A comparative analysis of girls' and boys' behavioral symptoms. *American Journal of Psychiatry, 143,* 74–77.

Janoff-Bulman, R. (1989). Assumptive worlds and the stress of traumatic events: Applications of the schema construct. *Social Cognition, 7,* 113–136.

Janoff-Bulman, R. (1992). *Shattered assumptions: Towards a new psychology of trauma.* New York: Free Press.

Jaycox, L., Stein, B. D., Kataoka, S. H., Wong, M., Fink, A., Escudero, P., et al. (2002). Violence exposure, posttraumatic stress disorder, and depressive symptoms among recent immigrant schoolchildren. *Journal of the American Academy of Child and Adolescent Psychiatry, 41,* 1104–1110.

Johnson, J. H., & McCutcheon, S. M. (1980). Assessing life stress in older children and adolescents: Preliminary findings with the Life Events Checklist. In I. G. Sarason & C. D. Spielberger (Eds.), *Stress and anxiety* (pp. 111–125). Washington, DC: Hemisphere.

Jones, J. C., & Barlow, D. H. (1990). The etiology of post-traumatic stress disorder. *Clinical Psychology Review, 10,* 299–328.

Jones, M. C., Dauphinais, P., Sack, W. H., & Somervell, P. D. (1997). Trauma-related symptomatology among American Indian adolescents. *Journal of Traumatic Stress, 10,* 163–173.

Jones, R. T. (1996). Psychometric review of Child's Reaction to Traumatic Events Scale (CRTES). In B. H. Stamm (Ed.), *Measurement of stress, trauma, and adaptation* (pp. 78–80). Lutherville, MD: Sidran Press.

Jones, R. T., Fletcher, K., & Ribbe, D. R. (2000). *Child's Reaction to Traumatic Events Scale—Revised (CRTES-R): A self-report traumatic stress measure.* Available from R. T. Jones upon request.

Jones, R. T., Fletcher, K. E., & Ribbe, D. P. (2003, October). *Child's Reaction to Traumatic Events Scale: Sensitivity and specificity.* Paper to presented at the 19th Annual Meeting of the International Society for Traumatic Stress Studies, Chicago.

Jones, R. T., Hadder, J. M., Carvajal, F., Chapman, S., & Alexander, A. (2006). Conducting research in diverse, minority, and marginalized communities. In F. H. Norris, S. Galea, M. J. Friedman, & P. J. Watson (Eds.), *Methods for disaster mental health research* (pp. 265–277). New York: Guilford Press.

Jones, R. T., & Ribbe, D. P. (1991). Child, adolescent and adult victims of residential fire. *Behavior Modification, 15,* 560–580.

Jones, R. T., Ribbe, D. P., & Cunningham, P. B. (1994). Psychosocial correlates of fire disaster among children and adolescents. *Journal of Traumatic Stress, 7,* 117–122.

Kaplan, L. M., & Reich, W. (1991). *Manual for Diagnostic Interview for Children and Adolescents—Revised (DICA-R).* St. Louis, MO: Washington University.

Kardiner, A. (1941). *The traumatic neurosis of war.* New York: Hoeber.

Kassam-Adams, N. (2006). The Acute Stress Checklist for Children (ASC-Kids): Development of a child self-report measure. *Journal of Traumatic Stress, 19,* 129–139.

Kassam-Adams, N., & Winston, F. K. (2004). Predicting child PTSD: The relationship between acute stress disorder and PTSD in injured children. *Journal of the American Academy of Child and Adolescent Psychiatry, 43,* 403–411.

Kaufman, J., Birmaher, B., Brent, D., Rao, U., Flynn, C., Moreci, P., et al. (1997). Schedule for Affective Disorders and Schizophrenia for School-age Children—Present and Lifetime Version (K-SADS-PL): Initial reliability and validity data. *Journal of the American Academy of Child and Adolescent Psychiatry, 36,* 980–988.

Keane, T. M. (1993). Symptomatology of Vietnam veterans with posttraumatic stress disorder. In J. R. T. Davidson & E. B. Foa (Eds.), *Posttraumatic stress disorder: DSM-IV and beyond* (pp. 99–111). Washington, DC: American Psychiatric Association.

Keane, T. M., & Kaloupek, D. G. (1997). Comorbid psychiatric disorders in PTSD: Implications for research. *Annals of the New York Academy of Sciences, 821,* 4–34.

Kendall-Tackett, K. A., Williams, L. M., & Finkelhor, D. (1993). Impact of sexual abuse on children: A review and synthesis of recent empirical studies. *Psychological Bulletin, 113,* 164–180.

Kilpatrick, D. G., Acierno, R., Saunders, B. E., Resnick, H. S., Best, C. L., & Schnurr, P. P. (2000). Risk factors for adolescent substance abuse and dependence: Data from a national sample. *Journal of Consulting and Clinical Psychology, 68,* 19–30.

Kilpatrick, D. G., Resnick, H. S., Freedy, J. R., Pelcovitz, D., Resick, P. A., Roth, S., et al. (1998). Posttraumatic stress disorder field trial: Evaluation of the PTSD construct—Criteria A through E. In T. A. Widiger, A. J. Frances, H. A. Pincus, R. Ross, M. B. First, W. Davis, & M. Kline (Eds.), *DSM-IV sourcebook* (Vol. 4, 4th ed., pp. 803–844).

Kilpatrick, D. G., Ruggiero, K. J., Acierno, R., Saunders, B. E., Resnick, H. S., & Best, C. L. (2003). Violence and risk of PTSD, major depression, substance abuse/dependence and comorbidity: Results from the National Survey of Adolescents. *Journal of Consulting and Clinical Psychology, 71,* 692–700.

Kindlon, D., Wright, B., Raudenbush, S., & Earls, F. (1996). The measurement of children's exposure to violence: A Rasch analysis. *International Journal of Methods in Psychiatric Research, 6,* 187–194.

Kiser, L. J., Ackerman, B. J., Brown, E., Edwards, N. B., McColgan, E., Pugh, R., et al. (1988). Post-traumatic stress disorder in young children: A reaction to purported sexual abuse. *Journal of the American Academy of Child Adolescent Psychiatry, 27,* 645–649.

Ko, S. (2005). *Culture and trauma brief.* The National Child Traumatic Stress Network. Retrieved August 31, 2006, from *www.nctsnet.org/nccts/nav.do?pid=ctr_top_srvc_pub*

Koenen, K. C. (2003). A brief introduction to genetics research in PTSD. *PTSD Research Quarterly, 14,* 1–3.

Korol, M., Green, B. L., & Gleser, G. C. (1999). Children's responses to a nuclear waste disaster: PTSD symptoms and outcome prediction. *Journal of the American Academy of Child and Adolescent Psychiatry, 38,* 368–375.

Kovacs, M. (1992). *The Children's Depression Inventory.* North Tonowanda, NY: Multi-Health Systems.

Kovacs, M., & Beck, A. T. (1977). An empirical-clinical approach toward a definition of childhood depression. In J. G. Schulterbrandt & A. Raskin (Eds.), *Depression in childhood: Diagnosis, treatment, and conceptual models* (pp. 1–25). New York: Raven Press.

La Greca, A. M., Silverman, W. K., Vernberg, E. M., & Prinstein, M. J. (1996). Symptoms of posttraumatic stress in children after Hurricane Andrew: A prospective study. *Journal of Consulting and Clinical Psychology, 64,* 712–723.

Lanktree, C. B., & Briere, J. (1995). *Early data on the new Sexual Concerns and Dissociation subscales of the TSCC.* Unpublished manuscript, Department of Psychiatry, University of Southern California School of Medicine, Los Angeles.

Lazarus, R. S., & Folkman, S. (1984). *Stress, appraisal and coping.* New York: Springer.

Lecrubier, Y., Sheehan, D., Weiller, E., Amorim, P., Bonora, I., Sheehan, K., et al. (1997). The MINI International Neuropsychiatric Interview (M.I.N.I.): A short diagnostic structured interview: Reliability and validity according to the CIDI. *European Psychiatry, 12,* 224–231.

Levendosky, A. A., Huth-Bocks, A. C., Semel, M. A., & Shapiro, D. L. (2002). Trauma symptoms in preschool-age children exposed to domestic violence. *Journal of Interpersonal Violence, 17,* 150–164.

Lindholm, K. J., & Willey, R. (1986). Ethnic differences in child abuse and sexual abuse. *Hispanic Journal of Behavioral Sciences, 8,* 111–125.

Lonigan, C. J., Shannon, M. P., Finch, A. J., Jr., Daugherty, T. K., & Taylor, C. M. (1991). Children's reactions to a natural disaster: Symptom severity and degree of exposure. *Advances in Behavioral Therapy, 13,* 135–154.

Maccoby, E. E., & Martin, J. A. (1983). Socialization in the context of the family: Parent–child interaction. In P. H. Mussen (Series Ed.) & E. M. Hetherington (Vol. Ed.), *Handbook of child psychology: Vol. 4. Socialization, personality, and social development* (4th ed., pp. 1–101). New York: Wiley.

Mannarino, A. P., Cohen, J. A., & Berman, S. R. (1994). The relationship between preabuse factors and psychological symptomatology in sexually abused girls. *Journal of Interpersonal Violence, 6,* 494–511.

Manson, S. M. (1997). Cross-cultural and multiethnic assessment of trauma. In J. P. Wilson & T. M. Keane (Eds.), *Assessing psychological trauma and PTSD* (pp. 239–266). New York: Guilford Press.

March, J. S. (1999). Assessment of pediatric posttraumatic stress disorder. In P. Saigh & D. Bremner (Eds.), *Post-traumatic stress disorder* (pp. 199–218). Washington, DC: American Psychological Press.

March, J. S., Amaya-Jackson, L., Murry, M. C., & Schulte, A. (1998). Cognitive-behavioral psychotherapy for children and adolescents with posttraumatic stress disorder after a single-incident stressor. *Journal of the American Academy of Child Psychiatry, 37,* 585–593.

March, J. S., Amaya-Jackson, L., Terry, R., & Costanzo, P. (1997). Posttraumatic symptomatology in children and adolescents after an industrial fire. *Journal of the American Academy of Child Psychiatry, 36,* 1080–1088.

March, J. S., Parker, J. D. A., Sullivan, K., Stallings, P., & Conners, K. (1997). The Multidimensional Anxiety Scale for Children (MASC): Factor structure, reliability, and validity. *Journal of the American Academy of Child and Adolescent Psychiatry, 36,* 554–565.

Marsella, A., Friedman, M., Gerrity, E., & Scurfield, R. (Eds.). (1996). *Ethnocultural variation in trauma and PTSD.* New York: American Psychological Association Press.

Marshall, R. D., Spitzer, R., & Liebowitz, M. R. (1999). Review and critique of the new DSM-IV diagnosis of acute stress disorder. *American Journal of Psychiatry, 156,* 1677–1685.

Martinez, P., & Richters, J. E. (1993). The NIMH community violence project: II. Children's distress symptoms associated with violence exposure. *Psychiatry, 56,* 22–35.

McCann, I. L., & Pearlman, L. A. (1990a). *Through a glass darkly: Understanding and treating the adult trauma survivor through constructivist self-development theory.* New York: Brunner/Mazel.

McCann, I. L., & Pearlman, L. A. (1990b). Vicarious traumatization: A framework for understanding the psychological effects of working with victims. *Journal of Traumatic Stress, 3,* 131–149.

McLeer, S., Deblinger, E., Henry, D., & Orvaschel, H. (1992). Sexually abused children at high risk for post-traumatic stress disorder. *Journal of the American Academy of Child and Adolescent Psychiatry, 31,* 876–879.

Mezzich, J. E. (1995). Cultural formulation and comprehensive diagnosis. *Psychiatric Clinics of North America, 18,* 649–657.

Milgram, N., & Toubiana, Y. H. (1996). Children's selective coping after a bus disaster: Confronting behavior and perceived support. *Journal of Traumatic Stress, 9,* 687–702.

Moller-Thau, D., & Fletcher, K. E. *Diagnosing child PTSD with two self-report measures: The Childhood PTSD Reaction Index and the When Bad Things Happen Scale.* Unpublished manuscript, University of Massachusetts Medical School, Worcester, MA.

Moran, P. B., & Eckenrode, J. (1992). Protective personality characteristics among adolescent victims of maltreatment. *Child Abuse and Neglect, 16,* 743–754.

Nader, K. (1991). *Posttraumatic stress assessment following a tornado at a school.* An unpublished report to a school district February 29, 1991.

Nader, K. (1993). *Instruction manual, Childhood PTSD Reaction Index, revised, English version.* Cedar Park, TX: Author.

Nader, K. (1995). *Childhood Post-Traumatic Stress Reaction, Parent Inventory (CPTSR-PI)* (3rd ed.). A copyrighted instrument. (Original work published 1984)

Nader, K. (1997). Assessing traumatic experiences in children. In J. P. Wilson & T. M. Keane (Eds.), *Assessing psychological trauma and PTSD* (pp. 291–348). New York: Guilford Press.

Nader, K. (1999). *Instruction manual, Childhood PTSD Reaction Index, revised, English version.* Cedar Park, TX: Author.

Nader, K. (in press). *Understanding and assessing trauma in children and adolescents: Measures, methods, and youth in context.* New York: Routledge.

Nader, K., & Fairbanks, L. (1994). The suppression of reexperiencing: Impulse control and somatic symptoms in children following traumatic exposure. *Anxiety, Stress, and Coping, 7,* 229–239.

Nader, K., Pynoos, R., Fairbanks, L., Al-Ajeel, M., & Al-Asfour, A. (1993). A preliminary study of PTSD and grief among the children of Kuwait following the Gulf crisis. *British Journal of Clinical Psychology, 32,* 407–416.

Nader, K., Pynoos, R., Fairbanks, L., & Frederick, C.

(1990). Children's PTSD reactions one year after a sniper attack at their school. *American Journal of Psychiatry, 147*, 1526–1530.

National Center for Study of Corporal Punishment and Alternatives in Schools. (1992). *My Worst Experience Survey.* Philadelphia: Temple University Press.

Nelson-Gardell, D. (1995). *Validation of a treatment outcome measurement tool: Research for and with human service agencies.* Paper presented at the 35th Annual Workshop of the national Association for Welfare Research and Statistics, Jackson, NY.

Newman, E., McMackin, R., Morrissey, C., & Erwin, B. (1997). Addressing PTSD and trauma-related symptoms among criminally involved male adolescents. *Traumatic StressPoints, 11*, 7.

Newman, E., Weathers, F. W., Nader, K. O., Kaloupek, D. G., Pynoos, R. S., Blake, D. D., et al. (2004). *Clinician-Administered PTSD Scale for Children and Adolescents (CAPS-CA) Interviewer's Guide.* Los Angeles: Western Psychological Services.

Norris, F. H., & Alegria, M. (2005). Mental health care for ethnic minority individuals and communities in the aftermath of disasters and mass violence. *CNS Spectrums, 10*, 1–9.

Norris, F. H., Byrne, C., Diaz, E., & Kaniasty, K. (2002). *50,000 disaster victims speak: An empirical review of the empirical literature, 1981–2001.* Unpublished technical report, National Center for PTSD, Dartmouth Medical School, Hanover, NH.

Norris, F. H., & Kaniasty, K. (1991). The psychological experience of crime: A test of the mediating role of beliefs in explaining the distress of victims. *Journal of Social and Clinical Psychology, 10*, 239–261.

Ohan, J. L., Myers, K., & Collett, B. R. (2002). Ten-year review of rating scales: IV. Scales assessing trauma and its affects. *Journal of the American Academy of Child and Adolescent Psychiatry, 41*, 1401–1422.

Ohmi, H., Kojima, S., Awai, Y., Kamata, S., Sasaki, K., Tanaka, Y., et al. (2002). Post-traumatic stress disorder in pre-school aged children after a gas explosion. *European Journal of Pediatrics, 161*, 643–648.

Orvaschel, J., Puig-Antich, J., Chambers, W., Tabrizi, M. A., & Johnson, R. (1982). Retrospective assessment of prepubertal major depression with the Kiddie-SADS-E. *Journal of the American Academy of Child and Adolescent Psychiatry, 21*, 392–397.

Osofsky, J. D., Wewers, S., Hann, D. M., & Fick, A. C. (1993). Chronic community violence: What is happening to our children? *Psychiatry, 56*, 36–45.

Pain, C. (2002, August). PTSD and comorbidity or disorder of extreme stress not otherwise specified? *Bulletin of the Canadian Psychiatric Association*, pp. 12–14.

Pelcovitz, D., Libov, B. G., Mandel, F., Kaplan, S., Weinblatt, M., & Septimus, A. (1998). Posttraumatic stress disorder and family functioning in adolescent cancer. *Journal of Traumatic Stress, 11*, 205–221.

Pelcovitz, D., van der Kolk, B., Roth, S., Mandel, F., Kaplan, S., & Resick, P. (1997). Development of a criteria set and a structured interview for disorders of

extreme stress (SIDES). *Journal of Traumatic Stress, 10*, 3–16.

Perry, B. D. (2001). The neurodevelopmental impact of violence in childhood. In D. Schetky & E. Benedek (Eds.), *Textbook of child and adolescent forensic psychiatry* (pp. 221–238). Washington, DC: American Psychiatric Press.

Perry, B. D., Pollard, R., Blakley, T., Baker, W. L., & Vigilante, D. (1995). Childhood trauma, the neurobiology of adaptation and "use-dependent" development of the brain: how "states" become "traits." *Infant Mental Health Journal, 16*, 271–291.

Peterson, C., & Seligman, M. E. P. (1983). Learned helplessness and victimization. *Journal of Social Issues, 2*, 103–116.

Pfefferbaum, B., Doughty, D. E., Reddy, C., Patel, N., Gurwitch, R. H., Nixon, S. J., et al. (2002). Exposure and peritraumatic response as predictors of posttraumatic stress in children following the 1995 Oklahoma City bombing. *Journal of Urban Health: Bulletin of the New York Academy of Medicine, 79*, 354–363.

Pfefferbaum, B., Seale, T. W., McDonald, N. B., Brandt, E. N., Jr., Rainwater, S. M., Maynard, B. T., et al. (2000). Posttraumatic stress two years after the Oklahoma City bombing in youths geographically distant from the explosion. *Psychiatry, 63*, 358–370.

Pierce, L. H., & Pierce, R. L. (1984). Race as a factor in the sexual abuse of children. *Social Work Research Abstracts, 20*, 9–14.

Praver, F. (1996). *Validation of a child measure for posttraumatic stress responses to interpersonal abuse.* Unpublished doctoral dissertation, St. John's University, Jamaica, NY.

Praver, F., DiGiuseppe, R., Pelcovitz, D., Mandel, F., & Gaines, R. (2000). A preliminary study of a cartoon measure for children's reactions to chronic trauma. *Child Maltreatment, 5*, 273–285.

Praver, F., & Pelcovitz, D. (1996). Psychometric review of Angie/Andy Child Rating Scales: A cartoon-based measure for post traumatic stress responses to chronic interpersonal abuse. In B. H. Stamm (Ed.), *Measurement of stress, trauma, and adaptation* (pp. 65–70). Lutherville, MD: Sidran Press.

Praver, F., Pelcovitz, D., & DiGiuseppe, R. (1993). *The Angie/Andy Parent Rating Scales.* An unpublished, copyrighted instrument.

Praver, F., Pelcovitz, D., & DiGiuseppe, R. (1998). *The Angie/Andy Child Rating Scales.* Toronto: Multi-Health Systems.

Putnam, F. W. (1998). Trauma models of the effects of childhood maltreatment. *Journal of Aggression, Maltreatment, and Trauma, 2*, 51–66.

Putnam, F. W., Helmers, K., & Trickett, P. K. (1993). Development, reliability, and validity of a child dissociation scale. *Child Abuse and Neglect, 17*, 519–531.

Pynoos, R. S., & Eth, S. (1985). Developmental perspective on psychic trauma in childhood. In C. R. Figley (Ed.), *Trauma and its wake* (Vol. 1, pp. 36–52). New York: Brunner/Mazel.

Pynoos, R. S., Frederick, C., Nader, K., Arroyo, W., Steinberg, A., Eth, S., et al. (1987). Life threat and posttraumatic stress in school-age children. *Archives of General Psychiatry, 44,* 1057–1063.

Pynoos, R., Goenjian, A., Tashjian, M., Karakashian, M., Manjikian, R., Manoukian, G., et al. (1993). Post-traumatic stress reactions of children after the 1988 Armenian earthquake. *British Journal of Psychiatry, 163,* 239–247.

Pynoos, R. S., Rodriguez, N., Steinberg, A. M., Stuber, M., & Frederick, C. (1998). *UCLA PTSD Index for DSM-IV (Revision 1).* Los Angeles: UCLA Trauma Psychiatry Program.

Quay, H. C., & Peterson, D. R. (1996). *Revised Behavior Problem Checklist: Manual.* Odessa, FL: Psychological Assessment Resources.

Rao, K., DiClemente, R. J., & Ponton, L. E. (1992). Child sexual abuse of Asians compared with other populations. *Journal of the American Academy of Child and Adolescent Psychiatry, 31,* 880–886.

Raviv, A., Erel, O., Fox, N. A., Leavitt, L. A., Raviv, A., Dor, I., et al. (2001). Individual measurement of exposure to everyday violence among elementary schoolchildren across various settings. *Journal of Community Psychology, 29,* 117–140.

Realmuto, G. M., Mastern, A., Carole, L. F., Hubbard, J., Groteluschen, A., & Chhun, B. (1992). Adolescent survivors of massive childhood trauma in Cambodia: Life events and current symptoms. *Journal of Traumatic Stress, 4,* 589–599.

Reich, W. (2000). Diagnostic Interview for Children and Adolescents (DICA). *Journal of the American Academy of Child and Adolescent Psychiatry, 39,* 59–66

Reich, W., Leacock, N., & Shanfeld, C. (1994). *Diagnostic Interview for Children and Adolescents—Revised (DICA-R).* St. Louis, MO: Washington University.

Reich, W., & Todd, R. D. (2002). *MAGIC Missouri Assessment of Genetics Interview for Children: Specifications manual.* St. Louis, MO: Washington University School of Medicine.

Reynolds, C. R., & Richmond, B. O. (1978). *Revised Children's Manifest Anxiety Scale manual.* Los Angeles: Western Psychological Services.

Richters, J. E., & Martinez, P. (1990a). *Checklist of Child Distress Symptoms: Parent report.* Rockville, MD: National Institute of Mental Health.

Richters, J. E., & Martinez, P. (1990b). *Things I Have Seen and Heard: A structured interview for assessing young children's violence exposure.* Rockville, MD: National Institute of Mental Health.

Richters, J. E., & Martinez, P. (1993). The NIMH community violence project: I. Children as victims of and witnesses to violence. *Psychiatry, 56,* 7–21.

Richters, J. E., Martinez, P., & Valla, J.-P. (1990). *Levonn: A cartoon-based structured interview for assessing young children's distress symptoms.* Rockville, MD: National Institute of Mental Health.

Richters, J. E., & Saltzman, W (1990). *Survey of Children's Exposure to Community Violence: Parent Report.* Rockville, MD: National Institute of Mental Health.

Rodriguez, N. (2001, December). *Youth PTSD assessment: Psychometric investigation of PTSD self-report instruments.* Paper presented at the 17th Annual International Society for Traumatic Stress Studies Meeting, New Orleans, LA.

Rodriguez, N. (in press). Psychometric analysis of a child and adolescent PTSD self-report assessment instrument. *Journal of Interpersonal Violence.*

Rodriguez, N., Steinberg, A. S., Saltzman, W. S., & Pynoos, R. S. (2001a, December). *PTSD Index: Preliminary psychometric analyses of the adolescent versions.* Symposium conducted at the Annual Meeting of the International Society for Traumatic Stress Studies. New Orleans, LA.

Rodriguez, N., Steinberg, A. S., Saltzman, W. S., & Pynoos, R. S. (2001b, December). *PTSD Index: Preliminary psychometric analyses of child and parent versions.* Symposium conducted at the Annual Meeting of the International Society for Traumatic Stress Studies. New Orleans, LA.

Rooney, M. T., Fristad, M. A., Weller, E. B., & Weller, R. A. (1999). *Administration manual for the ChIPS.* Washington, DC: American Psychiatric Press.

Rossman, B. B. R. (1992). School-age children's perceptions of coping with distress: Strategies for emotion regulation and the moderation of adjustment. *Journal of Child Psychology and Psychiatry, 33,* 1373–1397.

Rossman, B. B. R., Bingham, R. D., & Emde, R. N. (1997). Symptomatology and adaptive functioning for children exposed to normative stressors, dog attack, and parental violence. *Journal of the American Academy of Child and Adolescent Psychiatry, 36,* 1089–1097.

Rothbaum, B. O., & Foa, E. B. (1993). Subtypes of posttraumatic stress disorder and duration of symptoms. In J. R. T. Davidson & E. B. Foa (Eds.), *DSM-IV and beyond* (pp. 23–35). Washington, DC: American Psychiatric Association.

Rubel, A. J., O'Nell, C. W., & Collado-Ardon, R. (1984). *Susto, a folk illness.* Berkeley: University of California Press.

Rutter, M. (1983). Stress, coping, and development: Some issues and questions. In N. Garmezy & M. Rutter (Eds.), *Stress, coping, and development in children* (pp. 1–41). New York: McGraw-Hill.

Saigh, P. A. (1985). Adolescent anxiety following varying degrees of war exposure. *Journal of Clinical Child Psychology, 14,* 311–314.

Saigh, P. A. (1991). The development of posttraumatic stress disorder following four different types of traumatization. *Behaviour Research and Therapy, 29,* 213–216.

Saigh, P. A. (1998a). *Children's PTSD Inventory (DSM-IV Version).* New York: Author.

Saigh, P. A. (1998b). *Test manual for the Children's PTSD Inventory (DSM-IV Version).* New York: Author.

Saigh, P. A., Yasik, A. E., Oberfield, R. A., Green, B. L., Halamandaris, P. V., Rubenstein, H., et al. (2000). The Children's PTSD Inventory: Development and reliability. *Journal of Traumatic Stress, 13,* 369–380.

Saigh, P. A., Yasik, A. E., Sack, W. H., & Koplewicz, H. S. (1999). Child–adolescent posttraumatic stress disorder: Prevalence, risk factors, and comorbidity. In P. A. Saigh & J. D. Bremner (Eds.), *Posttraumatic stress disorder* (pp. 18–43). Needham Heights, MA: Allyn & Bacon.

Sattler, D., Preston, A., Kaiser, C., Olivera, V., Valdez, J., & Schlueter, S. (2002). Hurricane George: A cross-national study examining preparedness, resource loss, and psychological distress in the U.S. Virgin Islands, Puerto Rico, Dominican Republic, and the United States. *Journal of Traumatic Stress, 15,* 339–350.

Saunders, B. E., Arata, C. M., & Kilpatrick, D. G. (1990). Development of a crime-related post-traumatic stress disorder scale for women within the Symptom Checklist–90—Revised. *Journal of Traumatic Stress, 3,* 439–448.

Saylor, C. F., Swenson, C. C., Reynolds, S. S., & Taylor, M. (1999). The Pediatric Emotional Distress Scale: A brief screening measure for young children exposed to traumatic events. *Journal of Clinical Child Psychology, 28,* 70–81.

Saxe, G. N. (2001). *Child Stress Disorders Checklist (v. 4.0—11/01).* Unpublished measure, National Child Traumatic Stress Network and Boston University School of Medicine.

Saxe, G. N., & Bosquet, M. (2004). *Child Stress Disorders Checklist—Screening Form (CSDC-SF) (v. 1.0– 3/04).* Unpublished measure, National Child Traumatic Stress Network & Boston University School of Medicine.

Saxe, G., Chawala, N., Stoddard, F., Kassam-Adams, N., Courtney, D., Cunningham, K., et al. (2003). Child Stress Disorders Checklist: A Measure of ASD and PTSD in children. *Journal of the American Academy of Child and Adolescent Psychiatry, 42,* 972–978.

Scheeringa, M. S., Peebles, C. D., Cook, C. A., & Zeanah, C. H. (2001). Toward establishing procedural, criterion, and discriminant validity for PTSD in early childhood. *Journal of the American Academy of Child and Adolescent Psychiatry, 40,* 52–60.

Scheeringa, M. S., & Zeanah, C. H. (1994). *Posttraumatic stress disorder semi-structured interview and observational record for infants and young children.* Unpublished measure, Tulane University, New Orleans, LA.

Scheeringa, M. S., & Zeanah, C. H. (1995). Symptom expression and trauma variables in children under 48 months of age. *Infant Mental Health Journal, 16,* 259–270.

Scheeringa, M. S., & Zeanah, C. H. (2003). New findings on alternative criteria for PTSD in preschool children. *Journal of the American Academy of Child and Adolescent Psychiatry, 42,* 561–570.

Scheeringa, M. S., Zeanah, C. H., Drell, M. J., & Larrieu, J. A. (1995). Two approaches to the diagnosis of posttraumatic stress disorder in infancy and early childhood. *Journal of the American Academy of Child and Adolescent Psychiatry, 34,* 191–200.

Scheeringa, M. S., Zeanah, C. H., Myers, L., & Putnam, F. (2003). New findings on alternative criteria for PTSD in preschool children. *Journal of the American Academy of Child and Adolescent Psychiatry, 42,* 561–570.

Scheeringa, M. S., Zeanah, C. H., Myers, L., & Putnam, F. (2005). Predictive validity in a prospective follow-up in preschool children. *Journal of the American Academy of Child and Adolescent Psychiatry, 44,* 899–906.

Schneider-Rosen, K., & Cicchetti, D. (1984). The relationship between affect and cognition in maltreated infants: Quality of attachment and the development of visual self-recognition. *Child Development, 55,* 648–658.

Schwarz, E. D., & Kowalski, J. M. (1991). Posttraumatic stress disorder after a school shooting: Effects of symptom threshold selection and diagnosis by DSM-III, DSM-III-R, or proposed DSM-IV. *American Journal of Psychiatry, 148,* 592–597.

Seifer, R., Sameroff, A. J., Baldwin, C. P., & Baldwin, A. (1992). Child and family factors that ameliorate risk between 4 and 13 years of age. *Journal of the American Academy of Child and Adolescent Psychiatry, 31,* 893–903.

Selner-O'Hagan, M. B., Kindlon, D. J., Buka, S. L., Raudenbush, S. W., & Earls, F. J. (1998). Assessing exposure to violence in urban youth. *Journal of Child Psychology and Psychiatry and Allied Disciplines, 39,* 215–224.

Shaffer, D., Fisher, P., & Lucas, C. (2000). NIMH Diagnostic Interview Schedule for Children Version IV (NIMH DISC-IV): Description, differences from previous versions, and reliability of some common diagnoses. *Journal of American Academy of Child and Adolescent Psychiatry, 39,* 28–38.

Shaffer, D., Schwab-Stone, M., Fisher, P., Cohen, P., Piacentini, J., Davies, M., et al. (1993). The Diagnostic Interview Schedule for Children—Revised version (DISC-R): I. Preparation, field testing, interrater reliability, and acceptability. *Journal of American Academy of Child and Adolescent Psychiatry, 32,* 643–650.

Shaffer, D., Schwab-Stone, M., Fisher, P., Davies, M., Piacentini, J., & Gioia, P. (1988). *A revised version of the Diagnostic Interview Schedule for Children (DISC-R): Results of a field trial and proposals for a new instrument (DISC-R).* Rockville, MD: Epidemiology and Psychopathology Research Branch, National Institute of Mental Health.

Shahinfar, A., Fox, N. A., & Leavitt, L. A. (2000). Preschool children's exposure to violence: Relation of behavior problems to parent and child reports. *American Journal of Orthopsychiatry, 70,* 115–25.

Shannon, M. P., Lonigan, C. J., Finch, A. J., Jr., & Taylor, C. M. (1994). Children exposed to disaster: I. Epidemiology of post-traumatic symptoms and symptom profiles. *Journal of the American Academy of Child and Adolescent Psychiatry, 33,* 80–93.

Sharrer, V., & Ryan-Wenger, N. (2002). School-age children's self-reported stress symptoms. *Pediatric Nursing, 28,* 21–27.

Sheehan, D. V., Lecrubier, Y., Harnett-Sheehan, K., Amorim, P., Janavs, J., Weiller, E., et al. (1998). The Mini International Neuropsychiatric Interview (M.I.N.I.): The development and validation of a structured diagnostic psychiatric interview. *Journal of Clinical Psychiatry, 59*(Suppl. 20), 22–33.

Sheehan, D. V., Lecrubier, Y., Harnett-Sheehan, K., Janavs, J., Weiller, E., Bonara, I., et al. (1997). Reliability and Validity of the MINI International Neuropsychiatric Interview (M.I.N.I.): According to the SCID-P. *European Psychiatry, 12,* 232–241.

Silva, R. R., Alpert, M., Munoz, D. M., Singh, S., Matzner, F., & Dummit, S. (2000). Stress and vulnerability to posttraumatic stress disorder in children and adolescents. *American Journal of Psychiatry, 157,* 1229–1235.

Singer, M. I., Anglin, T. M., Song, L. Y., & Lunghofer, L. (1995). Adolescents' exposure to violence and associated symptoms of psychological trauma. *Journal of the American Medical Association, 273,* 477–482.

Skidmore, G. L., & Fletcher, K. E. (1997, November). *Assessing trauma's impact on beliefs: The World View Survey.* Paper presented at the 13th Annual Meeting of the International Society for Traumatic Stress Studies, Montreal, Canada.

Skybo, T. (2005). Witnessing violence: Biopsychosocial impact on children. *Pediatric Nursing, 31,* 263–270.

Slater, M. A., & Power, T. G. (1987). Multidimensional assessment of parenting in single-parent families. In J. P. Vincent (Ed.), *Advances in family intervention, assessment and theory* (Vol. 4, pp. 197–228). Greenwich, CT: JAI Press.

Smith, D. W., Saunders, B. E., Swenson, C. C., & Crouch, J. (1995). *Trauma Symptom Checklist for Children and Children's Impact of Traumatic Events—Revised scores in sexually abused children.* Unpublished manuscript, Medical University of South Carolina, Charleston, SC.

Smith, D. W., Swenson, C. C., Hanson, R. F., & Saunders, B. E. (1994, May). *The relationship of abuse and disclosure characteristics to Trauma Symptom Checklist for Children's scores: A preliminary construct validity analysis.* Poster session presented at the Second Annual Colloquium of the American Professional Society on the Abuse of Children, Boston.

Smith, P., Perrin, S., Dyregrov, A., & Yule, W. (2003). Principal components analysis of the Impact of Event Scale with children in war. *Personality and Individual Differences, 34,* 315–322.

Spilsbury, J. C., Drotar, D., Burant, C., Flannery, D., Creeden, R., & Friedman, S. (2005). Psychometric properties of the Pediatric Emotional Distress Scale in a diverse sample of children exposed to interpersonal violence. *Journal of Clinical and Child and Adolescent Psychology, 34,* 758–764.

Spitzer, R. L., Williams, J. B. W., Gibbon, M., & First, M. B. (1990). *Structured Clinical Interview for DSM-III-R, Patient Edition/Non-Patient Edition (SCID-P/SCID-NP).* Washington, DC: American Psychiatric Press.

Stallard, P., Velleman, R., Langsford, J., & Baldwin, S. (2001). Coping and psychological distress in children involved in road traffic accidents. *British Journal of Clinical Psychology, 40,* 197–208.

Stamm, B. H., & Friedman, M. J. (2000). Cultural diversity in the appraisal and expression of trauma. In A. Y. Shalev, R. Yehuda, & A. C. McFarlane (Eds.), *International handbook of human response to trauma* (pp. 69–85). New York: Kluwer Academic.

Stedman, R., Yule, W., Smith, P., Glucksman, E., & Dalgleish, T. (2005). Acute stress disorder and posttraumatic stress disorder in children and adolescents involved in assaults and motor vehicle accidents. *American Journal of Psychiatry, 162,* 1381–1383.

Stein, B., Comer, D., Gardner, W., & Kelleher, K. (1999). Prospective study of displaced children's symptoms in wartime Bosnia. *Social Psychiatry and Psychiatric Epidemiology, 334,* 464–469.

Steinberg, A. M., Brymer, M. J., Decker, K. B., & Pynoos, R. S. (2004). The University of California at Los Angeles Post-Traumatic Stress Disorder Reaction Index. *Current Psychiatry Report, 6,* 96–100.

Steiner, H., Garcia, I. G., & Matthews, Z. (1997). Posttraumatic stress disorder in incarcerated juvenile delinquents. *Journal of the Academy of Child and Adolescent Psychiatry, 36,* 357–365.

Stoddard, F., & Saxe, G. N. (2001). Childhood injuries: A review of the last 10-years. *Journal of American Academy of Child and Adolescent Psychiatry, 40,* 1128–1145.

Stokes, S. J., Saylor, C. F., Swenson, C. C., & Daugherty, T. K. (1995). A comparison of children's behaviors following three types of stressors. *Child Psychiatry and Human Development, 26,* 113–123.

Stover, C. S., & Berkowitz, S. (2005). Assessing violence exposure and trauma symptoms in young children: A critical review of measures. *Journal of Traumatic Stress, 18,* 707–717.

Straus, M. A. (1979). Measuring introfamily conflict and violence: The Conflict Tactics (CT) scales. *Journal of Marriage and the Family, 41,* 75–88.

Suliman, S., Kaminer, D., Seedat, S., & Stein, D. J. (Accessed March 1, 2005). Assessing post-traumatic stress disorder in South African adolescents: Using the Child and Adolescent Trauma Survey (CATS) as a screening tool. *Annals of General Psychiatry, 4.* Available online at *www.annals-general-psychiatry.com/contents/4/2*

Swenson, C. C., Saylor, C. F., Paige Powell, M., Stokes, S. J., Foster, K. Y., & Belter, R. W. (1996). Impact of a natural disaster on preschool children: Adjustment 14 months after a hurricane. *American Journal of Orthopsychiatry, 66,* 122–130.

Task Force on Research Diagnostic Criteria: Infancy and Preschool. (2003). Research diagnostic criteria for infants and preschool children: The process and empirical support. *Journal of the Academy of Child and Adolescent Psychiatry, 42,* 1504–1512. Available for download at *www.infantinstitute.org*

Teicher, M. H., Andersen, S. L., Pocari, A., Anderson, C. M., Navalta, C. P., & Kim, D. M. (2003). The neurological consequences of early stress and childhood maltreatment. *Neuroscience and Biobehavioral Reviews, 27,* 33–44.

Terr, L. C. (1981). "Forbidden games": Post-traumatic child's play. *Journal of the American Academy of Child Psychiatry, 20,* 741–760.

Thabet, A. A. M., & Vostanis, P. (1999). Post-traumatic stress responses in children of war. *Journal of Child Psychology and Psychiatry, 40,* 385–391.

Todd, R. D., Joyner, C. A., Heath, A. C., Neuman, R. J., & Reich, W. (2003). Reliability and stability of a semistructured DSM-IV interview designed for family studies. *Journal of the American Academy of Child and Adolescent Psychiatry, 42,* 1460–1468.

Udwin, O., Boyle, S., Yule, W., Bolton, D., & O'Ryan, D. (2000). Risk factors for long-term psychological effects of a disaster experienced in adolescence: Predictors of posttraumatic stress disorder. *Journal of Child Psychology and Psychiatry, 41,* 969–979.

Ursano, R. J., Fullerton, C. S., & McCaughey, B. G. (1994). Trauma and disaster. In R. J. Ursano, B. G. McCaughey, & C. S. Fullerton (Eds.), *Individual and community responses to trauma and disaster* (pp. 3–27). New York: Cambridge University Press.

U.S. Department of Health and Human Services, Administration for Children and Families. (2002). *Child Maltreatment 2002.* Washington, DC: Author.

Valla, J.-P. (1989). *Dominique: A cartoon interview for assessing young children's psychiatric symptoms.* Montreal, Canada: University of Montreal.

van der Kolk, B. A., & Courtois C. A. (2005). Editorial comments: Complex development trauma. *Journal of Traumatic Stress, 18,* 385–388.

van der Kolk, B. A., Pelcovitz, D., Roth, S., Mandel, F., McFarlane, A., & Herman, J. L. (1996). Dissociation, somatization, and affect dysregulation: The complexity of adaptation to trauma. *American Journal of Psychiatry, 153,* 83–93.

van der Kolk, B. A., Roth, S., Pelcovitz, D., Sunday, S., & Spinazzola, J. (2005). Disorders of extreme stress: The empirical foundation of a complex adaptation to trauma. *Journal of Traumatic Stress, 18,* 389–399.

Verducci, J. S., Mack, M. E., & DeGroot, M. H. (1988). Estimating multiple rater agreement for a rare diagnosis. *Journal of Multivariate Analysis, 27,* 512–535.

Vernberg, E. M., La Greca, A. M., Silverman, W. K., & Prinstein, J. J. (1996). Prediction of posttraumatic stress symptoms in children after Hurricane Andrew. *Journal of Abnormal Psychology, 105,* 237–248.

Vila, G., Porche, L., & Mouren-Simeoni, M. (1999). An 18-month longitudinal study of posttraumatic disorders in children who were taken hostage in their school. *Psychosomatic Medicine 61,* 746–754.

Vila, G., Witowski, P., Tondini, M. C., Perez-Diaz, F., Mouren-Simeoni, M. C., & Jouvent, R. (2001). A study of posttraumatic stress disorders in children who experienced an industrial disaster in the Briey region. *European Child and Adolescent Psychiatry, 10,* 10–18.

Wasserstein, S. B., & La Greca, A. M. (1998). Hurricane Andrew: Parent conflict as a moderator of children's adjustment. *Hispanic Journal of Behavioral Sciences, 20,* 212–224.

Weathers, F. W. (2004). *Clinician-Administered PTSD Scale (CAPS): Technical manual.* Los Angeles: Western Psychological Services.

Weathers, F. W., Newman, E., Blake, D. D., Nagy, L. M., Schnurr, P. P., Kaloupek, D. G., et al. (2004). *Clinician-Administered PTSD Scale (CAPS): Interviewer's guide.* Los Angeles: Western Psychological Services.

Weiss, D. S., & Marmar, C. R. (1997). The Impact of Event Scale—Revised. In J. P. Wilson & T. M. Keane (Eds.), *Assessing psychological trauma and PTSD.* New York: Guilford Press.

Weller, E. B., Weller, R. A., Fristad, M. A., Rooney, M. T., & Schecter, J. (2000). Children's Interview for Psychiatric Syndromes (ChIPS). *Journal of the American Academy of Child and Adolescent Psychiatry, 39,* 76–84.

Weller, E. B., Weller, R. A., Rooney, M. T., & Fristad, M. A. (1999). *Children's Interview for Psychiatric Syndroms: ChIPS.* Washington, DC: American Psychiatric Press.

Werner, E. E., & Smith, R. S. (1982). *Vulnerable but invincible: A longitudinal study of resilient children and youth.* New York: McGraw-Hill.

Williamson, D. E., Birmaher, B., Ryan, N. D., Shiffrin, T. P., Lusky, J. A., Protopapa, J., et al. (2003). The Stressful Life Events Schedule for children and adolescents: Development and validation. *Psychiatry Research, 119,* 225–241.

Winje, D., & Ulvik, A. (1998). Long-term outcome of trauma in children: The psychological consequences of a bus accident. *Journal of Child Psychology and Psychiatry, 39,* 635–642.

Winokur, A., Winokur, D. F., Rickles, K., & Cox, D. (1984). Symptoms of emotional stress in family planning service: Stability over a four-week period. *British Journal of Psychiatry, 144,* 395–399.

Wolfe, V. V., & Birt, J. H. (1993). *The Children's Peritraumatic Experiences Questionnaire.* Unpublished assessment instrument, Child and Adolescent Centre, London Health Sciences Centre, London, Ontario.

Wolfe, V. V., & Birt, J. H. (2002a). *The Children's Impact of Traumatic Events Scale—Revised (CITES-R): Scale structure, internal consistency, discriminant validity, and PTSD diagnostic patterns.* Manuscript submitted for publication.

Wolfe, V. V., & Birt, J. H. (2002b). *The Children's*

Peritraumatic Experiences Questionnaire: A measure to assess DSM-IV PTSD criterion A2.

Wolfe, V. V., Gentile, C., & Bourdeau, P. (1987). *History of Victimization Form.* Unpublished assessment instrument, Child and Adolescent Centre, London Health Sciences Centre, London, Ontario.

Wolfe, V. V., Gentile, C., Michienzi, T., Sas, L., & Wolfe, D. A. (1991). The Children's Impact of Traumatic Events Scale: A measure of post–sexual-abuse PTSD symptoms. *Behavioral Assessment, 13,* 359–383.

Wolfe, V. V., Gentile, C., & Wolfe, D. A. (1989). The impact of sexual abuse on children: A PTSD formulation. *Behavior Therapy, 20,* 215–228.

Wolfe, V. V., Wolfe, D. A., Gentile, C., & Larose, L. (1986). *Children's Impact of Traumatic Events Scale (CITES).* A copyrighted instrument, London, Ontario, Canada: London Health Sciences Center.

World Health Organization. (1992). *ICD-10 classification of mental and behavioural disorders: Clinical descriptions and diagnostic guidelines.* Geneva: Author.

Yasik, A. E., Saigh, P. A., Oberfield, R. A., Green, B., Halamandaris, P., & McHugh, M. (2001). The validity of the Children's PTSD Inventory. *Journal of Traumatic Stress, 14,* 81–94.

Yasik, A. E., Saigh, P. A., Oberfield, R. A., Rubenstein, H., Halamandaris, P., Nester, J., et al. (1998, November). *The reliability and validity of the Diagnostic Interview for Children and Adolescents—Revised PTSD module.* Poster presented at the annual meeting of the International Society for Traumatic Stress Studies Conference, Washington, DC.

Yule, W. (1992). Post Traumatic stress disorder in child survivors of shipping disasters: The sinking of the "Jupiter." *Journal of Psychotherapy and Psychosomatics, 57,* 200–205.

Yule, W. (1997). Anxiety, Depression and Post-Traumatic Stress in Childhood. In I. Sclare (Ed.), *Child Psychology Portfolio.* Windsor: NFER-Nelson.

Yule, W., Ten Bruggencate, S., & Joseph, S. (1994). Principal components analysis of the Impact of Event Scale in children who survived a shipping disaster. *Personality and Individual Differences, 16,* 685–691.

Zero to Three. (2005). *Diagnostic Classification of Mental Health and Developmental Disorders of Infancy and Early Childhood: Revised edition (DC:0–3R).* Washington, DC: Author.

Zlotnick, C., Zakriski, A. L., Shea, M. T., Costello, E., Begin, A., Pearlstein, T., et al. (1996). The long-term sequelae of sexual abuse: Support for a complex posttraumatic stress disorder. *Journal of Traumatic Stress, 9,* 195–205.

ADMINISTERED TO CHILD

Child and Adolescent Psychiatric Assessment (CAPA) Life Events Scale (Angold & Costello, 2000)

Brief Description: This Life Events Scale is part of the PTSD module of the CAPA, a semistructured psychiatric assessment interview (see Appendix 9.3 for a description of the full interview) that assesses both high- and low-magnitude stressors. High-magnitude stressors are assessed for child's whole life; low-magnitude stressors, for past 3 months. Training is required. Interviewer qualifications: Bachelor's degree or higher. Age range: 9–17 years. Languages available: English and Spanish.

Evidence of Reliability: For high-magnitude stressors, the intraclass correlation (ICC) within 2 weeks = .72. For low-magnitude stressors, ICC within 2 weeks = .62 (Costello, Angold, March, & Fairbank, 1998). For seven events that were reported by 4 or more children, the test–retest kappa ranged from .25 for learned about a traumatic event to .88 for diagnosis of a serious illness.

Evidence of Validity: Evidence of validity has yet to be published.

Contact Information: Developmental Epidemiology Program, Duke University Medical Center, Attention: Juné Rogers, DUMC Box 3454, Durham, NC 27710. Telephone: (919) 687-4686, extension 273. E-mail: *jrogers@psych.duhs.duke.edu.*

Children's Report of Exposure to Violence (CREV; Cooley, Turner, & Beidel, 1995)

Brief Description: The CREV is a self-report assessment of children's exposure to violence through four modes: media (television or film), reported (people's reports of occurrence), witnessed (directly witnessed), and victim (directly experienced). The CREV includes three categories of victims: the self, strangers, and familiar persons. This report comprises 32 items, 29 of which ask children to indicate the frequency of exposure to violent events in the community during their lifetime. Children rate the frequency of ever being exposed to each type of violence using a 5-point Likert-like scale: *No/Never* (0), *One time* (1), *A few times* (2), *Many times* (3), or *Every day* (4). The final three items, which are open-ended questions that allow children to describe any other kinds of violent experiences not already described, are not scored. Scores are based on the first 29 questions. Age range: 9–15 years.

Evidence of Reliability: In a sample of 228 children (Cooley et al., 1995) ages 9–15 (M = 11.4, SD = 1.37), attending grades 4 through 7, 50.9% girls, 74.1% African American, 19.7% European American, 1.8% Hispanic, 1.3% Native American, 1.3% Asian, and 1.8% biracial, Cronbach's alpha for the total score was .78, and it was .93 for the Direct Exposure factor (see "Evidence of Validity" below) and .75 for Media Exposure. Test–retest reliability was examined for a sample of 42 children who were retested 2 weeks later. The test–retest reliability Pearson correlation for the total score was .75, and it was .78 for the Direct Exposure and .52 for the Media Exposure factors.

Evidence of Validity: Factor analysis identified two factors on which all but 5 of the items loaded: Direct Exposure (21 items) and Media Exposure (3 items; Cooley et al., 1995). This factor analysis is frequently referred to as evidence of the validity of the CREV. Such "evidence" is incomplete. Although Cooley-Quille, Turner, and Beidel (1995) also are frequently cited as providing evidence for the validity of the CREV, in actuality they provide very little evidence of validity for the scale. This does not necessarily mean the CREV is not a valid instrument; however, the authors chose only to examine correlations between the CREV and general reports of depression, temperament, and internalizing and externalizing behavior, not its association with symptoms of PTSD. Moreover, they examined those correlations separately within two groups: those who scored in the upper and the lower quarters of the CREV. Not only did this reduce their sample sizes drastically but it also reduced the variance associated with exposure to violence within each of the groups, thus limiting the magnitude of any correlation that might be found.

Contact Information: Michele R. Cooley-Quille, PhD, Department of Psychology, George Mason University, Fairfax, VA 22030-4444. Telephone: (703) 993-1363. Fax: (703) 993-1359.

Juvenile Victimization Questionnaire (JVQ)—Child Report (Finkelhor, Hamby, Ormrod, & Turner, 2005)

Brief Description: The JVQ Child Report version (see below for the Caregiver Proxy Report version) asks screening questions about 34 acts of violence against children, related to five general areas: (1) conventional crime, (2) child maltreatment, (3) peer and sibling victimization, (4) sexual victimization, and (5) witnessing and indirect victimization. Questions association with each of the five areas are contained in their own module, each of which was designed for use on their own in stand-alone form. However, Finkelhor and colleagues (2005) note, "For theoretical and practical reasons, however, it is preferable to administer the full instrument" (p. 385). Events that are endorsed are followed up with questions about the number of times the child has been victimized in this manner, who victimized the child, whether or not the child was hurt, and questions specific to the type of victimization reported (e.g., the value of stolen items). The JVQ can be used without the follow-up questions, at the expense of eliciting detailed information about the different experiences. The JVQ asks about the occurrence of events in the previous year, but it can be adapted for asking about lifetime exposure. Early testing of the JVQ included extensive reviews by experts in the field of juvenile victimization. Draft versions were critiqued by focus groups of youth and parents to refine the wording. A series of cognitive interviews with 24 children between the ages of 6 and 15 were conducted to ensure comprehensibility of the questions. Administration time: 20 minutes on average. Age range: As an interview, it can be used with children 8 years and older. It can be administered in a self-report format with juveniles 12 years and older.

Evidence of Reliability: To conduct test–retest evaluation of the JVQ, 100 youth ages 10–17 were recontacted 3–4 weeks after their original telephone interviews and readministered the JVQ. The overall agreement for the total JVQ was 95%, with a range for the individual screener items of 77–100% (Finkelhor et al., 2005). The mean kappa of the items was. 63, with a range of .22–1.0. Small response rates for many items were associated with small kappas. Noting that there are good reasons to question the utility of tests of internal consistency among questions designed to assess actual experiences, the authors reported the values for the total of the 34 JVQ items (alpha = .80), as well as for each of the individual summary subscales: .61 for Conventional Crime (8 items), .64 for Physical Assault (10 items), .38 for Property Victimization (3 items), .39 for Child Maltreatment (4 items), .51 for Sexual Victimization (7 items), .35 for Sexual Assault (4 items), .55 for Peer or Sibling Victimization (9 items), and .35 for Peer or Sibling Assault (.35).

Evidence of Validity: Among 992 children and adolescents ages 10–17 who participated in a national telephone survey, most of the single items on the JQV correlated significantly with the Trauma Checklist for Children (TSCC—Briere, 1996b; see Appendix 9.5) subscales of Anxiety, Depression, and Anger, and all of the subscale totals correlated significantly with each of these subscales of the TSCC.

Contact Information: David Finkelhor, PhD, Crimes Against Children Research Center, University of New Hampshire, 126 Horton Social Science Center, Durham, NH 03824. Example items from the questionnaire are available as an appendix to Finkelhor and colleagues (2005).

KID-SAVE (Flowers, Hastings, & Kelley, 2000; Hastings & Kelley, 1997a)

Brief Description: The KID-SAVE measures the frequency of exposure to violence in the home, school, and neighborhood (Hastings & Kelley, 1997a). The scale comprises 34 items with three subscales derived from factor analysis: (1) Traumatic Violence—witnessing a shooting or murder, or being the victim of an assault with a deadly weapon (12 items); (2) Indirect Violence—witnessing less severe interpersonal violence or hearing about violent events (16 items); (3) Physical/Verbal Abuse—hitting among peers, and grownups hitting/screaming at child (6 items). The content of the items is identical to the adolescent version, the Screen for Adolescent Violence Exposure (SAVE; Hastings & Kelley, 1997b; see below, this appendix), although violence in three different settings is not assessed in the KID-SAVE as it is in the SAVE. Each item is rated by the child on frequency of exposure: *Never*, 0; *Sometimes*, 1; or *A lot*, 2. The impact of endorsed incidents—how upsetting they were to the child when they occurred—was rated with the following responses accompanied by faces: *Not at all, with a happy face*, 0; *Somewhat, with a "frowning face,"* 1; and *Very, with a "very upset" face*, 2, for a total possible score of 0–68. Readability was established at the fourth-grade level, so items must be read to children in the third grade. Age range: 8–12 years; grades 3–7. A Caretaker version also is available (P-KID-SAVE—Flowers, Lanclos, & Kelley, 2002; see below, this appendix).

Evidence of Reliability: Among 470 primarily (90%) African American children, 48% boys, ages 7–15 (M = 10.69, SD = 1.71), who lived in neighborhoods of high crime, Cronbach's alpha for the Frequency scale was .91 for the total, .86 for the Indirect Violence, .87 for the Traumatic Violence, and .66 for the Physical/Verbal Abuse subscales. The alphas are similar for the Impact totals and subscales: .88 for the total, .85 for Indirect Violence, .77 for Traumatic Violence, and .62 for Physical/Verbal Abuse. The correlation between Impact and Frequency scale scores was .69, and the correlations for subscales were as follows: .84 for Traumatic Violence; .60 for Indirect Violence; and .77 for Physical/Verbal Abuse. A 3-week test–retest reliability was conducted in a subsample of 22 children (55% girls) ages 8–11 (M = 9.5, SD = 0.91); reliability coefficients for Frequency were .86 for the total, .67 for Indirect Violence, .76 for Traumatic Violence, and .62 for Physical/Verbal Abuse subscales; and for Impact, they were .81 for the total, .73 for Indirect Violence, .82 for Traumatic Violence, and .58 for Physical/Verbal Abuse subscales (Hastings & Kelley, 1997a). Cronbach's alpha for the Flowers and colleagues (2000) sample was .89 for the Frequency scale. There was insufficient variability in responses on the Impact scale to calculate a Cronbach's alpha.

Evidence of Validity: Construct validity was established in a subsample of 187 primarily (87%) African American children, 47% boys, ages 7–15 (M = 10.28, SD = 1.72; Hastings & Kelley, 1997a) by correlating scores on the KID-SAVE with scores on the TSCC (Briere, 1996a, 1996b; see Appendix 9.5). Significant correlations for the frequency scale and subscales ranged from r = .20, p < .05 to r = .54, p < .001. Scores on the Impact scale and TSCC also were significantly correlated and ranged from r = .17, p < .05 to r = .43, p < .001. In a separate study (Flowers et al., 2002), children in higher grades indicated they experienced greater frequency of exposure to indirect violence, whereas the younger children reported more frequent physical/verbal abuse, and they reported significantly greater impact of their exposure to physical/verbal abuse. Scores on the frequency of exposure to traumatic violence were associated with scores on the Child Behavior Checklist (CBCL; Achenbach, 1991a) Withdrawn, Anxious–Depressed, Delinquent, and Aggression subscales. Frequency of indirect violence was associated with Social Problems on the CBCL. Reports of higher frequency of exposure to indirect violence, physical/verbal abuse, and traumatic violence were associated with higher Anxiety scores on the TSCC. TSCC Depression was associated with child reports of frequency of exposure to physical/verbal abuse and indirect violence. Both the Posttraumatic Stress and Anger scales of the TSCC were associated with frequency of exposure to indirect violence, traumatic violence, and physical/verbal abuse. The Dissociative scale of the TSCC was associated with the frequency of indirect violence and physical/verbal abuse. Total scores on the KID-SAVE were significantly associated with total TSCC scores.

Contact Information: Anise L. Flowers, PhD, Tarrow Center for Self-Management, 1001 West Loop South, #215, Houston, TX 77027. E-mail: doctorflower@email.com. Instructions and items for the child version are included in the original article (Hastings & Kelley, 1997a).

Lifetime Incidence of Traumatic Events (LITE), Student form (Greenwald & Rubin, 1999)

Brief Description: The LITE assesses exposure to 16 potentially traumatic stressors, such as a car accident or the death of someone in the family. It measures the frequency of exposure, age at time of exposure, and how upset the child was at the time of the event and currently on a 3-point scale (*None, Some, Lots*). Age range: 8+. Languages available: English, Spanish, German, Persian, and Swedish.

Evidence of Reliability: Evidence of reliability has yet to be published.
Evidence of Validity: Evidence of validity has yet to be published.
Contact Information: Sidran Institute, 200 E. Joppa Road, Suite 207, Towson, MD 21286. Telephone: (410) 825-8888. E-mail: sidran@sidran.org. Website: www.sidran.org.

My Exposure to Violence (My ETV; Buka, Selner-O'Hagan, Kindlon, & Earls, 1996; Selner-O'Hagan, Kindlon, Buka, Raudenbush, & Earls, 1998)

Brief Description: My ETV is a highly structured interviewer-administered instrument designed to cover lifetime and past-year exposure to 18 different violent events that have either been witnessed or personally experienced by a child or adolescent. It also ascertains the location of the violence (e.g., school, home, neighborhood), identifies both perpetrators and victims of violence (e.g., family member, stranger), and whether the exposure was gang-related. The instrument measures lifetime exposure ("ever") and prevalence ("in the past year"). Frequency of exposure is measured on a 6-point scale (*Never, Once, 2 or 3 times, 4 to 10 times, 11 to 50 times,* and *More than 50 times*). Six subscales are defined: (1) Witnessing Violent Events, (2) Victimization, and (3) Total Exposure (witnessing and victimization), obtaining scores for both lifetime and past-year exposure.

Age Range: 9 years and older.

Evidence of Reliability: The ICC test–retest reliability for the six subscales was .88 for the total My ETV Lifetime, .75 for the Victimization Lifetime, .85 for the Witnessing Lifetime, .81 for the Past-Year Total My ETV, .94 for the Past-Year Victimization, and .75 for the Past-Year Witnessing (Selner-O'Hagan et al., 1998). Internal consistency for the scales, as measured by Cronbach's alpha, was .93 for Total Lifetime My ETV, .89 for Total Past-Year My ETV, .79 for Lifetime Victimization, .68 for Past-Year Victimization, .92 for Lifetime Witnessing, and .91 for Past-Year Witnessing subscales.

Evidence of Validity: A theoretical underlying unidimensional latent construct of exposure to violence has been demonstrated using item response theory (IRT; Kindlon, Wright, Raudenbush, & Earls, 1996; Selner-O'Hagan et al., 1998). Neighborhoods with higher rates of crime were associated with significantly higher reports of exposure to past-year violence on the My ETV, but lifetime rates did not differ significantly (Selner-O'Hagan et al., 1998). Children, adolescents, and young adults who reported committing at least one violent event themselves had significantly higher My ETV scores for both the past year and over their lifetime (Selner-O'Hagan et al., 1998). Lifetime My ETV scores were positively correlated with age, with higher scores among older youth. However, there was also a significant quadratic association between age groups, with the two middle ages (15 and 18) reporting more lifetime exposure than the youngest (9–12) and oldest (21–24) age groups. For past-year scores, there was no linear association between age and scores, but there was again a significant quadratic association, with the two middle age groups again reporting more exposure to violence over the past year. African American children and adolescents reported significantly more exposure in the past year than European Americans, but there was no difference in reports of lifetime exposure. Boys reported higher levels of exposure over the lifetime and in the past year than girls, both in terms of witnessing and victimization.

Contact Information: Mary Beth Selner-O'Hagan, PhD, Department of Maternal and Child Health, Harvard School of Public Health, 677 Huntington Ave., Boston, MA 02115. E-mail: mohagan@phdcn.harvard.edu.

Post-Traumatic Stress Disorder Index (Diehl, Zea, & Espino, 1994)

Brief Description: Languages available: Spanish.
Evidence of Reliability: Evidence of reliability has yet to be published.
Evidence of Validity: Evidence of validity has yet to be published.
Contact Information: The measure is included as an appendix to Diehl and colleagues (1994).

Screen for Adolescent Violence Exposure (SAVE; Hastings & Kelley, 1997a)

Brief Description: The SAVE is a 32-item, Likert-type scale assessing violence exposure in school, home, and neighborhood on corresponding settings scales. Each setting scale comprises three subscale scores: Traumatic Violence, Indirect Violence, and Physical/Verbal Abuse, for a total of 9 subscales. Response categories for each question included 1, *Never;* 2, *Hardly ever;* 3, *Sometimes;* 4, *A lot;* and 5, *Almost always.* Total setting scores range from 32 to 160, with higher scores indicative of greater violence exposure (Hastings & Kelley, 1997a).

Evidence of Reliability: Coefficient alphas ranged from .58 to .91 for the nine subscales (mean alpha = .78). The lowest alphas were for the Physical/Verbal Abuse subscales (.58 for School Violence, .68 for Home Violence, and .61 for Neighborhood Violence; mean alpha = .62). The highest alphas were for the Indirect Violence subscales (.84 for School Violence, .89 for Home Violence, and .91 for Neighborhood Violence; mean alpha = .88). Alphas for the Trauma Violence subscales were almost as high (.78 for School Violence, .84 for Home Violence, and .85 for Neighborhood Violence; mean alpha = .82). Cronbach's alphas for the three settings (sums of the three subscales within each setting) were .90 for School Violence, .93 for Home Violence, and .94 for Neighborhood Violence. Two-week test–retest correlations varied from .53 to .91 (*M* = .76). The lowest test–retest correlations were again for the Physical/Verbal Abuse subscales (.53 for School Violence, .60 for Home Violence, and .61 for Neighborhood Violence; mean alpha = .58). The highest test–retest correlations were again for the Indirect Violence subscales (.87 for School Violence, .88 for Home Violence, and .91 for Neighborhood Violence; mean alpha = .89). Test–retest correlations for the Trauma Violence subscales were almost as high (.78 for School Violence, .81 for Home Violence, and .82 for Neighborhood Violence; mean alpha = .80). Test–retest coefficients for the three settings were .91 for School Violence, .92 for Home Violence, .92, and .92 for Neighborhood Violence (Hastings & Kelley, 1997b).

Evidence of Validity: Principal components factor analysis with a varimax rotation was conducted separately for each of the three settings in a sample of 1,036 adolescents, 94.2% African American, ages 11 to 19 years (M = 14.84, SD = 1.86) in grades 6 through 12. Each analysis produced three factor subscales: "(1) Traumatic Violence, relating to severe victimization experiences (12 items), (2) Indirect Violence, relating to the witnessing of or being informed of less severe interpersonal violence (14 items), and (3) Physical/Verbal Abuse, relating to the actual or threatened violent harm directed at the participant (six items)" (Hastings & Kelley, 1997b, p. 515). A separate sample of 214 adolescents, ranging in age from 13 to 18 years (M = 14.62, SD = 1.11), participated in validity studies of the measure. Confirmatory factor analysis indicated that the three-factor solution provided a reasonable fit for each of the three settings. Known-groups validity was assessed by dividing one group of adolescents according to police zones of low (n = 262) and high (n = 250) rates of reported violent crime to assess the Neighborhood setting subscales; scores of the upper (n = 98) and lower (n = 98) quartiles of the Conflict Tactics Scales (CTS; Straus, 1979) to assess the Home setting subscales; and schools reporting low (n = 238) and high (n = 214) levels of student aggression to assess the School setting subscales. All scales successfully discriminated between high- and low-violence groups. According to these analyses, the Neighborhood scale demonstrated sensitivity of .78 and specificity of .87; the School scale, sensitivity of .76 and specificity of .94; and the Home scale, sensitivity of .68 and specificity of .92. Convergent validity was demonstrated for the Neighborhood scale, with significant correlations between each of its subscales and violence scores for neighborhoods based on local crime data (r = .28 for the Traumatic Violence subscale; r = .38 for the Indirect Violence subscale; and r = .35 for the Physical/Verbal Abuse subscale of the Neighborhood setting scales). Divergent validity was demonstrated for most of the subscales of the Home and School settings based on nonsignificant correlations between the neighborhood violence scores, except for significant correlations with Indirect Violence for each setting (r = .24 and .27, respectively). Convergent validity was demonstrated for the Home Traumatic Violence and Physical/Verbal Abuse subscales through significant correlations with parental CTS Verbal Aggression (r = .43 for both) and CTS Violence (r's = .48 and .33, respectively). Divergent validity was demonstrated for the Home subscales, with nonsignificant correlations with the CTS Parent Reasoning scale. Construct validity was demonstrated with significant correlations between the nine SAVE subscales and subscales of the TSCC (Brier, 1996a, 1996b; see Appendix 9.5), the Impact of Event Scale (IES; Horowitz, Wilner, & Alvarez, 1979), and the Youth Self-Report (YSR; Achenbach, 1991b). All nine subscales correlated significantly with the Intrusion and Avoidance subscales of the IES, the Internalizing and Externalizing scales of the YSR, and the Anger subscale of the TSCC (with correlations ranging from .21 to .52). The TSCC Posttraumatic Stress subscale correlated significantly with the Home Indirect Violence subscale (.32), Home Physical/Verbal Abuse subscale (.34), the total Home setting scale (.27), the Neighborhood Physical/Verbal Abuse subscale (.23), the School Physical/Verbal Abuse subscale (.32), and the total School setting scale (.22). The TSCC Dissociation subscale correlated significantly with the Home Indirect Violence subscale (.32), Physical/Verbal Abuse subscale (.38), the total Home setting scale (.33), the Neighborhood Physical/Verbal Abuse subscale (.27), the total Neighborhood scale (.25), the School Physical/Verbal Abuse subscale (.33), and the total School scale (.24). The TSCC Anxiety and Depression subscales correlated significantly with Home Indirect Violence (.22 and .27), Home Physical/Verbal Abuse (.29 and .31), total Home setting scale (.22 and .27), and the School Physical/Verbal Abuse subscale (.32 and .27). The total School setting scale correlated .22 with the TSCC Anxiety subscale (Hastings & Kelley, 1997b).

Contact Information: Teresa L. Hastings, PhD, P.O. Box 95606, Seattle, WA 98145-2606. The items are listed in Hastings and Kelley (1997b).

Stressful Life Events Checklist (SLE; Bean, Eurelings-Bontekoe, Derluyn, & Spinhover, 2004c)

Brief Description: The SLE, a checklist of 12 stressful events "commonly experienced by refugee minors," includes one open-ended question and a space for comments. The experiences assessed, however, appear to be applicable to other children as well. Responses are yes–no. The SLE was written as a companion assessment tool to the Reactions of Adolescents to Traumatic Stress (RATS—Bean et al., 2004b; see Appendix 9.6). Some questions may require explanation. The manual supplies short answers for those questions that posed problems during the original testing. Age range: 12–18 years. Languages available: Amhars, Albans, Arabic, Bandini, Chinese (Mandarin), Croation, Dari, Dutch, English, French, German, Mongols, Portuguese, Russian, Servo-Croation, Spanish (presumably European Spanish rather than Central or South American Spanish), Soerani, Somali, and Turkish.

Evidence of Reliability: Evidence of reliability has yet to be published.

Evidence of Validity: The SLE correlated significantly with the RATS (Bean et al., 2004b; see Appendix 9.6 for details) in four different large samples: r's ranged from .45 to .52 for the total RATS, from .43 to .53 for the Intrusion scale, from .36 to .44 for the Numbing/Avoidance scale, and from .38 to .45 for the Hyperarousal scale.

Contact Information: All versions of the SLE, along with the manual, may be downloaded from *www.centrum45. nl/research/amaenggz/ukamtool.php*. Tammy Bean, PhD, may be contacted via e-mail at t.bean@centrum45.nl.

Stressful Life Events Schedule—Child Version (SLES; Williamson et al., 2003)

Brief Description: To assess stressors in children and adolescents, the SLES comprises 61 potentially stressful events in the life of the child or the child's important others. It also allows for the inclusion of additional events not covered. Events are categorized into domains of education, work, money, housing, crime, health, deaths, romantic relationships, and other relationships. Events are rated on subjective stressfulness on a 4-point scale: *Little or none*, *Some*, *Moderate*, and *High*. Memory aids help the child date the occurrence of each endorsed event. Duration of the event is also recorded. Events also are rated on whether they are behavior-dependent or independent; that is, whether or not the child was actively involved in creating the stressful event. Time required: 15–120 minutes (M = 35.5 ± 18.9, for nonpsychiatrically ill children; M = 55.5 ± 26.7, for psychiatrically ill children—Williamson et al., 2003).

Evidence of Reliability: Ratings for six raters of more than 1,000 events elicited from 60 children and adolescents (half of whom were psychiatrically ill) showed moderate to excellent agreement, with kappas of .67 for exact ratings of objective threat, .84 for behavior-dependence/independence, and .93 for the focus of the event (Williamson et al., 2003). For events labeled severe (rated 3 or 5 on objective threat) agreement was higher (kappa = .70). On an event rated behavior-dependent (3 or 4 on the dependence scale), kappa was .92. Age, gender, and diagnostic status did not significantly impact the reliability estimates. Fifty-nine of the children were reinterviewed approximately 1 week after their initial interview to examine the test–retest reliability of the interview. The ICC for the number of events reported in each interview was .93; for children age 12 or under, ICC was .91, and for those over age 12, it was .94. Normal children had higher intraclass reliability for nonsevere events than did children with psychopathology (.93 vs..83). The test–retest reliability of events with high objective threat was substantially lower, with an ICC of .70. Adolescents had higher test–retest reliability than younger children for severe events (.86 vs..43). The test–retest kappa for any event was .68, and girls had higher kappas (.74) than boys (.62). Test–retest for all events also was higher for adolescents (kappa = .72) than for younger children (.61). For severe events, test–retest reliability was higher, with a kappa of .80. For nonsevere events, kappa was .67, and girls again had higher kappas (.78) for these events than boys (.60).

Evidence of Validity: Children with psychiatric disorders reported more stressful events in the past year than normal children (M's = 8.1 ± 4.0 vs. 4.9 ± 3.5). Children with psychiatric disorders also reported more behavior-dependent events, more behavior-independent events, more severe events, and higher levels of stressful responses to the events. Adolescents were more likely to report behavior-dependent events and to score higher on the total sum of objective and subjective stress. Total stressful life events assessed with the SLES agreed with those assessed by the Life Events Checklist (Johnson & McCutcheon, 1980), with an ICC of .83 (Williamson et al., 2003).

Contact Information: Douglas E. Williamson, PhD, Department of Psychiatry, Western Psychiatric Institute and Clinic, University of Pittsburgh School of Medicine, 3811 O'Hara Street, Room E-723, Pittsburgh, PA 15213. Telephone: (412) 624-4526. E-mail: williamsonde@msx.upmc.edu.

Survey of Exposure to Community Violence—Self-Report Version (SECV-SR; Richters & Saltzman, 1990)

Brief Description: This self-report measure evaluates children's exposure to 20 forms of severe violence (shootings, stabbings, and rapes), less severe violence (beatings and chases), and moderately severe violence (threats, accidents, drug deals, and arrests). Children report on whether they have been the victim of, witnessed, and simply heard about each kind of event. The frequency of each exposure is assessed on a 9-point scale, ranging from *No exposure* (0) to *Exposed every day* (8). Also known as Survey of Children's Exposure to Community Violence. For the Parent Report Version, see below, this appendix.

Evidence of Reliability: Evidence of reliability has yet to be published.

Evidence of Validity: Children's reports of exposure to stressors on the SECV-SR (Martinez & Richters, 1993) were significantly correlated with their Checklist of Child Distress Symptoms (CCDS—Richters & Martinez, 1990a; see Appendix 9.5) scores, whether they were themselves victims of community violence ($r_{(37)}$ = .37) or witnessed it ($r_{(37)}$ = .39), or they witnessed violence in the home ($r_{(37)}$ = .33).

Contact Information: John E. Richters, PhD, Department of Human Development and Institute for Child Study, University of Maryland, Benjamin Building, Room 4104, College Park, MD 20742. Telephone: (301) 405-7354. E-mail: jrichter@nih.gov.

Tough Times Checklist (Fletcher, 1996f)

Brief Description: The Tough Times Checklist is a 70-item, paper-and-pencil assessment of lifetime and past-year exposure to low-, moderate-, and high-magnitude stressors, based on the Life Events and Coping Inventory (LECI; Dise-Lewis, 1988) with very minor or general stressors ("You felt angry or upset," "You felt rushed or pressured") excluded. Higher magnitude stressors have been added. Explicit questions about sexual abuse are excluded, although the child is asked whether any peers, adult strangers, or known adults ever made him or her do "something horrible." Assessors are required to inquire as to the nature of that event, if the child endorses it. If a measure that inquires about explicit sexual abuse experience is desired, see the Young Adult Upsetting Times Checklist below, this appendix. Response format is as follows: *Never happened*; *Happened, but the worst time was not upsetting*; *Happened, and the worst time was somewhat upsetting*; and *Happened, and the worst time was very upsetting*. Adolescents are also asked to describe the most upsetting event experienced in the past year, then rate it on how upsetting it was—*A little, Very much, Totally*. Then the child is asked to describe the most upsetting event experienced prior to last year, and to rate how upsetting it was. Age range: 7 and older. Third-grade reading level required.

Evidence of Reliability: Evidence of reliability has yet to be published.

Evidence of Validity: Evidence of validity has yet to be published.

Contact Information: Kenneth E. Fletcher, PhD, Department of Psychiatry, University of Massachusetts Medical School, 55 Lake Avenue North, Worcester, MA 01655. Telephone: (508) 856-8630. E-mail: kenneth.fletcher@umassmed.edu.

Things I Have Seen or Heard (Richters & Martinez, 1990b)

Brief Description: In this 15-question, simply worded, structured interview designed to assess the frequency of young children's exposure to violence and violence-related themes (Richters & Martinez, 1993), each question is described on a separate page. Response categories are depicted as five stacks of balls, with a different and increasing number of balls in each stack, ranging from none to five, labeled *Never/0 times*, *1 time*, *2 times*, *3 times*, and *Many times*. For the *Never/0 times* response, the ball is empty, and for the others the balls are filled. For times 1 through 3, an equivalent number of filled balls is shown. For *Many times*, five filled balls are shown. Children are taught to use the proper stack of balls to indicate the frequency of their exposure to each event prior to the interview. Age range: 6–10 years.

Evidence of Reliability: Test–retest correlation for the total score among 21 children over one week is .81, with no significant difference between scores at the two times ($t_{(2)}$ = 1.34, ns; Richters & Martinez, 1993).

Evidence of Validity: Among 111 first and second graders (Martinez & Richters, 1993) correlations between experiences of violent victimization in the community, as reported on the Things I Have Seen or Heard, and symptoms of distress, as measured by the Levonn, were significant ($r_{(31)}$ =.28, p < .01). Children's reports of witnessing violence in the community also correlated significantly with their total scores on the Levonn ($r_{(81)}$ = .30, p < .01). Children's reports of the frequency of seeing guns or drugs also correlated significantly with total distress scores on the Levonn, regardless of where that occurred ($r_{(81)}$ = .30).

Contact Information: John E. Richters, PhD, Department of Human Development and Institute for Child Study, University of Maryland, Benjamin Building, Room 4104, College Park, MD 20742. Phone: (301) 405-7354. E-mail: jrichter@nih.gov.

Traumatic Events Screening Inventory for Children (TESI-C; Ford et al., 2002)

Brief Description: On the TESI-C, a 16-item, structured interview regarding high-magnitude stressors, questions are arranged so that the lowest magnitude stressors are asked first and sexual abuse is at the end, to help the child tolerate the potentially stressful nature of the questions. Probes assist the interviewer to determine whether endorsed events meet both parts of criterion A of DSM-IV PTSD diagnosis. If criterion A is met for a particular type of stressor, the interviewer asks for more specifics about the event(s), the child's age at its occurrence, who else was involved, and whether anyone was hurt and needed medical attention. Age range: 8–17 years. Requires a qualified mental health professional or advanced trainee supervised by a qualified mental health professional.

Evidence of Reliability: Interrater reliability kappas for summary scores ranged from .73 to 1.00 in a sample of pediatric injury patients (Ford & Rogers, 1997). Test–retest reliability kappas for the TESI-C and TESI-P (the parent form; see below) summary scores ranged from .50 to .70 over a 2- to 4-month period. Test–retest kappas for specific events at assessments 1 month or more apart were .83 for sexual abuse, .69 for family arguments, .56 for domestic violence, .51 for physical abuse, .49 for witnessing a death or serious illness, .40 for verbal abuse, .25 for witnessing an accident, and –.07 for exposure to a natural disaster. Kappas of parent–child agreement on trauma on specific events ranged from .64 to .79.

Evidence of Validity: Evidence of validity has yet to be published.

Contact Information: Julian D. Ford, PhD, Director of Behavioral Healthcare Outcomes Research, Director of Outpatient Services, Department of Psychiatry 6410, University of Connecticut School of Medicine, University of Connecticut Health Center, 10 Talcott Notch Rd., Farmington, CT 06032. Telephone: (860) 679-6709/6732. Fax: (860) 679-6736. E-mail: ford@psychiatry.uchc.edu.

Violence Exposure Scale for Children—Preschool Version (VEX; Fox & Leavitt, 1995; Shahinfar, Fox, & Leavitt, 2000)

Brief Description: The VEX, a 23-item, cartoon-based interview to assess children's self-reports of exposure to violence, is based on the Things I Have Seen and Heard scale designed by Richters and Martinez (1990b; see above, this appendix). The preschool version consists of 15 items. Whereas the violent events are described verbally in the Things I have Seen and Heard scale, the VEX scale depicts each event in cartoons. Eight of the cartoons show a central character, Chris, witnessing violent events, and 6 cartoons depict Chris as the victim of violent events. "The violent incidents assessed by the preschool version of the VEX scale are beating, chasing, robbery, threat with a weapon, shooting, stabbing, pushing or shoving, and slapping. The children were asked about witnessing all of them, and about victimization by all but shooting or stabbing, partly because of the low probability that preschoolers would be victims of such events, partly out of concern for keeping the traumatic valence of the cartoon depictions at a minimum. Following the interviewer's explanation of what Chris is witnessing or experiencing in each picture, the children are asked how often they have been exposed to the same incident. Below each cartoon is a picture of four thermometers, each with the mercury at one of four labeled levels: never, once, a few times, and lots of times. For those incidents to which the child responds positively, the interviewer probes for information regarding where the event occurred, who was with the child at the time, and when the event occurred. The probing is intended to assess the veracity of the child's report on the basis of its relevance to the cartoon depiction. At the same time, the questions are designed to allow comparison between specific parent- and child-reported events" (Shahinfar et al., 2000, p. 117). A revised version was created by Shahinfar and colleagues (2000) based in part on preliminary testing. This resulted in removing several items that lacked clarity and adding new items designed to assess innocuous events to which the child was likely to have been exposed (e.g., watching television or seeing a child sitting on Santa's lap) to provide a "psychological break" from the more stressful events and to act as a test of a child's understanding of the questions. Gender-differentiated versions of the full, revised measure were created, wherein the test remained the same in both versions except for the gender of the main character. Shahinfar and colleagues found that children could be divided into three levels of comprehension of the measure: 73 (47.1%) of 155 children appeared to understand the interview; the level of comprehension was either unclear or variable for 56 (36.1%) children; and 26 (16.8%) children were unwilling or unable to complete the interview. Those who understood the VEX scored significantly higher on the Peabody Picture Vocabulary Test—Revised (PPVT-R; Dunn & Dunn, 1981). They also reported significantly lower levels of total violence exposure and symptoms of distress (as measured by a revised, preschool version of the Levonn; see Appendix 9.4), as reported by the children. No group differences were found for parent reports of violence exposure or CBCL behavior problems. In this study of primarily (98.8%) African American children between ages 3.5 and 4.5, the authors carefully debriefed children after administering the revised Levonn (Shahinfar et al., 2000). They reported that very few of the children indicated, either verbally or behaviorally, that they had been upset by the interview. The authors divided the items into two types: exposure to mild violence (beating, chasing, pushing or shoving, and slapping) and exposure to severe violence (robbery, threats with a weapon, shooting, and stabbing). A Hebrew version is available. It consists of 12 pairs of drawings, one depicting a child witnessing a violent events and the other depicting a child named Nitzan, in this version, as a victim of the same act of violence (Raviv et al., 2001). That version was administered to each child three times in three different settings: home, school, and neighborhood. Responses were depicted as stacks of balls, with *Never* depicted as a white or empty ball, *Once* depicted as a filled or black ball, *2 times* as 2 filled balls, *3 times* as 3 filled balls, and *Many times* as 5 filled balls. Cartoons of extremely violent events were shown only in the witness situation. Age range: Preschool. Languages: English and Hebrew.

Evidence of Reliability: A reliability study of a revised version for school-age children (age 14 and younger) of the VEX-R, used in the National Survey of Child and Adolescent Well-Being (NSCAW; Administration for Children and Families, 2006) reported a Cronbach's alpha of .96 in a sample of 2,738 children whose families had been investigated (but not necessarily supported) for reported maltreatment, and alphas of .86 for a subscale of items related to witnessing mild violence, .88 for items regarding mild violence victimization, and .92 for items related to witnessing severe violence. Among 73 children ages 3.5 to 4.5 who appeared to understand the VEX Preschool Version questions, Cronbach's alphas were .80 for children's reports of exposure to mild violence (8 items) and .86 for exposure to severe violence (6 items; Shahinfar et al., 2000). Parent and child reports showed no significant association with each other in this study. In the Raviv and colleagues (2001) study of Israeli children's exposure to violence, associations between child and parent report versions of the VEX tended to be significant, especially for episodes of mild violence, with correlations of .34 for the total of witnessing items and .47 for the total of victimization items.

Evidence of Validity: Small but significant correlations were found between symptoms of distress (as measured by the preschool version of the Levonn; see Appendix 9.4) and Witnessing Mild Violence ($r = .29$, $p < .05$), Victimization by Mild Violence ($r = .22$, $p = .05$), and Witnessing Severe Violence ($r = .25$, $p < .05$; Shahinfar et al., 2000). No significant association was found between child reports of distress and victimization by severe violence ($r = .14$, ns). Moreover, among the 73 children who appeared to understand the measures, those who reported witnessing mild violence were rated by their parents as displaying more internalizing problems on the CBCL (Achenbach, 1991a) than children who did not report such exposure. Those who reported victimization by mild violence were rated with higher externalizing behavior by their parents. Parents of children reporting exposure to extreme violence did not report any significantly different behavior problems on the CBCL than parents of children who did not report exposure to extreme violence. A factor analysis of the Hebrew version (Raviv et al., 2001) resulted in two factors: Mild Violence (six items: yell, chase, slap, push, beat up, throw something at) and Severe Violence (six items: threaten with a knife or gun, stab, shoot, arrest, deal drugs, rob). In the same study, responses of children from a low-violence neighborhood (LVN) were compared to those of children from a high-violence neighborhood (HVN). Children in the HVN group reported more exposure to violence than children in the LVN. In the same study, the correlations between child and parent reports of severe violence exposure were lower but still significant for the totals of the witnessing (.22) and the victimization items (.37). Mothers of children with more experiences of violent victimization reported that they had more behavior problems, as measured by the CBCL (Achenbach, 1991a). All reports of violent experiences on the VEX also correlated significantly with scores on a revised version of the Levonn (see description of Levonn and the Hebrew version, this appendix).

Contact Information: For revised preschool version: Ariana Shahinfar, PhD, Department of Psychology, University of North Carolina, Charlotte, NC 28223-0001. E-mail: ashahinf@email.unc.edu. For Hebrew version: A. Raviv, PhD, Department of Psychology, Tel Aviv University, Ramat Aviv, Tel Aviv 69978, Israel. Telephone: 972-3-640-8969. E-mail: raviv@post.tau.ac.il.

Young Adult Psychiatric Assessment (YAPA) Life Events Scale (Angold & Costello, 2000)

Brief Description: This Life Events Scale is a module of the full YAPA (Angold & Costello, 2000; see Appendix 9.6). Similar to the CAPA, with which the measure is associated, it assesses both high- and low-magnitude stressors. High-magnitude stressors are assessed for child's whole life; low-magnitude stressors, for past 3 months. Training is required for this semistructured interview. Age range: 18+. Interviewer qualifications: Bachelor's degree or higher. Languages available: English and Spanish.

Evidence of Reliability: Evidence of reliability has yet to be published.

Evidence of Validity: Evidence of validity has yet to be published.

Contact Information: Developmental Epidemiology Program, Duke University Medical Center, Attention: Juné Rogers, DUMC Box 3454, Durham, NC 27710. Telephone: (919) 687-4686, extension 273. E-mail: jrogers@psych.duhs.duke.edu.

Young Adults Upsetting Times Checklist (Fletcher, 1996f; Fletcher & Skidmore, 1997)

Brief Description: The Young Adults Upsetting Times Checklist, a paper-and-pencil assessment of lifetime and past-year exposure to low-, moderate-, and high-magnitude stressors, is based on the Life Events and Coping Inventory (LECI; Dise-Lewis, 1988), with minor stressors ("You felt angry or upset," "You felt rushed or pressured") excluded. Higher magnitude stressors have been added. Unlike the related measures, the Teen Tough Times Checklist, the Tough Times Checklist (both described earlier in this appendix), and the Child's Upsetting Times Checklist (a parent report version is described in this appendix), several explicit questions about sexual and physical abuse have been *included*. There are many questions about the occurrence of abuse before the age of 18, then again, after the age of 18. To accommodate the extra abuse questions, some of the lowest magnitude stressor questions included on the related stressor checklists have been omitted. Response format is as follows: *Never happened; Happened, but the worst time was not upsetting; Happened, and the worst time was somewhat upsetting; Happened, and the worst time was very* *upsetting*; and *Happened, and the worst time was extremely upsetting.* Two additional items ask respondents to describe and rate (1) the worst thing that happened to them in the past year, and (2) the worst thing that ever happened to them prior to the last year, using the same response format. Age range: 13 years and older. Ability of younger adolescents to comprehend the items need to be assessed, and questions referring to occurrences after the age of 18 should be omitted. Number of items: 76, with item 74 rated twice. Languages available: English; Spanish.

Evidence of Reliability: Among 295 undergraduate college students, ages 17–41 ($M = 19.9$, $SD = 2.8$, median = 19), Cronbach's alphas for the total of all stressors prior to the previous year was .96, and for the total of all stressors in the previous year, .97 (reanalysis of data is reported in Fletcher & Skidmore, 1997). Alphas for the six subscales of the lifetime stressors (see below for description of subscales) were .98 for the High-Magnitude Stressors, .78 for the Peer Social Stressors, .85 for the Home Life Stressors, .67 for the Alienation Stressors, .80 for Demoralizing Stressors, and .80 for Home Life Disruptions Stressors. Alphas were .98 for the Major Stressors of the previous year, and .88 for the Minor Stressors of the previous year.

Evidence of Validity: Factor analysis (Fletcher & Skidmore, 1997) of scores on the lifetime stressors prior to the previous year produced seven subscales: High-Magnitude Stressors (e.g., sexual or physical abuse, being shot at or stabbed), Peer Social Stressors (friend in hospital, know someone not family in bad accident, friend died, someone in family died), Home Life Stressors (had to go live with relatives, sibling moved out of house, parent lost job, house robbed), Alienation Stressors (does not like teacher, sent to principal, fight with friend, friend stops hanging out), Demoralizing Stressors (suspended from school, punished, sent back a grade), and Home Life Disruption Stressors (moved, a parent moved out, parents divorced, parent remarried). The total score for lifetime stressors, including the previous year, correlated significantly (.26) with the Impact of Event Scale (Horowitz et al., 1979), as did the total for lifetime prior to the previous year (.28), and total for just the previous year (.13; Fletcher & Skidmore, 1997). Each total also correlated significantly (.28, .25, and .22, respectively; Fletcher & Skidmore, 1997) with a PTSD score based on the Symptom Checklist 90 (SCL-90—Derogatis & Melisaratos, 1983; Saunders, Arata, & Kilpatrick, 1990).

Contact Information: Kenneth E. Fletcher, PhD, Department of Psychiatry, University of Massachusetts Medical School, 55 Lake Avenue North, Worcester, MA 01655. Telephone: (508) 856-8630. E-mail: kenneth.fletcher@ umassmed.edu.

ADMINISTERED TO CARETAKER OR OTHER ADULTS

Child and Adolescent Psychiatric Assessment (CAPA) Life Events Scale (Angold & Costello, 2000)

Brief Description: This Life Events Scale is a module of the CAPA general psychiatric assessment interview (see Appendix 9.3). It assesses both high- and low-magnitude stressors: High-magnitude stressors for the child's whole life; low-magnitude, for past 3 months. Training is required for this semistructured interview. Age range: 9–17 years. Interviewer qualifications: Bachelor's degree or higher. Languages available: English and Spanish.

Evidence of Reliability: For high-magnitude stressors, ICC within 2 weeks = .83. For low-magnitude stressors, ICC within 2 weeks = .58.

Evidence of Validity: For seven events reported by four or more children, kappas ranged from .16 for a serious accident to .81 for sexual abuse.

Contact Information: Developmental Epidemiology Program, Duke University Medical Center, Attention: Juné Rogers, DUMC Box 3454, Durham, NC 27710. Telephone: (919) 687-4686, extension 273. E-mail: jrogers@psych.duhs.duke.edu.

Child's Upsetting Times Checklist (Fletcher, 1996f)

Brief Description: The Child's Upsetting Times Checklist, a paper-and-pencil assessment of lifetime and past-year exposure to both low- and high-magnitude stressors, is based on the LECI (Dise-Lewis, 1988), with minor stressors ("You felt angry or upset," "You felt rushed or pressured") excluded. Explicit questions about sexual abuse are *excluded*, although the parent is asked if peers, an adult stranger, or a known adult ever made the child do "something horrible." Assessors then inquire as to the nature of that event if the parent endorses it. Response format is as follows: *Never happened*; *Happened, but the worst time was not upsetting*; *Happened, and the worst time was somewhat upsetting*; and *Happened, and the worst time was very upsetting.* The adult is also asked to describe the most upsetting event experienced in the past year, then rate it on how upsetting it was—*A little, Very much, totally.* Then the adult is asked to describe the most upsetting event experienced prior to last year and rate how upsetting it was. Age range: all ages. Number of items: 70. Languages available: English; Spanish.

Evidence of Reliability: Evidence of reliability has yet to be published.

Evidence of Validity: Significant correlations were found between the number of stressors endorsed by the parent on the Child's Upsetting Times Checklist and four measures of childhood PTSD (Fletcher, 1996b): the CPTSDI (.40), the Parent's CPTSDI (.47), the Parent's Report of the Child's Reaction to Stress (.50), and the post hoc CBCL PTSD scale (.52).

Contact Information: Kenneth E. Fletcher, PhD, Department of Psychiatry, University of Massachusetts Medical School, 55 Lake Avenue North, Worcester, MA 01655. Telephone: (508) 856-8630. E-mail: kenneth.fletcher@ umassmed.edu.

The History of Victimization Form (HVF; Wolfe, Gentile, & Bourdeau, 1987)

Brief Description: The History of Victimization Form is an interview with the caretaker or guardians and/or social worker that assesses timing, frequency, duration, time of cessation, number of perpetrators and their relationship to the child, of physical abuse, sexual abuse, neglect, emotional maltreatment, and family violence. A review of clinical and protective agency records also is considered. Age range: 8–16 years. Format: yes–no.

Evidence of Reliability: Evidence of reliability has yet to be published.

Evidence of Validity: Evidence of validity has yet to be published.

Contact Information: Vicky Veitch Wolfe, PhD, Child and Adolescent Centre, 346 South Street, London Health Sciences Centre, London, Ontario, Canada, N6A 4G5. Telephone: (519) 685-8500. E-mail: vicky.wolfe@lhsc.on.ca.

Juvenile Victimization Questionnaire—Caregiver Proxy Report Version (JVQ-CPR; Finkelhor, Hamby, Ormrod, & Turner, 2005)

Brief Description: The JVQ-CPR (see above for the self-report version for children 10 and older) comprises screening questions about 34 acts of violence against children related to five general areas: (1) conventional crime, (2) child maltreatment, (3) peer and sibling victimization, (4) sexual victimization, and (5) witnessing and indirect victimization. Questions association with each of the five areas are contained in their own module, each of which was designed to be used in its own stand-alone form. Finkelhor and colleagues (2005, p. 385) note, "For theoretical and practical reasons, however, it is preferable to administer the full instrument." Events that are endorsed are followed up with questions about the number of times the child has been victimized in this manner, who victimized the child, whether or not the child was hurt, and questions specific to the type of victimization reported (e.g., the value of stolen items). The JVQ-CPR can be used without the follow-up questions, at the expense of eliciting detailed information about the different experiences. It asks about the occurrence of events in the previous year, but it can be adapted to query about lifetime exposure. Early testing of the JVQ-CPR included extensive reviews by experts in the field of juvenile victimization. Draft versions were critiqued by focus groups of youth and parents to refine the wording. Administration time: 20 minutes on average. Ages: Intended to assess the experiences of children age 2 years and older.

Evidence of Reliability: To conduct test–retest evaluation of the JVQ-CPR, 100 caregivers of children ages 2–9 were recontacted 3–4 weeks after their original telephone interviews and readministered the JVQ-CPR. The overall agreement for the caregiver proxies was 95%, with a range of 80–100% for the individual items (Finkelhor et al., 2005). The mean kappa was .50, with a range of –.03 to 1.0. Most of the small kappas were associated with items that had a low response rate. Noting that there are good reasons to question the utility of tests of internal consistency among questions designed to assess actual experiences, the authors reported the values for the total of the 34 JVQ items (alpha = .80), as well as for each of the individual summary subscales: .61 for Conventional Crime (8 items), .64 for Physical Assault (10 items), .38 for Property Victimization (3 items), .39 for Child Maltreatment (4 items), .51 for Sexual Victimization (7 items), .35 for Sexual Assault (4 items), .55 for Peer or Sibling Victimization (9 items), and .35 for Peer or Sibling Assault (.35).

Evidence of Validity: Among 1,026 caregivers of young children ages 2–9 years who participated in a national telephone survey, most of the single items and all of the subscale totals of their measure of the JVQ-CPR correlated significantly with the Trauma Symptom Checklist for Young Children (TSCYC—Briere, 2000; see Appendix 9.4 below) Anxiety, Depression, and Anger subscales (Finkelhor et al., 2005).

Contact Information: David Finkelhor, PhD, Crimes Against Children Research Center, University of New Hampshire, 126 Horton Social Science Center, Durham, NH 03824. Example items from the questionnaire are available as an appendix to Finkelhor and colleagues (2005).

Lifetime Incidence of Traumatic Events (LITE), Parent Form (Greenwald & Rubin, 1999)

Brief Description: The LITE Parent Form assesses exposure to 16 potentially traumatic stressors, such as a car accident or death of someone in the family. It measures the frequency of exposure, age at time of exposure, and how upset the child was by the event at the time and currently on a 3-point scale (*None, Some, Lots*). Age range: 8+. Languages available: English, Spanish, German, Persian, Swedish.

Evidence of Reliability: Evidence of reliability has yet to be published.

Evidence of Validity: Evidence of validity has yet to be published.

Contact Information: Sidran Institute, 200 E. Joppa Road, Suite 207, Towson, MD 21286. Telephone: (410) 825-8888. E-mail: sidran@sidran.org. Website: *www.sidran.org*.

My Exposure to Violence (MyETV)—Parent/Caregiver Report Version (Selner-O'Hagan, Kindlon, Buka, Raudenbush, & Earls, 1998)

Brief Description: MyETV, Parent/Caregiver Report Version is a highly structured interview designed to cover a child's lifetime and past-year exposure to 18 different violent events that the child has either witnessed or personally experienced. It also ascertains location of violence (e.g., school, home, neighborhood), identifies both perpetrators and victims of violence (e.g., family member, stranger), and whether the exposure was gang-related. MyETV measures lifetime exposure (*Ever*) and annual prevalence (*In the past year*). Frequency of exposure is measured on a 6-point scale (*Never, Once, 2 or 3 times, 4 to 10 times, 11 to 50 times*, and *More than 50 times*). Six subscales are defined: (1) Witnessing violent events, (2) Victimization, and (3) Total Exposure (witnessing and victimization), obtaining scores for both lifetime and past-year exposure.

Evidence of Reliability: The version of MyETV for children, adolescents, and young adult respondents (see above, this appendix) had high internal consistency (r = .68–.93) and test–retest reliability (r = .75–.94). But psychometrics for the parent form are not available.

Evidence of Validity: The authors also provide evidence of construct validity for children, adolescents, and young adult respondents.

Contact Information: Mary Beth Selner-O'Hagan, PhD, Department of Maternal and Child Health, Harvard School of Public Health, 677 Huntington Avenue, Boston, MA 02115. E-mail: mohagan@phdcn.harvard.edu.

Parent Version of KID-SAVE (P-KID-SAVE; Flowers, Lanclos, & Kelley, 2002)

Brief Description: The P-KID-SAVE, a reworded version of the KID-SAVE (Hastings & Kelley, 1997a; see above, this appendix), allows administration to caregivers of children. The P-KID-SAVE has yet to be empirically validated.

Evidence of Reliability: Internal consistency among parents of 182 young children (48% girls), in grades 3 through 7 (average age = 9.88 years, SD = 1.65), was demonstrated with Cronbach's alphas of .88 for the frequency scale for Indirect Violence, .65 for frequency of Traumatic Violence, and .66 for frequency of Physical/Verbal Abuse; the alphas were .87 for the impact of Indirect Violence scale, .79 for impact of Traumatic Violence, and .69 for impact of Physical/Verbal Abuse. Alphas for the totals of the two domains, frequency and impact, were not reported.

Evidence of Validity: Correlations between parent and child responses to the P-KID-SAVE and the KID-SAVE on five of the six subscales were low (.26 to .30) but significant. The correlation between parent and child ratings on the impact of Indirect Violence were nonsignificant (.15). Paired t-tests resulted in only one significant difference between parent and child ratings on the six subscales. Children reported significantly greater frequency of exposure to physical/verbal abuse than did the parents. Parent reports of their children's frequency of physical/verbal abuse was significantly associated with their ratings of their children's Withdrawn, Anxious–Depressed, Social Problems, Attention Problems, Delinquent, and Aggression subscale scores, as well as the Internalizing and Externalizing scores on the CBCL (Achenbach, 1991a). Parent ratings of their children's frequency of traumatic violence also was associated with the Social Problems subscale on the CBCL. Anxiety scores on the Trauma Symptom Checklist for Children (TSCC—Briere, 1996a, 1996b; see Appendix 9.5) were associated with parent's ratings of the frequency of their children's exposure to indirect violence. However, only children's self-reports were associated with the Posttraumatic Stress subscale of the TSCC (see above, this appendix).

Contact Information: Anise Flowers, PhD, Tarnow Center for Self-Management, 1001 West Loop South, No. 215, Houston, Texas 77027. E-mail: doctorflowers@email.com.

Preschool Age Psychiatric Assessment (PAPA) Life Events Scale (Egger & Angold, 2004)

Brief Description: This is the life events form of a module of the full PAPA (Egger & Angold, 2004; see Appendix 9.3). The Life Events Scale is a semistructured interview that assesses stressors affecting this age group. High-magnitude stressors include physical and sexual abuse and death of a parent. Low-magnitude stressors include reduction in standard of living and attending unsafe day care. PAPA includes detailed history of accidents, as well as hospitalization, separation from significant attachment figures for more than 1 week, and becoming homeless. Training is required. Age range: 3–6 years. Interviewer qualifications: Bachelor's degree or higher. Languages available: English and Spanish.

Evidence of Reliability: Evidence of reliability has yet to be published.

Evidence of Validity: Evidence of validity has yet to be published.

Contact Information: Developmental Epidemiology Program, Duke University Medical Center, Attention: Juné Rogers, DUMC Box 3454, Durham, NC 27710. Telephone: (919) 687-4686, extension 273. E-mail: jrogers@psych.duhs.duke.edu.

Survey of Exposure to Community Violence—Parent Report Version (SECV-P; Richters & Saltzman, 1990)

Brief Description: The SECV-P is a self-report measure that evaluates children's exposure to 20 forms of severe violence (shootings, stabbings, and rapes), less severe violence (beatings and chasings), and moderately severe violence (threats, accidents, drug deals, and arrests). Parents report on whether the child has been the victim of, witnessed, or simply heard about each kind of event. The frequency of each exposure is assessed on a 9-point scale, ranging from *No exposure* (0) to *Exposed every day* (8). "For each positive response, the questionnaire includes context questions about (1) where the violence took place (in or near school versus home), (2) who perpetrated the violence (ranging from stranger to family member), (3) who, if not the child, was victimized (ranging from stranger to family member), and (4) when the incident occurred (ranging from 1 week ago to more than 5 years ago)" (Richters & Martinez, 1993, p. 9). The SECV is also known as the Survey of Children's Exposure to Community Violence. The Child Self-Report Version was presented earlier in this appendix.

Evidence of Reliability: Evidence of reliability has yet to be published.

Evidence of Validity: Among 53 mothers (Osofsky, Wewers, Hann, & Fick, 1993), their ratings of their children's distress using the CCDS (Richters & Martinez, 1990a; see Appendix 9.5) correlated significantly with the parent's report on the SECV-P child's witnessing community violence (r = .42), simply hearing about such violence (.48), minor family conflicts (.39), and severe family conflicts (.61). Moreover, the magnitude of the correlations was associated with the magnitude of the stressor. Thus, the CCDS correlated .35 with moderate types, .29 with the less than severe types of community violence, and .51 with the most severe (a shooting, a stabbing, or rape).

Contact Information: John E. Richters, PhD, Department of Human Development and Institute for Child Study, University of Maryland, Benjamin Building, Room 4104, College Park, MD 20742. Telephone: (301) 405-7354. E-mail: jrichter@nih.gov.

Traumatic Events Screening Inventory—Parent Report (TESI-P; Ghosh Ippen et al., 2002)

Brief Description: Based on TESI-C (presented earlier in this appendix), the TESI-P is a semistructured interview or self-completion instrument for parents. It is recommended that it be administered as an interview. Two stages are employed to the interview. Stage I comprises only questions about whether the child was exposed to each type of event. In Stage II, detailed follow-up questions, similar to those used in the TESI-C, are asked only for events endorsed positively by the parent. Age range: 0–18 years. Languages available: English, Spanish.

Evidence of Reliability: See TESI-C, this appendix.
Evidence of Validity: Evidence of validity has yet to be published.
Contact Information: Chandra Ghosh Ippen, PhD, Child Trauma Research Project, University of California, San Francisco, CA 94143. Telephone: (415) 206-5312. E-mail: chandra.ghosh@ucsf.edu.

Violence Exposure Scale for Children—Parent Version (VEX-R; Fox & Leavitt, 1995; Shahinfar et al., 2000)

Brief Description: The VEX-R parallels the preschool version (presented earlier in this appendix). For every event to which a caregiver responds positively, the interviewer probes for information regarding the location of the event, the identity of the perpetrators and victims, who was with the child at the time, and how long ago the exposure took place.

Evidence of Reliability: Among 155 parents of children ages 3.5 to 4.5, Cronbach's alpha was .72 for parent reports of their children's exposure to mild violence (8 items; Shahinfar et al., 2000). Too few parents (0.6%) reported that their children had been exposed to severe violence to allow the internal consistency of that set of items to be assessed. Parent and child reports showed no significant association with each other in this study. In the Raviv and colleagues (2001) study of Israeli children's exposure to violence, associations between child and parent reports on respective versions of the VEX tended to be significant, especially for episodes of mild violence, with correlations of .34 for the total of witnessing items, and .47 for the total of victimization items.

Evidence of Validity: No significant associations were found between parent reports of children's exposure to violence and children's distress, as assessed by the CBCL (Achenbach, 1991a). However, when analyses were restricted to children who appeared to understand the measures, parents who reported that their children had witnessed mild violence rated their children as having significantly higher levels of internalizing behavior problem. Parents who reported that their children had been victims of mild violence rated their children as having had higher levels of externalizing behavior problems than did the parents who indicated their children had not had such exposure. No significant association was found between parent reports of children's exposure to severe violence and reports of children's problem behaviors on the CBCL. In a study of the violence experiences of Israeli children (Raviv et al., 2001), the correlations between child and parent reports of severe violence exposure were lower but still significant for the totals of the witnessing items (.22) and the victimization items (.37). Children reporting more experiences of violent victimization were reported by their mothers to have more behavior problems, as measured by the CBCL.

Contact Information: Ariana Shahinfar, Department of Psychology, University of North Carolina, Charlotte, NC 28223-0001. E-mail: ashahinf@email.unc.edu.

APPENDIX 9.2. Assessments of the Level and Quality of Exposure

ADMINISTERED TO CHILD

Children's Peritraumatic Experiences Questionnaire (CPEQ; Wolfe & Birt, 1993)

Brief Description: The CPEQ is a 33-item self-report scale to assess children's emotional reactions during sexual abuse experiences, or for nonabused children, their most negative life experience. Feelings and thoughts related to DSM-IV criterion A2 are assessed, including helplessness, fear, terror, sadness, and anger. Items are divided into five scales derived from a principal components analysis: Extreme Reactions (e.g., thoughts of being killed or killing perpetrator, fear of death and injury, becoming ill, wanting to throw something, terror, or fainting), Fear/Anxiety, Negative Affect, Dissociation, and Guilt. Each question is rated on a 3-point Likert-like response set: None, Some, and A lot. Age range: 8–16 years. The CPEQ is now included with the Children's Impact of Traumatic Events Scale–II (CITES-II; Wolfe, Gentile, Michienzi, Sas, & Wolfe, 1991; see Appendix 9.5).

Evidence of Reliability: Internal consistency alphas are .89 for Extreme Reactions, .86 for Fear/Anxiety, .88 for Negative Affect, .81 for Dissociation, and .54 for Guilt (Wolfe & Birt, 2002a).

Evidence of Validity: Sexual abuse survivors scored significantly higher than both agency-referred and community children on all but the Guilt scale of the CPEQ. The scales correlated significantly with both child and parent ratings of the child's PTSD responses. Frequency of abuse correlated with the Dissociation scale at the .05 level, but not at the Bonferroni-corrected level of .003 (Wolfe & Birt, 2002a).

Contact Information: Vicky Veitch Wolfe, PhD, Child and Adolescent Centre, London Health Sciences Centre, 346 South Street, London, Ontario N6A 4G5. Telephone: (519) 685-8500. E-mail: vicky.wolfe@lhsc.on.ca.

Exposure Questionnaire (EQ; Nader, 1993, 1999)

Brief Description: The EQ assesses aspects of the event(s) that are associated with increased PTSD symptomatology—such as whether there was threat to life, threat of injury, subjective proximity to the events, relationship to victims, worries about others, property damage, and helping efforts—and the child's or adolescent's emotional reactions—such as helplessness, fear, horror, panic, guilt—both during and after the traumatic experience. Inquires are made about frequency and intensity of the reactions. Space is given for a description of the child's experience. Two questionnaires are included, one for Postwar questions and one for Postdisaster or Violence questions. Responses are either yes–no or based on a 5-point Likert-like scale. Age range: 7–17 years. Languages available: English, Croatian, Kuwaiti Arabic.

Evidence of Reliability: Evidence of reliability has not yet been published.

Evidence of Validity: Scores on the EQ have been shown to be associated with exposure and severity levels of children exposed to war (Nader & Fairbanks, 1994; Nader, Pynoos, Fairbanks, Al-Ajeel, & Al-Asfour, 1993).

Contact Information: Kathleen Nader, DSW. Fax: (512) 219-0486. E-mail: measures@twosuns.org.

ADMINISTERED TO CARETAKER OR OTHER ADULTS

Dimensions of Stressful Events (DOSE) Scale (Fletcher, 1996d)

Brief Description: The DOSE scale is designed to assess the characteristics or dimensions of high-magnitude stressor events suggested by the literature to increase the likelihood of a child or adolescent responding with PTSD symptomatology. Items are divided into two sections. The first section contains 25 items that assess things such as the child's proximity to the event, viewing of blood, and whether anyone was injured or died; whether or not the child was separated from caretakers; relationship of the child to any perpetrator and victims; the child's sense of stigmatization; the suddenness and unexpectedness of the event(s); the perceived uncontrollability of the event(s); duration and frequency of exposure to the event(s); whether the source of the event(s) was human rather than nature; whether the adverse consequences of the event(s) are long-lasting, irreversible, liable to recur, or involved moral conflicts for the child; whether the child perceived the event(s) as a threat to family or friends; and whether the event(s) originated within the family. The second section contains 24 items that assess the frequency and degree of child abuse experiences, as well as experiences that may mitigate the child's responses, such as the extent to which the parents support the child's claim. A suggested scoring key accompanies the scale. The measure is in the public domain. The interviewer or clinician completes the measure with information from the child, caretakers, and records. Age range: all ages.

Evidence of Reliability: Internal consistency alpha was .60 among 326 school-age and younger children exposed to domestic violence (Fletcher, Spilsbury, Creedan, & Friedman, 2006).

Evidence of Validity: The DOSE correlated significantly with school-age children's self-reported PTSD symptomatology, as measured by both the When Bad Things Happen scale (.70; Fletcher, 1996g; see Appendix 9.5) and the CPTSDI—Child Form (.77; Fletcher, 1996b, 1996c; see Appendix 9.5). It also correlated significantly with parent reports of the child's PTSD symptomatology, whether measured by the Parent Report of the Child's Reaction to Stress (.54; Fletcher, 1996e; see Appendix 9.5), the CPTSDI—Parent Form (.66; Fletcher, 1996b, 1996c; see Appendix 9.5), or an ad hoc CBCL PTSD scale (.47). When regressing the child's PTSD symptomatology on gender, family income, stressful life experiences, and the DOSE, the DOSE tended to be a significant predictor, whereas stressful life experiences were not (Fletcher, 1996c). Among adolescent psychiatric inpatients, the DOSE correlated significantly with the When Bad Things Happen scale (.45–.54), the CPTSDI—Child Form (.34), and the Child's Reaction to Traumatic Events Scale (CRTES—Jones, 1996; see Appendix 9.5) (.42). The DOSE again tended to predict PTSD symptomatology significantly in statistical regression tests, whereas lifetime stressors did not (Fletcher, Cox, Skidmore, Janssens, & Render, 1997). In a sample of 1,277 children (50.4% female, 44.7% African American, 29.4% European American, 3.1% Hispanic; mean age 7.6 ± 4.4 years) participating in a community-based intervention for children exposed to interpersonal violence, DOSE scores were normally distributed (mean score = 21.2 ± 5.7, median = 21.0, range 1–38; Fletcher et al., 2006). DOSE scores did not differ by gender. European American children scored slightly higher than African American children [21.9 vs. 21.1, $t(943) = 2.097$, $p = .030$]. The DOSE correlated significantly with Briere's (1996b) Trauma Symptom Checklist for Children (TSCC; see Appendix 9.5) Posttraumatic Symptom (PTS) scale (.42), Anxiety (.42), Depression (.35), and Dissociation (.26), as well as Saylor, Swenson, Reynolds, and Taylor's (1999) Pediatric Emotional Distress Scale (PEDS; Appendix 9.4) total (.28), and Quay and Peterson's (1996) Revised Behavior Problem Checklist (RBPC) Anxiety (.19) and Conduct Disorder (.20) scales, with TSCC correlations generally higher among girls, and PEDS and RBPC correlations only significant for boys. After adjusting for gender, age, and ethnicity, the DOSE significantly predicted TSCC PTS, Depression, Dissociation, Anxiety, Anger, and Sexual Concerns scales scores (in linear regressions) and clinical cutoffs (in logistic regressions). Receiver operating characteristic (ROC) analysis indicated that a total DOSE score of 22.5 or higher provides the best sensitivity–specificity trade-off when predicting the TSCC PTS scale (area under the curve [AUC] = .74, $p \leq .001$).

Contact Information: Kenneth E. Fletcher, PhD, Department of Psychiatry, University of Massachusetts Medical School, 55 Lake Avenue North, Worcester, MA 01655. Telephone: (508) 856-8630. E-mail: kenneth.fletcher@umassmed.edu.

Peritraumatic Response Scale (Pfefferbaum et al., 2002)

Brief Description: The Peritraumatic Response Scale contains 12 items addressing the participant's peritraumatic responses of fear, arousal, and dissociation at the time of the incident.

Evidence of Reliability: Evidence of reliability has yet to be published.

Evidence of Validity: Evidence of validity has yet to be published.

Contact Information: Betty Pfefferbaum, MD, JD, Department of Psychiatry and Behavioral Sciences, College of Medicine, University of Oklahoma Health Sciences Center, 920 Stanton L. Young Boulevard, WP-3470, Oklahoma City, OK 73104. Telephone: (405) 271-5251. E-mail: betty-pfefferbaum@ouhsc.edu.

APPENDIX 9.3. General Child Psychiatric Assessment Interviews with a PTSD Module

ADMINISTERED TO CHILD

Child and Adolescent Psychiatric Assessment (CAPA) Scale (Angold & Costello, 2000)

Brief Description: The CAPA is a general child and adolescent, glossary-based interview that includes a PTSD module. There are both child and parent report versions. Criteria A1 and A2 are assessed with the Life Events Scale. Other diagnoses covered include disruptive behavior disorders (including attention-deficit/hyperactivity disorder, on the parent version only, and conduct disorder), mood disorders (including depression and mania), anxiety disorders (including generalized anxiety disorder, separation anxiety, panic disorder, and obsessive–compulsive disorder), eating disorders, sleep disorders, elimination disorders, substance use/abuse/dependence, tic disorders, and others (including adjustment disorders, reactive attachment disorder of childhood, and somatization symptoms). Frequency and duration of symptoms are assessed for many symptoms. Psychosocial impairment related to the presence of a symptom is rated in 19 domains related to life at home, school, and elsewhere. There are two alternate forms for different ages: the PAPA for preschool-age children (see below, this appendix) and the YAPA for young adults (see Appendix 9.6). Age range: 9–17 years. Time period covered: Previous 3 months, except for select symptoms involving infrequent acts, such as firesetting or suicide attempts. Interviewer qualifications: bachelor's degree and up. Languages available: English, Spanish.

Evidence of Reliability: Test–retest reliability kappas for DSM-III-R diagnosis using the Child version (CAPA-C) with 77 clinically referred children ages 10–16 years ranged from .50 for conduct disorder to .90 for major depression. ICC for DSM-III-R PTSD symptom scale scores was >.90 (Angold & Costello, 1995). The ICC for level of psychosocial impairment by child self-report (on the CAPA-C) was .77 (Angold & Costello, 1995). A kappa coefficient of .64 for interrater reliability on PTSD diagnosis using the CAPA-C was found in another study (Costello et al., 1998). The same study found an ICC for interrater reliability of .94 for the overall CAPA-C. This same study found a kappa of .54 for interrater reliability for PTSD diagnosis using the parent version (CAPA-P), whereas an ICC for interrater reliability on the overall CAPA-P was .99.

Evidence of Validity: The PTSD module of both the Child (CAPA-C) and Parent (CAPA-P) versions differentiated between a clinical sample and a community sample based on PTSD diagnosis (Costello et al., 1998).

Contact Information: Developmental Epidemiology Program, Duke University Medical Center, Attention: Juné Rogers, DUMC Box 3454, Durham, NC 27710. Telephone: (919) 687-4686, extension 273. E-mail: jrogers@psych.duhs.duke.edu.

Children's Interview for Psychiatric Syndromes (ChIPS; Rooney, Fristad, Weller, & Weller, 1999; Weller, Weller, Rooney, & Fristad, 1999, 2000)

Brief Description: The ChIPS is a highly structured interview that screens for 20 DSM-IV Axis I disorders, as well as psychosocial stressors such as emotional, physical, or sexual abuse and neglect. Questions use simple language and short sentence structure to enhance subject comprehension and cooperation. The interview is based on DSM-IV, and results are presented in a concise, easy-to-interpret manner. The Stress Disorders section assesses both ASD and PTSD. Exposure to a high-magnitude stressor is assessed by one question asking whether anything very bad has happened to the child, such as being kidnapped or attacked, and if yes, what? A second question asks whether the child has ever witnessed something bad happening to someone else, but not on TV, and if so, what? If the child does not describe an experience that meets criterion A in one of these questions, no more Stress Disorder questions are asked. Otherwise, five questions attempt to ascertain the child's reactions to the experience(s) and whether or not they satisfy the second half of criterion A. If not, the rest of the Stress Disorder questions are skipped. Otherwise, the child is asked how long ago the event(s) took place. If it happened within 4 weeks of the interview, six questions are asked to assess whether the child reacted with symptoms of dissociation or derealization. If so, children are asked if they have felt as if they were not themselves, as if they were no longer real (depersonalization), and if they have trouble remembering things about the event(s). Then seven questions are asked to assess reexperiencing symptoms, two to assess feeling "upset" by reminders of the experience(s), and one to assess physical reactions to reminders, such as stomachaches or trouble breathing. If none of these symptoms are endorsed, the rest of the Stress Disorder questions are skipped. Otherwise, 10 questions are asked to assess symptoms of avoidance and withdrawal. If none of these are endorsed the rest of the questions are skipped. Otherwise, one question is asked about changes in moods or emotions since the event(s), one about feelings of numbness since the event(s), and two about feelings of foreshortened future. Six questions are then asked about symptoms of overarousal, anger, and difficulty concentrating. If none of these questions are endorsed, one question is asked about a tendency to startle easily. Then the interviewer is given two algorithms to determine whether the child meets criteria for ASD or PTSD, or neither. Next children are asked when the symptoms began and whether they are still troubled by the symptoms, and if not, the interviewer attempts to determine when the symptoms stopped. Children who meet criteria for ASD are asked if the symptoms began within 4 weeks of the event(s), if they lasted more than 2 days, and if they have lasted for less than 4 weeks. Those who meet criteria for PTSD are asked if the symptoms have lasted longer than 1 month. Finally, children are asked whether "these problems cause you trouble" at home, at school, and with other kids. If duration of symptoms can be determined, the interviewer can indicate whether or not the PTSD can be classified as being of acute or chronic duration, and whether symptoms had a regular onset (within 6 months of the event(s) or a delayed onset (more than 6 months after the event(s). Age range: 6–18 years, with an IQ over 70. Administration time: 49 minutes for inpatients, 30 minutes for outpatients, 21 minutes for a community-based sample (Weller et al., 2000). Training: ChIPS is designed to be administered by people with at least a bachelor's degree in a field associated with mental health. It is recommended that lay interviewers be trained by a clinician familiar with DSM-IV who has undergone similar training on ChIPS.

Evidence of Reliability: Evidence of reliability has yet to be published.

Evidence of Validity: Among 18 girl and 22 boy psychiatric inpatients (Fristad, Cummings, et al., 1998) agreement between the ChIPS and the Diagnostic Interview for Children and Adolescents—Revised (DICA-R; Kaplan & Reich, 1991; see below, this appendix) for diagnosis of PTSD was .77 for girls (using low-base-rate kappa; Verducci, Mack, & DeGroot, 1988), representing an 89% agreement rate, with the two interviews agreeing that 4 girls had PTSD and 12 did not, while disagreeing on 2 girls' PTSD diagnoses; whereas, the low-base-rate kappa for boys was .49, representing 95% agreement that 21 boys did not have PTSD, while there was disagreement on one boy's PTSD diagnosis. The same data indicated that the two interviews agreed 100% of the time on diagnosis for children ages 6–12 (with 1 yes and 20 no), whereas agreement was 84%, with a low-base-rate kappa of .67 for adolescents ages 13–17 (3 yes and 13 no) and disagreeing on three diagnoses. Among a community sample of 40 children and adolescents ages 6–18, agreement was 100% that none had PTSD (Fristad, Glickman, et al., 1998).

Contact Information: Available from American Psychiatric Publishing Group. Telephone: (800) 368-5777. Website: *www.appi.org*. Elizabeth Weller, MD, Department of Child Psychiatry, Children's Hospital of Philadelphia, 34th Street and Civic Center Boulevard, Philadelphia, PA 19104; E-mail: weller@email.chop.edu.

Diagnostic Interview for Children and Adolescents—Revised (DICA-R; Kaplan & Reich, 1991; see MAGIC below)

Brief Description: The DICA-R, a semistructured interview, has been replaced by the Missouri Assessment of Genetics Interview for Children (MAGIC—Reich & Todd, 2002; see below). It is included here primarily because so many other measures have used the interview to establish validity. The DICA-R is a modification of the Diagnostic Interview for Children and Adolescents (DICA; Herjanic & Reich, 1983a, 1983b), developed for the assessment of diagnoses in children 6–17 years old. The DICA-R modified the DICA to allow for assessment of DSM-III-R criteria. Questions were rephrased to be more conversational in manner, and questions related to DSM-III-R diagnoses were added (Kaplan & Reich, 1991), including a PTSD module. The DICA-R was revised to allow assessment of DSM-IV diagnoses. The PTSD module included four questions to assess criterion A (exposure to a high magnitude stressor), seven questions for criterion B (reexperiencing), nine for criterion C (denial and numbing), and five questions for criterion D (overarousal). Questions are asked to determine duration (criterion E) and intensity of endorsed symptoms, and to assess changes in social interactions and school behavior (criterion F). Response categories are *No*, *Rarely*, *Sometimes or Somewhat*, and *Yes*. Determination of criterion is accomplished by adding these ratings and meeting specific thresholds. Difficulties have been reported among 7-year-olds in understanding some of the DICA-R questions intended for use with 6- to 12-year-olds (reported in Nader, 1997). Age range: 6–17 years. Available languages: English, Spanish, and Arabic. A computerized version is available. Time required for administration of the full DICA-R is 1½ hours. Training is required. The interview may be administered by research assistants with no more than a bachelor's degree. There are versions for younger children ages 6–12 years, for adolescents, and for parents.

Evidence of Reliability: Cronbach's alphas on the PTSD module among 37 stress-exposed inner-city children were .44, .87, .83, and .87 for criteria A–D, respectively (Yasik et al., 1998). Test–retest reliability for diagnosis of PTSD per the module among 90 children was .79 (reported in Nader, 1997). Interrater reliability averaged .91 among interviewers of adolescents exposed to a residential fire (Jones & Ribbe, 1991).

Evidence of Validity: Agreement between DICA-R PTSD diagnoses and clinical diagnoses was 100% among 86 children; sensitivity was 1.00, and specificity was .86 (reported in Nader, 1997). When Yasik and colleagues (1998) compared DICA-R PTSD diagnoses and clinical diagnoses among 37 stress-exposed and 12 non-stress-exposed inner-city children, 9 of 15 PTSD cases were identified correctly (sensitivity = .60), and 33 of 34 non-PTSD cases were identified correctly (specificity = .97). Overall, the PTSD status of 85.7% of the children was identified correctly. Adolescents exposed to a residential fire reported significantly more symptoms of PTSD when interviewed with the DICA-R PTSD module than did those not exposed to the fire (Jones & Ribbe, 1991). On the other hand, the PTSD module was unable to distinguish between adolescents exposed to wildfires and those not exposed (Jones et al., 1994).

Contact Information: Wendy Reich, PhD, Department of Psychiatry, Washington University in St. Louis School of Medicine, 660 S. Euclid Ave., Campus Box 8134, St. Louis, MO 63110. Telephone: (314) 286-2263. E-mail: Wendyr@twins.wustl.edu.

Diagnostic Interview Schedule for Children (DISC; Shaffer et al., 1988, 1993, 2000)

Brief Description: The DISC is a structured interview that assesses more than 30 DSM-IV childhood psychiatric disorders. The PTSD module includes three questions to establish criterion A, exposure to a traumatic event. If none are endorsed, no more questions are asked. Responses are *No* (0), *Sometimes/somewhat* (1), and *Yes* (2). The presence of a symptom in the past month and the past year is assessed. Training recommended for interviewers usually takes 3 days.

Evidence of Reliability: Evidence of reliability has yet to be published.

Evidence of Validity: Among 671 children and adolescents ages 9–17 years and their parents residing in housing units, only 8 (1.2%) met DSM-III criteria for PTSD per child report using an earlier version of the DISC, and only 4 (0.6%) met PTSD criteria per parent report (Fisher et al., 1993; cited in Nader, 1997). But when the two reports were combined using an algorithm, 21.2% met two or more of the four diagnostic criteria. "There were strong associations between major depression, generalized anxiety disorder, conduct disorder, and substance-use disorders with increased risk of PTSD" (Nader, 1997, p. 321).

Contact Information: David Shaffer, MD, Division of Child and Adolescent Psychiatry, Columbia University Medical Center, Lawrence C. Kolb Research Building, Room 263A Unit/Box 78, 40 Haven Avenue, New York, NY 10032. Telephone: (212) 305-6001. E-mail: shafferd@childpsych.columbia.edu.

Schedule for Affective Disorders and Schizophrenia for School-Age Children (6–18 years)–IV–Revised (K-SADS-IV-R; Ambrosini & Dixon, 2000; Kaufman et al., 1997; Orvaschel, Puig-Antich, Chambers, Tabrizi, & Johnson, 1982)

Brief Description: The K-SADS-IV-R was developed from the adult interview, the Schizophrenia and Affective Disorder Scales. The semistructured versions are the K-SADS-E (Epidemiological version) and the K-SADS-PL (Present and Lifetime versions). This interview is primarily for use in research settings and is to be administered by a clinician trained in its use, so it is rarely used in ordinary clinical settings. It covers a broad spectrum of most child psychiatric diagnoses, with the exception of pervasive development disorders and personality disorders, and is used with children ages 6–18 years. For younger children it is recommended that a single clinician interview the parent(s) first, then repeat the interview with the child. It is recommended that adolescents be interviewed first. The scale includes questions about school performance and other issues relevant to children and adolescents. According to the K-SADS-PL website (see URL in contact information), "The K-SADS-PL was adapted from the K-SADS-P (Present Episode Version), which was developed by William Chambers, M.D., and Joaquim Puig-Antich, M.D., and later revised by Joaquim Puig-Antich, M.D., and Neal Ryan, M.D. The K-SADS-PL was written by Joan Kaufman, Ph.D., Boris Birmaher, M.D., David Brent, M.D., Uma Rao, M.D., and Neal Ryan, M.D. The K-SADS-PL was designed to obtain severity ratings of symptomatology, and assess current and lifetime history of psychiatric disorders, including several disorders not surveyed in the K-SADS-P. The current instrument is greatly indebted to several other existing structured and semi-structured psychiatric instruments, including the K-SADS-E (Orvaschel & Puig-Antich), the SADS-L (Spitzer and Endicott), the SCID ([Structured Clinical Interview for DSM-III-R] Spitzer, Williams, Gibbon, and First), the DIS ([Diagnostic Interview Schedule] Robins and Helzer), the ISC ([Interview Schedule for Children] Kovacs), the DICA (Reich, Shayka, and Taibleson), and the DUSI ([Drug Use Screening Inventory] Tarter, Laird, Bukstein, and Kaminer). . . . The K-SADS-PL is a semi-structured diagnostic interview designed to assess current and past episodes of psychopathology in children and adolescents according to DSM-III-R and DSM-IV criteria. Probes and objective criteria are provided to rate individual symptoms. The primary diagnoses assessed with the K-SADS-PL include: Major Depression, Dysthymia, Mania, Hypomania, Cyclothymia, Bipolar Disorders, Schizoaffective Disorders, Schizophrenia, Schizophreniform Disorder, Brief Reactive Psychosis, Panic Disorder, Agoraphobia, Separation Anxiety Disorder, Avoidant Disorder of Childhood and Adolescence, Simple Phobia, Social Phobia, Overanxious Disorder, Generalized Anxiety, Obsessive Compulsive Disorder, Attention Deficit Hyperactivity Disorder, Conduct Disorder, Oppositional Defiant Disorder, Enuresis, Encopresis, Anorexia Nervosa, Bulimia, Transient Tic Disorder, Tourette's Disorder, Chronic Motor or Vocal Tic Disorder, Alcohol Abuse, Substance Abuse, Post-Traumatic Stress Disorder, and Adjustment Disorders." The PTSD module first asks whether the child has ever experienced or witnessed something "very frightening, terrible or upsetting." If the answer is no, the remainder of the questions in the section are skipped. If yes, the child is asked how it made him or her feel. Again, if the response does not meet DSM-IV criterion A2, the remainder of the questions are skipped. If the answer meets criterion A2, questions are asked to assess the presence or absence of the 17 symptoms of DSM-IV PTSD criteria B through D. The interviewer then rates the overall severity of symptoms on a scale from 1 (*Not at all*) to 6 (*Extreme: almost all the time experience symptomatic trauma. Is impaired daily in all functional areas*). The month, day, and year of the onset and offset of PTSD is then estimated based on reports of the child and parent. Training: A semi-structured interview, the K-SADS-PL requires intensive training relative to the instrument, diagnostic classification, and differential diagnostic. Time required: For normal controls, the child and parent interviews required 35–45 minutes each. With psychiatric patients, they can required 1.5 hours or longer, depending on the range and severity of psychopathology of the child.

Evidence of Reliability: Psychometric properties of the K-SADS-PL were assessed in a sample of 55 psychiatric outpatients and 11 normal controls ages 7–17 years ($M = 12.4$, $SD = 2.6$; Kaufman et al., 1997). Parents and children were both interviewed. Interrater reliability among one Master's-level and four Bachelor's-level interviewers in scoring screens and diagnoses for 15 children was high, ranging between 93 and 100%. The test–retest reliability kappa coefficient ($n = 20$) for present PTSD diagnosis over an average of 18 days between administrations was .67. Using an earlier version, K-SADS-E, interrater (parent–child) agreement was 87.5% (McLeer, Deblinger, Henry, & Orvaschel, 1992).

Evidence of Validity: Evidence of validity has yet to be published.

Contact Information: K-SADS-P-IV-R: Paul J. Ambrosini, MD, MCP Hahnemann University, EPPI, 3200 Henry Avenue, Philadelphia, PA 19129. Telephone: (215) 842-4402. E-mail: paul.ambrosini@drexel.edu. K-SADS-PL: Joan Kaufman, PhD, Department of Psychology, Yale University, P.O. Box 208205, New Haven, CT 06520. E-mail: jk279@pantheon.yale.edu. The K-SADS-PL is available for free download at *www.wpic.pitt.edu/ksads/default.htm.*

Mini-International Neuropsychiatric Interview for Children and Adolescents (MINI Kids; Amorim et al., 1998; Lecrubier et al., 1997; Sheehan et al., 1997; Sheehan, Lecrubie, Weiller, Hergueta, & Sheehan, et al., 1998)

Brief Description: The MINI Kids is an abbreviated psychiatric interview for children. A parent version is available. Unfortunately, the PTSD module does not assess all of the DSM-IV symptoms. Criteria A1, A2, and B1 are all assessed with one question each. Six questions assess criterion C; five questions assess criterion D; and one question assesses whether the endorsed symptoms have upset the child a lot and caused him or her problems at school, at home, or with friends. All questions are answered yes or no.

Evidence of Reliability: Current psychometrics appear to be restricted to the adult version of the MINI. The interrater reliability kappa for the PTSD module for adults is .95, and the test–retest kappa is .73 (Sheehan et al., 1998).

Evidence of Validity: The psychometrics for the adult version look good, with agreement between the adult clinician rated MINI and the SCID-P (Spitzer, Williams, Gibbon, & First, 1990) diagnosis of PTSD, with a kappa of .78, a sensitivity of .85, specificity of .96, a positive predictive value of .82, and a negative predictive value of .97 (Sheehan et al., 1998).

Contact Information: Free download available online (after free registration) at *www.medical-outcomes.com/ indexssl.htm.*

Missouri Assessment of Genetics Interview for Children (MAGIC; Reich & Todd, 2002)

Brief Description: MAGIC, a semistructured interview with a glossary for interpreting responses, is based on the DSM-IV version of the DICA (Reich, 2000) and DICA-R (discussed earlier, this appendix). Unlike many interviews, most skip patterns have been removed from the different diagnostic modules to allow complete information to be gathered on the number of symptoms per diagnostic category, regardless of whether DSM-IV criteria are met for the diagnostic category. Versions are available for children (MAGIC-C), adolescents (MAGIC-A), and parents about their children (MAGIC-P). The initial question of the PTSD module asks whether the child has ever had something really awful happen to him or her. Many example probes are provided for the interviewer. If the answer is no, the PTSD module is skipped; otherwise, three questions attempt to establish criterion A2 (whether the child's reaction was one of terror, horror, or feeling completely helpless). A further question allows for a description of the child's feelings in his or her own words. Single questions are asked regarding four of the five DSM-IV symptoms of reexperiencing; three questions are asked about feeling as if the event were recurring, flashbacks, and playing games or drawing pictures about the event. Single questions are asked for six of the seven criterion C symptoms, and two questions are asked regarding feelings of detachment and restricted affect. Single questions are asked for four of the five criterion D symptoms, and two questions are asked about increased irritability and loss of temper. If at least one positive response is given to questions regarding criteria B–D, an attempt is made to determine how soon after the traumatic event the symptoms began, how long they lasted, and how much the symptoms have "interfered with her or his life" to assess criteria E and F. Questions are then asked about how much the child had the endorsed symptoms prior to the event, whether or not the child was taken to a doctor or counselor, or other professional because the parent was worried about the child, and if so, who the child saw and whether any medication was prescribed. Then the parent is asked whether he or she was worried about the child because of the event, whether the child stayed in his or her room because of the event, and whether the child ever attempted to "get out of doing things with the family" because of the event. Responses are *No* (0), *Sometimes/somewhat* (1), and *Yes* (2). *Sometimes* is considered an endorsement of a symptom for the PTSD module. Presence of symptoms is assessed for the past year and for the lifetime prior to the previous year. Age range: 9–17 for child and adolescent interviews, and for parents of children ages 7–17.

Evidence of Reliability: Although Todd, Joyner, Heath, Neuman, & Reich (2003) demonstrated good interrater and test–retest reliability for several of the disorders assessed by MAGIC, the reliability of the PTSD module has yet to be examined.

Evidence of Validity: Evidence of the validity of the PTSD module is currently unavailable.

Contact Information: Wendy Reich, PhD, Department of Psychiatry, Washington University in St. Louis School of Medicine, 660 S. Euclid Ave., Campus Box 8134, St. Louis, MO 63110. Telephone: (314) 286-2263. E-mail: Wendyr@twins.wustl.edu.

ADMINISTERED TO CARETAKER OR OTHER ADULTS

The Preschool Age Psychiatric Assessment (PAPA; Egger & Angold, 2004; Egger, Ascher, & Angold, 1999; Egger et al., 2004)

Brief Description: The PAPA is a substantial rewrite of the CAPA for preschool-age children, which included changing DSM-IV and ICD-10 criteria to better reflect experiences of younger children; symptoms and diagnoses were included from the *Diagnostic Classification of Mental Health and Developmental Disorders of Infancy and Early Childhood, Revised Edition* (CD:0–3R; Zero to Three, 2005); relevant items were added from other preschool measures not covered by the CAPA; appropriate changes were made to the family functioning and relationships sections; and alternative diagnostic criteria for some disorders were used, among other changes. Alternate PTSD and reactive attachment disorder diagnostic criteria were based on criteria suggested by Zeanah, Boris, and Scheeringa (Boris et al., 1998; Scheeringa et al., 1995, 2001; Scheeringa & Zeanah, 1995). In the PTSD module, detailed information is gathered regarding 21 changes in child's behaviors, emotions, or relationships that might have occurred due to the event, such as new fears or anxieties, increased crying, increased aggression, regression of toileting skills or language, and changes in the interactions with others (Egger & Angold, 2004). Each symptom is rated for frequency, intensity, duration, and date of onset. If the caregiver indicates that at least one high-magnitude stressor has occurred in the child's life, and believes that experience is related to at least one symptom (new fears, separation anxiety, etc.), then the interviewer asks the questions in the PTSD section. The PAPA includes the following sections: Family Structure and Function; Play and Peer and Sibling Relationships; Daycare/School Experiences and Behaviors; and Other Food-Related Behaviors; Sleep Behaviors; Elimination Problems; Somatization; Accidents; Oppositional Defiant Disorder/Conduct Disorder; Attention-Deficit/Hyperactivity Disorder; Separation Anxiety; Anxious Affect; Worries; Rituals and Repetitions; Tics; Stereotypes; Reactive Attachment; Depression; Mania; Dysregulation; Life Events; PTSD; Disabilities; Parental Psychopathology; Marital Satisfaction; and Socio-Economic Status. Interviewers must have at least a bachelor's level degree. PAPA training requires 1–2 weeks of classroom work and 1–2 weeks of practice, including at least four practice interviews. Didactic training on the glossary and interview methods is interspersed with role playing, taped and live interviews, and feedback. Certification by a qualified PAPA trainer is required before using the PAPA in the field. Age range: 3–6 years. Respondent: caregiver. Languages available: English and Spanish.

Evidence of Reliability: Test–retest kappa for PTSD diagnosis is .73 (Egger et al., 2004).

Evidence of Validity: Evidence of validity has yet to be published.

Contact Information: Developmental Epidemiology Program, Duke University Medical Center, Attention: Juné Rogers, DUMC Box 3454, Durham, NC 27710; Telephone: (919) 687-4686, extension 273. E-mail: jrogers@psych.duhs.duke.edu.

ADMINISTERED TO CHILD

Levonn: A Cartoon-Based Structured Interview for Assessing Young Children's Distress Symptoms (Martinez & Richters, 1993; Richters, Martinez, & Valla, 1990). A version for preschool children has been devised by Shahinfar and colleagues (2000; see the VEX scale in Appendix 9.1 for contact information)

Brief Description: Levonn is a 39-item, cartoon-based, structured interview of children's distress symptoms based on an earlier cartoon-based interview of general psychiatric symptoms, Dominique (Valla, 1989). The Dominique interview was revised so that the main character, Levonn, represents an urban child. The new interview includes cartoons of symptoms associated with PTSD, 2–3 sentence scripts are included for each cartoon, and the response format was changed to three thermometers filled to varying degrees of mercury, indicating increasing levels of frequency. The thermometers are labeled *Never*, *Some of the time*, and *A lot of the time*. Before administration of the PTSD interview, children are taught how to use the thermometer response format correctly. Each cartoon is described by the interviewer, after which children circle a thermometer to indicate how often they have felt like Levonn. On one page, for example, the three thermometers take up the top one-third of the page. On the right half of the lower portion of the page are three cartoons, laid out vertically one over the other. In the top cartoon, a frowning young boy, with a white face, is shown in his pajamas walking away from a bed, somewhat slouched over, with his head slightly bent down. The middle cartoon shows the boy, now dressed for school, walking, again slouched over, head bent, and frowning, dragging a book bag along the ground. In the bottom cartoon, Levonn is again in pajamas, standing facing his bed, head bent, and frowning. In the middle of the left bottom half of the page is the following script, which the interviewer reads to the child being interviewed, "Here is Levonn feeling very sad for a whole day. He gets up in the morning feeling sad, he feels sad all day, and he still feels sad at bedtime. How many times have you felt like Levonn?" (Martinez & Richters, 1993, p. 26). The scale comprises four subscales measuring Depression, Anxiety/Recurring Thoughts, Sleep Problems, and Impulsiveness. In the revised version for preschoolers (Shahinfar et al., 2000), the symptoms assessed include sadness, lack of appetite, fear of going outside because of possible violence, intrusive traumatic memories, and having nightmares. In a study of 155, primarily (98.8%) African American children between ages 3.5 and 4.5 years, the authors carefully debriefed children after administering the revised Levonn (Shahinfar et al., 2000). They reported that very few of the children indicated either verbally or behaviorally that they had been upset by the interview. A Hebrew version, with the main character named Sharon, exists (Raviv et al., 2001; see VEX, Appendix 9.1 for contact information).

Evidence of Reliability: Test–retest reliability over a 1-week period of the total was measured with Pearson's correlation, with $r_{(22)} = .81$ among children in first and second grades (Martinez & Richters, 1993). Cronbach's alphas among 111 first and second graders in the same study were .78 for the 10-item Depression subscale, .84 for the 14-item Anxiety/Intrusive Thoughts subscale, and .71 for the 7-item Depression subscale. The number of items in the Impulsiveness subscale was not reported, nor was the subscale's alpha. The alpha was not reported for the full scale.

Evidence of Validity: Among 111 children in the first and second grades (Martinez & Richters, 1993), the total score correlated significantly with parent ratings of their children's distress, as rated by the Checklist of Child Distress Symptoms (CCDS—Richters & Martinez, 1990a; see Appendix 9.5). Correlations among the subscales ranged from .64 to .85, which justified combining them into a total score. Scores on the Levonn correlated significantly ($r_{(76)} = .32$, $p < .01$) with parent reports of their child's distress on the Parent Form of the CCDS (Richters & Martinez, 1990a; see Appendix 9.5). Although parent–child agreement was significant for boys ($r_{(38)} = .41$, $p < .01$), it was not significant for girls ($r_{(38)} = .19$, ns). However, because girls reported significantly more exposure to intrafamilial violence, the agreement was assessed between just mother and daughters within families with levels of intrafamilial violence similar to that reported in the boys' families, and this agreement was significant ($r_{(31)} = .34$, $p < .05$). Correlations between experiences of violent victimization in the community and symptoms of distress as measured by the Levonn were significant ($r_{(31)} = .28$, $p < .01$). Children's reports of witnessing violence in the community also correlated significantly with their total scores on the Levonn ($r_{(81)} = .30$, $p < .01$). Children's reports of the frequency of seeing guns or drugs also correlated significantly with total distress scores on the Levonn, regardless of where that occurred ($r_{(81)} = .30$). In a study of violent experiences among school-age (second- and fourth-grade) Israeli children (Raviv et al., 2001), the Hebrew version of Levonn correlated significantly with the Hebrew version of the VEX (see description in Appendix 9.1) regardless of whether the violence was mild or severe, and whether the experience was as a victim, a witness, or seen on TV, with correlations ranging from .24 (for mild violence on TV) to .46 (for victimization by mild violence). Small but significant correlations were found between symptoms of distress (as measured by the preschool version of the Levonn) and witnessing mild violence ($r = .29$, $p < .05$), victimization by mild violence ($r = .22$, $p = .05$), and witnessing severe violence per reports on the VEX ($r = .25$, $p < .05$; see Appendix 9.1; Shahinfar et al., 2000).

Contact Information: John E. Richters, PhD, Department of Human Development and Institute for Child Study, University of Maryland, Benjamin Building, Room 4104, College Park, MD 20742. Telephone: (301) 405-7354. E-mail: jrichter@nih.gov.

Posttraumatic Symptom Inventory for Children (PT-SIC; Eisen, 1997)

Brief Description: The PT-SIC (Eisen, 1997, cited in Stover & Berkowitz, 2005), a 30-item questionnaire that assesses PTSD symptoms based on DSM-IV criteria, includes a checklist to screen for 11 high-magnitude stressors (e.g., car crashes, sexual abuse, witnessing or being a victim of community violence). Questions are addressed in two stages. A child is first asked whether a symptom ever occurs. If he or she answers affirmatively, the child is asked to indicate the frequency of such occurrences: *A real lot—like everyday* (scored 2) or *Just sometimes* (scored 1). Age range: 4–8 years.

Evidence of Reliability: The full scale had an internal consistency alpha of .91 among 220 children ages 4–17, and a test–retest kappa for diagnosis of .87. It is unclear how many of these children were under 6 years old (reported in Stover & Berkowitz, 2005).

Evidence of Validity: The PT-SIC correlated .64 with the TSCC (Briere, 1996; see Appendix 9.5); however, the TSCC is designed for use only with children age 8 years and older (reported in Stover & Berkowitz, 2005).

Contact Information: M. L. Eisen, PhD, Department of Psychology, California State University, 5151 State University Drive, Los Angeles, CA 90032-8227. Telephone: (323) 343-5006. E-mail: meisen@calstatela.edu.

ADMINISTERED TO CARETAKER OR OTHER ADULTS

Pediatric Emotional Distress Scale (PEDS; Saylor et al., 1999)

Brief Description: Although the 21-item PEDS was designed to assess behaviors theoretically and empirically associated with trauma in children, it does not assess DSM-IV criteria for PTSD. However, it has been used successfully to assess the responses of children ages 2–7 to traumatic events (Saylor et al., 1999; Spilsbury, Drotar, Burant, Flannery, Creeden, & Friedman, 2005; Stokes, Saylor, Swenson, & Daugherty, 1995; Swenson, Saylor, Paige Powell, Stokes, Foster, & Belter, 1996). The scale's first 17 items form three subscales: Anxious/Withdrawn, Fearful, and Acting Out. The sum of these 17 items produces an overall distress score. The additional four items are questions about the child's communication relative to the event or avoidance of reminders of the event. For each item, the frequency of the behavior is rated on a 4-point scale, ranging from *Almost never* to *Very often.* Saylor and colleagues (1999) found that to maximize discrimination between traumatized and nontraumatized children, cutoff scores for the PEDS and its subscales were best adjusted according to the mother's education. Thus, although a PEDS total greater than 27.5 appeared to provide the best sensitivity/specificity trade-off, for mothers with a high school education or less, a PEDS total of 16.5 provided the best cutoff; for mothers with some college or an Associate's degree, the best cutoff was 23.5, and for mothers with a Bachelor's degree or higher, the best cutoff was 36.5. Similar cutoffs for the subscales, overall and adjusted for the mothers' education, are presented in Saylor and colleagues (1999). Overall, the use of such adjusted cutoffs allowed "78% of the cases to be correctly classified, with a false positive rate of 9.5% and a false negative rate of 12.5%" (p. 77). Administration time: 5–8 minutes.

Evidence of Reliability: Among a sample of parents of 475 children ages 2–10, Saylor and colleagues (1999) reported an internal consistency alpha of .85 for the 17-item PEDS total, and alphas of .72 for the Fearful subscale, .74 for the Anxious/Withdrawn subscale, and .78 for the Acting Out subscale. Interrater reliability correlation between mothers' and test–retest fathers' ratings was .65 for the total, .47 for the Fearful subscale, .58 for the Anxious/Withdrawn subscale, and .64 for the Acting Out subscale. Over a 6- to 8-week test–retest period, scores for the two time periods correlated .56 for the total, .55 for the Fearful subscale, .58 Anxious/Withdrawn subscale, and .61 for the Acting Out subscale. In a sample of 383 children ages 2–7 years who received services from the Children Who Witness Violence Program of Cuyahoga County, Ohio, which provides mental health services to children who have witnessed domestic violence, assault, or other violent and traumatic events, exploratory and confirmatory factor analysis suggested the PEDS may actually be better conceived of as a having a two-factor structure, with an Act Out factor and an Internalize factor (see discussion in section on validity of evidence for this measure for more detail; Spilsbury et al., 2005). Cronbach's alpha was .80 for the revised total 13-item version, .80 for the Internalize subscale, and .82 for the Act Out subscale.

Evidence of Validity: Children exposed to a Class IV hurricane 14 months earlier scored significantly higher on overall behavioral problems, anxiety, and withdrawal than did children who had no known history of exposure to natural disaster (Swenson et al., 1996). In another study (Stokes et al., 1995), children with a history of negative life events or exposure to high-magnitude stressors scored significantly higher than those with no known trauma on the total PEDS and the Acting Out, Anxious/Withdrawn, and Fearful factors. Moreover, children evaluated due to allegations of sexual abuse scored significantly higher than the other groups on the total and all subscales. Evidence of convergent and discriminant validity in Saylor and colleagues' (1999) study was indicated by significant correlations between the PEDS total (.62) and Acting Out (.86), Anxious/Withdrawn (.42), and Fearful (.32) subscale scores, with scores on the Eyberg Child Behavior Inventory (Eyberg & Ross, 1978). The Reaction Index (Frederick, 1985b) correlated with the total PEDS (.62), and the Anxious/Withdrawn (.62) and Fearful (.59) subscales, but was not significantly correlated with the Acting Out subscale. Spilsbury and colleagues (2005), in a confirmatory factor analysis on 383 children ages 2–7, found that the three-factor solution could not be satisfactorily reproduced. Therefore, the sample was split in half, and an exploratory factor analysis was conducted on half the sample. Four items failed to load on any factor and were removed from further consideration: "Acts younger than used to for age," "Has trouble going to bed/falling asleep," "Clings to adults, doesn't want to be alone," and "Refuses to sleep alone." The final solution comprised two factors, one of which replicated Saylor and colleagues' (1999) Acting Out factor, except for the addition of one item: "Cries without good reason." The second factor, labeled Internalize, combined items from the original two factors of Anxious/Withdrawn and Fearful. A confirmatory factor analysis of the modified two-factor structure on the other half of the sample showed fairly good fit. Convergent and discriminant validity of the two factors was demonstrated by showing that they correlated differently with different subscales of the Revised Behavior Problem Checklist (RBPC; Quay & Peterson, 1996): The PEDS modified Acting Out factor correlated .21 with the RBPC Anxiety/Withdrawal T-score, .73 with the Conduct Disorder T-score, and .52 with Socialized Aggression, whereas the PEDS modified Internalize factor correlated .57, .18, and .21, respectively, with these RBPC subscales, and no significant correlations were found between either the PEDS modified factor or conceptually unrelated RBPC factors. Small but significant differences were found by gender, ethnicity, and chronicity of the violence in some of the revised PEDS scores. In a subsample of 192 children, both a caregiver and a mental health specialist completed the 17-item PEDS. Correlations between the two ratings were significant, ranging from .46 to .63, indicating good interrater reliability of the measure.

Contact Information: Conway F. Saylor, PhD, Department of Psychology, The Citadel, 171 Moultrie Avenue, Charleston, SC 29409. The items of the PEDS are listed in a table in Saylor and colleagues (1999).

Posttraumatic Stress Disorder Semistructured Interview and Observational Record for Infants and Young Children (PSDSIORIYC; Scheeringa & Zeanah, 1994)

Brief Description: The PSDIORIYC, a 37-item semistructured interview for the parent or guardian of infants or young children (generally 0–3 years of age) based on the authors' suggested alternate criteria for PTSD in preschool children (Scheeringa et al., 2003), has also been incorporated in both the Research Diagnostic Criteria for Infancy and Preschool (RDC:IP; Task Force on Research Diagnostic Criteria: Infancy and Preschool, 2003) and the Diagnostic Classification of Mental Health and Developmental Disorders of Infancy and Early Childhood: Revised Edition (DC:0–3R; Zero to Three, 2005). Both the RDC:IP and DC:0–3 slightly amend the DSM-IV overall criteria for PTSD, still requiring that both A1 and A2 criteria, one symptom of reexperiencing, but only one or more symptom of avoidance or numbing, and two symptoms of overarousal be met. The interviewer first asks the parent or guardian whether the preschooler or infant has been exposed to one of seven different high-magnitude stressors—an automobile accident or plane crash, an attack by a large animal, other man-made disasters, experiencing or witnessing a natural disaster, witnessing another person being violently abused, physical or sexual abuse—or ever accused someone of physical or sexual abuse. The parent or guardian is given an opportunity to identify an eighth possible high-magnitude stressor. The date of each event described is noted, along with a brief description. For each event, parents or guardians are asked whether the event was traumatic for the preschooler or infant, and whether the child's response was apparent intense fear, helplessness, horror, or disorganized or agitated behavior. Six questions are then asked about symptoms of reexperiencing, seven about symptoms of avoidance or numbing, and five about overarousal. Questions regarding four associated symptoms are asked next: loss of acquired developmental skills, new fears, new separation anxiety, and new aggressive behaviors. The parent or guardian is then asked whether the child has been bothered by most of his or her symptoms for as long as 1 month. Finally, five questions address the child's functioning in the family, among peers, at school, with caregivers, and whether the symptoms upset the child. Possible responses to the questions assessing criteria A–D are *No*, *Possibly*, and *Yes* relative to the symptom's presence. Possible responses for the final five questions on functioning are *A lot of the time*, *Some of the time*, and *Hardly ever or none of the time*. The interview with the caretaker is conducted with the child in the room. Observing the child's behavior during the interview allows the interviewer to include the child's behavior in scoring the interview. Interviewer training required: A high degree of clinical skill is required. Languages available: English, German, Hebrew.

Evidence of Reliability: Mean interrater reliability kappa among four raters of 12 children younger than 48 months for the individual symptoms was .67 (Scheeringa & Zeanah, 2003). Kappas ranged from .81 to 1.00 for the symptom clusters. The mean kappa for PTSD diagnosis was .75.

Evidence of Validity: Scheeringa and Zeanah (2003) compared 62 traumatized children ages 20 months through 6 years with 63 healthy control children of the same age. Mean duration between the traumatic experience and assessment was 11.3 months, with a median of 7.5 months and a 2- to 52-month range. The authors judged that requiring three symptoms of avoidance was too strict a criterion for this age group, and revised this criterion to just one symptom of avoidance to diagnose PTSD. With this revision, 26% (16) of the 62 traumatized children were diagnosed with PTSD, leaving 46 traumatized children with no PTSD. The PTSD group had significantly higher rates of separation anxiety disorder (SAD) and oppositional defiant disorder (ODD) and scored higher on the CBCL Internalizing and total scales compared to the trauma/no-PTSD group. The PTSD group scored higher on 9 of 11 comorbid conditions. Within the traumatized group, regardless of PTSD diagnosis, younger children (1–3 years) exhibited more symptoms of reexperiencing than older children (4–6 years). They also manifested more symptoms of PTSD, SAD, major depressive disorder, and higher Internalizing, Externalizing, and total scores on the CBCL. These children were followed up for at least 2 years (Sheeringa et al., 2005); at the 2-year follow-up assessment, of the 16 children diagnosed with PTSD at time 1 using the PSDSIORIYC, 8(50%) were diagnosed with PTSD 2 years later with the DISC (Shaffer et al., 1988; see Appendix 9.3), whereas 8.7% of the non-PTSD group received a PTSD diagnosis at the 2-year follow-up. Age range: 3–5 years.

Contact Information: Michael Scheeringa, MD, 1440 Canal Street, TB52, New Orleans, LA 70112. Telephone: (504) 588-5402. E-mail: mscheer@tulane.edu.

PTSD Symptoms in Preschool-Age Children (PTSD-PAC; Levendosky, Huth-Bocks, Semel, & Shapiro, 2002)

Brief Description: The PTSD-PAC is an 18-item questionnaire completed by caregivers, based on the DSM-IV PTSD criteria and with additional, young-child-focused questions based on the PSDSIORYC (Scheeringa & Zeanah, 1994; see this appendix). The first 5 items assess symptoms of DSM-IV criterion B; the next five assess criterion C; and the final eight items assess criterion D. Caregivers indicate the *Presence* or *Absence* of each symptom. The items are listed in Levendosky and colleagues (2002, Table 1).

Evidence of Reliability: Internal consistency alpha was .79 for the full scale (Levendosky et al., 2002).

Evidence of Validity: The PTSD-PAC did not correlate with CBCL post hoc "PTSD" scale (Achenbach, 1991a; the CBCL post hoc "PTSD" scale was created by Wolfe, Gentile, & Wolfe, 1989), perhaps because the so-called "PTSD" scale of the CBCL may actually measure general dysphoria more than PTSD. This possibility is supported by the fact that mothers' kinds of domestic violence experiences were significantly correlated with scores on the PTSD-PAC. Total scores ranged from .38 for "mild violence" experiences to .55 for threats of violence (although they were only .39 with sexual violence). Scores on the Reexperiencing (criterion B) subscale ranged from .45 for exposure to "mild violence" to .61 for exposure to threats of violence (.50 with sexual violence). Scores on the Hyperarousal (criterion D) subscale correlated significantly with three of the four types of domestic violence experiences assessed in the study, with correlations ranging from .27 with experiences of sexual violence to .50 with threats of violence. This subscale was not significantly correlated (.20) with experiences of "severe violence," although this may have something to do with the small sample size (62 children). On the other hand, the Avoidance (criterion C) subscale did not correlate significantly with any of the four types of the mothers' domestic violence experiences.

Contact Information: Alytia A. Levendosky, PhD, Department of Psychology, Michigan State University, 107C Psychology Building, East Lansing, MI 48824. Telephone: (517) 353-6396. E-mail: levendo1@msu.edu.

Trauma Symptom Checklist for Young Children (TSCYC; Briere, 2000)

Brief Description: The TSCYC, a 90-item caretaker report, may be used for children ages 3–12. Each symptom is rated on frequency of occurrence in the last month on a 4-point scale, from *Not at all* (1) to *Very often* (4). It contains eight subscales: Posttraumatic Stress–Intrusion (PTS-I), Posttraumatic Stress–Avoidance (PTS-AV), Posttraumatic Stress–Arousal (PTS-AR), Sexual Concerns (SC), Dissociation (DIS), Anxiety (ANX), Depression (DEP), and Anger/Aggression (ANG). A total Posttraumatic Stress scale is created by summing the PTS items. Unlike the Trauma Symptom Checklist for Children (TSCC; Briere, 1996a, 1996b; see Appendix 9.5), the TSCYC is capable of offering a possible diagnosis of PTSD and includes a scale of the validity of the caretaker report response level (RL), a measure of the tendency to endorse very unusual and unrelated behaviors, and atypical response (ATR), a measure of the tendency to deny even normal, minor problematic behavior in one's child. It also contains an item that asks, "On average, how many hours do you spend in the same place (for example, at home) with him or her each week, not counting when he or she is asleep?" which is rated on a scale from 1 (*0–1 hour*) to 7 (*Over 60 hours*). Examples of items on the TSCYC are looking sad, bad dreams or nightmares, living in a fantasy world, pretending to have sex, drawing pictures about an upsetting thing that happened to him or her, and throwing things at friends or family members. The English version of the scale has recently been tested with 750 children, which allows for the calculation of standard *T*-scores to be computed based on the age and gender of the child. So children's scores can be compared to normative scores, although the manual states that the normative sample included only 149 children (3- to 4-year-olds), so using the TSCYC to diagnose PTSD with this age group is not appropriate. Languages available: English and Spanish.

Evidence of Reliability: Among a sample of 219 children ages 3–12 ($M = 7.1 \pm 2.6$; 62.8% girls; 38% European American, 27.8% Hispanic, and 25.4% African American) internal consistency alphas were .87 for the total score, and .82 for the PTS-I, .85 for the PTS-AV, .93 for the PTS-AR, .93 for the PTS-Total, .81 for the SC, .86 for the ANX, .84 for the DEP, .91 for the DIS, and .91 for the ANG subscales (Briere, 2000; Briere et al., 2001). For the validity scales, alpha was .73 for the RL but only .36 for the ATR.

Evidence of Validity: Gilbert (2004, as cited in Stover & Berkowitz, 2005) found that the subscales had significant correlations, ranging from .55 to .82 with several other parent reports. The TSCYC ANX and DEP subscales correlated most strongly with the CBCL (Achenbach, 1991a) Anxiety–Depression subscale. The TSCYC ANG subscale correlated most strongly with the CBCL Aggression subscale. The TSCYC SC scale correlated most strongly with Friedrich's (1998) Child Sexual Behavior Inventory (CSBI). The TSCYC DIS scale was most strongly correlated with the Child Dissociation Checklist (CDC; Putnam, Helmers, & Trickett, 1993). Finkelhor and colleagues (2005) found that among 1,026 parents of young children ages 2–9 years, assessed in a national survey, most of the single items and all of the subscale totals of their measure of victimization in young children, the JVQ-CPR (see Appendix 9.1), correlated significantly with the TSCYC ANX, DEP, and ANG subscales. In a sample of 219 children being seen by therapists for abuse (Briere, 2000; Briere et al., 2001), hierarchical multiple regression analyses, which adjusted for children's age, gender, and ethnicity, indicated that childhood sexual abuse was associated with ratings of PTS-I, PTS-AV, PTS-Total, and SC on the TSCYC. Childhood physical abuse was related to PTS-I, PTS-AR, PTS-Total, and DIS. Witnessing domestic violence was related to PTS-I, PTS-AV, PTS-AR, PTS-Total, and negatively with SC.

Contact Information: John Briere, PhD, Department of Psychiatry and the Behavioral Sciences, Keck School of Medicine, University of Southern California, IRD Building, 2020 Zonal Avenue, Los Angeles, CA 90033. E-mail: info@johnbriere.com.

APPENDIX 9.5. PTSD-Specific Measures for Children Ages 7–18

ADMINISTERED TO CHILD

Checklist of Children's Distress Symptoms, Child Form (CCDS; Martinez & Richters, 1993; Richters & Martinez, 1990a)

Brief Description: The CCDS is a 28-item, self-report scale that asks questions associated with traumatic responses to high-magnitude stressors. Questions examine anxiety, memory problems, sleeping problems, self-esteem, school performance, and feelings of depression, isolation, or hopelessness. Responses are rated on a 1- to 4-point scale, ranging from *Never* (1) to *A lot of the time* (4). The CCDS comprises two subscales measuring Depression and Anxiety, but the two subscales' high correlation (.64) justifies combining them for the total score. Age range: 10 years and older.

Evidence of Reliability: Among 54 fifth and sixth graders, Cronbach's alphas for the Depression subscales and Anxiety were .71 and .72, respectively.

Evidence of Validity: Parents reported significantly lower levels of child distress than was reported by their children on both the Depression and Anxiety subscales, as well as on many of the individual items (Martinez & Richters, 1993). Agreement between parents and their daughters was nonsignificant ($r_{(17)} = .06$), whereas agreement between parents and their sons was significant, moderately high, and negative ($r_{(18)} = -.56$), which the authors note was not attributable to outliers (p. 30). They suggest that the negative correlation may be attributable to a tendency of the boys to deny their symptoms, at least in part. At the same time, children's reports of exposure to stressors were significantly correlated with their CCDS scores, whether they were themselves victims of community violence ($r_{(37)}$ = .37) or witnessed it ($r_{(37)}$ = .39), or witnessed violence in the home ($r_{(37)}$ = .33).

Contact Information: John E. Richters, PhD, Department of Human Development and Institute for Child Study, University of Maryland, Benjamin Building, Room 4104, College Park, MD 20742. Telephone: (301) 405-7354. E-mail: jrichter@nih.gov.

Child and Adolescent Trauma Survey (CATS—March, Amaya-Jackson, Terry, et al., 1997; March et al., 1998)

Brief Description: This 12-item, paper-and-pencil self-report measure is modeled on the CPTS-RI (see below, this appendix) and the Multidimensional Anxiety Scale for Children (MASC; March, Parker, Sullivan, Stallings, & Conners, 1997). It assesses DSM-IV PTSD symptomatology (March, Amaya-Jackson, Terry, et al., 1997; March et al., 1998). This measure has also been referred to as the Kiddie Posttraumatic Symptomatology Scale (March, 1999) and the Self-Reported Posttraumatic Symptomatology scale (SRPTS; March, Amaya-Jackson, Terry, et al., 1997). The CATS is currently undergoing further psychometric testing, and its final form is not yet determined. The CATS first assesses exposure to high-magnitude stressors (13 were included in the original version), which includes witnessing stressful events. Children and adolescent respondents are asked how often they experienced each symptom during the last month, using a 4-point Likert scale—*Never, Rarely, Sometimes,* or *Often.* Each DSM-IV PTSD criterion variable is represented by at least two questions (March, Amaya-Jackson, Terry, et al., 1997). A total score of 27 or above on the CATS is considered a clinically significant level of PTSD (Suliman, Kaminer, Seedat, & Stein, 2005), but PTSD diagnosis is not possible with the CATS (March, Amaya-Jackson, Terry, et al., 1997).

Evidence of Reliability: The CATS reportedly has excellent internal and test–retest reliability, but the actual values have not been published (March et al., 1998). However, Cronbach's alphas among 176 children and adolescents ages 8–17 (*M* = 11.8 years) within 1 month of a recent injury or intensive care unit admission (thus, not yet eligible for a PTSD diagnosis) were .84 at first administration, and then .82 among 146 of the young patients contacted 3 months later (Kassam-Adams, 2006).

Evidence of Validity: Among a sample of 1,327 children and adolescents in the fourth through ninth grades in Hamlet, North Carolina, where an industrial fire at a local chicken-processing plant caused loss of life among family, friends, and/or neighbors, factor analysis supported a three-factor solution (*n* = 1,327), with factors associated with symptoms of reexperiencing, avoidance, and hyperarousal (March, Amaya-Jackson, Terry, et al., 1997). An expected fourth factor, numbing, was highly correlated with the reexperiencing factor (.94), so the two factors were merged. Avoidance and reexperiencing were strongly correlated (*r* = .64), and hyperarousal was weakly correlated with reexperiencing/avoidance (.105). Thus, three subscales emerged from the factor analysis. The items were submitted to an item response theory (IRT)–model analysis, which allowed each item to be weighted optimally to reflect the domain of interest. In the "IRT analyses, information regarding reexperiencing/avoidance clustered at the high or 'symptomatic' end of the distribution of the latent PTS variable. In contrast, hyperarousal followed a bimodal distribution . . . [with] most of the 'information' in the hyperarousal questions [coming] from those with and without hyperarousal (an inverted U-shaped curve). If present, hyperarousal suggested PTS; if absent, it predicted no PTS as marked by reexperiencing/avoidance, but the effect was weak enough to be a distinction without a difference" (p. 1082). The IRT analysis suggested a *T*-score ≥ 65 on the reexperiencing factor indicative of PTS. Using this analysis, 9.7% of the children met criteria for PTSD, while 11.9% met PTSD DSM-III-R criteria. Agreement between the IRT and DSM-III-R criteria was moderate (kappa = .56), and the difference between the two methods was significant (McNemar's chi-square [1, 1015] = 5.56, *p* < .018). Increasing exposure to victims of the fire strongly predicted increased risk for posttraumatic stress symptomatology as assessed by the CATS. When an IRT-derived *T*-score > 65 was used to classify children as positive for posttraumatic stress, 3.0% of the children not exposed to the fire, 10.5% of the visually exposed, 15.8% of those with a friend or relative involved, and 30.4% with both visual and friend/relative exposure rose above the cutoff score ($F_{(3,1019)}$ = 35.15, *p* < .001; March, Amaya-Jackson, Terry, et al., 1997). The CATS has been demonstrated to be responsive to change (in the total score and in each subscale) over time due to an effective cognitive-behavioral treatment intervention (March et al., 1998). The CATS correlated significantly (.77) with the ASC-Kids (Kassam-Adams, 2006; see Appendix 9.7), a measure of ASD.

Contact Information: John March, PhD, Department of Psychiatry, DUMC Box 3527, Durham, NC 27710. Telephone: (919) 416-2400. E-mail: jsmarch@acpub.duke.edu.

Childhood PTSD Interview—Child Form (Fletcher, 1996b, 1996c)

Brief Description: The Childhood PTSD Interview—Child Form is a semistructured interview of the child that allows the interviewer to assess DSM-III-R (APA, 1987) and DSM-IV criteria and to make a diagnosis. It contains items that allow the interviewer to rate the child's willingness to describe the stressor(s), to indicate whether there is evidence that the events did not occur or that the child misperceived or described details inaccurately, and to rate how well the child's description of the event(s) matches that of the caregiver. Fifty-seven questions assess DSM-III-R PTSD criteria A–D. Four questions assess criterion A. Four questions assess the first symptom of criterion B (B1), three assess B2, four assess B3 (two of which ask for clarification of endorsed questions), and three assess B4. Five questions assess C1; three assess C2; one question assesses C3, with a follow-up question, if the first is answered in the negative (both require elaboration for positive responses); three assess C4 (with elaboration required for positive responses); three assess C5, two questions and a rater question regarding possible flat affect of the child assess C6; and 6 questions assess C7 (because C7 concerns a sense of foreshortened future, and few studies support the presence of this symptom in children, the author believes these six questions can be skipped). Two questions, with required elaborations for positive responses, assess D1; two questions, one of which is a follow-up question to establish changed behavior since ex-

467

posure to the stressor assess D2; four questions assess D3; four questions assess D4; and two questions assess D5. Two questions assess complaint of physiological reactions, which is D6 according to DSM-III-R, and B5 according to DSM-IV. An optional, additional 28 questions assess associated symptoms. Interviewers may choose to ask some, all, or none of these questions. Five questions assess symptoms of anxiety (three require elaboration for positive responses, and one asks the rater to indicate whether breathing problems may be due to asthma). Three questions assess symptoms of depression. Two questions, with required elaboration for positive responses, assess indications of whether the child perceives certain prestressor events as omens. Two questions, with required elaboration for positive responses, assess symptoms of survivor guilt. Two questions, with required elaboration for positive responses, assess symptoms of guilt or self-blame. The interviewer is asked to indicate to what extent the child actually might be considered to have some responsibility for events. Two questions, with required elaboration for positive responses, assess indications of fantasy denial. Three questions, two with required elaboration for positive responses, assess possible self-destructive or suicidal thoughts and behaviors. Four questions assess symptoms of dissociation. Three questions assess antisocial behavior. Two assess risk-taking behavior, and two assess changed eating habits. Age range: 7 or 8+, depending on the child's cognitive abilities. Items are answered *Yes* or *No*. *Don't know*s are allowed on many questions and are scored as *No*.

Evidence of Reliability: Cronbach's alpha = .91 for the full PTSD section of the interview, with alphas = .52 for the four questions of criterion A, .80 for criterion B, .76 for criterion C, and .78 for criterion D (Fletcher, 1996b).

Evidence of Validity: The interview correlated significantly with other measures of childhood PTSD: .87 with the When Bad Things Happen scale (see this appendix), .69 with the Childhood PTSD Interview—Parent Form (see this appendix), .60 with the Parent Report of the Child's Reaction to Stress (see this appendix), and .52 with an ad hoc CBCL PTSD scale. It correlated significantly (.40) with the total number of lifetime stressors the parent indicated the child had experienced, .53 with the parent's ratings of the child's stressful reactions to those events, and .77 with an assessment of the potentially traumatizing dimensions of the immediate stressor(s) for which the child's reactions were being assessed, according to the DOSE scale (see Appendix 9.2). The interview also correlated significantly with the Internalizing score of the CBCL (.40) but not the Externalizing score (.31), and it correlated significantly with the following CBCL subscales: Anxiety (.48), Thought Problems (which include obsessing on certain thoughts, problems concentrating, repetition of certain acts, and staring blankly; r = .60), Somatic Complaints (.39), Attention Problems (.39), and Social Problems (.49) (Fletcher, 1996b). The fact that the interview's correlations with other PTSD measures are all higher than its correlations with measures of other problems indicates its discriminant validity. Scores differentiated between traumatized and nontraumatized children (Fletcher, 1996b). Sensitivity in identifying probable cases of traumatized children, as assessed by the DOSE was 75%, and specificity was 90% (Fletcher, 1996b).

Contact Information: Kenneth E. Fletcher, PhD, Department of Psychiatry, University of Massachusetts Medical School, 55 Lake Avenue North, Worcester, MA 01655. Telephone: (508) 856-8630. E-mail: kenneth.fletcher@ umassmed.edu.

Child Posttraumatic Stress Reaction Index and Additional Questions (CPTS-RI—Frederick, Pynoos, & Nader, 1992; also known as the PTSD—Reaction Index and the Child PTSD—Reaction Index)

Brief Description: The CPTS-RI has been administered in several different forms. However, the primary version is a 20-item scale that assess some, but not all, of the DSM-IV PTSD symptoms from each of the three core criteria B–D and two associated features (guilt and regression). 11 Additional Questions have been added (Nader, 1999). Response format is 5-point, Likert-like frequency ratings for each symptom, from *None* (0) to *Most of the time* (4). DSM diagnosis of PTSD is not possible directly, although several studies have attempted to divide the symptoms into criteria B–D and dichotomize the 5-point response categories to provide provisional information on possible diagnostic caseness. Designed as a semistructured interview, the CPTS-RI has been used as a paper-and-pencil, self-report measure as well. The authors recommend using the three following thresholds: A total score of 12–24 indicates a mild level of PTS reaction; 25–39 indicates a moderate level; 40–59, a severe level; and 60+, a very severe level. A revised version has been created, the UCLA PTSD Index for DSM-IV (Pynoos et al., 1998; see this appendix). Another revision is being undertaken by Nader and Fletcher. Age range: 7–17 years. Languages available: English, Canadian French, Croatian, Kuwaiti Arabic, Norwegian, Vietnamese. Administration time: 20–45 minutes to administer and score (Ohan et al., 2002).

Evidence of Reliability: Pynoos and colleagues (1987) reported Cronbach's alphas for three subscales of Reexperiencing/Numbing, Fear/Anxiety, and Concentration/Sleep that ranged from .69 to .80. Cronbach's alphas for the total scale = .78 (Nader et al., 1993), .83 (Lonigan et al., 1991), and .89 (Vernberg, La Greca, Silverman, & Prinstein, 1996), respectively. Interrater reliability has been measured at a kappa of .89 (Nader, Pynoos, Fairbanks, & Frederick, 1990). Test–retest reliability over a 1-week period was .93 (Nader et al., 1990).

Evidence of Validity: The CPTS-RI correlated significantly (.51) with the Clinician-Administered PTSD Scale for Children and Adolescents (CAPS-CA; Carrion, Weems, Ray, & Reiss, 2002; see this appendix), .72 with the UCLA PTSD Index for DSM-IV (Pynoos et al., 1998; see this appendix), .84 with the When Bad Things Happen Scale (Fletcher, 1996g) and .80 with the Child PTSD Symptom Scale (CPSS; Foa et al., 2001; see this appendix). Factor analysis revealed three factors: Reexperiencing/Numbing, Fear/Anxiety, and Concentration/Sleep Problems (Pynoos et al., 1987). Level of exposure to or dosage of high-magnitude stressors has been repeatedly demonstrated to be correlated significantly with scores on the CPTS-RI (Nader et al., 1993; Rossman et al., 1997; Thabet & Vostanis, 1999). Levels of exposure to war-related experiences among children in Kuwait (Nader et al., 1993), as measured by the EQ (Nader, 1993, 1999; see Appendix 9.2) were correlated .38 with the total CPTSD-RI, .29 with the Reexperiencing subscale, .31 with the Avoidance subscale, and .36 with the Overarousal subscale.

Contact Information: Kathleen Nader, MSW. Fax: (512) 219-0486. E-mail: measures@twosuns.org. Robert Pynoos, MD, Trauma Psychiatry Service, University of California at Los Angeles, 300 UCLA Medical Plaza, Los Angeles, CA 90024. E-mail: rpynoos@npih.medsch.ucla.edu.

Child PTSD Symptom Scale (CPSS; Foa, Johnson, Feeny, & Treadwell, 2001)

Brief Description: The CPSS is based on the Posttraumatic Diagnostic Scale (Foa et al., 1997), a measure of PTSD in adults. The language of the adult scale was modified to be more appropriate for children. The 26-item scale includes 2 items assessing criterion A, 17 items assessing criteria B–D, and 7 items assessing criterion F, disruption of functioning. Children and adolescents are asked to indicate how often the 17 PTSD symptoms bothered them in the past month, with responses of *Not at all* (0), *Once a week or less* (1), *2 to 4 times a week* (2), and *5 or more times a week* (3). Children indicate whether their symptoms cause them difficulty in each of the following seven areas of functioning: prayers, chores and duties, relationships with friends, fun and hobbies, schoolwork, relationships with family, and general happiness. The seven questions about daily functioning are scored as either *Absent* (0) or *Present* (1). Age range: 8–18 years. Administration time: 15 minutes.

Evidence of Reliability: Psychometrics were assessed in a sample of 75 school-age children and adolescents ages 8–15 years (*M* = 11.8 years; 49% girls, 89% European American, in grades 3 through 8) 25 months after the 1994 Northridge, California, earthquake. Children were asked about their reactions to that event (Foa et al., 1997). All children lived within 3 miles of the epicenter of the earthquake and were asleep when it struck at 4:31 in the morning. Their homes sustained moderate to severe earthquake damage, the region was without water or electricity for 3 or more days, 30% of the children were displaced from their homes, and their school was condemned for more than 8 months. The scale and the other measures used in the study were read aloud to groups of 6–8 children. Cronbach's alphas were .89 for the total of the 17 PTSD criterion B–D items, .80 for reexperiencing, .73 for avoidance, and .70 for overarousal. The CPSS was readministered to 65 of the children and adolescents 1–2 weeks after the first administration. The test–retest reliability of PTSD symptom diagnosis according to the CPSS was moderate, with a kappa of .55. Percentage of agreement between the two time points was 84%. It is unclear what kind of reliability coefficients were used to report the test–retest reliability of the PTSD symptom severity scores, but they appear to have been Pearson correlations, with coefficients of .84 for the total score, .85 for reexperiencing, .63 for avoidance, and .76 for overarousal. The internal consistency alpha for the seven functional impairment items was .35, but when one item that was not related to the other items, "general happiness with life," was removed, the alpha for the remaining six items was .89. The test–retest coefficient for the total functional impairment score was .70. It is unclear whether this included all seven items or only the six that contributed to the internal consistency of this measure.

Evidence of Validity: The CPSS correlated .80 with the CPTSD-RI, demonstrating good convergent validity (Foa et al., 1997). When scored according to DSM-IV PTSD criteria, 24% of the children reported scores consistent with a PTSD diagnosis. Setting a cutoff score of 11 or higher on the CPSS as an indication of extreme distress yielded 95% sensitivity and 96% specificity when compared to the CPTSD-RI high-distress category. Of the children identified as having high PTSD scores on the CPTSD-RI, 70% met criteria for a PTSD diagnosis per the CPSS, and 17% of the children scoring low on the CPTSD-RI met PTSD criteria per the CPSS. The CPSS correlated .58 with the Depression Self-Rating Scale for Children (Birleson, 1981) and .48 with the MASC (March et al., 1997), demonstrating discriminant validity, because these correlations are substantially smaller than that with the CPTSD-RI. Functional impairment scores correlated .42 with the total of 17 PTSD items, .37 with reexperiencing, .39 with avoidance, and .36 with overarousal. Those children who met DSM-IV PTSD criteria per the CPSS also reported significantly more functional impairment than those who did not. Of those who met DSM-IV PTSD criteria per the CPSS, 70% endorsed at least one functional impairment item, whereas only 14% of those who did not meet PTSD criteria endorsed at least one functional impairment item.

Contact Information: Edna Foa, PhD, Center for the Treatment and Study of Anxiety, Department of Psychiatry, University of Pennsylvania School of Medicine, 3535 Market Street, Sixth Floor, Philadelphia, PA 19104-3309. Telephone: (215) 746-3327. E-mail: foa@mail.med.upenn.edu.

Children's Revised Impact of Event Scale (13 items) (CRIES-13; Children and War Foundation, 1998)

Brief Description: The CRIES-13 is based on one of the first adult measures of PTSD, the Impact of Event Scale (IES; Horowitz et al., 1979), which comprises 13 items that assess symptoms of reexperiencing and avoidance or withdrawal (DSM-IV criteria B and C). Although it was not designed to be used with children, it has been fairly successful in several studies of traumatized children age 8 and older. However, two large studies (the Yule [1992, 1997; Yule, Ten Bruggencate, & Joseph, 1994] study of 334 adolescent survivors of the Jupiter disaster and the Dyregrov, Kuterovac, & Barath [1996] study of traumatized children in Croatia) found that children misinterpreted several of the questions. Two separate factor analyses of children's responses to the IES (Dyregrov et al., 1996; Yule et al., 1994) revealed identical factor structures for the measure. This led to the creation of a shortened, 8-item version, the IES-8, for children. Weiss and Marmar (1997) added items to the IES reflecting symptoms of overarousal (criterion D), which were not represented in the original IES. So five additional items assessing symptoms of overarousal were created and added to the IES-8 to create the current version of the CRIES-13, which comprises four items measuring reexperiencing, four measuring avoidance, and five measuring overarousal. Respondents rate the frequency with which they experienced each of the 13 items during the past 7 days, using a 4-point Likert-like scale: *Not at all* (0), *Rarely* (1), *Sometimes* (3), or *Often* (5). Note that scoring for the last two response categories increases 2 points over the previous response category. The authors note that few studies have used the 13-item version to date; therefore, they recommend that screening be based on the 8-item version, with a score of 17 or greater indicating possible PTSD. Available languages: Arabic, Bosnian, Chinese, Dari, Dutch (Flemish and Dutch Netherlands, and a version for very young children for parents to complete), English, Finnish, German, Norwegian, Pashto, Swedish, and Tamil.

Evidence of Reliability: Psychometric data for the 8-item version reported in Yule (1997) indicated that the total score on the 8-item version correlated .95 with the original 15-item version. The CRIES-13 was used by Smith, Perrin, Dyregrov, and Yule (2003) to assess traumatic reactions of 2,976 children ages 9–14 years who had experienced war in Mostar, Bosnia. Cronbach's alphas were .70 for the Intrusion subscale, .73 for the Avoidance subscale, .60 for the Overarousal subscale, and .80 for the total.

Evidence of Validity: Yule (1997) reported that the 15-item and the 8-item versions of the IES correlated significantly with a symptom count of DSM-IV PTSD symptoms in adolescents following an acute trauma (15-item = .76, 8-item = .70). Factor analysis of the CRIES-13 (Smith et al., 2003) revealed a three-factor solution corresponding to the three hypothesized subscales.

Contact Information: The measure is available free online at *www.childrenandwar.org.*

Children's Impact of Traumatic Event Scale–II (CITES-II; Wolfe et al., 1991)

Brief Description: The CITES-II is a 78-item measure, 24 items of which assess DSM-IV PTSD symptoms. The remaining 54 items assess other symptoms, particularly those associated with interpersonal violence or sexual abuse. Questions assessing symptoms associated with DSM-IV PTSD criteria B and C are based on the Impact of Event Scale (IES; Horowitz et al., 1979); questions assessing hyperarousal are included. The remaining 54 items are from the original version of the measure, the CITES (Wolfe, Wolfe, Gentile, & Larose, 1986). Its 11 subscales are divided into four dimensions: PTSD (Intrusive Thoughts, Avoidance, Hyperarousal, and Sexual Anxiety), Abuse Attributions (Self-Blame/Guilt, Empowerment, Distrust, and Dangerous World), Eroticism, and Social Relations (Negative Reactions to Others, Social Support). Originally designed to assess reactions to childhood sexual abuse, the CITES-II can now be used with youth exposed to any kind of potentially traumatic event. Because it was originally used with abused children, the CITES-II assesses many of the symptoms associated with complex PTSD. Many of the items refer to sexual abuse. It can be scored for a DSM-IV diagnosis or as a continuous measure. The measure continues to evolve. Norms are available for adolescent girls, and research is planned to gather norms for adolescent boys. Psychometric analyses suggested that the Personal Vulnerability scale be replaced by a Distrust scale, and the Hyperarousal scale items are being changed, as well. Age range: 8–16 years. Recommended for use as a semistructured interview, the CITES-II can be used as a paper-and-pencil self-report with children with good reading skills. The 3-point scale response categories are *Not true, Somewhat true,* or *Very true.*

Evidence of Reliability: Cronbach's alphas are .89 for the full scale, .89 for PTSD, .78 for Abuse Attributions, .57 for Eroticism, and .87 for Social Relations (Wolfe et al., 1991). Alphas greater than.70 were found for the Reexperiencing, Hyperarousal, Sexual Anxiety, Negative Reactions, and Self-Blame/Guilt scales, and alphas less than .60, for the Dangerous World and Personal Vulnerability scales in a sample of 80 sexual abuse survivors ages 8–17 years (Crouch, Smith, Ezzell, & Saunders, 1999). In another study of 158 sexual abuse survivors ages 7–12 (Chaffin & Shultz, 2001), average alpha was .69 for the scales, whereas alphas for subscales were as follows: .79 for Intrusive Thoughts, .56 for Avoidance, .67 for Hyperarousal, .79 for Negative Reactions by Others, .73 for Self-Blame/Guilt, .67 for Empowerment, .66 for Personal Vulnerability, .73 for Social Support, .72 for Sexual Anxiety, .68 for Eroticism, and .57 for Dangerous World.

Evidence of Validity: Significant, though low, correlations were found between the ad hoc CBCL PTSD scale and the scales of the CITES-II: .28 with Intrusive Thoughts scale, .17 with Avoidance, .28 with Hyperarousal, .17 with Sexual Anxiety, .17 with Dangerous World, .18 with Negative Reactions, .24 with Personal Vulnerability, and .22 with Self-Blame/Guilt (Wolfe & Birt, 2002b). The PTSD scale correlated significantly (.72) with the Trauma Symptom Checklist for Children (TSCC; see below, this appendix) PTS scale among 80 survivors of sexual abuse, ages 8–17 years, whereas the Sexual Anxiety score correlated .65 with the Sexual Distress scale, .49 with the Sexual Concerns scale, .50 with the PTS scale, .62 with the Depression scale, and .38 with the Dissociation scale (Crouch et al., 1999). In a different study of the psychometrics of the measure (Chaffin & Schultz, 2001), no aspects of the abuse for which children were being seen, as measured by the Abuse Dimensions Inventory (ADI; Chaffin, Wherry, Newlin, Crutchfield, & Dykman, 1997), predicted any of the CITES-II subscales, though the ADI did correlate significantly with the DICA-R (Kaplan & Reich, 1991; see Appendix 9.3) PTSD scale. CITES-II scores on the Intrusive Thoughts subscale were significantly associated with the child's (eta = .50) but not the parent's DICA-R PTSD reexperiencing symptoms. The Avoidance subscale was associated with the child's (eta = .38) but not the parent's DICA-R avoidance symptoms. The Hyperarousal subscale was associated with the child's (eta = .45) but not the parent's DICA-R hyperarousal symptoms. The Sexual Anxiety subscale was associated with the child's (eta = .25) but not the parent's DICA-R Total Anxiety score, and it was associated with neither parent report on the CBCL Anxiety and Depression scale nor on the Teacher's Report Form Anxiety and Depression scale. Correlations between the CITES-II Personal Vulnerability and Dangerous World scales were small but significant, with similar alternate measures. The CITES-II Social Support scale did not correlate with any child or parent alternate report of social support. The Negative Reactions by Others subscale was significantly correlated with an alternate parent report of similar behaviors (*r* = .18), and the Eroticism subscale was significantly associated with the parent CBCL report of the child's Sexual Problems (.22). The CITES-II was found to be responsive to pre- to postintervention change (Chaffin & Shultz, 2001), although significant changes over time were found only for the Intrusive Thoughts, Avoidance, Hyperarousal, Self-Blame/Guilt, and Eroticism subscales.

Contact Information: Vicky Veitch Wolfe, PhD, Child and Adolescent Centre, London Health Sciences Centre, 346 South Street, London, Ontario N6A 4G5. Telephone: (519) 685-8500. E-mail: vicky.wolfe@lhsc.on.ca.

Children's PTSD Inventory (CPTSDI; Saigh, 1998a, 1998b)

Brief Description: The CPTSDI is a 47-question interview designed to provide a DSM-IV diagnosis of childhood PTSD. The child is first read a list of sample traumatic events, then is asked four questions intended to examine exposure to high-magnitude stressors, and four questions to assess possible traumatic reactivity to the exposure, per PTSD criterion A in DSM-IV. If this criterion is not met, the interview terminates. Eleven questions examine the presence or absence of symptoms of intrusion (criterion B in DSM-IV). Sixteen questions address criterion C, avoidance and numbing symptoms. Seven questions address criterion C, symptoms of overarousal. Five questions assess duration of symptoms (criterion E) and significant impairment in functioning (criterion F). Each item is scored as *Present* or *Absent*. Age range: 7–18 years. Training: May be administered by an individual with a bachelor's degree following approximately 2 hours of professionally supervised analogue training with corrective feedback (Saigh et al., 2000). Time: For youth with trauma history, the CPTSDI requires 15–20 minutes; for youths with no trauma history, less than 5 minutes (Saigh et al., 2000).

Evidence of Reliability: In a sample of 51 girls and 53 boys ages 7–18 ($M = 13.8$), with 30% in elementary school, 25% in junior high school, and 46% in high school, 66% Hispanic, 10% European American, 17% African American, and 8% Asian, Cronbach's alphas were .95 for overall diagnosis, .53 for the Situational Reactivity (criterion A) subscale, .89 for the Reexperiencing subscale, .89 for Avoidance and Numbing subscale, .80 for the Overarousal subscale, and .69 for the Significant Impairment subscale (criterion F; Saigh et al., 2000). All children were diagnosed by two examiners to assess interrater reliability. Agreement was 98.1% on overall diagnosis (kappa = .96). Kappas were 1.00 for judgments of meeting the criterion for the Exposure subscale, .66 for Reactivity, .84 for Reexperiencing, .93 for Avoidance/Numbing, and .95 for Significant Impairment. Based on independent administrations (twice for each child), comparisons of the total symptoms endorsed by the two examiners resulted in an ICC of .98 for the total scale, .89 for Exposure, .88 for Reactivity, .95 for Reexperiencing, .96 for Avoidance/Numbing, .96 for Overarousal, and .94 for Significant Impairment. Forty-two children were readministered the scale 2 weeks apart to assess test–retest reliability. Agreement on the total scale was 97.6%. Kappas for overall diagnosis were .91, 1.0 for both Exposure and Situational Reactivity, .81 for Reexperiencing, .86 for Avoidance/Numbing, .78 for Overarousal, and .66 for Significant Impairment. ICCs for the number of symptoms endorsed both times were .88 overall, .94 for Exposure, .93 for Reactivity, .87 for Reexperiencing, .93 for Avoidance/Numbing, .74 for Overarousal, and .66 for Significant Impairment.

Evidence of Validity: Content validity was shown by high levels of correspondence with DSM-IV diagnostic criteria by three child PTSD experts (Saigh et al., 2000). In a sample of 56–62 youth exposed to high-magnitude stressors (Yasik et al., 2001), CPTSDI scores correlated .92 with the number of PTSD items endorsed on the DICA-R (Reich, Leacok, & Shanfeld, 1994) and .91 with the number of items endorsed on the PTSD module of the Structured Clinical Interview for the DSM-IV (SCID; First, Gibbon, Williams, & Spitzer, 1996). The correlations between the CPTSDI and the DICA-R and SCID PTSD module and subscales was .85 and .87 (respectively) for Reexperiencing, .80 and .87 for Avoidance/Numbing, and .84 and .81 for Overarousal. The CPTSDI correlated .70 with the Revised Children's Manifest Anxiety Scale (RCMAS; Reynolds & Richmond, 1978) but not with the Lie Scale of the RCMAS (.08), providing evidence of discriminant validity. It also correlated .59 with the Children's Depression Inventory (CDI; Kovacs, 1992). It correlated significantly (.55) with the CBCL (Achenbach & Edelbrock, 1983) Internalizing subscale but not with the Externalizing subscale (.21), which, the authors contend, provides evidence of discriminant validity. PTSD diagnosis with the CPTSDI has a sensitivity of .87 with clinician-derived diagnosis, 1.00 with DICA-R diagnosis, and .93 with the SCID diagnosis. It has a specificity of .99 with clinician-derived diagnosis, .92 with the DICA-R diagnosis, and .95 with the SCID diagnosis.

Contact Information: Harcourt Assessment, Inc., 19500 Bulverde Road, San Antonio, TX 78259. Telephone: (800) 211-8378. Website: *harcourtassessment.com*.

Children's Stress Symptom Scale (CSSS; Sharrer, & Ryan-Wenger, 2002)

Brief Description: The CSSS assesses 24 cognitive–emotional and physiological stress symptoms in children 7–12 years of age. Items were generated by children, based on Lazarus's theory that individual appraisal is the most relevant perspective (Sharrer & Ryan-Wenger, 2002). Occurrence of items are rated as *Yes* (1) or *No* (0). Frequency of occurrence of endorsed items is rated as follows: *Once in a while* (0), *A lot* (1), and *Most of the time* (2), for a total possible score of 0 to 48. An impact scale, which assesses "how bad this feeling is for you," is scored as follows: *Not bad* (0), *Pretty bad* (1), and *Terrible* (2), for a total possible score of 0 to 48 (Sharrer & Ryan-Wenger, 2002).

Evidence of Reliability: Based on the data from a pilot study of 14 inner-city children, Cronbach alphas were .79 for the Occurrence scale, .92 for the Frequency scale, and .91 for the Impact scale (Sharrer & Ryan-Wenger, 2002). Cronbach alphas for another sample of 63 children (32% girls) between ages 7 and 14 years ($M = 9$) were .99 for the Occurrence scale, .99 for the Frequency scale, and .85 for the Impact scale (Skybo, 2005).

Evidence of Validity: The total CSSS score was not significantly correlated (.22) with the total Impact score of the KID-SAVE (Hastings & Kelley, 1997a; Flowers et al., 2000; see Appendix 9.1) or with the total KID-SAVE Frequency score (.15). However, it was significantly correlated (.27) with the total number of violent encounters reported. On the other hand, although the total Impact score of the CSSS was not significantly correlated with the total Frequency score of the KID-SAVE (.25), it was significantly correlated with both the total Impact score of the KID-SAVE (.39) and the total number of violent encounters reported (.29). Similarly, although the total Frequency score of the CSSS was not significantly correlated with the total Frequency score of the KID-SAVE (.27), it also was significantly correlated with both the Impact score of the KID-SAVE (.29) and the total number of violent encounters (.34).

Contact Information: Vicki W. Sharrer, MS, RN, CPNP, Department of Nursing, Ohio University, 1425 Newark Road, Zanesville, OH. Telephone: (740) 588-1514. E-mail: sharrer@ohio.edu. Nancy A. Ryan-Wenger, PhD, RN, CPNP, Ohio State University College of Nursing, 1585 Neil Avenue, Columbus, OH 43210. Telephone: (614) 292-4078. E-mail: ryan-wengen10@osu.edu.

Child Report of Post-Traumatic Symptoms (CROPS—Greenwald, 1997; Greenwald & Rubin, 1999)

Brief Description: The CROPS is a 26-item child interview that includes DSM-IV symptoms of PTSD and additional symptoms. Items are based on DSM-IV (APA, 1994) criteria for PTSD and Fletcher's (1996a, 2003) meta-analysis of the empirical literature on children's responses to high-magnitude stressors. It can be used with or without an identified stressor. Scores are continuous rather than keyed to diagnostic categories. The child rates how true each statement is on a 3-point scale: *None*, *Some*, and *Lots*. Age range: 5–17 years. Languages available: English, Spanish, Bosnian, Dutch, German, Italian, Persian.

Evidence of Reliability: Cronbach's alpha was .89 in a community sample of 206 children, grades 3–8 (Greenwald & Rubin, 1999). Preliminary results in a study of incarcerated youth (*n* = 300; Greenwald, Satin, Azubuike, Borgen, & Rubin, 2001) indicated an alpha of .92, and a test–retest reliability correlation for a 6-month interval was .70 for 177 of the youth.

Evidence of Validity: The CROPS significantly correlated (.60) with the LITE measure of exposure to stressful events (see Appendix 9.1) in a community sample of 206 children, grades 3–8. Scores increased with increases in traumatic experience and loss (Greenwald & Rubin, 1999). Associations remained strong after controls for age, gender, ethnicity, parent education, and location (urban vs. rural). Preliminary results in a study of incarcerated youth (*n* = 300; Greenwald et al., 2001) indicated that CROPS scores correlated with history of trauma (.48–.52), the TSCC (see below, this appendix), with *r* = .53–.56 using one scoring system and *r* = .63–.80 for the subscales (and *r* = .83 for the total scale) and *r* = .74 with the Adolescent Dissociative Experiences Scale (A-DES; Armstrong, Putnam, & Carlson, 1993).

Contact Information: Sidran Institute, 200 E. Joppa Road, Suite 207, Towson, MD 21286. Telephone: (410) 825-8888. Fax: (410) 337-0747 or (888) 825-8249. Website: *www.sidran.org*. E-mail: sidran@sidran.org.

Child's Reaction to Traumatic Events Scale—Revised (CRTES-R—Jones, 1996; Jones, Fletcher, & Ribbe, 2000)

Brief Description: The CRTES-R (Jones, Fletcher, & Ribbe, 2000) is a 23-item revision of the CRTES (Jones, 1996). The CRTES (originally called the Horowitz Impact of Event Scale for Children) was a 15-item self-report measure based on Horowitz's Impact of Event Scale (IES; Horowitz et al., 1979). As such, it measured symptoms of intrusive thoughts (criterion A), and avoidance and denial (criterion B). The CRTES was revised by the addition of eight items assessing overarousal. Wording used in the IES has been substantially rewritten, making the questions more appropriate for children and adolescents. The CRTES-R is a paper-and-pencil self-report for children and adolescents that can also be administered as a semistructured interview. Respondents indicate how often they have experienced each symptom in the past week, using responses of *Not at all* (0), *Rarely* (1), *Sometimes* (3), and *Often* (5). Note the weighting of the last two responses. Age range: 6–18 years. The CRTES-R must be administered as an interview to younger children and to children with reading disabilities. Scoring the CRTES was based on threshold scores. The CRTES-R allows the use of both thresholds and tentative DSM-IV caseness for PTSD based on criteria B–D. Currently, data are not available for the CRTES-R, but, based on ROC analysis responses of 118 children ages 8–18 who survived residential fires, using DICA PTSD diagnosis as the gold standard, the recommended thresholds for the 15-item CRTES are as follows: Scores of 0–14 indicate low distress; 15–27, moderate distress; and 28+, high distress (Jones, Fletcher, & Ribbe, 2003). Languages available: English and Spanish.

Evidence of Reliability: Psychometrics have yet to be done for the CRTES-R. However, in a sample of African American children living in a low-income, high-crime neighborhood, Cronbach's alphas were .73 for the total 15 items of the original HIES-C, .68 for the Intrusion subscale, and .73 for the Avoidance subscale (Cunningham, Jones, & Yang, 1984). Among children who had experienced a hurricane, alphas were = .85 for the total 15-item HIES-C, .84 for Intrusion, and .72 for Avoidance (Jones et al., 1993). In a sample of 167 children and adolescents ages 4–18, who lived through residential fires, alphas were .86 for the total 15-item CRTES, .85 for Intrusion, and .77 for Avoidance (Jones et al., 2003).

Evidence of Validity: A principle axis factor analysis with a varimax rotation followed by a promax rotation of the CRTES responses of 167 children who had survived residential fires (Jones, Fletcher, & Ribbe, 2003) produced two factors that accounted for 46.54% of the variance: (1) Intrusion (35.49% of the variance) and (2) Avoidance (11.04% of the variance). These results support the theoretical structure of the CRTES, although several items loaded well on both factors and two items did not achieve the .40 threshold on either factor. A higher order factor analysis resulted in a single factor, providing support for the assumption that both factors measure the single underlying dimension of PTSD. Age was associated with neither the total or either of the subscales. Girls and boys did not differ on their total score or on their Avoidance score, but girls scored significantly higher on Intrusion. Among 118 children and adolescents ages 8–18 who survived residential fires, those diagnosed with DSM-IV PTSD per the DICA had significantly higher CRTES scores than those not diagnosed with PTSD (Jones et al., 2003). ROC analysis (Jones et al., 2003) revealed that if children who scored 28 or higher were considered to have PTSD, compared to DSM-IV diagnosis with the DICA (Reich et al., 1994), the sensitivity of this diagnosis would be .83 and the specificity would be .70.

Contact Information: Russell T. Jones, PhD, Department of Psychology, Stress and Coping Lab, Virginia Tech University, 137 Williams Hall, Blacksburg, VA 24060. Telephone: (540) 231-5934. E-mail: rtjones@vt.edu.

Clinician-Administered PTSD Scale for Children and Adolescents (CAPS-CA; Newman et al., 2004)

Brief Description: The CAPS-CA, a structured interview with the child, comprises approximately 53 items, most of which require additional questions to assess such things as the intensity and duration of the experience. Most of the PTSD-specific items are questions about the occurrence, intensity, and frequency of endorsed symptoms both for the past month and over the lifetime. The interview begins with a script for establishing the meaning of a month's time for younger children who might have trouble with the concept. To establish criterion A, 17 different types of high-magnitude stressors are described one by one, and the child or adolescent is asked to indicate whether each event actually happened to him or her, or whether he or she *Saw it*, *Learned about it*, is *Not sure*, or it *Never happened*. If none of the 17 events is endorsed, four additional prompts are provided to attempt to elicit an experience of a high-magnitude stressor. If three or more events are endorsed, the interviewer tries to determine whether the experience evoked fear or terror, a sense of helplessness, horror, or disorganized agitation. The various means of eliciting this information use wording that is appropriate for children and adolescents. The interviewer rates whether each event was a life threat, whether a serious injury or threat to physical integrity occurred, and whether each of the four listed emotional reactions occurred. After the interviewer uses a practice question to teach the child or adolescent how to respond to the questions about frequency and intensity of events, questions related to each PTSD symptom listed in DSM-IV are then administered to those who met criterion A. Two questions related to the duration of symptoms (criterion E) are asked, then four questions regarding subjective distress and social, scholastic, and developmental (loss of acquired skill) functioning (criterion F). Three global rating scales are available: one that rates the overall validity of the responses, another that rates the overall severity of PTSD symptoms, and still another that rates global improvement for instances of repeated administration of the interview over time. Six items examine the presence of seven associated features: guilt over acts of commission or omission, survivor guilt when there were multiple victims, shame, reduction of awareness of surroundings, derealization, depersonalization, and changes in attachment. Three open-ended questions determine how the child or adolescent thinks the event has affected his or her life, what has helped him or her to feel better since the event, and coping strategies. Three optional rating sheets provide different graphical representations of the ratings for frequency and intensity of reactions to each symptom. One represents the five categories of frequency as a calendar grid, with increasing numbers of days crossed off, from none to 2, 6, 12, and 24. A second sheet illustrates increasing levels of intensity with a drawing of the top half of a young person who could be either male or female. The facial expression changes from a smile to a slight frown and slightly furrowed eyebrows; to a deeper frown with more deeply furrowed eyebrows; to a partially open mouth, gritted teeth and very furrowed eyebrows, with three drops of sweat flying off the top of the head; to an opened-mouthed gasp with very deeply furrowed eyebrows and five drops of sweat flying off the head. In addition, although the first illustration indicating "no problem" had no lines across the person's stomach, the illustrations that follow have three increasingly darker, wavy lines across the stomach. The final, optional rating sheet contains two rows of five "smiley" faces; those in the top row illustrate increasing levels of distress, whereas those in the bottom row illustrate increasing levels of pleasure. The interview's guide and summary scoring sheet for the CAPS-CA include scoring for ASD, although no algorithms are provided that actually derive a diagnosis of ASD. In addition, because the CAPS-CA assesses the DSM-IV associated symptoms, it should be possible to at least screen for complex PTSD, which might be indicated if the symptoms of ASD last longer than 1 month. In addition to the ability to make a DSM-IV diagnosis, the CAPS-CA also allows the interviewer to make judgments about the level of severity of PTSD, based on the total CAPS-CA scores. Five "rationally derived" categories range from *Minimal PTSD: Asymptomatic or few symptoms* (scores of 0–19) to *Extreme PTSD symptoms* (scores of 80–136). No research supports the use of these categories, however, although empirically derived rules are available for adults assessed with the CAPS. Clinicians should be wary of applications to children until these rules receive empirical support.

Evidence of Reliability: In a study of 50 incarcerated adolescent males (Newman, McMackin, Morrissey, & Erwin, 1997), Cronbach's alpha was found to be .81 for the Reexperiencing subscale, .75 for Numbing and Avoidance, and .79 for Arousal. Among children hospitalized after an injury (Daviss, Mooney, Racusin, Ford, et al., 2000) alphas for these subscales were .78, .73, and .78, respectively. Interrater reliability for 23 hospitalized children was 100% (Daviss, Mooney, Racusin, Ford, et al., 2000), and among 10 children with histories of traumatic stress the interrater kappa reliability was .97 (Carrion et al., 2002). Among a sample of traumatized adolescents, interrater reliability was .54 for the lifetime diagnosis and .84 for current diagnosis (reported in Ohan et al., 2002).

Evidence of Validity: The mean Intensity rating across the 17 diagnostic items correlated .64 with a child self-report measure of PTSD, the Child PTSD Checklist (Amaya-Jackson, McCarthy, Newman, & Cherney, 1995; cited in Weathers, 2004) and .51 with the CPTS-RI (Carrion et al., 2002). The CAPS-CA has been demonstrated to be responsive to change over time due to an effective cognitive behavioral treatment intervention (March et al., 1998).

Contact Information: Western Psychological Services (WPS), 12031 Wilshire Blvd., Los Angeles, CA 90025-1251. Telephone: (800) 648-8857 or (310) 478-2061. Fax: (310) 478-7838. Website: *www.wpspublish.com*.

Kauai Recovery Index (KRI—Hamada, Kameoka, & Yanagida, 1996; Hamada, Kameoka, Yanagida, & Chemtob, 2003)

Brief Description: The KRI, a 24-item, paper-and-pencil self-report measure based on the CPTS-RI (discussed earlier, this appendix), was originally developed to assess children's posttraumatic responses to Hawaii's Hurricane Iniki, a Category 4 storm that affected the islands. It also was used as an outcome measure in a study of the effectiveness of treatment on children affected by Hurricane Iniki (Chemtob, Nakashima, Hamada, & Carlson, 2002). The scale has been used with children as young as second graders. It comprises six reexperiencing items, seven avoidance items, six arousal items, two age-specific items, and three associated features items that do not pertain to PTSD symptoms (Hamada et al., 2003). The KRI was designed as a screening device to help identify children with substantial traumatic reactions to large-scale critical incidents such as natural disasters of large magnitude. Therefore, the guiding principles of its developers were brevity and ease of administration, while preserving reliability and validity. Children rate the frequency of each symptom in the past week by marking each item on a 3-point scale: *No, Sometimes,* or *Almost all the time.* The scale is currently suggested for children exposed to Type I (acute) traumas only.

Evidence of Reliability: Ratings of 3,732 children ages 6–15 years ($M = 9.49$, $SD = 1.55$), in grades 2–6 (53% boys, 38% Asian, 28% Hawaiians or part-Hawaiian, 22% white, and 12% from other ethnic backgrounds) were taken about 2 years after the hurricane. When subscales were rationally derived, based on the DSM-IV diagnostic criteria, the Cronbach alphas were .84 for the total scale, .78 for criterion B, .52 for criterion C, and .64 for criterion D (Hamada et al., 2003). Test–retest reliability for 43 students over a 4-week period was .77 for the total score and .44, .29, and .64 for criteria B, C, and D, respectively (Hamada et al., 1996).

Evidence of Validity: Children who thought they would "die or get hurt" during the hurricane had significantly higher scores on the KRI than children who did not think they might die or get hurt. Children who feared for the lives of family members had significantly higher scores than did those who did not. Children whose home suffered greater damage had significantly higher scores than those whose homes had less damage, and those who reported greater fear during the hurricane had higher scores than those who did not (Hamada et al., 2003). Principal axis factor analysis with promax rotation on the 24 items resulted in a four-factor solution. The first three factors corresponded to reexperiencing, arousal, and avoidance symptoms. The fourth factor comprised two items that could not be labeled, one originally associated with avoidance and the other associated with overarousal.

Contact Information: Claude M. Chemtob, PhD, Department of Psychiatry, Mount Sinai School of Medicine, One Austave L, Levy Place, Box 1230, New York, NY 10029. Telephone: (212) 987-0559. E-mail: claude.chemtob @mssm.edu.

Kiddie Post-Traumatic Symptomatology Scale (see CATS, this appendix).

My Worst Experience Scale (MWES); My Worst School Experience Scale (MWSES—Hyman, Zelikoff, & Clarke, 1988; National Center for Study of Corporal Punishment and Alternatives in Schools, 1992)

Brief Description: The MWES and the MWSES are self-report scales that assess the reactions of children and adolescents to high-magnitude stressors. Respondents describe their worst experience, answer questions about the experience, then rate the frequency and duration of 105 possible responses. The MWES provides a list of possible high-magnitude stressors. The MWSES provides a list of 39 high-magnitude stressors that might occur at school. Both scales allow DSM-III and DSM-IV diagnoses of PTSD. Factor analysis extracted seven factors that became the seven subscales: Reexperiencing/Intrusive Thoughts, Dissociation/Disturbing Dreams, Depression/Withdrawal, Hopelessness/ Suicidal, Avoidance/Hypervigilance, Somatic Symptoms, Oppositional/Defiant, and an overall scale of General Maladjustment. Age range: 9–18 years. No special training is required. Time to administer: 20–30 minutes.

Evidence of Reliability: Internal consistency for the subscales of the MWES ranges from .68 to .91. Test–retest Pearson correlations range from .88 to .95 (Hyman, Snook, Lurkis, Phan, & Britton, 2001).

Evidence of Validity: Evidence of validity has yet to be published.

Contact Information: Western Psychological Services, 12031 Wilshire Blvd., Los Angeles, CA 90025-1251. Telephone: (800) 646-8857. Fax: (310) 478-7838. E-mail: custsvc@spspublish.com. Website: *www.wpspublish.com.*

Trauma Symptom Checklist for Children (TSCC; Briere, 1996a, 1996b)

Brief Description: The TSCC is a 54-item scale that "evaluates traumatic symptomatology in children, including the effects of child abuse (sexual, physical, and psychological) and neglect, other interpersonal violence, witnessing trauma to others, major accidents, and disasters" (Briere, 1996a, p. 378). It assess symptoms of posttraumatic stress and associated responses on six subscales: Anger (ANG), Anxiety (ANX), Depression (DEP), Dissociation (DIS), Posttraumatic Stress (PTS), and Sexual Concerns (SC). Dissociation itself has two subscales (Overt and Fantasy). The TSCC also contains eight critical items. The subscales do not provide diagnosis of disorders, including PTSD. Two validity scales are included, one assessing a tendency to underreport and the other assessing a tendency to overreport symptoms. Some symptoms are shared by more than one subscale. The TSCC is available in two versions: the full 54-item test, which includes 10 items tapping sexual symptoms and preoccupation, and a 44-item alternate version (TSCC-A) that makes no reference to sexual issues. The items are written to be understood by children 8 years or older. Each item is rated according to "how often it happens to you," on a 4-point response scale ranging from *Never* to *Almost all of the time.* Time required: 15–20 minutes.

Evidence of Reliability: The internal consistency and reliability of the TSCC and subscales have been studied in a large (*n* = 3,008) normative, standardization sample (Brier, 1996b), as well as in several samples of sexually abused children (*n* = 105, Lanktree & Briere, 1995; *n* = 399, Elliot & Briere, 1994; *n* = 103, Nelson-Gardell, 1995). In the normative sample, alpha was .82 for ANX, whereas in the three clinical samples, it ranged from .83 to .86. For ANG, alpha was .89 in the normative sample and ranged from .87 to .89 in the clinical samples. For DEP, the respective alphas were .86 and .85–.89. For PTS alphas were .87 and .85–.87, respectively. For SC, they were .77 and .67–.78, respectively. For DIS, alphas were .83 and .80–.89, respectively, with .81 for the Overt DIS subscale and .58 for the Fantasy DIS subscale, in the normative sample. The two validity scales were only reported in the normative sample, where alphas were .85 for the Underresponse subscale and .66 for the Hyperresponse subscale.

Evidence of Validity: Convergent and discriminant validity of the scales have been demonstrated through correlations between the TSCC subscales and the relevant scales of the CBCL (Briere & Lanktree, 1995), where similar scales correlated more highly than did dissimilar scales. Evans, Briere, Boggiano, and Barrett (1994) found that TSCC scores correlated significantly with the CDI (Kovacs & Beck, 1977) and the RCMAS: ANX, .45 and .63; DEP, .68 and .63; ANG, .57 and .51; PTS, .51 and .60; DIS, .51 and .56, respectively. In a study of 39 children identified as sexual abuse victims, Smith, Saunders, Swenson, and Crouch (1995) found that the TSCC scale correlated highest with the Intrusive Thoughts of the CITES-II (discussed earlier, this appendix) scale, the TSCC DEP scale correlated highest (positively and negatively respectively) with the CITES-II Self-Blame and Empowerment scales, the TSCC SC scale correlated highest with the CITES-II Sexual Anxiety and Eroticism scales, and the CITES-II Avoidance scale correlated second highest with the TSCC DIS scale, (*r* = .60). Freidrich and Jaworski (1995) found that the TSCC SC was significantly related to CSBI (Friedrich, 1991) but not to CDC scores, whereas the TSCC DIS scale related to CDC scores but not to CSBI scores. Finkelhor and colleagues (2005) found that among 992 children ages 10–17 years in a national telephone survey, most of the single items and all of the subscale totals of their measure of youth victimization, the JVQ (see Appendix 9.1), correlated significantly with the TSCC ANX, DEP, and ANG subscales. Evidence that the TSCC assesses posttraumatic stress was demonstrated by Smith, Swenson, Hanson and Saunders (1994), who found that each of the subscales related to specific aspects of childhood trauma: PTS, DIS, and ANX correlated with stressors involving perceptions of life threat; ANG and DEP correlated negatively with clinician ratings of parental support following abuse disclosure; and sexual assault victims who had experienced penetration had higher SC scores. Briere and Lanktree (1995) found that sexual penetration correlated most highly with TSCC scales related to trauma and sexual distress: PTS, SC and DIS. The TSCC subscales also discriminated between 81 sexually abused girls and 151 controls (Diaz, 1994). The TSCC has also discriminated between groups of adolescents exposed to violence and controls (Singer, Anglin, Song, & Lunghofer, 1995).

Contact Information: Psychological Assessment Resources, Inc. (PAR). Telephone: (800) 331-TEST. John Briere, PhD, Department of Psychiatry and the Behavioral Sciences, Keck School of Medicine, University of Southern California Medical Center, FRD Building, 2020 Zonal Ave., Los Angeles, CA 90033. E-mail: info@johnbriere.com.

UCLA PTSD Reaction Index for DSM-IV (UPRID Child and Parent report forms—Pynoos, Rodriguez, Steinberg, Stuber, & Frederick, 1998; Steinberg, Brymer, Decker, & Pynoos, 2004)

Brief Description: The UPRID is a 49-item scale purportedly derived from the CPTS-RI (this appendix); however, its provenance appears to be related more to intention than to direct derivation. The DSM PTSD-specific symptoms cover all 17 symptoms, unlike the CPTS-RI, and the items are much better written. The items were written by Rodriguez and Steinberg (Rodriguez, in press). A panel of youth PTSD experts reviewed them for their readability and comprehension by youth, a pilot study led to some refinement of the items, and items reflecting fear of recurrence of the traumatic event and posttraumatic guilt were added given the apparent high incidence of these experience among traumatized youth, as reported by Fletcher (1996a). The first 13 items assess exposure to different high-magnitude stressors for children. Each item is rated either *Present* or *Absent*. Stressors assessed include community violence, natural disaster, medical trauma, and abuse. These are followed by an item that asks children to select the experience that bothers them the most and rate how bothersome it is on a 3-point scale: *A little* (1), *somewhat* (2), or *A lot* (3). The next 13 items assess different responses to the experience that children might have had at the time. These items are intended to establish whether children responded with fear, helplessness, or horror, per DSM-IV criterion A2, but one item also asks about reactions of confusion, one about upset or disorganized behavior, and one about feelings of unreality. These are rated either *Yes* or *No*. Of the final 22 questions, 20 assess the presence of symptoms related to DSM-IV criteria B–D; in addition, fear of recurrence of the trauma and trauma-related guilt are assessed by one item each. These item ratings range from *None of the time* (0) to *Most of the time* (4). The questionnaire is accompanied by a frequency rating sheet that visually assists children in providing accurate responses about how often the reaction has occurred over the past month. Although the instrument was not created to be a diagnostic tool, there is also a score sheet that allows the interviewer to make a preliminary DSM-IV diagnosis. The UPRID has been selected to be the primary PTSD screening measure for the National Child Traumatic Stress Network. Age range: 7–18 years. It is recommended that the instructions and questions be read aloud to children under the age of 12 or to youth with reading comprehension problems. A parent version is available. An original adolescent version (Rodriguez, Steinberg, Saltzman, & Pynoos, 2001a) was eventually merged with the child version (Steinberg et al., 2004). Two shorter versions, one with seven items and one with nine, are available for screening. Training required: Licensed Master's-level clinician, with experience in assessment of trauma exposure and PTSD in children. The measure is designed to be administered three different ways: (1) as a self-report; (2) as a one-on-one "interview," wherein the items are read to the child; and (3) group administration. Time for administration: 20–30 minutes. When criterion A is met, and when sufficient endorsement in each of the B–D criteria categories is made at the top two rating categories (*Much of the time* or *Most of the time*), a likely diagnosis of PTSD is made. When criterion A is met and children meet criteria for only two symptoms of criteria B–D, they are scored as "partial" PTSD. A cutoff of 38 or greater has the greatest sensitivity and specificity for detecting PTSD (Rodriguez et al., 2001a, 2001b).

Evidence of Reliability: In a sample of 46 children, 29 of whom had been exposed to high-magnitude stressors, internal consistency alpha for the child version total score was .87, whereas it was .82 for the Intrusion scale, .72 for the Avoidance scale, and .67 for the Hyperarousal scale (Rodriguez, 2001). The test–retest Pearson correlation for the total was .86, whereas it was .86 for Intrusion, .92 for Avoidance, and .59 for Overarousal. In a sample of 73 adolescents, the internal consistency alpha for the adolescent version total was .92, whereas it was .80 for Intrusion, .84 for Avoidance, and .73 for Hyperarousal. The test–retest correlation among 25 of the adolescents was .84 for the total, .78 for Intrusion, .78 for Avoidance, and .73 for Hyperarousal (Rodriguez et al., 2001a, 2001b). In another sample of 75 youthful clients of school-based trauma clinics (53% boys; 51% Hispanic, 32% African American, and 17% European American [mean age = 13 years, SD = 2.0 years] in grades 5–11), Rodriguez (in press) reported interrater kappas were 1.0 for PTSD diagnosis, reexperiencing (DSM-IV criterion B), and overarousal (criterion D) and .57 for withdrawal and numbing (criterion C). In this study, Cronbach's alphas were .72 for criterion D, .75 for criterion C, .76 for criterion B, and .89 for the total PTSD severity score.

Evidence of Validity: A pilot study (Rodriguez et al., 2001b) indicated that the first 13 trauma exposure questions demonstrated poor validity and high rates of false-negative and false-positive responses when compared with prior information about the youth trauma histories. The UPRID child version correlated .82 with the CAPS-CA intensity scale (this appendix), and traumatized children had significantly higher scores than nontraumatized ones. The adolescent version correlated .70 with the K-SADS PTSD module (Rodriguez, 2001; Rodriguez et al., 2001a, 2001b). The authors report that numerous studies have found consistently higher UPRID scores among traumatized children compared to nontraumatized children, as well as clear "dose–response" relationships of scores across exposure groups (Steinberg et al., 2004). However, because the UPRID was developed from the CPTS-RI (this appendix), it seems that the authors have a tendency to report psychometrics that were actually based on various versions of the CPTS-RI, while implying that those results apply to the UPRID as well. For example, Steinberg and colleagues in the purported psychometric study of the UPRID, reported that in studies after the 1988 earthquake in Armenia (Pynoos et al., 1993), a cutoff of 40 or higher correctly identified 78% of children who met DSM-III-R criteria for PTSD, and 79% of those who did not. Of those who scored 40 or higher, 90% had PTSD. However, the actual measure used to assess PTSD in that study was a version of the CPTS-RI, not the UPRID. Despite the fact that the former was a forerunner of the latter, they are not the same measure. In fact, the two differ very much. Therefore, psychometrics on versions of the

CPTS-RI cannot just be assumed to reflect the psychometrics of the UPRID. In a study of 75 youth receiving services for traumatic responses, Rodriguez (in press) found significant Spearman's rho correlations of .73 between the UPRID subscales reflecting DSM-IV criteria B–D and the total PTSD severity score, and the respective subscales of the K-SADS PTSD module (Kaufman et al., 1997; see Appendix 9.3). Using the K-SADS PTSD diagnosis as the "gold standard" in a ROC analysis, Rodriguez determined that an optimal cutoff score is 37 or greater, which provides a sensitivity of .82 and a specificity of .87. This cutoff score resulted in a positive predictive power of .67, a negative predictive power of .94, and an overall diagnostic efficiency of .86. Rodriguez also suggested that a cutoff score of 27 or greater would be best for purposes of screening for possible PTSD, providing a sensitivity of .94 and a specificity of .66. A cutoff score of 50 or higher leads to a nearly definitive diagnosis of PTSD, with a specificity of .97 and a sensitivity of .65.

Contact Information: Robert Pynoos, MD, UCLA Trauma Psychiatry Service, 300 UCLA Medical Plaza, Suite 2232, Los Angeles, CA 90025. Telephone: (310) 206-8973. E-mail: rpynoos@mednet.ucla.edu.

When Bad Things Happen Scale (WBTH; Fletcher, 1996g)

Brief Description: The WBTH scale is a 90-item, paper-and-pencil report by the child regarding his or her reactions to exposure to a high-magnitude stressor. The first 58 questions allow the assessment of DSM-IV PTSD criteria A–D. The first four questions assess criterion A; three questions assess recurrent and intrusive recollections of the event(s) (symptom B1); four questions assess distressing dreams (B2); four questions assess acting or feeling as if the event were recurring (B3); three assess intense distress at reminders (B4); two assess psychological reactivity to reminders (B5); five assess avoidance of thoughts, feelings, or conversations that serve as reminders of the event(s) (C1); three assess avoidance of other reminders (C2); two assesses the child's inability to recall important aspects of the event (C3); two assess lost of interest in previous activities or loss of recently acquired skills (C4); three assess feelings of estrangement from others (C5); two assess restricted affect (C6); six assess a sense of foreshortened future (C7); two assess sleep problems (D1); three assess increased irritability (D2); four assess difficulties concentrating (D3); four assess hypervigilance (D4); and two questions assess exaggerated startle response (D5). Associated symptoms are assessed by an additional 32 items, five of which assess anxiety; three assess depressive symptoms; two assess superstitious beliefs related to the event(s); two assess survivor guilt; two assess self-blame; two assess fantasy denial; three assess self-destructive behavior, including attempted suicide; four assess symptoms of dissociation; three assess aggressive, antisocial behavior; two assess risk-taking behavior; and four assess changes in eating habits since the occurrence of the event(s). Response to all items is rated on a 3-point scale: *Never, Some,* and *Lots.* It is possible with the WBTH to derive DSM-II-R and DSM-IV diagnoses of PTSD and a total PTSD severity score, either for the first 58 DSM PTSD symptoms questions or for the full 90 questions, including the additional 32. Age range: 4 or 5 years to 19 years. Available languages: English and Spanish.

Evidence of Reliability: In a sample of 10 clinically referred children diagnosed with PTSD, 10 community children exposed to high-magnitude stressors, and 10 community children with no reported exposure to high-magnitude stressors (Fletcher, 1996), internal consistency alphas were .92 for the total 58 PTSD items .70 for the four criterion A items, .89 for the criterion B (reexperiencing) items, .70 for the criterion C (avoidance/numbing) items, and .82 for the criterion D (overarousal) items. Among a sample of 40 adolescent psychiatric inpatients, 24 of whom had a diagnosis of PTSD, the WBTH scale was administered two times, 1–2 weeks apart. The test–retest ICC was .78 (Fletcher et al., 1997). The inpatient adolescents with a diagnosis of PTSD reported significantly higher WBTH total PTSD severity scores than did those without a PTSD diagnosis. Among these adolescents, the WBTH had a sensitivity of 78% and a specificity of 54%. Scores on the WBTH appeared to be associated with IQ in these adolescents.

Evidence of Validity: In the same study referred to earlier (Fletcher, 1996), the WBTH scale correlated .87 with scores on the Childhood PTSD Interview—Child Form (this appendix). It also demonstrated unusually high agreement with parent reports of PTSD. It correlated .60 with the parent's paper-and-pencil self-report on the Parent Report of the Child's Reaction to Stress scale (see below, this appendix), .59 with the Childhood PTSD Interview—Parent Form (see below, this appendix), and .54 with an ad hoc CBCL PTSD scale completed by the parent. The WBTH also correlated .70 with a measure of the potentially stressful characteristics of the child's individual high-magnitude stressor (assessed with the DOSE, see Appendix 9.2), .30 ($p > .05$, ns) with the parent's report of the number of stressors to which the child had been exposed in his or her lifetime, and .42 ($p < .05$) with the parent's ratings of the severity of the child's distress at exposure to each of the stressors on the Child's Upsetting Times Checklist (Fletcher, 1996f; see Appendix 9.1). The WBTH correlated .48 with the CBCL Internalizing and .36 ($p > .05$, ns) with the CBCL Externalizing scales. It correlated .57 with the CBCL Anxiety scale, .43 with the Withdrawn scale, .55 with the Thought Problems scale, .21 ($p > .05$, ns) with the Somatic Complaints scale, .37 with the Attention Problems scale, .49 with the Social Problems scale, .33 ($p > .05$, ns) with the Aggression scale, 36 ($p > .05$, ns) with the Delinquent Behavior scale, and .03 ($p > .05$, ns) with the Sexual Problems scale (none of the children had been sexually abused). The fact that WBTH correlations with other PTSD measures and the DOSE tend to be higher than its correlations with measures of other problems provides evidence of the scale's discriminant validity. Scores differentiated between traumatized and nontraumatized children (Fletcher, 1996b). Sensitivity in identifying probable cases of traumatized children, as assessed by the DOSE scale, was 40%, and specificity was 100% (Fletcher, 1996b). Among a sample of 40 adolescents psychiatric inpatients, 24 of whom had a diagnosis of PTSD, the WBTH scale correlated .78 with the Childhood PTSD Interview—Child Form (this appendix), .79 with the CRTES (this appendix), .38 with scores on the Teen Tough Times Checklist (see Appendix 9.1), .45 with the DOSE (see Appendix 9.1), and .54 with the A-DES (Armstrong, Putnam, & Carlson, 1993), and did not correlate significantly with any of the scales of the Brief Symptom Inventory (Derogatis & Melisaratos, 1983), providing evidence of the convergent and discriminant validity of the scale (Fletcher et al., 1997). Among 15 sexually abused children (Moller-Thau & Fletcher, unpublished), the WBTH scale correlated .84 with the CPTS-RI (this appendix). The kappa for agreement between the two measures for diagnosis of PTSD was .67. The WBTH classified two children with PTSD that the CPTS-RI did not classify.

Contact Information: Kenneth E. Fletcher, PhD, Department of Psychiatry, University of Massachusetts Medical School, 55 Lake Avenue North, Worcester, MA 01655. Telephone: (508) 856-8630. E-mail: kenneth.fletcher@umassmed.edu.

ADMINISTERED TO CARETAKER OR OTHER ADULTS

Checklist of Child Distress Symptoms, Parent Form (CCDS—Martinez & Richters, 1993; Richters & Martinez, 1990a) (also known as the Survey of Children's Distress Symptoms)

Brief Description: The CCDS Parent Form, is a 28-item, self-report scale that asks questions associated with traumatic responses to high-magnitude stressors. Questions examine anxiety, memory problems, sleeping problems, self-esteem, school performance, and feelings of depression, isolation, or hopelessness. Thus, it does not allow diagnosis of PTSD to be made. Responses are rated on a 4-point scale, ranging from *Never occurs* (1), *Seldom occurs* (2), *Occurs once in a while* (3), or *Occurs lot of the time* (4). The CCDS comprises two subscales measuring Depression and Anxiety, although the two subscales' very high correlation (.80) justifies combining them for the total score. Age range: 6–10 years.

Evidence of Reliability: Among parents of 54 fifth and sixth graders, Cronbach's alphas were .75 for the Depression subscale, and .70 for the Anxiety subscale.

Evidence of Validity: Parents reported significantly lower levels of their children's distress than were reported by their children on both the Depression and Anxiety subscales, as well as on many of the individual items (Martinez & Richters, 1993). Agreement between parents and their daughters was nonsignificant ($r_{(17)} = .06$), whereas agreement between parents and their sons was significant, moderately high, and negative ($r_{(18)} = -.56$), which the authors note was not attributable to outliers (p. 30). They suggest that the negative correlation may be attributable at least in part to a tendency of the boys to deny their symptoms. Total parent ratings of their children's distress on the CCDS did not correlate significantly with any type of exposure to violence reported by the children, neither for younger children (first and second graders) or older children (fifth and sixth graders). However, another study that examined ratings of 53 children's exposure to potentially traumatizing stressors and ratings on the CCDS by mothers found significant correlations between these ratings (Osofsky et al., 1993). Although the parents' CCDS ratings correlation with the parents' reports of their children's victimization (r = .21) was nonsignificant, the parents' CCDS correlations with the child's witnessing community violence (r = .42), and the correlations with simply hearing about such violence (.48), minor family conflicts (.39), and severe family conflicts (.61) were all significant. Moreover, the magnitude of the correlations were associated with the magnitude of the stressor. Thus, the CCDS correlated .35 with moderate types, .29 with the less than severe types of community violence, and .51 with the most severe (a shooting, a stabbing, or rape).

Contact Information: John E. Richters, PhD, Department of Human Development and Institute for Child Study, University of Maryland, Benjamin Building, Room 4104, College Park, MD 20742. Telephone: (301) 405-7354. E-mail: jrichter@nih.gov.

Childhood PTSD Interview—Parent Form (Fletcher, 1996b, 1996c)

Brief Description: The Childhood PTSD Interview—Parent Form, a semistructured interview of the caretaker regarding the child's reactions to the stressor(s), allows the interviewer to assess DSM-III-R and DSM-IV criteria and to make a diagnosis. It contains 1 item that allows the interviewer to rate how well the caregiver's description of the event(s) matches the description of the child. Sixty-two questions assess DSM PTSD criteria A–D. Four questions assess criterion A. Of the six questions that assess the first symptom of criterion B (B1), one requires elaboration for positive responses; four assess B2, with a follow-up to a positive response to the first question; four questions assess B3 (two of which ask for clarification of endorsed questions); and three questions assess B4 (with elaboration required for a positive response to the first question). Five questions assess C1, four assess C2, one question assesses C3 with a follow-up question if the first is answered in the negative (both require elaboration for positive responses), three assess C4 (with elaboration required for positive responses), three assess C5, two questions and a rater question regarding possible flat affect of the child assess C6, and six questions assess C7 (because C7 concerns a sense of foreshortened future, and few studies support the presence of this symptom in children, the author believes these six questions can be skipped). Two questions with required elaborations for positive responses assess D1, three questions assess D2, four questions assess D3, four questions assess D4, and two questions assess D5. Two questions assess complaint of physiological reactions, which is D6 according to DSM-III-R, and B5 according to DSM-IV.

An optional additional 26 questions assess associated symptoms. Interviewers may choose to ask some, all, or none of these questions. Five questions assess symptoms of anxiety (two require elaboration for positive responses, and one asks the rater to indicate whether breathing problems may be due to asthma). Three questions assess symptoms of depression. Two questions with required elaboration for positive responses assess indications of whether the child perceives certain prestressor events as omens. Two questions with required elaboration for positive responses assess symptoms of survivor guilt. Two questions, one of which requires elaboration for positive responses, assess symptoms of guilt or self-blame. The interviewer is asked to indicate to what extent the child actually might be considered to have some responsibility for events. Two questions, with required elaboration for positive responses, assess indications of fantasy denial. Three questions, one of which requires elaboration for positive responses, assess possible self-destructive or suicidal thoughts and behaviors. Four questions assess symptoms of dissociation. Three questions assess antisocial behavior. Two questions assess risk-taking behavior, and two assess changed eating habits. Items are answered *Yes* or *No*. *Don't know*s are allowed on many questions and are scored as *No*. Age range: 5–7 years and older.

Evidence of Reliability: Cronbach's alphas were .94 for the full PTSD section of the interview, .60 for the four questions on criterion A, .86 for questions on criteria B and C, and .83 for questions on criterion D (Fletcher, 1996b).

Evidence of Validity: The interview correlated significantly with other measures of childhood PTSD: .59 with the WBTH scale (this appendix), .69 with the Childhood PTSD Interview—Child Form (this appendix), .93 with the Parent Report of the Child's Reaction to Stress (this appendix), and .78 with an ad hoc CBCL PTSD scale. The first two correlations demonstrate unusually high agreement between the parent and child reports. The interview also correlated significantly (.50) with the total number of lifetime stressors the parent indicated the child had experienced, .63 with the parent's ratings of the child's stressful reactions to those events, and .54 with an assessment of the potentially traumatizing dimensions of the immediate stressor(s) for which the child's reactions were being assessed, as measured by the DOSE scale (see Appendix 9.1). The interview also correlated significantly with the Internalizing score (.68) and the Externalizing score (.48) of the CBCL and the following CBCL subscales: Anxiety (.52), Withdrawn (.49), Thought Problems (which include obsessing on certain thoughts, problems concentrating, repetition of certain acts, and staring blankly; $r = .62$), Somatic Complaints (.78), Attention Problems (.45), Social Problems (.63), Aggression (.45), Delinquent Behavior (.40), and Sexual Problems (.41) (Fletcher, 1996b). The fact that the interview's correlations with other PTSD measures are, for the most part, higher than its correlations with measures of other problems indicates its discriminant validity. Scores differentiated between clinically referred traumatized children and traumatized children in the community, and between both of those groups and nontraumatized children (Fletcher, 1996b). Sensitivity in identifying probable cases of traumatized children, as assessed by the DOSE, was 55%, and specificity was 100% (Fletcher, 1996b).

Contact Information: Kenneth E. Fletcher, PhD, Department of Psychiatry, University of Massachusetts Medical School. 55 Lake Avenue North, Worcester, MA 01655. Telephone: (508) 856-8630. E-mail: kenneth.fletcher@umassmed.edu.

Childhood Post-Traumatic Stress Reaction—Parent Inventory (CPTSR-PI; Nader, 1984/1995)

Brief Description: The CPTSR-PI is a parent interview that assesses trauma-related responses and additional symptoms in five sections: (1) Pretrauma descriptors of family background, child's behaviors, and personality (e.g., moods, self-confidence, social behaviors) before and after the event; (2) prior trauma history of child and family; (3) parents' description of the child's reported experience of the event and parents' reactions to the child's initial responses; (4) child's reactions after the event, especially in the previous month; and (5) associated symptoms similar to those asked about in the Additional Questions of the CPTS-RI (this appendix). DSM-IV symptoms are assessed. Similarities with the CPTS-RI are identified.

Evidence of Reliability: Evidence of reliability has yet to be published.

Evidence of Validity: The CPTSR-RI has been found to differentiate between traumatized and nontraumatized children (Nader, 1991). In a sample of youth exposed to a hurricane, the CPTSR-PI correlated .55 with the RCMAS (Lonigan et al., 1991). In a sample of sexually and/or physically abused adolescents, it correlated .64 with the RCMAS and .70 with the CDI (Kovacs, 1992).

Contact Information: Kathleen Nader, DSW. Fax: (512) 219-0486. E-mail: measures@twosuns.org.

Child Stress Disorders Checklist (CSDC; Saxe, 2001) and Child Stress Disorders Checklist—Screening Form (CSDC-SF; Saxe & Bosquet, 2004)

Brief Description: The CSDC, a 42-item, paper-and-pencil scale, asks parents, guardians, or other observers to report on the child's reaction to high-magnitude stressors. The respondent is first asked to indicate whether and at what age the child has been exposed to eight kinds of high-magnitude stressors (an "Other" category is included). The next five questions ask about the child's emotional reactions to the experience(s). Then, seven items assess symptoms of reexperiencing, five assess avoidance, eight assess numbing and dissociation, six assess increased arousal, and four assess functional impairment. Responses to each questions can be *Not true (as far as you know)*, *Somewhat true*, or *Very true*. The Screening Form (CSDC-SF) includes the same first eight kinds of high-magnitude stressors, followed by just four questions about the child's reactions during the past month: whether the child gets upset at reminders, experiences physical complaints at reminders, does not want to talk about the experience, or startles easily. Unlike most other child PTSD measures to date, the CSDC allows assessment of symptoms of both DSM-IV PTSD and ASD.

Evidence of Reliability: Among a sample of 84 children, which included 43 children with acute burns and 41 who had experienced a traffic crash (Saxe et al., 2003), the internal consistency alpha for the 84 parent respondents was .84. The ICC between total scores reported by the burned children's parents and primary nurse was 0.44 ($n = 37$). For the individual scales of the measure, alpha was .45 for the reexperiencing items, .28 for avoidance, .24 for numbing and dissociation, .36 for arousal, and .27 for functioning. Test–retest reliability (Pearson correlations) over a 2-day period was .84 for the total scale, .89 for reexperiencing, .85 for avoidance, .70 for numbing and dissociation, .74 for arousal, and .63 for functioning. Cronbach's alpha among 176 children and adolescents ages 8–17 ($M = 11.8$ years) on the 30 ASD symptom items within a month of a recent injury or intensive care unit admission was .87 (Kassam-Adams, 2006).

Evidence of Validity: Concurrent, convergent, and discriminant validity were assessed among both parent and nurse reporters for child burn victims ($n = 19$–43; Saxe et al., 2003). Total body surface area burned was measured and shown to correlate .56 with parent reports and .43 with nurse reports on the total CSDC scores. Parent total scores also correlated significantly (.39) with the children's reports of their own symptomatology on the CPTS-RI (this appendix), but nurse reports did not correlate significantly (.26) with the CPTS-RI scores, although the *p*-value was < .10 for this correlation. The total score correlated .49 with a CBCL post hoc PTSD scale for parent reporters and .33 for nurse reporters. It also correlated with the CDC (Putnam, Helmers, & Trickett, 1993) .49 for parent reports and

.33 for nurse reports. Discriminant validity was demonstrated with nonsignificant correlations between the CSDC and the CBCL Thought Disorder subscale.

Contact Information: Glenn Saxe, MD, Department of Psychiatry, Children's Hospital Boston, Karp Family Research Building, 300 Longwood Avenue, Boston, MA 02115. Telephone: (617) 414-7504. E-mail: glenn.saxe@ childrens.harvard.edu.

The CSDC is available online for download at *www.nctsnet.org/nctsn_assets/acp/hospital/csdc.pdf*. The CSDC-SF is available online for download at *www.nctsnet.org/nctsn_assets/acp/hospital/csdc-Screening%20Form2.pdf*.

Parent Report of the Child's Reaction to Stress (PRCRS; Fletcher, 1996e)

Brief Description: The PRCRS is a 78-item, paper-and-pencil parent report about the child's reaction to exposure to a high-magnitude stressor. The first 51 questions allow the assessment of DSM-IV PTSD criteria A–D. The first four questions assess criterion A, then six questions assess recurrent and intrusive recollections of the event(s) (symptom B1); three assess distressing dreams (B2); one assesses acting or feeling as if the event was recurring (B3); three assess intense distress at reminders (B4); two assess psychological reactivity to reminders (B5); four assess avoidance of thoughts, feelings, or conversations that serve as reminders of the event(s) (C1); three assess avoidance of other reminders (C2); one assesses the child's inability to recall important aspects of the event (C3); four assess loss of interest in previous activities or loss of recently acquired skills (C4); three assess feelings of estrangement from others (C5); one assesses restricted affect (C6); five assess a sense of foreshortened future (C7); two assess sleep problems (D1); two assess increased irritability (D2); three assess difficulties concentrating (D3); three assess hypervigilance (D4); and two questions assess exaggerated startle response (D5). Associated symptoms are assessed by an additional 27 items, five of which assess anxiety; two assess depressive symptoms; two assess superstitious beliefs related to the event(s); two assess survivor guilt; two assess self-blame; two assess fantasy denial; two assess self-destructive behavior; three assess symptoms of dissociation; three assess aggressive, antisocial behavior; two assess risk-taking behavior; and two assess changes in eating habits since the occurrence of the event(s). Most items have 6-point Likert-like responses, ranging from *Never* to *Always*, and a seventh *Don't know* category. Some positive responses are followed by a request for further information. Scorers of the responses are cautioned to consider these explanations carefully before rating the response. For example, parent or guardians are asked to explain what makes them believe their child behaves in new and unusual ways since the event(s). Age range: 4 or 5 years to 19 years. Available languages: English and Spanish.

Evidence of Reliability: In a sample of 10 clinically referred children diagnosed with PTSD, 10 community children exposed to high-magnitude stressors, and 10 community children with no reported exposure to high-magnitude stressors (Fletcher, 1996b), internal consistency alphas were .89 for the total 51 PTSD items, .81 for the four criterion A items, .86 for the criterion B (Reexperiencing) items, .70 for the criterion C (Avoidance/Numbing) items, and .81 for the criterion D (Overarousal) items.

Evidence of Validity: In the same study referred to earlier (Fletcher, 1996b), the PRCRS correlated .93 with scores on the Childhood PTSD Interview—Parent Form (this appendix), .54 with the child's own paper-and-pencil self-report on the WBTH scale (this appendix), .60 with the Childhood PTSD Interview—Child Form (this appendix), and .80 with an ad hoc CBCL PTSD scale completed by the parent. The PRCRS also correlated .54 with a measure of the stressfulness of the experience (the DOSE, see Appendix 9.2), .50 with the parent's report of the number of stressors to which the child had been exposed in his or her lifetime, and .63 with the parent's ratings of the severity of the child's distress at exposure to each of the stressors. The PRCRS correlated .70 with the CBCL Internalizing and .53 with the CBCL Externalizing scales, .56 with the CBCL Anxiety scale, .50 with the Withdrawn scale, .59 with the Thought Problems scale, .77 with the Somatic Complaints scale, .43 with the Attention Problems scale, .63 with the Social Problems scale, .53 with the Aggression scale, 39 with the Delinquent Behavior scale, and .46 with the Sexual Problems scale.

Scores differentiated between traumatized and nontraumatized children (Fletcher, 1996b). Sensitivity in identifying probable cases of traumatized children, as assessed by the DOSE scale was 35%, and specificity was 80% (Fletcher, 1996b).

Contact Information: Kenneth E. Fletcher, PhD, Department of Psychiatry, University of Massachusetts Medical School, 55 Lake Avenue North, Worcester, MA 01655. Telephone: (508) 856-8630. E-mail: kenneth.fletcher@ umassmed.edu.

Parent Report of Post-Traumatic Symptoms (PROPS; Greenwald, 1997; Greenwald & Rubin, 1999)

Brief Description: The PROPS, a 32-item report based on the CITES (see CITES-II, this appendix) and the CBCL (Achenbach & Edelbrock, 1983), includes items that assess symptoms of DSM-IV PTSD criteria, as well as associated symptoms. Although a companion measure to the child version (CROPS; this appendix), the two measures do not ask parallel questions, but they do share some content. The scale is scored as a continuous measure rather than providing DSM-IV diagnosis. A tentative "clinical" threshold of 16 indicates possible PTSD (Greenwald & Rubin, 1999). The PROPS can be administered as either a paper-and-pencil self-report or a structured telephone interview. Frequency of symptoms during the past week is rated on a 3-point scale: *None*, *Some*, or *Lots*.

Evidence of Reliability: Cronbach's alpha was .93 in a community sample of 206 children in grades 3–8 (Greenwald & Rubin, 1999). Test–retest correlation was .79 in the same study.

Evidence of Validity: PROPS correlates significantly with the LITE measure of exposure to stressors (see Appendix 9.1), with $r = .56$.

Contact Information: Sidran Institute, 200 E. Joppa Road, Suite 207, Towson, MD 21286. Telephone: (410) 825-8888. Fax: (410) 337-0747 or (888) 825-8249. E-mail: sidran@sidran.org. Website: *www.sidran.org*.

APPENDIX 9.6. PTSD-Specific Measures for Adolescents and Young Adults

ADMINISTERED TO ADOLESCENT OR YOUNG ADULT

Reactions of Adolescents to Traumatic Stress Questionnaire (RATS; Bean, Eurelings-Bontekoe, Derluyn, & Spinhover, 2004b)

Brief Description: The RATS, a multicultural self-report measure of PTSD for adolescents exposed to high-magnitude stressors, has been translated into 19 languages. The 22 items were derived from the 17 DSM-IV symptoms of criteria B, C, and D of PTSD, with symptoms B3, C1, C5, D1, and D2 divided into two items each. Each of these symptoms has two components, because division into two related questions makes the intent of each question clearer to respondents. Each item is rated by the adolescent or young adult using three response categories: *Not much*(1), *Some* (2), *Much* (3), and *Very much* (4). Each response category is illustrated with a colored circle that increases in size and changes color from *Not much* (small green circle) to *Very much* (large red circle). Items are written to be readable by 12-year-olds. Each question is written both in English and in another language, because the researchers found that many immigrants had limited knowledge of their own written language but had learned their new language (Dutch, in this case) quickly (Bean, Derluyn, Eurelings-Bontekoe, Broekaert, & Spinhoven, 2006). No written back-translations were made, but the "translated questionnaires were reviewed orally with professional interpreters who were regularly involved in treatment sessions of traumatized adult refugees to control the quality of the translations, to ensure that the original meaning was conveyed in the items, and to attempt to achieve semantic equivalence" (Bean et al., 2006, p. 245). Age range: 12–18 years. Languages available: Amhars, Albans, Arabic, Bandini, Chinese (Mandarin), Croatian, Dari, Dutch, English, French, German, Mongols, Portuguese, Russian, Servo-Croatian, Spanish (presumably European Spanish rather than Central or South American Spanish), Soerani, Somali, and Turkish.

Evidence of Reliability: Internal consistency is excellent for all versions of the RATS, with alphas ranging from .81 to .93 for the different versions (Bean et al., 2006). Test–retest reliability was conducted on a sample of 519 adolescents over a 12-month period, which is an exceedingly long time period for assessing test–retest reliability. Nonetheless, the "stability coefficients" (which kind was not specified) were .63 for the total RATS score, .61 for the Intrusion subscale, .44 for the Numbing/Avoidance subscale, and .55 for the Hyperarousal subscale. These low "coefficients" and the extraordinarily long time between first and second assessments make this test of the stability of the RATS over time of little worth.

Evidence of Validity: Validity of the RATS was assessed among 4 separate, large youth samples: 771 unaccompanied refugee minors in the Netherlands, 1,058 Dutch pupils from schools throughout the Netherlands, 939 Belgian immigrant and refugee adolescents, and 617 Belgian schoolchildren (Bean et al., 2006). The RATS correlated significantly with a measure of exposure to high-magnitude stressors created by the authors, the Stressful Life Events Checklist (SLE; Bean et al., 2004c; see Appendix 9.1), among all four samples (r's ranged from .45 to .52 for the total RATS, from .43 to .53 for the Intrusion scale, from .36 to .44 for the Numbing/Avoidance scale, and from .38 to .45 for the Hyperarousal scale). The RATS consistently demonstrated dose–response relationships. Adolescents who reported exposure to four or more high-magnitude stressors on the SLE were more likely to meet DSM-IV criteria for PTSD according to the RATS (odds ratio [OR] = 8.95, 95% confidence interval [CI] = 7.06–11.35). Those who reported sexual abuse were more likely to meet PTSD criteria (OR = 4.47, 95% CI = 3.57–5.58), as were those who had been separated from their families (OR = 6.18, 95% CI = 5.14–7.42). The RATS was significantly and strongly correlated with the Internalizing scale of the Hopkins Symptom Checklist–37 for Adolescents (HSCL-37A—Bean et al., 2004a; an adaptation of the HSCL-25 of Winokur, Winokur, Rickles, & Cox, 1984) in all four samples (r's ranged from .66 to .79 for the total RATS, from .56 to .70 for the Intrusion scale, from .55 to .67 for the Numbing/Avoidance scale, and .58 to .73 for the Hyperarousal scale). At the same time it correlated significantly but far less strongly with the Externalizing scale of the HSCL-37A (r's ranged from .23 to .33 for the total, from .12 to .23 for the Intrusion scale, from .10 to .27 for the Numbing/Avoidance scale, and from .34 to .40 for the Hyperarousal scale). The authors argue that the lower correlations between the RATS and the Externalizing scale of the HSCL-37A provide evidence of the discriminant validity of the RATS.

Contact Information: Tammy Bean, PhD, Centrum 45, Rijnzichtweg 35, 2342 AX Oegstageest, Netherlands. Telephone: 071-519-1500. E-mail: t.bean@centrum45.nl. All versions of the RATS, along with the manual, and SPSS code for computing scale scores can be downloaded at *www.centrum45.nl/research/amaenggz/ukamtool.php.*

Young Adult Psychiatric Assessment (YAPA; Angold & Costello, 2000)

Brief Description: The YAPA, a modification of the CAPA, is suitable for use with young adults, providing a focus on diagnoses, living situations, relationships, and areas of functioning relevant to this age group (Angold & Costello, 2000). Age range: 18+.

Evidence of Reliability: Evidence of reliability has yet to be published.

Evidence of Validity: Evidence of validity has yet to be published.

Contact Information: Developmental Epidemiology Program, Duke University Medical Center, Attention: Juné Rogers, DUMC Box 3454, Durham, NC 27710. Telephone: (919) 687-4686, extension 273. E-mail: jrogers@psych.duhs.duke.edu.

ADMINISTERED TO CHILD

Acute Stress Checklist for Children (ASC-Kids; Kassam-Adams, 2006)

Brief Description: The ASC-Kids is a 29-item self-report, with 25 items assessing ASD according to DSM-IV criteria: four items assess whether the experience was horrible, frightening, beyond the child or adolescent's control, or the child feared for his or her life; four assess emotional numbing, derealization, and dissociation; 15 items assess the remaining DSM-IV criteria; one item assesses the degree to which the child or adolescent was emotionally upset by the experience; one assesses disruptions to social interaction with meaningful others; two items assess social functioning at school and with the immediate family; one item assesses social support; and one assesses self-perceived coping skill. Most response categories are rated *Never/Not true* (0), *Sometimes/Somewhat* (1), and *Often/Very true* (2). Items rated 2 can be counted as indicating a DSM-IV symptom is present. Symptom category subscales include Dissociation, Reexperiencing, Avoidance, and Overarousal/Anxiety. Age range: 8–17; items should be read to children 9 years and younger, and to any 10- or 11-year-old who appears to require assistance. Languages: English and Spanish.

Evidence of Reliability: Based on the responses of 176 recently injured children and adolescents (mean age = 11.8; Kassam-Adams, 2006), internal consistency alpha for the 19 ASD items (questions 5–23) was .85, whereas it was .86 for all 29 items, and .64 for the Dissociation, .74 for the Reexperiencing, .73 for the Avoidance, and .73 for the Overarousal/Anxiety subscales. Test–retest correlations among 111 children and adolescents over a 1-week period on the 19 ASC-Kids symptom items were .76, and for total 29 items, .83, whereas it was .72 for the Dissociation, .75 for the Reexperiencing, .59 for the Avoidance, and .68 for the Overarousal/Anxiety subscales.

Evidence of Validity: The ASD-Kids total correlated .77 with the CATS (March, Amaya-Jackson, et al., 1997; see Appendix 9.5) PTSD subscale immediately after the injury occurred and .61 among 147 children and adolescents contacted 3 months later, and .37 with the CSDC (Saxe et al., 2003; see Appendix 9.5) caretaker report of the child's ASD symptoms immediately after the injury. Discriminant validity was demonstrated by lower, though significant, correlations of .49 with the Internalizing *T*-score on the YSR (Achenbach, 1991b) and .30 with the Externalizing *T*-score of the YSR. It correlated even less, but still significantly, with the parent report of Internalizing behavior on the CBCL (.23; Achenbach, 1991a) and of Externalizing behavior (.25). Factor analysis resulted in four factors that "correspond fairly well to the four symptom categories" (p. 136) of DSM-IV ASD.

Contact Information: Nancy Kassam-Adams PhD, Children's Hospital of Philadelphia, TraumaLink 3535 10th Floor, 34th Street and Civic Center Boulevard, Philadelphia, PA 19104. Telephone: (215) 590-1000. E-mail: nlkaphd@mail.med.upenn.edu. A listing of the ASC-Kids items can be found in Kassam-Adams (2006).

Angie/Andy Cartoon Trauma Scales (Praver & Pelcovitz, 1996; Praver, Pelcovitz, & DiGiuseppe, 1998)

Brief Description: Based on the cartoon-based child interview, Levonn: A Cartoon-Based Structured Interview for Assessing Young Children's Distress Symptoms (Richters et al., 1990), this interview is a child version of the Structured Interview for Disorders of Extreme Stress (SIDES; this appendix). It contains 44 full-page cartoons illustrating DSM-IV symptomatic responses to high-magnitude stressors plus the additional symptoms associated with complex PTSD (see Table 9.3). As such, it is primarily a measure of reactions to prolonged, repeated abuse; thus, it is probably more appropriate for assessing complex PTSD among young children. However, it does allow assessment of posttraumatic stress symptomatology. Two summary scores are computed: one for Posttraumatic Stress symptoms and the other for Total Associated symptoms. The associated items are relevant for the assessment of complex PTSD in addition to PTSD. See description of the parallel Angie/Andy Parent Rating Scales below for more detail about which associated symptoms are measured. The child rates how often he or she feels like the child in the drawing by using four separate thermometers filled to levels that correspond to responses of *Never, Just a few times, Some of the time,* and *A lot of the time*. Age range: 3 or 4 years to adolescence, depending on verbal ability. May be appropriate for children with lower IQs or learning problems as well.

Evidence of Reliability: Cronbach's alphas ranged from .70 to .95 for the scales (Praver & Pelcovitz, 1996).

Evidence of Validity: Among 208 children in three trauma groups—Intrafamilial Violence, Extrafamilial Violence, and Combined Violence—all scored higher than a nontrauma group on the six scales of the interview (Praver & Pelcovitz, 1996). The number of violence and abuse experiences to which a child was exposed correlated with the six subscales, from .44 to .57. The six subscales correlated from .71 to .81 with the Behavioral Assessment System for Children (BASC; Praver & Pelcovitz, 1996). It also significantly correlated with the BASC Parent Report Scale (*r* = .55). The Posttraumatic Stress scale had a sensitivity of .72 and specificity of .94 when differentiating between chronically traumatized and nontraumatized children (Praver, 1996; Praver, DiGiuseppe, Pelcovitz, Mandel, & Gaines, 2000).

Contact Information: Lisa Ayoung, Multi-Health Systems, P.O. Box 950, North Tonawanda, NY 14120-0950. Telephone: (800) 456-3003. Fax: (888) 540-4484. E-mail: r_d@mhs.com. Website: *www.mhs.com*. Francis Praver, PhD, 5 Marseilles Drive, Locust Valley, NY 11560. Telephone: (516) 671-8531. E-mail: drfranpraver@cs.com.

Structured Interview for Disorders of Extreme Stress Not Otherwise Specified (SIDES; Pelcovitz, van der Kolk, Roth, Mandel, & Kaplan, 1997)

Brief Description: This 48-item interview, which can be administered as a paper-and-pencil self-report measure, assesses the suggested criteria for complex PTSD (also known as disorder of extreme stress not otherwise specified, or

DESNOS). The SIDES was the instrument used to investigate the viability of a separate diagnostic category for complex PTSD during the DSM-IV field trials (Kilpatrick, et al., 1998; van der Kolk et al., 1996). Several questions assess specific symptoms of the domains of complex PTSD. In the domain of alteration in regulation of Affect and Impulses, three questions assess problems with affect regulation in general, four assess problems modulating anger, three assess self-destructive behaviors, one assesses suicidal preoccupation, seven assess difficulty modulating preoccupation with sexual involvement, and one question assesses excessive risk-taking behavior. In the domain of alterations in Attention or Consciousness, one item assesses amnesia and four items assess transient dissociative episodes and depersonalization, and one assesses a sense of ineffectiveness. In the domain of alteration in Self-Perception, one item assesses a sense of ineffectiveness, one assesses a sense of permanent damage to the self, one assesses guilt and responsibility, one assesses shame, one assesses a feeling that nobody can understand, and one item assesses minimizing the traumatic experience(s). In the domain of alterations in Perception of the Perpetrator, one item assesses the adoption of distorted beliefs about the perpetrator, one assesses idealization of the perpetrator, and one assesses preoccupation with hurting the perpetrator. In the domain of alterations in relations with others, three items assess the inability to trust others, one assesses the occurrence of revictimization experiences, and one assesses the tendency to victimize others. In the domain of Somatization, problems with the digestive system and chronic pain are assessed by one question each; cardiopulmonary symptoms are assessed with one item, wherein the respondent can indicate whether any of four different symptoms have been experienced; conversion symptoms are assessed with one item, wherein the respondent can indicate whether any of nine different symptoms have been experienced; and sexual symptoms are assessed with one item, wherein up to four symptoms can be endorsed. In the domain of alterations in Systems of Meaning, three items assess a pessimistic attitude toward the future (also known as a sense of foreshortened future), and two items assess a loss of previously sustaining beliefs. Endorsement of complex PTSD is met when criteria for all scales, except that assessing alterations in perceptions of the perpetrator (see reliability evidence below for details) are met (Pelcovitz et al., 1997).

Evidence of Reliability: In the DSM-IV field trials, a sample of 520 adults was assessed with the SIDES; 395 of the adults were seeking treatment, whereas the rest were from the community; 149 of them had been physically or sexually abused as children; 87 adults were victims of interpersonal abuse as adolescents or adults, 58 witnessed a disaster, and 226 reported on other stressors (Pelcovitz et al., 1997). Cronbach's alphas were .96 for the full scale, .90 for the items assessing alteration in regulation of Affect and Impulses, .76 for alterations in Attention or Consciousness, .77 for alterations in Self-Perception, .53 for alterations in Perception of the Perpetrator, .77 for alterations in Relations with Others, .88 for Somatization, and .78 for alterations in Systems of Meaning. Due to the low internal consistency, the authors did not include the scale intended to assess alterations in Perceptions of the Perpetrator in analyses of validity, and they recommend not requiring evidence for that set of symptoms when assessing complex PTSD. The kappa for interrater reliability for the full scale among 10 raters was .81.

Evidence of Validity: In the DSM-IV field trials (Pelcovitz et al., 1997), endorsement rates were compared between the various abuse groups (see reliability evidence for details). Out of 34 comparisons, differences between the early-onset interpersonal violence group and the disaster group were significant for all but one subscale, Symptoms of Ineffectiveness. Moreover, 23 of 34 differences in endorsement rates between the late-onset interpersonal violence group and the disaster group were significant.

Contact Information: David Pelcovitz, PhD, Azrieli School of Jewish Education, Yeshiva University, 500 West 185th St., New York, NY 10033. Telephone: (212) 960-0196. E-mail: depelcovi@yu.edu.

World View Survey (Fletcher, 1996h; Skidmore & Fletcher, 1997)

Brief Description: The World View Survey, a 50-item paper-and-pencil self-report, assesses important beliefs that may be changed by traumatic experience. The psychometrics of the scale were tested in a sample of 295 college students. Factor analysis (Skidmore & Fletcher, 1997) extracted nine factors, and a secondary factor analysis of these nine factors resulted in two second-order factors. The first factor concerns Trauma Reactive Beliefs and comprises five subscales: (1) Anxious Uncertainty (exemplified by beliefs such as "Life does not seem to make much sense anymore"); (2) Inadequacy (e.g., "I am a jinx"); (3) Dangerous World (e.g., "The world is a dangerous place to live"); (4) Self-Abnegation (e.g., "Sometimes I think I am not a very good person"); and (5) Lack of Control (e.g., "I feel like I have control over my life"—if disagreed with). The second higher-order factor concerns Negative Beliefs and comprises four subscales: (1) Poor Ego-Strength (e.g., "Since I have lived through some bad times, I have a better idea of what is important to me and what is not"); (2) Lack of Personal Empowerment (e.g., "I feel like nothing can keep me from getting what I want out of life anymore"—if disagreed with); (3) Negative Outlook (e.g., "Nowadays I feel like every new day I am alive is a gift"); and (4) Poor Attachment (e.g., "It is easy for me to make friends"—if disagreed with). The total of all items is not used, because the Trauma Reactive scale correlates only moderately with the Negative Beliefs scale ($r = .57$; Skidmore & Fletcher, 1997). Age range: 13 years and older.

Evidence of Reliability: The nine subscales had the following alphas: Anxious Uncertainty, .90; Inadequacy, .85; Dangerous World, .71; Self-Abnegation, .76; Lack of Control, .64; Poor Ego-Strength, .70; Poor Attachment, .74; Lack of Personal Empowerment, .63; and Negative Outlook, .61 (Skidmore & Fletcher, 1997). Alphas were .90 for the Trauma Reactive and .71 for the Negative Beliefs subscales.

Evidence of Validity: Correlations among the five Trauma Reactive subscales with theoretically related measures were all significant, whereas those between the Negative Beliefs scales with these same measures tended to be nonsignificant (Skidmore & Fletcher, 1997), providing further evidence that the two types of scales measure different domains. Thus, the overall Trauma Reactive and Negative Beliefs subscales are correlated .23 ($p < .001$) and .12 ($p < .05$), respectively, with the Young Adults Upsetting Times Checklist (see Appendix 9.1), a measure of exposure to lifetime stress; .34 ($p < .001$) and .02 (ns), respectively, with traumatic reactions as assessed by the IES (Horowitz et al., 1979); .61 ($p < .001$) and .27 ($p < .001$), respectively, with another measure of traumatic reactions derived from the Symptom Checklist–90—Revised (SCL-90-R; Derogatis, 1977; Saunders et al., 1990). Comparisons of scores on the

World View Survey of the 295 college students and 40 adolescent psychiatric inpatients, many of whom had diagnoses of PTSD (Skidmore & Fletcher, 1997), demonstrated that the inpatient adolescents scored significantly higher than the college students on the Trauma Reactive subscale (M = 72.41 ± 14.22 vs. 89.18 ± 16.35) and the Negative Beliefs subscale (M = 38.09 ± 6.84 vs. 42.58 ± 9.94). The inpatient adolescents scored significantly higher than the college students on all five subscales of the Trauma Reactive subscale, but on only two of the four subscales of the Negative Beliefs subscale. The two groups did not differ significantly on the Poor Ego-Strength subscale or on the Negative Outlook subscale.

Contact Information: Kenneth E. Fletcher, PhD, Department of Psychiatry, University of Massachusetts Medical School, 55 Lake Avenue North, Worcester, MA 01655. Telephone: (508) 856-8630. E-mail: kenneth.fletcher@umassmed.edu.

ADMINISTERED TO CARETAKER OR OTHER ADULTS

Angie/Andy Parent Rating Scales (Praver, Pelcovitz, & DiGiuseppe, 1993)

Brief Description: Forty-four items on these scales parallel the Angie/Andy Cartoon Trauma Scales (this appendix), minus the cartoons. As noted in the description for that scale, these two measures were designed to assess reactions to prolonged, repeated abuse; they are therefore more suitable for assessing complex PTSD than simple PTSD in young children. Scales include Attention and Consciousness, Dysregulation of Affect and Impulses, Relations with Others, Self-Perception, Somatization, and Systems of Meaning. Symptoms such as despair, hopelessness, and loss of previously sustained beliefs are included. Two summary scores are also computed: one for Posttraumatic Stress symptoms and one for Total Associated symptoms. Age range: 3 or 4+ years.

Evidence of Reliability: Cronbach's alphas ranged from .75 to .95 for the scales (Praver et al., 1993).

Evidence of Validity: Correlated significantly with the BASC-PRS (r = .71 to .81; Praver, 1996).

Contact Information: Lisa Ayoung, Multi-Health Systems, P.O. Box 950, North Tonawanda, NY 14120-0950. Telephone: (800) 456-3003. Fax: (888) 540-4484. E-mail: r_d@mhs.com. Website: http://www.mhs.com. Frances Praver, PhD, 5 Marseilles Drive, Locust Valley, NY 11560. Telephone: (516) 671-8531. E-mail: drfranpraver@cs.com.

Child Stress Disorders Checklist (CSDC; Saxe, 2004) and Child Stress Disorders Checklist—Screening Form (CSDC-SF; Saxe & Bosquet, 2004)

Brief Description: Unlike most other child PTSD measures to date, the CSDC allows assessment of symptoms of both DSM-IV PTSD and ASD. See full description in Appendix 9.5.

PART V

Developmental Disorders

CHAPTER 10

Autism Spectrum Disorders

Sally Ozonoff
Beth L. Goodlin-Jones
Marjorie Solomon

In this chapter, we review issues and methods relevant to the assessment of autism spectrum disorders (ASDs). We begin with some background about these disorders, including their diagnostic criteria, associated features, developmental course, epidemiology, etiologies, and outcomes. This information is used as a foundation for understanding and evaluating assessment strategies and instruments used with this population of children. Next we provide an overview of the assessment process, common referral questions, and special issues relevant to ASD that must be considered. We then describe the components of a core assessment battery, followed by additional domains that might be considered in a more comprehensive assessment. Domains covered include autism symptomatology, intelligence, language, adaptive behavior, neuropsychological functions, comorbid psychiatric illnesses, and family functioning. Throughout these sections, we discuss the feasibility of particular methods and highlight those that are practical for use in a typical clinical setting. We end with a discussion of the utility of specific instruments for treatment planning and evaluation, outcome assessment, and sensitivity to change.

DIAGNOSTIC CRITERIA

The fourth edition, text revision of the *Diagnostic and Statistical Manual of Mental Disorders* (DSM-IV-TR; American Psychiatric Association [APA], 2000) lists five pervasive developmental disorders (PDDs)[1]: autistic disorder, Asperger's disorder, Rett's disorder, childhood disintegrative disorder, and pervasive developmental disorder not otherwise specified. Symptoms of autistic disorder fall into three domains (see Table 10.1): social relatedness, communication, and behaviors and interests, with delays or abnormal functioning in at least one of these areas evident in children prior to 3 years of age. In the social domain, symptoms include impaired use of nonverbal behaviors (e.g., eye contact, facial expression, gestures) to regulate social interaction, failure to develop age-appropriate peer relationships, little seeking to share enjoyment or interests with other people, and limited social–emotional reciprocity. Communication deficits include delay in or absence of spoken language,

---

[1] This term is used synonymously with ASD in this chapter.

TABLE 10.1. DSM-IV-TR Criteria for Autistic Disorder

DSM-IV-TR symptoms	Examples
Deficits in reciprocal social interaction	
(1a) Difficulty using nonverbal behaviors to regulate social interaction	• Poor eye contact • Little use of gestures while speaking • Few or unusual facial expressions • Unusual intonation or voice quality
(1b) Failure to develop age-appropriate peer relationships	• Lack of interest in peers • Few or no same-age friends • Trouble interacting in groups and following cooperative rules of games
(1c) Little sharing of pleasure, achievements, or interests with others	• Delay in or failure to develop joint attention • Does not point to show • Enjoys activities alone, without involving others
(1d) Lack of social or emotional reciprocity	• Does not respond to others; appears indifferent • Strongly prefers solitary activities • Does not notice when others are hurt or upset; does not offer comfort
Deficits in communication	
(2a) Delay in or total lack of development of language	• No use of words to communicate by age 2 • No simple phrases (e.g., "more milk") by age 3 • After speech develops, immature grammar
(2b) Difficulty holding conversations	• Trouble knowing how to start, maintain, and/or end a conversation • Little back-and-forth; may talk on and on in a monologue • Failure to respond to the comments of others; response only to direct questions • Difficulty talking about topics not of special interest
(2c) Unusual or repetitive language	• Repeating what others say to them (echolalia) • Repeating from videos, books, or commercials at inappropriate times or out of context • Using words or phrases that the child has made up or that have special meaning only to him/her • Overly formal, pedantic style of speaking (sounds like "a little professor")
(2d) Play that is not appropriate for developmental level	• Little acting out scenarios with toys • Rarely pretends an object is something else (e.g., a banana is a telephone) • Prefers to use toys in a concrete manner (e.g., building with blocks, arranging dollhouse furniture) rather than pretending with them • When young, little interest in social games like peekaboo, ring-around-the-rosie, etc.
Restricted, repetitive behaviors, interests, or activities	
(3a) Interests that are narrow in focus, overly intense, and/or unusual	• Very strong focus on particular topics to the exclusion of other topics • Interest in topics that are unusual for age (sprinkler systems, movie ratings, astrophysics, radio station call letters) • Excellent memory for details of special interests • Interference with other activities (e.g., delays eating or toileting due to focus on activity)
(3b) Unreasonable insistence on sameness and following familiar routines	• Wants to perform certain activities in an exact order (e.g., close car doors in specific order) • Need for advanced warning of even minor changes • Becomes highly anxious and upset if routines or rituals not followed

(continued)

TABLE 10.1. (continued)

DSM-IV-TR symptoms	Examples
Restricted, repetitive behaviors, interests, or activities (continued)	
(3c) Repetitive motor mannerisms	• Flaps hands when excited or upset • Flicks fingers in front of eyes • Odd hand postures or other hand movements • Spins or rocks for long periods of time
(3d) Preoccupation with parts of objects	• Uses objects in unusual ways (e.g., flicks doll's eyes, repeatedly opens and closes doors on toy car), rather than as intended • Interest in sensory qualities of objects (e.g., likes to sniff objects or look at them closely) • Attachment to unusual objects (orange peel, string)
Onset criteria	• Delays or abnormal functioning must be present before 3 years of age.

Note. From American Psychiatric Association. Copyright 2000 by the American Psychiatric Association. Adapted by permission.

difficulty with conversational reciprocity, idiosyncratic or repetitive language, and imitation and pretend play deficits. In the behaviors and interests domain, there are often encompassing, unusual interests, inflexible adherence to nonfunctional routines, stereotyped body movements, and preoccupation with parts or sensory qualities of objects (APA, 2000). To meet criteria for autistic disorder, an individual must demonstrate at least 6 of 12 symptoms—at least two from the social domain, and one each from the communication and restricted behaviors/interests categories.

Asperger's disorder (or Asperger syndrome, as it is often called) shares the social disabilities and restricted behaviors and interests of autism, but language abilities are well developed and intellectual functioning is not impaired.[2] Symptoms of Asperger syndrome are identical to those just listed for autistic disorder except that there is no requirement that the child demonstrate any difficulties in the second category, communication. The main point of differentiation from autistic disorder, especially the higher-functioning subtype, is that those with Asperger syndrome do not exhibit significant delays in the onset or early course of language. As specified in the DSM-IV-TR, nonechoed, communicative use of single words must be demonstrated by age 2 and meaningful phrase speech, by age 3. Most parents of children with

Asperger syndrome are not concerned about early language development and may even report precocious language abilities, such as a large vocabulary and adult-like phrasing from an early age. Autistic disorder must be ruled out before a diagnosis of Asperger syndrome is justified. DSM-IV-TR mandates that the diagnosis of autism always take precedence over that of Asperger syndrome. Thus, if a child meets criteria for autistic disorder, the diagnosis must be autism even if he or she displays excellent language, average or better cognitive skills, and other "typical" features of Asperger syndrome.

Individuals who meet criteria for autistic disorder and are intellectually normal are considered "high functioning." Research comparing Asperger syndrome and high-functioning autism (HFA) provides mixed evidence of their external validity. Early history differences are evident between the disorders, with children with Asperger syndrome showing fewer and less severe symptoms, and better language in the preschool years than children with HFA, but these group differences are likely artifacts of the diagnostic definitions (Ozonoff, South, & Miller, 2000). Follow-up studies demonstrate similar trajectories in outcome (Ozonoff et al., 2000; Szatmari et al., 2000). Neuropsychological research suggests that the two conditions are more similar than different, and consensus has not been achieved on the validity of their distinction (Howlin, 2003; Macintosh & Dissanayake, 2004). Whether the two conditions are different enough to warrant sepa-

---

[2] Generally defined as IQ scores above 69, although no operational definition exists and other thresholds, such as IQ > 84, are sometimes used.

rate names is of more than academic interest, because resources in many states are provided differentially to children based on the particular autism spectrum diagnosis they receive.

Two other conditions also appear in the DSM-IV-TR PDD category: Rett's disorder and childhood disintegrative disorder. Both involve a period of typical development, followed by a loss of skills and regression in development. The classic symptoms of Rett's disorder, seen primarily in females, include lack of typical social interaction; lack of language; very frequent stereotyped hand movements, including repetitive wringing, "washing," twisting, clapping, or rubbing of the hands in the midline (often leading to lack of functional hand use); unsteady gait; and severe to profound mental retardation. A gene on the X chromosome, *MECP2*, causes most cases of Rett's disorder (Amir et al., 1999).

In childhood disintegrative disorder (CDD), an abrupt and severe regression occurs after at least 2 (and up to 10) years of normal development. After the loss of skills, the child has all the characteristics of severe autism and severe mental retardation. Without taking a history of early development and onset, it is difficult to distinguish between the behavioral phenotype of CDD and autism, and treatments for the two conditions are similar. It is not clear whether the cause(s) of CDD differ from those of autism. There appears to be relatively less improvement over time than occurs in autism, and the condition continues as a chronic, severe, developmental disability throughout life. CDD is a very rare condition, occurring in only 1 in 100,000 individuals (Fombonne, 2002). Given the low incidence of both CDD and Rett's disorder, these conditions are not considered further in this chapter. The interested reader is referred to recent comprehensive reviews for more information (Van Acker, Loncola, & Van Acker, 2005; Volkmar, Koenig, & State, 2005).

The fifth and final condition that falls within the PDD category is pervasive developmental disorder not otherwise specified (PDD NOS). This label is used for children who experience difficulties in at least two of the three autism-related symptom clusters, but who do not meet criteria for any of the other PDDs. The same list of 12 symptoms outlined earlier is used to diagnose PDD NOS, but only one difficulty within the "reciprocal social interaction" domain and one symptom from either the "communication deficits" or "repetitive, restricted behaviors" domains are required. Thus, this is a very heterogeneous category (Walker et al., 2004). Children with PDD NOS demonstrate autistic-like behaviors and difficulties but display either too few symptoms or a different pattern of symptoms than other conditions in the PDD category. For example, a child might be diagnosed with PDD NOS if he displayed only four of the DSM-IV-TR symptoms (ruling out autistic disorder), displayed a delay in language onset (ruling out Asperger syndrome), and showed no regression in development (ruling out both Rett's disorder and CDD). The diagnosis is often misused, with substantial proportions of children carrying this label either meeting full criteria for autism or not meeting criteria for any ASD (Buitelaar, Van der Gaag, Klin, & Volkmar, 1999). Thus, it is always worth reevaluating a child who presents with a diagnosis of PDD NOS made by another clinician or agency, to examine the accuracy of the initial diagnosis.

ASSOCIATED FEATURES

ASDs can co-occur with a variety of other difficulties. Best appreciated is the high comorbidity rate of autism and mental retardation. Most studies have found that the majority of individuals with autism (roughly 75%) are intellectually handicapped, with approximately half of the group functioning in the range of mild to moderate mental retardation, and half in the severe to profound range. However, recent epidemiological investigations focusing on the preschool period found a decrease (down to 25–50%) in the percentage of those with mental retardation (Chakrabarti & Fombonne, 2001; Honda, Shimizu, Misumi, Niimi, & Ohashi, 1996). This trend is consistent with increasing recognition of milder cases. Rising IQ may also reflect the effect of early intervention.

Another commonly associated symptom is seizures. Up to one-third of children with autism develop seizures, although rates tend to be higher in clinic-based studies (e.g., Rossi, Posar, & Parmeggiani, 2000) and may be closer to 10–15% in larger, community-based samples (Tharp, 2004). Seizures are more common in children who have both autism and mental retardation (Danielsson, Gillberg, Billstedt, Gillberg, & Olsson, 2005). Epilepsy onset is often during the preschool years, but there is lack of consensus on whether there is a second peak onset period for seizures after puberty (Danielsson et al., 2005; Rossi et al., 2000).

Other nonspecific abnormalities have been found in children with autism, including dysregulation of both eating and sleeping patterns. Food sensitivities and selective food intake are widely reported and are a cause of significant concern for many parents, although the nutritional and behavioral impact of these patterns is far from clear at this time. It has been hypothesized that allergies to dairy and wheat byproducts may cause or exacerbate symptoms of autism (Erickson et al., 2005), but insufficient empirical study has been conducted to evaluate the validity of such hypotheses. Several studies have found that sleep problems in ASD are approximately double (55%) or higher the prevalence in typically developing children and adolescents (Honomichl, Goodlin-Jones, Burnham, Gaylor, & Anders, 2002; Oyane & Bjorvatn, 2005; Schreck & Mulick, 2000). These findings are consistent across studies that use a variety of methods, including objective measures, such as actigraphy, as well as parental report. However, the impact of the sleep disturbances on daytime functioning in the ASD population is largely unknown (Oyane & Bjorvatn, 2005).

PSYCHIATRIC AND BEHAVIORAL COMORBIDITIES

ASDs can co-occur with a variety of additional psychiatric and behavioral disturbances. Accurate identification of these comorbidities is of great importance for treatment planning and educational interventions. In a study of school-age children who were consecutive cases at an ASD clinic, 85% of those with Asperger syndrome and 65% of those with HFA exhibited clinically significant behavioral and emotional issues (Tonge, Brereton, Gray, & Einfeld, 1999).

Mood and Anxiety Disorders

The most common comorbid conditions in the ASD population are anxiety disorders and depressed mood (Kim, Szatmari, Bryson, Streiner, & Wilson, 2000; Lainhart & Folstein, 1994). There is general agreement that rates are higher than expected (e.g., greater than the 10% lifetime rate in the general population), but epidemiological studies of comorbidity prevalence

have not been done. Risk for anxiety and mood disorders may be especially elevated at the higher functioning end of the autism spectrum (Howlin, Goode, Hutton, & Rutter, 2004; Klin, Pauls, Schultz, & Volkmar, 2005; Towbin, 2005) and may in some cases be secondary to stressful peer interactions and teasing (Howlin et al., 2004; Klin & Volkmar, 1997). In a well-designed study comparing high-functioning children with ASD to a community sample (Kim et al., 2000), individuals with Asperger syndrome and HFA both scored in the clinically concerning range on scales measuring depression (17% of the total sample) and generalized anxiety (13.6% of total). There were no differences between the Asperger syndrome and HFA diagnostic groups in comorbidity rates, but children with higher verbal than nonverbal abilities had more anxiety and mood problems (Kim et al., 2000). Significantly higher rates of phobias and specific fears in children with ASD relative to children with Down syndrome and typical development have also been reported by Evans, Canavera, Kleinpeter, Maccubin, and Taga (2005).

Behavioral Problems

Children with undiagnosed, higher-functioning ASDs are sometimes first identified in a general psychiatry clinic (Towbin, 2005) after referral for nonspecific behavioral problems. Longitudinal studies illustrate that behavior problems are relatively common in children with ASDs, even in higher-functioning individuals. For example, in a large follow-up study of adults with ASD, Ballaban-Gil, Rapin, Tuchman, and Shinnar (1995) found that 69% of participants exhibited behavioral difficulties. Even among individuals with average intelligence, close to half were reported by their families to have behavioral problems. Approximately 25% of individuals with ASD have a history of aggressive outbursts and irritability that bring them to the attention of a mental health clinic (Gillberg & Coleman, 2000). Comorbid mania and bipolar disorder have been described in children with ASD (Frazier, Doyle, Chiu, & Coyle, 2002; Wozniak et al., 1997). Tantum (2003) reported that individuals with Asperger syndrome, like patients with frontal lobe disorders, may experience "catastrophic reactions" or extreme emotional or behavioral responses to apparently ordinary stressors, such as failure or sensory overstimulation. Such reactions can include screaming, shouting, swearing, and/or running away. Levels of irritability, temper tantrums, and defiance comparable to those seen in conduct disorder have been found in samples of children with Asperger syndrome (Gilmour, Hill, Place, & Skuse, 2004; Green, Gilchrist, Burton, & Cox, 2000).

Despite the apparently elevated rate of behavioral and conduct difficulties just described, the vast majority of individuals with ASDs are not violent toward others (Ghaziuddin, Tsai, & Ghaziuddin, 1991). There have been occasional reports of antisocial acts such as fire setting (e.g., Everall & LeCouteur, 1990), but it appears that such behavior is often driven by social naivete and lack of understanding of consequences or social norms. For example, a child with ASD may not realize the necessity of paying for things in a store or appreciate that interest in a member of the opposite sex is unreciprocated.

Attention and Activity Level

Tsai (2000) reported that 60% of individuals with ASD have poor attention and concentration and that 40% are hyperactive. Similarly, Goldstein and Schwebach (2004) completed a retrospective chart review of 27 children with ASD and found that almost 60% met criteria for attention-deficit/hyperactivity disorder (ADHD). In this sample, 26% met the criteria for ADHD combined type and 33% met criteria for ADHD inattentive type. Ghaziuddin, Weidmer-Mikhail, and Ghaziuddin (1998) reported that approximately 30% of individuals with Asperger syndrome meet diagnostic criteria for ADHD. Despite these research reports and the clinical experience of many practitioners, DSM-IV-TR criteria do not permit the diagnosis of ADHD in individuals with ASD. It has been suggested that this exclusion should change in future DSM versions, and many clinicians do diagnose both conditions in the same individual (Frazier et al., 2001; Ghaziuddin, Tsai, & Alessi, 1992), particularly when symptoms that are not part of the autism spectrum, such as hyperactivity, are evident. It is more challenging to distinguish between ASD and the inattentive subtype of ADHD, and the validity of this differential diagnosis has not been adequately studied.

It has been suggested that attention problems in the context of ASD differ qualitatively from those found in ADHD. "Overfocus" of

attention and internal distractibility are said to be more characteristic of ASDs, whereas underfocused attention and distractibility by external events and stimuli are the hallmarks of ADHD (Hendren, 2003; Jensen, Larrieu, & Mack, 1997). It has also been suggested that hyperactivity may be more prominent in children with ASD at younger ages but diminish with age, so that only inattention and distractibility remain in adulthood (Klin, Sparrow, Marans, Carter, & Volkmar, 2000; Tantum, 2003). Others have found that occasionally children present with ASD in preschool but appear to "grow out" of their social symptoms and present later in childhood very much like children with primary ADHD (Fein, Dixon, Paul, & Levin, 2005).

Psychosis

Another psychiatric condition important in the differential diagnosis of ASD is schizophrenia (see McDonell & McClellan, Chapter 11, on early-onset schizophrenia, this volume). For many years, the prevailing belief was that autism and schizophrenia shared a common etiology (Volkmar & Cohen, 1991); in fact, the terms "autism" and "childhood schizophrenia" were used interchangeably for the first several decades after Kanner's (1943) description of the syndrome. More recent research has, however, established clear diagnostic boundaries for autism and schizophrenia, and suggests that they do not co-occur more often than expected by chance. One well-known, large study found only one individual with schizophrenia and autism in a sample of 163 adolescents and adults (Volkmar & Cohen, 1991). In another 22-year prospective follow-up study of 38 individuals with autism, none went on to develop schizophrenia as adults (Mouridsen, Rich, & Isager, 1999).

The differentiation between ASD and psychosis is less clear, however, when considering symptoms that exist on the diagnostic boundaries of both the autism and schizophrenia spectrums. Clinically, it can occasionally be quite challenging to disentangle the ritualistic behaviors, unusual verbalizations, and social withdrawal that are part of autism from signs of psychosis, such as formal thought disorder, delusional beliefs, and affective flattening. Studies have documented signs of formal thought disorder (e.g., illogical statements, loose associations, disorganized thinking) and other negative symptoms of schizophrenia in individuals with ASD (Dykens, Volkmar, & Glick, 1991; Ghaziuddin, Leininger, & Tsai, 1995; Konstantareas & Hewitt, 2001; Van der Gaag, Caplan, van Engeland, Loman, & Buitelaar, 2005). It is not clear whether these are just superficial similarities in presentation or whether a subgroup of individuals with ASD also shows signs of psychosis (Clark, Baxter, Perry, & Prasher, 1999). Several groups have described complicated clinical cases in which symptoms of ASD, such as gross impairments in peer relationships, circumscribed interests, and deficits in conversational reciprocity, exist alongside delusions, paranoia, formal thought disorder, poor attention and impulse control, and affective instability (Kumra et al., 1998; Towbin, Dykens, Pearson, & Cohen; 1993; Van der Gaag et al., 1995). Consistent with this, a National Institute of Mental Health study of 75 children with childhood-onset schizophrenia found that 25% had a lifetime diagnosis of ASD (mostly PDD NOS; Sporn et al., 2004).

DEVELOPMENTAL COURSE

The onset of autistic disorder always occurs before age 3, at two peak periods. The majority of children (approximately two-thirds) display developmental abnormalities within the first 2 years of life. A smaller group of children with autism display a period of normal or mostly normal development, followed by a loss of communication and social skills, and onset of autism (Kurita, 1985). Onset, parental recognition, and clinical diagnosis do not always (or even usually) coincide. The average age of diagnosis of autism is currently right around the third birthday (Lingam et al., 2003; Mandell, Novak, & Zubritsky, 2005). For example, in a large epidemiological study in the United Kingdom, the child's age at the time of first symptom recognition by parents was 18.6 months, age at referral was 32.4 months, and age at diagnosis was 37.8 months (Chakrabarti & Fombonne, 2005). Parents often begin to be concerned when language fails to develop as expected (De Giacomo & Fombonne, 1998). However, several other behavioral differences, particularly social ones, appear to predate the child's language abnormalities that parents report at the time of recognition, including less looking at faces, responding to his or her name,

pointing, and sharing enjoyment and interests with others (Baron-Cohen et al., 1996; Lord, 1995; Osterling & Dawson, 1994; Trevarthen & Daniel, 2005; Wetherby et al., 2004; Wimpory, Hobson, Williams, & Nash, 2000; Zwaigenbaum et al., 2005).

In the regressive pattern of onset, there is a period of normal development, followed by a change in or loss of previously acquired behavior and the onset of autistic symptoms (Kurita, 1985). The average onset of regression is consistently described across studies as between 14 and 24 months of age (Fombonne & Chakrabarti, 2001; Hoshino et al., 1987; Kurita, 1985; Shinnar et al., 2001). Regression typically progresses gradually, although onset can be sudden in a minority of cases. It is important to distinguish between regression and a developmental plateau, in which children fail to progress as expected and do not gain new skills. This form of onset is not considered a regression, because there is no loss of previously acquired skills. Loss of language is the most commonly described and perhaps most salient manifestation of regression (Goldberg et al., 2003; Siperstein & Volkmar, 2004), but even within the communication domain, the nature and extent of loss is heterogeneous. Some children stop talking altogether, whereas others lose only some words and retain others; still others lose only nonverbal means of communication. Virtually all children who lose language lose social behaviors as well, such as eye contact, interest and engagement with others, and social games such as peekaboo (Lord, Shulman, & DiLavore, 2004; Ozonoff, Williams, & Landa, 2005). By definition, the regression that occurs in approximately one-third of children with autistic disorder occurs earlier than that in children with CDD. It is not yet known whether autism and CDD are on a continuum, or whether they differ in important ways other than onset.

The onset of Asperger syndrome and PDD NOS is less well understood. Children with these disorders usually present at older ages (Mandell et al., 2005), and parent report of early development may not be as accurate when more time has passed. Additionally, the symptoms of Asperger syndrome and PDD NOS may be far subtler in preschool than those of autism and difficult to detect even by professionals. In a large sample of children with ASD identified at 2–3 years of age, less than 3% met criteria for Asperger syndrome (McConachie,

Le Couteur, & Honey, 2005). This may reflect that one of the most common symptoms to bring children to early clinical attention is language delay (Mandell et al., 2005), which is an exclusion for the diagnosis of Asperger syndrome. Many parents of children with Asperger syndrome and PDD NOS do retrospectively report social symptoms before age 3, but this criterion is not required by the DSM-IV-TR for a diagnosis of Asperger syndrome or PDD NOS, as it is for autistic disorder. No prospective studies of these higher-functioning forms of ASD have addressed this question, but at present it is assumed that onset is usually early in life for these conditions, too.

ASDs are considered lifelong, chronic conditions. There may be periods of waxing or waning of particular symptoms, and improvement with age and development, however. Some studies suggest that improvement is most marked in preschool and early childhood, with functioning levels remaining stable and sometimes even worsening in adolescence and adulthood (Eaves & Ho, 1996; Sigman & McGovern, 2005). Once diagnosed with an ASD, the vast majority of children retain this diagnosis into adulthood (Gonzalez, Murray, Shay, Campbell, & Small, 1993; Piven, Harper, Palmer, & Arndt, 1996) and present with functional impairment throughout life (Billstedt, Gillberg, & Gillberg, 2005; Howlin, 2003; Seltzer et al., 2003). In a very small proportion of cases, children appear to "grow out of" an ASD diagnosis (Lovaas, 1987; Perry, Cohen, & DeCarlo, 1995), although some do retain difficulties in other areas (Fein et al., 2005). Diagnosis at age 2 is remarkably reliable and stable, with 85–90% of children diagnosed at this age retaining the diagnosis over time (Lord, 1995; Moore & Goodson, 2003; Stone et al., 1999).

There have been several large longitudinal studies of individuals with autism. As summarized by Howlin (2005), outcomes for adults with ASD have improved over the last 25 years. Results of studies conducted after 1980 (e.g., Ballaban-Gil et al., 1995; Howlin, 2003; Kobayashi, Murata, & Yashinaga, 1992; Venter, Lord, & Schopler, 1992) suggest that approximately 20% of adults have good outcomes. Although highly variable across studies, the average percentage of individuals with ASD attending college in these studies was 12%. Enrollment ranged from 0 to 50%, with the highest rates found among those with the highest cognitive abilities. In these same studies, ap-proximately 24% of individuals with ASD were employed. Most of their jobs were relatively menial and included food service, unskilled factory, and warehouse work. Employment stability also was low. Again, individuals with higher cognitive abilities fared better. Some of these individuals secured jobs in the computer and electronics industries. Howlin (2005) also points out that there also has been a drop in individuals with poor outcomes over time, from 65% prior to 1980 to 46% after 1980.

In contrast to the relatively optimistic portrait painted by Howlin's (2005) review, a recent Scandinavian study published the results of a prospective, population-based, follow-up study of 120 individuals diagnosed with autism in childhood (Billstedt et al., 2005). This sample of largely mentally retarded and/or nonverbal individuals was followed 13–22 years after initial contact. The mortality rate was unexpectedly high (5%). The rate of epilepsy was over 40%. Approximately 80% of the sample had poor or very poor outcomes, defined as displaying obvious, severe handicaps, without the possibility of independent living or satisfying social relationships.

Several inferences may be drawn from these studies. First, outcome is highly related to overall cognitive ability. Across all studies conducted to date, the most powerful predictors of outcome continue to be two factors identified over 20 years ago: IQ scores and verbal ability at age 5 (Lotter, 1974; Rutter, 1984). Howlin and colleagues (2004) found that a minimum IQ of 70 was required for a positive outcome. Even above this IQ cutoff, however, outcomes were mixed, with over 40% of individuals having poor or very poor outcomes. Educational, vocational, community, and family supports appear to play an important role in promoting positive adaptation and may be important factors in explaining variability in outcome. For example, the strength of the local economy and availability of vocational assistance programs may impact the employment outlook for persons with autism (Shea & Mesibov, 2005). Finally, it is important to remember that longitudinal studies of the least severely impaired individuals on the autism spectrum have not yet been undertaken. Given their lack of language delay, these individuals may be diagnosed later in life, and not in time to be included in longitudinal studies. Additionally, the availability of high-quality, intensive early intervention has increased in the last decade, and children who were provided such treatment have not yet reached adulthood. For these reasons, we really do not yet know what "best outcomes" for ASD may be and how often they might be achieved. It is important for clinicians to represent accurately our current state of knowledge about outcome as they counsel families over time, and not inadvertently dampen their hopes, aspirations, and enthusiasm for interventions.

EPIDEMIOLOGY

Early research suggested that autism (strictly defined, meeting full criteria for the disorder) occurred at the rate of 4–6 affected individuals per 10,000 (Lotter, 1966; Wing & Gould, 1979). An influential study in the mid-1980s broadened diagnostic criteria somewhat, and found a rate of 10 per 10,000 in a total population screening of a circumscribed geographical region in Canada (Bryson, Clark, & Smith, 1988). Newer studies that have utilized standardized diagnostic measures of established reliability and validity employed active ascertainment techniques. These surveys have given prevalence estimates of 60–70 per 10,000 or approximately 1 in 150 across the spectrum of autism, and 1 in 500 for children with the full syndrome of autistic disorder (Chakrabarti & Fombonne, 2001). One obvious reason for the rise in rates is that more recent research has examined all ASDs, whereas early surveys looked only at rates of strictly defined autism. However, in studies that have broken down the rates by specific PDD subtypes, it is clear that the prevalence of classic autism itself is higher. Chakrabarti and Fombonne (2001) reported a rate of 16.8 per 10,000 for autistic disorder, which is three to four times higher than the rate suggested in the 1960s and 1970s, and over 1.5 times the rate reported in the 1980s and 1990s. Thus, ASDs are no longer rare conditions, and it is likely that many or most practitioners will encounter individuals with suspected ASD in their practices.

Several reasons for the rising prevalence rates have been proposed, from methodological artifacts to newly emerging environmental and biological risk factors. The first category includes increased awareness among clinicians and the general public, better identification and referral practices, more sensitive diagnostic tools, broader classification systems, and more active methods of case ascertainment in epidemiological studies. No doubt, the ability of clinicians to identify more subtle manifestations of ASD and to discriminate between autism and mental retardation has improved; it is also clear that the DSM-IV-TR diagnostic system casts a broader net than previous classification systems. Diagnostic criteria and methods of ascertainment (e.g., active case finding vs. registry screening) have also influenced estimates of prevalence (Kielinen, Linna, & Moilanen, 2000). Whether changes in referral, case ascertainment, and diagnostic criteria alone can account for the large increase is uncertain, and hypotheses abound about environmental factors that may have emerged in the last few decades to put infants and young children at greater risk for developing autism. These are covered, along with other etiological factors, in the next section.

Very few studies have examined the prevalence of autism as a function of race and ethnic group. It has occasionally been suggested that the rate of ASD is higher in immigrant than in native populations (Gillberg, Steffenburg, & Schaumann, 1991). For example, one study observed an elevated rate of autism in immigrants from Pakistan to the United Kingdom (Morton, Sharma, Nicholson, Broderick, & Poyser, 2002), suggesting that the increase was due to high (60%) rates of consanguinity. However, a large California study with a similar database analysis of the prevalence rate of autism across race and ethnic groups (white, Hispanic, black, Asian, or other) described the rates as very similar during an 8-year period (Croen, Grether, Hoogstrate, & Selvin, 2002). Fombonne (2005) suggests that there is no relationship between ethnicity or race and ASD in large studies with adequate sampling and statistical control.

Kanner (1943), who provided the first description of autism, was the first to identify the much greater preponderance of affected boys. A meta-analysis suggests that the widely reported 4:1 ratio of boys to girls is quite consistent across studies, geographical regions, ethnicities, and time (Fombonne, 2003). Sex differences in autism have received little attention except for the purpose of examining differences in prevalence. Of the few studies, most describe greater severity in females. For example, studies of intelligence consistently report lower IQ (Kurita, Osada, & Miyake, 2004;

Tsai, Stewart, & August, 1981; Volkmar, Szatmari, & Sparrow, 1993) and mental age (Pilowsky, Yirmiya, Shulman, & Dover, 1998) in females than in males with autism. Other studies have reported more pronounced behavioral abnormalities in females with autism (Steinhausen & Metzke, 2004). Some investigators have suggested that females with autism have a different phenotype and present with different referral issues than boys (Gillberg & Rastam, 1992; Kopp & Gillberg, 1992), but this position is controversial and has not been studied enough. More attention to the area of gender differences in prevalence, presentation, functioning, treatment needs, and outcome is clearly needed (Koenig & Tsatsanis, 2005; Thompson, Caruso, & Ellerbeck, 2003).

ETIOLOGIES

Kanner suggested that children with autism are born with "an innate inability to form the usual, biologically provided affective contacts with people" (Kanner, 1943, p. 250). Later, however, his thinking came into line with that of his contemporaries trained in the psychoanalytic tradition that was predominant at the time. He and others suggested (incorrectly) that autism was the result of inadequate nurturance by emotionally cold, rejecting parents (Bettelheim, 1967), a theory that prevailed until the late 1960s. Rimland (1964) did a tremendous service to the field when he provided powerful arguments that autism had an organic etiology. It is now clear that biological mechanisms produce brain changes that lead to the symptoms of autism. There are no viable social–environmental hypotheses of autism etiology.

Genetic factors play a strong role in the development of autism (Bailey et al., 1995; Veenstra-Vanderweele, Christian, & Cook, 2004). The recurrence risk for autism after the birth of one child with the disorder is at least 3–6% (Bailey, Palferman, Heavey, & LeCouteur, 1998) and perhaps as high as 10–15% (Zwaigenbaum et al., 2005), far exceeding that of the general population rate. The concordance rate for autism in monozygotic (MZ) twins is greatly elevated relative to that for dizygotic (DZ) twins. The most recent twin studies, which used standardized diagnostic measures and total population screening, found concordance rates for strictly defined au-

tistic disorder of 60% in MZ pairs (up to 90% concordance for broader ASD symptoms), but only 5% in DZ pairs (Bailey et al., 1998). These figures yield a heritability estimate greater than .90 for ASD (Bailey et al., 1995; Le Couteur et al., 1996). There is also evidence of familial transmission of an extended set of cognitive and social anomalies that are milder than, but qualitatively similar to, autism (the so-called "broader autism phenotype"; Bailey et al., 1998). Family members also have higher than average rates of anxiety and affective disorders, and learning disabilities. Collectively, these features of the broader autism phenotype have been found in 15–45% of family members of people with ASD (Bailey et al., 1998).

Advances in the molecular genetics of autism have been rapid, but the results so far are inconclusive. One reason is that the inheritance pattern appears far from simple, with statistical models suggesting that several, and perhaps as many as 10, genes are involved in conferring susceptibility (Pickles et al., 1995; Risch et al., 1999). Case reports have demonstrated a link between autism and a wide variety of chromosomal anomalies, with one review (Gillberg, 1998) reporting associations with all but three chromosomes. It is not yet clear which associations are random and which may provide clues about etiology. The one cytogenetic abnormality that has been consistently replicated in a small proportion of children with autism is a duplication of material on chromosome 15 (Rutter, 2000).

Twin studies also make it clear that autism is not a purely genetic disorder, since the concordance rate for identical twins falls short of 100%, and there can be tremendous phenotypic variability even among MZ twins. The search for nongenetic factors that influence the development and severity of autism is intense and has received much media attention. It has been suggested that environmental factors, including immunizations, heavy metal or pesticide exposures, viral agents, and food products, may interact with genetic susceptibility to trigger autism, to cause it alone, or to mediate the expression and severity of the disorder (Hornig & Lipkin, 2001). The potential environmental etiological agent that has received the most attention is immunization. Wakefield and colleagues (1998) described a case series of 12 children with gastrointestinal disturbances that were reported to begin around the time that autistic behaviors became evident. He postulated that these children had a new subtype of "regressive autism" induced by the measles–mumps–rubella (MMR) vaccination. The postulated mechanism was a persistent measles virus infection resulting in damage to the intestinal lining, increased permeability, and absorption of toxic peptides that caused central nervous system dysfunction and behavioral regression. Recent studies do not support this hypothesis, however. Taylor and colleagues (1999, 2002) identified 498 children with autism, born since 1979, and linked clinical records to independently recorded immunization data. No evidence of a change in trend in incidence or age at diagnosis was associated with the introduction of the MMR vaccine in 1988. Other recent studies that have examined large cohorts of children born in Japan and Denmark failed to find any increase in vaccinated relative to unvaccinated children, and any temporal clustering of autism cases after immunization (Honda, Shimizu, & Rutter, 2005; Madsen et al., 2002).

A related hypothesis about environmental risks for autism concerns mercury exposure, through either environmental exposures or thimerosal, an ethyl-mercury-based preservative included in some vaccines to prevent bacterial contamination. MMR, polio, and varicella vaccines have never contained thimerosal, but it was included in other, multiple-use vaccines since the 1930s. Concerns have been raised recently that the cumulative exposure to ethyl-mercury, via thimerosal, is far greater now than in the past, due to the increased number of vaccines given to children before age 2. This controversial theory has provoked strong reactions on both sides, but current scientific evidence does not clearly support a link between autism and thimerosal exposure (Madsen et al., 2003).

Several decades of research have demonstrated conclusively that the brains of people with autism are both structurally and functionally different from normal. Kanner's original description (1943) noted unusually large head size in a proportion of children, and macrocephaly (head circumference > 97th percentile) has been confirmed in approximately 20% of individuals with autism (Fombonne, Roge, Claverie, Courty, & Fremolle, 1999; Lainhart et al., 1997). The increase in head volume reflects an increase in brain volume, which is not apparent at birth but is present by the first birthday (Courchesne, Carper, & Akshoomoff, 2003) and is hypothesized to be due to both

overgrowth and the failure of normal pruning mechanisms (Piven et al., 1996). Recent studies have suggested that excessive growth may be followed by a period of abnormally slow or arrested growth later in childhood (Courchesne, 2004), although not all studies support this conclusion.

Aside from macrocephaly, structural neuroimaging studies have yielded inconsistent results, possibly stemming from methodological issues: small samples, inappropriate or no control groups, and inconsistent use of covariates, such as gender, IQ, and total brain volume, in statistical analyses. Studies have demonstrated decreased volume of the cerebellar vermis, particularly lobules VI and VII (Courchesne, Yeung-Courchesne, Press, Hesselink, & Jernigan, 1988), but this finding has not always been replicated by other research teams (Hardan, Minshew, Harenski, & Keshavan, 2001; Piven, Bailey, Ranson, & Arndt, 1997). Bauman and Kemper (1985, 1988) published seminal findings of normal volume but smaller neuron size and increased cell density in the amygdala and several other brain regions of autopsied brains of people with autism. More studies have found abnormalities of amygdala volume, including both increased (Howard et al., 2000; Sparks et al., 2002) and decreased size (Abell et al., 1999; Aylward et al., 1999; Pierce, Mueller, Ambrose, Allen, & Courchesne, 2001). More recently, Schumann and colleagues (2004) reported that group differences in amygdala volume may be related to age. They found larger volume in children under age 12.5 years with autism than in controls, but no difference in amygdala volume between adolescents over age 12.5 with autism and typical controls.

Structural magnetic resonance imaging (MRI) results are variable across studies and do not point to any signature abnormality characteristic of ASD. Because regional volumetric changes do not directly measure brain function, they are not the most sensitive index of the brain-level mechanisms operative in ASD. Functional brain imaging studies have more consistently demonstrated differences in samples of children with autism. In activation studies that examine brain regions used during performance of specific tasks, several research groups have found that individuals with autism show reduced or different patterns of brain activity than do controls. In one study in which participants had to identify facial expressions of emotion, those with autism activated the fusiform gyrus (part of the temporal lobes), the left amygdala, and the left cerebellum significantly less than did controls (Critchley et al., 2000). Other researchers have found reduced or absent activation of similar brain regions in children with autism during social reasoning tasks (Baron-Cohen et al., 1999; Schultz et al., 2000).

In summary, it is now abundantly clear that early psychogenic theories of etiology have no merit and that ASDs have biological underpinnings. There is ample evidence that the disorder is genetically influenced and that the brain is both structurally and functionally different, but specific causes (e.g., particular genes or brain defects) are not yet clear, and there is likely to be substantial etiological heterogeneity among affected individuals. In the remainder of the chapter, we examine concepts and methods relevant to the evaluation of individuals with ASD.

ASSESSMENT OF ASDs

Specific practice parameters for the assessment of ASD have been published by the American Academy of Neurology (Filipek et al., 2000), the American Academy of Child and Adolescent Psychiatry (Volkmar, Cook, Pomeroy, Realmuto, & Tanguay, 1999), and a consensus panel with representation from multiple professional societies (Filipek et al., 1999). These practice parameters describe two levels of screening/evaluation. Level 1 screening involves routine developmental surveillance by providers of general services for young children, such as pediatricians. Level 2 evaluation involves a comprehensive diagnostic assessment by experienced clinicians for children who fail the initial screening (Filipek et al., 1999, 2000; Volkmar et al., 1999). These publications have been significant milestones in the field of autism, because they provide, for the first time, consensus guidelines for ASD assessment. We cover Level 2 evaluation in this chapter.

Special Issues in Assessment of ASDs

Several important considerations should inform the assessment process. First, a developmental perspective must be maintained (Burack, Iarocci, Bowler, & Mottron, 2002). Autism is a lifelong disorder. It is first diag-

nosed in early childhood and continues to be apparent throughout a person's life. It is characterized by unevenness in development that differs over the lifespan of the individual. Studying a child within a developmental framework provides a benchmark for understanding the severity and quality of delays and/or deficits. Delays in one developmental achievement can significantly impact the acquisition of later developmental milestones, such as when early levels of joint attention (i.e., focus on an object shared with another person) predict later language acquisition (Mundy, Sigman, & Kasari, 1990) and theory of mind abilities (Baron-Cohen, 1991). Autism symptoms are usually at their worst in preschool and may substantially improve over time. Children who have very poor eye contact and make few social initiations at this age may have quite different social symptoms when they are teenagers. They may be somewhat more interested in social engagement by this later stage and may have acquired some more advanced social skills. Their social difficulties may now be manifest as awkwardness or inappropriateness rather than the lack of interest seen in young childhood. Thus, the form and quality of symptoms change with age. There are also characteristic patterns of delays in ASD that differ across domain and developmental levels. For example, a child with autism may have meaningful expressive language, a large vocabulary, and adequate syntactic abilities but not be able to participate in a conversation or even adequately answer questions.

A second important consideration is that the evaluation of a child with ASD should include information from multiple sources and contexts, because symptoms of ASD may be dependent on characteristics of the environment. For example, children with HFA and Asperger syndrome may present as charming, precocious, and highly intelligent when provided with one-on-one attention and conversational scaffolding from a well-meaning adult professional. The same child may look much more symptomatic with peers on a playground or in a distracting classroom situation, where individual adult attention is unavailable. Conversely, children with severe learning and behavioral deficits may seem much more competent in a known environment, such as the classroom, than in an evaluation room without familiar, well-practiced routines. Thus, parent and teacher reports; child observation across settings; cognitive and adaptive behavior assessments; and clinical judgments may all be part of the most comprehensive ASD assessment (Filipek et al., 1999).

Third, it is recommended that assessments of ASD be multidisciplinary whenever possible, including professionals from psychology, speech–language pathology, and medical specialties as needed (e.g., pediatrics, psychiatry, neurology). On interdisciplinary teams, it is important that one member act as the evaluation coordinator. The person in this role communicates with parents and referring professionals before the evaluation to understand the referral questions, organizes appropriate team members, plans the components of the assessment, establishes contact with the service providers in the community who will implement the recommendations from the evaluation, and perhaps monitors later treatment. This type of coordination is critical for the successful outcome of an evaluation.

Common Referral Questions

As one might expect, the types of concerns that prompt clinical referrals depend on both the age and cognitive abilities of the child. Concerns about language development in toddlers constitute the most common reason for referral (DeGiacomo & Fombonne, 1998). Parental concerns about a toddler's hearing and lack of response to his or her name or verbal commands are also frequent reasons for referral for assessment of ASD. In school-age children, the most frequent reasons for referral revolve around unexpected academic and social problems.

Children with ASD frequently present with academic underperformance. Although some of them may be quite bright, their cognitive profiles are usually uneven (Stewart, 2002). They tend to have spared rote memory, mechanical, and visual–spatial processes and deficient higher-order conceptual processes such as abstract reasoning (Minshew, Goldstein, & Siegel, 1997). Children with ASD who have average cognitive ability may do well in early elementary grades, when success relies largely on vocabulary, reading decoding, simple reading comprehension, and rote memorization. Some children, especially those who possess a great deal of knowledge about specific topics and who display adult-like language with advanced vocabulary, may be perceived as intellectually gifted; only some of these children will actually perform in the superior range of intelligence on

an IQ test, however. When abstract reasoning becomes a more important part of academic work (approximately in fourth grade), children with ASD exhibit greater than anticipated problems with reading comprehension, understanding the "gist" of written and verbally presented material, math concepts that rely on abstract principles, and organizational skills. At this juncture, their academic performance decline may confuse parents and teachers. The children may present with internalizing or externalizing problems symptomatic of stress due to increased academic challenges (Goodlin-Jones & Solomon, 2003). Referral to a psychologist or neuropsychologist can help to illuminate the exact nature of the child's strengths and weaknesses, and assist those working with the child to adjust their expectations and the academic program accordingly. Suggestions for educational accommodations and other considerations related to school environments may be found in Ozonoff, Dawson, and McPartland (2002).

Impairments in reciprocal social interaction are among the defining features of ASD; thus, social issues and peer problems comprise another common set of presenting problems. Everyday social interactions that require "give and take" (i.e., maintaining friendships, solving social problems, responding to others empathically, and having mutually enjoyable conversations) are challenging for children with ASD. As discussed earlier in the section "Behavioral Problems," these children also may have difficulty managing frustration and anger, creating additional obstacles to interpersonal relationships.

A third type of referral question revolves around differential diagnosis. As discussed earlier, there is both overlap between the symptoms of ASD and the symptoms of other conditions (e.g., social withdrawal that is a part of autism, some anxiety disorders, and schizophrenia), and comorbidity between ASD and other psychiatric disorders. Thus, referral questions are sometimes explicitly related to differential diagnosis (e.g., Is it ASD or ADHD or both?), whereas at other times, the need to distinguish conditions is inherent in the referral (e.g., What is the appropriate diagnosis for this child?). Differential diagnosis within the autism spectrum is another common referral question (Is it HFA or Asperger syndrome?).

Another reason for referral is to determine appropriate treatments given a child's unique combination of strengths and weaknesses, both for symptoms of autism and for the associated problems that often co-occur, such as eating, sleeping, behavior, and discipline problems. Related to this is the referral to evaluate progress and response to treatment.

In the sections below, we discuss assessment approaches that address these common referral questions. First, we describe the components of a "core" assessment battery necessary for almost any referral concern (diagnosis, treatment planning, annual or other regularly scheduled assessment, evaluation of treatment progress, program admission or discharge, eligibility for entitlements, etc.). Then we discuss other domains that might be part of a more comprehensive assessment and/or necessary for a particular individual, depending on the referral question and/or evaluation goals.

A Core Autism Assessment Battery

The first step of the core assessment process is to review with parents the child's early developmental history and their current concerns. The critical aspects of this history taking are reviews of communication, social, and behavioral development; additionally, brief screening of potential medical and psychiatric issues, such as anxiety and depression, should be conducted at this stage to determine the need for more detailed evaluation (possibly including referral to specialists). A review of available records (e.g., medical, school, previous testing, intervention reports) rounds out the history-taking aspect of the evaluation. Combined with this review is direct observation of and interaction with the child. Whenever feasible, teachers should be consulted to provide their observations about the child's functioning in the less structured, socially challenging school setting.

Autism Diagnostic Measurement

There is general agreement in North America and Europe on the primary characteristics of autism, as evidenced by close overlap of the diagnostic criteria laid out in DSM-IV-TR and the 10th edition of the International Classification of Diseases (ICD-10) (Sponheim, 1996). All professional practice parameters state the necessity of collecting data from both parents (i.e., interviews) and the child (i.e., observation and direct testing; Filipek et al., 1999, 2000; Volkmar et al., 1999), ideally using the types of standardized instruments we review below. In the relatively short observation of the child that

is feasible in most clinical settings, the full range of difficulties he or she experiences will likely not be evident, so parent report is vital. Parents, however, do not have the professional expertise and experience to recognize or interpret all difficulties, so observation and testing by informed practitioners in a controlled setting are also necessary. The information gained from these sources can then be integrated into a diagnosis. We describe the parent report, then the direct assessment tools available for use in the diagnosis of ASD.

Clinical impression, oral traditions, and subjective observations dominated the assessment process of ASD until fairly recently (Klinger & Renner, 2000). Use of standard diagnostic criteria, and recognition and interpretation of symptoms differed across settings (university clinics, private practice settings, research projects). The publication of two standardized assessment tools—the parent interview, Autism Diagnostic Interview—Revised (Lord, Rutter, & LeCouteur, 1994; Rutter, LeCouteur, & Lord, 2003) and the performance-based Autism Diagnostic Observation Schedule (ADOS; Lord et al., 2000)—have ended many of these disparities and are currently considered "gold standards" for diagnosis of ASD. Use of these and other tools described below has advanced scientific progress and improved the accuracy and reliability of diagnostic assessment (Filipek et al., 1999).

PARENT INTERVIEWS AND QUESTIONNAIRES

The Autism Diagnostic Interview—Revised (ADI-R; Lord et al., 1994; Rutter et al., 2003) is a comprehensive parent interview that probes for symptoms of autism. It is administered by a trained clinician using a semistructured interview format. The "long" version of the ADI-R requires approximately 3 hours for administration and scoring, and is used primarily for research purposes. A short form of the ADI-R, which includes only the items on the diagnostic algorithm, may be used for clinical assessment and takes less time, approximately 90 minutes (Lord et al., 1994). The use of the ADI-R for research purposes requires attending a 3-day training seminar by a certified trainer and completion of reliability testing with the developers of the instrument. Training to use the ADI-R as a clinical tool is also available; it is helpful, but not required, for routine use by practitioners who do not participate in research protocols.

The ADI-R elicits information from the parent on current behavior and developmental history. It is closely linked to the diagnostic criteria set forth in the DSM-IV-TR and ICD-10. The significant developmental time point on the ADI-R is age 4 to 5 years for most behaviors. The rationale for the focus on this age period is that children are old enough to provide an adequate range of behavior but young enough not to have undergone major changes that may occur with age (Lord et al., 1994). The items that empirically distinguish between children with autism and those with other developmental delays are summed into three algorithm scores measuring social difficulties, communication deficits, and repetitive behaviors. The algorithm scores discriminate well between autism and other developmental disorders, such as severe receptive language disorders (Mildenberger, Sitter, Noterdaeme, & Amorosa, 2001) and general developmental delays (Cox et al., 1999; Lord et al., 1994). There are no thresholds yet established for other autism spectrum disorders (e.g., Asperger syndrome or PDD NOS).

The ADI-R is a very helpful tool, but it does have some limitations. Because it is not sensitive to differences among children with mental ages below 20 months or IQs below 20 (Cox et al., 1999; Lord, 1995), it is not advised for use with such children. Its sensitivity to the milder ASDs in children (Asperger syndrome and PDD NOS) is low early in the preschool period (McConachie et al., 2005) but improves by age 4. It is not designed to assess change through repeated administrations and is best suited to confirm the initial diagnosis of autism (Arnold et al., 2000). Finally, and perhaps most importantly, it is labor intensive and requires more administration time than most practitioners can spend. The Social Communication Questionnaire (SCQ, formerly known as the Autism Screening Questionnaire or ASQ; Berument, Rutter, Lord, Pickles, & Bailey, 1999; Rutter, Bailey, & Lord, 2003) is a short parent report questionnaire based on the ADI-R. It contains the same questions included on the ADI-R algorithm, presented in a briefer, yes–no format that parents can complete on their own in 10 minutes or less. Its agreement with the more labor-intensive ADI-R on diagnostic categorization is high (Bishop & Norbury, 2002); thus, it is an efficient way to obtain information from parents about autism symptoms. Two versions are available—one for current behavior and the other for lifetime behavior. The life-time version is recommended for diagnostic purposes, whereas the current version is more appropriate for assessment of change over time in an individual. A cutoff score of 15 differentiates between ASD and other diagnoses for children age 4 years and older, whereas a cutoff of 22 discriminates between children with autistic disorder and those with other ASDs (PDD NOS or Asperger syndrome). Using these cutoffs, sensitivity of .85 and specificity of .75 have been reported in a large sample of children and adults with autism and other developmental disorders (Berument et al., 1999). In summary, this measure, which has excellent psychometric properties, is useful for treatment monitoring, is feasible for use in general clinical settings, and is highly recommended.

The Autism Behavior Checklist (ABC; Krug, Arick, & Almond, 1988), an informant report questionnaire, was once widely used in both clinics and schools, but is based on conceptualizations of ASD that are no longer current (e.g., emphasizing sensory dysfunction and motor stereotypies). Several studies have demonstrated that the rate of both false positives and false negatives produced by the ABC is quite high and that most children with HFA or Asperger syndrome are not identified by the cutoff of 67 (Sevin, Matson, Coe, Fee, & Sevin, 1991; Sponheim & Spurkland, 1996; Volkmar et al., 1988; Wadden, Bryson, & Rodger, 1991). Therefore, it is not recommended for use.

The Modified Checklist for Autism in Toddlers (M-CHAT; Dumont-Mathieu & Fein, 2005; Robins, Fein, Barton, & Green, 2001) is a 23-item parent checklist designed to be used at well-baby 24-month visits to screen quickly for symptoms of autism. There are six critical items on the M-CHAT (pointing, following a point, response to name, showing, interest in other children, imitation); any child who fails two or more requires a more comprehensive evaluation. The sensitivity (.87) and specificity (.99) of this instrument are quite impressive, but the original population-based sample has not been followed long enough to gauge the false-negative rate. As discussed in a later section, the M-CHAT's predecessor, the CHAT, appeared to be an excellent screening measure in initial studies with short follow-up periods, only to demonstrate a high rate of failed identification once the population was rescreened in middle childhood. Thus, it is not yet possible to evaluate fully the utility of this measure. In particular, low scores that are not consistent with parent concerns or clinical judgment may represent false negatives. Therefore, this instrument should not be used as the sole measure of parent report about autism symptoms.

The Gilliam Autism Rating Scale (GARS; Gilliam, 1995), another informant-report instrument that has rapidly come into wide use in schools and diagnostic clinics, is appropriate for rating the behavior of children and young adults ages 3–22 years. It consists of four subscales measuring Social Interaction, Communication, Stereotyped Behaviors, and Developmental Disturbances. Ratings made on a 4-point scale are summed and converted to standard scores based on the reference sample (but not broken down by age or gender). The primary score of interest is the Autism Quotient, which is intended to measure "the likelihood that a child has autism" (Gilliam, 1995). Reference data are from over 1,000 North American children with informant-reported (but not verified) diagnoses of autism. Enthusiasm for the GARS stems from its ease of use, its recent norms, and its explicit relationship to DSM-IV-TR symptoms. However, the only two reports of the psychometric properties of the GARS both raise significant questions about its utility. In a sample of children with autism, verified by ADI-R, ADOS, and expert clinical consensus, over half were rated as having below average or very low likelihood of autism by the GARS in one study (sensitivity of .48; South et al., 2002). This high false-negative rate was replicated in the second study (Lecavalier, 2005) and is seriously troubling, because it may result in many missed diagnoses when used by practitioners with little ASD expertise. Therefore, the GARS, in its current form, is not recommended for routine clinical use.

The Parent Interview for Autism (PIA; Stone, Coonrod, Pozdol, & Turner, 2003) is an instrument developed specifically for the purpose of measuring change in autistic symptomatology over time. It is appropriate for preschool children ages 2–6. It has good internal consistency and is able to differentiate between autism and nonautism developmental delays (Stone et al., 2003). Change in PIA scores after 2 years of intervention correlated highly with clinical ratings of behavioral and diagnostic improvement (Stone et al., 2003). Another informant report instrument developed to measure behavioral change in response to treatment is the PDD Behavior Inventory (Cohen & Sudhalter, 2005). Norms exist for children ages 1.5 to 12.5 years. The questionnaire covers both autism symptoms and adaptive and maladaptive behaviors that might be altered by treatment. It demonstrates a high degree of internal consistency, provides adequate test–retest reliability (Cohen, Schmidt-Lackner, Romanczyk, & Sudhalter, 2003), and correlates highly with both the ADI-R and the Childhood Autism Rating Scale (CARS; Cohen, 2003). These measures appear both feasible and useful for practitioners who wish to track the progress of patients enrolled in treatment programs.

ASPERGER SYNDROME DIAGNOSTIC TOOLS

The differential diagnosis of HFA and Asperger syndrome is both difficult and of questionable nosological validity (Miller & Ozonoff, 2000; Prior, 2000). While at one time it was proposed that individuals with Asperger syndrome differed from those with autism in several meaningful ways (Klin, Volkmar, Sparrow, Cicchetti, & Rourke, 1995; Ozonoff, Rogers, & Pennington, 1991), research has largely failed to confirm this, and most studies conclude that the two are more similar than different (Howlin, 2003). Differences, when present, are most distinct in early childhood (Ozonoff et al., 2000), and the two conditions appear to converge phenomenologically at older ages (Howlin, 2003; Starr, Szatmari, Bryson, & Zwaigenbaum, 2003). This conclusion has not yet been incorporated into clinical practice, however, and many clinicians are convinced that the two are distinct conditions.

Asperger syndrome was included for the first time in DSM-IV (APA, 1994). As described at the beginning of the chapter, Asperger syndrome is differentiated from autism in DSM-IV-TR primarily by age of onset of speech. Precedence is given to the diagnosis of autism, so if an individual meets criteria for both conditions, autistic disorder is the diagnosis that must be made. Prior to DSM-IV, clinical and research diagnoses were made according to a variety of different proposed criteria. Diagnostic assignment (HFA vs. Asperger syndrome) was highly dependent on which diagnostic criteria were used (Ghaziuddin, Tsai, & Ghaziuddin, 1992; Klin, Pauls, Schultz, & Volkmar, 2005), complicating significantly the interpretation of research conducted before DSM-IV. Despite the appeal of the standardized criteria for Asperger syndrome outlined in DSM-IV-TR, there has been dissatisfaction with it on several grounds, particularly the narrowness of the criteria that lead to even Asperger's original cases meeting criteria for autism when applied rigorously (Miller & Ozonoff, 2000; see also Woodbury-Smith, Klin, & Volkmar, 2005 for a different perspective). In clinical practice, it appears that DSM-IV-TR criteria are often ignored, with Asperger syndrome used synonymously with autism without mental retardation or autism without language delay (Klin et al., 2005; Mayes, Calhoun, & Crites, 2001).

In recent years, several parent report measures have been developed to assist with the Asperger syndrome diagnosis, but all suffer from the current lack of consensus in the field about the definition and boundaries of the condition. As summarized recently in an excellent review by Campbell (2005), three commercially available instruments with published psychometric data have been developed to diagnose Asperger syndrome. The Gilliam Asperger Disorder Scale (GADS; Gilliam, 2001), a 32-item, informant report rating scale based on DSM-IV-TR criteria, is widely used in some settings, such as schools. It was standardized on a large, multicultural sample with unverified diagnoses of Asperger syndrome. Internal consistency reliability is somewhat lower than desirable standards. The Asperger Syndrome Diagnostic Scale (ASDS; Myles, Bock, & Simpson, 2001) is a 50-item, informant report rating scale appropriate for children and adolescents ages 5–18. The standardization sample recruited through mailings and conferences was not evaluated by the test authors for independent diagnostic verification. Reliability is below a .90 criterion for internal consistency considered by Campbell (2005) to be adequate (see also Goldstein, 2002). The *Krug Asperger's Disorder Index* (KADI; Krug & Arick, 2003), a 32-item rating scale, can be completed by anyone in daily contact with the individual being rated. Two forms, an elementary and a secondary version, are available and may be used for individuals from ages 6–21. The KADI has the strongest psychometric properties of the published Asperger syndrome measures. However, as with the GADS and ASDS, the diagnoses of individuals in the standardization sample were not confirmed by the test developers.

As Campbell (2005) states succinctly, "Any instrument that claims to diagnose [Asperger syndrome] must be able to discriminate between [Asperger syndrome] and HFA, given the considerable overlap of diagnostic features"

(p. 34). However, none of the three commercially available measures verified the Asperger syndrome diagnoses of individuals in the standardization sample, examined classification accuracy in samples with HFA, or examined directly the ability to differentiate between the two conditions. Thus, these measures should never be used for differential diagnosis of Asperger syndrome versus HFA. In summary, at the time this volume went to press, no parent report measures alone should be used to diagnose Asperger syndrome. The best the field currently has to offer is measures, such as the SCQ, that can differentiate between ASDs as a group (e.g., Asperger syndrome, HFA, PDD NOS) and non-ASD conditions.

DIRECT TESTING AND OBSERVATIONAL DIAGNOSTIC INSTRUMENTS

In the ADOS (Lord et al., 2000; Lord, Rutter, DiLavore, & Risi, 2002), a semistructured interactive assessment of ASD symptoms, four different modules, graded according to language and developmental level, make possible administration to a wide range of patients, from very young children with no language to verbal, high-functioning adults. Most diagnostic observation instruments are hampered by the short time period of assessment. One cannot always be sure that a behavior is deficient after only an hour of observation, but this is often all the time a professional has with a patient. The ADOS minimizes this problem by including multiple opportunities or "presses" for social interaction and communication that elicit spontaneous behaviors in standardized contexts. There are, for example, a number of different activities and situations during administration of the ADOS that, in a typical child, consistently elicit eye contact. Once a child misses several chances to display this typical social behavior, a clinician can be reasonably certain that the behavior in question is difficult for the child being assessed. The algorithm for the ADOS includes only social and communication symptoms; because there are no "presses" for repetitive and stereotyped behaviors, their presence or absence cannot be reliably assessed. Two empirically defined cutoff scores, one for autistic disorder and the other for broader ASDs (e.g., PDD NOS or Asperger syndrome), are provided.

For children with younger mental and chronological ages, items from Modules 1 and 2 of the ADOS assess social interest, joint attention, communicative behaviors, symbolic play, and atypical behaviors (e.g., excessive sensory interest, motor stereotypies). For older and more capable individuals, Modules 3 and 4 of the ADOS focus on conversational reciprocity, empathy, insight into social relationships, and special interests. Until recently, there was a gap in coverage of the ADOS for older, lower-functioning individuals. Specifically, the materials and activities of the first two modules, such as bubbles and dolls, may be appropriate for the mental age of older children, teens, and adults with severe-to-profound mental retardation, but were experienced by clinicians, parents, and sometimes even the individuals themselves as inappropriate for their chronological age. Recently, activities in ADOS Modules 1 and 2 have been adapted to make them more developmentally appropriate for older individuals (Berument et al., 2005). As with the ADI-R, use of the ADOS for research purposes requires attending a training workshop and establishing reliability with a certified trainer. Shorter clinical training available for clinicians not involved in research, like that for the ADI-R, is very helpful but not required for routine clinical use of the instrument.

Lord and colleagues (2000) published a study of the psychometric properties of the four modules of the ADOS. Excellent interrater reliability, internal consistency, and test–retest reliability were reported for each module. Diagnostic validity (sensitivity and specificity) for autism versus nonspectrum disorders was also excellent. The ADOS is used widely in empirical studies of autism and as an outcome measure in several treatment studies (e.g., Owley et al., 2001). In summary, the ADOS is highly recommended. It is considered a "gold standard" method of assessment in both research and clinical practice, and is feasible for use in typical clinical settings provided that appropriate training has taken place.

The Childhood Autism Rating Scale (CARS; Schopler, Reichler, & Renner, 1988), a 15-item structured observation instrument, is appropriate for children over 24 months of age. Items are scored on a 7-point scale (from *Typical* to *Severely deviant*) and summed into a composite score that ranges from 0 to 60. Scores above 30 are consistent with a diagnosis of autism, although slightly lower cutoffs have been recommended for adolescents (Garfin, McCallon, & Cox, 1988). Several studies report high internal

consistency, interrater and test–retest reliability, and criterion-related validity (DiLalla & Rogers, 1994; Eaves & Milner, 1993; Sevin et al., 1991), even when used by raters with little training on the measure or sophistication about ASD (Schopler et al., 1988). The CARS total score correlates highly with the ADI-R ($r = .81$; Saemundsen, Magnusson, Smari, & Sigurdardottir, 2003) but overidentifies autism relative to the ADI-R, occasionally classifying children with mental retardation as having autism (Lord, 1997; Saemundsen et al., 2003). It was developed as a tool to rate behavior observed during developmental evaluation, but it has also been adapted for use as a parent questionnaire (Tobing & Glenwick, 2002). The CARS is a frequently used measure (Luiselli et al., 2001), but it is based on pre-DSM-IV conceptualizations of autism (Van Bourgondien, Marcus, & Schopler, 1992) and does not measure some constructs now considered important to autism diagnosis and/or to have prognostic significance (e.g., joint attention). Therefore, it is not as highly recommended as the ADOS.

The Checklist for Autism in Toddlers (CHAT; Baron-Cohen, Allen, & Gillberg, 1992; Baron-Cohen et al., 1996, 2000) was developed for use in primary care settings to screen children for possible autism before their second birthday. There are two sections: a brief (nine-question) parent interview and a set of five items administered by a clinician to the child. It appears to work best for children who meet full criteria for autism and to be less sensitive to those with milder presentations. Although initially this instrument appeared very promising for use in general clinical settings, sensitivity was quite low (.38) when the initial screened population was followed to age 7 years, with a high false-negative rate (Baird et al., 2000). Thus, this instrument is not recommended for routine clinical use. It is currently undergoing revision by the authors.

The Screening Tool for Autism in Two-Year-Olds (STAT; Stone Coonrod, & Ousley, 2000) is an interactive measure for children between ages 24 and 36 months. Similar in purpose and scope to the ADOS Module 1 but slightly briefer to administer, the STAT consists of a 20-minute play session in which several different activities are presented to the child to assess symbolic play, reciprocal social behavior, joint attention, imitation, and communication. The STAT differentiates well between autism and other forms of developmental delay. This promising instrument, because of its relatively recent development, is not yet used as routinely as the ADOS.

SUMMARY

Several measures are available to collect information from parents and directly assess children suspected of ASD, each with its own strengths and weaknesses. Few studies compare these instruments; thus, there are few empirical data to guide clinicians in choosing among them. In many cases, practical constraints dictate choices. Table 10.2 lists all measures recommended for use, with information on dimensions such as format, administration time, training requirements, and applicable age ranges to assist examiners in choosing among them. One limitation of all diagnostic observational measures for autism is their reliance on current behavior. Deviancies and delays typical of autism are most apparent in early childhood and occasionally may be missed or not recog-

TABLE 10.2. Recommended Measures of a Core Assessment Battery for ASDs

Measure	Format	Age range[a]	Administration/ completion time	Training need[b]
Autism diagnosis: Parent report				
ADI-R	Interview	18 months–adult	1.5–3 hours	Intensive
SCQ	Questionnaire	4 years–adult	10 minutes	Minimal
M-CHAT	Questionnaire	18–30 months	10 minutes	Minimal
PIA	Questionnaire	2–6 years	20–30 minutes	Minimal
PDDBI	Questionnaire	1–17 years	10–15 minutes	Minimal
Autism diagnosis: Direct observation				
ADOS	Direct testing	2 years–adult	30–50 minutes	Intensive
CARS	Observation	2 years–adult	5–10 minutes	Moderate
Intelligence				
MSEL	Direct testing	Birth–68 months	15–60 minutes	Moderate
DAS	Direct testing	2.5–17 years	25–65 minutes	Moderate
WISC-IV	Direct testing	6–16 years	50–70 minutes	Moderate
Stanford–Binet V	Direct testing	2–85 years	45–75 minutes	Moderate
Leiter—Revised	Direct testing	2–20 years	25–90 minutes	Moderate
Language				
CELF	Direct testing	3–21 years	30–45 minutes	Moderate
PPVT	Direct testing	2.5–90+	10–15 minutes	Moderate
EOWPVT-2000	Direct testing	2–18 years	10–15 minutes	Moderate
TLC	Direct testing	5–18 years	< 60 minutes	Moderate
CCC	Questionnaire	5–17 years	10–15 minutes	Minimal
Adaptive behavior				
Vineland	Interview	Birth–18 years	20–60 minutes	Moderate

Note. ADI-R, Autism Diagnostic Interview—Revised; ADOS, Autism Diagnostic Observation Schedule; CARS, Childhood Autism Rating Scale; CCC, Children's Communication Checklist; CELF, Clinical Evaluation of Language Fundamentals; DAS, Differential Abilities Scale; EOWPVT, Expressive One-Word Picture Vocabulary Test–2000; M-CHAT, Modified Checklist for Autism in Toddlers; MSEL, Mullen Scales of Early Learning; PDDBI, Pervasive Developmental Disorders Behavior Inventory; PIA, Parent Interview for Autism; PPVT, Peabody Picture Vocabulary Test; SCQ, Social Communication Questionnaire; TLC, Test of Language Competence; WISC-IV, Wechsler Intelligence Scale for Children, 4th edition.
[a] Inclusive (e.g., 2–6 years = from 2 years, 0 months through 6 years, 11 months).
[b] Minimal: little to no training required, but presumes familiarity with instrument; moderate: presumes prior basic interviewing/cognitive assessment training; intensive: additional specialized training, such as workshop attendance, suggested.

nized at an older age (Bolte & Poustka, 2000). In addition, some characteristics of ASD are low base-rate behaviors that are not always apparent during an observation or structured interaction with a practitioner. Thus, for diagnosis, it is critical both to observe the child directly and to obtain information from parents; we recommend choosing one measure of each type from the list in Table 10.2. On occasion, when these measures provide discordant information (de Bildt et al., 2004; Mildenberger et al., 2001), we recommend that further data be collected from teachers (see below) and other informants in an attempt to resolve the discrepancy.

Intellectual Assessment

A second important domain that must be part of the assessment is intellectual functioning. Intellectual assessment helps to frame the interpretation of many observations about the child. Level of intellectual functioning is associated with severity of autistic symptoms, ability to acquire skills, and level of adaptive function, and is one of the best predictors of outcome (Harris & Handleman, 2000; Lotter, 1974; Rutter, 1984; Stevens et al., 2000; Venter et al., 1992). Major goals of intellectual assessment include generating a profile of the child's cognitive strengths and weaknesses, facilitating educational planning, determining eligibility for certain IQ-related services (e.g., state-funded developmental disability services), and suggesting prognosis. Measured IQ is more stable and predictive the older the age of the child at assessment (Lord & Schopler, 1989). Scores can and do change with development and intervention (Freeman et al., 1991; Mayes & Calhoun, 2003a), and also as a function of the assessment instrument chosen (Magiati & Howlin, 2001).

The child suspected of having ASD often presents an assessment challenge due to social difficulties, unusual use of language, frequent off-task behaviors, high distractibility, and variable motivation. Motivation can have a tremendous influence on test results, and assessments that incorporate reinforcement procedures can result in very different test scores (Koegel, Koegel, & Smith, 1997). It is important to enhance motivation as much as possible, without altering the standard administration of the instrument, and to consider the motivational element when interpreting scores.

More frequent breaks may be needed, and testing may need to be conducted over multiple, shorter sessions. When experienced clinicians evaluate children with autism, few should be "untestable." Untestability reflects primarily lack of availability of appropriate tests or clinician inexperience. There are special concerns about the validity of testing younger, lower-functioning, and nonverbal children, and care must be taken in choosing appropriate tests. It is important that the test chosen (1) be appropriate for both the chronological *and* the mental age of the child, (2) provide a full range (in the lower direction) of standard scores, and (3) measure verbal and nonverbal skills separately (Filipek et al., 1999).

There are several commonly used tests for children with lower mental ages (e.g., those who are younger, nonverbal, and/or who have moderate to severe mental retardation). The Leiter International Performance Scales—Revised (Roid & Miller, 1997; Tsatsanis et al., 2003) is appropriate for individuals with a mental age of 2 years or higher and requires no expressive or receptive language skills. The Differential Abilities Scales (DAS; Elliott, 1990), which assess both intellectual and academic skills, have grown in popularity and use, and may be administered to children across a wide chronological and mental age range (2.5–17 years), making these scales ideal for repeat administrations, for tracking progress, and for research projects in which the developmental range of participants may vary considerably. Especially helpful for the ASD population is the option of out-of-range testing (i.e., administration of tests usually given to children of a different age): Norms for school-age children are available for the preschool battery, permitting use of the test with older children with significant intellectual limitations. For younger children (below age 5) or those with skills that fall below the entry levels of the tests just described, a few additional choices for assessment of intellectual functioning include the Bayley Scales of Infant Development–II (for ages 1–42 months—Bayley, 1993) and the Mullen Scales of Early Learning (MSEL; for ages 1–60 months—Mullen, 1995). For children suspected of having an ASD, the MSEL is often chosen over the Bayley due to its wider age range and five distinct scales that allow separate assessment of verbal and nonverbal abilities. The Bayley has a longer research tradition than the MSEL but yields less detailed information, with one score averaging memory, problem-solving, communication, and other abilities. These instruments provide both standard scores and developmental age equivalents. Thus, they may be used to evaluate children who are older than the test norms but whose developmental skills are not high enough to administer more age-appropriate instruments.

For children capable of spoken language, the Wechsler Intelligence Scales for Children are the most widely used intellectual instruments. There are not yet any published studies of the most recent revision, the WISC-IV (Wechsler, 2003), but in studies of earlier editions (i.e., WISC-R, WISC-III), individuals with ASD often exhibit uneven subtest profiles. Performance IQ (PIQ) is often higher than Verbal IQ (VIQ; Lincoln, Allen, & Kilman, 1995), but the verbal–performance discrepancy is severity dependent, and the majority of individuals with ASD do not show a significant split (> 12 points; Siegel, Minshew, & Goldstein, 1996). When present, a PIQ > VIQ pattern may have important implications for how the child learns best and what activities may be most and least enjoyable. One study suggests that children with significantly uneven intellectual development (in favor of nonverbal skills) are more socially impaired than those with similar overall intelligence but smaller or reversed nonverbal–verbal discrepancies (Joseph, Tager-Flusberg, & Lord, 2002). As a group, they also demonstrate larger head circumference and brain volume than children without large nonverbal > verbal discrepancies (Tager-Flusberg & Joseph, 2003), suggesting potentially an etiologically distinct subtype of autism.

Children with Asperger syndrome may exhibit the opposite intellectual test profile, with VIQ significantly higher than PIQ (Klin et al., 1995), but this is by no means universal and has not been replicated in all studies (see Ozonoff & Griffith, 2000, for a review). Thus, intellectual test profiles should *never* be used for diagnostic confirmation or differential diagnosis of ASD subtypes (e.g., between Asperger syndrome and HFA). However, when a VIQ > PIQ profile is evident, the child may prefer verbally based leisure activities, benefit from verbal explanations, and excel in subjects that require good verbal processing (Klin et al., 1995), unlike a child with the opposite (PIQ > VIQ) intellectual profile.

There are fewer published studies of the Stanford–Binet Intelligence Scale with children

with ASD, but they suggest similar patterns (e.g., PIQ > VIQ, particularly in young children; Mayes & Calhoun, 2003b). One benefit of the Stanford–Binet is the very wide age range of individuals for whom it is appropriate (2–85 years). The standardization study of the revised fifth edition (Roid, 2003) included 108 children with autism in the normative sample and added entry items, improving measurement of young children, lower-functioning older children, and adults with mental retardation. It is appropriate for both verbal and nonverbal individuals, because half the subtests utilize a nonverbal mode of testing. The Stanford–Binet V may be a good choice when examiners must select an instrument before knowing a child's abilities, or when planning a longitudinal assessment.

Short forms of intelligence tests are often used in clinical settings, because they reduce both the economic burden of assessment for families and the stress of testing for the individual. Because autism involves significant behavioral disturbances that might limit compliance during testing, short forms are especially appealing for this group. A recent study demonstrated that short forms of intelligence tests provide very good estimates of IQ for individuals with autism (Minshew, Turner, & Goldstein, 2005). Prediction accuracy was high for both high-functioning individuals and those with significant levels of mental retardation. Even when there was significant intersubtest variability and the subtest profile was atypical relative to individuals without autism, short forms provided excellent estimates of IQ. Administration of full intelligence scales is recommended for initial assessment, particularly when placement decisions or treatment plans are being formulated, but short forms appear useful for purposes such as educational reassessment, research, or assessment with significant time constraints.

Language Assessment

Expressive language level, along with IQ, is the other best predictor of long-term outcome, so it is another important characteristic to measure (Lotter, 1974; Rutter, 1984; Stone & Yoder, 2001). A variety of general instruments, such as the third edition of the Peabody Picture Vocabulary Test (PPVT-III; Dunn & Dunn, 1997), the Expressive One-Word Picture Vocabulary Test–2000 (EOWPVT-2000; Brownell, 2000), the fourth edition of the Clinical Evaluation of Language Fundamentals (CELF-4; Semel, Wiig, & Secord, 2003), and the fourth edition of the Preschool Language Scales (PLS-4; Zimmerman, Steiner, & Pond, 2002), have been used to measure receptive and expressive language abilities in children with ASD, but referral for a more comprehensive evaluation by a speech–language pathologist, who can give detailed language recommendations, is also often helpful (Filipek et al., 1999). Children with adequate spoken language who score in the average range on these tests may still exhibit deficits in the use of language in a social context. Pragmatic communication includes nonverbal behaviors (e.g., eye contact, gestures, facial expression, "body language"), turn taking, and understanding of inferences and figurative expressions. Tests that examine pragmatic language include the Test of Language Competence (TLC; Wiig & Secord, 1989) and the Children's Communication Checklist (CCC; Bishop & Baird, 2001).

Adaptive Behavior Assessment

This domain comprises the final component of the core autism assessment. It is an essential component for three reasons. First, assessment of adaptive behavior should always accompany intellectual testing, because a diagnosis of mental retardation cannot be made unless functioning is compromised across both standardized tests of intelligence and measures of adaptive function and daily living. Second, measuring adaptive behavior is also important for setting appropriate treatment goals. Adaptive abilities largely determine whether an individual requires constant supervision or is capable of some independence. Finally, it is an important measure of outcome that has been used in many longitudinal and treatment studies (e.g., Freeman, Del'Homme, Guthrie, & Zhang, 1999; Szatmari, Bryson, Boyle, Streiner, & Duku, 2003). Children with autism consistently demonstrate lower adaptive behavior levels than their intelligence levels, and this pattern is most pronounced for individuals with HFA and Asperger syndrome and those with normal IQ (Bolte & Poustka, 2002).

The most widely used adaptive measure with children suspected of having an ASD (Luiselli et al., 2001) is the Vineland Adaptive Behavior Scales (Sparrow, Cicchetti, & Balla, 2006). Domains of functioning include communication, daily living skills, socialization, and, for children under age 5, motor skills. The Vineland is completed during an interview with a parent or teacher and is appropriate for children up to age 19 and for mentally retarded adults (separate norms are provided for each population). In a recent study, the Vineland was moderately sensitive to changes due to developmental progress (Charman, Howlin, Berry, & Prince, 2004). The Vineland has just undergone restandardization and now includes supplemental norms for children with ASD (Sparrow et al., 2006; see also Carter et al., 1998). There are no published studies that used other adaptive measures, such as the Scales of Independent Behavior—Revised (SIB-R; Bruininks, Woodcock, Weatherman, & Hill, 1996) or the second edition of the Adaptive Behavior Assessment System (ABAS-2; Harrison & Oakland, 2003), with individuals with ASD, but these may be reasonable choices when time is a constraint, because they are questionnaires completed by parents, rather than interviews, and require little or no training to score and interpret.

Additional Domains of Assessment: Beyond the Core Battery

Depending on the referral question(s), goals of the assessment, and practical constraints such as finances, insurance reimbursements, and waiting lists, a more comprehensive evaluation might include a number of additional components.

Neuropsychological Assessment

The neuropsychology of ASD has been studied extensively. As reviewed earlier, children with ASD often exhibit spared rote, mechanical, and visual–spatial processes, and deficient higher-order processes, such as organization, reasoning, and interpretation (Minshew et al., 1997). They often perform acceptably on simple language, memory, and perspective-taking tasks but show deficits when tasks become more complex. Data from neuropsychological testing may be able to provide greater clarity about the individual's profile of strengths and weaknesses, an important foundation for treatment and educational planning. However, neuropsychological testing is costly and time-consuming, and its use may be impacted by managed care concerns (Piotrowski, 1999).

The decision to carry out neuropsychological assessment, the choice of domains to evaluate, and the selection of instruments should be done thoughtfully and emphasize instruments with the most relevance for educational and treatment plans (Groth-Marnat, 1999; Klin & Shepard, 1994; Ozonoff, Dawson, et al., 2002). Space issues preclude a comprehensive review of all domains of neuropsychology; below, we discuss three areas of particular interest with this population. Neuropsychological assessment is not usually useful (or even possible) with nonverbal and/or mentally retarded children with ASD. It may be warranted for higher-functioning individuals when there are unexplained discrepancies or weaknesses in school performance, behavioral difficulties that appear to stem from undiagnosed learning disorders, and suspected organic problems. For example, neuropsychological assessment of children with unexpected school failure or behavioral issues at school may reveal attention, flexibility, or organization problems that cause frustration, anxiety, or disorganization, and significantly interfere with school function.

ATTENTION

Children with ASDs do not usually have problems with sustained attention (Garretson, Fein, & Waterhouse, 1990). They do, however, have difficulty with focused attention. In particular, they tend to overfocus their attention on extraneous details, while missing meaning, a difficulty that has also been called "impaired central coherence" (Frith & Happé, 1994). Some children with ASD do exhibit classic ADHD symptoms of distractibility and hyperactivity, as discussed earlier (Noterdaeme, Amorosa, Mildenberger, Sitter, & Minow, 2001; Perry, 1998). For these children, a traditional ADHD workup is indicated (see Smith, Barkley, & Shapiro, Chapter 2, this volume). Along with parent and teacher ratings of attention problems, measures such as continuous performance tests may be helpful in examining treatment response in such children (Aman et al., 2004) but should never be the sole basis for determining medication response.

EXECUTIVE FUNCTION

One of the most consistently replicated cognitive deficits in individuals with ASD is executive dysfunction (Pennington & Ozonoff,

1996; Russell, 1997). The executive function domain includes the many skills required to prepare for and execute complex behavior, such as planning, inhibition, organization, self-monitoring, cognitive flexibility, and set shifting. Because executive functions are important to school success (Clark, Prior, & Kinsella, 2002), predict response to treatment (Berger, Aerts, van Spaendonck, Cools, & Teunisse, 2003) and long-term outcome (Szatmari, Bartolucci, Bremner, Bond, & Rich, 1989), and are associated with "real-world" adaptive skills (Clark et al., 2002; Gilotty, Kenworthy, Sirian, Black, & Wagner, 2002), they are important skills to measure.

The "gold standard" executive function task, the Wisconsin Card Sorting Test (WCST; Grant & Berg, 1948; Heaton, Chelune, Talley, Kay, & Curtiss, 1993), measures cognitive flexibility and set shifting. It is available in both an examiner- and a computer-administered version. Individuals with ASD often perform better on the computer-administered version of the test (Ozonoff, 1995). If this executive function test is being given to document deficits for the purposes of treatment eligibility, it may therefore be best to use the examiner-administration format. If, however, the examiner wants to evaluate achievement under supportive conditions or to see how well the child is potentially capable of performing, then the computer-administration format may be preferable (Ozonoff, South, & Provencal, 2005). Computer administration is also more time- and cost-efficient, so when evaluators face such practical constraints, as they often do (Groth-Marnat, 1999), it may be an acceptable choice.

The Delis–Kaplan Executive Function System (D-KEFS; Delis, Kaplan, & Kramer, 2001) provides a battery of tests that assess cognitive flexibility, concept formation, planning, impulse control, and inhibition in children and adults. The D-KEFS was standardized on a sample of over 1,700 children and adults ages 8–89. Most of its nine subtests are adaptations of traditional research measures of executive function that have been refined to examine skills more precisely, with fewer confounding variables. Subtests include Trail Making, Verbal Fluency, Design Fluency, Color–Word Interference (similar to a Stroop test), Sorting (similar to the WCST), Twenty Questions, Tower (similar to the Towers of Hanoi or London), Word Context, and Proverbs. The only published study in which this instrument was used with children with ASD (Lopez, Lincoln, Ozonoff, & Lai, 2005) demonstrates the familiar pattern of deficits (e.g., deficits in cognitive flexibility and planning, with intact inhibitory processes). The NEPSY (Korkman, Kirk, & Kemp, 1998) is a test like the D-KEFS that includes several measures of executive function, but it can be used with younger children (ages 3–12) and has been used successfully with children with autism (Joseph, McGrath, & Tager-Flusberg, 2005).

The Behavioral Rating Inventory of Executive Function (BRIEF; Gioia, Isquith, Guy, & Kenworthy, 2000), a parent- or teacher-rated questionnaire for children ages 5–18 years, has 86 questions and takes about 10 minutes to complete. Clinical subscales measure Inhibition, Cognitive Flexibility, Organization, Planning, Metacognition, Emotional Control, and Initiation. Specific items tap everyday behaviors indicative of executive dysfunction that may not be captured by performance measures, such as organization of the school locker or the home closet, monitoring of homework for mistakes, or trouble initiating leisure activities. Thus, this measure may have more ecological validity than other executive function tests. It may be especially useful to document the impact of executive function deficits on the child's "real-world" function and to plan treatment and educational accommodations. Correlational analyses with other behavior rating scales and executive function tests provide evidence of both convergent and divergent validity (Gioia et al., 2000), and the BRIEF has been used empirically in samples with autism (Gilotty et al., 2002).

Assessment of Academic Functioning

Assessment of academic ability, even in younger children, is helpful for the purposes of educational decision making. It is often an area of strength that may go unrecognized. Many children with ASD have precocious reading skills and can decode words at a higher level than others of the same age and functional ability. Reading and other academic strengths may be used to compensate for weaknesses, such as when a written schedule is provided to facilitate transitions (Bryan & Gast, 2000) or written directions are supplied to improve compliance. The good memory of children with ASD may mean that they learn spelling lists and multiplication tables more easily (Mayes &

Calhoun, 2003a). Conversely, specific areas of weakness also exist, most consistently in reading comprehension. This academic profile is quite different from the problem patterns most teachers and school psychologists are trained to detect (e.g., the poor decoding but good comprehension seen in dyslexia). Thus, it is important to include appropriate test batteries that highlight both academic strengths and weaknesses in the comprehensive evaluation, to interpret the learning patterns they suggest in the feedback to parents and in the written report, and to make appropriate educational recommendations. For young children, the Bracken Basic Concepts Scale (Bracken, 1998), the Young Children's Achievement Test (YCAT; Hresko, Peak, Herron, & Bridges, 2000), and the Psychoeducational Profile—Revised (PEP-R; Schopler, Reichler, Bashford, Lansing, & Marcus, 1990) are useful instruments that highlight both the strengths and the challenges typical of ASD. For older children who are verbal, the most frequently used academic tests are the Woodcock–Johnson Tests of Achievement (Mather & Woodcock, 2001) and the Wechsler Individual Achievement Test (WIAT; Wechsler, 2002).

Some children with ASD may exhibit a so-called nonverbal learning disability profile (NLD; Rourke, 1995). Children with NLD have difficulties in tactile perception, psychomotor coordination, mathematic reasoning, visual–spatial organization, and nonverbal problem solving. They have well-developed rote verbal skills, as well as strong verbal memory and auditory linguistic capabilities. Some children with Asperger syndrome and HFA display an NLD profile (Klin et al., 1995). They may require additional interventions, such as occupational therapy and math tutoring. NLD is an academic diagnosis that does not take the place of the primary ASD diagnosis, which is a more complete description of the full range of the child's behavioral and developmental limitations.

Assessment of Psychiatric and Other Comorbidities

Over the course of development, children with ASD may exhibit symptoms and behaviors not directly attributable to their autism that disrupt their daily functioning. These include problems with sleep, appetite, mood, anxiety, activity level, anger management, aggression, tics, mood instability, psychosis, and/or thought disorder. Many factors influence the presentation of psychiatric disorders in individuals with ASD and complicate their assessment. The decrement in functioning associated with having an ASD means that baseline is already lower than average and that a change in behavior has to be relatively marked to be identifiable. Autism, by itself, causes a variety of psychosocial deficits and maladaptive behaviors, and their presence may "mask" other psychiatric symptoms or make them difficult to identify. Cognitive limitations may mean that the range and quality of symptoms differ or that presentation is atypical. For example, anxiety may be manifest as obsessive questioning or insistence on sameness rather than rumination or somatic complaints. Individuals with ASD may not demonstrate certain symptoms, such as the feelings of guilt often seen in depression, or the grandiosity and inflation of self-esteem typical of mania. The diminished ability to think abstractly, communicate effectively, and be aware of and describe internal states also means that interview and self-report measures are often of less use. People with autism may lack the self-insight to recognize symptoms, or the motivation and social relatedness needed to report them (Perry, Marston, Hinder, Munden, & Roy, 2001). Some behaviors, including complex motor mannerisms and self-injury, may be responses to potentially painful medical problems that the individual is unable to describe. These can include gastrointestinal issues (e.g., reflux, esophageal scarring, constipation); endocrine imbalances, such as those occurring with the onset of menstruation; and/or metabolic disorders (Bauman, 2005). When the clinician can find no reason for a problem, referral to a gastroenterologist or endocrinologist may be helpful. Thus, the assessment of coexisting psychiatric illness and behavioral problems can be quite tricky. Nevertheless, it is important to add to an evaluation whenever significant behavioral issues outside the autism spectrum (inattention, mood instability, anxiety, sleep disturbance, aggression, etc.) are evident or when major changes in behavior from the typical baseline are reported. Comorbidity should also be carefully investigated when severe or worsening symptoms do not respond to traditional methods of treatment (Lainhart, 1999).

As reviewed earlier, depression and anxiety disorders are the most common coexisting psychiatric problems observed in individuals with ASD, particularly individuals with HFA and Asperger syndrome, who can describe their difficulties (Kim et al., 2000; Lainhart & Folstein, 1994; Muris, Steerneman, Merckelback, Holdrinet, & Meesters, 1998). Assessment of these problems is challenging, because no specific tools for the autism spectrum have been developed. The validity of existing inventories (e.g., the Children's Depression Inventory [Kovacs, 1992] or the Multidimensional Anxiety Scale for Children [March, 1997]) is uncertain, because these are self-report measures. Given the limited self-insight of children with ASD, reports of "no problems" should be interpreted with caution, and careful interviews of parents should also be included in the assessment. No empirical studies of the use of these instruments with ASD have been performed.

The Child Behavior Checklist (CBCL; Achenbach & Rescorla, 2001) is widely used to identify child behavioral and mental health issues, but it has only rarely been used with children with ASD. It does not provide an autism factor, but a few studies have suggested that certain patterns, such as high scores on the Social Problems and Thought Problems subscales, may be associated with an ASD diagnosis (Bolte, Dickhut, & Poustka, 1999; Duarte, Bordin, de Oliveira, & Bird, 2003). The CBCL's utility in identifying comorbid internalizing and externalizing problems in children with ASD is not yet known, but it may well be useful as a screening tool given its excellent psychometric properties.

Another measure for assessing several symptom profiles simultaneously, the Behavioral Assessment System for Children–2 (BASC-2), includes parent report, teacher report, and self-report questionnaires for children ages 8–18 years (Kamphaus, Reynolds, & Hatcher, 1999). There are subscales for Internalizing, Externalizing, and Adaptive Behaviors. Subscales assess school, clinical, and personal adjustment. The self-report form also measures Sense of Inadequacy and Sense of Atypicality, which in our experience are helpful for understanding the struggles of children with ASD who can validly report on their internal states (Ozonoff, Provencal, & Solomon, 2002), and these subscales may also prove helpful for measuring treatment effects in ASD. Importantly, each form provides caution indices to inform the clinician of overly positive or negative responses and to provide a measure of the consistency of the respondent's profile.

Another multisymptom scale often used with ASD, the Aberrant Behavior Checklist (Aman, Singh, Stewart, & Field, 1985), is a global behavior checklist completed by a caregiver or teacher familiar with the child in different settings. It was initially designed as a scale for rating inappropriate and maladaptive behavior of individuals with mental retardation in residential settings. However, the scale has been used often to monitor the effects of a variety of pharmacological, behavioral, dietary, and other treatments that may be expected to alter behavior, and the instrument appears sensitive to change in ASD samples (Arnold et al., 2000). There are five subscales (Irritability, Lethargy, Stereotypy, Hyperactivity, and Inappropriate Speech). The published validity and reliability studies report excellent test–retest reliability, internal consistency, and construct validity (Aman et al., 1985).

Another method of assessing problem behaviors that often coexist with ASD, such as aggression, destructiveness, tantrums, stereotypies, or self-injury, is functional analysis (Horner, 1994; O'Neill, Horner, Albin, Sprague, & Storey, 1997). Such challenging behaviors are rarely random and usually serve a purpose. Functional analysis is a systematic approach to determine the function or communicative equivalent of the behavior. Some common functions of problem behaviors include gaining access to a desired object, asking for help or attention, escaping a situation (e.g., schoolwork), and expressing a sensation (e.g., hunger, illness), emotion, or state (e.g., confusion, frustration). The ultimate goal of functional analysis is to provide the child with a more appropriate means of expressing the message (also called "functional communication training"; Carr & Durand, 1985). Although the functions of a particular problem behavior may seem obvious, the perceptions of informants who work with the child may not be confirmed through direct observations and analogue probes that replicate the environmental antecedents of the problem behavior (Calloway & Simpson, 1998). Thus, functional assessment may require referral of the child to a professional trained in these methods, such as a certified behavior analyst, who will also be able to assist in development of a behavioral support plan.

Upon collecting information about various potential comorbid conditions and associated problems, the clinician must finish the process of case formulation by figuring out whether the child has an ASD only, another disorder, or both. The first step is to determine whether the child meets criteria for an ASD. The clinician examines information collected from parents and direct testing, and determines whether cutoffs or thresholds for ASD have been exceeded. Although this sounds deceptively simple, the instruments reviewed in this chapter have very good reliability and validity when used by trained personnel, and the diagnosis may be straightforward in many cases. More difficult is evaluating children who present with subclinical symptoms or behaviors that may be part of multiple conditions (e.g., the poor eye contact that might be seen in both autism and depression). Again, however, the answer is relatively simple. Children with depression alone do not exhibit the pervasive difficulties in social interaction, communication, and behavior that are characteristic of ASDs. If a child presents with both low mood and impaired peer relationships, lack of empathy, few gestures, pedantic speech, echolalia, and unusual interests, he or she likely has both a depressive disorder and an ASD. The package of social and communication limitations, combined with odd or repetitive behaviors, should alert the clinician that an ASD must be part of the differential diagnosis. No other condition includes all of these difficulties. Then, if additional problems not encompassed by ASD criteria are present, such as low mood, tics, or anxiety, the clinician can examine diagnostic criteria for these conditions and determine whether comorbidity is present.

The School Context

Since the goal of assessment should be to understand how ASDs affect individuals in the course of daily life, when feasible, it is helpful to augment the evaluation by obtaining information from teachers or others who interact with the child in the challenging and relatively unstructured school setting (Klin et al., 2000). Teachers may be excellent sources of information about the child's adaptive, social, and emotional functioning outside of home and thereby enrich the clinician's understanding of the child. For example, in typically developing children, as well as those with ADHD, teacher reports of peer relationships correspond more closely to ratings completed by peers than to parent ratings (Glow & Glow, 1980; Hinshaw

& Melnick, 1995). Information from the school setting may be obtained through interviews, questionnaires, and direct clinician observations. Measures include the classroom/teacher editions of the Vineland Adaptive Behavior Scales (Sparrow et al., 2006), the PDD Behavior Inventory (Cohen et al., 2003), the BASC-2, and the Aberrant Behavior Checklist. Although not specifically designed for children on the autism spectrum, the teacher report form of the Social Skills Rating System (Gresham & Elliott, 1989) has been used successfully in research to assess social skills in children with ASDs (Bauminger, 2002). In addition to questionnaires, school-based observations may yield a richer perspective on child social functioning and/or may be part of a functional analysis of behavioral problems (e.g., Dunlap & Kern, 1993; Wood, 1995). In many clinical settings, the resources required to conduct a school visit are not available; thus, this should be considered an optional, albeit helpful, addition to a comprehensive evaluation.

When information on a child is from multiple sources, there may be disagreements in reports of the severity of the disorder, the level of daily adaptive behaviors, and the level of compliance or disruptive behaviors (Offord et al., 1996; Szatmari, Archer, Fisman, & Streiner, 1994). High levels of family stress appear to contribute to higher parent than teacher reports of autistic behavior (Szatmari et al., 1994). Because these well-known discrepancies exist and may well reflect setting-dependent expression of symptoms, our recommendation is to conceptualize them as separate types of information, without attempting to reconcile them by considering one more or less accurate than another, as suggested by Offord and colleagues (1996).

Assessment of Family Functioning

Assessment of the family system may also be important (Hauser-Kram, Warfield, Shonkoff, & Krauss, 2001). Many studies have documented increased stress and depression in parents of children with ASDs (Bristol, 1984; Wolf, Noh, Fisman, & Speechley, 1989) that exceed that of parents of children with other disabilities (Olsson & Hwang, 2001). Stress levels are strongly correlated with severity of the child's disorder (Tobing & Glenwick, 2002). Of the several instruments that measure the impact of a disabled child on the family,

those with established psychometric properties that have been used with the ASD population include the Parenting Stress Index (Abidin, 1995), the Questionnaire on Resources and Stress (Holroyd, 1974; Konstantareas, Homatidis, & Plowright, 1992), and the Stress Index for Parents of Adolescents (Sheras, Abidin, & Konold, 1998).

Evaluation of Response to Treatment

One of the most practical contributions of assessment is the planning and evaluation of intervention (Hayes, Nelson, & Jarrett, 1987). We have highlighted this purpose frequently in this chapter, evaluating certain domains and specific instruments in terms of their sensitivity to change. There are, however, no widely agreed-upon skills that must change, nor any degree of change, for treatment effects to be considered clinically significant. There is general consensus that intervention outcomes should have social validity, making a genuine (functional, noticeable) difference in everyday life for the person treated or those who live with him or her (Foster & Mash, 1999; Kazdin, 1999). There is less agreement on the magnitude of change that must be shown to be considered clinically significant. It is often measured as an effect size, a percentage decline in symptoms, a change from baseline (pretreatment), or an attainment of functioning within the normal range (Kendall, Marrs-Garcia, Nath, & Sheldrick, 1999). Kazdin (1999), however, argues that when change does not meet such criteria, it may nevertheless be meaningful if it helps the person become more functional, even if symptoms remain well outside the normal range. Even no change in symptoms at all may be significant, if the treatment improves coping skills and the ability to deal with symptoms. These examples are particularly relevant to ASD, a lifelong condition in which functioning within the normative range may be possible for only a small proportion of affected individuals. Change in quantity, quality, or severity of autistic behaviors may be minimal, and many treatment studies do not consider this domain the primary target of the therapy (Kasari, 2002). Many drug studies, for example, focus on change in aberrant behaviors, such as irritability and aggression, or other target symptoms that make life difficult for individuals and families (e.g., Arnold et al., 2000, 2003). Therefore, domains of central importance in the evaluation of response to treatment are adaptive behavior, comorbid symptoms, quality of life, and family functioning (Wolery & Garfinkle, 2002).

CONCLUSION

In this chapter, we have reviewed the components of a core assessment battery and a more comprehensive evaluation of suspected ASD. In choosing the components of these batteries, we focused on their utility and relevance to identification, differential diagnosis, service delivery, and treatment response. We focused on assessment strategies and tools with good psychometric properties that are also practical for use in clinical settings (Luiselli et al., 2001). Few studies have directly compared different instruments; thus, there is little empirical evidence to guide practitioners' selections among different assessment tools. Therefore, we have highlighted features such as length of administration and training requirements, in addition to validity and reliability, to assist in instrument selection. We also highlighted several widely used but seriously flawed instruments, with some cautions about their real-world applications. Although challenges remain, this chapter summarizes the tremendous growth that has taken place in the last decade in evaluation methods for ASD. As recently as 10 years ago, autism was not considered a spectrum disorder and was thought to be very rare. Few clinicians knew how to evaluate it or considered it in a differential diagnosis. ASD was diagnosed through subjective clinical opinion, without the use of objective measures of development or behavior. As consensus about the diagnosis has been achieved, a number of standardized interviews and observational measures have been developed. In the next decade, the area that most needs refinement is the evaluation and differential diagnosis of the highest end of the autism spectrum (Asperger syndrome vs. HFA). Another pressing challenge is the paucity of professionals capable of evaluating suspected ASD, leading to very long waiting lists and delays in diagnosis. This chapter is an attempt to address these challenges and, we hope, to continue to broaden the preparation of trainees so that future professionals feel more competent to undertake this important area of assessment.

ACKNOWLEDGMENTS

Our comments in this chapter have been influenced by the membership of Sally Ozonoff on the National Institute of Mental Health's Workgroups on Interventions Research in Autism Spectrum Disorders (September 5–6, 2002, Rockville, Maryland, and May 6, 2004, Sacramento, California). Sally Ozonoff was supported during the writing of this chapter by funding from the National Institutes of Health (Grant Nos. R01-MH068398 and U19-HD35468). Beth L. Goodlin-Jones was supported by Grant No. R01 MH068232. Marjorie Solomon was supported by a Health Services Research Award from the University of California Davis School of Medicine. The opinions expressed here do not necessarily represent those of the funding institutes.

REFERENCES

Abell, F., Krams, M., Ashburner, J., Passingham, R., Friston, K., Frackowiak, R., et al. (1999). The neuroanatomy of autism: A voxel-based whole brain analysis of structural scans. *NeuroReport, 10*, 1647–1651.

Abidin, R. R. (1995). *Parenting stress index* (3rd ed.). Odessa, FL: Psychological Assessment Resources.

Achenbach, T. M., & Rescorla, L. A. (2001). *Manual for the ASEBA school-age forms and profiles.* Burlington: University of Vermont, Research Center for Children, Youth, and Families.

Aman, M. G., Novotny, S., Samango-Sprouse, C., Lecavalier, L., Gadow, K. D., King, B. H., et al. (2004). Outcome measures for clinical drug trials in autism. *CNS Spectrums, 9*, 36–47.

Aman, M. G., Singh, N. N., Stewart, A. W., & Field, C. J. (1985). The Aberrant Behavior Checklist: A behavior rating scale for the assessment of treatment effects. *American Journal of Mental Deficiency, 89*, 485–491.

American Psychiatric Association (APA). (1994). *Diagnostic and statistical manual of mental disorders* (4th ed.). Washington, DC: Author.

American Psychiatric Association (APA). (2000). *Diagnostic and statistical manual of mental disorders* (4th ed., text rev.). Washington, DC: Author.

Amir, R. E., Van Den Veyver, I. B., Wan, M., Tran, C. Q., Franke, U., & Zoghbi, H. (1999). Rett syndrome is caused by mutations in X-linked MECP2, encoding methyl CpG binding protein 2. *Nature Genetics, 23*, 185–188.

Arnold, L. E., Aman, M. G., Martin, A., Collier-Crespin, A., Vitiello, B., Tierney, E., et al. (2000). Assessment in multi-site randomized clinical trials of patients with autistic disorder: The autism RUPP network. *Journal of Autism and Developmental Disorders, 30*, 99–111.

Arnold, L. E., Vitiello, B., McDougle, C., Scahill, L., Shah, B., Gonzalez, N. M., et al. (2003). Parent-defined target symptoms respond to risperidone in the RUPP autism study: Customer approach to clinical trials. *Journal of the American Academy of Child and Adolescent Psychiatry, 42,* 1443–1450.

Aylward, E. H., Minshew, M. J., Goldstein, G., Honeycutt, N. A., Augustine, A. M., Yates, K., et al. (1999). MRI volumes of amygdala and hippocampus in non-mentally retarded autistic adolescents and adults. *Neurology, 52,* 2145–2150.

Bailey, A., LeCouteur, A., Gottesman, I., Bolton, P., Simonoff, E., Yuzda, E., et al. (1995). Autism as a strongly genetic disorder: Evidence from a British twin study. *Psychological Medicine, 25,* 63–77.

Bailey, A., Palferman, S., Heavey, L., & LeCouteur, A. (1998). Autism: The phenotype in relatives. *Journal of Autism and Developmental Disorders, 28,* 369–392.

Baird, G., Charman, T., Baron-Cohen, S., Cox, A., Swettenham, J., Wheelwright, S., et al. (2000). A screening instrument for autism at 18 months of age: A 6-year follow-up study. *Journal of the American Academy of Child and Adolescent Psychiatry, 39,* 694–702.

Ballaban-Gil, K., Rapin, I., Tuchman, R., & Shinnar, S. (1995). Longitudinal examination of the behavioral, language, and social changes in a population of adolescents and young adults with autistic disorder. *Pediatric Neurology, 15,* 217–223.

Baron-Cohen, S. (1991). Precursors to a theory of mind: Understanding attention in others. In A. Whiten (Ed.), *Natural theories of mind: The evolution, development and simulation of everyday mindreading* (pp. 233–251). Oxford, UK: Blackwell.

Baron-Cohen, S., Allen, J., & Gillberg, C. (1992). Can autism be detected at 18 months? The needle, the haystack, and the CHAT. *British Journal of Psychiatry, 161,* 839–843.

Baron-Cohen, S., Cox, A., Baird, G., Swettenham, J., Nightingale, N., Morgan, K., et al. (1996). Psychological markers in the detection of autism in infancy in a large population. *British Journal of Psychiatry, 168,* 158–163.

Baron-Cohen, S., Ring, H. A., Bullmore, E. T., Wheelwright, S., Ashwin, C., & Williams, S. C. (2000). The amygdala theory of autism. *Neuroscience and Biobehavioral Review, 24,* 355–364.

Baron-Cohen, S., Ring, H., Wheelwright, S., Bullmore, E., Brammer, M., Simmons, A., et al. (1999). Social intelligence in the normal and autistic brain: An fMRI study. *European Journal of Neuroscience, 11,* 1891–1898.

Bauman, M. (2005, May). *The autism spectrum disorders: Beyond behavior—implications for research and treatment.* Paper presented at the International Meeting for Autism Research (IMFAR), Boston.

Bauman, M., & Kemper, T. L. (1985). Histoanatomic observations of the brain in early infantile autism. *Neurology, 35,* 866–874.

Bauman, M., & Kemper, T. L. (1988). Limbic and cere-bellar abnormalities: Consistent findings in infantile autism. *Journal of Neuropathology and Experimental Neurology, 47,* 369.

Bauminger, N. (2002). The facilitation of social–emotional understanding and social interaction in high-functioning children with autism: Intervention outcomes. *Journal of Autism and Developmental Disorders, 32,* 283–298.

Bayley, N. (1993). *The Bayley Scales of Infant Development* (2nd ed.). San Antonio, TX: Psychological Corporation.

Berger, H. J., Aerts, F. H., van Spaendonck, K. P., Cools, A. R., & Teunisse, J. P. (2003). Central coherence and cognitive shifting in relation to social improvement in high-functioning young adults with autism. *Journal of Clinical and Experimental Neuropsychology, 25,* 502–511.

Berument, S. K., Rutter, M., Lord, C., Pickles, A., & Bailey, A. (1999). Autism screening questionnaire: Diagnostic validity. *British Journal of Psychiatry, 175,* 444–451.

Berument, S. K., Starr, E., Pickles, A., Tomlins, M., Papanikolauou, K., Lord, C., et al. (2005). Prelinguistic Autism Diagnostic Observation Schedule adapted for older individuals with severe to profound mental retardation: A pilot study. *Journal of Autism and Developmental Disorders, 35,* 821–829.

Bettelheim, B. (1967). *The empty fortress.* New York: Free Press.

Billstedt, E., Gillberg, C., & Gillberg, C. (2005). Autism after adolescence: Population-based 13- to 22-year follow-up study of 120 individuals with autism diagnosed in childhood. *Journal of Autism and Developmental Disorders, 35,* 351–360.

Bishop, D. V., & Baird, G. (2001). Parent and teacher report of pragmatic aspects of communication: Use of the Children's Communication Checklist in a clinical setting. *Developmental Medicine and Child Neurology, 43,* 809–818.

Bishop, D. V., & Norbury, C. F. (2002). Exploring the borderlands of autistic disorder and specific language impairment: A study using standardized instruments. *Journal of Child Psychology and Psychiatry, 43,* 917–930.

Bolte, S., Dickhut, H., & Poustka, F. (1999). Patterns of parent-reported problems indicative in autism. *Psychopathology, 32,* 93–97.

Bolte, S., & Poustka, F. (2000). Diagnosis of autism: The connection between current and historical information. *Autism, 4,* 382–390.

Bracken, B. A. (1998). *Bracken Basic Concept Scale— Revised.* San Antonio, TX: Psychological Corporation.

Bristol, M. M. (1984). Family resources and successful adaptation in families of autistic children. In E. Schopler & G. Mesibov (Eds.), *The effects of autism on the family* (pp. 289–310). New York: Plenum Press.

Brownell, R. (2000). *Expressive One-Word Picture Vo-*

cabulary Test—2000. Novato, CA: Academic Therapy Publications.

Bruininks, R. H., Woodcock, R. W., Weatherman, R. E., & Hill, B. K. (1996). *Scales of Independent Behavior—Revised.* Itasca, IL: Riverside.

Bryan, L. C., & Gast, D. L. (2000). Teaching on-task and on-schedule behaviors to high-functioning children with autism via picture activity schedules. *Journal of Autism and Developmental Disorders, 30,* 553–567.

Bryson, S. E., Clark, B. S., & Smith, I. M. (1988). First report of a Canadian epidemiological study of autistic syndromes. *Journal of Child Psychology and Psychiatry and Allied Disciplines, 29,* 433–445.

Buitelaar, J. K., Van der Gaag, R., Klin, A., & Volkmar, F. (1999). Exploring the boundaries of pervasive developmental disorder not otherwise specified: Analyses of data from the DSM-IV Autistic Disorder Field Trial. *Journal of Autism and Developmental Disorders, 29,* 33–43.

Burack, J. A., Iarocci, G., Bowler, D., & Mottron, L. (2002). Benefits and pitfalls in the merging of disciplines: The example of developmental psychopathology and the study of persons with autism. *Development and Psychopathology, 14,* 225–237.

Calloway, C. J., & Simpson, R. (1998). Decisions regarding functions of behavior: Scientific versus informal analyses. *Focus on Autism and Other Developmental Disabilities, 13,* 167–175.

Campbell, J. M. (2005). Diagnostic assessment of Asperger's disorder: A review of five third-party rating scales. *Journal of Autism and Developmental Disorders, 35,* 25–35.

Carr, E. G., & Durand, V. M. (1985). Reducing behavior problems through functional communication training. *Journal of Applied Behavior Analysis, 18,* 111–126.

Carter, A. S., Volkmar, F. R., Sparrow, S. S., Wang, J. J., Lord, C., Dawson, G., et al. (1998). The Vineland Adaptive Behavior Scales: Supplementary norms for individuals with autism. *Journal of Autism and Developmental Disorders, 28,* 287–302.

Chakrabarti, S., & Fombonne, E. (2001). Pervasive developmental disorders in preschool children. *Journal of the American Medical Association, 285,* 3093–3099.

Chakrabarti, S., & Fombonne, E. (2005). Pervasive developmental disorders in preschool children: Confirmation of high prevalence. *American Journal of Psychiatry, 162,* 1133–1141.

Charman, T., Howlin, P., Berry, B., & Prince, E. (2004). Measuring developmental progress of children with autism spectrum disorders on school entry using parent report. *Autism, 8,* 89–100.

Clark, D., Baxter, M., Perry, D., & Prasher, V. (1999). The diagnosis of affective and psychotic disorders in adults with autism: Seven case reports. *Autism, 3,* 149–164.

Clark, C., Prior, M., & Kinsella, G. (2002). The relationship between executive function abilities, adap-

tive behavior, and academic achievement in children with externalizing behavior problems. *Journal of Child Psychology and Psychiatry, 43,* 785–796.

Cohen, I. L. (2003). Criterion-related validity of the PDD Behavior Inventory. *Journal of Autism and Developmental Disorders, 33,* 47–54.

Cohen, I. L., Schmidt-Lackner, S., Romanczyk, R., & Sudhalter, V. (2003). The PDD Behavior Inventory: A rating scale for assessing response to intervention in children with pervasive developmental disorder. *Journal of Autism and Developmental Disorders, 33,* 31–46.

Cohen, I. L., & Sudhalter, V. (2005). *PDD Behavior Inventory (PDDBI) manual.* Lutz, FL: Psychological Assessment Resources.

Courchesne, E. (2004). Brain development in autism: Early overgrowth followed by premature arrest of growth. *Mental Retardation Developmental Disabilities Review, 10,* 106–111.

Courchesne, E., Carper, R., & Akshoomoff, N. (2003). Evidence of brain overgrowth in the first year of life in autism. *Journal of the American Medical Association, 290,* 337–344.

Courchesne, E., Yeung-Courchesne, R., Press, G. A., Hesselink, J. R., & Jernigan, T. L. (1988). Hypoplasia of cerebellar vermal lobules VI and VII in autism. *New England Journal of Medicine, 26,* 1349–1354.

Cox, A., Klein, K., Charman, T., Baird, G., Baron-Cohen, S., Swettenham, J., et al. (1999). Autism spectrum disorders at 20 and 42 months of age: Stability of clinical and ADI-R diagnosis. *Journal of Child Psychology and Psychiatry, 40,* 719–732.

Critchley, H. D., Daly, E. M., Bullmore, E. T., Williams, S. C, Van Amelsvoort, T., Robertson, D. M., et al. (2000). The functional neuroanatomy of social behaviour: Changes in cerebral blood flow when people with autistic disorder process facial expressions. *Brain, 123,* 2203–2212.

Croen, L. A., Grether, J. K., Hoogstrate, J., & Selvin, S. (2002). The changing prevalence of autism in California. *Journal of Autism and Developmental Disorders, 32,* 207–215.

Danielsson, S., Gillberg, I. C., Billstedt, E., Gillberg, C., & Olsson, I. (2005). Epilepsy in young adults with autism: A prospective population-based follow-up study of 120 individuals diagnosed in childhood. *Epilepsia, 46,* 918–923.

de Bildt, A., Sytema, S., Ketelaars, C., Kraijer, D., Mulder, E., Volkmar, F., et al. (2004). Interrelationships between the ADOS, ADI-R, and DSM-IV-TR classification in children and adolescents with mental retardation. *Journal of Autism and Developmental Disorders, 34,* 129–137.

De Giacomo, A., & Fombonne, E. (1998). Parental recognition of developmental abnormalities in autism. *European Child and Adolescent Psychiatry, 7,* 131–136.

Delis, D. C., Kaplan, E., & Kramer, J. H. (2001). *Delis–Kaplan Executive Function System.* San Antonio, TX: Psychological Corporation.

DiLalla, D. L., & Rogers, S. J. (1994). Domains of the Childhood Autism Rating Scale: Relevance for diagnosis and treatment. *Journal of Autism and Developmental Disorders, 24*, 115–128.

Duarte, C. S., Bordin, I. A. S., Oliveira, A., & Bird, H. (2003). The CBCL and the identification of children with autism and related conditions in Brazil: Pilot findings. *Journal of Autism and Developmental Disorders, 33*, 703–707.

Dumont-Mathieu, T., & Fein, D. (2005). Screening for autism in young children: The modified checklist for autism in toddlers (M-CHAT) and other measures. *Mental Retardation and Developmental Disabilities Research Reviews, 11*, 253–262.

Dunlap, G., & Kern, L. (1993). Assessment and intervention for children within the instructional curriculum. In J. Reichle & D. Wacker (Eds.), *Communicative alternatives to challenging behavior: Integrating functional assessment and intervention strategies* (pp. 106–126). San Diego, CA: College Hill Press.

Dunn, L. M., & Dunn, L. M. (1997). *Peabody Picture Vocabulary Test* (3rd ed.). Circle Pines, MN: American Guidance Service.

Dykens, E., Volkmar, F., & Glick, M. (1991). Thought disorder in high-functioning autistic adults. *Journal of Autism and Developmental Disorders, 21*, 291–301.

Eaves, L. C., & Ho, H. H. (1996). Stability and change in cognitive and behavioral characteristics of autism through childhood. *Journal of Autism and Developmental Disorders, 26*, 557–570.

Eaves, R. C., & Milner, B. (1993). The criterion-related validity of the Childhood Autism Rating Scale and the Autism Behavior Checklist. *Journal of Abnormal Child Psychology, 21*, 481–491.

Elliott, C. (1990). *Differential Abilities Scales.* San Antonio, TX: Psychological Corporation.

Erickson, C. A., Stigler, K. A., Corkins, M. R., Posey, D. J., Fitzgerald, J. F., & McDougle, C. J. (2005). Gastrointestinal factors in autistic disorder: A critical review. *Journal of Autism and Developmental Disorders, 35*, 713–727.

Evans, D. W., Canavera, K., Kleinpeter, F. L., Maccubin, E., & Taga, K. (2005). The fears, phobias, and anxieties of children with autism spectrum disorders and Down syndrome: Comparisons with developmentally and chronologically age matched children. *Child Psychiatry and Human Development, 36*, 3–26.

Everall, I. P., & LeCouteur, A. (1990). Firesetting in an adolescent boy with Asperger's syndrome. *British Journal of Psychiatry, 157*, 284–287.

Fein, D., Dixon, P., Paul, J., & Levin, H. (2005). Pervasive developmental disorder can evolve into ADHD: Case illustrations. *Journal of Autism and Developmental Disorders, 35*, 525–534.

Filipek, P. A., Accardo, P. J., Ashwal, S., Baranek, G. T., Cook, E. H., Jr., Dawson, G., et al., (2000). Practice parameter: Screening and diagnosis of autism. *Neurology, 55*, 468–479.

Filipek, P. A., Accardo, P. J., Baranek, G. T., Cook, E. H., Jr., Dawson, G., Gordon, B., et al. (1999). The screening and diagnosis of autistic spectrum disorders. *Journal of Autism and Developmental Disorders, 29*, 439–484.

Fombonne, E. (2002). Prevalence of childhood disintegrative disorder. *Autism, 6*, 149–157.

Fombonne, E. (2003). Epidemiological surveys of autism and other pervasive developmental disorders: An update. *Journal of Autism and Developmental Disorders, 33*, 365–382.

Fombonne, E. (2005). Epidemiological studies of pervasive developmental disorders. In F. R. Volkmar, R. Paul, A. Klin, & D. Cohen (Eds.), *Handbook of autism and pervasive developmental disorders* (3rd ed., pp. 42—69). Hoboken, NJ: Wiley.

Fombonne, E., & Chakrabarti, S. (2001). No evidence for a new variant of measles–mumps–rubella-induced autism. *Pediatrics, 108*, 1–8.

Fombonne, E., Roge, B., Claverie, J., Courty, S., & Fremolle, J. (1999). Microcephaly and macrocephaly in autism. *Journal of Autism and Developmental Disorders, 29*, 113–119.

Foster, S. L., & Mash, E. J. (1999). Assessing social validity in clinical treatment research: Issues and procedures. *Journal of Consulting and Clinical Psychology, 67*, 308–319.

Frazier, J. A., Biederman, J., Bellordre, C. A., Garfield, S. B., Geller, D. A., Coffey, B. J., et al. (2001). Should the diagnosis of attention-deficit/hyperactivity disorder be considered in children with pervasive developmental disorder? *Journal of Attention Disorders, 4*, 203–211.

Frazier, J. A., Doyle, R., Chiu, S., & Coyle, J. T. (2002). Treating a child with Asperger's disorder and comorbid bipolar disorder. *American Journal of Psychiatry, 159*, 13–21.

Freeman, B. J., Del'Homme, M., Guthrie, D., & Zhang, F. (1999). Vineland Adaptive Behavior Scale scores as a function of age and initial IQ in 210 autistic children. *Journal of Autism and Developmental Disorders, 29*, 379–384.

Freeman, B. J., Rahbar, B., Ritvo, E. R., Bice, T. L., Yokota, A., & Ritvo, R. (1991). The stability of cognitive and behavioral parameters in autism: A 12-year prospective study. *Journal of the American Academy of Child and Adolescent Psychiatry, 30*, 479–482.

Frith, U., & Happé, F. (1994). Autism: Beyond theory of mind. *Cognition, 50*, 115–132.

Garfin, D. G., McCallon, D., & Cox, R. (1988). Validity and reliability of the Childhood Autism Rating Scale with autistic adolescents. *Journal of Autism and Developmental Disorders, 18*, 367–378.

Garretson, H. B., Fein, D., & Waterhouse, L. (1990). Sustained attention in children with autism. *Journal of Autism and Developmental Disorders, 20*, 101–114.

Ghaziuddin, M., Leininger, L., & Tsai, L. (1995). Thought disorder in Asperger syndrome: Comparison with high-functioning autism. *Journal of Autism and Developmental Disorders, 25,* 311–317.

Ghaziuddin, M., Tsai, L. Y., & Alessi, N. (1992). ADHD and PDD. *Journal of the American Academy of Child and Adolescent Psychiatry, 31,* 567.

Ghaziuddin, M., Tsai, L. Y., & Ghaziuddin, N. (1991). Violence in Asperger syndrome: A critique. *Journal of Autism and Developmental Disorders, 21,* 349–354.

Ghaziuddin, M., Tsai, L. Y., & Ghaziuddin, N. (1992). A comparison of the diagnostic criteria for Asperger syndrome. *Journal of Autism and Developmental Disorders, 22,* 643–649.

Ghaziuddin, M., Weidmer-Mikhail, E., & Ghaziuddin, N. (1998). Comorbidity of Asperger syndrome: A preliminary report. *Journal of Intellectual Disability Research, 4,* 279–283.

Gillberg, C. (1998). Chromosomal disorders and autism. *Journal of Autism and Developmental Disorders, 28,* 415–425.

Gillberg, C., & Coleman, M. (2000). *The biology of autistic syndromes* (3rd ed.). London: MacKeith.

Gillberg, C., & Rastam, M. (1992). Do some cases of anorexia nervosa reflect underlying autistic-like conditions? *Behavioral Neurology, 5,* 27–32.

Gillberg, C., Steffenburg, S., & Schaumann, H. (1991). Is autism more common now than ten years ago? *British Journal of Psychiatry, 158,* 403–409.

Gilliam, J. E. (1995). *Gilliam Autism Rating Scale.* Austin, TX: PRO-ED.

Gilliam, J. E. (2001). *Gilliam Asperger Disorder Scale.* Austin, TX: PRO-ED.

Gilmour, J., Hill, B., Place, M., & Skuse, D. H. (2004). Social communication deficits in conduct disorder: a clinical and community survey. *Journal of Child Psychology and Psychiatry and Allied Disciplines, 45,* 967–978.

Gilotty, L., Kenworthy, L., Sirian, L., Black, D. O., & Wagner, A. E. (2002). Adaptive skills and executive function in autism spectrum disorders. *Child Neuropsychology, 8,* 241–248.

Gioia, G. A., Isquith, P. K., Guy, S. C., & Kenworthy, L. (2000). *Behavior Rating Inventory of Executive Function (BRIEF).* Lutz, FL: Psychological Assessment Resources.

Glow, R. A., & Glow, P. H. (1980). Peer and self-rating: Children's perception of behavior relevant to hyperkinetic impulse disorder. *Journal of Abnormal Child Psychology, 8,* 397–404.

Goldberg, W. A., Osann, K., Filipek, P. A., Laulhere, T., Jarvis, K., Modahl, C., et al. (2003). Language and other regression: Assessment and timing. *Journal of Autism and Developmental Disorders, 33,* 607–615.

Goldstein, S. (2002). Review of the Asperger Syndrome Diagnostic Scale. *Journal of Autism and Developmental Disorders, 32,* 611–614.

Goldstein, S., & Schwebach, A. J. (2004). The comorbidity of pervasive developmental disorder and attention deficit hyperactivity disorder: Results of a retrospective chart review. *Journal of Autism and Developmental Disorders, 34,* 329–339.

Gonzalez, N. M., Murray, A., Shay, J., Campbell, M., & Small, A. M. (1993). Autistic children on follow-up: Change of diagnosis. *Psychopharmacology Bulletin, 29,* 353–358.

Goodlin-Jones, B., & Solomon, M. (2003). Contributions of psychology. In S. Ozonoff, S. J. Rogers, & R. Hendren (Eds.), *Autism spectrum disorders: A research review for practitioners* (pp. 55–85). Arlington, VA: American Psychiatric Publishing.

Grant, D. A., & Berg, E. A. (1948). A behavioral analysis of degree of reinforcement and ease of shifting to new responses in a Weigle-type card-sorting problem. *Journal of Experimental Psychology, 32,* 404–411.

Green, J., Gilchrist, A., Burton, D., & Cox, A. (2000). Social and psychiatric functioning in adolescents with Asperger syndrome compared to conduct disorder. *Journal of Autism and Developmental Disorders, 30,* 279–293.

Gresham, F. M., & Elliot, S. N. (1989). Social skills assessment technology for the learning disabled student. *Learning Disability Quarterly, 12,* 141–152.

Groth-Marnat, G. (1999). Financial efficacy of clinical assessment: Rational guidelines and issues for future research. *Journal of Clinical Psychology, 55,* 813–824.

Hardan, A. Y., Minshew, N. J., Harenski, K., & Keshavan, M. S. (2001). Posterior fossa magnetic resonance imaging in autism. *Journal of the American Academy of Child and Adolescent Psychiatry, 40,* 666–672.

Harris, S. L., & Handleman, J. S. (2000). Age and IQ at intake as predictors of placement for young children with autism: A four- to six-year follow-up. *Journal of Autism and Developmental Disorders, 30,* 137–142.

Harrison, P., & Oakland, T. (2003). *Adaptive Behavior Assessment System* (2nd ed.). San Antonio, TX: Psychological Corporation.

Hauser-Kram, P., Warfield, M. E., Shonkoff, J. P., & Krauss, M. W. (2001). Children with disabilities: A longitudinal study of child development and parent well-being. *Monographs of the Society for Research in Child Development, 66,* 1–131.

Hayes, S. C., Nelson, R. O., & Jarrett, R. B. (1987). The treatment utility of assessment: A functional approach to evaluating assessment quality. *American Psychologist, 42,* 963–974.

Heaton, R. K., Chelune, G. J., Talley, J. L., Kay, G. G., & Curtiss, G. (1993). *Wisconsin Card Sorting Test manual: Revised and expanded.* Odessa, FL: Psychological Assessment Resources.

Hendren, R. L. (2003). Contributions of the psychiatrist. In S. Ozonoff, S. J. Rogers, & R. L. Hendren (Eds.), *Autism spectrum disorders* (pp. 37–53). Arlington, VA: American Psychiatric Publishing.

Hinshaw, S. P., & Melnick, S. M. (1995). Peer relationships in boys with attention deficit hyperactivity disorder with and without comorbid aggression. *Developmental Psychopathology, 7,* 627–647.

Holroyd, J. (1974). The Questionnaire on Resources and Stress: An instrument to measure family response to a handicapped member. *Journal of Humanistic Psychology, 37,* 1–11.

Honda, H., Shimizu, Y., Misumi, K., Niimi, M., & Ohashi, Y. (1996). Cumulative incidence and prevalence of childhood autism in children in Japan. *British Journal of Psychiatry, 169,* 228–235.

Honda, H., Shimizu, Y., & Rutter, M. (2005). No effect of MMR withdrawal on the incidence of autism: A total population study. *Journal of Child Psychology and Psychiatry and Allied Disciplines, 46,* 572–570.

Honomichl, R. D., Goodlin-Jones, B. L., Burnham, M., Gaylor, E., & Anders, T. F. (2002). Sleep patterns of children with pervasive developmental disorders. *Journal of Autism and Developmental Disorders, 32,* 553–561.

Horner, R. H. (1994). Functional assessment: Contributions and future directions. *Journal of Applied Behavior Analysis, 27,* 401–404.

Hornig, M., & Lipkin, W. I. (2001). Infectious and immune factors in the pathogenesis of neurodevelopmental disorders: Epidemiology, hypotheses, and animal models. *Mental Retardation and Developmental Disabilities Research Reviews, 7,* 200–210.

Hoshino, Y., Kaneko, M., Yashima, Y., Kumashiro, H., Volkmar, F. R., & Cohen, D. J. (1987). Clinical features of autistic children with setback course in their infancy. *Japanese Journal of Psychiatry and Neurology, 41,* 237–246.

Howard, M. A., Cowell, P. E., Boucher, J., Broks, P., Mayes, A., Farrant, A., et al. (2000). Convergent neuroanatomical and behavioural evidence of an amygdala hypothesis of autism. *NeuroReport, 11,* 2931–2935.

Howlin, P. (2003). Outcome in high-functioning adults with autism with and without early language delays: Implications for the differentiation between autism and Asperger syndrome. *Journal of Autism and Developmental Disorders, 33,* 3–14.

Howlin, P. (2005). Outcomes in autism spectrum disorders. In F. R. Volkmar, R. Paul, A. Klin, & D. Cohen (Eds.), *Handbook of autism and pervasive developmental disorders* (3rd ed., pp. 201–220). Hoboken, NJ: Wiley.

Howlin, P., Goode, S., Hutton, J., & Rutter, M. (2004). Adult outcome for children with autism. *Journal of Child Psychology and Psychiatry and Allied Disciplines, 45,* 212–229.

Hresko W. P., Peak, P. K., Herron, S. R., & Bridges, D. L. (2000). *Young Children's Achievement Test.* Austin, TX: PRO-ED.

Jensen, V. K., Larrieu, J. A., & Mack, K. K. (1997). Differential diagnosis between attention-deficit/hyperactivity disorder and pervasive developmental disorder–not otherwise specified. *Clinical Pediatrics, 36,* 555–561.

Joseph, R. M., McGrath, L. M., & Tager-Flusberg, H. (2005). Executive dysfunction and its relation to language ability in verbal school-age children with autism. *Developmental Neuropsychology, 27,* 361–378.

Joseph, R. M., Tager-Flusberg, H., & Lord, C. (2002). Cognitive profiles and social-communicative functioning in children with autism spectrum disorders. *Journal of Child Psychology and Psychiatry and Allied Disciplines, 43,* 807–821.

Kamphaus, R. W., Reynolds, C. R., & Hatcher, N. M. (1999). Treatment planning and evaluation with the Behavior Assessment System for Children. In M. E. Maruish (Ed.), *The use of psychological testing for treatment planning and outcomes assessment* (2nd ed., pp. 563–597). Mahwah, NJ: Erlbaum.

Kanner, L. (1943). Autistic disturbances of affective content. *Nervous Child, 2,* 217–250.

Kasari, C. (2002). Assessing change in early intervention programs for children with autism. *Journal of Autism and Developmental Disorders, 32,* 447–461.

Kazdin, A. E. (1999). The meanings and measurement of clinical significance. *Journal of Consulting and Clinical Psychology, 67,* 332–339.

Kendall, P. C., Marrs-Garcia, A., Nath, S. R., & Sheldrick, R. C. (1999). Normative comparisons for the evaluation of clinical significance. *Journal of Consulting and Clinical Psychology, 67,* 285–299.

Kielinen, M., Linna, S. L., & Moilanen, I. (2000). Autism in Northern Finland. *European Child and Adolescent Psychiatry, 9,* 162–167.

Kim, J. A., Szatmari, P., Bryson, S. E., Streiner, D. L., & Wilson, F. J. (2000). The prevalence of anxiety and mood problems among children with autism and Asperger syndrome. *Autism, 4,* 117–132.

Klin, A., Pauls, D., Schultz, R., & Volkmar, F. (2005). Three diagnostic approaches to Asperger syndrome: Implications for research. *Journal of Autism and Developmental Disorders, 35,* 221–234.

Klin, A., & Shepard, B. A. (1994). Psychological assessment of autistic children. *Child and Adolescent Psychiatric Clinics of North America, 3,* 53–70.

Klin, A., Sparrow, S. S., Marans, W. D., Carter, A., & Volkmar, F. R. (2000). Assessment issues in children and adolescents with Asperger syndrome. In A. Klin, F. R. Volkmar, & S. S. Sparrow (Eds.), *Asperger syndrome* (pp. 309–339). New York: Guilford Press.

Klin, A., & Volkmar, F. R. (1997). The pervasive developmental disorders: Nosology and profiles of development. In S. S. Luthar, J. A. Burack, D. Cicchetti, & J. R. Weisz (Eds.), *Developmental psychopathology: Perspectives on adjustment, risk, and disorder* (pp. 208–226). New York: Cambridge University Press.

Klin, A., Volkmar, F. R., Sparrow, S. S., Cicchetti, D. V., & Rourke, B. P. (1995). Validity and neuropsychological characterization of Asperger syndrome: Convergence with nonverbal learning disabilities syndrome. *Journal of Child Psychology and Psychiatry and Allied Disciplines, 36,* 1127–1140.

Klinger, L. G., & Renner, P. (2000). Performance-based measures in autism: Implications for diagnosis, early detection, and identification of cognitive profiles. *Journal of Clinical Child Psychology, 29,* 479–492.

Kobayashi, R., Murata, T., & Yashinaga, K. (1992). A follow-up study of 201 children with autism in Kyushu and Yamaguchi areas, Japan. *Journal of Autism and Developmental Disorders, 22,* 395–411.

Koegel, L. K., Koegel, R. L., & Smith, A. (1997). Variables related to differences in standardized test outcomes for children with autism. *Journal of Autism and Developmental Disorders, 27,* 233–243.

Koenig, K., & Tsatsanis, K.D. (2005). Pervasive developmental disorder in girls. In D. J. Bell, S. L. Foster, & E. J. Mash (Eds.), *Handbook of emotional and behavioral disorders in girls* (pp. 211–237). New York: Kluwer.

Konstantareas, M. M., & Hewitt, T. (2001). Autistic disorder in schizophrenia: Diagnostic overlaps. *Journal of Autism and Developmental Disorders, 31,* 19–28.

Konstantareas, M. M., Homatidis, S., & Plowright, C. M. (1992). Assessing resources and stress in parents of severely dysfunctional children: The Clarke modification of Holroyd's Questionnaire on Resources and Stress. *Journal of Autism and Developmental Disorders, 22,* 217–234.

Kopp, S., & Gillberg, C. (1992). Girls with social deficits and learning problems: Autism, atypical Asperger syndrome or a variant of these conditions. *European Child and Adolescent Psychiatry, 1,* 89–99.

Korkman, M., Kirk, U., & Kemp, S. (1998). *NEPSY manual: A developmental neuropsychological assessment.* San Antonio, TX: Psychological Corporation.

Kovacs, M. (1992). *Children's Depression Inventory.* North Tonawanda, NY: Multi-Health Systems.

Krug, D. A., & Arick, J. R. (2003). *Krug Asperger's Disorder Index.* Austin, TX: PRO-ED.

Krug, D. A., Arick, J. R., & Almond, P. J. (1988). *Autism Behavior Checklist.* Austin, TX: PRO-ED.

Kumra, S., Jacobsen, L. K., Lenane, M., Zahn, T. P., Wiggs, E., Alaghband-Rad, J., et al. (1998). Multidimensionally impaired disorder: Is it a variant of very early-onset schizophrenia? *Journal of the American Academy of Child and Adolescent Psychiatry, 37,* 91–99.

Kurita, H. (1985). Infantile autism with speech loss before the age of thirty months. *Journal of the American Academy of Child and Adolescent Psychiatry, 24,* 191–196.

Kurita, H., Osada, H., & Miyake, Y. (2004). External validity of childhood disintegrative disorder in comparison with autistic disorder. *Journal of Autism and Developmental Disorders, 34,* 355–362.

Lainhart, J. E. (1999). Psychiatric problems in individuals with autism, their parents and siblings. *International Review of Psychiatry 11,* 278–298.

Lainhart, J. E., & Folstein, S. E. (1994). Affective disorders in people with autism: A review of published cases. *Journal of Autism and Developmental Disorders, 24,* 587–601.

Lainhart, J. E., Piven, J., Wzorek, M. M., Landa, R., Santangelo, S. L., Coon, H., et al. (1997). Macrocephaly in children and adults with autism. *Journal of the American Academy of Child and Adolescent Psychiatry, 36,* 282–288.

Lecavalier, L. (2005). An evaluation of the Gilliam Autism Rating Scale. *Journal of Autism and Developmental Disorders, 35,* 795–805.

Le Couteur, A., Bailey, A., Goode, S., Pickles, A., Robertson, S., Gottesman, I., et al. (1996). A broader phenotype of autism: The clinical spectrum of twins. *Journal of Child Psychology and Psychiatry and Allied Disciplines, 37,* 785–801.

Lincoln, A. J., Allen, M. H., & Kilman, A. (1995). The assessment and interpretation of intellectual abilities in people with autism. In E. Schopler & G. B. Mesibov (Eds.), *Learning and cognition in autism* (pp. 89–117). New York: Plenum Press.

Lingam, R., Simmons, A., Andrews, N., Miller, E., Stowe, J., & Taylor, B. (2003). Prevalence of autism and parentally reported triggers in a northeast London population. *Archives of Disease in Children, 88,* 666–670.

Lopez, B. R., Lincoln, A. J., Ozonoff, S., & Lai, Z. (2005). Examining the relationship between executive functions and restricted, repetitive symptoms of autistic disorder. *Journal of Autism and Developmental Disorders, 35,* 445–460.

Lord, C. (1995). Follow-up of two-year-olds referred for possible autism. *Journal of Child Psychology and Psychiatry and Allied Disciplines, 36,* 1365–1382.

Lord, C. (1997). Diagnostic instruments in autism spectrum disorders. In D. J. Cohen & F. R. Volkmar (Eds.), *Handbook of autism and pervasive developmental disorders* (2nd ed., pp. 460–483). New York: Wiley.

Lord, C., Risi, S., Lambrecht, L., Cook, E. H., Leventhal, B. L., DiLavore, P. C., et al. (2000). The Autism Diagnostic Observation Schedule—Generic: A standard measure of social and communication deficits associated with the spectrum of autism. *Journal of Autism and Developmental Disorders, 30,* 205–223.

Lord, C., Rutter, M., DiLavore, P. C., & Risi, S. (2002). *Autism Diagnostic Observation Schedule manual.* Los Angeles: Western Psychological Services.

Lord, C., Rutter, M., & LeCouteur, A. (1994). Autism Diagnostic Interview—Revised: A revised version of a diagnostic interview for caregivers of individuals with possible pervasive developmental disorders. *Journal of Autism and Developmental Disorders, 24,* 659–685.

Lord, C., & Schopler, E. (1989). The role of age at assessment, developmental level, and test in the stability of intelligence scores in young autistic children. *Journal of Autism and Developmental Disorders, 19,* 483–499.

Lord, C., Shulman, C., & DiLavore, P. (2004). Regression and word loss in autistic spectrum disorders. *Journal of Child Psychology and Psychiatry and Allied Disciplines, 45,* 936–955.

Lotter, V. (1966). Epidemiology of autistic conditions in

young children: Prevalence. *Social Psychiatry, 1,* 124–137.

Lotter, V. (1974). Factors related to outcome in autistic children. *Journal of Autism and Childhood Schizophrenia, 4,* 263–277.

Lovaas, O. I. (1987). Behavioral treatment and normal educational and intellectual functioning in young autistic children. *Journal of Consulting and Clinical Psychology, 55,* 3–9.

Luiselli, J. K., Campbell, S., Cannon, B., DiPietro, E., Ellis, J. T., Taras, M., et al. (2001). Assessment instruments used in the education and treatment of persons with autism: Brief report of a survey of national service centers. *Research in Developmental Disabilities, 22,* 389–398.

Macintosh, K. E., & Dissanayake, C. (2004). The similarities and differences between autistic disorder and Asperger disorder: A review of the empirical evidence. *Journal of Child Psychology and Psychiatry and Allied Disciplines, 45,* 410–434.

Madsen, K. M., Hviid, A., Vestergaard, M., Schendel, D., Wohlfahrt, J., Thorsen, P., et al. (2002). A population-based study of measles, mumps, and rubella vaccination and autism. *New England Journal of Medicine, 347,* 1477–1482.

Madsen, K. M., Lauritsen, M. B., Pedersen, C. B., Thorsen, P., Plesner, A. M., Andersen, P. H., et al. (2003). Thimerosal and the occurrence of autism: Negative ecological evidence from Danish population-based data. *Pediatrics, 112,* 604–606.

Magiati, I., & Howlin, P. (2001). Monitoring the progress of preschool children with autism enrolled in early intervention programs: Problems in cognitive assessment. *Autism, 5,* 399–406.

Mandell, D. S., Novak, M. M., & Zubritsky, C. D. (2005). Factors associated with age of diagnosis among children with autism spectrum disorders. *Pediatrics, 11,* 1480–1486.

March, J. S. (1997). *Multidimensional Anxiety Scale for Children.* North Tonawanda, NY: Multi-Health Systems.

Mather, N., & Woodcock, R. W. (2001). *Woodcock–Johnson III Tests of Achievement.* Chicago: Riverside.

Mayes, S., & Calhoun, S. (2003a). Ability profiles in children with autism: Influence of age and IQ. *Autism, 6,* 83–98.

Mayes, S. D., & Calhoun, S. L. (2003b). Analysis of WISC-III, Stanford–Binet:IV, and academic achievement test scores in children with autism. *Journal of Autism and Developmental Disorders, 33,* 329–341.

Mayes, S. D., Calhoun, S., & Crites, D. L. (2001). Does DSM-IV Asperger's disorder exist? *Journal of Abnormal Child Psychology, 29,* 263–271.

McConachie, H., Le Couteur, A. L., & Honey, E. (2005). Can a diagnosis of Asperger syndrome be made in very young children with suspected autism spectrum disorder? *Journal of Autism and Developmental Disorders, 35,* 167–176.

Mildenberger, K., Sitter, S., Noterdaeme, M., &

Amorosa, H. (2001). The use of the ADI-R as a diagnostic tool in the differential diagnosis of children with infantile autism and children with receptive language disorder. *European Child and Adolescent Psychiatry, 10,* 248–255.

Miller, J. N., & Ozonoff, S. (2000). The external validity of Asperger disorder: Lack of evidence from the domain of neuropsychology. *Journal of Abnormal Psychology, 109,* 227–238.

Minshew, N. J., Goldstein, G., & Siegel, D. J. (1997). Neuropsychologic functioning in autism: Profile of a complex information processing disorder. *Journal of the International Neuropsychological Society, 3,* 303–316.

Minshew, N. J., Turner, C. A., & Goldstein, G. (2005). The application of short forms of the Wechsler Intelligence Scales in adults and children with high functioning autism. *Journal of Autism and Developmental Disorders, 35,* 45–52.

Moore, V., & Goodson, S. (2003). How well does early diagnosis of autism stand the test of time?: Follow-up study of children assessed for autism at age 2 and development of an early diagnostic service. *Autism, 7,* 47–63.

Morton, R., Sharma, V., Nicholson, J., Broderick, M., & Poyser, J. (2002). Disability in children from different ethnic populations. *Child: Care, Health and Development, 28,* 87–93.

Mouridsen, S. E., Rich, B., & Isager, T. (1999). Psychiatry morbidity in disintegrative psychosis and infantile autism: A long-term follow-up study. *Psychopathology, 32,* 177–183.

Mullen, E. M. (1995). *Mullen Scales of Early Learning.* Circle Pines, MN: American Guidance Service.

Mundy, P., Sigman, M., & Kasari, C. (1990). A longitudinal study of joint attention and language development in autistic children. *Journal of Autism and Developmental Disorders, 20,* 115–128.

Muris, P., Steerneman, P., Merckelback, H., Holdrinet, I., & Meesters, C. (1998). Comorbid anxiety symptoms in children with pervasive developmental disorders. *Journal of Anxiety Disorder, 12,* 387–393.

Myles, B. S., Bock, S. J., & Simpson, R. (2001). *Asperger Syndrome Diagnostic Scale.* Austin, TX: PRO-ED.

Noterdaeme, M., Amorosa, H., Mildenberger, K., Sitter, S., & Minow, F. (2001). Evaluation of attention problems in children with autism and children with a specific language disorder. *European Child and Adolescent Psychiatry, 10,* 58–66.

Offord, D., Boyle, M., Racine, Y., Szatmari, P., Fleming, J., Sanford, M., et al. (1996). Integrating assessment data from multiple informants. *Journal of the American Academy of Child and Adolescent Psychiatry, 35,* 1078–1085.

Olsson, M. B., & Hwang, C. P. (2001). Depression in mothers and fathers of children with intellectual disability. *Journal of Intellectual Disability Research, 45,* 535–543.

O'Neill, R. E., Horner, R. H., Albin, R. W., Sprague, J.

R., & Storey, K. (1997). *Functional assessment and program development for problem behavior* (2nd ed.). Pacific Grove, CA: Brooks/Cole.

Osterling, J., & Dawson, G. (1994). Early recognition of children with autism: A study of first birthday home video tapes. *Journal of Autism and Developmental Disorders, 24,* 247–259.

Owley, T., McMahon, W., Cook, E. H., Laulhere, T. M., South, M., Mays, L. Z., et al. (2001). A multi-site, double-blind, placebo-controlled trial of porcine secretin in autism. *Journal of the American Academy of Child and Adolescent Psychiatry, 40,* 1293–1299.

Oyane, N. M. F., & Bjorvatn, B. (2005). Sleep disturbances in adolescents and young adults with autism and Asperger syndrome. *Autism, 9,* 83–94.

Ozonoff, S. (1995). Reliability and validity of the Wisconsin Card Sorting Test in studies of autism. *Neuropsychology, 9,* 491–500.

Ozonoff, S., Dawson, G., & McPartland, J. (2002). *A parent's guide to Asperger syndrome and high-functioning autism: How to meet the challenges and help your child thrive.* New York: Guilford Press.

Ozonoff, S., & Griffith, E. M. (2000). Neuropsychological function and the external validity of Asperger syndrome. In A. Klin, F. R. Volkmar, & S. S. Sparrow (Eds.), *Asperger syndrome* (pp. 72–96). New York: Guilford Press.

Ozonoff, S., Provencal, S., & Solomon, M. (2002, October). *The effectiveness of social skills training programs for autism spectrum disorders.* Paper presented at the annual meeting of the American Academy of Child and Adolescent Psychiatry, San Francisco.

Ozonoff, S., Rogers, S. J., & Pennington, B. F. (1991). Asperger syndrome: Evidence of an empirical distinction from high-functioning autism. *Journal of Child Psychology and Psychiatry and Allied Disciplines, 32,* 1107–1122.

Ozonoff, S., South, M., & Miller, J. (2000). DSM-IV-defined Asperger syndrome: Cognitive, behavioral and early history differentiation from high-functioning autism. *Autism, 4,* 29–46.

Ozonoff, S., South, M., & Provencal, S. (2005). Executive functions. In F. R. Volkmar, R. Paul, A. Klin, & D. Cohen (Eds.), *Handbook of autism and pervasive developmental disorders* (3rd ed., pp. 606–627). Hoboken, NJ: Wiley.

Ozonoff, S., Williams, B. J., & Landa, R. (2005). Parental report of the early development of children with regressive autism. *Autism, 9,* 461–486.

Pennington, B. F., & Ozonoff, S. (1996). Executive functions and developmental psychopathologies. *Journal of Child Psychology and Psychiatry and Allied Disciplines, 37,* 51–87.

Perry, R. (1998). Misdiagnosed ADD/ADHD: Rediagnosed PDD. *Journal of the American Academy of Child and Adolescent Psychiatry, 37,* 113–114.

Perry, R., Cohen, I., & DeCarlo, R. (1995). Case study: Deterioration, autism, and recovery in two siblings.

Journal of the American Academy of Child and Adolescent Psychiatry, 34, 232–237.

Perry, D. W., Marston, G. W., Hinder, S. A., Munden, A. C., & Roy, A. (2001). The phenomenology of depressive illness in people with learning disability and autism. *Autism, 5,* 265–275.

Pickles, A., Bolton, P. F., MacDonald, H., Bailey, A., LeCouteur, A., Sim, C. H., et al. (1995). Latent-class analysis of recurrence risks for complex phenotypes with selection and measurement error: A twin and family history study of autism. *American Journal of Human Genetics, 57,* 717–726.

Pierce, K., Muller, R. A., Ambrose, J., Allen, G., & Courchesne, E. (2001). Face processing occurs outside the fusiform "face area" in autism: Evidence from functional MRI. *Brain, 124,* 2059–2073.

Pilowsky, T., Yirmiya, N., Shulman, C., & Dover, R. (1998). The Autism Diagnostic Interview—Revised and the Childhood Autism Rating Scale: Differences between diagnostic systems and comparison between genders. *Journal of Autism and Developmental Disorders, 28,* 148–151.

Piotrowski, C. (1999). Assessment practices in the era of managed care: Current status and future directions. *Journal of Clinical Psychology, 55,* 787–796.

Piven, J., Bailey, J., Ranson, B. J., & Arndt, S. (1997). An MRI study of the corpus callosum in autism. *American Journal of Psychiatry, 154,* 1051–1056.

Piven, J., Harper, J., Palmer, P., & Arndt, S. (1996). Course of behavioral change in autism: A retrospective study of high-IQ adolescents and adults. *Journal of the American Academy of Child and Adolescent Psychiatry, 35,* 523–529.

Prior, M. (2000). Guest editorial: Special issue on Asperger syndrome. *Autism, 4,* 5–8.

Rimland, B. (1964). The etiology of infantile autism: The problem of biological versus psychological causation. *Infantile autism: The syndrome and its implications for a neural theory of behavior* (pp. 39–66). Englewood Cliffs, NJ: Prentice-Hall.

Risch, N., Spiker, D., Lotspeich, L., Nouri, N., Hinds, D., Hallmayer, J., et al. (1999). A genomic screen of autism: Evidence for a multilocus etiology. *American Journal of Human Genetics, 65,* 493–507.

Robins, D. L., Fein, D., Barton, M. L., & Green, J. A. (2001). The modified checklist for autism in toddlers: An initial study investigating the early detection of autism and pervasive developmental disorders. *Journal of Autism and Developmental Disorders, 31,* 131–144.

Roid, G., & Miller, L. (1997). *Leiter International Test of Intelligence—Revised.* Chicago: Stoelting.

Roid, G. H. (2003). *Stanford–Binet Intelligence Scale manual* (5th ed.). Itasca, IL: Riverside.

Rossi, P. G., Posar, A., & Parmeggiani, A. (2000). Epilepsy in adolescents and young adults with autistic disorder. *Brain Development, 22,* 102–106.

Rourke, B. P. (Ed.). (1995). *Syndrome of nonverbal learning disabilities: Neurodevelopmental manifestations.* New York: Guilford Press.

Russell, J. (Ed.). (1997). *Autism as an executive disorder.* New York: Oxford University Press.

Rutter, M. (1984). Autistic children growing up. *Developmental Medicine and Child Neurology, 26,* 122–129.

Rutter, M. (2000). Genetic studies of autism: From the 1970s into the millennium. *Journal of Abnormal Child Psychology, 28,* 3–14.

Rutter, M., Bailey, A., & Lord, C. (2003). *Social Communication Questionnaire (SCQ) manual.* Los Angeles: Western Psychological Services.

Rutter, M., LeCouteur, A., & Lord, C. (2003). *Autism Diagnostic Interview—Revised manual.* Los Angeles: Western Psychological Services.

Saemundsen, E., Magnusson, P., Smari, J., & Sigurdardottir, S. (2003). Autism Diagnostic Interview—Revised and the Childhood Autism Rating Scale: Convergence and discrepancy in diagnosing autism. *Journal of Autism and Developmental Disorders, 33,* 319–328.

Schopler, E., Reichler, R., & Renner, B. (1988). *The Childhood Autism Rating Scale (CARS).* Los Angeles: Western Psychological Services.

Schopler, E., Reichler, R. J., Bashford, A., Lansing, M. D., & Marcus, L. M. (1990). *Psychoeducational Profile—Revised (PEP-R).* Austin, TX: PRO-ED.

Schreck, K. A., & Mulick, J. A. (2000). Parental report of sleep problems in children with autism. *Journal of Autism and Developmental Disorders, 30,* 127–135.

Schultz, R. T., Gauthier, I., Klin, A., Fulbright, R. K., Anderson, A. W., Volkmar, F., et al. (2000). Abnormal ventral temporal cortical activity during face discrimination among individuals with autism and Asperger syndrome. *Archives of General Psychiatry, 57,* 331–340.

Schumann, C. M., Hamstra, J., Goodlin-Jones, B. L., Lotspeich, L. J., Kwon, H., Buonocore, M. H., et al. (2004). The amygdala is enlarged in children but not adolescents with autism; the hippocampus is enlarged at all ages. *Journal of Neuroscience, 24,* 6392–6401.

Seltzer, M. M., Krauss, M. W., Shattuck, P. T., Orsmond, G., Swe, A., & Lord, C. (2003). The symptoms of autism spectrum disorders in adolescence and adulthood. *Journal of Autism and Developmental Disorders, 33,* 565–581.

Semel, E., Wiig, E. H., & Secord, W. A. (2003). *Clinical Evaluation of Language Fundamentals* (4th ed.). San Antonio, TX: Psychological Corporation.

Sevin, J. A., Matson, J. L., Coe, D. A., Fee, V. E., & Sevin, B. M. (1991). A comparison and evaluation of three commonly used autism scales. *Journal of Autism and Developmental Disorders, 21,* 415–432.

Shea, V., & Mesibov, G. B. (2005). Adolescents and adults with autism. In F. R. Volkmar, R. Paul, A. Klin, & D. Cohen (Eds.), *Handbook of autism and pervasive developmental disorders* (3rd ed., pp. 288–311). Hoboken, NJ: Wiley.

Sheras, P. L., Abidin, R. R., & Konold, T. R. (1998). *The Stress Index for Parents of Adolescents: Professional manual.* Odessa, FL: Psychological Assessment Resources.

Shinnar, S., Rapin, I., Arnold, S., Tuchman, R. F., Shulman, L., Ballaban-Gil, K., et al. (2001). Language regression in childhood. *Pediatric Neurology, 24,* 185–191.

Siegel, D. J., Minshew, N. J., & Goldstein, G. (1996). Wechsler IQ profiles in diagnosis of high-functioning autism. *Journal of Autism and Developmental Disorders, 26,* 389–406.

Sigman, M., & McGovern, C. W. (2005). Improvement in cognitive and language skills from preschool to adolescence in autism. *Journal of Autism and Developmental Disorders, 35,* 15–23.

Siperstein, R., & Volkmar, F. (2004). Parental reporting of regression in children with pervasive developmental disorders. *Journal of Autism and Developmental Disorders, 34,* 731–734.

South, M., Williams, B. J., McMahon, W. M., Owley, T., Filipek, P. A., Shernoff, E., et al. (2002). Utility of the Gilliam Autism Rating Scale in research and clinical populations. *Journal of Autism and Developmental Disorders, 32,* 593–599.

Sparks, B. F., Friedman, S. D., Shaw, D. W., Aylward, E. H., Echelard, D., Artru, A. A., et al. (2002). Brain structural abnormalities in young children with autism spectrum disorder. *Neurology, 25,* 184–192.

Sparrow, S., Cicchetti, D. V., & Balla, D. A. (2006). *Vineland–II Adaptive Behavior Scales* (2nd ed.). Circle Pines, MN: American Guidance Service.

Sponheim, E. (1996). Changing criteria of autistic disorders: A comparison of ICD-10 research criteria and DSM-IV with DSM-III-R, CARS, and ABC. *Journal of Autism and Developmental Disorders, 26,* 513–525.

Sponheim, E., & Spurkland, I. (1996). Diagnosing childhood autism in clinical practice: An inter-rater reliability study of ICD-10, DSM-III-R, Childhood Autism Rating Scale, and Autism Behavior Checklist. *Nordic Journal of Psychiatry, 50,* 5–9.

Sporn, A. L., Addington, A. M., Gogtay, N., Ordonez, A. E., Gornick, M., Clasen, L., et al. (2004). Pervasive developmental disorder and childhood-onset schizophrenia: Comorbid disorder or a phenotypic variant of a very early onset illness? *Biological Psychiatry, 55,* 989–994.

Starr, E., Szatmari, P., Bryson, S., & Zwaigenbaum, L. (2003). Stability and change among high-functioning children with pervasive developmental disorders: A 2-year outcome study. *Journal of Autism and Developmental Disorders, 33,* 15–22.

Steinhausen, H. C., & Metzke, C. W. (2004). Differentiating the behavioral profile in autism and mental retardation and testing of a screener. *European Child and Adolescent Psychiatry, 13,* 214–220.

Stevens, M. C., Fein, D. A., Dunn, M., Allen, D., Waterhouse, L. H., Feinstein, C., et al. (2000). Subgroups of children with autism by cluster analysis: A longitudinal examination. *Journal of the American Academy of Child and Adolescent Psychiatry, 39,* 346–352.

Stewart, K. (2002). *Helping a child with nonverbal learning disorder or Asperger's syndrome: Parent's guide.* Oakland, CA: New Harbinger.

Stone, W. L., Coonrod, E. E., & Ousley, O. Y. (2000). Screening Tool for Autism in Two-Year-Olds (STAT): Development and preliminary data. *Journal of Autism and Developmental Disorders, 30,* 607–612.

Stone, W. L., Coonrod, E. E., Pozdol, S. L., & Turner, L. M. (2003). The Parent Interview for Autism—Clinical version (PIA-CV): A measure of behavioral change for young children with autism. *Autism, 7,* 9–30.

Stone, W. L., Lee, E. B., Ashford, L., Brissie, J., Hepburn, S. L., Coonrod, E. E., et al. (1999). Can autism be diagnosed accurately in children under 2 years? *Journal of Child Psychology and Psychiatry and Allied Disciplines, 40,* 219–226.

Stone, W. L., & Yoder, P. J. (2001). Predicting spoken language level in children with autism spectrum disorders. *Autism, 5,* 341–361.

Szatmari, P., Archer, L., Fisman, S., & Streiner, D. L. (1994). Parent and teacher agreement in the assessment of pervasive developmental disorders. *Journal of Autism and Developmental Disorders, 24,* 703–717.

Szatmari, P., Bartolucci, G., Bremner, R., Bond, S., & Rich, S. (1989). A follow-up study of high-functioning autistic children. *Journal of Autism and Developmental Disorders, 19,* 213–225.

Szatmari, P., Bryson, S. E., Boyle, M. H., Streiner, D. L., & Duku, E. (2003). Predictors of outcome among high functioning children with autism and Asperger syndrome. *Journal of Child Psychology and Psychiatry and Allied Disciplines, 44,* 520–528.

Szatmari, P., Bryson, S. E., Streiner, D. L., Wilson, F., Archer, L., & Ryerse, C. (2000). Two-year outcome of preschool children with autism or Asperger's syndrome. *American Journal of Psychiatry, 157,* 1980–1987.

Tager-Flusberg, H., & Joseph, R. M. (2003). Identifying neurocognitive phenotypes in autism. *Philosophical Transactions of the Royal Society of London, 358,* 303–314.

Tantum, D. (2003). The challenge of adolescents and adults with Asperger syndrome. *Child and Adolescent Psychiatric Clinics of North America, 12,* 143–163.

Taylor, B., Miller, E., Farrington, C. P., Petropoulos, M. C., Favot-Mayaud, I., Li, J., et al. (1999). Autism and measles, mumps, and rubella vaccine: No epidemiological evidence for a causal association. *Lancet, 353,* 2026–2029.

Taylor, B., Miller, E., Lingam, R., Andrews, N., Simmons, A., & Stowe, J. (2002). Measles, mumps, and rubella vaccination and bowel problems or developmental regression in children with autism: Population study. *British Medical Journal, 324,* 393–396.

Tharp, B. R. (2004). Epileptic encephalopathies and their relationship to developmental disorders: Do spikes cause autism? *Mental Retardation and Developmental Disabilities Research Reviews, 10,* 132–134.

Thompson, T., Caruso, M., & Ellerbeck, K. (2003). Sex matters in autism and other developmental disabilities. *Journal of Learning Disabilities, 7,* 345–362.

Tobing, L. E., & Glenwick, D. S. (2002). Relation of the Childhood Autism Rating Scale-Parent Version to diagnosis, stress, and age. *Research in Developmental Disabilities, 23,* 211–223.

Tonge, B. J., Brereton, A. V., Gray, K. M., & Einfeld, S. L. (1999). Behavioural and emotional disturbance in high-functioning autism and Asperger syndrome. *Autism, 3,* 117–130.

Towbin, K. E. (2005). Pervasive developmental disorder not otherwise specified. In F. R. Volkmar, R. Paul, A. Klin, & D. Cohen (Eds.), *Handbook of autism and pervasive developmental disorders* (3rd ed., pp. 165–200). Hoboken, NJ: Wiley.

Towbin, K. E., Dykens, E. M., Pearson, G. S., & Cohen, D. J. (1993). Conceptualizing "borderline syndrome of childhood" and "childhood schizophrenia" as a developmental disorder. *Journal of the American Academy of Child and Adolescent Psychiatry, 32,* 775–782.

Trevarthen, C., & Daniel, S. (2005). Disorganized rhythm and synchrony: Early signs of autism and Rett syndrome. *Brain Development, 27,* S25–S34.

Tsai, L. (2000). Children with autism spectrum disorder: Medicine today and in the new millennium. *Focus on Autism and other Developmental Disabilities, 15,* 138–145.

Tsai, L., Stewart, M. A., & August, G. (1981). Implication of sex differences in the familial transmission of infantile autism. *Journal of Autism and Developmental Disorders, 11,* 165–173.

Tsatsanis, K. D., Dartnall, N., Cicchetti, D., Sparrow, S. S., Klin, A., & Volkmar, F. R. (2003). Concurrent validity and classification accuracy of the Leiter and Leiter-R in low-functioning children with autism. *Journal of Autism and Developmental Disorders, 33,* 23–30.

Van Acker, R., Loncola, J. A., & Van Acker, E. Y. (2005). Rett syndrome: A pervasive developmental disorder. In F. R. Volkmar, R. Paul, A. Klin, & D. Cohen (Eds.), *Handbook of autism and pervasive developmental disorders* (3rd ed., pp. 126–164). Hoboken, NJ: Wiley.

Van Bourgondien, M., Marcus, L., & Schopler, E. (1992). Comparison of DSM-III-R and Childhood Autism Rating Scale diagnoses of autism. *Journal of Autism and Developmental Disorders, 22,* 493–506.

Van der Gaag, R. J., Buitelaar, J., Van den Ban, E., Bezemer, M., Njio, L., & Van Engeland, H. (1995). A controlled multivariate chart review of multiple complex developmental disorder. *Journal of the American Academy of Child and Adolescent Psychiatry, 34,* 1096–1106.

Van der Gaag, R. J., Caplan, R., van Engeland, H., Loman, F., & Buitelaar, J. K. (2005). A controlled study of formal thought disorder in children with autism and multiple complex developmental disorders. *Journal of Child and Adolescent Psychopharmacology, 15*, 465–476.

Veenstra-Vanderweele, J., Christian, S. L., & Cook, E. H., Jr. (2004). Autism as a paradigmatic complex genetic disorder. *Annual Review of Genomics of Human Genetics, 5*, 379–405.

Venter, A., Lord, C., & Schopler, E. (1992). A follow-up study of high-functioning autistic children. *Journal of Child Psychology and Psychiatry and Allied Disciplines, 33*, 489–507.

Volkmar, F. R., Cicchetti, D. V., Dykens, E., Sparrow, S. S., Leckman, J. F., & Cohen, D. J. (1988). An evaluation of the Autism Behavior Checklist. *Journal of Autism and Developmental Disorders, 16*, 81–97.

Volkmar, F. R., & Cohen, D. J. (1991). Comorbid association of autism and schizophrenia. *American Journal of Psychiatry, 148*, 1705–1707.

Volkmar, F. R., Cook, E. H., Jr., Pomeroy, J., Realmuto, G., & Tanguay, P. (1999). Practice parameters for the assessment and treatment of children, adolescents, and adults with autism and other pervasive developmental disorders. *Journal of the American Academy of Child and Adolescent Psychiatry, 38*, 32S–54S.

Volkmar, F. R., Koenig, K., & State, M. (2005). Childhood disintegrative disorder. In F. R. Volkmar, R. Paul, A. Klin, & D. Cohen (Eds.), *Handbook of autism and pervasive developmental disorders* (3rd ed., pp. 70–87). Hoboken, NJ: Wiley.

Volkmar, F. R., Szatmari, P., & Sparrow, S. S. (1993). Sex differences in pervasive developmental disorders. *Journal of Autism and Developmental Disorders, 23*, 579–591.

Wadden, N. P., Bryson, S. E., & Rodger, R. S. (1991). A closer look at the Autism Behavior Checklist: Discriminant validity and factor structure. *Journal of Autism and Developmental Disorders, 21*, 529–541.

Wakefield, A. J., Murch, S. H., Anthony, A., Linnell, J., Casson, D. M., Malik, M., et al. (1998). Ileal-lymphoid-nodular hyperplasia, non-specific colitis, and pervasive developmental disorder in children. *Lancet, 351*, 637–641.

Walker, D. R., Thompson, A., Zwaigenbaum, L., Goldberg, J., Bryson, S. E., Mahoney, W. J., et al. (2004). Specifying PDDNOS: A comparison of PDDNOS, Asperger syndrome and autism. *Journal of the American Academy of Child and Adolescent Psychiatry, 43*, 172–180.

Wechsler, D. (2002). *Wechsler Individual Achievement Test, second edition.* San Antonio, TX: Psychological Corporation.

Wechsler, D. (2003). *Wechsler Intelligence Scale for Children*, fourth edition (WISC-IV). San Antonio, TX: Psychological Corporation.

Wetherby, A. M., Woods, J., Allen, L., Cleary, J., Dickinson, H., & Lord, C. (2004). Early indicators of autism spectrum disorders in the second year of life. *Journal of Autism and Developmental Disorders, 34*, 473–493.

Wiig, E., & Secord, W. (1989). *Test of Language Competence—Expanded edition.* San Antonio, TX: Psychological Corporation.

Wimpory, D. C., Hobson, R. P., Williams, J. M., & Nash, S. (2000). Are infants with autism socially engaged?: A study of recent retrospective parental reports. *Journal of Autism and Developmental Disorders, 30*, 525–536.

Wing, L., & Gould, J. (1979). Severe impairments of social interaction and associated abnormalities in children. *Journal of Autism and Developmental Disorders, 9*, 11–29.

Wolery, M., & Garfinkle, A. N. (2002). Measures in intervention research with young children who have autism. *Journal of Autism and Developmental Disorders, 32*, 463–478.

Wolf, L., Noh, S., Fisman, S. N., & Speechley, M. (1989). Psychological effects of parenting stress on parents of autistic children. *Journal of Autism and Developmental Disorders, 19*, 157–166.

Wood, M. (1995). Parent–professional collaboration and the efficacy of the IEP process. In R. L. Koegel & L. K. Koegel (Eds.), *Teaching children with autism* (pp. 147–174). Baltimore: Brookes.

Woodbury-Smith, M., Klin, A., & Volkmar, F. (2005). Asperger's syndrome: A comparison of clinical diagnoses and those made according to the ICD-10 and DSM-IV. *Journal of Autism and Developmental Disorders, 35*, 235–240.

Wozniak, J., Biederman, J., Faraone, S. V., Frazier, J., Kim, J., Millstein, R., et al. (1997). Mania in children with pervasive developmental disorder revisited. *Journal of the American Academy of Child and Adolescent Psychiatry, 36*, 1552–1560.

Zimmerman, I. L., Steiner, V. G., & Pond, R. E. (2002). *Preschool Language Scales, fourth edition.* San Antonio, TX: Psychological Corporation.

Zwaigenbaum, L., Bryson, S., Rogers, T., Roberts, W., Brian, J., & Szatmari, P. (2005). Behavioral manifestations of autism in the first year of life. *International Journal of Developmental Neuroscience, 23*, 143–152.

CHAPTER 11

Early-Onset Schizophrenia

Michael G. McDonell
Jon M. McClellan

Schizophrenia is often a chronic, debilitating neuropsychiatric disorder with enormous individual, family, and societal burden. Early-onset schizophrenia (EOS) is defined as onset before age 18 years. The onset of schizophrenia in children is very rare, with the incidence increasing during adolescence. Some symptoms of schizophrenia may be difficult to differentiate from other psychiatric disorders or even normative childhood experiences. As with other low base rate disorders, comprehensive multi-informant, multimethod assessment is key to accurate diagnosis.

Accurate assessment of schizophrenia in children and adolescents can be a challenge. Historically the definition of childhood schizophrenia has varied. Rare cases of schizophrenia in children, described by Kraepelin (1919) in the early 1900s, were similar to the adult form of the disorder, and distinct from autism and pervasive developmental disorders (Werry, 1979). Beginning with the works of Bender, Kanner, and others (Fish & Ritvo, 1979), childhood schizophrenia was equated with the broader construct of childhood psychoses, including infantile autism. Whereas psychotic speech and thought were considered inherent components of childhood schizophrenia, hallucinations and delusions were not required criteria (Fish & Ritvo, 1979). The second edition of the *Diagnostic and Statistical Manual for Men-*

tal Disorders (DSM-II; American Psychiatric Association [APA], 1968) adopted this nosology by grouping all childhood psychoses under childhood schizophrenia, resulting in diagnostic overlap with that of autism and other psychotic disorders. However, seminal studies by Kolvin (1971) and Rutter (1972) demonstrated that autism and childhood-onset schizophrenia are distinct entities. Therefore, beginning with DSM-III (APA, 1980), the diagnosis of schizophrenia in childhood has used the same criteria as those for adults, regardless of age of onset.

DEFINITIONS

Diagnostic Criteria for Schizophrenia

Psychotic Symptoms

The diagnosis of EOS is made when DSM-IV-TR (APA, 2000) or *International Classification of Diseases* (ICD-10; World Health Organization [WHO], 1992) criteria are met (Tables 11.1 and 11.2). Psychotic symptoms are the hallmark of the disorder. In terms of DSM-IV-TR, active psychotic symptoms (e.g., hallucinations, delusions, disorganized speech, disorganized or catatonic behavior) and/or negative symptoms must be present for at least a period of 1 month.

TABLE 11.1. DSM-IV-TR Diagnostic Criteria for Schizophrenia

A. *Characteristic symptoms:* Two (or more) of the following, each present for a significant period of time during a 1-month period (or less if successfully treated):

(1) delusions
(2) hallucinations
(3) disorganized speech (e.g., frequent derailment or incoherence?)
(4) grossly disorganized or catatonic behavior
(5) negative symptoms (i.e., affective flattening, alogia, or avolition)

Note: Only one Criterion A symptom is required if delusions are bizarre or hallucinations consist of a voice keeping up a running commentary on the person's behavior or thoughts, or two or more voices are conversing with each other.

B. *Social/occupational dysfunction*: For a significant portion of the time since onset of the disturbance, one or more major areas of functioning such as work, interpersonal relations, or self-care are markedly below the level achieved prior to the onset (or when onset is in childhood or adolescence, failure to achieve expected level of interpersonal, academic, or occupational achievement).

C. *Duration*: Continuous signs of the disturbance persist for at least 6 months. This 6-month period must include at least 1 month of symptoms (or less if successfully treated) that meet Criterion A (i.e., active-phase symptoms) and may include periods of prodromal or residual symptoms. During these prodromal or residual periods, the signs of the disturbance maybe manifested by only negative symptoms or two or more symptoms listed in Criterion A present in the attenuated form (e.g., odd beliefs, unusual perceptual experiences).

D. *Schizoaffective and Mood Disorder exclusion*: Schizoaffective Disorder and Mood Disorder with Psychotic Features have been ruled out because either (1) no Major Depressive, Manic, or Mixed Episodes have occurred concurrently with the active-phase symptoms; or (2) if mood episodes have occurred concurrently with the active-phase symptoms, their total duration has been brief relative to the duration of the active and residual periods.

E. *Substance/general medical condition exclusion*: The disturbance is not due to the direct physiological effects of a substance (e.g., a drug of abuse, a medication) or a general medical condition.

F. *Relationship to Pervasive Developmental Disorder:* If there is a history of Autistic Disorder or another Pervasive Developmental Disorder, the additional diagnosis of Schizophrenia is made only if prominent delusions or hallucinations are also present for at least a month (or less if successfully treated).

Note. From American Psychiatric Association (2000). Copyright 2000 by the American Psychiatric Association. Reprinted by permission.

Hallucinations may occur in any sensory modality, including olfactory or tactile. Auditory hallucinations are the most common and often are experienced as voices separate from a person's thoughts (APA, 2000; American Psychiatric Association, Steering Committee on Practice Guidelines [APASCPG], 2004). Delusions are often bizarre and unrealistic in the context of one's life experience and culture. Delusions may be persecutory (e.g., being followed by the CIA), referent (e.g., receiving special messages from the television), grandiose (e.g., believing in special powers), somatic (e.g., believing that one suffers from a terminal illness despite medical evidence to the contrary), or religious (e.g., believing that one is a religious prophet) (APA, 2000; APASCPG,

2004). Delusions may also involve thought withdrawal or insertion, or the belief that one is controlled by an outside force (APA, 2000; APASCPG, 2004).

Disorganized speech includes loosening of associations (i.e., frequent, sudden, and apparently unrelated changes in the subject of conversation), as well as tangential or incoherent speech (APA, 2000; APASCPG, 2004). Persons with schizophrenia may often change subjects suddenly or provide oblique responses to questions. Similar to disorganized speech, disorganized behavior is often characterized as difficulty in sustaining goal-oriented behavior (APASCPG, 2004). As a result, a range of activities, from planning a meal to personal hygiene, may be impaired. Catatonic behavior, which

TABLE 11.2. ICD-10 Diagnostic Criteria for Schizophrenia

The schizophrenic disorders are characterized in general by fundamental and characteristic distortions of thinking and perception, and affects that are inappropriate or blunted. Clear consciousness and intellectual capacity are usually maintained, although certain cognitive deficits may evolve in the course of time. The most important psychopathological phenomena include thought echo, thought insertion or withdrawal, thought broadcasting, delusional perception and delusions of control, influence or passivity, hallucinatory voices commenting or discussing the patient in the third person, and thought disorders and negative symptoms.

The course of schizophrenic disorders can be either continuous or episodic with progressive or stable deficit, or there can be one or more episodes with complete or incomplete remission. The diagnosis of schizophrenia should not be made in the presence of extensive depressive or manic symptoms unless it is clear that schizophrenic symptoms antedate the affective disturbance. Nor should schizophrenia be diagnosed in the presence of overt brain disease or during states of drug intoxication or withdrawal. Similar disorders developing in the presence of epilepsy or other brain disease should be classified under F06.2, and those induced by psychoactive substances under F10–F19 with common fourth character .5.

Excludes:
1. Acute schizophrenia-like disorder (F23.2), symptoms persisting for less than 1 month
2. Schizoaffective disorder, mixed type (F25.2)
3. Schizotypal disorder (F21)

Note. From WHO (1992). Copyright 1992 by the World Health Organization. Adapted by permission.

involves a general lack of response to one's environment, may present as motor immobility, mutism, posturing or stereotyped behavior, excessive motor behavior, echolalia, or echopraxia (APA, 2000; APASCPG, 2004).

Negative symptoms describe a variety of deficit symptoms, such as avolition, alogia, and affective flattening (APA, 2000). "Avolition" is defined as difficulties initiating and maintaining motivation to complete tasks necessary for successful functioning. Alogia typically manifests itself as poverty in the content and amount of speech. Persons with schizophrenia may also demonstrate a limited range of facial affective expression (affective flattening). Limited eye contact and "body language" are also indicative of affective flattening. Persons

with schizophrenia may also have a general lack of interest in previously enjoyable activities (anhedonia). Negative symptoms may be difficult to differentiate from comorbid depression or the side effects of antipsychotic medications (APASCPG, 2004).

Social–Occupational Dysfunction

The symptoms listed earlier must be associated with a marked decline in the level of social, occupational, and self-care functioning below preonset levels. In children and adolescents, this may include the failure to achieve age-appropriate levels of interpersonal, academic, or occupational development. This decline in functioning should be pervasive rather than limited to one or two specific situations (e.g., quitting a job because of a persecutory delusion). Although functioning may improve with treatment, deficits are often chronic and functioning may not return to premorbid levels (APA, 2000).

Duration

The disturbances must be present for a period of at least 6 months. This period must include an active phase of illness (i.e., psychotic symptoms) with or without a prodromal or residual phase. The prodromal phase involves deterioration in functioning prior to the onset of psychotic symptoms. The residual phase typically involves an improvement of psychotic symptoms and follows the active phase of illness. Prodromal and residual phases may include lower intensity psychotic symptoms, such as social isolation, deterioration in occupational functioning, peculiar behavior, blunted or inappropriate affect, disordered thought processes (tangentiality, circumferentiality), poverty of speech or speech content, odd beliefs or perceptions, and lack of energy (anergia).

Differential Diagnosis

Schizoaffective disorder and mood disorders with psychotic features should be ruled out. For a diagnosis of schizophrenia, psychotic symptoms must persist when the episodes of depression and mania remit. If psychotic symptoms persist for at least 2 weeks in the absence of mood disturbance and criteria for a major depressive, manic, or mood episode are met for a substantial portion of the active and residual phase of the illness, then a diagnosis of schizoaffective disorder should be made (APA, 2000). Persons with a chronic and debilitating disorder such as schizophrenia are likely to experience difficulties with mood. If these difficulties with mood neither meet criteria for a depressive, manic, or mixed episode, nor present for a substantial portion of the period of the disorder, then a diagnosis of schizophrenia is appropriate.

Psychosis as a result of other general medical conditions, substance use, or medications also should be ruled out. A thorough medical evaluation is necessary to rule out psychosis secondary to a general medical condition, such as acute intoxication or delirium. Prolonged abstinence from a substance or medication often differentiates between substance- or medication-induced psychosis and schizophrenia. A diagnosis of schizophrenia should be made when psychotic symptoms persist despite prolonged abstinence from the substance believed to have caused psychotic symptoms.

In cases where diagnostic criteria are met for autism or other pervasive developmental disorders, symptoms of active psychosis (e.g., overt hallucinations and/or delusions) must be present for at least 1 month, and other explanations for psychotic symptoms must have been ruled out (e.g., belief in fantasy vs. delusions or hallucinations, a lack of interest in social relationships vs. negative symptoms).

ICD-10 Criteria for Schizophrenia

ICD-10 diagnostic criteria are similar to DSM-IV-TR criteria except that the diagnosis can be made once sufficient symptoms have been present for a period of 1 month or more, rather than 6 months (WHO, 1992). Armenteros and colleagues (1995) found a high rate of diagnostic agreement between DSM-III-R, DSM-IV, and ICD-10 in hospitalized psychotic adolescents.

Schizophrenia Subtypes

Subtypes of schizophrenia are found in both DSM-IV-TR and ICD-10, including paranoid, disorganized (hebephrenic), catatonic, undifferentiated, and residual. The paranoid subtype is characterized by hallucinations and persecutory delusions, without substantial disorganized behavior or speech. Persons with disorganized or hebephrenic schizophrenia demonstrate predominately disorganized thought and/or behavior, and may be too con-

fused to provide descriptions of organized delusions and hallucination. Catatonic schizophrenia is rare, especially in EOS, and is marked by unresponsiveness to one's environment. Undifferentiated schizophrenia characterizes individuals who meet criteria for schizophrenia but do not meet criteria for paranoid, catatonic, or disorganized subtypes. The residual subtype describes persons with schizophrenia who no longer manifest symptoms consistent with an active phase of illness (e.g., hallucinations, disorganized speech and behavior) but still manifest negative symptoms, and other symptoms of the illness in an attenuated form.

In addition, the subtypes simple and postschizophrenic depression are found in ICD-10, but not in DSM-IV-TR. Simple schizophrenia, as defined by ICD-10, is a form of the illness with an insidious onset of decreased functioning and residual symptoms of schizophrenia (e.g., blunting of affect and avolition), without previous overt psychotic symptoms. Postschizophrenic depression describes the presence of a depressive episode after onset of the schizophrenic illness. Symptoms of schizophrenia must persist during episodes of depression (WHO, 1992).

Reports vary as to whether the paranoid subtype (Eggers, 1978) or the undifferentiated subtype (McClellan, Werry, & Ham, 1993; Werry, McClellan, & Chard, 1991) is more common in EOS. Furthermore, an individual's subtype may vary, depending in part on response to treatment. Therefore, it is not clear whether these subtypes represent truly distinct clinical or biological entities. There is not sufficient evidence currently to justify categorizing EOS as a separate diagnostic subcategory (Werry, 1992).

Developmental Factors and DSM-IV-TR and ICD-10 Criteria

Although the criteria for the diagnosis of schizophrenia are the same for children and adolescents as for adults (APA, 2000), developmental factors still need to be considered in the assessment of EOS. In general, the extant research has defined "early onset" as onset prior to age 18 years, with childhood onset, prior to age 12 years. Some developmental differences in symptom presentation are noted. Children with EOS are more likely to present with hallucinations, thought disorder, and negative symptoms, and are less likely to experience complex or systematized delusions (Pavuluri, Herbener, & Sweeney, 2004). An earlier age of onset is also generally associated with other developmental delays and a high rate of premorbid problems (Ropcke & Eggers, 2005). These differences are mostly qualitative and likely relate to the timing of the illness with regard to neural development. Younger children in general have less abstract thinking; therefore, not surprisingly, those with schizophrenia are less likely to have complex delusions. The timing of the onset of the illness may be in part a "dose effect." Therefore, the association between greater premorbid and cognitive difficulties, and earlier onset may simply reflect a greater neurodevelopmental insult.

Appropriate developmental assessment includes determining whether symptom reports suggestive of schizophrenia represent the underlying diagnosis as opposed to normative developmental experiences or symptoms of other psychiatric disorders. Distinguishing psychotic symptoms from other developmental issues can be challenging, especially in children. Very young children's idiosyncratic logical reasoning, overactive perceptions, or magical belief systems may be misinterpreted as psychosis by clinicians that apply adult criteria without developmental accommodations. True psychosis is exceedingly rare in very young children. Therefore, clinicians need to be very cautious when interpreting psychotic-like reports in this age group.

Most children and adolescents reporting psychotic symptoms do not actually have a psychotic disorder (Del Beccaro, Burk, & McCauley, 1988; Garralda, 1984a, 1984b). Atypical psychotic symptoms may represent a number of phenomena, including posttraumatic stress disorder (PTSD), factitious or conversion disorders, personality disorders, or developmental delays that interfere with the accurate reporting of internal experiences; difficulty distinguishing fantasy from reality; and/or misunderstanding the questions asked by the clinician (Hlastala & McClellan, 2005; Hornstein & Putnam, 1992; McClellan et al., 1993; McClellan & McCurry, 1999). In these cases the psychotic symptom reports are often atypical in the following manner: (1) The reports are inconsistent, and there is no other documented evidence of a psychotic process (e.g., thought disorder, bizarre disorganized behavior); (2) the qualitative nature of the reports are not typical of psychotic symptoms

(e.g., greatly detailed descriptions or reports more suggestive of fantasy or imagination); and/or (3) the reported symptoms only occur in specific situations (e.g., hearing voices only after an aggressive outburst) (Hlastala & McClellan, 2005).

EPIDEMIOLOGY

The prevalence of schizophrenia in the general population is approximately 1% and occurs worldwide in all known cultural and ethnic groups. Although the prevalence of EOS has not been adequately studied, the few studies available, plus clinical experience, suggest that onset prior to age 13 years is quite rare. In children younger than 15 years of age, the prevalence rate has been estimated at 14 per 100,000 (Beitchman, 1985; Volkmar, Cohen, Hoshino, Rende, & Paul, 1988). Gillberg (1984) estimated the prevalence of very early-onset schizophrenia (VEOS) in Sweden at 1.6 per 100,000. Thomsen (1996) reported that only 1% of hospitalized youth with schizophrenia were younger than 13 years of age, and only 9% were younger than 15 years of age. The rate of onset increases during adolescence, with onset for the disorder typically ranging from 15 to 30 years (APA, 2000). Although the onset of puberty has been theorized to play some type of neurobiological role, pubertal status was not associated with the onset of psychosis in a study of youth with childhood schizophrenia (Frazier et al., 1997).

EOS occurs predominantly in males (Bettes & Walker, 1987; Green & Padron-Gayol, 1986; Green, Padron-Gayol, Hardesty, & Bassiri, 1992; Kolvin, 1971; McClellan & McCurry, 1998; Russell, Bott, & Sammons, 1989; Werry et al., 1991). Because the adult literature suggests that the average age of onset in males is 5 years earlier than that in females (Loranger, 1984), the male predominance in EOS may be a cross-sectional effect.

CLINICAL PRESENTATION

Symptomatology

Historically, schizophrenia has been characterized as having positive and negative symptoms. Positive symptoms of schizophrenia refer to florid hallucinations and delusions, whereas negative symptoms refer to deficits (i.e., flat affect, anergy, and paucity of speech and thought; APA, 2000). Hallucinations, especially auditory hallucinations, thought disorder (e.g., loose associations), and flattened affect all have been consistently found in EOS, whereas systematic delusions and catatonic symptoms are less frequent (Biederman, Petty, Faraone, & Seidman, 2004; Green et al., 1992; McClellan, McCurry, Speltz, & Jones, 2002; Pavuluri et al., 2004; Russell et al., 1989; Werry et al., 1991). Social deficits, such as withdrawal and social isolation, have also been observed in EOS and are correlated with negative symptoms (Hollis, 2003; McClellan, Breiger, McCurry, & Hlastala, 2003).

Youth with schizophrenia also display evidence of formal thought disorder. In comparison to normal children, those with schizophrenia have three characteristic communication deficits: loose associations, illogical thinking, and impaired discourse skills (Caplan, Guthrie, Gish, Tanguay, & David-Lando, l989; Pavuluri et al., 2004). Rates of incoherence and poverty of speech content are low (Caplan et al., 1989). When assessing a child's thinking, it is important to differentiate between the thought disorder of psychosis and language disorders or developmental delays. For instance, typical language difficulties in EOS (i.e., disorganized speech, loose associations) are manifestations of disorganized thought rather than language difficulties, such as word finding or word recognition.

Associated Cognitive Symptoms

Neuropsychological studies suggest that children with schizophrenia have global impairments across tasks that require greater capacity for information processing rather than deficits isolated to specific functions or areas of the brain (Asarnow, Tompson, & Goldstein, 1994; McClellan, Prezbindowski, Breiger, & McCurry, 2004). However, it is important to recognize that there are no specific neuropsychological profiles diagnostic of schizophrenia (Kumra et al., 2000; McClellan et al., 2004). Youth with EOS who have identified genetic disorders, such as velocardiofacial syndrome, may demonstrate greater neuroanotomical and neuropsychological abnormalities (Rapoport & Inoff-Germain, 2000; Usiskin et al., 1999).

Language and communication and global cognitive deficits are common in youth with schizophrenia (Baltaxe & Simmons, 1995;

Caplan, Guthrie, & Komo, 1996; Helgeland & Torgersen, 2005; McClellan et al., 2004). Of those with EOS, 10–20% have IQs in the borderline to mentally retarded range (Asarnow & Ben-Meir, 1988; Eggers, 1978; Goldberg, Karson, Leleszi, & Weinberger, 1988; Green et al., 1992; Kenny et al., 1997; McClellan et al., 1993; McClellan & McCurry, 1998; Werry et al., 1991). Because many research studies have excluded patients with mental retardation, these rates may actually be lower than what otherwise would be found in a clinical population.

Developmental and Cognitive Influences on Symptom Presentation

Developmental differences in language and cognition may affect the range and quality of symptom presentation (Caplan et al., 1989; Volkmar et al., 1988; Watkins, Asarnow, Tanguay, & Perdue, 1988; Werry, 1992). Bettes and Walker (1987) found that among youth with EOS and other psychiatric disorders, positive symptoms increased linearly with age and were associated with IQs greater than 85. Young children are also less likely to present with systematic delusions. Thus, the complexity of psychotic symptoms appears to be correlated with cognitive development, with the capacity for more systematic delusional beliefs and complex hallucinations linked to the capacity for abstract thinking and a general fund of knowledge. This is not surprising, because psychotic thought emanates from an individual's own experiences and belief systems.

Course of Illness

Schizophrenia is a phasic disorder, with a great deal of individual variability. As a result of the fluctuation of symptoms across phases, accurate assessment must take into account these variations in clinical presentation.

Premorbid Functioning

The majority of patients with EOS (with some reports as high as 90%) have premorbid developmental and/or behavioral abnormalities (Alaghband-Rad et al., 1995; Asarnow & Ben-Meir, 1988; Eggers, 1978; Green & Padron-Gayol, 1986; Helgeland & Torgersen, 2005; Hollis, 1995, 2003; Kolvin, 1971; McClellan et al., 2003; McClellan & McCurry, 1998; Russell et al., 1989; Schaeffer & Ross, 2002; Vourdas, Pipe, Corrigal, & Frangou, 2003; Watkins et al., 1988; Werry et al., 1991). A wide range of premorbid difficulties is described, including idiosyncratic or bizarre preoccupations, unusual behaviors, social withdrawal and isolation, deteriorating self-care, disruptive behavior disorders, academic difficulties, speech and language problems, and developmental delays (Hollis, 1995; McClellan et al., 2003; McClellan & McCurry, 1998). Autism and pervasive developmental disorders also have been reported (Alaghband-Rad et al., 1995; Nicolson et al., 2001; Russell et al., 1989), although these conditions should be considered distinct and separate from schizophrenia (American Academy of Child and Adolescent Psychiatry [AACAP], 2001; Cantor, Evans, Pearce, & Pezzot-Pearce, 1982; Watkins et al., 1988). McClellan and colleagues (2003) found that greater premorbid global impairment, social withdrawal and schizoid/schizotypal personality types differentiate between youth with EOS and those with bipolar disorder or atypical psychosis. Hollis (2003) also found that impaired premorbid social functioning differentiates between youth with EOS and those with other psychotic disorders.

Prodromal Phase

The prodromal phase represents a significant decline from baseline functioning or a worsening of premorbid personality/behavioral characteristics. In general, this phase is characterized by changes in social, cognitive, and/or academic functioning. Presentations can include the development of odd or idiosyncratic beliefs, worsening school performance, social isolation and withdrawal, and/or worsening hygiene. The duration of the prodromal phase can vary from an acute change (days to weeks) to chronic impairment (months to years) (AACAP, 2001). Children generally have an insidious onset (Asarnow & Ben-Meir, 1988; Green & Padron-Gayol, 1986; Kolvin, 1971; Rapoport & Inoff-Germain, 2000). In young adolescents, both acute onset (less than 1 year) and insidious onset are noted (Kolvin, 1971; McClellan et al., 1993; McClellan & McCurry, 1998; Ropcke & Eggers, 2005; Werry et al., 1991). Insidious onset has been found to be predictive of a more severe course of illness (Ropcke & Eggers, 2005). Furthermore, because many youth with EOS have an insidious onset, it is often difficult to distinguish between premorbid personality/cognitive abnormalities and the onset of the disorder.

Acute Phase

Diagnosis is most common in this phase of the illness, because the acute phase is marked by a predominance of positive symptoms (i.e., hallucinations, delusions, disorganized speech and behavior), as well as a significant deterioration in functioning. This phase generally lasts 1 to 6 months or longer, depending in part on the response to treatment (AACAP, 2001). Most youth with EOS will have subsequent acute episodes (Ropcke & Eggers, 2005).

Recovery Phase

Following the acute phase, with remission of the acute psychosis, the patient generally continues to experience a significant degree of impairment for several months (AACAP, 2001), primarily due to negative symptoms (flat affect, anergia, social withdrawal), although some psychotic symptoms may persist (Remschmidt, Martin, Schulz, Gutenbrunner, & Fleischhaker, 1991). In addition, some patients may develop a postschizophrenic depression characterized by dysphoria and flat affect.

Residual Phase

Youth with EOS may have prolonged periods (several months or more) between acute phases, in which they do not experience significant positive symptoms. However, most patients continue to be at least somewhat impaired by negative symptoms.

Longitudinal Outcome

In the adult literature, schizophrenia typically follows a pattern characterized by cycles of the previously discussed phases, with increasing deterioration after each cycle. However, after approximately 10 years, the acute phases of the disorder tend to remit, leaving a residual state (predominately negative symptoms) with varying disability (AACAP, 2001). Further research is needed to clarify whether this long-term pattern holds for EOS. Some youth with schizophrenia may have only one cycle, although most have more (Asarnow et al., 1994; Eggers, 1978; Hollis, 2003; McClellan et al., 1993; Ropcke & Eggers, 2005; Werry et al., 1991). Others remain chronically symptomatic despite adequate treatment (Asarnow et al., 1994; Eggers & Bunk, 1997; Maziade, Gingras, et al., 1996; McClellan et al., 1993; Werry et al., 1991). These patients are generally the most severely impaired and require the most comprehensive treatment resources.

Generally, the literature suggests moderate to severe impairment across the lifetime (Eggers, 1978, 1989; Eggers & Bunk, 1997; Hollis, 2000; Jarbin, Ott, & von Knorring, 2003; Maziade, Bouchard, et al., 1996; Maziade, Gingras, et al., 1996; McClellan et al., 1993; Ropcke & Eggers, 2005; Werry et al., 1991). Premorbid characteristics, such as cognitive ability, treatment response, and adequacy of therapeutic resources invariably influence short-term outcome (Remschmidt et al., 1991). Poor long-term outcome is predicted by family history of nonaffective psychosis, low premorbid functioning, insidious onset, diagnosis prior to adolescence, low intellectual functioning, and severe symptoms during acute phases (Eggers, 1989; Jarbin et al., 2003; Maziade, Bouchard, et al., 1996; Ropcke & Eggers, 2005; Werry, 1992). When followed into adulthood, youth with EOS demonstrated greater social deficits, lower levels of employment, and were less likely to live independently relative to those with other childhood-onset psychotic disorders (Hollis, 2000; Jarbin et al., 2003).

Individuals with EOS also have a high risk of eventual suicide. The risk of suicide or accidental death directly due to behaviors caused by psychotic thinking appears to be at least 5% (Eggers, 1978; Werry, 1991), although the numbers studied are small and the follow-up periods are short in some subjects. In adults with schizophrenia, there is an increased risk for medical illnesses and mortality, including a suicide rate of approximately 10% (APA, 2000). Adults with schizophrenia are also at higher risk for other morbidities, such as heart disease, obesity, human immunodeficiency virus, hepatitis, and diabetes (Goff et al., 2005).

ETIOLOGY AND PATHOGENESIS

Genetic and Environmental Factors

Current research suggests that schizophrenia is a neurodevelopmental disorder that stems from both genetic and environmental risk factors. The phenotype is heterogeneous and complex, with multiple genes and environmental exposures likely involved. Identifying preventable causes and means to avert the disorder remains a public health priority. Furthermore, unraveling molecular mechanisms underlying schizophrenia may shed light on factors responsible for the development of other mental illnesses.

In the general population, family, twin, and adoption studies all support a strong genetic component for schizophrenia. The lifetime risk of developing the illness is 5–20 times higher in first-degree relatives of affected probands compared to the general population (Cardno & Murray, 2003; Thaker & Carpenter, 2001). The rate of concordance among monozygotic twins is approximately 40–60%, whereas the rate of concordance in dizygotic twins and other siblings is 5–15% (Cardno & Gottesman, 2000).

Large, collaborative studies evaluating linkage of schizophrenia in multiply affected families have identified multiple-candidate chromosomal regions (Straub et al., 1995; Zammit, Lewis, & Owen, 2003). Regions best supported by genome-wide scans include 6p22–p24 (Straub et al., 1995), 1q21–q22 (Brzustowicz et al., 2000), and 13q32–q34 (Blouin et al., 1998). Other regions with positive linkage findings include 1q42, 5q21–q33, 6q21–q25, 8p21–p22, 10p15–p11, and 22q11–q12 (Owen, Williams, & O'Donovan, 2004). These regions combined represent a substantial portion of the genome. This is not surprising given genetic heterogeneity and the complexity of neural development.

Candidate genes have been suggested in several of these regions, including dysbindin on 6p22, neuregulin on 8p22, *G72* on 13q34, *COMT* on 22q11, *RGS4* on 1q21, *DISC1* on 1q42, and *GRM3* on 7q21 (see review, Harrison & Weinberger, 2005). Each of these genes is biologically plausible (Harrison & Weinberger, 2005). However, for each candidate gene, both positive and negative associations have been reported; strengths of effects are generally weak; the specific allele or haplotype associated with the illness varies across studies; and definitive causative mutations for the most part have not been identified.

Etiological research for EOS remains limited, although the National Institute of Mental Health's (NIMH) Childhood-Onset Schizophrenia Program has contributed substantially to this area. In its cohort of youth with adolescent-onset schizophrenia, positive associations have been reported for several candidate genes of interest, including dysbindin (Gornick et al., 2005), *GAD1* (Addington et al., 2005) and *G72* (Addington et al., 2004). Furthermore, in this series, the rate of cytogenetic abnormalities, including 22q11 deletion (which is associated with an elevated rate of schizophrenia) appears to be higher than that in reports of adults (Nicolson et al., 1999; Usiskin et al., 1999).

In addition to genetic contributions, environmental factors likely play a role in the development of schizophrenia. Disruptions in prenatal brain development may contribute to the illness. Individuals with schizophrenia have higher rates of minor physical anomalies (Gourion et al., 2004; Hata, Iida, Iwasaka, Negoro, & Kishimoto, 2003; Ismail, Cantor-Graae, & McNeil, 1998; McGrath et al., 2002), deficits in smooth pursuit eye movements (Frazier et al., 1996; Jacobsen & Rapoport, 1998; Jacobsen et al., 1997; Karp et al., 2001; Zahn et al., 1997), developmental disturbances in childhood (Bearden et al, 2000; Cannon et al., 1999; Crow, Done, & Sacker, 1995; Jones, Rogers, Murray, & Marmot, 1994), and structural anomalies on brain imaging (Collinson et al., 2003; Gogtay et al., 2004; James, James, Smith, & Javaloyes, 2004; Keller et al., 2003; Kumra et al., 2004; Kumra, Ashtari, et al., 2005; Lawrie & Abukmeil, 1998; Matsumoto et al., 2001; Sporn et al., 2003).

At the onset of illness, many affected individuals already have ventricular enlargement and decreased hippocampal volume, with some evidence suggesting that individuals with earlier onset have more progressive neuroanatomical changes (Gogtay et al., 2004). Relative to normal controls, greater longitudinal decreases in overall volume of gray matter (Sporn et al., 2003), in frontal lobe (Gogtay et al., 2004), prefrontal cortex (James et al., 2004), temporal lobe (Gogtay et al., 2004), parietal lobe (Gogtay et al., 2004), and thalamus (James et al., 2004) have been described. Deficits in white matter have also been noted in the frontal lobe, anterior and posterior commissures, anterior cingulate, corpus callosum, and the right occipital lobe (Keller et al., 2003; Kumra, Ashtari, et al., 2005). Rapoport and Inoff-Germain (2000) suggest that these changes may peak in adolescence, representing critical neurodevelopmental delay during this time.

In the adult literature, gestational exposures, including maternal starvation, are also suspected risk factors for schizophrenia (Brown, Cohen, Greenwald, & Susser, 2000; Brown et al., 2004; Buka et al., 2001; Neugebauer, 2005; Opler et al., 2004; Smil, 2005; St. Clair et al., 2005; Susser et al., 1996). These putative risk exposures may interact with genetic factors in susceptible individuals.

Psychological and Social Factors

There is no evidence that psychological or social factors cause schizophrenia. Rather, environmental factors interact with biological risk factors to mediate the timing of onset, course, and severity of the disorder. Psychosocial stressors, including family expressed emotion, influence the onset and/or exacerbation of acute episodes, and relapse rates (APA, 2000). Communication deficits are often found in families of youth with EOS, although these may be shared phenotypic traits rather than etiological agents (Asarnow & Ben-Meir, 1988). Similarly, family members of youth with EOS appear to have subtle deficits in neuropsychological functioning (Gochman et al., 2004) that may contribute to increased communication and social difficulties. The interactions between psychological, social, and illness-related factors are complex. Therefore, causal mechanisms cannot be inferred based on positive associations. In terms of social factors, adults with schizophrenia typically have lower socioeconomic status (SES). Overall, adult research has suggested that this is likely a result of the illness causing disability and lower SES, rather than vice versa (Munk-Jorgensen & Mortensen, 1992). Available studies investigating the link between EOS and economic factors have a selection bias toward inpatient samples, with higher rates of low SES found in some studies (Green et al., 1992; Kolvin, 1971; McClellan et al., 1993), but not others (Russell et al., 1989; Werry et al., 1991).

COMORBID DISORDERS

As with other chronic conditions, children and adolescents with EOS have a number of comorbid conditions, including depression, anxiety, and externalizing disorders (McClellan et al., 2003; Russell et al., 1989). In adolescents with EOS, substance abuse is also a major concern (Kumra, Thaden, & Kranzler, 2005; McClellan et al., 2003). Finally, youth with EOS also have a high rate of developmental delays and cognitive difficulties. Many youth with EOS are diagnosed with pervasive developmental disorders.

ASSESSMENT

A diagnosis of schizophrenia is made in youth when DSM-IV-TR, or ICD-10, criteria are met, and other pertinent disorders have been ruled out. The standard principles and procedures of psychological and psychiatric assessment, outlined in this volume, apply to the assessment of EOS. Although a variety of assessment tools (e.g., checklists, rating scales, neuropsychological measures) may be helpful in the assessment of children with EOS, multi-informant interviews, observation and mental status examinations, symptom rating scales, record reviews, and a comprehensive medical evaluation comprise the "gold standard." Long-term monitoring and reassessment are also needed to ensure diagnostic accuracy (AACAP, 2001). Comprehensive assessment techniques are necessary, because the clinical complexity of youth who present with possible EOS often leads to misdiagnosis and inadequate treatment (AACAP, 1998a; Schaeffer & Ross, 2002; Stayer et al., 2004). Assessment of comorbid diagnoses and other domains of functioning (e.g., cognitive, academic, social) are also important for treatment planning.

The procedures for reliable and valid assessment of EOS outlined below should be administered by clinicians using an informed hypothesis-testing approach. The information presented earlier, regarding epidemiology, symptomatology, and course of illness help to guide assessment. Perhaps most importantly, clinicians should remember that EOS, especially childhood onset, is rare, and most children who present with symptoms suggestive of psychosis have neither EOS nor, for that matter, a psychotic illness. Therefore, the diagnosis of EOS requires that clinicians establish the validity of psychotic symptoms while ruling out other, possible conditions with similar presentations (see "Differential Diagnosis" section below).

Typical Referral Questions

Youth with possible EOS may present with psychotic symptoms (i.e., hallucinations, delusions), disorganized behavior or speech, social impairment, academic difficulties, and/or aggression (McClellan et al., 2003; Schaeffer & Ross, 2002; Vourdas et al., 2003). Schaeffer and Ross (2002) found that among youth with schizophrenia, the most frequent initial clinical concerns were school failure and aggressive behavior. Although important issues, these nonspecific concerns present with a number of different clinical situations.

Referrals from medical and mental health professionals typically require accurate diagnostic assessment. The first step of the diagnostic process involves determining whether psychotic symptoms are present (vs. atypical reports concurrent with nonpsychotic disorders or normative childhood phenomena). The second step entails determining the type of psychotic disorder present (EOS vs. other psychotic disorders). Other referral questions include assessing comorbid diagnoses, neuropsychological strengths and weaknesses, and functional impairment; and determining treatment recommendations.

Appropriate treatment is dependent upon an accurate diagnosis. For instance, Schaeffer and Ross (2002) found that prior to an accurate diagnosis of EOS, the majority of children received inappropriate or insufficient treatment (88% received individual psychotherapy, 77% were prescribed stimulant medications). Treatment planning may also be informed by assessment of neuropsychological, academic, social, vocational, and other areas of functioning associated with EOS.

Assessment Procedures

Multi-Informant Assessment

Interviews with the child, caregivers, teachers, and other relevant adults provide rich and ecologically valid data that aid in diagnosis and treatment planning. Involving parents and other important adults in the assessment process is key, because youth at risk for EOS may have difficulty reporting on current symptomatology and relevant history. The multi-informant assessment can provide information relevant to current and previous clinical presentation and course, as well as comorbid conditions. A multi-informant assessment also rules out the possibility of single informant bias.

The interview with the child or adolescent with EOS provides an opportunity to obtain his or her description of current symptoms, as well as to observe the youth's mental status. Youth with EOS can generally describe relevant aspects of their psychotic symptoms, although acutely ill youth may be too disorganized and confused to provide a cogent history. In those cases, however, clinician observations and the mental status exam (see section below) are the best evidence of the disorder. Similarly, negative symptoms, and disorganized speech and thought, may be best assessed through observation and by interviewing other informants.

Involving parents or caregivers in assessment is particularly important when gathering information about developmental, psychological, medical, and family psychiatric history. In addition, caregivers are typically able to provide information about the child's functioning in a variety of settings. Caregiver interview and observation also provide information about important family factors, such as expressed emotion, social support, caregiver burden, and overall caregiver functioning. Because EOS appears to be related to genetic factors, assessment of family psychiatric history is important. Whenever possible, diagnostic verification of an affected family member from a third party (e.g., an affected family member's psychiatrist) is advisable.

Involving other important adults in the assessment is optimal. Teachers, therapists, medical providers, and other professionals can often provide information to supplement child and caregiver interviews. The teacher interview is particularly important, because school is the primary area of functioning for most youth, and data obtained from teachers inform later academic, behavioral, and social intervention. Interviews of teachers should focus on academic performance and social functioning.

STRUCTURED INTERVIEWS

In terms of assessment procedures, diagnostic accuracy of EOS may be substantially improved through the use of structured diagnostic interviews (Carlson Bromet, & Sievers, 2000). Diagnoses made in clinical settings are notorious for being unreliable (McClellan & Werry, 2000). Structured interviews are particularly helpful in the assessment of EOS, as a result of the complexity of the illness. While these tools have been used primarily in epidemiological and clinical research (McClellan & Werry, 2000), they provide a format for reliably assessing both schizophrenia and comorbid conditions. For a full review of structured diagnostic interviews see Doss (2005) and the special issue of the *Journal of the American Academy of Child and Adolescent Psychiatry* edited by McClellan and Werry (2000). Table 11.3 summarizes characteristics of structured interviews

for youth that contain either screening items for psychosis or complete diagnostic criteria for schizophrenia.

It is important to remember that although structured interviews improve reliability, validity is more difficult to establish (McClellan & Werry, 2000). This is a major limitation in all psychiatric research given the lack of biological or other markers for disorders. For complex illnesses such as EOS, it is important for the clinician administering the interview to be familiar with both the illness and, more broadly, developmental psychopathology in youth. Clinician-based structured diagnostic interviews, such as the K-SADS and Kid SCID, are recommended when assessing EOS. These assessments are being used in clinical research (McClellan et al., 2002, Sikich, Hamer, Bashford, Sheitman, & Lieberman, 2004). Clinician-based tools balance structure and flexibility, and provide a structure for the diagnostic interview while allowing for clinician probes, rewording of items, and clinical judgment.

Screening interviews, or nonclinician-based interviews, are not sufficient for the diagnosis of EOS, because the complexity of psychotic symptom presentation in children and adolescents makes it necessary that clinicians, not laypersons or computers, determine the veracity of psychotic symptoms. However, they may be useful screening tools and help to identify youth at risk for EOS and other comorbid disorders.

Clinician familiarity with developmental psychopathology is key, because structured interviews with youth have demonstrated a substantial rate of false-positive results related to psychosis (Breslau, 1987). In general, most youth may not understand the wording of questions relevant to psychosis; therefore, they respond based on their own normal experiences. Few children and adolescents have familiarity with the concept of psychosis. Therefore, they may respond honestly in trying to describe normal mentation. Furthermore, many traumatized youth report unusual sensory experiences that may relate to dissociative symptoms (Hlastala & McClellan, 2005). Although important clinically, these symptoms should not be equated with true psychosis.

When utilizing structured diagnostic interviews, clinicians must be aware of the general nature of psychosis. In general, psychotic symptoms are confusing to the individual and are experienced as external phenomena beyond

TABLE 11.3. Characteristics of Structured Diagnostic Interviews That Assess Psychotic Symptoms in Children and Adolescents

Instrument	Disorders covered	Informant	Age range (years)	Type	Time (minutes)	Interviewer qualifications	Special issues
Child and Adolescent Psychiatric Assessment (CAPA; Angold & Costello, 2000)	BEH, ANX, MOOD, EAT, ELIM, SUB, TIC, SCH, SOM	Child Parent	9–17	Interviewer	60–150	Bachelor plus training program	Glossary used to define symptoms and severity ratings; Spanish version available
Related instruments YAPA (young adult) PAPA (preschool age)		Patient Parent	18+ 3–6				
Diagnostic Interview Schedule for Children—Version IV (DISC-IV; Shaffer et al., 2000) Versions DISC-Y (youth) DISC-P (parent)	BEH, ANX, MOOD, EAT, ELIM, SUB, TIC, SCH	Child Parent	6–17 9–17 6–17	Respondent	70–120	Trained lay interviewers	Self-administered computer and Spanish versions available
Schedule for Affective Disorders and and Schizophrenia for School-Age Children (K-SADS; Ambrosini, 2000) K-SADS-E (epidemiological) K-SADS-PL (present and lifetime) K-SADS-P (present state) Washington University K-SADS	BEH, ANX, MOOD, EAT, SUB, SCH Also assesses TIC and ELIM Expands definitions of mania	Child Parent	6–18	Interviewer	75–90	Trained clinicians	Although designed for clinicians, many researchers use trained interviewers
Diagnostic Interview for Children and Adolescents (DICA; Reich, 2000)	BEH, ANX, MOOD, EAT, ELIM, SUB, SOM, TIC, PSYCH	Child Parent	6–17	Respondent/ interviewer	60–120	Trained lay interviewers	Used both as structured and semistructured interview
Structured Clinical Interview for DSM-IV, Childhood Diagnoses (KID-SCID; Matzner et al., 1997)	BEH, ANX, MOOD, SUB, SCH, SOM	Child Parent	?–17	Interviewer	60–120	Clinicians	Only preliminary data available
Interview Schedule for Children and Adolescents (ISCA; Sherrill & Kovacs, 2000)	BEH, ANX, MOOD, EAT, ELIM, SUB, SOM, TIC, PSYCH	Child Parent	8–17	Interviewer	120 (parent) 60 (child)	Clinicians	Organized around symptom reports
Follow-Up Schedule for Adults (FISA)		Young adults	18+		60–120		Designed for longitudinal research
Children's Interview for Psychiatric Syndromes (ChIPS; Weller et al., 2000)	BEH, ANX, MOOD, EAT, ELIM, SUB, SCH	Child Parent	6–18	Respondent	40	Trained lay interviewers	Primarily a screening tool

Note. Disorders: BEH, disruptive behavior disorders; MOOD, mood disorders (depressive and bipolar); ANX, anxiety disorders (often includes posttraumatic stress disorder); ELIM, encopresis and enuresis; SUB, substance abuse/dependence; TIC, Tic disorders; SCH, schizophrenia and psychotic disorders; PSYCH, nondiagnostic screen for psychotic symptoms; SOM, somatoform disorders. Type of interview: Respondent, answers coded based on response, also described as structured; Interviewer, interviewer allowed to make clinical judgments regarding respondents answers, also called semistructured. Interview times are approximates, and may vary depending on the case and interviewer. From McClellan (2005). Copyright 2005 by American Psychiatric Publishing, Inc. Adapted by permission.

537

his or her control. The more detailed, organized, or ego-syntonic the symptom reports, the less likely such symptoms represent true psychosis. Moreover, psychosis is a process, not just a positive response to a question. When individuals develop psychotic illnesses, there are a number of associated symptoms, including disorganized thinking and behavior, and a deterioration in functioning. Without such symptoms, the validity of psychotic-like symptom reports needs to be scrutinized carefully.

Finally, clinicians should be cautious when investigating psychosis, with or without structured interviews, in children younger than age 12. Among young children and youth with cognitive delays, it is a challenge to identify true psychotic symptoms. In these cases, the clinician must not only ensure that the child understands the context of the question but also take developmental considerations into account. Extrapolating adult symptom definitions onto children's experiences may result in misdiagnosis.

Observation and Mental Status Examination

Observation and mental status examination are key components of a comprehensive evaluation of EOS. Observation should take place during the interview, and whenever possible, in the child's natural environment (e.g., school, home). Observation and mental status examination provide information regarding psychotic, negative, and disorganized symptoms. It is important to observe and assess the structure and form of the youth's speech and language, and also to assess overt behavioral evidence of psychosis, such as responding to internal stimuli. Negative symptoms, such as flat and inappropriate affect, poverty of amount and content of speech, and anhedonia should also be assessed as part of the mental status examination. Disorganized speech and behavior are also observable behavior. Assessment of attention (e.g., serial sevens or fives), problem solving (e.g., "What would you do if you were lost in the forest?"), abstract reasoning (e.g., similarities: "How are . . . and . . . alike?"), and memory should also be assessed. Difficulty with attention, problem solving, abstract reasoning, and memory functioning may suggest a need for neuropsychological assessment. Mental status examination and observation should be conducted in a developmentally appropriate fashion, especially when assessing cognitive function.

Symptom Rating Scales

Brief clinician-administered rating scales may also be used to assess EOS. Scales developed for adults with schizophrenia and administered by clinicians, such as Scale for the Assessment of Positive Symptoms (SAPS; Andreasen & Olsen, 1982), Scale for the Assessment of Negative Symptoms (SANS; Andreasen & Olsen, 1982), and the Positive and Negative Syndrome Scale (PANSS; Kay, Fiszbein, & Opler, 1987) are widely used in research and clinical practice to assess the treatment effects. These rating scales have also been used in studies with juveniles (e.g., McClellan et al., 2002). In addition, utilizing a modified version of the PANSS, Fields and colleagues (1994) found acceptable internal consistency and interrater reliability. Finally, there are also general ratings of psychopathology, such as the Brief Psychiatric Rating Scale for Children (BPRS-C—Hughes, Rentelmann, Emslie, Lopez, & MacCabe, 2001; Lachar et al., 2001), that include questions regarding psychotic symptoms.

McClellan and colleagues (2002) used the SAPS and SANS (Andreasen & Olsen, 1982) and the BPRS-C to assess adolescents with psychotic disorders. Factor analysis of these items identified four factors: negative symptoms, positive symptoms, behavior, and dysphoria. Scores on the negative symptoms factor differentiated between youth with EOS and those with other a bipolar or psychotic disorder, not otherwise specified, suggesting that negative symptoms, as measured by clinician rating scales, may be clinically useful in differential diagnosis. Tools such as the PANSS, SAPS, SANS, and BPRS-C may be helpful in differential diagnosis and assessment. These tools have also been used to measure treatment outcomes (e.g., Kumra et al., 1996, Sikich et al., 2004). Clinician rating scales are recommended, because they are relatively brief tools that can differentiate between children with EOS and those with other psychiatric disorders.

Record Review

Record review is an informative and often neglected assessment tool. Accurate diagnostic assessment requires a longitudinal overview of the pattern of illness rather than a sole focus on cross-sectional symptom presentation. Record review is a helpful tool that provides detailed information that may have been forgotten by the youth and his or her family (e.g., when the child first qualified for special education). In this sense, it can corroborate or question the veracity of a child's and his or her parents' historical report. The clinician should focus on identifying a pattern of declining function and a prodromal phase of illness.

All school-age youth have academic records that provide a measure of school and often social–emotional functioning (e.g., level of class participation, discipline record, social functioning). Academic records of children and adolescents who have been evaluated for or have received special education services may include intellectual, achievement, and social–emotional testing, as well as a functional behavior analysis and other assessments. Youth who qualify for special education services may also have received documented academic, behavioral, emotional, speech and hearing, and occupational interventions.

Outside of the academic setting, because youth who present with possible EOS often have a long history of psychological and, possibly, medical difficulties, they may have received psychological, psychiatric, developmental, neurological, speech and hearing, and other relevant types of assessment. A review of these assessments may be helpful in establishing onset and characterizing the prodromal phase of illness. In addition, a medical record review is likely to be helpful in the current medical evaluation.

Treatment history should also be investigated, because youth with EOS are likely to have received a variety of psychiatric treatments prior to accurate diagnosis (Schaeffer & Ross, 2002). Information on development, premorbid functioning, onset of illness, and the effectiveness of previous treatments should be collected.

Comprehensive Medical Examination

Before a diagnosis of EOS can be made, organic causes must be ruled out. The list of potential exposures or neuropsychiatric conditions associated with psychosis is lengthy. However, entities that should be considered include (1) delirium, (2) seizure disorders, (3) central nervous system lesions (e.g., brain tumors, congenital malformations, head trauma),

(4) neurodegenerative disorders (e.g., Huntington's chorea, lipid storage disorders), (5) metabolic disorders (e.g., endocrinopathies, Wilson's disease), (6) developmental disorders (e.g., velocardiofacial syndrome), (7) toxic encephalopathies (e.g., substances of abuse, such as amphetamines, cocaine, hallucinogens, phencyclidine, alcohol, marijuana, and solvents; medications, such as stimulants, corticosteroids, or anticholinergic agents; and other toxins, such as heavy metals), and (8) infectious diseases (e.g., encephalitis, meningitis, and/or HIV-related syndromes).

Laboratory and neuroimaging procedures are not helpful for making a diagnosis of schizophrenia but may be indicated to rule out other neurological or medical problems. Tests and procedures should be justified based on the clinical presentation and significant findings in either the history or physical examination. As part of the basic medical evaluation (and for medication monitoring), laboratory tests to be considered include blood counts, serum chemistries, thyroid functions, and toxicology screens. If the risk factors are present, HIV testing should be done. Chromosomal analysis may be indicated for patients with clinical presentations/features suggestive of a developmental syndrome. Evidence of neurological dysfunction warrants a more thorough evaluation, including consideration of neuroimaging studies, electroencephalography (EEG), and/or a neurological consultation.

Other Recommended Assessment Procedures

Other assessment tools may be helpful in assessing clinical features associated with EOS and assist in treatment planning, but they are not necessary for diagnosis. Assessment of the youth should include cognitive, academic, and functional measures, as indicated by the clinical presentation. These assessments are particularly helpful in formulating effective psychiatric, academic, social, and vocational interventions.

Behavioral checklists provide useful and efficient methods of screening youth at risk for psychotic disorders and assessing comorbid conditions. Multi-informant checklists such as the Achenbach System of Empirically Based Assessment (ASEBA; Achenbach & Rescorla, 2001), the Behavioral Assessment System for Children–2 (BASC–2; Reynolds & Kamphaus, 2004), the Conners Scales—Revised (Conners,

1997) and the Personality Inventory for Children–2 and Personality Inventory for Youth (PIC-2, PIY; Lachar & Gruber, 2001) are standardized self-report, parent report, and teacher report measures of social and emotional functioning. These measures have acceptable psychometric properties and efficiently assess global psychopathology. They are designed to identify typical DSM-IV-TR disorders of childhood and adolescence. Most include subscales relevant to the assessment of EOS that measure social and cognitive functioning and atypical behavior. Youth with EOS scored higher on subscales of the Child Behavior Checklist (CBCL) that measure social functioning, thought and attention problems, and school competencies (Muratori, Salvadori, Arcangelo, Viglione, & Picchi, 2005). Among youth at a high risk of developing schizophrenia, CBCL ratings in adolescence were found to discriminate between youth who went on to develop the disorder and those who did not (Miller, Byrne, Hodges, Lawrie, & Johnstone, 2002). Despite these data, the CBCL and other checklists are not diagnostically specific to psychotic disorders, much less EOS. Therefore, checklists can identify children and adolescents who may be at risk for EOS, provide information about global psychological functioning, allow for comparison of informants, and assess comorbid conditions. Although neither necessary nor sufficient for a diagnosis of EOS, checklists can be efficient and informative assessment tools. Checklists may also be helpful in treatment planning and in measuring treatment effects.

Cognitive testing can identify specific deficits that may require remediation or accommodation. For EOS, measures of attention, intelligence, memory, and executive functioning (i.e., problem solving, inhibition, working memory) may be particularly relevant. Self-, parent and teacher report checklists, such as the Behavioral Rating Inventory of Executive Functioning (BRIEF; Gioia, Isquith, Guy, & Kenworthy, 2000) may also be helpful in assessing cognitive functioning.

Academic assessment, a primary area of concern for most youth with EOS, is also recommended. A comprehensive assessment of academic achievement through standardized academic skills measures is necessary to identify academic strengths and weaknesses, and to screen for specific learning disabilities. In addition, a behavioral assessment in structured (i.e.,

classroom) and unstructured (i.e., playground, lunchroom) environments may assist in identifying behaviors that interfere with academic functioning. Other assessments relevant to the school setting, such as assessments by occupational and speech therapists, may also be helpful. Based on these assessments, an individualized educational program may then be formulated to improve academic functioning. Academic assessment and remediation are also important, because academic skills may form the foundation for later vocational functioning.

In terms of functional abilities, interviews such as the Vineland Adaptive Behavior Scales, Second Edition (Sparrow, Cicchetti, & Balla, 2005) and checklists such as the Adaptive Behavior Assessment System, Second Edition (Harrison & Oakland, 2000) provide comprehensive measures of adaptive skills. These assessments assist in identifying specific skills deficits that may require remediation. More specifically, they provide specific assessment of social and communication skills.

Although schizophrenia is not caused by family functioning, research suggests that family functioning influences the outcome of the disorder (Leff & Vaughn, 1985). Therefore, assessment of family functioning is important for treatment planning. Assessment of parenting stress, caregiver burden, social support, and expressed emotion is recommended. The Parenting Stress Index, Third Edition (Abidin, 1995) is a brief parent report measure of distress related to parenting. Measures of burden and expressed emotion, such as the Child and Adolescent Burden Assessment (CABA; Messer, Angold, Costello, & Burns, 1996) and the Five Minute Speech Sample (FMSS; Magana, 1993) may also be helpful in measuring caregiver functioning. Although measures such as the CABA and FMSS have been utilized primarily in research, measurement of expressed emotion may be particularly important, because it has been shown to impact relapse rates in adults (Leff & Vaughn, 1985) and is positively correlated with outcomes for a variety of childhood psychiatric and medical disorders (Wamboldt & Wamboldt, 2000).

Other Assessment Issues

Personality assessments are standard components of psychological practice. However, no evidence supports the discriminative validity of objective or projective measures of personality when assessing EOS. Whereas measures such as the Rorschach Inkblot Test or the Thematic Apperception Test have been used by many clinicians to identify psychotic thinking processes, no projective assessment has demonstrated an ability to increase the diagnostic accuracy of EOS. Objective personality tests, including the Minnesota Multiphasic Personality Inventory—Adolescent Edition (MMPI-A) and the Millon Adolescent Clinical Inventory (MACI), are also of limited clinical utility in terms of diagnosis. Instead, they may provide information about comorbid diagnoses and global personality functioning.

Differential Diagnosis

When assessing a child or adolescent with symptoms suggestive of schizophrenia, a thorough diagnostic evaluation is needed to rule out other conditions that present with similar symptomatology and to identify comorbid disorders. Overall, an accurate assessment includes a thorough review of presenting symptoms, course and premorbid functioning, adherence to DSM-IV-TR or ICD-10 criteria, familiarity with how psychotic symptoms present in this youth age group, and determination of family psychiatric history. However, discriminating among these various disorders still may be difficult, especially at the initial presentation, and periodic diagnostic reassessments are always indicated (AACAP, 2001).

Schizophreniform Disorder

Schizophreniform disorder is diagnosed when the duration of illness has not yet reached 6 months. Most of the cases are presumed to meet full criteria eventually for a schizophrenia spectrum disorder, and are treated accordingly.

Psychotic Disorder Not Otherwise Specified

A diagnosis of psychotic disorder not otherwise specified (PD NOS) simply implies that criteria for a defined psychotic illness have not been met. This term is used broadly in clinical settings, perhaps in part based on reticence to label youth with schizophrenia (McClellan, McCurry, Speltz, & Jones, 1999). However, this classification has also been used in research to describe youth with transient or atypical reports of psychotic symptoms, some of whom likely do not have a true psychotic illness. In

the NIMH Childhood Schizophrenia Study, adolescents with PD NOS had similar significant overall impairment, and risk factor profiles and neurobiological abnormalities to those with EOS (Kumra, Jacobsen, et al., 1998; Kumra, Wiggs, et al., 1998; Kumra et al., 2000). Half of those with PD NOS received a later diagnosis of a psychotic mood disorder (e.g., schizoaffective disorder, bipolar disorder, major depressive disorder with psychotic features; Nicolson et al., 2001).

In a prospective study of youth with psychotic disorders, subjects with PD NOS were more likely to have been abused and to have a diagnosis of PTSD in comparison to those with EOS or bipolar disorder (Hlastala & McClellan, 2005). This suggested that their psychotic symptoms may be posttraumatic phenomena, and, clinically, these cases often met criteria for borderline personality disorder. In this study, none of the subjects with PD NOS went on to develop schizophrenia.

Schizoaffective Disorder and Mood Disorders

Schizophrenia, schizoaffective, and psychotic mood disorders (especially bipolar disorder) may present with psychotic symptoms (AACAP, 2001). In children and adolescents with schizophrenia, negative symptoms may be mistaken for depression, especially since it is common for patients to experience dysphoria with their illness. Alternatively, mania in teenagers often presents with florid psychosis, including hallucinations, delusions, and thought disorder (Pavuluri et al., 2004). Psychotic depression may present with mood congruent or incongruent hallucinations or delusions (AACAP, 1998a).

This overlap in symptoms increases the likelihood of misdiagnosis at the time of onset. Historically, approximately one-half of adolescents with bipolar disorder were originally misdiagnosed as having schizophrenia (AACAP, 1997). Awareness of the phenomenon changed diagnostic practices, but did not necessarily improve accuracy (McClellan et al., 1993, 1999). Longitudinal reassessment is needed to ensure accuracy of diagnosis. Family psychiatric history may also be a helpful differentiating factor. Psychotic illnesses have a strong familial component. Therefore, if a youth with psychosis has a close relative with a psychotic disorder, then it is likely that he or she has the same illness.

Youth with bipolar disorder tend to have more mood-congruent delusions and a lower percentage of hallucinations, loosening of associations, and negative symptoms than those with schizophrenia (Calderoni et al., 2001; McClellan et al., 2002; Pavuluri et al., 2004). Bipolar disorder is also more likely to be associated with grandiose delusions, pressured speech, irritability, depression, and elevated mood (Pavuluri et al., 2004). In addition to differences during the acute phase of illness, youth with schizophrenia have higher rates of premorbid social withdrawal and global impairments than do youth with bipolar disorder (McClellan et al., 2003). Furthermore, psychotic symptoms, by definition, must only present during active periods of depression or mania for a diagnosis of bipolar disorder (see Youngstrom, Chapter 6, this volume).

Schizoaffective disorder and major depression with psychotic features may be the most difficult disorders to distinguish from schizophrenia (Calderoni et al., 2001). Negative symptoms of EOS are sometimes mistaken for depression, especially because dysphoria is commonly experienced as a part of EOS. Although an accurate picture of the temporal overlap between mood episodes and psychotic symptoms can be extremely difficult to obtain, this retrospective understanding is necessary to distinguish between EOS and other psychotic disorders. For a diagnosis of depression with psychotic features, psychosis is only present in the context of a severe major depressive episode.

A diagnosis of schizoaffective disorder requires that one meet diagnostic criteria for both schizophrenia and mood disorders independently, over the course of illness. Early-onset schizoaffective disorder has not been well studied in this age group. Follow-up studies of psychotic youth have found low rates of this condition (McClellan et al., 1993; Stayer et al., 2005; Werry et al., 1991). However, the diagnosis is commonly used in clinical settings, perhaps unreliably, since many youth with mood and behavioral dysregulation problems are now characterized as having schizoaffective disorder without clear evidence of true psychosis (McClellan & Hamilton, 2006).

General Medical Conditions

As described earlier, all youth who are evaluated for EOS should receive a comprehensive medical evaluation to rule out a medical cause of symptoms. Given the significant rates of comorbid substance abuse in adolescents with schizophrenia (as high as 50% comorbidity in some studies), it is common to obtain a history of substance abuse at the first onset of psychotic symptoms (Kumra, Thaden, et al., 2005; McClellan et al., 1993, 2002; McClellan & McCurry, 1998). Patients with a substance-induced psychosis generally present with an acute onset of psychotic symptoms that are temporally related to the intake of the drug. Psychostimulants can produce paranoid delusions and disorientation, whereas hallucinogens may produce vivid hallucinations and delusions. Substance intoxication and/or withdrawal can also induce delirium, which is associated with fluctuating mental status, varied levels of consciousness, and altered short-term memory. If psychotic symptoms persist significantly beyond documented detoxification from the abused substance(s), the clinician must consider the diagnosis of a primary psychotic disorder. In adolescents, it is not uncommon for the first psychotic break to occur with comorbid substance abuse, which may be an exacerbating (and possibly a triggering) factor rather than a primary etiological agent (Kumra, Thaden, et al., 2005).

Nonpsychotic Behavioral and/or Emotional Disorders

Youth with conduct disorder and other nonpsychotic emotional disorders may report psychotic-like symptoms and, as a result, be improperly diagnosed as having a primary psychotic disorder (Del Beccaro et al., 1988; Garralda, 1984a, 1984b; Hlastala & McClellan, 2005; Hornstein & Putnam, 1992; McClellan et al., 1993; McClellan & Hamilton, 2006). When compared to youth with psychotic disorders, these youth have lower rates of negative symptoms, bizarre behavior, and thought disorder (Hlastala & McClellan, 2005). At follow-up, an increase in personality dysfunction, including personality disorders but not psychotic disorders, has been found (Garralda, 1984a, 1984b; Lofgren et al., 1991; McClellan et al., 1993; Thomsen, 1996).

Youth who report atypical, psychotic-like phenomena may have problems with tumultuous relationships, and behavioral and affective dysregulation, and are often described as having borderline characteristics (McClellan & Hamilton, 2006). At follow-up, these youth do not seem to have an increased risk for schizophrenia or affective disorders (Lofgren, Bemporad, King, Lindem, & O'Driscoll, 1991; Hlastala & McClellan, 2005). Their reported hallucinations and delusions may be associated with dissociative symptoms, especially when there is a history of abuse or neglect (Altman, Collins, & Mundy, 1997; Hlastala & McClellan, 2005; Hornstein & Putnam, 1992). Maltreated youth, especially those with PTSD, report significantly higher rates of psychotic symptoms than controls (Famularo, Kinscherff, & Fenton, 1992). However, the lack of observable psychotic phenomena, such as formal thought disorder, plus the characteristics of their relationship skills help to distinguish between such youth and those with schizophrenia.

Pervasive Developmental Disorders and Autism

Autism and pervasive developmental disorder (PDD) are distinguished by the absence or transitory nature of psychotic symptoms and the predominance of the characteristic deviant language patterns, aberrant social relatedness, and other key symptoms that characterize these disorders (see Ozonoff, Goodlin-Jones, & Solomon, Chapter 10, this volume; Kolvin, 1971; Volkmar et al., 1988; Volkmar & Cohen, 1991). The onset of schizophrenia is later than that of autism, although some youth with schizophrenia have early premorbid histories of developmental delays (Alaghband-Rad et al., 1995; Russell et al., 1989; Watkins et al., 1988). However, compared to autism, the premorbid abnormalities in EOS tend to be less pervasive and severe. It is important to recognize that symptoms of schizophrenia include social withdrawal and communication problems, which are also criteria for PDD. Schizophrenia is an exclusion criterion for autism and, when present, supercedes the diagnosis of PDD.

Obsessive–Compulsive Disorder

Youth with obsessive–compulsive disorder have intrusive thoughts and repetitive ritualistic behaviors, symptoms that may be difficult to differentiate from psychosis. Patients with obsessive–compulsive disorder generally recognize their symptoms as unreasonable and excessive products of their own thinking (although this may not be the case for young

children) (AACAP, 1998b). Conversely, psychotic symptoms are usually experienced as phenomena occurring independently of the patient's own cognitive processes. However, some obsessive–compulsive symptoms are so severe that distinguishing them from delusions is difficult. Conversely, patients with schizophrenia may have significant obsessive–compulsive features. Therefore, assessment of disorganized thought and behavior, negative symptoms, and other psychotic symptoms is key to differentiating between these disorders.

Other Disorders

Other disorders that need to be differentiated from schizophrenia include speech problems, language disorders, and developmental disorders. Youth with language and communication problems may be mistakenly diagnosed as having a thought disorder. Such children and adolescents do not, however, have other prerequisite symptoms of schizophrenia, such as hallucinations, delusions, or odd social relatedness (Baker & Cantwell, 1991).

TREATMENT

An accurate diagnostic assessment is needed for appropriate treatment. Effective treatment of schizophrenia requires both intensive psychopharmacological and psychosocial interventions (Lehman et al., 2004). In adults, early diagnosis and treatment improve outcome (Harrison et al., 2001). Therefore, it is important that the diagnosis be made when the illness first presents (Shaeffer & Ross, 2002). As Shaeffer and Ross also highlight, misdiagnosis and inadequate treatment are common in children with EOS.

A comprehensive multidisciplinary approach is generally required to address adequately the complexity of the disorder (AACAP, 2001), with the goals of reducing symptomatology, morbidity, and relapse rates, while maintaining patients in their homes and communities. Only a few randomized studies have demonstrated the efficacy of either typical or atypical antipsychotic medications for EOS (Kumra et al., 1996; Pool, Bloom, Mielke, Roniger, & Gallant, 1976; Realmuto, Erikson, Yellin, Hopwood, & Greenberg, 1984; Sikich et al., 2004; Spencer, Kafantaris, Padron-Gayol, Rosenberg, & Campbell, 1992). Thus, current pharmacological practices are largely informed by clinical experience, case reports, and the adult literature (AACAP, 2001). Psychosocial interventions such as cognitive-behavioral psychotherapy (Rector & Beck, 2001) and family psychoeducation and support interventions (for a review, see McDonell & Dyck, 2004) may also be effective in reducing symptoms in youth with EOS. The one study that has investigated the efficacy of a psychosocial treatment in those with EOS yielded promising results (Rund, Moe, Sollien, & Fjell, 1994).

The diagnostic assessment dictates other important domains of treatment planning, including comorbid disorders, cognitive functioning, and academic functioning. Treatments are needed to address these associated areas. Finally, systematic assessment is also important when measuring treatment effectiveness.

SUMMARY AND CONCLUSION

EOS is a neurodevelopmental disorder associated with significant morbidity and chronic impairment. Assessment should include clinician interview with multiple informants, observation and mental status examination, clinician rating scales, record review, and comprehensive medical evaluation. In addition, cognitive, academic, functional, and family assessments may assist in treatment planning. Future research is needed to improve the reliability, validity, and feasibility of assessment tools designed to measure EOS. As advancements in genome and neurodevelopmental sciences occur, mechanisms underlying the disorder are likely to be elucidated, leading to improved diagnostic, treatment, and prevention strategies.

REFERENCES

Abidin, R. R. (1995). *Parenting Stress Index, third edition, professional manual*. Odessa, FL: Psychological Assessment Resources.

Achenbach, T. M., & Rescorla, L. A. (2001). *Manual for the ASEBA school-age forms and profiles*. Burlington: University of Vermont, Research Center for Children, Youth, and Families.

Addington, A. M., Gornick, M., Duckworth, J., Sporn, A., Gogtay, N., Bob, A., et al. (2005). GAD1 (2q51.1), which encodes glutamic acid decarboxylase (GAD67), is associated with childhood-onset schizophrenia and cortical gray matter volume loss. *Molecular Psychiatry, 10*, 581–588.

Addington, A. M., Gornick, M., Sporn, A., Gogtay, N., Bob, A., Greenstein, D., et al. (2004). Polymorphisms in the 13q33.2 gene G72/G30 are associated with childhood-onset schizophrenia and psychosis not otherwise specified. *Biological Psychiatry, 55*, 976–980.

Alaghband-Rad, J., McKenna, K., Gordon, C. T., Albus, K. E., Hamburger, S. D., Rumsey, J. M., et al. (1995). Childhood-onset schizophrenia: The severity of premorbid course. *Journal of the American Academy of Child and Adolescent Psychiatry, 34*, 1273–1283.

Altman, H., Collins, M., & Mundy, P. (1997). Subclinical hallucinations and delusions in nonpsychotic adolescents. *Journal of Child Psychology and Psychiatry, 38*, 413–420.

Ambrosini, P. J. (2000). Historical development and present status of the Schedule for Affective Disorders and Schizophrenia for School-Age Children (K-SADS). *Journal of the American Academy of Child and Adolescent Psychiatry, 39*, 49–58.

American Academy of Child and Adolescent Psychiatry (AACAP). (1997). Practice parameters for the assessment and treatment of children and adolescents with bipolar disorder. *Journal of the American Academy of Child and Adolescent Psychiatry, 36*(Suppl. 10), 177–193.

American Academy of Child and Adolescent Psychiatry (AACAP). (1998a). Practice parameters for the assessment and treatment of children and adolescents with depressive disorders. *Journal of the American Academy of Child and Adolescent Psychiatry, 37*, 63–83.

American Academy of Child and Adolescent Psychiatry (AACAP). (1998b). Practice parameters for the assessment and treatment of children and adolescents with obsessive–compulsive disorder. *Journal of the American Academy of Child and Adolescent Psychiatry, 37*, 27–45.

American Academy of Child and Adolescent Psychiatry (AACAP). (2001). Practice parameters for the treatment of children and adolescents with schizophrenia. *Journal of the American Academy of Child and Adolescent Psychiatry, 40*, 4S–23S.

American Psychiatric Association (APA). (1968). *Diagnostic and statistical manual of mental disorders* (2nd ed.). Washington, DC: Author.

American Psychiatric Association (APA). (1980). *Diagnostic and Statistical Manual of Mental Disorders* (3rd ed.). Washington, DC: Author.

American Psychiatric Association (APA). (2000). *Diagnostic and Statistical Manual of Mental Disorders* (4th ed., text rev.). Washington, DC: Author.

American Psychiatric Association, Steering Committee on Practice Guidelines (APASCPG). (2004). Practice guideline for the treatment of patients with schizophrenia, second edition. *American Journal of Psychiatry, 161*(Suppl. 2), 1–56.

Andreasen, N. C., & Olsen, S. (1982). Negative v positive schizophrenia: Definition and validation. *Archives of General Psychiatry, 39*, 789–794.

Angold, A., & Costello, E. (2000). The Child and Adolescent Psychiatric Assessment (CAPA). *Journal of the American Academy of Child and Adolescent Psychiatry, 39,* 39–48.

Armenteros, J. L., Fennelly, B. W., Hallin, A., Adams, P. B., Pomerantz, P., Michell, M., et al. (1995). Schizophrenia in hospitalized adolescents: Clinical diagnosis, DSM-III-R, DSM-IV, and ICD-10 criteria. *Psychopharmacology Bulletin, 31,* 383–387.

Asarnow, J. R., & Ben-Meir, S. (1988). Children with schizophrenia spectrum and depressive disorders: A comparative study of premorbid adjustment, onset pattern and severity of impairment. *Journal of Child Psychology and Psychiatry, 29,* 477–488.

Asarnow, J. R., Tompson, M. C., & Goldstein, M. J. (1994). Childhood onset schizophrenia: A follow-up study. *Schizophrenia Bulletin, 20,* 647–670.

Baker, L., & Cantwell, D. P. (1991). Disorders of language, speech, and communication. In M. Lewis (Ed.), *Child and adolescent psychiatry: A comprehensive textbook* (pp. 516–521). Baltimore: Williams & Wilkins.

Baltaxe, C. A. M., & Simmons, J. Q., III. (1995). Speech and language disorders in children and adolescents with schizophrenia. *Schizophrenia Bulletin, 21,* 677–692.

Bearden, C. E., Rossom I. M., Hollister, J. M., Sanchez, L. E., Hadley, T., & Cannon, T.D. (2000). A prospective cohort study of childhood behavioral deviance and language abnormalities as predictors of adult schizophrenia. *Schizophrenia Bulletin, 26,* 395–410.

Beitchman, J. H. (1985). Childhood schizophrenia: A review and comparison with adult-onset schizophrenia. *Psychiatric Clinics of North America, 8,* 793–814.

Bettes, B., & Walker, E. (1987). Positive and negative symptoms in psychotic and other psychiatrically disturbed children. *Journal of Child Psychology and Psychiatry and Allied Disciplines, 28,* 555–567.

Biederman, J., Petty, C., Faraone, S. V., & Seidman, L. (2004). Phenomenology of childhood psychosis: Findings from a large sample of psychiatrically referred youth. *Journal of Nervous and Mental Disease, 192,* 607–614.

Blouin, J. L., Dombroski, B. A., Nath, S. K., Lasseter, V. K., Wolyniec P. S., Nestadt, G., et al. (1998). Schizophrenia susceptibility loci on chromosomes 13q32 and 8p21. *Nature Genetics, 20,* 70–77.

Breslau, N. (1987). Inquiring about the bizarre: False positives in Diagnostic Interview Schedule for Children (DISC), ascertainment of obsessions, compulsions and psychotic symptoms. *Journal of the American Academy of Child and Adolescent Psychiatry, 26,* 639–655.

Brown, A. S., Begg, M. D., Gravenstein, S., Schaefer, C. A., Wyatt, R. J., Bresnahan, M., et al. (2004). Serologic evidence of prenatal influenza in the etiology of schizophrenia. *Archives of General Psychiatry, 61,* 774–780.

Brown, A. S., Cohen, P., Greenwald, S., & Susser, E. (2000). Nonaffective psychosis after prenatal exposure to rubella. *American Journal of Psychiatry, 157,* 438–443.

Brzustowicz, L. M., Hodgkinson, K. A., Chow, E. W., Honer, W. G., & Bassett, A. S. (2000). Location of a major susceptibility locus for familial schizophrenia on chromosome 1q21–q22. *Science, 288,* 678–682.

Buka, S. L., Tsuang, M. T., Torrey, E. F., Klebanoff, M. A., Bernstein, D., & Yolken, R. H. (2001). Maternal infections and subsequent psychosis among offspring. *Archives of General Psychiatry, 58,* 1032–1037.

Calderoni, D., Wudarsky, M., Bhangoo, R., Dell, M. L., Nicolson, R., Hamburger, S. D., et al. (2001). Differentiating childhood-onset schizophrenia from psychotic mood disorders. *Journal of the American Academy of Child and Adolescent Psychiatry, 40,* 1190–1196.

Cannon, M., Jones, P., Huttunen, M. O., Tanskanen, A., Huttunen, T., Rabe-Hesketh, S., et al. (1999). School performance in Finnish children and later development of schizophrenia: A population-based longitudinal study. *Archives of General Psychiatry, 56,* 457–463.

Cantor, S., Evans, J., Pearce, J., & Pezzot-Pearce, P. (1982). Childhood schizophrenia, present but not accounted for. *American Journal of Psychiatry, 139,* 758–762.

Caplan, R., Guthrie, D., Gish, B., Tanguay, P., & David-Lando, G. (1989). The Kiddie Formal Thought Disorder Scale: Clinical assessment, reliability, and validity. *Journal of the American Academy of Child and Adolescent Psychiatry, 28,* 408–416.

Caplan, R., Guthrie, D., & Komo, S. (1996). Conversational repair in schizophrenic and normal children. *Journal of the American Academy of Child and Adolescent Psychiatry, 35,* 950–958.

Cardno, A. G., & Gottesman, I. I. (2000). Two studies of schizophrenia: From bow-and-arrow concordances to star wars Mx and functional genomics. *American Journal of Medical Genetics, 97,* 12–17.

Cardno, A., & Murray, R. M. (2003). The "classical" genetic epidemiology of schizophrenia. In R. M. Murray, P. B. Jones, E. Susser, J. van Os, & M. Cannon (Eds.), *Epidemiology of schizophrenia* (pp. 195–219). New York: Cambridge University Press.

Carlson, G. A., Bromet, E. J., & Sievers, S. (2000). Phenomenology and outcome of subjects with early- and adult-onset psychotic mania. *American Journal of Psychiatry, 157,* 213–219.

Collinson, S. L., Mackay, C. E., James, A. C., Quested, D. J., Phillips, T., Roberts, N., et al. (2003). Brain volume, asymmetry and intellectual impairment in the relation to sex in early-onset schizophrenia. *British Journal of Psychiatry, 183,* 114–120.

Conners, C. K. (1997). *Conners's Rating Scales—Revised user's manual.* North Tonawanda, NY: Multi-Health Systems.

Crow, T. J., Done, D. J., & Sacker, A. (1995). Childhood precursors of psychosis as clues to its evolutionary origins. *European Archives of Psychiatry and Clinical Neuroscience, 245,* 61–69.

Del Beccaro, M. A., Burk, P., & McCauley, E. (1988). Hallucinations in children: A follow-up study. *Journal of the American Academy of Child and Adolescent Psychiatry, 27,* 462–465.

Doss, A. J. (2005). Evidence-based diagnosis: Incorporating diagnostic instruments into clinical practice. *Journal of the American Academy of Child and Adolescent Psychiatry, 44,* 947–952.

Eggers, C. (1978). Course and prognosis in childhood schizophrenia. *Journal of Autism and Childhood Schizophrenia, 8,* 21–36.

Eggers, C. (1989). Schizo affective psychosis in childhood: A follow-up study. *Journal of Autism and Developmental Disorders, 19,* 327–334.

Eggers, C., & Bunk, D. (1997). The long-term course of childhood-onset schizophrenia: A 42-year follow-up. *Schizophrenia Bulletin, 23,* 105–117.

Famularo, R., Kinscherff, R., & Fenton, T. (1992). Psychiatric diagnoses of maltreated children: Preliminary findings. *Journal of the American Academy of Child and Adolescent Psychiatry, 31,* 863–867.

Fields, J. H., Grochowski, B. A., Lindenmayer, J. P., Kay, S. R., Grosz, D., Hyman, R. B., et al. (1994). Assessing positive and negative symptoms in children and adolescents. *American Journal of Psychiatry, 151,* 249–253. ·

Fish, B., & Ritvo, E. (1979). Psychoses of childhood. In J. D. Noshpitz & I. Berlin (Eds.), *Basic handbook of child psychiatry* (pp. 249–304). New York: Basic Books.

Frazier, J. A., Alaghband-Rad, J., Jacobsen, L., Lenane, M. C., Hamburger, S., Albus, K., et al. (1997). Pubertal development and onset of psychosis in childhood onset schizophrenia. *Psychiatry Research, 70,* 1–7.

Frazier, J. A., Giedd, J. N., Hamburger, S. D., Albus, K. E., Kaysen, D., Vaituzis, A. C., et al. (1996). Brain anatomic magnetic resonance imaging in childhood-onset schizophrenia. *Archives of General Psychiatry, 53,* 617–624.

Garralda, M. E. (1984a). Hallucinations in children with conduct and emotional disorders: I. The clinical phenomena. *Psychological Medicine, 14,* 589–596.

Garralda, M. E. (1984b). Hallucinations in children with conduct and emotional disorders: II. The follow-up study. *Psychological Medicine, 14,* 597–604.

Gillberg, C. (1984). Infantile autism and other childhood psychoses in a Swedish urban region: Epidemiological aspects. *Journal of Child Psychology and Psychiatry and Allied Disciplines, 25,* 35–43.

Gioia, G. A., Isquith, P. K., Guy, S. C., & Kenworthy, L. (2000). *Behavior Rating Inventory of Executive Functioning, professional manual.* Lutz, FL: Psychological Assessment Resources.

Gochman, P. A., Greenstein, D., Sporn, A., Gogtay, N., Nicolson, R., Keller, A., et al. (2004). Childhood onset schizophrenia: Family neurocognitive measures. *Schizophrenia Research, 71,* 43–47.

Goff, D. C., Cather, C., Evins, A. E., Henderson, D. C., Freudenreich, O., Copeland, P. M., et al. (2005). Medical morbidity and mortality in schizophrenia: Guidelines for psychiatrists. *Journal of Clinical Psychiatry, 66,* 183–194.

Gogtay, N., Sporn, A., Clasen, L. S., Nugen, T. F., Greenstein, D., Nicolson, R., et al. (2004). Comparison of progressive cortical gray matter loss in childhood-onset schizophrenia with that in childhood-onset atypical psychoses. *Archives of General Psychiatry, 61,* 17–22.

Goldberg, T. E., Karson, C. N., Leleszi, J. P., & Weinberger, D. R. (1988). Intellectual impairment in adolescent psychosis: A controlled psychometric study. *Schizophrenia Research, 1,* 261–266.

Gornick, M. C., Addington, A. M., Sporn, A., Gogtay, N., Greenstein, D., Lenane, M., et al. (2005). Dysbindin (DTNBP1, 6p22.3) is associated with childhood-onset psychosis and endophenotypes measured by the Premorbid Adjustment Scale (PAS). *Journal of Autism and Developmental Disorders 10,* 1–8.

Gourion, D., Goldberger, C., Bourdel, M. C., Bayle, F. J., Loo, H., & Krebs, M. O. (2004). Minor physical anomalies in patients with schizophrenia and their parents: Prevalence and pattern of craniofacial abnormalities. *Psychiatric Research, 125,* 21–28.

Green, W. H., Padron-Gayol, M., Hardesty, A. S., & Bassiri, M. (1992). Schizophrenia with childhood onset: A phenomenological study of 38 cases. *Journal of the American Academy of Child and Adolescent Psychiatry, 31,* 968–976.

Harrison, G., Hopper, K., Craige, T., Laska, E., Siegel, C., Wanderling, J., et al. (2001). Recovery from psychotic illness: A 25-year international follow-up study. *British Journal of Psychiatry, 178,* 506–517.

Harrison, P. J., & Weinberger, D. R. (2005). Schizophrenia genes, gene expression, and neuropathology: On the matter of their convergence. *Molecular Psychiatry, 10,* 40–68.

Harrison, P. L., & Oakland, T. (2003). *Adaptive Behavior Assessment System, second edition, manual.* San Antonio, TX: Harcourt Assessment.

Hata, K., Iida, J., Iwasaka, H., Negoro, H., & Kishimoto, T. (2003). Association between minor physical anomalies and lateral ventricular enlargement in childhood and adolescent onset schizophrenia. *Acta Psychiatrica Scandinavica, 108,* 147–151.

Helgeland, M. I., & Torgersen, S. (2005). Stability and prediction of schizophrenia from adolescence to adulthood. *European Child and Adolescent Psychiatry, 14,* 83–94.

Hlastala, S. A., & McClellan, J. (2005). Phenomenology and diagnostic stability of youths with atypical psychotic symptoms. *Journal of Child and Adolescent Psychopharmacology, 15,* 497–509.

Hollis, C. (1995). Child and adolescent (juvenile onset)

schizophrenia: A case control study of premorbid developmental impairments. *British Journal of Psychiatry, 166*(4), 489–495.

Hollis, C. (2000). Adult outcomes of child- and adolescent-onset schizophrenia: Diagnostic stability and predictive validity. *American Journal of Psychiatry, 157*, 1652–1659.

Hollis, C. (2003). Developmental precursors of child- and adolescent-onset schizophrenia and affective psychoses: Diagnostic specificity and continuity with symptom dimensions. *British Journal of Psychiatry, 182*, 37–44.

Hornstein, J. L., & Putnam, F. W. (1992). Clinical phenomenology of child and adolescent dissociative disorders. *Journal of the American Academy of Child and Adolescent Psychiatry, 31*, 1077–1085.

Hughes, C. W., Rentelmann, J., Emslie, G. J., Lopez, M., & MacCabe, N. (2001). A revised anchored version of the BPRS-C for childhood psychiatric disorders. *Journal of Child and Adolescent Psychopharmacology, 11*, 77–93.

Ismail, B., Cantor-Graae, E., & McNeil, T. F. (1998). Minor physical anomalies in schizophrenic patients and their siblings. *American Journal of Psychiatry, 155*, 1695–1702.

Jacobsen, L. K., Giedd, J. N., Berquin, P. C., Krain, A. L., Hamburger, S. D., Kumra, S., et al. (1997). Quantitative morphology of the cerebellum and fourth ventricle in childhood-onset schizophrenia. *American Journal of Psychiatry, 154*, 1663–1669.

Jacobsen, L. K., & Rapoport, J. L. (1998). Research update: Childhood-onset schizophrenia: Implications of clinical and neurobiological research. *Journal of Child Psychology and Psychiatry and Allied Disciplines, 39*, 101–113.

James, A. C., James, S., Smith, D. M., & Javaloyes, A. (2004). Cerebellar, prefrontal cortex, and thalamic volumes over two time points in adolescent-onset schizophrenia. *American Journal of Psychiatry, 161*, 1023–1029.

Jarbin, H., Ott, Y., & von Knorring, A. L. (2003). Adult outcome of social functioning in adolescent-onset schizophrenia and affective psychosis. *Journal of the American Academy of Child and Adolescent Psychiatry, 42*, 176–183.

Jones, P., Rodgers, B., Murray, R., & Marmot, M. (1994). Child development risk factors for adult schizophrenia in the British 1946 birth cohort. *Lancet, 344*, 1398–1402.

Karp, B. I., Garvey, M., Jacobsen, L. K., Frazier, J. A., Hamburger, S. D., Bedwell, J. S., et al. (2001). Abnormal neurological maturation in adolescents with early-onset schizophrenia. *American Journal of Psychiatry, 158*, 118–122.

Kay, S. R., Fiszbein, A., & Opler, L. A. (1987). The Positive and Negative Syndrome Scale (PANSS) for schizophrenia. *Schizophrenia Bulletin, 13*, 261–176.

Keller, A., Jeffries, N. A., Blumenthal, J., Clasen, L. S.,

Liu, H., Giedd, J. N., et al. (2003). Corpus callosum development in childhood-onset schizophrenia. *Schizophrenia Research, 62*, 105–114.

Kenny, J. T., Friedman, L., Findling, R. L., Swales, T. P., Strauss, M. E., Jesberger, J. A., et al. (1997). Cognitive impairment in adolescents with schizophrenia. *American Journal of Psychiatry, 154*, 1316–1325.

Kolvin, I. (1971). Studies in the childhood psychoses. *British Journal of Psychiatry, 6*, 209–234.

Kraepelin, É. (1919). Dementia praecox and paraphrenia. In R. M. Barclay (Trans.), *Textbook of psychiatry* (8th ed., Vol. 3, part 2). Edinburgh, UK: Livingstone.

Kumra, S., Ashtari, M., Cervellione, K. L., Henderson, I., Kester, H., Roofeh, D., et al. (2005). White matter abnormalities in early-onset schizophrenia: A voxel-based diffusion tensor imaging study. *Journal of the American Academy of Child and Adolescent Psychiatry, 44*, 934–941.

Kumra, S., Ashtari, M., McMeniman, M., Vogel, J., Augusin, R., Becker, D. E., et al. (2004). Reduced frontal white matter integrity in early-onset schizophrenia: A preliminary study. *Biological Psychiatry, 55*, 1138–1145.

Kumra, S., Frazier, J. A., Jacobsen, L. K., McKenna, K., Gordon, C., Lenane, M. C., et al. (1996). Childhood-onset schizophrenia: A double-blind clozapine–haloperidol comparison. *Archives of General Psychiatry, 53*, 1090–1097.

Kumra, S., Jacobsen, L. K., Lenane, M., Zahn, T. P., Wiggs, E., Alaghband-Rad, J., et al. (1998). "Multidimensionally impaired disorder": Is it a variant of very early-onset schizophrenia? *Journal of the American Academy of Child and Adolescent Psychiatry, 37*, 91–99.

Kumra, S., Thaden, E., & Kranzler, H. (2005). Correlates of substance abuse in adolescents with treatment-refractory schizophrenia and schizoaffective disorder. *Schizophrenia Research, 73*, 369–371.

Kumra, S., Wiggs, E., Bedwell, J., Smith, A. K., Arling, E., Albus, K., et al. (2000). Neuropsychological deficits in pediatric patients with childhood-onset schizophrenia and psychotic disorder not otherwise specified. *Schizophrenia Research, 42*, 135–144.

Kumra, S., Wiggs, E., Krasnewich, D., Meck, J., Smith, A. C., Bedwell, J., et al. (1998). Brief report: Association of sex chromosome anomalies with childhood-onset psychotic disorders. *Journal of the American Academy of Child and Adolescent Psychiatry, 37*, 292–296.

Lachar, D. & Gruber, C. P. (2001). *Personality Inventory for Children, second edition, manual.* Los Angeles: Western Psychological Services.

Lacher, D., Randle, S. L., Harper, R. A., Scott-Gurnell, K. C., Lewis, K. R., Santos, C. W., et al. (2001). The Brief Psychiatric Rating Scale for Children (BPRS-C): Validity and reliability of an anchored version. *Journal of the American Academy of Child and Adolescent Psychiatry, 37*, 333–340.

Lawrie, S. M., & Abukmeil S. S. (1998). Brain abnormality in schizophrenia: A systematic and quantitative review of volumetric magnetic resonance imaging studies. *British Journal of Psychiatry, 172,* 1110–1120.

Leff, J., & Vaughn, C. (1985). *Expressed emotion in families: Its significance for mental illness.* New York: Guilford Press.

Lehman, A. F., Kreyenbuhl, J., Buchanan, R. W., Dickerson, F. B., Dixon, L. A., Goldberg, R., et al. (2004). The schizophrenia Patient Outcomes Research Team (PORT): Updated treatment recommendations 2003. *Schizophrenia Bulletin, 30,* 193–217.

Lofgren, D. P., Bemporad, J., King, J., Lindem, K., & O'Driscoll, G. (1991). A prospective follow-up study of so-called borderline children. *American Journal of Psychiatry, 148,* 1541–1547.

Loranger, A. (1984). Sex differences in age at onset of schizophrenia. *Archives of General Psychiatry, 41,* 157–161.

Magana, A. B. (1993). *Manual for coding expressed emotion from the Five Minute Speech Sample.* Los Angeles: UCLA Family Project.

Matsumoto, H., Simmons, A., Williams, S., Hadjulis, M., Pipe, R., Murray, R., et al. (2001). Superior temporal gyrus in early-onset schizophrenia: Similarities and differences with adult-onset schizophrenia. *American Journal of Psychiatry, 158,* 1299–1304.

Matzner, F., Silva, R., Silvan, M., Chowdhury, M., & Nastasi, L. (1997). *Preliminary test–retest reliability of the KID-SCID.* Proceedings of the American Psychiatric Association Meeting. Available online at *cpmcnet.columbia.edu/dept/scid/kidscid. htm*

Maziade, M., Bouchard, S., Gingras, N., Charron, L., Cardinal, A., Roy, M. A., et al. (1996). Long-term stability of diagnosis and symptom dimensions in a systematic sample of patients with onset of schizophrenia in childhood and early adolescence, II: Positive/negative distinction and childhood predictors of adult outcome. *British Journal of Psychiatry, 169,* 371–378.

Maziade, M., Gingras, N., Rodrigue, C., Bouchard, S., Cardinal, A., Gauthier, B., et al. (1996). Long-term stability of diagnosis and symptom dimensions in a systematic sample of patients with onset of schizophrenia in childhood and early adolescence, I: Nosology, sex and age of onset. *British Journal of Psychiatry, 169,* 361–370.

McClellan, J. M. (2005). Diagnostic Interviews. In J. Wiener & M. K. Dulcan (Eds.), *The American Psychiatric Publishing textbook of child and adolescent psychiatry* (3rd ed., pp. 137–148). Washington, DC: American Psychiatric Publishing.

McClellan, J. M., Breiger, D., McCurry, C., & Hlastala, S. A. (2003). Premorbid functioning in early onset psychotic disorders. *Journal of the American Academy of Child and Adolescent Psychiatry, 42,* 666–672.

McClellan, J. M., & Hamilton, J. D. 2006). An evidence-based approach to an adolescent with emo-

tional and behavioral dysregulation. *Journal of the American Academy of Child and Adolescent Psychiatry, 45,* 489–493.

McClellan, J. M., & McCurry, C. (1998). Neurocognitive pathways in the development of schizophrenia. *Seminars in Clinical Neuropsychiatry, 3,* 320–322.

McClellan, J. M., & McCurry, C. (1999). Early onset psychotic disorders: Diagnostic stability and clinical characteristics. *European Child and Adolescent Psychiatry, 8*(Suppl. 2), 1S–7S.

McClellan, J. M., McCurry, C., Snell, J., & DuBose, A. (1999). Early onset psychotic disorders: Course and outcome over a two year period. *Journal of the American Academy of Child and Adolescent Psychiatry, 38,* 1380–1389.

McClellan, J. M., McCurry, C., Speltz, M. L., & Jones, K. (2002). Symptom factors in early-onset psychotic disorders. *Journal of the American Academy of Child and Adolescent Psychiatry, 41,* 791–789.

McClellan, J. M., Prezbindowski, A., Breiger, D., & McCurry, C. (2004). Neuropsychological functioning in early onset psychotic disorders. *Schizophrenia Research, 68,* 21–26.

McClellan, J. M., & Werry, J. S. (2000). Introduction: Research psychiatric diagnostic interviews for children and adolescents. *Journal of the American Academy of Child and Adolescent Psychiatry, 39,* 19–27.

McClellan, J. M., Werry, J. S., & Ham, M. (1993). A follow-up study of early onset psychosis: Comparison between outcome diagnoses of schizophrenia, mood disorders and personality disorders. *Journal of Autism and Developmental Disorders, 23,* 243–262.

McDonell, M. G., & Dyck, D. G. (2004). Multiple family group treatment as an effective intervention for children suffering from psychological disorders. *Clinical Psychology Review, 24,* 685–706.

McGrath, J., El-Saadi, O., Grim, V., Cardy, S., Chapple, B., Chant, D., et al. (2002). Minor physical anomalies and quantitative measures of the head and face in patients with psychosis. *Archives of General Psychiatry, 59,* 458–464.

Messer, S. C., Angold, A., Costello, E. J., & Burns, B. J. (1996). The child and adolescent burden assessment (CABA): Measuring the family impact of emotional and behavioral problems. *International Journal of Methods in Psychiatric Research, 6,* 261–284.

Miller, P. M., Byrne, M., Hodges, A., Lawrie, S. M., & Johnstone, E. C. (2002). Childhood behaviour, psychotic symptoms and psychosis onset in young people at risk of schizophrenia: Early findings from the Edinburgh High Risk Study. *Psychological Medicine, 32,* 173–179.

Munk-Jorgensen, P., & Mortensen, P. B. (1992). Social outcome in schizophrenia: A 13-year follow-up. *Social Psychiatry and Psychiatric Epidemiology, 27,* 129–134.

Muratori, F., Salvadori, F., D'Arcangelo, G., Viglione, V., & Picchi, L. (2005). Childhood psychopathological antecedents in early onset schizophrenia. *European Psychiatry, 20*, 309–314.

Neugebauer, R. (2005). Accumulating evidence for prenatal nutritional origins of mental disorders. *Journal of the American Medical Association, 294*, 621–623.

Nicolson, R., Giedd, J. M., Leane, M., Hamburger, S., Singarachariu, S., Badwell, J., et al. (1999). Clinical and neurobiological correlates of cytogenetic abnormalities in childhood-onset schizophrenia. *American Journal of Psychiatry, 156*, 1575–1579.

Nicolson, R., Leane, M., Brookner, F. B., Gochman, P., Kumra, S., Spechler, L., et al. (2001). Children and adolescents with psychotic disorder not otherwise specified: A 2-to 8- year follow up study. *Comprehensive Psychiatry, 42*, 319–325.

Opler, M. G., Brown, A. S., Graziano, J., Desai, M., Zheng, W., Schaefer, C., et al. (2004). Prenatal lead exposure, delta-aminolevulinic acid, and schizophrenia. *Environmental Health Perspective, 112*, 548–552.

Owen, M. J., Williams, N. M., & O'Donovan, M. C. (2004). The molecular genetics of schizophrenia: New findings promise new insights. *Molecular Psychiatry, 9*, 14–27.

Pavuluri, M. N., Herbener, E. S., & Sweeney, J. A. (2004). Psychotic symptoms in pediatric bipolar disorder. *Journal of Affective Disorders, 80*, 19–28.

Pool, D., Bloom, W., Mielke, D. H., Roniger, J. J., Jr., & Gallant, D. M. (1976). A controlled evaluation of loxitane in seventy-five adolescent schizophrenia patients. *Current Therapeutic Research, 19*, 99–104.

Rapoport, J. L., & Inoff-Germain, G. (2000). Update on childhood-onset schizophrenia. *Current Psychiatric Reports, 2*, 410–415.

Realmuto, G. M., Erikson, W. D., Yellin, A. M., Hopwood, J. H., & Greenberg, L. M. (1984). Clinical comparison of thiothixene and thioridazine in schizophrenic adolescents. *American Journal of Psychiatry, 141*, 440–442.

Rector, N. A., & Beck, A. T. (2001). Cognitive behavioral therapy for schizophrenia: An empirical review. *Journal of Nervous and Mental Disease, 189*, 278–287.

Reich, W. (2000). Diagnostic Interview for Children and Adolescents (DICA). *Journal of the American Academy of Child and Adolescent Psychiatry, 39*, 59–66.

Remschmidt, H., Martin, M., Schulz, E., Gutenbrunner, C., & Fleischhaker, C. (1991). The concept of positive and negative schizophrenia in child and adolescent psychiatry. In A. Marneros, N. C. Andreasen, & M. T. Tsuang (Eds.), *Positive versus negative schizophrenia* (pp. 219–242). Berlin: Springer-Verlag.

Reynolds, C. R., & Kamphaus, R. W. (2004). *Behavior Assessment System for Children, second edition (BASC-2), manual*. Circle Pines, MN: American Guidance Services.

Ropcke, B., & Eggers, C. (2005). Early-onset schizophrenia: A 15-year follow-up. *European Journal of Child and Adolescent Psychiatry, 14*, 341–350.

Rund, B. R., Moe, L., Sollien, T., & Fjell, A. (1994). The psychosis project: Outcome and cost-effectiveness of a psychoeducational treatment programme for schizophrenic adolescents. *Acta Psychiatrica Scandinavica, 89*, 211–218.

Russell, A. T., Bott, L., & Sammons, C. (1989). The phenomenology of schizophrenia occurring in childhood. *Journal of the American Academy of Child and Adolescent Psychiatry, 28*, 399–407.

Rutter, M. (1972). Childhood schizophrenia reconsidered. *Journal of Autism and Child Schizophrenia, 2*, 315–337.

Schaeffer, J., & Ross, R. G. (2002). Childhood-onset schizophrenia: Premorbid and prodromal diagnosis and treatment histories. *Journal of the American Academy of Child and Adolescent Psychiatry, 41*, 538–545.

Shaffer, D., Fisher, P., Lucus, C. P., Dulcan, M. K., & Schwab-Stone, M. E. (2000). NIMH Diagnostic Interview Schedule for Children—Version IV (NIMH DISC-IV): Description, differences from previous versions and reliability of some common diagnoses. *Journal of the American Academy of Child and Adolescent Psychiatry, 39*, 28–38.

Sherrill, J. T., & Kovacs, M. (2000). Interview Schedule for Children and Adolescents (ISCA). *Journal of the American Academy of Child and Adolescent Psychiatry, 39*, 67–75.

Sikich, L., Hamer, R. M., Bashford, R. A., Sheitman, B. B., & Lieberman, J. A. (2004). A pilot study of risperidone, olanzapine, and haloperidol in psychotic youth: A double-blind, randomized, 8-week trial. *Neuropsychopharmacology, 29*, 133–145.

Smil, V. (2005). China's great famine: 40 years later. *British Medical Journal, 319*, 1619–1621.

Sparrow, S. S., Cicchetti, D. V., & Balla, D. A. (2005). *Vineland Adaptive Behavior Scales, second edition*. Circle Pines, MN: American Guidance Services.

Spencer, E. K., Kafantaris, V., Padron-Gayol, M. V., Rosenberg, C., & Campbell, M. (1992). Haloperidol in schizophrenic children: Early findings from a study in progress. *Psychopharmacology Bulletin, 28*, 183–186.

Sporn, A. L., Greenstein, D. K., Gogtay, N., Jeffries, N. O., Leane, M., Gochman, P., et al. (2003). Progressive brain volume loss during adolescence in childhood-onset schizophrenia. *American Journal of Psychiatry, 160*, 2181–2189.

St. Clair, D., Xu, M., Wang, P., Yu, Y., Fang, Y., Zhang, F., et al. (2005). Rates of adult schizophrenia following prenatal exposure to the Chinese famine of 1959–1961. *Journal of the American Medical Association, 294*, 557–562.

Stayer, C., Sporn, A., Gogtay, N., Tossell, J. W., Leane, M., Gochman, P., et al. (2005). Multidimensionally impaired: The good news. *Journal of Child and Adolescent Psychopharmacology, 15*, 510–519.

Stayer, C., Sporn, A., Gogtay, N., Tossell, J. W., Leane, M., Gochman, P., et al. (2004). Looking for childhood schizophrenia: Case series of false positives.

Journal of the American Academy of Child and Adolescent Psychiatry, 43, 1026–1029.

Straub, R. E., MacLean, C. J., O'Neill, F. A., Burke, J., Murphy, B., Duke, F., et al. (1995). A potential vulnerability locus for schizophrenia on chromosome 6p24–22: Evidence for genetic heterogeneity. *Nature Genetics, 11*, 287–293.

Susser, E. S., Neugebauer, R., Hoek, H. W., Brown, A. S., Lin, S., Labovitz, D., et al. (1996). Schizophrenia after prenatal famine. Further evidence. *Archives of General Psychiatry, 53*, 25–31.

Thaker, G. K., & Carpenter, W. T. (2001). Advances in schizophrenia. *Nature Medicine, 7*, 667–671.

Thomsen, P. H. (1996). Schizophrenia with childhood and adolescent onset: A nationwide register-based study. *Acta Psychiatrica Scandinavica, 94*, 187–193.

Usiskin, S. I., Nicolson, R., Krasnewich, D. M., Yan, W., Lenane, M., Wudarsky, M., et al. (1999). Velocardio-facial syndrome in childhood-onset schizophrenia. *Journal of the American Academy of Child and Adolescent Psychiatry, 38*, 1536–1543.

Volkmar, F. R., & Cohen, D. J. (1991). Comorbid association of autism and schizophrenia. *American Journal of Psychiatry, 148*, 1705–1707.

Volkmar, F. R., Cohen, D. J., Hoshino, Y., Rende, R. D., & Paul, R. (1988). Phenomenology and classification of the childhood psychoses. *Psychological Medicine, 18*, 191–201.

Vourdas, A., Pipe, R., Corrigal, R., & Frangou, S. (2003). Increased developmental deviance and premorbid dysfunction in early onset schizophrenia. *Schizophrenia Research, 62*, 13–22.

Wamboldt, M. Z., & Wamboldt, F. S. (2000). Role of the family in the onset and outcome of childhood disorders: Selected research findings. *Journal of the American Academy of Child and Adolescent Psychiatry, 39*, 1212–1219.

Watkins, J. M., Asarnow, R. F., Tanguay, P., & Perdue, S. (1988). Symptom development in childhood onset schizophrenia. *Journal of Child Psychology and Psychiatry and Allied Disciplines, 29*, 865–878.

Weller, E. B., Weller, R. A., Fristad, M., Rooney, M. T., & Schecter, J. (2000). Children's Interview for Psychiatric Syndromes (ChIPS). *Journal of the American Academy of Child and Adolescent Psychiatry, 39*, 76–84.

Werry, J. S. (1979). Psychoses. In H. C. Quay & J. S. Werry (Eds.), *Psychopathological disorders of childhood* (2nd ed., pp. 43–89). New York: Wiley.

Werry, J. S. (1992). Child and adolescent (early onset) schizophrenia: A review in light of DSM-III-R. *Journal of Autism and Developmental Disorders, 22*, 601–624.

Werry, J. S., McClellan, J., & Chard, L. (1991). Early-onset schizophrenia, bipolar and schizoaffective disorders: A clinical follow-up study. *Journal of the American Academy of Child and Adolescent Psychiatry, 30*, 457–465.

World Health Organization (WHO). (1992). *The ICD-10 classification of mental health and behavioural disorders: Clinical descriptions and diagnostic guidelines.* Geneva: Author.

Zahn, T. P., Jacobsen, L. K., Gordon, C. T., McKenna, K., Frazier, J. A., & Rapoport, J. L. (1997). Autonomic nervous system markers of psychopathology in childhood-onset schizophrenia. *Archives of General Psychiatry, 54*, 904–912.

Zammit, S., Lewis, G. G., & Owen, M. J. (2003). Molecular genetics and epidemiology in schizophrenia: A necessary partnership. In R. M. Murray, P. B. Jones, E. Susser, J. van Os, & M. Cannon (Eds.), *Epidemiology of schizophrenia* (pp. 220–234). New York: Cambridge University Press.

CHAPTER 12

Intellectual Disability (Mental Retardation)

Benjamin L. Handen

The field of intellectual disability, or mental retardation, went through a number of sweeping changes during the latter half of the 20th century. The catalyst for such changes began in the 1960s, with the movement to deinstitutionalize residents in State schools for individuals with intellectual disability. Today, almost 50 years later, a significant number of institutions have closed, and it is the exception rather than the rule that a child or adult with intellectual disability is placed in such a large group setting. Over this same period of time, an important series of laws were enacted, guaranteeing appropriate educational services for children with intellectual disability, beginning with Public Law 94-142 in 1975, in which the concepts of normalization and least restrictive environment were stressed. Others, such as Public Law 99-457, enacted in 1986, recognized the need for comprehensive early intervention and enhanced educational services for infants and young children with disabilities (including intellectual disability). And most recently, we have seen a growing movement to include children with intellectual disability in our schools and communities (the Individuals with Disabilities Education Act [IDEA], 1990, 2004). This is exemplified by the inclusion of children with intellectual disability on a full-time basis in classrooms with typically developing peers.

With such significant changes in the field, assessing children with intellectual disability has become evermore challenging. It requires knowledge of the service delivery system, and etiological and developmental issues; the ability to work with families; experience in using and adapting standardized assessment tools; and an understanding of the legal rights of children and their families, and best clinical practices for assessment and intervention. My purpose in this chapter is to present best practices guidelines for the assessment of children with intellectual disability that take into account the rapidly changing service delivery system.

HISTORY

Treatment of individuals with intellectual disability and other disabilities has changed considerably during the past 200 years (Wolfensberger, 1969; Zigler & Hodapp, 1986). Significant changes in the field of intellectual disability in the United States began in the middle of the 19th century. This was motivated largely by the work of Edouard Seguin in France, who felt that individuals with a variety of handicapping conditions could be taught, if provided appropriate training. During this same period of time, a number of schools for children and adults with intellectual disability (as well as training centers for deaf, blind, or mentally ill individuals) were established. These early institutions were based on the principle of "moral education," which assumed that, through education, individuals with intellectual disability could be elevated to a level of normal human existence. However, only a small percentage of individuals with intellectual disability were able to return successfully to society and independent living situations. Gradually, institutions began to change in character, serving a less educational and a more custodial purpose to protect individuals with intellectual disability from society (Wolfensberger, 1969).

With the publication of Galton's work on genius across British families, Dugdale's (1910) study of the Juke family, and Goddard's (1913) study of the Kallikaks, there became greater acceptance of the role of heredity in intelligence. Related studies reported that adults with intellectual disability had higher than expected rates of illegitimacy, criminality, and poverty (see Baumeister, 1970). At around this same time, intelligence testing was introduced to the United States by Henry Goddard and quickly gained popularity. Repeated testing by Goddard of individuals with intellectual disability found little improvement in intellectual functioning over time (see Zigler & Hodapp, 1986). The number of institutions also grew, with placement farther from urban areas, as the role of the institution changed to that of protecting society from individuals with intellectual disability. As public fears grew, the first eugenics laws were passed in the early 20th century, requiring the forced sterilizations of men and women with intellectual disability. By 1936, 25 States had passed such laws (see Zigler & Hodapp, 1986). With the exception of a few experiments in the provision of community services, institutions and the number of individuals residing in them grew steadily until the 1960s.

According to Zigler and Hodapp (1986), the deinstitutionalization movement began in earnest in the 1960s, due in large part to four events and trends. First, a number of individuals made public the deplorable conditions in some of our nation's institutions. This included publication of Christmas in Purgatory (Blatt & Kaplan, 1966), a pictorial documentary of several institutions, as well as increased media attention (such as a television exposé of the Willowbrook facility in Staten Island by Geraldo Reviera). Second, the National Associ-

ation for Retarded Citizens began to apply increasing political pressure to change institutions. Third, was the development of the principle of "normalization," which promotes the idea that individuals have the right to experience a life-style that is as normal as possible. Finally, laws such as Public Law 94-142, were enacted, stressing the doctrine of "least restrictive environment." This law, known as the Education for All Handicapped Children Act of 1975, mandated "a free appropriate public education" as a right for all children, regardless of level of impairment of disability. All children were to be placed in the "least restrictive" school environment and provided with an Individual Education Program (IEP).

Today we have a wide continuum of services for children with intellectual disability: from early intervention programs for infants to developmental preschool programs, and from special education programs in regular public schools to full inclusion programs. The goal of today's service provider is to include children within the community in the least restrictive setting.

The enactment of recent laws affecting individuals with disabilities, as well as changes in the service provision model, have significantly influenced assessment practices. For example, with the enactment of Public Laws 94-142 (1975) and 99-457 (1986), families have been given a more central role in the assessment and decision-making process. Additionally, with the use of the IEP, children and adolescents with disabilities must receive programming designed to meet their individual needs rather than simply being fitted into existing programs or services. Consequently, assessment must focus on identifying a child's or adolescent's strengths and deficits to develop an appropriate educational program. As I discussed below, the definition of "intellectual disability" itself is now more functionally based, stressing both cognitive and functional deficits (American Association on Mental Retardation [AAMR], 2002).

DEFINITION OF INTELLECTUAL DISABILITY/ MENTAL RETARDATION

"Intellectual disability" (mental retardation) refers to a particular state of functioning that begins prior to age 18, characterized by significant limitations in both intellectual functioning and adaptive behavior (AAMR, 2002). The definition of "intellectual disability" has been revised a number of times during the past few decades as our understanding of the disorder has changed, and in response to various consumer, professional, political, and social forces. Even now, there is some controversy regarding how one defines and diagnoses intellectual disability (AAMR, 2002). Yet without an agreed-upon definition, it is difficult for professionals to understand fully the nature of this disorder and to make significant gains in improving the lives of children and adults with intellectual disability (Zigler & Hodapp, 1986). The confusion in this area can be illustrated by examining changes in the definition of "intellectual disability" adopted by the American Association on Intellectual and Developmental Disabilities (AAIDD; previously known as the American Association on Mental Deficiency [AAMD] and the American Association on Mental Retardation [AAMR]) during the past half-century.

In 1959 the AAIDD definition of "intellectual disability" specified that individuals with IQ scores one standard deviation or greater below the mean of 100 were considered to have intellectual disability (Heber, 1959). With most IQ tests having a mean of 100 and a standard deviation of 15–16 points, this placed a significant portion of the population (up to 16%, or 32 million people) in this group. The definition was amended in 1973 to a two standard deviation cutoff (IQ below 70), thereby lowering the incidence of intellectual disability to around 2–3%, or 6 million individuals. The subsequent 1983 revision of the AAIDD definition read as follows: "Mental retardation [intellectual disability] refers to significantly subaverage intellectual functioning resulting in or associated with impairments in adaptive behavior and manifested during the developmental period" (Grossman, 1983, p. 11). This definition involved three specific factors: (1) intellectual functioning below 70, (2) associated adaptive deficits, and (3) deficits occurring prior to age 18. Whereas this revision represented an improvement over earlier attempts to define intellectual disability, it also placed greater emphasis than did prior definitions on associated deficits in adaptive functioning. This created some difficulties, because few, if any, reliable and valid measures of adaptive functioning were available at the time, and there was little agreement over both the definition of "adap-

tive behavior" and how to assess it (Zigler & Hodapp, 1986).

Basing a diagnosis of intellectual disability on an IQ score alone was not without its problems as well. For example, the past few decades have seen much criticism of the use of intelligence tests for school placement purposes, because of concerns that such tests are biased against certain minorities (Hawkins & Cooper, 1990). Therefore, using a single factor, such as a score on an IQ test, to define intellectual disability may have resulted in a greater number of children from minority groups being labeled with intellectual disability and placed in special education classes. Such concerns were reflected in a 1974 court decision in California (*Larry P. v. Riles*, 1974), in which the use of IQ tests for purposes of special education placement by California school districts was eliminated.

1992 AAIDD Definition

In 1992, the AAIDD proposed and adopted a new definition that reads as follows:

> Mental retardation [intellectual disability] refers to substantial limitations in present functioning. It is characterized by significantly subaverage intellectual functioning, existing concurrently with related limitations in two or more of the following applicable adaptive skills areas: communication, self-care, home living, social skills, community use, self-direction, health and safety, functional academics, leisure, and work. Mental retardation manifests before age 18. (AAMR, 1992, p. 5)

Three aspects of this new definition were controversial. First, the IQ range had again been changed, this time suggesting "an IQ standard score of approximately 70 to 75 or below" (p. 5). The second concern about this new definition was the requirement that up to 10 areas of adaptive functioning be assessed. However, there continued to be no agreed-upon parameters for assessing adaptive behavior in a number of these areas (MacMillan, Gresham, & Siperstein, 1995). Finally, the new definition eliminated the previously used classification system that divided individuals with intellectual disability into four IQ categories based on level of cognitive functioning (*Mild*, *Moderate*, *Severe*, and *Profound*), opting instead for a classification system based the level and intensity of supports needed (*Intermittent*, *Limited*, *Extensive*, and *Pervasive*) by individuals across a range of domains.

With the elimination of IQ as a means of describing individuals' levels of functioning, there was no clear substitute terminology. Many researchers, educators, and providers criticized the elimination of the severity levels, because it was no longer possible to classify individuals with intellectual disability. Additionally, the use of levels of support had no psychometric properties, making them subjective and unreliable. At the same time, the use of intensity levels (i.e., levels of support) was felt to be cumbersome. The elimination of severity levels even affected teacher certification requirements in some states, where teachers were specifically certified in *Severe/Profound* or *Mild/Moderate* mental retardation. Although proponents argued that the intensity levels were not meant to be psychometrically sound, these levels were often used as if they were. Others were concerned that the number of individuals diagnosed with intellectual disability would increase when the IQ cutoff was raised from 70 to "70 to 75." It was feared that this would result in an overrepresentation of minorities diagnosed with intellectual disability. Finally, there were issues related to the imprecision of the 10 adaptive behavior domains, which had not been determined empirically.

2002 AAIDD Definition

The most recent, 2002, AAIDD definition of intellectual disability contains a number of noteworthy revisions. First, the 2002 revision resulted in a return to the two standard deviation IQ test cutoff for intellectual disability (lowering the cutoff from a standard score of "70 to 75" back to 70). Second, IQ range was once again deemed appropriate for use in describing individuals with intellectual disability (i.e., individuals could be described as having *Mild*, *Moderate*, *Severe*, or *Profound* levels of mental retardation). Third, a revision in the definition of adaptive behavior deficits was made. Whereas the 1992 AAIDD definition required specific deficits in at least 2 of 10 specific skills areas, the 2002 definition requires significant limitations in "adaptive behavior as expressed in conceptual, social and practical adaptive skills" (AAMR, 2002, p. 1). These three broader domains were felt to be more consistent with available research on adaptive behavior. However, the support intensity needs were retained as well, because feedback from many families and individuals with intellectual disability indicated a preference for the shift away from a focus on impairment to one describing the supports necessary for an individual; the focus on supports was also felt to provide guidance regarding the types of services needed (Polloway, 1997, p. 176).

As discussed in the newest AAIDD publication on definition, classification, and systems of support in mental retardation (AAMR, 2002), there was also some controversy regarding the names for the various subtypes of mental retardation, as well as pressure to explore an alternative to the term "mental retardation" itself. MacMillan, Siperstein, and Gresham (1996) proposed using the terms "cognitive impairment" or "general learning disability" for individuals with mild mental retardation. This same group recommended that the term "mental retardation" be reserved for individuals with organicity. Many European professional journals had been using the term "intellectual disability" in place of the term "mental retardation." This same terminology was recently accepted by the AAIDD Board of Directors, and in 2007 the name of the Association was officially changed from the AAMR to the AAIDD. In this chapter I use the terms "mental retardation" and "intellectual disability" interchangeably, because not all organizations and systems serving this population have accepted this new terminology.

CLASSIFICATION

A number of ways have been developed to classify children with intellectual disability during the past few decades. Such systems are clearly required due to the heterogeneous makeup of this group of individuals and serve a number of purposes. Most importantly they serve as a means of distinguishing between subgroups to determine level and intensity of required services and to examine long-term prognosis and treatment outcome. The two most common means of classification involve division by either functional ability or etiology. In some aspects, these two systems have considerable overlap.

Different professional groups have tended to develop their own classification systems. For example, as discussed earlier, in 1992, the AAIDD adopted a system based on level of support needed (*Intermittent*, *Limited*, *Extensive*, and *Pervasive*). Conversely, the American

Psychiatric Association chose to retain levels of cognitive functioning to describe individuals with intellectual disability (i.e., mild, moderate, severe, and profound mental retardation). Educators have used a separate system of classification based on IQ level, with associated deficits in adaptive functioning (e.g., Special Education Services, 1990; West Virginia Department of Education, 1985). Consequently, it is important that clinicians who assess children with intellectual disability both understand the different classification systems and be able to move comfortably among these systems, depending on the agency with which one is communicating.

The 1973 and 1983 AAIDD definitions of intellectual disability divided severity of disability into four categories (mild, moderate, severe, and profound mental retardation), a classification system that continues to have widespread acceptance and use (see Table 12.1). Children who function within the mild range of mental retardation comprise approximately 85% of children diagnosed with intellectual disability. Most children with mild mental retardation can be expected to succeed within an academic curriculum, although most will remain below their typically developing peers in terms of reading and arithmetic levels. Many of these children participate in vocational training and succeed in competitive employment, and live independent and self-supporting lives. Children with moderate mental retardation comprise approximately 10% of children with intellectual disability. The curriculum for these individuals often focuses on life skills and functional academics. With proper vocational training and community support, individuals with moderate mental retardation may be able to manage competitive, or semicompetitive, employment situations. Children with severe mental retardation make

up approximately 3.5% of the population of children with intellectual disability. These individuals typically have less extensive communication and social skills. A more life-skills, functional curriculum is often provided, with emphasis on self-help skills. Finally, less than 1.5% of children with intellectual disability fall in the category of profound mental retardation. These children tend to develop very basic communication skills and limited self-help skills.

Schools have tended to develop their own classification systems for purposes of educational placement. Terms such as "classrooms for the educable mentally retarded" (for children functioning in the mild range of mental retardation) or for the trainable mentally retarded (children functioning within the moderate range of mental retardation) have been used for some time. However, with the growing trend of inclusion practices, such educational labels may be of little use. Some districts have moved toward more functional descriptors for children's needs, because placement is less and less likely to be based on level of cognitive functioning. Instead, appropriate services follow the child, who may be served in any number of settings, including the regular education classroom.

An alternative classification system divides individuals based on etiology. It has been generally accepted that between 25 and 50% of individuals with intellectual disability have an organic etiology for their cognitive and adaptive skills deficits. Specific biomedical causes have been found in as many as 70% of individuals with severe/profound mental retardation (Shapiro, 2002). The remaining individuals are assumed to have intellectual disability due to psychosocial or familial factors. However, both the AAIDD (AAMR, 1992, 2002) publications on the definition and classification of intellectual disability suggested that this two-factor

TABLE 12.1. Classification of Mental Retardation

Level of mental retardation	IQ range	Approximate mental age in adulthood	% of persons with mental retardation at this level
Mild	55–69	8 years, 3 months to 10 years, 9 months	85.0
Moderate	36–51	5 years, 7 months to 8 years, 2 months	10.0
Severe	20–35	3 years, 2 months to 5 years, 6 months	3.5
Profound	<20	<3 years, 2 months	1.5

Note. From Sattler (2002, p. 337). Copyright 2002 by Jerome M. Sattler, Publisher. Adapted by permission.

classification system was no longer appropriate. First, as Masland (1988) argued, simply because there is no known cause for the presence of an intellectual disability does not necessarily mean that an organic etiological explanation does not exist. It may be that our knowledge and technology are not yet at an advanced enough stage to detect many of the causes of intellectual disability. For example, not until 1969 was fragile X syndrome discovered (Lubbs, 1969). This syndrome may account for a considerable number of males with intellectual disability and is caused by what appears to be a pinching of the tips of the long arm of the X chromosome. Similarly, during the past few decades, there has been a greater appreciation of the potential adverse effects of environmental teratogens, such as lead poisoning, even at subclinical levels (Mendola, Selevan, Gutter, & Rice, 2002). The current view is that intellectual disability has multiple causal factors, including genetic predisposition, environmental insults, developmental vulnerability, heredity, and environment (Harris, 2006). Consequently, the AAIDD proposed a multifactorial approach to etiology, involving the following four categories (AAMR, 2002, p. 127):

1. *Biomedical*: factors that relate to biological processes, such as genetic disorders or nutrition.
2. *Social*: factors that relate to social and family interaction, such as stimulation and adult responsiveness.
3. *Behavioral*: factors that relate to potentially causal behaviors, such as dangerous (injurious) activities or maternal substance abuse.
4. *Educational*: factors that relate to the availability of educational supports that promote mental development and the development of adaptive skills.

PREVALENCE OF INTELLECTUAL DISABILITY

There are about twice as many males as females among individuals with mild mental retardation; the male to female ratio decreases somewhat to 1.5:1.0 among those with severe mental retardation (Chiurazzi & Oostra, 2000). Historically, the incidence of intellectual disability in the United States has been estimated to be approximately 3% of the population (Heward, 2006). Based on the normal distribution of intelligence, approximately 2.3% of the population would be expected to fall two standard deviations below the mean IQ of 100 (i.e., IQ below 70). On the one hand, this could be seen as a slight underestimate, because it fails to take into account those individuals whose intellectual disability is due to organic factors that would not reflect normal variations in intelligence. On the other hand, basing estimates of the incidence of intellectual disability on IQ alone may result in a considerable *overestimate* of the true prevalence rate. Two recent studies suggest incidence rates of closer to 1% if significant deficits in both IQ and adaptive functioning are required for a diagnosis of intellectual disability (Fujiura, 2003; Larson et al., 2001). Another factor making it difficult to determine easily the "true" incidence of intellectual disability is that differences exist in reported rates across age groups. For example, infants, toddlers, and preschoolers are generally not diagnosed with intellectual disability unless a child evidences severe developmental delays. Conversely, the incidence of intellectual disability seems to be greatest at school age, when children having learning difficulties are typically assessed and diagnosed. Yet even recent estimates from the U.S. Office of Special Education Programs (2004) indicates that only around 1% of students receive special education due to cognitive deficits. McLaren and Bryson (1987) reported that the prevalence of intellectual disability in children peaks between 10 and 14 years of age, because children with milder impairments tend to be identified much later than children who are more severely involved. Once individuals reach adulthood, the reported rate of intellectual disability decreases, due in part to the fact that once the academic demands of school end, some adults with previous diagnoses of intellectual disability obtain jobs, evidence only minimal adaptive skills deficits, and need few, if any, supportive services. According to the 2002 AAIDD definition of mental retardation, such individuals may no longer meet criteria for a diagnosis of intellectual disability.

Clinicians are generally reluctant to make a diagnosis of intellectual disability in children under 5–6 years of age, preferring instead to use the term "development delay." The reasons for this are threefold, according to Fotheringhan (1983): (1) Measurement of intelligence in infants and preschoolers, which focuses primarily on developmental progress, is not always reliable; (2) other conditions (e.g., cerebral palsy, aphasia) may affect communication or motor skills required to assess intelligence; and (3) various family circumstances, such as neglect or abuse, may adversely affect functioning (whereas functioning may improve as these issues are addressed). Children with developmental delays should receive intervention services and periodic reassessment to assist in determining whether diagnosis of intellectual disability should eventually be made.

The reliability of early intelligence testing is highly dependent upon factors such as age of the child and level of cognitive functioning. Assessment of infants tends to focus on developmental progress, especially sensory–motor functions. Thus, infant tests do not assess the same factors as those designed for children at and above preschool age. Assessment results during infancy that suggest average or above functioning have little predictive power (Sattler, 2001). Conversely, for infants whose scores suggest a developmental disability, there is a much higher correlation with later functioning. For example, Brooks-Gunn and Lewis (1983) found that 73% of a group of infants who had tested within the moderate to profound range of mental retardation continued to be classified with intellectual disability 1 to 3 years later. However, this study did not include infants with milder delays. Sattler (2001) rightfully cautioned that such findings are based on group data, that no diagnosis should be based on a single score, and that infants may have very individualized rates of development. Test scores have been found to be rather unstable for otherwise normally developing preschoolers. Conversely, such scores tend to be fairly stable for preschoolers with disabilities in the cognitive domain (Kamphaus, 2001). In general, children's intelligence test scores appear to stabilize around 6 years of age (Kamphaus, 2001). It is around this period of time (which correlates with entry to school) that clinicians are likely to begin to use the term "intellectual disability" (rather than "developmental disability") for children who continue to evidence significant deficits in cognitive and adaptive functioning.

CAUSES OF INTELLECTUAL DISABILITY

Approximately 70% of individuals with severe mental retardation and 50% of individuals with mild mental retardation have an organic or biological basis for their disorder (McLaren & Bryson, 1987). Some children's cognitive deficits may simply reflect the lower end of the normal IQ distribution (Achenbach, 1982). In such cases, functioning represents an interaction of both genetic and environmental factors. Factors such as poverty, neglect, abuse, limited stimulation, and poor parent–child interactions are but a few of the psychosocial factors that have been found to be related to intellectual functioning (AAMR, 2002). In attempting to determine possible biological causes of intellectual disability in an individual, three time spans should be examined: prenatal onset, perinatal onset, and postnatal onset. Table 12.2 outlines the general hypotheses and strategies for determining possible causes of intellectual disability for each of these areas. It should be noted that the presence of a particular etiology in and of itself does not indicate that an individual will have an intellectual disability. For example, approximately 50% of individuals with cerebral palsy have intellectual disability. Other disorders, such as neurofibromatosis, involve a gradual regression in skills and cognitive functioning over time. Consequently, a child with this disorder may exhibit age-appropriate functioning during early assessments but will likely be diagnosed with intellectual disability at some later point in time.

According to the American Psychiatric Association (APA; 2000), heredity accounts for about 5% of cases of intellectual disability; inherited factors include metabolic errors present at conception (e.g., Tay–Sachs disease), single-gene anomalies with Mendelian inheritance patterns and varying expression (e.g., tuberous sclerosis), and chromosomal abnormalities (e.g., translocation Down syndrome). Early alterations of embryonic development account for approximately 30% of intellectual disability cases and include chromosomal aberrations (e.g., trisomy 21 Down syndrome) or toxin-induced prenatal injury (e.g., maternal alcohol consumption). Postnatal problems account for about 6% of cases; these include fetal malnutrition, hypoxia, various infections, and traumas. General medical conditions acquired in infancy or childhood account for approximately 5% of cases and include traumas, infections, and poisoning. Finally, environmental influences (e.g., deprivation) and other mental disorders (e.g., autism) account for approximately 15–20% of cases.

TABLE 12.2. Hypotheses and Strategies for Determining Etiology

Hypothesis	Possible strategies
I. Prenatal onset	
A. Chromosomal disorder	• Extended physical examination • Referral to geneticist • Chromosomal analysis, including fragile X study and high-resolution banding
B. Syndrome disorder	• Extended family history and examination of relatives • Extended physical examination • Referral to clinical geneticist or neurologist
C. Inborn error of metabolism	• Screening for amino acids and organic acids • Quantification of amino acids in blood, urine, and/or spinal fluid • Analysis of organic acids by gas chromatography–mass spectroscopy or other methods • Blood levels of lactate, pyruvate, carnitine, and long-chain fatty acids • Arterial ammonia and gases • Assays of specific enzymes • Biopsies of specific tissue for light and electron microscopic study and biochemical analysis
D. Developmental disorder	• Computed tomographic (CT) scan of brain formation • Magnetic resonance imaging (MRI) scan of the brain
E. Environmental influence	• Growth charts • Placental pathology • Maternal history and physical examination of mother • Toxicological screening of mother at prenatal visits of child at birth • Referral to clinical geneticist
II. Perinatal onset	• Review maternal records (prenatal care, labor, and delivery) • Review birth and neonatal records
III. Postnatal onset	
A. Head injury	• Detailed medical history • Skull X-rays, CT, or MRI scan (for evidence of sequelae)
B. Infection	• Detailed medical history
C. Demyelinating disorder	• CT or MRI scan
D. Degenerative disorder	• CT or MRI scan • Evoked potential studies • Assays of specific enzymes • Biopsy of specific tissue for light and electron microscopy and biochemical analysis
E. Seizure disorder	• Electroencephalography
F. Toxic–metabolic disorder	• See "Inborn error of metabolism" (IC) • Toxicological studies, heavy metal assays
G. Malnutrition	• Body measurements • Detailed nutritional history • Family history of nutrition
H. Environmental deprivation	• Detailed social history • Psychological evaluation • Observation in new environment
I. Hypoconnection syndrome	• Detailed morphological study of tissue (Huttenlocher, 1991)

Note. From AAMR (2002, pp. 133–134). Copyright 2002 by the American Association on Mental Retardation. Reprinted by permission.

Determining the etiology of intellectual disability may be useful for a number of reasons. First, families often have a desire to understand why their children have cognitive and adaptive skills deficits. This may help with the process of coming to accept a child's difficulties and allow the family to move ahead to ensure that the child's needs are appropriately met. Second, if a genetic basis for a child's disability is identified, there may be a need for other family members, such as siblings or parents, to pursue genetics counseling for future planning. Third, with a clear etiology, one may be able to provide information on long-term course and the types of supports a child will be likely to need. Fourth, there may be clear treatment implications if certain etiologies are determined (e.g., phenylketonuria, hydrocephalus, lead intoxication, seizure disorders). Finally, determining the etiological basis for intellectual disability in general allows individuals to be placed into more homogenous groupings and results in improved research in the field.

PSYCHIATRIC DISORDERS IN CHILDREN WITH INTELLECTUAL DISABILITY

Children and adolescents with intellectual disability can experience the entire range of psychiatric disorders and appear to be at greater risk than the general population for developing such disorders (Emerson, 2003; Quay & Hogan, 1999). In fact, the presence of behavioral and/or comorbid psychiatric disorders in children with intellectual disability may present the most significant obstacle toward inclusion in both educational and community settings (Johnson, 2002). A number of recent prevalence studies have documented that between 30 and 50% of children with intellectual disability have psychiatric diagnoses or behavior problems, which is up to three times that found among the typically developing population (Dekker & Koot, 2003a; Emerson, 2003; Linna et al., 1999; Stromme & Diseth, 2000). Such rates are consistent with those reported by Rutter, Tizard, Yule, Graham, and Whitmore (1976) in the Isle of Wight study. Whereas males and older children with intellectual disability appear to be at greatest risk for developing psychiatric disorders according to some studies (Emerson, 2003; Stromme & Diseth, 2000), this finding is less robust in others (Dekker & Koot, 2003a). Level of intellectual disability does not appear to increase an individual's risk of a psychiatric diagnosis (Dekker & Koot, 2003a; Emerson, 2003; Stromme & Diseth, 2000). Outcome predictors for continued mental health problems appear to include poor social competence and daily living skills, child health problems, negative life events, and parental mental health issues (Dekker & Koot, 2003b)

Externalizing disorders, such as attention-deficit/hyperactivity disorder (ADHD) and conduct disorders, appear to be among the most common behavioral disorders diagnosed in children with intellectual disability (Emerson, 2003). Surveys indicate that between 9 and 16% of children with intellectual disability meet diagnostic criteria for ADHD, a rate that is three to five times greater than that of the general population (Dekker & Koot, 2003a; Emerson, 2003; Stromme & Diseth, 2000). Longitudinal studies have found that the majority of children with intellectual disability and ADHD continue to exhibit symptoms 2–4 years posttreatment (Aman, Pejeau, Wolford, Rojahn, & Handen, 1996; Handen, Janosky, & McAuliffe, 1997). Between 17 and 25% of children with intellectual disability exhibit conduct problems, with oppositional defiant disorder being the most commonly reported diagnosis (Dekker & Koot, 2003a; Emerson, 2003).

Estimates regarding the rate of internalizing disorders (e.g., anxiety, depression) among children and adolescents with intellectual disability are quite variable. Whereas surveys have reported the rate of anxiety disorders to range from 3 to 8.7% (Emerson, 2003; Linna et al., 1999), studies using structured diagnostic interviews of parents have found rates approaching 22% (Dekker & Koot, 2003a). Similarly, survey data indicate that depression among children and adolescents with intellectual disability is around 1.5%, whereas structured parent interviews suggest a rate above 4% (Dekker & Koot, 2003a; Emerson, 2003; Linna et al., 1999). Although diagnosis of an externalizing disorder is generally based on observable behavior, diagnosis of anxiety or mood disorders often requires the description of internal states. Consequently, the rate of internalizing disorders among individuals with intellectual disability is likely to be an underestimate, because the available data are based solely on parental reports of observable symptoms (e.g., crying, loss of appetite, difficulty sleeping), without the additional benefit of a clinical interview of the child or adolescent.

In diagnosing psychiatric disorders in children and adolescents with intellectual disability, the clinician must often rely on observable behavior rather than self-report (MacLean, 1993). It is generally accepted that diagnostic criteria for psychiatric disorders, such as those found in DSM-IV-TR (APA, 2000) can be reasonably applied to children and adolescents functioning at IQs above 50. However, such criteria appear to be less appropriate for individuals functioning below that level (MacLean, 1993).

Numerous conditions with which the clinician should be familiar are often associated with specific maladaptive behavior disorders. For example, children with fragile X syndrome typically function in the mild to moderate range of mental retardation and often exhibit attentional deficits, hyperactivity, hand flapping, hand biting, perseverative speech, preoccupation with inanimate objects, shyness, and poor social interaction (Hagerman & Sobesky, 1989). Children with autism often engage in a range of maladaptive behaviors, such as stereotyped and repetitive motor mannerisms (e.g., hand or finger flapping), impairments in social interactions, and deficits in communication (e.g., delayed expressive language development, stereotyped and repetitive use of language) (APA, 2000). Finally, Prader–Willi syndrome is characterized by mild mental retardation, impaired satiety, food-seeking behavior, and obesity (AAMR, 2002). The presence of specific maladaptive behaviors during an assessment may suggest that a particular disorder or syndrome be considered. This further informs the progress of the assessment, including the types of questions to be asked, the possible need for more extended observation of the child or adolescent, and the need for evaluation by clinicians in other professional fields (e.g., genetics, endocrinology). Similarly, when a child or adolescent with a specific disorder or syndrome is referred for evaluation, knowledge of the associated behavioral indices is necessary to guide the evaluation.

LEGAL ISSUES AND STATE POLICIES

The past few decades have seen the enactment of a number of laws that have significantly affected the assessment and delivery of services for children and adolescents with intellectual disability. Among the most far-reaching pieces of legislation was the IDEA (Public Law 94-142), passed by Congress in 1975. This landmark piece of legislation resulted in significant changes in how children with intellectual and other disabilities are to be educated. The primary purpose of the IDEA is to "assure that all children with disabilities have available to them . . . a free appropriate public education which emphasizes special education and related services designed to meet their unique needs, to assure that the rights of children with disabilities and their parents or guardians are protected, to assist states and localities to provide for the education of all children with disabilities, and to assess and assure the effectiveness of efforts to educate children with disabilities" (IDEA, 1990, §1400[c]). The IDEA comprises six primary principles:

1. *Zero reject.* Schools were required to educate all children with disabilities, ages 6 through 17 years (states that provided educational services for children 3–5 and 18–21 years of age would also be required to provide educational services to children with disabilities in those age groups).

2. *Nondiscriminatory identification and evaluation.* All testing needed to be conducted in the student's native language, and students could not be discriminated against based on race, culture, or native language. Placement decisions could not be based on a single test score.

3. *Free, appropriate public education.* All children, regardless of disabilities, were entitled to a free, appropriate public education, with an IEP developed for each child with special needs.

4. *Least restrictive environment.* Students were to be educated in the least restrictive school environment. School districts were required specifically to justify why a student could not participate with typical peers in academic classes and nonacademic activities (e.g., lunch, gym, transportation). School districts were also mandated to provide a continuum of placement options to meet the least restrictive needs of each student.

5. *Due process safeguards.* Parents who disagreed with the results of an evaluation or placement decision could obtain a due process hearing.

6. *Parent and student participation and shared decision making.* Both parents and the identified student were to be involved in decisions regarding the design and implementation of services.

In addition, to these six principles, the IDEA required that a student be provided with related services and assistive technology, if the disability prevented the child from fully participating in educational activities. Such services included special transportation, speech and language therapy, physical and occupational therapy, and counseling.

The IDEA was reauthorized in 1997 (Pub. L. 105-17) and again in 2004 (Pub. L. 108-446). It is now referred to as the Individuals with Disabilities Education Improvement Act of 2004. In addition to maintaining most of the original provisions, the reauthorized bill includes a number of new regulations. For example, school districts are now allowed to use funds to provide early intervention services (i.e., services for students who have not yet been identified with disabilities but are in need of academic and/or behavioral support). Paperwork has been reduced to increase teacher instruction time. Additionally, the bill provides funds for the training of school staff in effective teaching strategies and outlines steps to be taken to prevent overidentification of minority students. Furthermore, both the definition of a learning disability and the process for amending IEPs has been revised (providing greater flexibility in identifying students with learning problems) (Council for Exceptional Children, 2005). Additional updates on the reauthorized bill may be found on websites hosted by advocacy groups such as the Council for Exceptional Children (2005).

Another law that has had a significant impact on the provision of services to children with special needs was Public Law 99-457 (enacted in 1986). An amendment to the 1975 Public Law 94-142, it extended IDEA rights and protections to children ages 3–5 with developmental disabilities. Additionally, early intervention services for infants and toddlers (birth to 2 years of age) with developmental disabilities and their families were authorized. Infants and toddlers were determined to be in need of early intervention services if they were diagnosed with a physical or mental condition with a high probability of resulting developmental delay, or if they exhibited developmental delays in one or more of the following areas (as measured by an appropriate diagnostic instrument): cognitive development, physical development, language and speech development, psychosocial development, or self-help skills. An individualized family service plan was to be developed for identified infants and toddlers.

The clinician must be well versed not only in the provisions of certain federal laws but also have a working knowledge of state legal decisions affecting the assessment and placement of children in special education programs. For example, two court cases in the early 1970s (*Pennsylvania Association of Retarded Children (PARC) v. Commonwealth of Pennsylvania*, 1971, and *Mills v. Board of Education*, 1972) were "class actions" that established the legal rights of children with intellectual disability to a free public education and as normalized an educational placement as possible. Such cases set the stage for the enactment of laws such as Public Law 94-142. In 1974, a California court decision (*Larry P. v. Riles*) disallowed the use of IQ tests for purposes of classroom placement in that state, because standardized intelligence tests were found by the court to be racially and culturally biased. A number of other states have been affected by similar court decisions regarding the assessment and placement of minority children in special education.

Other court cases, such as *Bales v. Clark* (1981) and *Battle v. Commonwealth of Pennsylvania* (1981), focused on a school district's responsibilities in meeting a child's educational needs. In the former case, the family of a 13-year-old girl who had sustained a head injury following an accident requested that the district provide funding for the girl to attend a specialized private school located outside the district. The Eighth U.S. Circuit Court of Appeals in Virginia sided with the school district by ruling that costs may be considered in placement decisions. The court also ruled that the family need not be reimbursed for the cost of a tutor over the summer. Only in cases where irreparable loss of progress during the summer months could be documented would districts be required to provide year-round schooling. Conversely, in the latter case in Pennsylvania, the U.S. Court of Appeals for the Third Circuit recognized that some children who are severely or profoundly impaired tend to acquire skills more slowly and to forget what has been learned more quickly than their typically developing peers. Consequently, a school year limited to 180 days may not meet the requirement of a free, appropriate public education for such individuals. Cases such as these impact a family's ability to obtain year-round services for their child and may require that all those working with a child with intellectual disability carefully document the impact of summer breaks on that child's or adolescent's progress.

In addition to delineating the types of services school districts must provide for children with intellectual disability, courts have also had an impact on districts' ability to manage disruptive students. For example, in *Honig v. Doe* (1988), the Supreme Court held that school systems could not unilaterally exclude a child from the classroom for dangerous or disruptive behavior resulting from his or her disability. For a more detailed description of both relevant court cases and federal legislation concerning the education and rights of children with disabilities, see Heward (2006).

Finally, states often use different terminology to describe the continuum of available special education services. For example, children in Pennsylvania with mild mental retardation are often placed in learning support classrooms. However, in the neighboring state of Ohio, the same child would be placed in a classroom for developmental handicaps. Older terms for programs serving children with intellectual disability, such as "educable mentally retarded" (for children with mild mental retardation) and "trainable mentally retarded" (for children with moderate mental retardation) tend to be outdated and are less often used (Beirne-Smith, Patton, & Kim, 2006). States also use different cutoff scores for determining eligibility for special education services. For example, in Pennsylvania a child with an IQ of up to 79 and significant deficits in adaptive functioning may be labeled as having an intellectual disability and be eligible for special education services (Special Education Services and Programs, 1990). However, if the same child's family moves across the state line to West Virginia, he or she might not be identified as needing special services and could be placed in a regular classroom without supports (West Virginia Department of Education, 1985). Therefore, it is incumbent upon clinicians to become well versed in their state's terminology, regulations, and relevant court decisions that affect the assessment and service provision of children and adolescents with intellectual disability.

APPROACH TO ASSESSMENT

Sattler (2001) defines *assessment* as "a way of gaining some understanding of the child in order to make informed decisions" (p. 3). A child may be referred for evaluation by families, school districts, or mental health agencies, typically for one of five possible reasons (Sattler, 2001): (1) *screening*: a relatively brief evaluation to determine eligibility for a certain program or the need for more thorough assessment; (2) *focused/problem-solving assessment*: a more in-depth evaluation to answer a specific question (e.g., does the child have obsessive–compulsive disorder?); (3) *diagnostic assessment*: a detailed evaluation to identify strengths and weaknesses in a range of areas (e.g., cognition, adaptive behavior, achievement) that may result in recommendation for specific services; (4) *counseling/rehabilitation assessment*: similar to a diagnostic assessment, but with an emphasis on a child's ability to manage daily responsibilities; and (5) *progress evaluation assessment*: a means of assessing treatment effectiveness and identifying needed changes in the intervention plan. Consequently, there is no standard battery of assessment tools and procedures for all individuals with intellectual disability. Instead, the assessment must be guided by the referral question.

Below are some guiding principles for assessing children with intellectual disability.

1. *Understand the referral question.* Obtain a clear understanding of what specific question(s) needs to be answered at the conclusion of the evaluation. Without such an understanding, even the most thorough assessment is of little value if it fails to answer the referral source's question. In cases where an unrealistic question may be posed, establishing the ground rules early on (e.g., "It is unlikely that we will be able to tell you exactly why your child has intellectual disability") facilitates discussion and helps the referral source to frame more appropriate questions. Only after the referral question is clear can the appropriate assessment tools and methods be selected. Some referral questions may have less to do with diagnosis or understanding the child's problems than with understanding the child's impact on parents or others within the family that led to the evaluation at this particular time.

2. *Use multiple sources.* Obtain information from as many sources as possible (e.g., parents,

schools, agencies, other clinicians), because children may behave differently across environments. There is some research evidence that parents and teachers describe the behaviors and skills of children with intellectual disability in different ways. For example, Handen, Feldman, and Honigman (1987) examined parent–teacher agreement on a questionnaire assessing self-help skills, speech and language, play skills, and behavior problems in a group of 98 children with developmental disabilities. Whereas significant levels of parent–teacher agreement were noted for 77% of items assessed, the mean level of agreement was only 68.1%. Additionally, when a specific behavior problem (e.g., temper tantrums, hitting others) was endorsed by either a parent or a teacher, the probability that the same problem would be endorsed by the other respondent was at or below chance levels. In another study of the reliability of parent and child reports of symptoms, parents were found to be more reliable informants (r's of .73 to .76) than their typically developing children (r's of .43 to .71) (Edelbrock, Costello, Dulcan, Kalas, & Conover, 1985). This same study found typically developing children under the age of 10 to be extremely unreliable informants (with the exception of reporting simple fears). Additionally, reliability of informant rating may be affected by population variables. For example, Havercamp (1986) found that internal and interrater reliability on the Reiss Screen for Maladaptive Behavior (RSMB; Reiss, 1994) and the Psychopathology Instrument for Mentally Retarded Adults (PIMRA; Matson, Kazdin, & Senatore, 1984) decreased significantly when used with individuals functioning within the profound range of mental retardation. Such findings cast suspicion upon the clinical utility of information provided by parents, children, or teachers alone, and suggest that additional information be gathered whenever conflicting reports are obtained from two or more sources.

3. *Use disorder-specific knowledge.* Whenever possible, use disorder-specific knowledge as a framework for organizing the approach to assessment. For example, if asked to assess a child with fragile X syndrome, one's focus might be on behaviors such as echolalia, social nonresponsiveness, and self-stimulation. Therefore, a behavioral assessment conducted as part of the evaluation would need to be designed to elicit such behaviors. Conversely, if

evaluating a child with Williams syndrome, one might expect feeding problems if the child is an infant or toddler. Therefore, the assessment would need to include observation of mealtime behavior. Other disorders often present with specific strengths and/or deficits that may influence the choice of assessment tools or the interpretation of results. For example, children with Down syndrome have a unique pattern of language development. Miller (1992) found that the vocabulary size and grammatical complexity of sentences of children with Down syndrome is smaller than expected in comparison to other children of the same mental age. Conversely, receptive language skills develop as expected for their cognitive abilities. Therefore, one may want to assess receptive and expressive language skills independently (i.e., use an assessment tool to measure receptive language skills that does not require an expressive language response).

4. *Use appropriate assessment strategies.* Use tools which are appropriate with respect to areas such as functional level, language skills, and motor skills. For example, a test such as the Wechsler Intelligence Scale for Children–IV (WISC-IV; Wechsler, 2003), which is standardized for children ages 6 years to 16 years, 11 months may be inappropriate for a 7-year-old child with suspected intellectual disability, because even the easiest test items might be below the child's ability level. A standardized IQ test such as the Kaufman Assessment Battery for Children (K-ABC-II; Kaufman & Kaufman, 2004c), which has an IQ floor of 60 for 6-year-olds would be inappropriate for a 6-year-old child with moderate mental retardation. A test of visual–motor skills, such as the Berry–Buktenica Developmental Test of Visual–Motor Integration, Third Edition (VMI; Beery, Buktenica, & Berry, 2004), will be of limited value when assessing a child with significant motor or visual impairments.

5. *Use a multiple assessment approach.* Sattler (2001) outlines "four pillars of assessment": norm-referenced tests (standardized tools), interviews (information from parents, teachers, the child, and other individuals familiar with the child), observations (both in the clinic and in settings such as the home or school), and informal assessment (nonstandardized tools, such as language samples or assessment of a child's ability to benefit from systematic cues). Significant discrepancies

among assessment findings require further investigation before a diagnosis and recommendations can be offered. For example, Sattler cited a case in which a child scored within the intellectual disability range on a test of cognitive functioning, but interviews and assessment of adaptive functioning suggested age-appropriate skills. Clearly, in such a case, a diagnosis of intellectual disability would not be made and additional assessment would be necessary.

6. *Collaborate with other professionals.* Refer to or include professionals from other disciplines (e.g., communication disorders, psychiatry, education, developmental pediatrics, genetics, occupational therapy) depending on the question being asked and the need to determine potential causes for a particular deficit or behavior problem. For example, a child's inattention may be due to a possible hearing loss (suggesting the need for an audiology evaluation), or the presence of a number of dysmorphic features may suggest the need for a genetics consultation. In a child with Down syndrome, receptive language skills that fall below expected levels may suggest the need for an audiology evaluation: About 50% of children with Down syndrome have some hearing loss due to ear infections or neurological impairment (Miller, 1992).

7. *Provide appropriate feedback.* Provide feedback at a level appropriate to the family with respect to language, education, and culture. Limit the use of overly professional language or simply stating numbers from various tests. When providing feedback regarding a diagnosis of intellectual disability, Shea (1984) recommends that the feedback session address three goals: (1) to provide specific information about the child's developmental functioning, and to answer all of the parents' questions about these findings; (2) to support and help parents as they begin to cope emotionally with the knowledge of their child's disability; and (3) to assist the parents in making plans to carry out specific recommendations and interventions. For schools, feedback should provide guidance about how best to meet the learning–behavioral–emotional needs of the student. Whereas a student may require additional academic support, for example, this might be accomplished in a variety of ways (depending on school resources, parental wishes, etc.), with a final determination made by the treatment team.

ASSESSMENT OF COGNITIVE FUNCTIONING

Despite the aforementioned issues regarding the role of adaptive behavior in children with intellectual disability, evaluation of cognitive functioning remains the first and primary step in assessing intellectual disability. Most school districts continue to overemphasize IQ testing for purposes of determining a child's eligibility for special needs services (Furlong & LeDrew, 1985; Reschly & Ward, 1991). Even among researchers in the field, the majority of published articles in the area of intellectual disability use IQ alone as an inclusionary or exclusionary criterion for entry into studies (Hawkins & Cooper, 1990). There are a range of cognitive assessment tools available to evaluate a child for the presence of intellectual disability. These tools are called norm-based or norm-referenced scales, in that they compare a child's test performance with others of similar age and gender (as well as possibly other dimensions, such as socioeconomic status or race). As a result, such tests must be standardized across a large group of individuals. Norm-referenced tests are able to assess relative performance across a wide range of developmental domains. These tests are almost exclusively individually administered and, according to Morgenstern and Klass (1991), meet a number of the following conditions:

1. The examiner must be skilled in test administration and have experience with a wide range of available tests.
2. The examiner must be knowledgeable about normal and abnormal development, and the needs of children with intellectual disability, in order to best interpret test results.
3. The tests given must be reliable and valid.
4. Tests are not valid for every purpose. Therefore, chosen tests must be appropriate for their purpose, particularly if they enhance the prediction of nontest behavior.
5. It is assumed that the child is giving his or her best performance. Problems with poor concentration, anxiety, or poor motivation compromise the reliability and validity of a test score.

Scales for Infants and Preschool-Age Children

Table 12.3 provides a summary of the most frequently used standardized cognitive assessment

TABLE 12.3. Frequently Used Standardized Tests for Cognitive Assessment

Test	Age range	Description/comments
Cognitive assessment options		
Bayley Scales of Infant Development, third edition (Bayley, 2005)	1 to 42 months	Provides indices of early cognitive and motor development. For children over 42 months, can use age equivalents.
Differential Ability Scales (DAS; Elliott, 1990)	2 years, 6 months to 17 years, 11 months	General Conceptual Ability and three subscale scores: Verbal Ability, Nonverbal Reasoning Ability, Spatial Ability.
Kaufman Assessment Battery for Children II (K-ABC-II; Kaufman & Kaufman, 2004c)	3 years, 0 months to 18 years, 11 months	Domains: Simultaneous Processing, Sequential Processing, Planning, Learning, and Knowledge. Includes a Mental Processing Index (IQ), Fluid Crystalized Index, as well as a Nonverbal Index.
Mullen Scales of Early Learning (Mullen, 1989)	0 to 42 months	Tests Language, Fine and Gross Motor, Cognitive, Personal–Social domains. For children over 42 months, must use age equivalents.
Stanford–Binet, fifth edition (Roid, 2003)	2 to 85+ years	Factor indexes: Fluid Reasoning, Knowledge, Quantitative Reasoning, Visual–Spatial Processing, and Working Memory. Both Verbal and Nonverbal IQ scores (as well as a Full-Scale IQ).
Wechsler Preschool and Primary Scale of Intelligence–III (Wechsler, 2002)	2 years, 6 months to 7 years, 3 months	Domains: Verbal, Performance, and Processing Speed (in addition to a Full Scale IQ). More of a screening tool for ages 2 years, 6 months to 3 years, 11 months. Best for IQs above 55.
Wechsler Intelligence Scale for Children (WISC-IV; Wechsler, 2003)	6 years to 16 years, 11 months	Four factors: Verbal Comprehension, Perceptual Reasoning, Working Memory, Processing Speed. Full-Scale IQ (40–160)
Nonverbal cognitive assessment options		
Blind Learning Aptitude Test (BLAT; Newland, 1971)	6 to 16 years	Assesses children with visual impairments, using a raised dot, braille-like format; directions are given verbally and require a pointing response.
Comprehensive Test of Nonverbal Intelligence (Hammill, Pearson, & Wiederholt, 1997)	6 to 90+ years	Three composite scores: Nonverbal Intelligence Quotient, Pictorial Nonverbal Intelligence Quotient, and Geometric Nonverbal Intelligence Quotient. Uses pictures of familiar objects and geometric designs; possible alternative for those with communication disorders, neurological impairments, autism, and mental retardation.
Leiter International Performance Scale—Revised (Leiter-R; Roid & Miller, 1997)	2 to 20 years	Comprised of two batteries (Visualization and Reasoning, Attention and Memory) and 20 subtests. A short form is also available.
Pictorial Test of Intelligence II (PTI-II; French, 2001)	3 to 8 years	No expressive language abilities required. As an untimed test, the PTI-II can be useful for children with a range of motor and developmental disorders.
Test of Nonverbal Intelligence (TONI-3; Brown, Sherbenou, & Johnson, 1997)	6 years to 89 years, 11 months	Requires no reading, writing, speaking, or listening. Is completely nonverbal and largely motor-free, requiring only a point, nod, or symbolic gesture to indicate response choices.
Universal Nonverbal Intelligence Test (UNIT, Bracken & McCallum, 1998)	5 years to 17 years, 11 months	Requires multiple response modes, including use of manipulatives, paper and pencil, and pointing.

tools for infants, preschool-age, and school-age children. As discussed earlier, infant and pre-school scales do not correlate well with later levels of cognitive functioning. Only in the case of infants and preschoolers with significant developmental delays are early test results predictive of future functioning (DuBose, 1981). The most commonly used infant–toddler scale is the Bayley Scales of Infant Development, Third Edition (Bayley, 2005). The Bayley was standardized for infants, toddlers, and preschoolers between 1 and 42 months of age. Five developmental domains are available to identify deficits in very young children, including cognitive, language, motor, adaptive behavior, and social–emotional domains, as well as an optional sixth, behavior rating scale, domain. In addition, there is a screening test to determine whether further testing is needed. Another option, the Infant Mullen Scales of Early Learning (Mullen, 1989), was standardized on a sample of 1,231 children ages birth to 68 months and has five scales (including motor, visual, and language areas).

As children approach preschool age, tests tend to emphasize more language-mediated tasks. The Stanford–Binet Intelligence Scales (fifth edition; Roid, 2003) and the Wechsler Preschool and Primary Scale of Intelligence–III (WPPSI-III; Wechsler, 2002) are the most commonly used cognitive tests for this age group. The Stanford–Binet was revised in 2003 and standardized on nationally representative sample of 4,800 children and adults between 2 and 85+ years of age. It assesses functioning across five factor indexes: Fluid Reasoning, Knowledge, Quantitative Reasoning, Visual–Spatial Processing, and Working Memory. In addition, there are both Verbal and Nonverbal IQ scores (as well as a Full Scale IQ). The latter may be useful in assessing individuals with communication disorders, autism, or traumatic brain injury. Scores are expressed as a deviation IQ, with a mean of 100 and a standard deviation of 15. However, the test is not appropriate for individuals functioning in the severe to profound range of mental retardation, because 40 is the lowest Full-Scale IQ given.

The WPPSI-III (Wechsler, 2002) is appropriate for preschoolers between 2 years, 6 months and 7 years, 3 months of age. The test was standardized on a sample of 1,700 preschoolers, with a mean score of 100 and a standard deviation of 15. The WPPSI-III assesses functioning across three domains: Verbal, Perfor-

mance, and Processing Speed (in addition to a Full Scale IQ). Children between 2 years, 6 months and 3 years, 11 months of age are given only two core subtests in the Verbal domain and two in the Performance domain. A fifth, supplemental subtest is available in the Processing Speed domain. Consequently, the WPPSI-III is more a screening instrument than a comprehensive cognitive test battery for this age group (Sattler & Dumont, 2004). For the 4 years to 7 years, 3 months age group, three core subtests are available within both the Verbal and Performance domains, and an additional core subtest in the Processing Speed domain. Five additional supplemental subtests and two optional subtests are available for this age range. Sattler and Dumont recommend against the use of the WPPSI-III for children with IQs below 55 (moderate range of mental retardation), because the instrument fails to assess cognitive ability adequately in this population.

Another available option for assessing children under the age of 6 years is the KABC-II (Kaufman & Kaufman, 2004), which comprises 20 subtests spanning the age range of 3 years to 18 years, 11 months and was standardized on a sample of 3,025 children. The KABC-II assesses a child's capabilities in five areas: (1) simultaneous processing, which taps an individual's ability to integrate inputs from multiple sources at the same time; (2) sequential processing, which taps an individual's ability to solve problems based on the arrangement of arrays of information; (3) planning; (4) learning; and (5) knowledge. In addition, this instrument provides a Mental Processing Index (IQ), Fluid Crystalized Index, as well as a Nonverbal Index. The Nonverbal scale of the KABC-II is particularly useful in assessing children with hearing impairments or language disorders. However, the KABC-II should not be used to classify intellectual disability across the entire age range of the scale. For example, the Mental Processing Index has a floor of 45 for a 3-year-old, 54 for a 4-year-old, and 48 for a 5-year-old.

Two other alternative preschool tests are the Differential Abilities Scales (DAS; Elliott, 1990) and the Woodcock–Johnson III Tests of Cognitive Abilities (WJ-III; Woodcock, McGrew, & Mather, 2001). The DAS was normed on a national sample of 3,475 children between 2 years, 6 months and 17 years, 11 months of age. It comprises 20 subtests (17 cognitive and 3 achievement), yielding a General Conceptual Ability score, as well as three subscale scores: Verbal Ability, Nonverbal Reasoning Ability, and Spatial Ability. The Nonverbal Reasoning Ability subscale can be useful when assessing children with communication disorders or autism. The DAS-II (second edition) was published in early 2007. The WJ-III is normed for individuals ages 2–90+ years. It comprises 10 tests in the standard battery and 10 in the extended battery (although younger children are not given the entire battery). The scale, which can only be scored by a computer software program, provides seven clusters: Comprehension–Knowledge, Long-Term Retrieval, Visual–Spatial Thinking, Auditory Processing, Fluid Reasoning, Processing Speed, and Short-Term Memory.

Recommendations

The Bayley Scales of Infant Development, Third Edition (Bayley, 2005) remains the most used developmental assessment for infants and toddlers. It is certainly a good choice for evaluating a child under 2 years of age with suspected developmental delays. The Infant Mullen Scales of Early Learning (Mullen, 1989) remains a strong option for children between birth and 68 months of age. Because the Mullen is standardized on children starting from birth, it also allows for assessment of a child who may be functioning below the 24-month developmental age. Finally, the Stanford–Binet (fifth edition; Roid, 2003) is felt to be the best option for preschoolers with intellectual disability. The Nonverbal subscale also makes this a useful tool for nonverbal children. However, the Mullen may need to be substituted for preschoolers functioning within the severe to profound range of mental retardation.

Tests for School-Age Children

The Stanford–Binet (fifth edition), school-age version of the Wechsler (WISC-IV), the KABC-II, WJ-III, and the DAS are the most commonly used tools for assessing cognitive functioning in school-age children. The Stanford–Binet (fifth edition), KABC-II, and DAS were discussed earlier. The WISC-IV (Wechsler, 2003) is structurally similar to the WPPSI-III, but spans the age range of 6–16 years. It comprises 10 primary and 5 supplemental subtests divided into four factors: Verbal Comprehension (Similarities, Vocabulary, Comprehension, Information, Word Reasoning), Perceptual Reasoning (Block Design, Picture Concepts, Matrix Reasoning, Picture Completion), Working Memory (Digit Span, Letter–Number Sequencing, Arithmetic), and Processing Speed (Coding, Symbol Search, Cancellation). The most recent revision was standardized on 2,200 children. The test has excellent reliability and validity. However, the full-scale IQ range of 40–160 does not meet the needs for assessing children who may function within the severe to profound range of mental retardation.

Nonverbal Cognitive Assessment Options

One option for assessing children who have limited expressive and receptive language skills, according to Morgenstern and Klass (1991), is to use a tool such as the Bayley to provide information on the course of growth and development across a range of areas (e.g., social, adaptive, language, and motor). It is often difficult to use measures such as the Stanford–Binet and the Wechsler tests to assess children with significant neuromotor or language-based disorders. These tools are also inappropriate for evaluating children functioning in the low end of the moderate to profound range of mental retardation, due to the limited IQ ranges covered by the tests. Additionally, tests such as the Stanford–Binet, WISC-IV, WJ-III, and KABC-II require the evaluator to present items in a highly standardized manner; deviations from this may significantly affect the validity of the test results. The option of making alterations in response modalities (e.g., using yes–no responses or gestures) or excluding those items that require responses a particular child is unable to provide (e.g., eliminating all verbal items or all items that require motor responses) may not allow for comparison with the standardization group. Therefore, alternative measures often need to be used that provide valid estimates of cognitive functioning for this group of children, that are normed for children with specific handicaps (e.g., visual or motor impairments), or that have standardized adaptations for children with intellectual disability (Neisworth & Bagnato, 1987).

There are a number of options for assessing children and adolescents with limited expressive language skills. One option is to use subtests comprising the nonverbal scales of some of the IQ tests discussed earlier (e.g., KABC-II, WISC-IV, DAS). However, most of these subtests are administered with the use of verbal directions and might best be described as "language-reduced instruments with verbal directions" (McCallum, 2003). There are a few alternative tools administered in a nonverbal manner that can be used to obtain estimates of cognitive functioning in children with severe language deficits. The Pictorial Test of Intelligence II (PTI-II; French, 2001) was designed to assess intellectual functioning in both typically developing and children with disabilities, ages 3–8 years. It includes three subtest areas (Verbal Abstraction, Form Discrimination, and Quantitative Concepts) that are combined to obtain a Pictorial Intelligence Quotient, as well as a global index of performance. Standardized with a sample of 972 children, the PTI-II does not require any expressive language abilities. However, individuals are required to have normal vision and hearing. As an untimed test, the PTI-II may be useful for children with a range of motor and developmental disorders.

The Comprehensive Test of Nonverbal Intelligence (Hammill, Pearson, & Wiederholt, 1997) was standardized on 2,500 individuals between 6 and 90+ years of age. It provides three composite scores: Nonverbal Intelligence Quotient, Pictorial Nonverbal Intelligence Quotient, and Geometric Nonverbal Intelligence Quotient. Stimuli that include pictures of familiar objects and geometric designs make it a possible alternative for school-age children and adolescents with communication disorders, neurological impairments, autism, and intellectual disability.

The Leiter International Performance Scale—Revised (Leiter-R; Roid & Miller, 1997) was designed to assess general cognitive functioning in children and adolescents between 2 and 20 years of age with language or motor deficits. The test depends on the use of visual demonstration to provide instructions. The Leiter-R comprises two batteries (Visualization and Reasoning, Attention and Memory) and 20 subtests. It was standardized on a sample of 1,719 individuals for the Visualization and Reasoning battery and 763 individuals for the Attention and Memory battery. A short form of the Leiter, called the Stoelting (Leiter) Brief Nonverbal Intelligence Tests (S-BIT; Roid & Miller, 1999) is also available for individuals between 6 and 20 years of age. Other nonverbal cognitive assessment options include the third edition of the Test of Nonverbal Intelligence (TONI-3; Brown, Sherbenou, & Johnson, 1997), which was standardized on individuals between 6 years and 89 years, 11 months of age, and the Universal Nonverbal Intelligence Test (UNIT, Bracken & McCallum, 1998), which was standardized for individuals between 5 years and 17 years, 11 months of age.

Finally, the Blind Learning Aptitude Test (BLAT; Newland, 1971) was specifically developed to assess children with visual impairments, using a raised dot, braille-like format; directions are given verbally and require a pointing response. Although this tool provides normative data for individuals 6–16 years of age, the standardization sample is over 30 years old. An additional option is to assess children and adolescents who have visual impairments using subtests from the verbal domains of tools such as the WISC-IV or WPPSI-III, to obtain a Verbal IQ score (Chaudry & Davidson, 2001). However, Van Hasselt and Sisson (1987) caution that variability among subtest scores is common among children with visual impairments; therefore, subtest scores are not necessarily indicative of a learning disability.

Recommendations

The WISC-IV and Stanford–Binet (fifth edition) remain the most commonly used tests of cognitive functioning for both typically developing children and children with intellectual disability. The challenge is selecting alternative tools for children who are nonverbal and for children whose IQs fall below 40. One option is to use the Nonverbal scales from the WISC-IV and Stanford–Binet (fifth edition), with the caveat that most of the items involve the use of verbal directions. The best known purely nonverbal assessment tool is the Leiter-R. Finally, for children functioning within the severe to profound range of mental retardation we often use the Infant Mullen Scales of Early Learning (for which an estimated age-equivalent score needs to be derived).

ASSESSMENT OF ACADEMIC ACHIEVEMENT

Table 12.4 includes a summary of the most frequently used tests to assess academic achievement skills. The assessment of academic achievement is the primary means of determin-

TABLE 12.4. Tests Frequently Used to Assess Achievement Skills

Test	Age range	Description/comments
Grey Oral Reading Test—Fourth Edition (GORT-4; Wiederholt & Bryant, 2001)	6 years to 18 years, 11 months	Assesses skills in reading rate, accuracy, fluency, comprehension, and overall reading ability. Two parallel forms available.
Kaufman Test of Educational Achievement II—Comprehensive Form (K-TEA-II; Kaufman & Kaufman, 2004a)	4 years, 6 months to 25 years	Individually administered comprehensive assessment of reading, mathematics, written language, and oral language.
Kaufman Test of Educational Achievement–II—Brief Form (Kaufman & Kaufman, 2004b)	4 years, 6 months to 90 years	Assesses skills in reading, mathematics, and written expression. Serves as a screening tool. Because items do not overlap with K-TEA-II, can be used for retesting.
KeyMath-R/NU (Connolly, 1998)	5 to 22 years	Assesses skills in basic concepts, operations, and applications. Absence of reading requirements makes this a good assessment tool for children with mental retardation. Two parallel forms available.
The Peabody Individual Achievement Test—Revised/Normative Update (PIAT-R/NU; Markwardt, 1998)	5 years to 22 years, 11 months	Requires that a child respond by pointing to the correct picture from an array of four items. Good choice for children with motor impairments, language deficits, or mental retardation.
Wechsler Individual Achievement Test–II (WIAT-II; Wechsler, 2001)	4 to 85 years	Seven subtests covering Oral Expression, Listening Comprehension, Written Expression, Basic Reading, Reading Comprehension, Mathematics Calculation, and Mathematics Reasoning.
Wechsler Individual Achievement Test–II—Abbreviated (WIAT-II-Abbreviated; Kaplan et al., 2001)	Kindergarten to adult	Assesses skills in word reading, spelling, and numerical operations. Serves as a screening tool.
Wide Range Achievement Test Expanded edition (WRAT-E; Robertson, 2002)	Grades 2–12: group administered; Ages 4–24 years: individually administered	Areas assessed include reading comprehension, mathematics, and nonverbal reasoning (for group administration only).
Wide Range Achievement Test 4 (WRAT-4; Wilkinson & Robertson, 2006)	5 to 94 years	Assesses skills in word reading, sentence comprehension, spelling, and math computation. Serves as a screening tool.
Woodcock–Johnson–III Tests of Achievement (WJ-III; Woodcock, McGrew, & Mather, 2001)	2 to 90+ years	Twenty-two subtests covering reading, mathematics, written language, and academic knowledge. A Total Achievement score can be derived.
Woodcock Reading Mastery Tests—Revised/Normative Update (WRMT-R/NU; Woodcock, 1998)	5 to 75+ years	Assesses skills: Visual–Auditory Learning, Letter Identification, Word Identification, Word Attack, Word Comprehension, and Passage Comprehension. Two parallel forms are available (last four subtests only).

ing how a child with intellectual disability is faring in school. Such data also allow for the comparison between a child's abilities (as estimated with a test of cognitive functioning) and actual school performance. A child who is achieving significantly below what would be expected based on IQ score may present with other problems that need to be investigated as part of the overall assessment. These might include psychiatric disorders (e.g., ADHD, depression) that may adversely affect the child's ability to concentrate and perform in school, significant family stressors, a specific learning disability, or inappropriate classroom placement and instruction.

Tests of academic achievement can serve as either a screening function or as a more comprehensive assessment of skills. Screening tests take considerably less time to administer and typically are used to determine whether a more comprehensive evaluation is required. For the child with an intellectual disability, however, a more comprehensive assessment is generally recommended to provide as much information as possible on the child's current levels of functioning and to assist in developing plans for remediation. Academic achievement tests may be designed to be given either individually or in a group format. However, it is generally recommended that a child with intellectual disability be evaluated individually. A good number of norm-referenced assessment tools are available to assess a child's abilities in reading, spelling, and mathematics.

The Wide Range Achievement Test–4 (WRAT-4; Wilkinson & Robertson, 2006), a screening tool that requires 20–30 minutes to administer, assesses skills in word reading, sentence comprehension, spelling, and math computation for ages 5 through 94. An Expanded edition (WRAT-E; Robertson, 2002) provides both group and individual assessment of academic achievement in reading comprehension, mathematics, and nonverbal reasoning. It can be group administered (for grades 2–12) with a multiple-choice format or individually administered (for ages 4–24) with a flipbook form of presentation. A second achievement measure, the WJ-III (Woodcock et al., 2001), includes 22 subtests (comprising 12 in the Standard battery and 10 in the Extended battery) covering a range of areas, such as reading, mathematics, written language, and academic knowledge. A Total Achievement score can be derived. The test was standardized on a sample of 8,818 in-

dividuals (including 1,143 preschoolers and 4,784 school-age children) ranging in age from 2 to 90+ years. Results can be presented as standard scores ($X = 100$, $SD = 15$), age/grade equivalents, percentile ranks, instructional ranges, discrepancy scores, and a Relative Proficiency Index.

Another option for assessing academic achievement, the Wechsler Individual Achievement Test–II (WIAT-II, Wechsler, 2001), is empirically linked with the WISC-IV and WPPSI-III. This test was normed with a sample of individuals ages 4–85 years and comprises seven subtests covering a range of areas, such as reading, oral and written expression, listening comprehension, and mathematics. An abbreviated version is also available (WIAT-II-Abbreviated; Kaplan, Fein, Kramer, Delis, & Morris, 2001), covering word reading, spelling, and numerical operations. The Peabody Individual Achievement Test—Revised/Normative Update (PIAT-R/NU; Markwardt, 1998) uses a somewhat different format than the tools discussed previously. Rather than providing paper-and-pencil tasks, the PIAT-R/NU requires that a child respond by pointing to the correct picture from an array of four items. Consequently, the PIAT-R/NU is a good choice for assessing children with motor impairments, language deficits, or intellectual disability. However, the Reading Comprehension subtest requires some memory skills as well. The test was recently restandardized on approximately 3,000 individuals from 5 years through 22 years, 11 months of age. The Kaufman Test of Educational Achievement—Second Edition, Comprehensive form (K-TEA-II; Kaufman & Kaufman, 2004c), covering ages 4 years, 6 months to 25 years, also remains an option. There is a companion screening version, the TEA-II Brief Form (Kaufman & Kaufman, 2004b) for ages 4 years, 6 months to 90 years.

Finally, there are achievement tests available that focus more specifically on either reading or mathematics. For example, the Woodcock Reading Mastery Tests—Revised/Normative Update (WRMT-R/NU; Woodcock, 1998), covering ages 5 years through 75+ years, as well as the Grey Oral Reading Test—Fourth Edition (GORT-4; Wiederholt & Bryant, 2001), covering ages 6 years through 18 years, 11 months, provide a more detailed assessment of reading skills. Similarly, the KeyMath—Revised/Normative Update: A Diagnostic Inventory of Essential Mathematics (KeyMath-R/

NU; Connolly, 1998) is an individually administered test of arithmetic skills. It provides considerably more depth than most other available tools, comprising 13 subtest areas. The test was standardized on over 3,000 individuals from 5 to 22 years of age. It was co-normed with the K-TEA/NU and PIAT-R/NU. The absence of reading requirements makes this a good assessment tool for children with intellectual disability. The availability of two parallel forms allows individuals to be pretested and retested at a later time.

Recommendations

The WRAT-4 (Wilkinson & Robertson, 2006) has always offered a means of providing a quick, but fairly narrow picture of current achievement. This can then provide guidance regarding the need for more in-depth assessment. The WJ-III, the only tool that assesses children as young as 2 years of age (most others start at age 5), may be helpful when evaluating younger school-age children with intellectual disability. The PIAT-R (Markwardt, 1998) uses a pointing response, which makes it also a reasonable choice with this population.

ASSESSMENT OF RELATED NEUROPSYCHOLOGICAL PROCESSES: LANGUAGE SKILLS, PERCEPTUAL–MOTOR SKILLS, AND MEMORY

There are a range of measures designed to assess specific neuropsychological processes such as language, attention, memory, and perception (see Table 12.5). Neisworth and Bagnato (1987) provide a number of reasons why the use of such tools may be helpful in assessing children with intellectual disability: (1) to define a child's strongest individual modality for learning, (2) to monitor medication efficacy, (3) to assess progress or deterioration in children with traumatic brain injuries, and (4) to better understand how the brain mediates control of behavior (e.g., verbal mediation and self-control). A wide range of options are available for assessing processes that reflect specific brain functions. Tools discussed previously, such as the KABC-II, can assess functions such as attention, memory, and processing. The study of patterns of subtest performance on the WISC-IV or Stanford–Binet (fifth edition) can also provide information on brain functions. A variety of assessment tools are also available to evaluate more specific areas.

Language Skills

For children who are nonverbal or have significant language-based deficits, a number of alternative assessment tools are available for assessing receptive language skills. One such tool, the Peabody Picture Vocabulary Test–4 (PPVT-4; Dunn & Dunn, 2006) requires an individual to point to one of four pictorial plates in response to an instruction from the evaluator (e.g., "Point to the ball"). The PPVT-4 was normed on 4,000 children and adults, and has excellent reliability and validity. Age range for the tool is 2 years, 6 months to 90+ years. The PPVT-4 should be considered a screening device for identifying language comprehension difficulties.

The Receptive–Expressive Emerging Language Scale, Third Edition (REEL-3; Bzoch, League, & Brown, 2003) is designed to assess children from birth to 3 years of age with language impairments or disabilities that affect language development. Results are based on parental report. The Preschool Language Scale 4 (PLS-4; Zimmerman, Steiner, & Pond, 2002) assesses expressive and receptive language skills for ages birth through 6 years. It combines screening of the child and a parental interview.

The Test of Auditory Comprehension of Language—Third Edition (TACL-III; Carrow-Woolfolk, 1999) is an individually administered test of auditory comprehension (receptive language functioning) that requires only a pointing response. It contains three subtests: Vocabulary, Grammatical Morphemes, and Elaborated Phrases and Sentences. The TACL-III was standardized on a sample of 1,102 children between the ages of 3 years and 9 years, 11 months. Reliability studies have been carried out with children with intellectual disability (Carrow-Woolfolk, 1999). The second edition of the Clinical Evaluation of Language Fundamentals—Preschool (CELF-2 Preschool; Wiig, Secord, & Semel 2004) and Clinical Evaluation of Language Fundamentals, Fourth Edition (CELF-4; Semel, Wiig, & Secord, 2003) may be used to assess a wide range of both receptive and expressive language functions in preschool and school-age children. The preschool version was standardized on 1,500 preschool children (ages 3 to 6

TABLE 12.5. Tests Frequently Used to Assess Language Skills, Perceptual–Motor Skills, and Memory

Test	Age range	Description/comments
	Language skills	
Clinical Evaluation of Language Fundamentals—Preschool, Second Edition (CELF-2 Preschool; Semel, Wiig, & Secord, 2004)	3 to 6 years	Provides a core language score, receptive language index, expressive language index, language content index, and language structure index.
Clinical Evaluation of Language Fundamentals–4 (CELF-4; Semel et al., 2003)	5 to 21 years	Provides composite scores in the areas of language structure, language content, language memory, and working memory.
Clinical Evaluation of Language Fundamentals–4—Screening Test (Semel et al., 2003)	5 to 21 years	A criterion-referenced screen used to determine whether further evaluation is needed.
Peabody Picture Vocabulary Test–III (PPVT-III; Dunn & Dunn, 1997)	2 years, 6 months to 90+ years	A screening device for identifying language comprehension difficulties.
Preschool Language Scale–4 (PLS-4; Zimmerman, Steiner, & Pond, 2002)	Birth to 6 years	Combines screening of the child, along with a parental interview.
Receptive–Expressive Emerging Language Scale, Third Edition (REEL-3; Bzoch, League, & Brown, 2003)	Birth to 3 years	Results are based on parental report.
Test of Auditory Comprehension of Language–III (TACL-III; Carrow-Woolfolk, 1999)	3 years and 9 years, 11 months	Assesses receptive language functioning, requiring only a pointing response. Contains three subtests: Vocabulary, Grammatical Morphemes, and Elaborated Phrases and Sentences.
	Perceptual–motor tests	
Beery–Buktenica Developmental Test of Visual–Motor Integration, Third Edition (VMI; Beery, Buktenica, & Beery, 2004)	2 years to 17 years, 11 months	Individually administered paper-and-pencil test. Child is asked to copy 24 geometric figures. Assesses visual–motor integration skills. A short form is available for use with children 2 to 8 years of age.
Bender Visual–Motor Gestalt Test, Second Edition (Braningan & Decker, 2003)	4 to 85 years	Individually administered paper-and-pencil test. Child is asked to copy up to 14 geometric figures. Assesses visual–motor memory and visual–motor skills.
Bruininks–Oseretsky Test of Motor Proficiency—second edition (Bruininks & Bruininks, 2005)	4 to 21 years	Assesses both fine and gross motor skills. Both short and long forms available, but age equivalents can be derived from the full battery only.
Full Range Test of Visual–Motor Integration (Hammill et al., 2005)	5 to 74 years	Includes norms for special education students in the 19- to 21-year age range.
Motor-Free Visual Perception Test, third edition (Colarusso & Hammill, 2002)	4 to 85 years	Useful for assessing children with motor impairments. Child is asked to point to one of four figures on a page that matches a target figure.

(continued)

TABLE 12.5. *(continued)*

Test	Age range	Description/comments
	Memory	
Children's Memory Scale (Cohen, 1997)	5 to 16 years	Comprises six subtests tapping immediate and delayed verbal memory, general memory, and immediate and delayed visual memory.
NEPSY (Korman, Kirk, & Kemp, 1990)	3 to 12 years	Assesses five functional domains, including Executive Functions, Language and Communication, Sensorimotor Functions, Visuospatial Functions, and Learning and Memory.
Test of Memory and Learning (TOMAL; Reynolds & Bigler, 1994)	5 to 19 years	Comprises 10 regular and four supplementary subtests. The three primary derived indices include a Verbal Memory Index, a Nonverbal Memory Index, and a Composite Memory Index.
Wide Range Assessment of Memory and Learning, second edition (WRAML-2; Sheslow & Adams, 2003)	5 to 90 years	Comprises six subtests and three indices (Verbal Memory, Visual Memory, and Attention/Concentration) as well as a General Memory Index. There is also an available screening battery.

years) and contains nine subtests (e.g., Expressive Vocabulary, Following Directions, Word Structure). The school-age version was standardized on 2,650 individuals (ages 5–21 years) and provides composite scores in the areas of Language Structure, Language Content, Language Memory, and Working Memory. The CELF-2-Preschool and CELF-4 both require a considerable amount of time to complete, if the entire battery is administered. A screening test for the CELF-4 is available (Semel et al., 2003).

Visual–Motor Skills

Evaluation of visual–motor perception and integration is particularly useful in assessing children with possible learning and neurological deficits (see Table 12.5). Children with intellectual disabilities also often have deficits in perceptual–motor skills. However, one must be cautious when interpreting test results for children with accompanying visual impairments or motor delays.

The most widely known visual–motor test is the Bender Visual–Motor Gestalt Test, Second Edition (Braningan & Decker, 2003). In this individually administered paper-and-pencil test, the child is asked to copy 14 geometric figures

drawn on template cards. The newly revised edition includes recall procedures to assess visual–motor memory, in addition to assessing visual–motor skills. It has been standardized for ages 4–85 years.

The VMI (Beery et al., 2004) is a paper-and-pencil test that provides scores in three areas: Motor Coordination, Visual–Motor Integration (in which the child is required to copy up to 24 geometric forms of increasing difficulty), and Visual Perception. The Visual–Motor Integration subtest provides somewhat greater structure than the Bender, in that forms are copied in clearly outlined spaces. The test was normed on a national sample of 2,512 children ages 2 years through 17 years, 11 months. Results can be presented as percentiles, standard scores (X = 10, SD = 3), or age equivalents. An available short form can be used with children 2 to 8 years of age. Another option, the Full Range Test of Visual–Motor Integration (Hammill, Pearson, Voress, & Reynolds, 2005), provides norms for both children and adults (ages 5–74 years).

The Motor-Free Visual Perception Test, Third Edition (Colarusso & Hammill, 2002) is a useful tool for assessing children who have significant motor impairments. The child is asked to point on a page to one of four figures that matches a target figure. The test was standardized for individuals between the ages of 4 and 85 years. Finally, the Bruininks–Oseretsky Test of Motor Proficiency, Second Edition (Bruininks & Bruininks, 2005) provides a comprehensive assessment both gross and fine motor skills. The test contains 53 items arranged into eight subtest areas. Four subtest scores are obtained: Fine Manual Control, Manual Coordination, Body Coordination, Strength and Agility, and a Total Motor Composite. There are both short and long forms, but age equivalents can be derived for the full battery only, which may take 45–60 minutes to complete. The test was standardized on a sample of children and adolescents ages 4–21 years of age.

Memory

There are a number of available assessment options that provide a more in-depth means of examining memory processes. Such information can be extremely helpful when developing specific treatment or instructional recommendations. The Wide Range Assessment of Memory and Learning, Second Edition (WRAML-2; Sheslow & Adams, 2003) provides a means of examining memory processes for individuals ages 5 to 90 years. The core battery, which requires less than 60 minutes to complete, comprises two verbal, two visual, and two attention/concentration subtests. Three indices are derived (Verbal Memory, Visual Memory, Attention/Concentration) as well as a General Memory Index. There is also a screening battery that comprises four subtests. The Children's Memory Scale (Cohen, 1997) is normed for ages 5–16 years and requires approximately 30 minutes to administer. The scale comprises six subtests tapping immediate and delayed verbal memory, general memory, and immediate and delayed visual memory.

Another option is the NEPSY (Korman, Kirk, & Kemp, 1990), a developmental neuropsychological assessment scale for children ages 3–12 years. The NEPSY assesses five functional domains, including Executive Functions, Language and Communication, Sensorimotor Functions, Visual–Spatial Functions, and Learning and Memory. Finally, The Test of Memory and Learning (TOMAL; Reynolds & Bigler, 1994), developed for ages 5–19 years, requires approximately 45 minutes to administer. The TOMAL comprises 10 regular and four supplementary subtests. The three primary derived indices include a Verbal Memory Index, a Nonverbal Memory Index, and a Composite Memory Index.

Recommendations

The assessment of specific language skills in a child with significant language-based deficits depends in part on the child's level of cooperation. For the child who is noncompliant or reluctant to respond, the REEL (which is based solely on parental report) and the PLS-4 (which includes parental report) are appropriate options. Although these tools were developed for the younger child, language age equivalents can still be calculated/estimated for the older child and relative areas of strength and weakness identified. The PPVT is fairly fast to administer and requires only a pointing response. The other options, such as the CELF-2 Preschool and CELF-4, are much more comprehensive. Only specific subtests might be used, depending on the question, or the entire battery might be administered if the assessment of language skills is deemed to be an area of considerable importance. In the area of visual–motor skills, the VMI is often the preferred option when assessing children with intellectual disability. It provides more structure than the Bender and also has normative data that begins at 2 years of age. For children with significant motor impairments, the Motor-Free Visual Perception Test is also an option. Finally, in the area of assessing memory, the NEPSY has a number of advantages for assessing children with intellectual disabilities. First, it can be used with children as young as 3 years of age (the other options start at 5 years of age). Second, it requires limited motor skills on the part of the child. However, the NEPSY is considerably better at assessing verbal memory than visual memory (for which there is only a single subscale). Finally, the Children's Memory Scale is also a good option for children who have some motor skills deficits.

ALTERNATIVE ASSESSMENT METHODS

Norm-referenced assessment tools present numerous problems for individuals with intellectual disability and other developmental disabilities. For many such children who are unable to sit still, to follow directions, or to attend to the types of tasks utilized in traditional assessments, the result is invalid measures of functioning and abilities. Additionally, many conventional tests have not been normed for either young children with disabilities or for older children functioning within the severe to profound range of mental retardation (Neisworth & Bagnato, 2004). Alternative tools, such as curriculum-based and performance-based assessments, typically allow evaluation of the child in a more natural environment, and often by individuals who know them best. This is in contrast to more traditional assessment situations, in which the child is taken to a separate room to be evaluated by a psychologist with whom he or she likely has had little, if any, prior interactions. Additionally, some alternative assessment tools involve a questionnaire or interview format for caregivers.

Curriculum-Based Assessment Tools

Whereas norm-referenced assessment tools are used primarily for diagnostic purposes, curriculum-based assessment tools allow test results, teaching, and progress evaluation to be merged within a single process (Neisworth & Bagnato, 1987). Instead of comparing a child's performance to a normative group of peers, criterion-based tools allow for the comparison of a child to him- or herself (once baseline levels are established). Consequently, these tools are used to monitor progress via performance on a range of task analyses of basic developmental skills. Based on a child's progress, a specific treatment or teaching plan can be devised. White and Haring (1978) noted that norm-referenced tests are relatively insensitive to developmental changes in children with IQs below 35. Even assessment measures that employ normal developmental scales may be inappropriate for this population, because the development of children with severe or profound mental retardation does not necessarily proceed like that of typically developing children (White & Haring, 1978).

Neisworth and Bagnato (1987) divided criterion-based assessment tools into two categories: (1) developmental measures (in which the content and objectives are developmentally sequenced), and (2) specialized curriculum measures (in which content and objectives have been designed and field-tested for distinct groups of children with developmental disabilities).

Developmental Curriculum-Based Assessment Tools

A number of curricula have been developed and field-tested specifically for preschool programs serving children with developmental disabilities. For example, the Carolina Curriculum (third edition) is an assessment and intervention program designed for use among children from birth to age 5 years with mild to severe disabilities (Johnson-Martin, Attermeier, & Hacker, 2004; Johnson-Martin, Jens, Attermeier, & Hacker, 2004). An Infant/Toddler version is available, covering children from birth to 36 months of age, and a Preschool version covers the period of 24–60 months of age. Both curricula comprise five areas: Cognition, Communication, Social Adaptation, Fine Motor, and Gross Motor. Similarly, the Assessment, Evaluation, and Programming System for Infants and Children, Second Edition (AEPS; Bricker, 2002) is both an evaluation tool and a curriculum for children (from birth to 6 years of age) with disabilities. Six developmental areas are assessed, including Fine Motor, Gross Motor, Cognitive, Adaptive, Social–Communication, and Social. The Hawaii Early Learning Profile (HELP; Parks, 1992) comprises 685 skills and behaviors within six domains for children with developmental disabilities from birth to age 36 months. Finally, the Brigance Diagnostic Inventory of Early Development II (Brigance, 2004) is both a diagnostic instrument and a criterion-referenced classroom assessment. It provides criterion-referenced task analyses across 11 domains for children from birth to age 84 months. However, unlike the previously discussed tools, the Brigance is not a curriculum, in that it does not provide specific teaching strategies or activities based on the test results.

Specialized Curriculum Measures

Specialized measures have also been developed to assess and provide curricula for specific subgroups of children. For example, the Oregon Project Curriculum for Visually Impaired and Blind Preschool Children (Brown, Simmons, & Methvin, 1986) assesses children with both visual and other impairments from birth to age 72 months. The Developmental Assessment for Students with Severe Disabilities, Second Edition (DASH-2; Dykes & Erin, 1999) is a criterion-referenced instrument that assesses performance in language, sensory–motor skills, activities of daily living, basic academic skills, and social–emotional skills in children whose developmental functioning falls between birth and 6 years, 11 months of age. It can serve as an initial assessment instrument, a tool for curriculum planning, and a means of monitoring progress. The Assessment of Basic Language and Learning Skills (ABLLS; Sundberg & Partington, 1998) is a language-based assessment tool and curriculum for young children with autism and other developmental disabilities. Twelve areas related to language are addressed, such as requests, motor imitation, labeling, and conversations. Finally, The Callier–Azusa Scale (Stillman, 1978; Stillman & Battle, 1985) was designed specifically for children who are deaf–blind, but it can also be used with most students with severe disabilities. The scale is based on direct observation of the child over a 2-week period and includes subscales assessing visual, auditory, and tactile development. Information on other specialized scales can be found in Bagnato, Neisworth, and Munson (1997).

Performance-Based Assessment Tools

Neisworth and Bagnato (2004) described a continuum of measurement contexts, including clinical (conducting the assessment in a highly scripted manner in a laboratory-like setting), simulated (using standardized administration, but in a setting that may better resemble the child's natural environment), analogue (presenting materials in the child's natural setting), and natural (observing play and learning behaviors in the child's natural setting). Some tools that can be used within an analogue contact include the Communication and Symbolic Behavior Scales—Developmental Profile (CSBS-DP; Wetherby & Prizant, 2002), the Developmental Observation Checklist System (DOCS; Hresko, Miguel, Sherbenou, & Burton, 1994), and the Work Sampling System (WSS; Meisels et al., 2002). The CSBS-DP, a norm-referenced tool, helps assess the communicative competence (use of eye gaze, gestures, sounds, words, understanding, and play) of children with a functional communication age between 6 months and 24 months (chronological age up to about 6 years). The DOCS, a parent-completed checklist, has been normed for birth to age 6 years and assesses language, social, motor, and cognitive functioning. The

WSS, a curriculum-embedded, performance assessment for preschool to grade 5, is highly correlated with individually administered psychoeducational batteries.

Some options for use in more natural contexts include the DOCS, the Pediatric Evaluation of Disability Inventory (PEDI; Feldman, Haley, & Coryell, 1990) and the second edition of the Ages and Stages Questionnaire (ASQ; Bricker & Squires, 1999). The PEDI, a parent report questionnaire, evaluates functioning in children with disabilities ages 6 months to 7 years, 6 months, and includes both functional performance and capability in three domains: Self-Care, Mobility, and Social Function. The ASQ is a parent-completed questionnaire about communication, gross motor, fine motor, problem solving, and personal–social skills for children up to 5 years of age. Table 12.6 provides a summary of selected criterion- and performance-based assessment tools.

Task Analysis

Another way to conduct a performance assessment involves the use of a task analysis, which is the breaking down of a complex skill or sequence of behaviors into its component behaviors (Sulzer-Azaroff & Mayer, 1991). Each component is listed in the order of occurrence. For example, an eight-step task analysis for washing hands follows:.

1. Turn on water.
2. Pick up soap.
3. Put hands under water.
4. Remove hands from water and rub hands with soap.
5. Put soap down.
6. Rub hands together.
7. Rinse soap off of hands.
8. Turn off water.

Once a task analysis is developed, individuals may be assessed on their level of independence for each step. Typically, a child's or adolescent's rating is based on the level of assistance required to complete a given step. Types of assistance include physical guidance, pointing, modeling, verbal cues, and visual cues. To conduct a skills assessment, an evaluator often uses a "least to most" prompting strategy. For example, the individual might simply be told to wash his or her hands. The evaluator waits a few seconds, and if the individual does not ini-

TABLE 12.6. Criterion-Based and Performance-Based Assessment Tools

Test	Age range	Description/comments
Ages and Stages Questionnaire, second edition (ASQ; Bricker & Squires, 1999)	Birth to 5 years	A parent-completed questionnaire on Communication, Gross Motor, Fine Motor, Problem Solving, and Personal–Social Skills.
Assessment, Evaluation, and Programming System for Infants and Children, second edition (AEPS; Bricker, 2002)	Birth to 6 years	An evaluation tool and curriculum for children with disabilities. Areas assessed include Fine Motor, Gross Motor, Cognitive, Adaptive, Social–Communication, and Social.
Assessment of Basic Language and Learning Skills (ABLLS; Sundberg & Partington, 1998)	NA	A language-based assessment tool and curriculum for young children with autism and other developmental disabilities.
Brigance Diagnostic Inventory of Early Development II (Brigance, 2004)	Birth to 84 months	Is both a diagnostic instrument and a criterion-referenced classroom assessment, but not a curriculum.
Callier–Azusa Scale (Stillman, 1978; Stillman & Battle, 1985)	NA	Designed for children who are deaf–blind, but can also be used with students with severe disabilities. Based on direct observation.
Carolina Curriculum (Johnson-Martin, Attermeier, & Hacker, 2004; Johnson-Martin, Jens, Attermeier, & Hacker, 2004)	Infant/Toddler version: birth to 36 months Preschool version: 24 to 60 months	Both curricula comprise five areas: Cognition, Communication, Social Adaptation, Fine Motor, and Gross Motor.
Communication and Symbolic Behavior Scales—Developmental Profile (CSBS-DP; Wetherby & Prizant, 2002)	6- to 24-month level of functioning (chronological age up to about 6 years)	A norm-referenced tool that assesses communicative competence (Use of Eye Gaze, Gestures, Sounds, Words, Understanding, and Play).
Developmental Assessment for Students with Severe Disabilities II (DASH-2; Dykes & Erin, 1999)	Birth and 6 years, 11 months (developmental functioning level)	A criterion-referenced instrument that assesses performance in Language, Sensory–Motor Skills, Activities of Daily Living, Basic Academic Skills, and Social–Emotional Skills.
Developmental Observation Assessment System (DOCS; Hresko, Miguel, Sherbenou, & Burton, 1994)	Birth to 6 years	A parent-completed checklist that assesses language, social, motor, and cognitive functioning.
Oregon Project Curriculum for Visually Impaired and Blind Preschool Children (Brown, Simmons, & Methvin, 1986)	Birth to 72 months	Assesses children with moderate to severe mental retardation.
Work Sampling System (WSS; Meisels et al., 2002)	Preschool to Grade 5	A curriculum-embedded performance assessment.
Pediatric Evaluation of Disability Inventory (PEDI; Feldman et al., 1990)	6 months to 7 years, 6 months	A parent report questionnaire of functional performance and capability in Self-Care, Mobility, and Social Function.

tiate the first step of the task analysis (e.g., turning on the water), the least intrusive prompt is given (e.g., "Turn on the water"). If the individual continues to require a greater level of assistance, a modeling or pointing prompt might be provided. Finally, physical guidance is given if less intrusive prompts are unsuccessful in assisting the individual to complete the step. This is repeated for every step of the task analysis.

Skills can also be broken down into more basic components, often in a developmental sequence. For example, the Carolina Curriculum for Preschoolers with Special Needs (second edition) (Johnson-Martin, Attermeier, & Hacker, 2004) provides curriculum sequences in a range of development areas, such as attention and memory, size and number concepts, and receptive language skills. Several published assessment tools and curricula provide task analyses for teaching a range of skills, such as preschool or preacademic skills (e.g., Johnson-Martin, Attermeier, & Hacker, 2004), language skills (Sundberg & Partington, 1998), and motor, cognitive, and adaptive skills (Bricker 2002).

Recommendations

It is difficult to provide specific recommendations or preferences regarding the previously mentioned alternative assessment methods. Most are used for assessment and educational planning. Choice of tool can be based on the age range covered and the desired response method. For example, the DASH-2 is appropriate for children 6–11 years of age, whereas many of the other scales focus on younger children. Some tools involve direct observation or assessment of the child (e.g., the Brigance); others rely on parental report (e.g., the DOCS). The ABLLS, which has become rather popular, can be extremely helpful in curriculum planning but is not norm based. Conversely, the Brigance, which is a popular, criterion-referenced assessment tool, does not provide a curriculum or educational guidance.

ASSESSMENT OF ADAPTIVE BEHAVIOR

Table 12.7 summarizes the most frequently used adaptive behavior scales. Adaptive behavior reflects an individual's ability independently to meet the needs and social demands of the en- vironment. Although the identification of deficits in adaptive functioning are a requirement for making a diagnosis of intellectual disability, there remains considerable disagreement within the field over what skills constitute adaptive behavior (AAMR, 2002). The current AAIDD definition of "intellectual disability" requires significant limitations in both intellectual functioning and adaptive behavior, as expressed in conceptual, social, and practical adaptive skills. This definition also focuses on an individual's ability to perform these skills versus his or her acquisition of such skills. Furthermore, the operational definition of "limitations in adaptive behavior" is falling at least two standard deviations below the mean for (1) one of the three types of adaptive behavior or (2) an overall score on a standardized measure of adaptive behavior. Although many of the available tools for measuring adaptive behavior do not contain domain names that directly match the three areas encompassed in the AAIDD definition, most commonly used tools have empirically derived factors that correspond to the three dimensions of adaptive behavior.

A number of available scales have a history of use in intellectual disability. Most involve the use of a clinical interview of an informant who knows the individual well. Some also include options for a simple questionnaire format. The Vineland Adaptive Behavior Scales–II (Sparrow, Cicchetti, & Balla, 2005), perhaps the best known tool, has recently been revised. The survey and expanded interview forms utilize a semistructured interview format to gather information on adaptive functioning from a parent/caregiver. Teacher and caregiver rating forms are also available as an alternative to the interview. The Vineland assesses areas of communication, daily living skills, socialization, and motor skills (for ages 6–11 years and younger). Results can be expressed as a standard score ($X = 100$, $SD = 15$), percentiles, or age equivalents of each area, as well as an Adaptive Behavior Composite. The Interview Edition Survey and Expanded Form were standardized on 3,695 individuals (birth to age 90 years). Validity of the Vineland was also established for individuals with mild, moderate, and severe/profound mental retardation, as well as those with emotional disorders and other disabilities.

A second frequently used scale, the second edition of AAMR Adaptive Behavior Scale— School, last revised in 1993 (Lambert, Nihira,

TABLE 12.7. Tests Frequently Used to Assess Adaptive Functioning

Test	Age range	Description/comments
AAMR Adaptive Behavior Scale—School 2 (Lambert, Nihira, & Leland, 1993)	3 to 21 years	Assesses personal independence and personal responsibility in daily living as well as problem behavior. Both school/community and residential/community versions.
Adaptive Behavior Assessment System, second edition (ABAS; Harrison & Oakland, 2000)	Birth to 89 years	Assesses 10 adaptive skills domains. Infant/Preschool, School Age, and Adult kits available.
Adaptive Behavior Evaluation Scale—Revised (second edition) (McCarney & Arthaud, 2006)	4 to 12 years; 13 to 18 years	Includes both home and school versions.
Battelle Developmental Inventory II (Newborg, 2004)	Birth to 8 years	Assesses Personal–Social, Adaptive, Motor, Communication, and Cognitive. Assesses through interview, direct testing, or observation. Screening test also available.
Comprehensive Test of Adaptive Behavior—Revised (CTAB-R; Adams, 1999)	Birth to 60 years	Assesses Self-Help Skills, Home Living Skills, Independent Living Skills, Social Skills, Sensory and Motor Skills, Language Concepts, and Academic Skills.
Developmental Profile II (Alpern et al., 1989)	Birth to 12 years, 6 months	Well-standardized tool that covers a number of dimensions and contains 186 items.
Scales of Independent Behavior—Revised (SIB-R, Bruininks et al., 1996)	Birth through adult	Assesses Social Interaction and Community Skills, Personal Living Skills, Community Living Skills, Motor Skills, and Problem Behavior.
Vineland Adaptive Behavior Scales II (Sparrow, Cicchetti, & Balla, 2005)	Caregiver Survey Interview Form: 0 to 90 years Teacher Rating Form: 3 years to 21 years, 11 months	'Assesses Communication, Daily Living Skills, Socialization, and Motor Skills (for ages 6–11 and younger). Caregiver survey and expanded interview forms and Teacher/Caregiver rating forms available.

& Leland, 1993), was normed on two groups: a sample of 2,000 students with intellectual disability and a sample of 1,000 typically developing students, ages 3–21 years. The scale should be completed by someone who knows the child or adolescent well; results are expressed as either standard scores ($X = 10$, $SD = 3$), percentiles, or age equivalents. There are nine skills domains and seven maladaptive behavior domains. The Scales of Independent Behavior—Revised (SIB-R, Bruininks, Woodcock, Weatherman, & Hill, 1996) contains a full-scale form, short form, and early development form, each of which also includes a Problem Behavior scale. Domains assessed include Social Interaction and Community Skills, Personal Living Skills, Community Living Skills,

and Motor Skills. The Comprehensive Test of Adaptive Behavior—Revised (CTAB-R; Adams, 1999) is normed for children and adults, covering areas such as self-help skills, home living skills, independent living skills, social skills, sensory and motor skills, language concepts, and academic skills. The teacher is typically the primary respondent, but information from other sources (e.g., a parent or guardian survey) can be used in order to complete the assessment tool.

The Adaptive Behavior Assessment System, Second Edition (ABAS; Harrison & Oakland, 2000) is a relatively new scale, based on the 10 adaptive skill domains identified in the 1992 AAIDD definition. Consequently, it is not possible to derive broader domains that correspond to the 2002 AAIDD definition (requiring the evaluator to use only the total score). The ABAS is normed across the age span (birth to 89 years) and includes infant/preschool, school age, and adults kits. Parent, teacher, and day care forms are available.

A number of alternative adaptive behavior scales are also worth considering. One well standardized tool is the Developmental Profile II (Alpern, Boll, & Shearer, 1989), a 186-item inventory covering birth to 12 years, 6 months of age. Another option is the second edition of the Adaptive Behavior Evaluation Scale–Revised (McCarney & Arthaud, 2006). This recently updated scale comprises separate versions for 4- to 12-year-olds and 13- to 18-year-olds. The scale also includes both a home and school version. Finally, the Battelle Developmental Inventory II (Newborg, 2004), designed for children from birth to 8 years of age, covers five domains: Personal–Social, Adaptive, Motor, Communication, and Cognitive. Whereas the assessment takes 1–2 hours to complete, there is a screening test that requires 10–30 minutes. Ratings can be obtained via interview with parents, direct assessment of the child, or through observation of the child in the natural environment.

Recommendations

Although there are a number of options available for assessing adaptive behavior, the Vineland Adaptive Behavior Scales (Sparrow et al., 2005) remains that most frequently used tool. However, the Vineland is based on parent and/or teacher report rather than direct observation of an individual's skills by an independent evaluator. Clinicians who desire to conduct their own observations of adaptive behavior (in addition to obtaining parent–teacher feedback) may find the Battelle Developmental Inventory II (Newborg, 2004) to be of use. However, the scale only goes up to age 8 and can require a considerable length of time to complete.

ASSESSING PSYCHOSOCIAL FACTORS

As discussed previously, a range of psychosocial factors place an individual at risk for intellectual disability. The AAIDD (2002) divides psychosocial risk factors into three categories: social (e.g., poverty, maternal malnutrition,

lack of pre- and perinatal care), behavioral (e.g., parental substance abuse, domestic violence, child abuse and neglect), and educational (e.g., inadequate early intervention and special education services, impaired parenting). It is important to assess such factors, both to increase the understanding of potential contributions to intellectual dysfunction and to assist in development of recommendations for treatment. A considerable literature indicates that families of children with intellectual disability experience significantly more parental stress than other families (Baker, Blacher, Crnic, & Edelbrock, 2002; Nachsehn & Minnes, 2005). The level of stress perceived by families may be influenced by a number of factors, such as a child's diagnosis (Crnic, Friedrich, & Greenberg, 1983), severity of the handicapping condition (Donovan, 1988), severity of behavior problems (Baker et al., 2002; Hassall, Rose, & McDonald, 2005; Margalit, Shulman, & Stuchiner, 1989), a child's age (Bristol, 1979), race (Flynt & Wood, 1989), maternal age (Flynt & Wood, 1989), family socioeconomic status (Rabkin & Streuning, 1976) and parental marital status (Salisbury, 1987). The additional caregiving requirements for children with developmental disabilities are often a significant source of stress to families, with level of stress positively associated with the caregiving demands placed on mothers (Beckman, 1991). The availability of informal supports also has been found to be negatively associated with mothers' stress levels (Beckman, 1991).

Interestingly, siblings of children with intellectual disability appear to experience fewer adjustment problems than their parents. For example, Dyson (1989) compared 55 older siblings of young children with handicaps and 55 matched siblings of nonhandicapped children. Results indicated similar levels of self-concept, behavior problems, and social competence in the two groups. Hannah and Midlarsky (1999) also found no overall differences between siblings of children with intellectual disability and siblings of typically developing children on measures of internalizing disorders, externalizing disorders, and self-esteem. In a further examination of sibling functioning based on type of handicap, siblings of children with intellectual disability evidenced the best adjustment levels. These findings are consistent with other reports (e.g., Breslau, Weitzman, & Messenger, 1981; Lobato, Barbour, Hall, & Miller, 1987).

A number of structured questionnaires are available to assess family functioning. For example, the Parenting Stress Index—Third Edition (PSI; Abidin, 1995), a 120-item questionnaire, assesses family stress related to child characteristics, parent characteristics, and life stressors. The tool was normed with 2,633 parents of children 1 month through 12 years of age. Referenced group profiles are provided for families of children with autism, as well as with developmental disabilities. A short form comprising 36 questions is also available. The PSI has received considerable use by researchers examining stress in families of children with developmental disabilities. For example, Hassall and colleagues (2005) recently documented a positive relationship between level of parental stress (as measured by the PSI) and parental locus of control, parenting satisfaction, and child behavior difficulties in a group of 46 mothers of children with intellectual disability. Nachshen and Minnes (2005) also documented that parents of children with developmental disabilities reported more stress and less well-being, as measured by the PSI, than parents of typically developing children.

A number of other assessment tools have been used in studies of families of children with developmental disabilities. For example, the Questionnaire on Resources and Stress—Short Form (Friedrich, Greenberg, & Crnic, 1983) is a 52-item self-report questionnaire developed primarily for assessing stress in families who care for children with developmental or intellectual disability. It is a psychometrically derived version of the 285-item Questionnaire on Resources and Stress (Holroyd, 1974) and uses a true–false format. This tool was used by Dyson, Edgar, and Crnic (1989) to examine adjustment in siblings of children with developmental disabilities. The Family Impact Questionnaire (FIQ; Donenberg & Baker, 1993), a 50-item questionnaire that assesses parents' perceptions and of a child's impact on the family, has been used in recent studies of maternal well-being and parenting stress in families of preschoolers with developmental delays (Baker et al., 2002; Eisenhower, Baker, & Blacher, 2005; Nachshen & Minnes, 2005). The Family Member Well-Being Index (McCubbin, Paterson, & Glynn, 1982), an eight-item measure of family members' well-being, assessing health, tension, energy, cheerfulness, fear, anger, sadness, and general concern, was recently used in a study by Nachshen and Minnes (2005) to ex-

amine parental empowerment of school-age children with developmental disabilities. Finally, scales such as the Family Environment Scale (Moos & Moos, 1994) have a long history of use in family research, including studies of families with child or sibling with intellectual disability (e.g., Hannah & Midlarsky, 1999).

Recommendations

Despite the availability of a number of options to assess family functioning, the PSI, third edition (Abidin, 1995) is still used frequently with this and other pediatric populations. However, it fails to provide information regarding parental mental health and possesses only a limited number of items related to marital issues.

ASSESSING PSYCHIATRIC PROBLEMS

Conducting a psychiatric assessment for an individual with intellectual disability remains challenging for a number of reasons: (1) Language deficits often make it difficult for a child with intellectual disability to report internal and feeling states; (2) some behaviors may be maladaptive, yet developmentally appropriate (e.g., an adolescent with intellectual disability takes an item from a peer, but has no concept of "stealing"); (3) few available assessment instruments have been normed for this population; (4) sensory and/or physical impairments may complicate diagnosis; and (5) the presence of "diagnostic overshadowing" (Benson & Aman, 1999). Diagnostic overshadowing refers to situations in which the presence of intellectual disability decreases the diagnostic significance of a psychiatric disorder. In other words, behaviors that might be seen as evidence of psychopathology in typically developing children and adolescents are attributed to cognitive deficits in individuals with intellectual disability.

Proper diagnosis also often requires that clinicians rely on observable behavior rather than self-report (MacLean, 1993). As with typically developing children who require mental health treatment, parent/caregiver and teacher reports provide an invaluable source of information. Despite the aforementioned challenges, it is generally accepted that diagnostic criteria for psychiatric disorders, such as those found in DSM-IV-TR (APA, 2000), can be reasonably applied to children and adolescents functioning at or above the mild range of mental retardation (IQs above 50). However, these criteria may be less appropriate or useful for those functioning within the severe to profound range of functioning (MacLean, 1993).

In assessing children and adolescents with intellectual disability, the clinician must be aware of certain symptom clusters that often may indicate the presence of a specific disorder associated with intellectual disability. For example, a child who exhibits regression in skills prior to 30 months of age, such as a loss of previously acquired language skills, along with unusual behaviors such as stereotyped hand movements, may be displaying symptoms consistent with Rett's disorder (APA, 2000). Lesch–Nyhan syndrome is often associated with severe self-injury (Nyhan, 1976). Children with Angelman syndrome typically display unprovoked laughter, hyperactivity, and sleep disorders, whereas children with Williams syndrome often have short attention spans but are quite social and often have strong musical skills (AAMR, 2002; Einfeld & Aman, 1995). Children with Smith–Magenis syndrome are often impulsive, have sleep disorders, and engage in stereotypical and self-injurious behaviors (AAMR, 2002).

Similarly, when evaluating a child or adolescent with a previously diagnosed medical disorder, it is important that the clinician be aware of any associated behavioral sequelae, because such behaviors are often the reason for referral. For example, when evaluating a child with intellectual disability secondary to lead poisoning, the clinician should ask questions regarding pica (the persistent eating of non-nutritive substances; APA, 2000). A child seen for evaluation with a diagnosis of Prader–Willi syndrome is likely exhibiting behaviors related to compulsive eating (Pueschel & Thuline, 1991).

Structured Diagnostic Interviews

To improve the reliability of open-ended psychiatric interviews, a number of structured psychiatric interview tools have been developed. Such interviews involve asking groups of questions in a standard manner and order. The rater indicates the presence or absence of each symptom, then tallies ratings at the conclusion of the interview and makes a diagnosis. Kamphaus and Frick (2002) reported a number of advantages to structured psychiatric interviews, in-

cluding (1) the ability to obtain important parameters of a child's behavior that are not typically assessed by most behavior rating scales, (2) the ability to provide temporal sequencing among behaviors (i.e., to determine whether a behavior suggestive of depression occurs contiguously with other behaviors associated with this diagnosis), (3) the ability to determine the level of impairment, (4) enhancement of the correspondence between the assessment technique and DSM diagnostic criteria, and (5) help in improving clinical assessors' competence in interviewing. Conversely, some specific weaknesses are also associated with structured psychiatric interviews: (1) the amount of time required to conduct such interviews, (2) the need to train interviewers to meet reliability standards, (3) lack of information from other sources (such as teachers), and (4) difficulty in accounting for age-related norms (i.e., being unable to account for age-appropriate differences in activity level between preschoolers and adolescents) (Kamphaus & Frick, 2002).

Three structured interview tools have received the most attention in the literature and have revised versions that include both DSM-III-R and DSM-IV criteria. Each has parent and child versions and takes up to 90 minutes to complete. None has been normed with children or adolescents with intellectual disability. The Schedule for Affective Disorder and Schizophrenia for School-Age Children—Present and Lifetime Version (K-SADS-PL; Kaufman, Birmaher, Brent, Rao, & Ryan, 1996), a semistructured diagnostic interview, assesses past and present psychopathology in children and adolescents ages 6–18. It covers all major DSM-III-R and DSM-IV diagnoses applicable to this age group, with separate parent and child interviews. The Diagnostic Interview for Children and Adolescents–IV (DICA-IV) (de la Osa, Ezpeleta, Domenech, Navarro, & Losilla, 1997; Reich, 2000) was similarly developed for children and adolescents ages 6–18 and has a more structured format than the K-SADS. It, too, assesses all major DSM-III-R and DSM-IV diagnoses for children and adolescents. It also includes separate interviews for parents and children/adolescents and is available in a computerized form. The Diagnostic Interview Schedule for Children–IV (DISC-IV; Shaffer, Fisher, Lucas, Dulcan, & Schwab-Stone, 2000) is a highly structured, standardized interview schedule with versions for both children and parents. It is based on DSM-IV criteria covering children ages 6–17 years in the parent version and ages 9–17 in the self-report version. A computerized interview version (C-DISC) is also available. A couple of additional tools provide a similar interview format for both parent and child. The Child and Adolescent Psychiatric Assessment (CAPA; Angold & Costello, 2000), developed for individuals 8–17 years of age, and the Children's Interview for Psychiatric Symptoms (ChIPS; Weller et al., 2000), covering individuals 6–18 years of age, both offer possible alternatives to the K-SADS-PL, DISC-IV, and DICA.

Some of the available self-report interviews may be of particular interest to clinicians who assess children and adolescents with intellectual disability. However, none of these tools has been normed for individuals with developmental, cognitive, or learning disorders, and all appear to be based on DSM-III-R diagnostic criteria. The Dominic—Revised (Dominic-R; Valla, Bergeron, & Smolla, 2000), a structured pictorial questionnaire, assesses DSM-III-R–based diagnoses in children ages 6–11 years. A child is shown a number of drawings of a peer in situations associated with various childhood psychiatric disorders and is simply asked whether the same kind of thing has happened to him or her ("Are you like this?"). The reliability and validity data are promising. A recent article has been published with preliminary data on an adolescent version of the Dominic-R for 12- to 16-year-olds, also using DSM-III-R–based diagnostic criteria (Smolla, Valla, Bergeron, Berthiaume, & St. Georges, 2004). The third edition of the Pictorial Instrument for Children and Adolescents—Revised (PICA-III-R; Ernst, Cookus, & Moravec, 2000) comprises 137 pictures organized in modules that cover five diagnostic categories, including disorders of anxiety, mood, psychosis, disruptive behavior, and substance abuse. Although the standardization sample was drawn from individuals whose ages ranged from 6 to 16 years, limited data are available on the tool's psychometric properties. Like the Dominic-R, it uses DSM-III-R–based diagnostic criteria.

A few structured psychiatric interview schedules have been developed specifically for children and adolescents with intellectual disability. The Structured Clinical Interview (Spragg, 1988) was designed for individuals with intellectual disability. It uses simple language, relying on open-ended questions and items with choice formats. However, there are limited available data on the scale's psychometric properties, and little evidence of its use for clinical or research purposes. The Schedule of Handicaps, Behaviour, and Skills (HBS)—Revised (Wing, 1982; Wing & Gould, 1978) was originally developed for children with intellectual disability or autism. Information is obtained from the caregiver in a semistructured interview. Although there are some psychometric data available (van Berckelaer-Onnes & van Duijn, 1993), it too does not appear to have received much attention in the literature.

Recommendations

The majority of tools reviewed here that were designed specifically for individuals with intellectual disability have seen limited use, and have minimal available data on psychometric properties. The clinical questionnaires with the strongest psychometric properties and history of use (e.g., K-SADS-PL, DISC-IV, DICA) require a greater amount of time to complete than is typically available within a clinical setting. Additionally, some require considerable training for staff to become skilled at proper administration (e.g., the K-SADS-PL). Consequently, most of these measures are used primarily for research purposes. Behavior problem checklists are an alternative option for assessing psychiatric problems in this population (discussed below).

Behavior Problem Checklists and Self-Report Scales

Behavior problem checklists have been used extensively to augment the diagnosis of psychiatric disorders in children with intellectual disability. Additionally, such tools have provided documentation of changes in behavior following a range of interventions, especially pharmacological treatment (e.g., Aman, De Smedt, Derivan, Lyons, & Findling, 2002; Handen & Hardan, 2006). Checklists can be completed by primary informants, such as teachers or parents, as well as by the child or adolescent. From an assessment standpoint, these tools allow one to obtain information from informants (e.g., teachers) who would otherwise not be available during the assessment. These tools also provide structure for informants and allow for comparison of the behavior of the child being evaluated with that of same-age and -gender peers.

The challenge facing the evaluator is whether to use a questionnaire that has been normed for children with intellectual disability or one that has been normed for typically developing children. From a diagnostic standpoint, the use of an appropriately normed tool is recommended. Such a tool takes into account population differences between typically developing individuals and those with intellectual disability. However, this is less of a concern for purposes of demonstrating a treatment effect (e.g., using either psychosocial or pharmacological treatment), because the individual can serve as his or her own control. However, the tool must be appropriate for individuals with intellectual disability. For example, a tool containing a high number of questions about con-duct problems (e.g., swearing, threatening others with weapons) would be inappropriate for an adolescent with severe mental retardation and no language skills. I summarize some of the tools used in intellectual disability research, most of which have been normed with atypical populations.

Table 12.8 summarizes the most commonly used behavior problem checklists and self-report scales for children and adolescents with intellectual disability. Among the best-known checklists is the Conners Rating Scales (Conners, 1997), which have been used extensively as a supplemental data source for assessing ADHD and also the efficacy of a wide range of psychotropic medications in children with intellectual disability and/or autism

TABLE 12.8. Behavior Problem Checklists

Test	Age range	Description/comments
Aberrant Behavior Checklist (ABC; Aman & Singh, 1986)[a]	6 years to adult	Comprises 58 items and five factors: Irritability, Lethargy, Stereotypical Behavior, Hyperactivity, and Inappropriate Speech.
Conners Rating Scales (Conners, 1997)	3 to 17 years	Includes Parent and Teacher versions, including long and short forms. All forms include the ADHD Index.
Developmental Behaviour Checklist II (DBD-II; Einfeld & Tonge, 2002)[a]	Children and adults	A 96-item parent and 93-item teacher rating scale. Comprises five subscales: Disruptive/Antisocial Behavior, Self-Absorbed, Communication Disturbance, Anxiety, and Social Relating Disturbance. Norms for both parents and teachers.
Fear Survey for Children with and without Mental Retardation (Ramirez & Kratochwill, 1990)[a]	10 to 13 years	A 60-item, self-report questionnaire, appropriate for children with mild mental retardation. A self-report scale.
Nisonger Child Behavior Rating Form (Tasse et al., 1996)[a]	3 to 16 years	Includes parent and teacher forms. Comprises 66 items and five subscales: Conduct Problems, Hyperactivity, Self-Injury/Stereotypy, Insecure/Anxious, Self-Isolated/ Ritualistic, Overly Sensitive (parent form), and Irritability (teacher form).
Reiss Scales for Children's Dual Diagnosis (Reiss & Valenti-Hein, 1990)[a]	4 to 21 years	Is a downward extension of the RSMB. Comprises 60 items with nine factors (e.g., Anger/Self-Control, Anxiety, Attention Disorder).
Reiss Screen for Maladaptive Behavior (RSMB; Reiss, 1988)[a]	Adolescents and adults	Comprises 38 items and seven clinical subscales: Aggressive Behavior, Psychosis, Paranoia, Depression (behavioral), Depression (physical), Dependent Personality Disorder, and Avoidant Disorder.
Repetitive Behavior Scale— Revised (RBS-R; Bodfish et al., 2000)[a]	NA	A 43-item rating scale with six factors: Stereotypical Behavior, Self-Injurious Behavior, Compulsive Behavior, Ritualistic Behavior, Sameness Behavior, and Restricted Behavior.

[a] Normed or developed for individuals with mental retardation.

(Aman, Marks, Turbott, Wilsher, & Merry, 1991; Handen et al., 1992; Jaselskis, Cook, Fletcher, & Leventhal, 1992). The current revision of the checklist comprises a 59-item teacher version and an 80-item parent version. In addition, short forms for both teachers (28 items) and parents (27 items) are available. Each item is rated on a 4-point scale based on frequency of occurrence (from *Not at all* to *Very often*). The parent version comprises 10 subscales, whereas the teacher version has nine subscales. All four long and short versions include an ADHD Index.

Whereas the Conners Rating Scales are normed with typically developing children, they continue to be used as both a tool to establish research criteria for ADHD in children with intellectual disability and to document medication efficacy (e.g., Aman, Kern, McGhee, & Arnold, 1993; Handen et al., 1992). A 1994 study by Pearson and Aman compared the results of mental versus chronological age when using the Conners norms for children with intellectual disability. The study was prompted by the recommendation of some researchers and clinicians that mental rather than chronological age be used when comparing the score of a child with an intellectual disability with the normal group (Barkley, 1990). However, Pearson and Aman found significant correlations in only 4 of 27 comparisons between scale ratings and mental age, lending little support to guidelines stating that mental age be used to determine which norms should be applied when children with intellectual disability are evaluated.

A number of additional available behavior problem checklists have been developed and specifically normed for children, adolescents, and adults with intellectual disability. The reader is also referred to a 2004 chapter by Lecavalier and Aman, as well as an article by Aman (1994), that reviewed many of the available behavior problem checklists for use with this population.

The most extensively validated tool is the Aberrant Behavior Checklist (ABC; Aman & Singh, 1986). A Community Version of the ABC was validated in 1992 (Marshburn & Aman, 1992). The ABC comprises a list of 58 behavioral items, rated on a 3-point scale. The Community Version has been normed on a group of 666 children (ages 6–15) and 1,024 adults. The factor analysis resulted in five subscales: Irritability, Agitation/Crying, Lethargy/

Social Withdrawal, Stereotypic Behavior, and Hyperactivity. There are separate norms for children by both age and gender. The Community Version is completed by teachers or other staff who work with individuals with intellectual disability. The Nisonger Child Behavior Rating Form (Tasse, Aman, Hammer, & Rojahn, 1996) comprises a list of 66 behavioral items rated on a 4-point severity scale. The Nisonger was originally standardized on a sample of 369 children (ages 3–16) who were seen consecutively at an interdisciplinary clinic for children with intellectual/developmental disabilities. The majority of the sample functioned within the mild range of mental retardation. Both parent and teacher forms are available. Subscales include Conduct Problems, Hyperactivity, Self-Injury/Stereotypy, Insecure/Anxious, Self-Isolated/Ritualistic, Overly Sensitive (parent form), and Irritability (teacher form).

Another option for assessing mental health problems in adolescents and adults with intellectual disability is the RSMB (Reiss, 1994). It comprises seven clinical subscales, based on a factor analysis of data from a sample of 306 individuals with intellectual disability and mental health problems. An alternative for children is a downward extension of the RSMB, the Reiss Scales for Children's Dual Diagnosis (RSCDD; Reiss & Valenti-Hein, 1990). The original factor analysis was based on data from 313 individuals with intellectual disability (ages 4–21 years) seen at community-based agencies. Using a 3-point rating scale, the RSCDD comprises 60 items resolving into nine factors (e.g., Anger/Self-Control, Anxiety, Attention Disorder). However, because no "Depression" subscale was identified via the factor analysis, the authors selected a set of items from the DSM and other sources on an a priori basis to create such a subscale.

One of the most psychometrically sound behavior scales for children and adults with intellectual disability is the Developmental Behaviour Checklist II (DBD-II; Einfeld & Tonge, 2002). The authors have recently renormed the scale (with a sample of 1,155 teachers and 1,536 parents), which was originally adapted from the Child Behavior Checklist (Achenbach, 1991). The scale seems to be particularly useful for individuals functioning within the moderate to severe range of mental retardation, but the recent revision includes a good number of items for individuals with mild mental retardation (see Lecavalier & Aman, 2004). Utilizing a 3-point rating scale, the DBD-II comprises 96 items for the Parent version and 93 items for the Teacher version. Five subscales were derived from the most recent factor analysis: (1) Disruptive and Antisocial Behavior, (2) Self-Absorbed, (3) Communication Disturbance, (4) Anxiety, and (5) Social Relating Disturbance. A total behavior problem score may also be tabulated.

An assessment tool that may be useful for work with individuals with repetitive behaviors (a common problem among individuals with intellectual disability) is the Repetitive Behavior Scale—Revised (RBS-R; Bodfish, Symons, Parker, & Lewis, 2000). This empirically derived scale was developed by combining items measuring repetitive behaviors contained in other scales, along with clinical experience. The 43 items are rated on a 4-point scale, resulting in six factors: Stereotypic Behavior, Self-Injurious Behavior, Compulsive Behavior, Ritualistic Behavior, Sameness Behavior, and Restricted Behavior. Few self-report scales have been normed with individuals with intellectual disability. One of the obvious problems with such scales is the validity of the responses. One option is the Fear Survey for Children with and without Mental Retardation (Ramirez & Kratochwill, 1990), a simplified 60-item revision of the Children's Fear Survey Schedule (Ryan & Dietiker, 1979). The survey involves asking the child to indicate whether an item makes him or her scared, afraid, or nervous. Although it appears to be appropriate for children with mild mental retardation, the study sample included only children in the 10- to 13-year age range with intellectual disability.

Recommendations

In summary, for children and adolescents functioning within the moderate to mild range of mental retardation, scales such as those by Conners, may be useful but should be interpreted cautiously. Supplementing or replacing these scales with one that is normed and developed specifically for individuals with intellectual disability may be the best practice. For children and adolescents functioning within the severe to profound range of mental retardation, scales specifically developed for this population should be used. Obtaining information from multiple sources (e.g., parents and teach-

ers) is also recommended. Finally, one should be particularly cautious in using a self-report scale as the sole or primary source of information during an assessment.

BEHAVIORAL OBSERVATION

Direct behavioral observation provides an important part of a multimethod assessment of a child's strengths and weaknesses. When the referral question relates to specific behavior problems (e.g., self-injury, inattention), direct observation becomes paramount. Unfortunately, an outpatient clinic is not necessarily the best setting in which to observe a child. A child experiences considerable reactivity when first seen in a new and strange place. Therefore, when possible, home or school visits are an effective (although not necessarily efficient) means of obtaining valid information regarding a child's behavior. Because this is not always possible, researchers and clinicians have developed a number of different analogue, in-clinic situations that attempt to replicate home and school settings as closely as possible. In doing so, they hope to elicit behaviors similar to those observed outside the clinic.

Once the target behaviors have been identified (e.g., noncompliance, out-of-seat behavior, aggression), children may be observed in a variety of different situations within the clinic. However, it may require some ingenuity on the part of the clinician to provide a specific setting in which the target behaviors can be elicited and observed. For the child who is noncompliant, having the parent work with him or her on both easy and demanding tasks (e.g., simulate a homework session) may provide an opportunity both to see the behavior and to observe how it is handled by the parent. Sometimes, the assessment situation itself can elicit the behavior of concern. Such might be the case for a child who uses aggression or other disruptive behaviors to obtain attention. The youngster may attempt to interrupt or disrupt when the parent is talking with the clinician. Observing such interactions between parent and child provides a rich database from which to understand the problem and recommend solutions.

A variety of methods are available for quantifying direct observations of children alone or interacting with their parents. The most commonly used strategy is frequency recording, which involves counting the number of occurrences of an event. For example, Kern, Mauk, Marder, and Mace (1995) examined the functional relationship between breath holding and various situations (e.g., being placed alone in a room, during play, being provided adult attention when breath holding) in a child with severe mental retardation and Cornelia de Lange syndrome. The dependent measure was the number of breath-holding episodes observed during each 10-minute observation. A second strategy involves recording the duration of an event. This might be useful when observing behaviors such as remaining seated or playing appropriately. The clinician simply records the total time a child engages in the target behaviors during the observation period. More complex observational strategies have involved the use of event sequences. For example, a clinician might track social interactions by scoring ongoing sequences of behavioral events, such as might occur during a mother–child interaction. Such data provide information on interactional patterns of behavior that can be used in treatment. Breiner and Forehand (1982) used such a tool to examine mother–child interactions in oppositional preschoolers with and without developmental disabilities. They found that mothers of the children with delays used significantly more commands, and the delayed children exhibited greater noncompliance than did the typically developing children. Similarly, Handen, Feldman, Lurier, and Husar (1999) observed mothers and their developmentally delayed preschoolers (all diagnosed with ADHD) during a clinic task, in which the mother asked the child to comply with 10 requests. Observations were conducted while the children were on both Ritalin and placebo. The preschoolers were found to be significantly more compliant and less disruptive during the Ritalin condition compared to the placebo condition.

A particular area of emphasis in behavior analysis has been to conduct a functional assessment of the target behaviors. Such an assessment can be done in a variety of ways. One strategy involves the taking data over a period of a few days or weeks (depending on the rate of the behavior of interest) by caregivers. When the target behavior occurs, information on possible antecedents (e.g., date, time, who was involved, what was occurring at the time), a description of the behavior, and the consequences

(i.e., how the behavior was managed) is gathered. With this information, the clinician can begin to develop hypotheses as to the function of the behavior and develop appropriate treatment interventions. Behavior analysts have typically divided the function of behavior into four categories: task avoidance, attention seeking, obtaining a tangible item, and obtaining sensory stimulation.

An alternative and more analytic approach is to conduct a functional analysis of a behavior. This involves the *direct manipulation of variables* to test the various functional relationships. One example is provided by Iwata, Dorsey, Slifer, Bauman, and Richman (1994), who used this model to better understand variables that either produced or maintained self-injury in nine children with developmental disabilities. Over a number of weeks, children were repeatedly observed for 15-minute periods in one of four experimental conditions: social disapproval for self-injury, academic demands in which the clinician turned away for 30 seconds following self-injury (with praise given for task completion), a no-demand play situation (with self-injury ignored), and an alone condition. Six of the nine subjects consistently evidenced higher levels of self-injury in specific stimulus conditions, suggesting that within-subject variability was a function of features of the environment. These findings have implications for the selection of appropriate treatment intervention. A number of other researchers have also used this model to assess children in a variety of settings. For example, Piazza and colleagues (2003) evaluated 15 children with feeding disorders (typically involving food refusal). Each child's behavior was observed under four different feeding conditions: (1) baseline: simply talking to the child throughout the meal and leaving a spoonful of food near the child's mouth; (2) attention: coaxing and other forms of adult attention following food refusal; (3) escape: removing the food following refusal to eat; and (4) tangible: providing tangible items (e.g., favorite toys, foods, or drinks) when the child refused to eat. Results found increased food refusal for 10 of the 15 children during one or more of the conditions, suggesting that environmental variables played a role in the feeding problem. Additionally, this information provided important information regarding possible treatment interventions for each child. Figure 12.1 shows in-

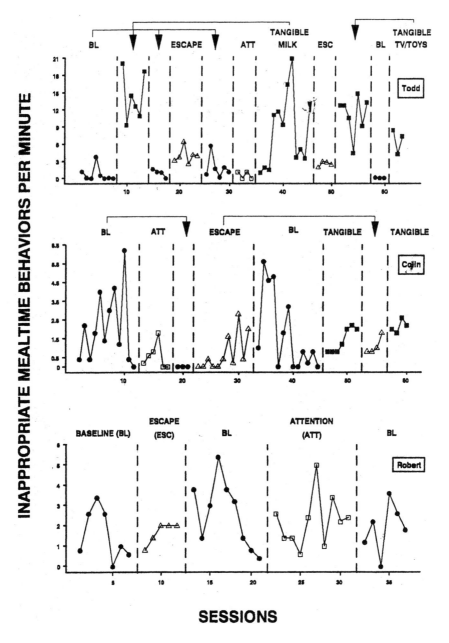

FIGURE 12.1. Inappropriate mealtime behaviors per minute for three children: Todd, Colin, and Robert. From Piazza et al. (2003). Copyright 2003 by the Society for the Experimental Analysis of Behavior. Reprinted by permission.

appropriate mealtime behaviors per minute in the attention and escape conditions for three children.

A number of clinicians and researchers have also developed complex observation systems to code behavior in the home or school. Such systems typically involve an interval recording strategy. This method divides time into small intervals (e.g., 10–15 seconds). Observers record as many as 25 possible behaviors (present–absent) during each interval. For example, Pierce and Schreibman (1997) used such a system to code social interactions between dyads of preschoolers with autism and typically developing peers. Daily sessions between two peers were videotaped and coded using 10-second intervals. Coded behaviors included maintaining interactions, initiating conversations, and initiating play. Computerized coding systems, such as the Social Interaction Code (SIC; Niemeyer & McEvoy, 1989), are also available. The SIC uses a laptop computer to code initiations, responses, and interactions of a target child with peers during play. A number of other software programs on the market allow clinicians/researchers to design their own coding schemes, depending on the target behaviors to be observed (e.g., The Observer XT, Procoder for Digital Video).

Recommendations

The type of direct observational method to utilize depends on the specific behavior problem, as well as the resources available. Determining the function of the target behavior is the first priority if an appropriate treatment plan is to be developed. A clinician working within a school or home setting may observe the child directly. The clinician who is limited to seeing individuals in a clinical setting can still obtain outside data or observe directly through simulation of various conditions (e.g., a demand situation, play condition, attention condition). The ability to conduct abbreviated functional assessments within a clinic setting has been demonstrated by a number of researchers (e.g., Cooper et al., 1990; Wacker et al., 1994).

SUMMARY OF BEST PRACTICES IN ASSESSMENT

The choice of tools to be used for an assessment of a child or adolescent with intellectual disability must match the question being posed. For example, a child who is referred for assessment and treatment of self-injurious behavior may not require IQ or achievement testing as part of the evaluation. Specific recommendations regarding assessment tools are provided at the end of each of the previous subsections. However, for a child referred for assessment of possible intellectual disability, a number of areas that represent current best practices should be thoroughly examined. These include a thorough developmental/medical history, use of a well-matched cognitive assessment tool, measurement of adaptive functioning, evaluation of achievement levels, assessment of related areas as appropriate (e.g., speech and language, motor, memory), the completion of behavior problem scale(s) (by both parent and teacher), and additional history and/or direct observation of behavioral concerns to assess the function of the behavior and to determine a possible comorbid psychiatric diagnosis. Referral to other specialists may also need to be considered (e.g., genetics, psychiatry, neurology, audiology, speech and language specialist, occupational therapy), depending on the possible role of other factors in the clinical picture (e.g., seizures, hearing loss, genetic disorder). Finally, the clinician needs to assess child and family strengths, and available resources to develop appropriate treatment recommendations.

INTEGRATING ASSESSMENT RESULTS

With data and information gathered from a wide array of sources, it may initially seem a formidable task to integrate the assessment results, let alone make treatment recommendations. Morgenstern and Klass (1991) suggest that the primary referral question should serve as a frame of reference for determining the answers to be provided during feedback to the family and in any subsequent report. Sattler (2001) recommends that a number of questions be considered that will guide the integration of information gathered during the assessment. Most important to consider is how the assessment results will help to answer the referral question and what questions remain. Once this is determined, the clinician must decide which major findings to interpret, which trends to develop in the feedback or report (i.e., Do the results suggest developmental delays across all areas? Do the results indicate consistent patterns of errors or relative weaknesses?), and which recommendations to make. Crnic (1988) provides a list of six questions that may be useful in integrating assessment results.

1. Is there significant test scatter across skills areas?
2. How do the results compare with previous assessment?
3. Did changes in the structure of testing (e.g., testing limits or allowing the use of alternative strategies) affect performance?
4. What behavioral factors were problems and what factors were strengths? Did they affect the assessment outcome?
5. Did performance or behavior vary across settings?
6. Are historical variables (e.g., developmental, medical, behavioral) relevant to the child's performance?

In formulating specific recommendations following the assessment of a child with intellectual disability, Sattler (1988) suggests that a number of questions be considered:

1. Do the results indicate a diagnosis of intellectual disability?
2. Is the child eligible for special services?
3. What are the least restrictive options for programming?
4. If mainstreaming or inclusion is possible, what additional supports will be needed?
5. What are the child's social skills strengths and weaknesses?
6. What skills will be needed for productive employment (for adolescents)?
7. As the individual reaches adulthood, what types of supports will he or she require to live independently? If this is not possible, what type of living arrangement will be needed?

PROVIDING FEEDBACK

The success of the feedback session depends in large part on how the initial interview was conducted and on the development of a shared referral question between clinician and family. Assisting the family to frame the proper question early on sets the stage for productive and useful feedback. One should be careful not to have the feedback focus solely on a child's or adolescent's deficits. Instead, it will be impor-

tant to stress strengths, as well as areas in which interventions will be focused. Perhaps the most difficult feedback to offer a family is that of a diagnosis of intellectual disability. It is not unusual to find that others who have already evaluated the child and found identical results have never used the terms "intellectual disability" or "mental retardation" when talking with the family. This places the clinician in an awkward and in some ways unfair position. Yet it is important that this information be shared with the family.

The clinician should also offer to meet again with the family to process the information and to ensure that the recommendations have been followed. Specific recommendations should be provided in writing at the time of feedback whenever possible. These should include whom to contact regarding obtaining appropriate services, names of parent support groups, local and state resources for services such as respite, summer camperships, and so forth. Providing reading materials at the time can also be helpful. It is also important that families receive a copy of your report as soon as possible. Assessment results should not simply be exchanged among professionals and agencies, but should be shared with families. In fact, reports should be written with families in mind, so that they are clear and understandable, with as little jargon as possible. Often, when a family hears stressful news, it is difficult for them to hear the remainder of the findings and recommendations. Written reports provide another chance for family members to react to the results and recommendations.

SUMMARY

Assessment of the child or adolescent with intellectual disability is a considerable challenge. It requires a number of important skills on the part of the clinician, including the ability to work with families, knowledge of developmental and etiological issues, experience in using a range of standardized and criterion-based assessment tools, understanding of the service delivery system, knowledge of the law as it pertains to developmental disabilities, and experience in providing clinical interventions with this population. The heterogeneity of this group of children makes this a particularly daunting task. Consequently, the clinician needs to gather data from as many sources as possible, assess a wide range of areas of functioning, and work closely with the family, as well as professionals from other disciplines. Finally, the clinician should work with the family to push the limits often placed upon individuals with intellectual disability. This means being open to suggesting the creative use of supports to enhance to the fullest the involvement of children and adolescents with intellectual disability in their schools, communities, and families.

REFERENCES

Abidin, R. R. (1995). *Parenting Stress Index—Third Edition*. Lutz, FL: Psychological Assessment Resources.

Achenbach, T. M. (1982). *Developmental psychopathology* (2nd ed.). New York: Ronald Press.

Achenbach, T. M. (1991). *Manual for the Child Behavior Checklist/4–18 and 1991 profile*. Burlington: University of Vermont, Department of Psychiatry.

Adams, G. L. (1999). *Comprehensive Test of Adaptive Behavior—Revised*. Seattle, WA: Educational Achievement Systems.

Alpern, G., Boll, T. J., & Shearer, M. (1989). *Developmental Profile II*. Aspen, CO: Psychological Development.

Aman, M. G. (1994). Instruments for assessing treatment effects in developmentally disabled populations. *Assessment in Rehabilitation and Exceptionality, 1*, 1–20.

Aman, M. G., De Smedt, G., Derivan, A., Lyons, B., & Findling, R. L. (2002). Risperidone Disruptive Behavior Study Group: Double-blind, placebo-controlled study of risperidone for the treatment of disruptive behaviors in children with subaverage intelligence. *American Journal of Psychiatry, 159*, 1337–1346.

Aman, M. G., Kern, R. A., McGhee, D. E., & Arnold, E. (1993). Fenfluramine and methylphenidate in children with mental retardation and ADHD: Clinical and side effects. *Journal of the American Academy of Child and Adolescent Psychiatry, 32*, 851–859.

Aman, M. G., Marks, R., Turbott, S., Wilsher, C., & Merry, S. (1991). The clinical effects of methylphenidate and thioridazine in intellectually subaverage children. *Journal of the American Academy of Child and Adolescent Psychiatry, 30*, 246–256.

Aman, M. G., Pejeau, C., Wolford, P., Rojahn, J., & Handen, B. L. (1996). Four-year follow-up of children with mental retardation and ADHD. *Research in Developmental Disabilities, 17*, 417–432.

Aman, M. G., & Singh, N. N. (1986). *Manual for the Aberrant Behavior Checklist*. East Aurora, NY: Slosson Educational.

American Association on Mental Retardation (AAMR). (1992). *Mental retardation: Definition, classification, and systems of supports* (9th ed.). Washington, DC: Author.

American Association on Mental Retardation (AAMR). (2002). *Mental retardation: Definition, classification, and systems of supports* (10th ed.). Washington, DC: Author.

American Psychiatric Association (APA). (2000). *Diagnostic and statistical manual of mental disorders* (4th ed., text rev.). Washington, DC: Author.

Angold, A., & Costello, J. (2000). The child and adolescent psychiatric assessment (CAPA). *Journal of the American Academy of Child and Adolescent Psychiatry, 39*, 49–58.

Bagnato, S. J., Neisworth, J. T., & Munson, S. M. (1997). *Linking assessment and early intervention: An authentic curriculum-based approach*. Baltimore: Brookes.

Baker, B. L., Blacher, J., Crnic, K. A., & Edelbrock, C. (2002). Behavior problems and parenting stress in families of three-year-old children with and without developmental delays. *American Journal on Mental Retardation, 107*, 433–444.

Bales v. Clark, 523 F. Supp. 1366 (8th Cir. Va. 1981).

Barkley, R. A. (1990). *Attention-deficit hyperactivity disorder: A handbook for diagnosis and treatment*. New York: Guilford Press.

Battle v. Commonwealth of Pennsylvania, 629 F.2d Pa.269 (3d Cir. 1980), cert. denied 452 U.S. 968 (1981).

Baumeister, A. (1970). American residential institution: Its history and character. In A. Baumeister & E. Butterfield (Eds.), *Residential facilities for the mentally retarded* (pp. 1–28) Chicago: Aldine.

Bayley, N. (2005). *Manual for the Bayley Scales of Infant Development* (3rd ed.). San Antonio, TX: Psychological Corporation.

Beckman, P. J. (1991). Comparison of mothers' and fathers' perceptions of the effect of young children with and without disabilities. *American Journal of Mental Retardation, 95*, 585–595.

Beery, K. E., Buktenica, N. A., & Beery, N. A. (2004). *The Berry–Buktenica Developmental Test of Visual–Motor Integration* (3rd ed.). Minneapolis, MN: Pearson Assessments.

Beirne-Smith, M., Patton, J. R., & Kim, S. H. (2006). *Mental retardation* (7th ed.). Upper Saddle River, NJ: Merrill/Prentice-Hall.

Benson, B. A., & Aman, M. G. (1999). Disruptive behavior disorders in children with mental retardation. In H. C. Quay & A. E. Hogan (Eds.), *Handbook of disruptive behavior disorders* (pp. 559–578). New York: Plenum Press.

Blatt, B., & Kaplan, F. (1966). *Christmas in purgatory*. Boston: Allyn & Bacon.

Bodfish, J. W., Symons, S. J., Parker, D. E., & Lewis, M. H. (2000). Varieties of repetitive behavior to autism: comparison with mental retardation. *Journal of Autism and Developmental Disorder, 30*, 237–243.

Bracken, B. A., & McCallum, R. S. (1998). *Universal Nonverbal Intelligence Test*. Itasca, IL: Riverside.

Braningan, G., & Decker, S. L. (2003). *Bender Visual–Motor Gestalt Test, second edition.* Itasca, IL: Riverside.

Breiner, J., & Forehand, R. (1982). Mother–child interactions: A comparison of a clinic-referred developmentally delayed group and two non-delayed groups. *Applied Research in Mental Retardation, 3,* 175–183.

Breslau, N., Weitzman, M., & Messenger, K. (1981). Psychologic functioning of siblings of disabled children. *Pediatrics, 67,* 344–353.

Bricker, D. (2002). *Assessment, Evaluation, and Programming System for Infants and Children, second edition (AEPS).* Baltimore: Brookes.

Bricker, D., & Squires, J., (1999) *Ages and Stages Questionnaire: A parent completed child-monitoring system* (2nd ed.). Baltimore: Brookes.

Brigance, A. H. (2004). *Brigance Diagnostic Inventory of Early Development II.* North Billerica, MA: Curriculum Associates.

Bristol, M. M. (1979). *Maternal coping with autistic children: Adequacy of interpersonal support and effect of child's characteristics.* Unpublished doctoral dissertation, University of North Carolina.

Brooks-Gunn, J., & Lewis, M. (1983). Screening and diagnosing handicapped infants. *Topics in Early Childhood Special Education, 3,* 14–28.

Brown, D., Simmons, V., & Methvin, J. (1986). *Oregon Project curriculum for visually impaired and blind preschool children.* Eugene, OR: Jackson County Education Service District.

Brown, L., Sherbenou, R. J., & Johnson, S. K. (1997). *Test of nonverbal Intelligence* (3rd ed.). Austin, TX: PRO-ED.

Bruininks, R. H., & Bruininks, B. D. (2005). *Bruininks–Oseretsky Test of Motor Proficiency—Second Edition.* Circle Pines, MN: American Guidance Service.

Bruininks, R. H., Woodcock, R., Weatherman, R., & Hill, B. (1996). *Scales of Independent Behavior—Revised.* Itasca, IL: Riverside.

Bzoch, K., League, R., & Brown, V. (2003). *The Receptive–Expressive Emerging Language Scale. Third Edition (REEL-3).* Austin, TX: PRO-ED.

Carrow-Woolfolk, E. (1999). *Test of Auditory Comprehension of Language—Third Edition.* Austin, TX: PRO-ED.

Chaudry, N. M., & Davidson, P. W. (2001). Assessment of children with visual impairment or blindness. In R. J. Simeonsson & S. L. Rosenthal (Eds.), *Psychological and developmental assessment: Children with disabilities and chronic conditions* (pp. 225–247). New York: Guilford Press.

Chiurazzi, P., & Oostra, B. A. (2000). Genetics of mental retardation. *Current Opinion in Pediatrics, 12,* 529–535.

Cohen, M. (1997). *Children's Memory Scale.* San Antonio, TX: Harcourt Assessment.

Colarusso, R. P., & Hammill, D. D. (2002) *The Motor-Free Visual Perception Test, 3rd edition.* Austin, TX: PRO-ED.

Conners, C. K. (1997). *Conners Rating Scales—Revised.* Minneapolis, MN: Pearson Assessments.

Connolly, A. J. (1998). *Manual for the KeyMath Revised/NU: A diagnostic inventory of essential mathematics.* Circle Pines, MN: American Guidance Service.

Cooper, L. J., Wacker, D. P., Sasso, G. M., Reimers, T. M., & Donn, L. K. (1990). Using parents as therapists to evaluate appropriate behavior of their children: Application to a tertiary diagnostic clinic. *Journal of Applied Behavior Analysis, 23,* 285–296.

Council for Exceptional Children. (2005). *IDEA law and resources.* Retrieved from *www.cec.sped.org*

Crnic, K. A. (1988). Mental retardation. In E. J. Mash & G. Terdal (Eds.), *Behavioral assessment of childhood disorders* (2nd ed., pp. 317–354). New York: Guilford Press.

Crnic, K. A., Friedrich, W., & Greenberg, M. (1983). Adaptation of families with mentally retarded children: A model of stress, coping, and family ecology. *American Journal of Mental Deficiency, 88,* 125–138.

Dekker, M. C., & Koot, H. M. (2003a). DSM-IV disorders in children with borderline to moderate intellectual disability: I. Prevalence and impact. *Journal of the American Academy of Child and Adolescent Psychiatry, 42,* 915–922.

Dekker, M. C., & Koot, H. M. (2003b). DSM-IV disorders in children with borderline to moderate intellectual disability: II. Child and family predictors. *Journal of the American Academy of Child and Adolescent Psychiatry, 42,* 923–931.

de la Osa, N., Ezpeleta, L., Domenech, J. M., Navarro, J. B., & Losilla, J. M. (1997). Convergent and discriminate validity of the Structured Diagnostic Interview for Children and Adolescents (DICA-R). *Psychology in Spain, 1,* 37–44.

Donenberg, G., & Baker, B. L. (1993). The impact of young children with externalizing behaviours on their families. *Journal of Abnormal Child Psychology, 21,* 179–198.

Donovan, A. (1988). Family stress and ways of coping with adolescents who have handicaps: Maternal perceptions. *American Journal on Mental Retardation, 92,* 502–509.

DuBose, R. (1981). Assessment of severely impaired young children: Problems and recommendations. *Topics in Early Childhood Special Education, 1*(2), 9–22.

Dugdale, R. L. (1910). *The Jukes: A study in crime, pauperism, disease and heredity.* New York: Putnam.

Dunn, L. M., & Dunn, L. M. (2006). *Peabody Picture Vocabulary Test—4.* Circle Pines, MN: American Guidance Service.

Dykes, M. K., & Erin, J. (1999). *The Developmental Assessment for Students with Severe Disabilities II (DASH-2).* Austin, TX: PRO-ED.

Dyson, L. L. (1989). Adjustment of siblings of handicapped children: A comparison. *Journal of Pediatric Psychology, 14,* 215–229.

Dyson, L. L., Edgar, E., & Crnic, K. (1989). Psychological predictors of adjustment by siblings of developmentally disabled children. *American Journal on Mental Retardation, 94,* 292–302.

Edelbrock, C. S., Costello, A. J., Dulcan, M. K., Kalas, R., & Conover, N. C. (1985). Age differences in the reliability of the psychiatric interview of the child. *Child Development, 56,* 265–275.

Education of the Handicapped Act Amendment, Pub. L. No. 99-457, 20, U.S.C. §1471 (1986).

Education for All Handicapped Children Act, Pub. L. No. 94-142, 20 U.S.C. §1401 (1975).

Einfeld, S. L., & Aman, M. G. (1995). Issues in the taxonomy of psychopathology in children and adolescents with mental retardation. *Journal of Autism and Developmental Disorders, 25,* 143–167.

Einfeld, S. L., & Tonge, B. J. (2002). *Manual for the Developmental Behaviour Checklist* (2nd ed.). Clayton, Melbourne, and Sydney: Monash University Center for Developmental Psychiatry and School of Psychiatry, University of New South Wales.

Eisenhower, A. S., Baker, B. L., & Blacher, J. (2005). Preschool children with intellectual disability: Syndrome specificity, behaviour problems, and maternal well-being. *Journal of Intellectual Disability Research, 49,* 657–671.

Elliot, C. D. (2007). *DAS-II* (2nd ed.). San Antonio, TX: Psychological Corporation.

Emerson, E. (2003). Prevalence of psychiatric disorders in children and adolescents with and without intellectual disability. *Journal of Intellectual Disability Research, 47,* 51–58.

Ernst, M., Cookus, B., & Moravec, B. C. (2000). Pictorial Instrument for Children and Adolescents. *Journal of the American Academy of Child and Adolescent Psychiatry, 39,* 94–99.

Feldman, A. B., Haley, S. M., & Coryell, J. (1990). Concurrent and construct validity of the Pediatric Evaluation of Disability Inventory. *Physical Therapy, 70,* 602–610.

Flynt, S. W., & Wood, T. A. (1989). Stress and coping of mothers of children with moderate mental retardation. *American Journal on Mental Retardation, 94,* 278–283.

Fotheringhan, J. B. (1983). Mental retardation and developmental delay. In K. D. Paget & B. A. Bracken (Eds.), *The psychoeducational assessment of preschool children* (pp. 207–223). New York: Grune & Stratton.

Friedrich, W., Greenberg, M., & Crnic, K. (1983). A short-form of the Questionnaire on Resources and Stress. *American Journal on Mental Deficiency, 88,* 41–48.

French, J. L. (2001). *Manual: Pictorial Test of Intelligence II.* Austin, TX: PRO-ED.

Fujiura, G. T. (2003). Continuum of intellectual disabilities: Demographic evidence for the "forgotten" generation. *Mental Retardation, 41,* 420–429.

Furlong, J. M., & LeDrew, L. (1985). IQ = 68 = mildly retarded?: Factors influencing multidisciplinary team recommendations on children with FS IQs between 63 and 75. *Psychology in the Schools, 22,* 5–9.

Goddard, H. H. (1913). *The Kallikak family: A study in heredity of feeble-mindedness.* New York: Macmillan.

Grossman, J. J. (Ed.). (1983). *Classification in mental retardation.* Washington, DC: American Association on Mental Deficiency.

Hagerman, R. J., & Sobesky, W. E. (1989). Psychopathology in fragile X syndrome. *American Journal of Orthopsychiatry, 59,* 142–152.

Hammill, D. D., Pearson, N. A., Voress, J. K., & Reynolds, C. R. (2005). *The Full Range Test of Visual–Motor Integration.* Austin, TX: PRO-ED.

Hammill, D. D., Pearson, N. A., & Wiederholt, J. L. (1997). *The Comprehensive Test of Nonverbal Intelligence.* Austin, TX: PRO-ED.

Handen, B. L., Breaux, A. M., Janosky, J., McAuliffe, S., Feldman, & Gosling, A. (1992). Effects and non-effects of methylphenidate in children with mental retardation and ADHD. *Journal of the American Academy of Child and Adolescent Psychiatry, 31,* 455–461.

Handen, B. L., Feldman, R. S., & Honigman, A. (1987). Comparison of parent and teacher assessments of developmentally delayed children's behavior. *Exceptional Children, 54,* 137–144.

Handen, B. L., Feldman, H., Lurier, M., & Husar, P. J. (1999). Efficacy of methylphenidate among preschoolers with developmental disabilities and ADHD. *Journal of the American Academy of Child and Adolescent Psychiatry, 38,* 805–812.

Handen, B. L., & Hardan, A. Y. (2006). Open label, prospective trial of olanzapine in adolescents with subaverage untelligence and disruptive behavioral disorders. *Journal of the American Academy of Child and Adolescent Psychiatry, 45,* 928–935.

Handen, B. L., Janosky, J., & McAuliffe, S. (1997). Long-term follow-up of children with mental retardation and ADHD. *Journal of Abnormal Child Psychology, 25,* 287–295.

Hannah, M. E., & Midlarsky, E. (1999). Competence and adjustment of siblings of children with mental retardation. *American Journal of Mental Retardation, 104,* 22–37.

Harris, J. C. (2006). *Intellectual disability: Understanding its development, causes, classification, evaluation, and treatment.* Oxford, UK: Oxford University Press.

Harrison, P. L., & Oakland, T. (2000). ABAS: Adaptive Behavior Assessment System. San Antonio: TX: Psychological Corporation.

Hassall, R., Rose, J., & McDonald J. (2005). Parenting stress in mothers of children with an intellectual disability: The effects of parental cognitions in relation to child characteristics and family support. *Journal of Intellectual Disability Research, 49,* 405–418.

Havercamp, S. M. (1986). Psychiatric symptoms and mental retardation: Reliability of rating scales as a function of IQ. Unpublished Master's thesis, Ohio State University, Columbus.

Hawkins, G. D., & Cooper, D. H. (1990). Adaptive behavior measures in mental retardation research: Subject description in AJMD/AJMR articles (1979–1987). *American Journal on Mental Retardation, 94,* 654–660.

Heber, R. (1959). A manual on terminology and classification in mental retardation. *American Journal of Mental Deficiency (Monograph Suppl.), 64*(2).

Heward, W. L. (2006). *Exceptional children: An introduction to special education* (8th ed.). Upper Saddle River, NJ: Pearson/Prentice-Hall.

Holroyd, J. (1974). The Questionnaire on Resources and Stress: An instrument to measure family response to a handicapped family member. *Journal of Community Psychology, 2,* 92–94.

Honig v. Doe, 108 S. Ct. 592 (1988).

Hresko, W., Miguel, S., Sherbenou, R., & Burton, S. (1994). *Developmental Observation Checklist System* (DOCS). Austin, TX: PRO-ED.

Huttenlocher, P. R. (1991). Dendritic and synaptic pathology in mental retardation. *Pediatric Neurology, 7,* 79–85.

Individuals with Disabilities Education Act, Pub. L. No. 101-476, 20, U.S.C. §1400. (1990).

Individuals with Disabilities Education Act, Pub. L. No. 105-17, 20, U.S.C. §1400. (1997).

Individuals with Disabilities Education Improvement Act, Pub. L. No. 108–446 (2004).

Iwata, B., Dorsey, M., Slifer, K., Bauman, K., & Richman, G. (1994). Toward a functional analysis of self-injury. *Journal of Applied Behavior Analysis, 27,* 197–210.

Jaselskis, C. A., Cook, E. H., Jr., Fletcher, K. E., & Leventhal, B. L. (1992). Clonidine treatment of hyperactive and impulsive children with autistic disorder. *Journal of Clinical Psychopharmacology, 12,* 322–327.

Johnson, C. R. (2002). Mental retardation. In M. Hersen (Ed.), *Clinical behavior therapy: Adults and children* (pp. 420–433). New York: Wiley.

Johnson-Martin, N., Attermeier, S., & Hacker, B. (2004). *The Carolina Curriculum for Preschoolers with Special Needs* (2nd ed.). Baltimore: Brookes.

Johnson-Martin, N., Jens, K., Attermeier, S., & Hacker, B. (2004). *The Carolina Curriculum for Infant and Toddlers with Special Needs* (3rd ed.). Baltimore: Brookes.

Kamphaus, R. W. (2001). *Clinical assessment of child and adolescent intelligence* (2nd ed.). Boston: Allyn & Bacon.

Kamphaus, R. W., & Frick, P. J. (2002). *Clinical assessment of child and adolescent personality and behavior* (2nd ed.). Boston: Allyn & Bacon.

Kaplan, E., Fein, D., Kramer, J., Delis, D., & Morris, R. (2001). *Wechsler Individual Achievement Test–II—Abbreviated*. San Antonio, TX: Harcourt Assessment.

Kaufman, A. S., & Kaufman, N. L. (2004a). *The Kaufman Assessment Battery for Children II (K-ABC-II)*. Circle Pines, MN: American Guidance Service.

Kaufman, A. S., & Kaufman, N. L. (2004b). *Kaufman Test of Educational Achievement II—Brief Form*. Circle Pines, MN: American Guidance Service.

Kaufman, A. S., & Kaufman, N. L. (2004c). *Kaufman Test of Educational Achievement II—Comprehensive form*. Circle Pines, MN: American Guidance Service.

Kaufman, J., Birmaher, B., Brent, D. A., Rao, U., & Ryan, N. (1996). *Revised Schedule for Affective Disorders and Schizophrenia for School Aged Children: Present and Lifetime version* (K-SADS-PL). Pittsburgh, PA: Western Psychiatric Institute and Clinic.

Kern, L., Mauk, J., Marder, T., & Mace, F. C. (1995). Functional analysis and intervention for breath holding. *Journal of Applied Behavior Analysis, 28,* 339–340.

Korman, M., Kirk, U., & Kemp, S. (1990). *NEPSY: A Developmental Neuropsychological Assessment*. San Antonio, TX: Psychological Corporation.

Lambert, N., Nihira, K., & Leland, H. (1993). *Manual for the Adaptive Behavior Scale—School* (2nd ed.). Austin, TX: PRO-ED.

Larry P. v. Riles, 343 F. Supp. 1306 (9th Cir. 1979).

Larson, S. A., Lakin, K. C., Anderson, L., Kwak, N., Hak Lee, J., & Anderson, D. (2001). Prevalence of mental retardation and developmental disabilities: Estimates from the 1994/1995 National Health Interview Survey Disability Supplements. *American Journal of Mental Retardation, 105,* 231–252.

Lecavalier, L., & Aman, M. (2004).Rating instruments. In J. L. Matson, R. B. Laud, & M. L. Matson (Eds.), *Behavior modification for persons with developmental disabilities: Treatments and support* (Vol. 1. 160–189). Kingston, NY: National Association for the Dually Diagnosed.

Linna, S. L., Moilanen, I., Ebeling, H., Piha, J., Kumpulainen, K., Tamminen, T., et al. (1999). Psychiatric symptoms in children with intellectual disability. *European Child and Adolescent Psychiatry, 8*(Suppl. 4), 77–82.

Lobato, D., Barbour, L., Hall, L. J., & Miller, C. T. (1987). Psychosocial characteristics of preschool siblings of handicapped and nonhandicapped children. *Journal of Abnormal Child Psychology, 15,* 329–338.

Lubbs, H. A. (1969). A marker-X chromosome. *American Journal of Human Genetics, 21,* 231–244.

MacLean, W. E., Jr. (1993). Overview. In J. L. Matson & R. P. Barrett (Eds.), *Psychopathology in the mentally retarded* (2nd ed., pp. 1–14). Needham Heights, MA: Allyn & Bacon.

MacMillan, D. L., Gresham, F. M., & Siperstein, G. N. (1995). Heightened concerns over the 1992 AAMR definition: Advocacy versus precision. *American Journal of Mental Retardation, 100,* 87–97.

MacMillan, D. L., Siperstein, G. N., & Gresham, F. M. (1996). A challenge to the viability of mild mental retardation as a diagnostic category. *Exceptional Children, 62,* 356–371.

Margalit, M., Shulman, S., & Stuchiner, N. (1989). Behavior disorders and mental retardation: The family system perspective. *Research in Developmental Disabilities, 10,* 315–326.

Markwardt, F. C., Jr. (1998). *Manual for the Peabody Individual Achievement Test—Revised/Normative Update.* Circle Pines, MN: American Guidance Service.

Marshburn, E., & Aman, M. (1992). Factor validity and norms for the Aberrant Behavior Checklist in a community sample of children with mental retardation. *Journal of Autism and Developmental Disorders, 22,* 357–373.

Masland, R. H. (1988, May). *Career research award address.* Paper presented at the annual meeting of the American Association on Mental Retardation, Washington, DC.

Matson, J., Kazdin, A., & Senatore, V. (1984). Psychometric properties of the Psychopathology Instrument for Mentally Retarded Adults. *Applied Research in Mental Retardation, 5,* 81–89.

McCallum, R. S. (2003). Context for nonverbal assessment of intelligence and related abilities. In R. S. McCallum (Ed.), *Handbook of nonverbal assessment* (pp. 3–21). New York: Kluwer Academic/Plenum Press.

McCarney, S., & Arthaud, T. (2006). *Adaptive Behavior Evaluation Scale—Revised* (2nd ed.). Columbia, MS: Hawthorne Education.

McCubbin, H. I., Paterson, J., & Glynn, T. (1982). Social support index (SSI). In H. I. McCubbin, A. I. Thompson, & M. A. McCubbin (Eds.), *Family assessment: Resiliency, coping and adaptation-inventories for research and practice* (pp. 357–389). Madison: University of Wisconsin.

McLaren, J., & Bryson, S. E. (1987). Review of recent epidemiological studies of mental retardation: Prevalence, associated disorders, and etiology. *American Journal of Mental Retardation, 92,* 243–254.

Meisels, S. J., Atkins-Burnett, S., Xue, Y., Nicholson, J., Bickel, D., & Son, S. (2002). Creating a system of accountability: The impact of instructional assessment on elementary children's achievement test scores. *American Educational Research Journal, 39,* 3–25.

Mendola, P., Selevan, S. G., Gutter, S., & Rice, D. (2002). Environmental factors associated with a spectrum of neurodevelopmental deficits. *Mental Retardation and Developmental Disabilities Research Reviews, 8,* 188–197.

Miller, J. F. (1992). Development of speech and language in children with Down syndrome. In I. T. Lott & E. E. McCoy (Eds.), *Down syndrome: Advances in medical care* (pp. 39–50). New York: Wiley.

Mills v. Board of Education, 348 F. Supp. 866 (1972).

Moos, R., & Moos, B. (1994). *Family Environment Scale.* Palo Alto, CA: Consulting Psychologists Press.

Morgenstern, M., & Klass, E. (1991). Standard intelligence tests and related assessment techniques. In J. L.

Matson & J. A. Mulick (Eds.), *Handbook of mental retardation* (2nd ed., pp. 195–210). Elmsford, NY: Pergamon Press.

Mullen, E. M. (1989). *Infant Mullen Scales of Early Learning.* Bloomington, MN: Pearson Assessments.

Nachshen, J. S., & Minnes, P. (2005). Empowerment in parents of school-aged children with and without developmental disabilities. *Journal of Intellectual Disability Research, 49,* 889–904.

Neisworth, J. T., & Bagnato, S. J. (1987). Developmental retardation. In V. Van Hasselt & M. Hersen (Eds.), *Psychological evaluation of the developmentally and physically disabled* (pp. 179–211). New York: Plenum Press.

Neisworth, J. T., & Bagnato, S. J. (2004). The mismeasure of young children: The authentic assessment alternative. *Infants and Young Children, 17,* 198–212.

Newborg, J. (2004). *Battelle Developmental Inventory II.* Scarborough, Ontario: Thomas Nelson Company.

Newland, T. E. (1971). *Blind Learning Aptitude Test.* Champaign: University of Illinois Press.

Niemeyer, J., & McEvoy, M. (1989). *Social interaction code.* Nashville, TN: Vanderbilt University.

Nyhan, W. L. (1976). Behavior in the Lesch–Nyhan syndrome. *Journal of Autism and Childhood Schizophrenia, 6,* 235–252.

Parks, S. (1992). *Hawaii Early Learning Profile (HELP).* Palo Alto, CA: VORT.

Pearson, D., & Aman, M. G. (1994). Ratings of hyperactivity and developmental indices: Should clinicians correct for developmental level? *Journal of Autism and Developmental Disorders, 24,* 395–404.

Pennsylvania Association of Retarded Children (PARC) v. Commonwealth of Pennsylvania, 334 F. Supp. 1257 (E.D. Pa. 1971).

Piazza, C. C., Fisher, W. W., Brown, K. A., Shore, B. A., Patel, M. R., Katz, R. M., et al. (2003). Functional analysis of inappropriate mealtime behaviors. *Journal of Applied Behavior Analysis, 36,* 187–204.

Pierce, K., & Schreibman, L. (1997). Multiple peer use of pivotal response training to increase social behaviors of classmates with autism: Results form training and untrained peers. *Journal of Applied Behavior Analysis, 30,* 157–160.

Polloway, E. (1997). Developmental principles of the Luckasson et al. (1992) AAMR definition of mental retardation. *Education and Training in Mental Retardation and Developmental Disabilities, 32,* 174–178.

Pueschel, S. M., & Thuline, H. C. (1991). Chromosome disorders. In J. L. Matson & J. A. Mulick (Eds.), *Handbook of mental retardation* (2nd ed., pp. 115–138). Elmsford, NY: Pergamon Press.

Quay, H. C., & Hogan, A. E. (1999). *Handbook of disruptive behavior disorders.* Dordrecht, The Netherlands: Kluwer Academic.

Rabkin, J. G., & Streuning, E. L. (1976). Life events, stress and illness. *Science, 194,* 1013–1020.

Ramirez, S. A., & Kratochwill, T. R. (1990). Development of the Fear Survey for Children with and without Mental Retardation. *Behavioral Assessment, 12,* 457–470.

Reich, W. (2000). Diagnostic Interview for Children and Adolescents—(DICA). *Journal of the American Academy of Child and Adolescent Psychiatry, 39,* 59–66.

Reiss, S. (1994). *Test manual for the Reiss Screen for Maladaptive Behavior* (2nd ed.). Worthington, OH: IDS.

Reiss, S., & Valenti-Hein, D. (1990). *Reiss Scales for Children's Dual Diagnosis: Test manual* (2nd ed.). Worthington, OH: International Diagnostic Services.

Reschly, D. J., & Ward, S. M. (1991). Use of adaptive behavior and overrepresentation of black students in programs for students with mild mental retardation. *American Journal of Mental Retardation, 96,* 257–268.

Reynolds, C., & Bigler, E. (1994). *TOMAL: Test of Memory and Learning.* Austin, TX: PRO-ED.

Robertson, G. J. (2002). *The Wide Range Achievement Test Expanded edition.* San Antonio, TX: Harcourt Assessment.

Roid, G. H. (2003). *Stanford–Binet Intelligence Scales, Fifth Edition.* Itasca, IL: Riverside Publishing

Roid, G. H., & Miller, L. J. (1997). *Leiter International Performance Scale—Revised.* Wood Dale, IL: Stoelting.

Roid, G. H., & Miller, L. J. (1999). *Leiter/Stoelting brief nonverbal intelligence scale manual (S-BIT).* Wood Dale, IL: Stoelting.

Rutter, M., Tizard, J., Yule, W., Graham, P., & Whitmore, K. (1976). Research report: Isle of Wright Studies 1964–1974. *Psychological Medicine, 6,* 313–332.

Ryan, M. R., & Dietiker, K. E. (1979). Reliability and clinical validity of the Children's Fear Survey Schedule. *Journal of Behavior Therapy and Experimental Psychiatry, 9,* 303–309.

Salisbury, C. (1987). Stressors of parents with young handicapped and nonhandicapped children. *Journal of the Division for Early Childhood, 11,* 154–160.

Sattler, J. M. (1988). *Assessment of children* (3rd ed.). San Diego, CA: Author.

Sattler, J. M. (2001). *Assessment of children: Cognitive applications* (4th ed.). San Diego, CA: Author.

Sattler, J. M. (2002). *Assessment of children: Behavioral and clinical applications* (4th ed.). San Diego, CA: Author.

Sattler, J. M., & Dumont, R. (2004). *Assessment of children: WISC-IV and WPPSI-III supplement.* San Diego, CA: Jerome M. Sattler.

Semel, E., Wiig, E., & Secord, W. (2003). *Manual for the Clinical Evaluation of Language Fundamentals (4th ed.)(CELF-4).* San Antonio, TX: Psychological Corporation.

Shaffer, D., Fisher, P., Lucas, C. P., Dulcan, M. K., & Schwab-Stone, M. E. (2000). NIMH Diagnostic Interview Schedule for Children Version IV (NIMH DISC-IV): Description, differences from previous versions, and reliability of some common diagnoses. *Journal of the American Academy of Child and Adolescent Psychiatry, 39,* 28–38.

Shapiro, B. K. (2002). Normal and abnormal development: Mental retardation. In M. L. Batshaw (Ed.), *Children with disabilities* (5th ed., pp. 287–305). Baltimore: Brookes.

Shea, V. (1984). Explaining mental retardation and autism to parents. In E. Schopler & G. B. Mesibov (Eds.), *The effects of autism on the family* (pp. 265–288). New York: Plenum Press.

Sheslow, D., & Adams, W. (2003). *Wide range assessment of memory and learning* (2nd ed.). Los Angeles: Western Psychological Services.

Smolla, N., Valla, J. P., Bergeron, L., Berthiaume, C., & St. Georges, M. (2004). Development and reliability of a pictorial mental disorders screen for young adolescents. *Canadian Journal of Psychiatry, 49,* 828–837.

Sparrow, S. S., Cicchetti, D. V., & Balla, D. A. (2005). *Vineland Adaptive Behavior Scales II.* Circle Pines, MN: American Guidance Service.

Special Education Services and Programs under General Provisions §342.1, 20 Pa. Bull. (1990).

Spragg, P. A. (1988). *Structured Clinical Interview.* Unpublished instrument, University of Colorado Health Sciences Center, Denver.

Stillman, R. D. (1978). *The Callier-Azusa Scale.* Unpublished instrument, University of Texas at Dallas.

Stillman, R. D., & Battle, C. (19850. *The Callier-Azusa Scale (H).* Unpublished instrument, University of Texas at Dallas.

Stromme, P., & Diseth, T. H. (2000). Prevalence of psychiatric diagnoses in children with mental retardation: Data from a population-based study. *Developmental Medicine and Child Neurology, 42,* 266–270.

Sulzer-Azaroff, B., & Mayer, G. R. (1991). *Behavior analysis for lasting change.* Fort Worth, TX: Harcourt Brace College.

Sundberg, M. L., & Partington, J. W. (1998). *The Assessment of Basic Language and Learning Skills (ABLLS).* Pleasant Hills, CA: Behavior Analysts.

Tasse, M. J., Aman, M. G., Hammer, D., & Rojahn, J. (1996). The Nisonger Child Behavior Rating Form: Age and gender effects and norms. *Research in Developmental Disabilities, 17,* 59–75.

U.S. Office of Special Education Programs. (2004). *Individuals with Disabilities Education Act (IDEA Data).* Washington, DC: Author. Available online at *www.ideadata.org*

Valla, J. P., Bergeron, L., & Smolla, N. (2000). The Dominic-R: A pictorial interview for 6- to 11-year-old children. *Journal of the American Academy of Child and Adolescent Psychiatry, 39,* 85–93.

Van Berckelaer-Onnes, I., & van Duijn, G. (1993). A comparison between the Handicaps, Behaviour and Skills Schedule and the Psychoeducational Profile. *Journal of Autism and Developmental Disorder, 23,* 263–272.

Van Hasselt, V. B., & Sisson, L. A. (1987). Visual impairment. In C. Frame & J. Matson (Eds.), *Handbook of assessment in child psychopathology: Applied issues in diagnosis and treatment evaluation* (pp. 593–618). New York: Plenum Press.

Wacker, D. P., Berg, W. K., Cooper, L. J., Derby, K., Steege, M., Northrup, J., et al. (1994). The impact of functional analysis methodology on outpatient clinic services. *Journal of Applied Behavior Analysis, 27,* 405–407.

Wechsler, D. (2001). *Manual for the Wechsler Individual Achievement Test–II.* San Antonio, TX: Psychological Corporation.

Wechsler, D. (2002). *WPPSI-III: Administration and scoring manual.* San Antonio, TX: Psychological Corporation..

Wechsler, D. (2003). *Wechsler Intelligence Scale for Children—Fourth Edition*: Administration and scoring manual. San Antonio, TX: Psychological Corporation.

Weller, E. B., Weller, R. A., Fristad, M. A., Rooney, M. T., & Schecter, J. (2000). Children's interview for psychiatric symptoms (ChIPS). *Journal of the American Academy of Child and Adolescent Psychiatry, 39,* 76–84.

West Virginia Department of Education. (1985). *Regulations for the education of exceptional students* (Office of Special Education, Policy No. 2419). Charleston, WV: Author.

Wetherby, A. M., & Prizant, B. M. (2002). *Communication and Symbolic Behavior Scales—Developmental Profile (CSBS-DP).* Baltimore: Brookes.

White, O. R., & Haring, N. G. (1978). Evaluating educational programs serving the severely and profoundly handicapped. In N. G. Haring & D. D. Bricker (Eds.), *Teaching the severely handicapped* (Vol. 3, pp. 153–200). Seattle, WA: American Association for the Education of the Severely/Profoundly Handicapped.

Wiederholt, J. L., & Bryant, B. R. (2001). *Grey Oral Reading Test—Fourth Edition.* Austin, TX: PRO-ED.

Wiig, E., Secord, W., & Semel, E. (2004). *Manual for the Clinical Evaluation of Language Fundamentals—Preschool* (2nd ed.). San Antonio, TX: Psychological Corporation.

Wilkinson, G. S., & Robertson, G. J. (2006). *Manual for the Wide Range Achievement Test—4.* Lutz, FL: Psychological Assessment Resources.

Wing, L. (1982). *Schedule of Handicaps, Behaviour and Skills.* Unpublished manuscript, MRC Social Psychiatry Unit, Institute of Psychiatry, London.

Wing, L., & Gould, J. (1978). Systematic recording of behaviors and skills of retarded and psychotic children. *Journal of Autism and Childhood Schizophrenia, 8,* 79–97.

Wolfensberger, W. (1969). The origin and nature of our institutional models. In R. B. Kugel & W. Wolfensberger (Eds.), *Changing patterns in residential services for the mentally retarded* (pp. 59–171). Washington, DC: U.S. Government Printing Office.

Woodcock, R. W. (1998). *Woodcock Reading Mastery Tests—Revised/Normative Update.* Circle Pines, MN: American Guidance Service.

Woodcock, R. W., McGrew, K. S., & Mather, N. (2001). *The Woodcock-Johnson III.* Itasca, IL: Riverside.

Zigler, E., & Hodapp, R. (1986). *Understanding mental retardation.* Cambridge, UK: Cambridge University Press.

Zimmerman, I., Steiner, V., & Pond, R. (2002). *Preschool Language Scale 4.* San Antonio, TX: Harcourt Assessment.

CHAPTER 13

Learning Disabilities

Deborah L. Speece
Sara J. Hines

It is an interesting and challenging time to consider the assessment of learning disabilities. The U.S. Congress recently passed legislation that modified regulations pertaining to identification of learning disabilities as part of the reauthorization of the Individuals with Disabilities Education Act (IDEA, 2004). Academics debate the merits of the changes and what they may portend for the field, while practitioners await state guidelines and, in some cases, apply new methods of identification. We assume that children and youth who struggle with learning the school curriculum continue to be identified and provided with services to assist their achievement despite the current ambiguity on identification procedures.

Our goal in this chapter is to identify, describe, and evaluate trends in the assessment of learning disabilities (LDs). The federal definition follows:

Sec. 602(30)(A)
SPECIFIC LEARNING DISABILITY.—

(A) IN GENERAL.—The term "specific learning disability" means a disorder in 1 or more of the basic psychological processes involved in understanding or in using language, spoken or written, which disorder may manifest itself in imperfect ability to listen, think, speak, read, write, spell, or do mathematical calculations.

(B) DISORDERS INCLUDED.—Such term includes such conditions as perceptual disabilities,

brain injury, minimal brain dysfunction, dyslexia, and developmental aphasia.

(C) DISORDERS NOT INCLUDED.—Such term does not include a learning problem that is primarily the result of visual, hearing, or motor disabilities, of mental retardation, of emotional disturbance, or of environmental, cultural, or economic disadvantage. (IDEA Amendments of 2004, Sec. 602(30), p. 118)

This statutory definition has survived 30 years of scrutiny. Although modifications have been proposed, with some changes generally accepted by the field (Hammill, 1990), the central concepts of psychological processing problems coupled with academic difficulties remain intact. The recently passed regulations change the guidelines for implementing the statutory definition. It is here that the debate begins. There are two primary issues. The first is the possibility of not requiring an aptitude–achievement discrepancy. We view the discrepancy criterion as a proxy for psychological processing problems. The second is allowing a process called response to intervention (RTI) to be used as one means of documenting LDs. We provide more detail later on the changes, but it is this dynamic that sets the stage for most of our discussion. Although the regulations explicitly allow the possibility of using either a discrepancy formula or RTI, comments in the regulations by the U.S. Department of Education suggest that RTI approaches are favored. In some sense, the train has left the station with RTI in the driver's seat. However, given the wiggle room in the current regulations and the need for any assessment to be valid regardless of backing by the federal government, we evaluate the merits (i.e., validity) of current identification standards. First we provide an historical perspective on LD assessment. A discussion of current issues that include overviews of exclusion factors, prevalence, and comorbidity follows this section. The primary emphasis in this section is the review of validity evidence for two major approaches to diagnosis: psychological/cognitive processing discrepancies and RTI. We end with recommendations and suggestions for future directions.

HISTORY OF LD ASSESSMENT

Historically the purpose of assessment of LD was not only to identify students with LDs but also to link assessment results to remediation. It seems that, over time, Federal involvement in the field resulted in an abandonment of the identification–assessment–remediation link. Therefore, we divide our analysis of historical issues into pre-Federal and Federal periods.

Hallahan and Mercer (2002) provide a detailed account of the history of LDs. Information for the current review relies heavily on that account, as well as those of Wiederholt (1974), Hammill (1993), Torgesen (1998, 2004), Shepherd, (2001), Hallahan and Mock (2003), and Lyon, Fletcher, and Barnes (2003).

Pre-Federal Involvement

Although the term "learning disabilities" was not coined until the 1960s, there is a long history of clinicians and researchers studying children and adults with related conditions. We highlight their major contributions to the identification and assessment of persons with LDs.

European Researchers

The contributions of Gall (ca. 1800) in Germany were integral to the development of the field of LDs (Hallahan & Mock, 2003; Hammill, 1993; Lyon et al., 2003). The systematic investigation of LDs began around 1800, with Gall's examination of adults who suffered head injuries resulting in loss of the ability to speak (aphasia) but not the ability to write. Gall introduced the concept of relative strengths and weaknesses within an individual. He also focused on the related concept of specific rather than general cognitive deficits as the result of brain damage. Furthermore, for Gall it was critical that the patient's problems were not caused by other conditions, such as mental retardation or deafness, an exclusionary clause that continues in present definitions (Hammill, 1993).

Gall's discussions of the localization of brain functions stimulated and influenced the investigation of other European researchers concerned with spoken language disorders (Wiederholt, 1974). Specifically, the work of Bouillaud, Broca, Jackson, Wernicke, and Head established the occurrence of very specific types of mental impairment as a result of damage to isolated regions of the brain (Torgesen, 2004).

Hinshelwood, a French researcher, investigated not only individuals with head injuries, resulting in reading and language problems, but also children with what he referred to as "congenital word blindness" (Hallahan & Mercer, 2002). Kussmaul (1877) had previously used the term "word-blindness" to describe an adult patient with no apparent disability other than difficulty with reading (cited in Hallahan & Mercer, 2002). Hinshelwood was among the first to assert that congenital, rather than acquired brain defects, might cause children to have developmental reading problems and to speculate about effective remedial reading methods for such children. This concept of a specific reading problem that was not the result of a known head injury was significant to the conceptualization and assessment of LDs, as was Hinshelwood's linking of that condition to remediation. According to Wiederholt (1974), "Hinshelwood's landmark publications offered the first major detailed attempt to present the etiology of disorders of written language and to describe educational intervention techniques" (p. 117).

U.S. Researchers

READING-RELATED DISORDERS

European researchers in the 1800s who investigated the effects of brain injury or congenital factors on speech and language functions had a significant impact on research in the United

States. Several prominent physicians, psychologists, and educators used the findings of Gall, Hinshelwood, and other Europeans as a springboard for further research (Hallahan & Mercer, 2002). Specifically, Samuel Orton, Grace Fernald, Marion Monroe, and Samuel Kirk impacted the development of the LD field in the United States through their investigations of language and reading disabilities (Hallahan & Mercer, 2002).

Samuel Orton, in the 1920s and 1930s, relied heavily on Hinshelwood's prior work with individuals with "congenital word blindness." Orton's views differed from Hinshelwood's, in that Orton viewed the condition as more prevalent (over 10% of school population) than did Hinshelwood (less than 1 in 1000 students). Current estimates are more in line with Orton's view. Orton renamed the condition "strephosymbolia," which means mixed symbols, and hypothesized that inherited mixed cerebral dominance was the cause of many cases of the condition. He theorized that the nondominant hemisphere of the brain stored mirror images of those stored in the dominant hemisphere. In individuals with complete hemispheric dominance, the mirrored images were suppressed. However, in children with mixed dominance, the mirrored images emerged, causing reversals of letters and words, or strephosymbolia. Although Orton's ideas of mixed dominance are no longer popular in the field of LDs, Lyon and colleagues (2003) credit Orton with being the first to stress that reading disabilities were related to cerebral dysfunction and that they did not occur strictly in persons with low intelligence.

Orton was one of the first researchers to suggest direct instruction in phonics for students with reading disabilities, including instruction in sound blending. Furthermore, he was one of the first to suggest multisensory instruction for students with such disabilities. His ideas regarding phonics instruction were reflected in the work of Anna Gillingham and Bessie Stillman. In fact, the Orton–Gillingham method of phonics instruction is still used in practice. This technique uses a multisensory, direct instruction approach to teach phonics. Samuel Orton was prophetic in his emphasis on direct phonics instruction. Researchers over the last 20 years have linked phonological awareness deficits and poor grapheme–phoneme correspondence as the core issues underlying reading disabilities (e.g., Adams, 1990; Torgesen et al., 1999).

Marion Monroe, who served as Orton's research associate, developed diagnostic tests based on the theories of Orton and Grace Fernald, and used the results to guide instruction. Monroe introduced two practices that are important in current theories of LD assessment (Hallahan & Mercer, 2002). First, she introduced the idea of discrepancy between actual and expected achievement as a means of identifying students with reading disabilities, calculating a reading index by comparison of the child's reading level (based on the average of four achievement tests) to an average of the child's chronological, mental, and arithmetic grades. Second, she advocated analyzing the specific types of reading errors children made on achievement tests to guide instruction, rather than focusing on the test scores. This practice introduced the notion of what would later be referred to as "diagnostic prescriptive instruction." Monroe also developed individual profiles of student errors to aid identification of students and selection of appropriate remedial tactics. The success of her instructional programs supported the optimistic belief that the reading problems of students could be remediated given the appropriate interventions based on diagnostic findings.

Influenced by Monroe's use of profiles, Samuel Kirk created the Illinois Test of Psycholinguistic Abilities (ITPA) as an instrument to provide profiles of intraindividual differences (Hallahan & Mercer, 2002). Results from the diagnosis of psycholinguistic strengths and weaknesses were used to inform remediation. Kirk's ITPA was the first formal attempt to measure cognitive processing and design remedial techniques based on the assessment findings. According to Barbara Bateman (2005), a student of Kirk in the 1960s, Kirk had a leading role in the field of LD as it emerged from its roots in language disorders, reading, and brain injury, because he distilled the three conceptual linchpins of LD: (1) the educability of intelligence; (2) pronounced intraindividual differences in cognitive abilities as the hallmark of children with LD, in contrast to the flat profiles of children with mental retardation; and (3) educational diagnosis of LD to inform recommendations of what and how to teach.

MORE GENERALIZED DISORDERS

The described work of Orton, Fernald, Monroe, and Kirk focused specifically on reading disabilities. It was the investigations of Heinz Werner and Alfred Strauss and colleagues during the period after World War II that led to the emergence of the more generalized category of LD as a formally recognized field (Lyon et al., 2003). Kurt Goldstein's work in Germany with soldiers with head injuries influenced that of Heinz Werner and Alfred Strauss, who both emigrated from Germany to the United States and were simultaneously employed at the Wayne County Training School (Hammill, 1993). Together Werner and Strauss investigated whether children classified as mentally retarded who had suffered brain injury were different from those with congenital mental retardation. They wanted to determine whether the children classified as mentally retarded following brain injury were similar to Goldstein's nonretarded adults with brain injuries. They differentiated between children with brain injuries and retardation and those with congenital retardation, with a description of their correlated disorders, such as perceptual problems, impulsivity, disorganization, distractibility, disinhibition, and perseveration (Hallahan & Mercer, 2002; Hammill, 1993). Strauss and another colleague, Lehtinen, assessing the performance of these children with brain injuries and retardation, reported that they exhibited problems in the areas of figure–ground perception, attention, concept formation, as well as hyperactivity (Lyon et al., 2003). Strauss and colleagues used the term "minimal brain injury" (MBI) for these children. From their studies, the concept of MBI or dysfunction that emerged in the 1960s assumed that the condition could be identified by behavioral signs in the absence of physical or neurological evidence (Lyon et al., 2003).

The Wayne County research team recommended differentiated educational programming for the group with brain injuries. They suggested a distraction-free environment, and the diagnosis and remediation of perceptual disturbances (Hallahan & Mercer, 2002). According to Torgesen (1998, 2004) the effect of Werner and Strauss on the field of LD was profound, in that they crystallized three concepts used repeatedly by earlier researchers that provided a rationale for the field of LD as a separate entity, identifying a core about what was unique about children with LD. Those concepts were as follows: (1) individual differences in learning could be understood by examining how children approached learning tasks; (2) educational practices should be tailored to individual strengths and weaknesses; and (3) children with deficient learning processes could

be helped to learn normally, if those processes were strengthened (Torgesen, 1998, 2004). Werner and Strauss also suggested that standardized test scores be interpreted cautiously, advocating that clinicians dig deeper to determine why a particular error was made (Hallahan & Mock, 2003).

William Cruickshank extended Werner and Strauss's work with students with mental retardation to children with normal intelligence (Hallahan & Mercer, 2002). Cruickshank's instructional program focused on controlling the learning environment and providing readiness training in the form of perceptual and perceptual motor exercises, because he believed that deficiencies in those areas were responsible for the child's learning problems. The program paid little attention to reading or phonics instruction (Hallahan & Mercer, 2002). Results after the first year indicated that the program was only effective in improving perceptual motor abilities and reducing distractibility for the short term, and had no effects on achievement or IQ (Hallahan & Mercer, 2002).

A number of other individuals developed training programs in the 1960s for visual–perceptual and/or visual–motor skills; prominent among them were Newell Kephart, Marianna Frostig, Glen Doman, and Carl Delacato (Hallahan & Mercer, 2002). Their programs were also eventually found to be ineffective in improving academic performance. However, at this point in time, researchers had discovered tools they considered effective for identifying and educating students with disabilities, and they had sufficient knowledge to claim the existence of a specific construct, a construct not yet referred to as LD (Hallahan & Mock, 2003).

By 1963 the new LD field was moving toward the formal definition of LD as a handicapping condition (Lyon et al., 2003), based largely on the beliefs of the previously discussed pioneers in the field: that children with LDs learned differently than children with mental retardation, that their learning difficulties resulted from intrinsic (i.e., neurobiological) rather than environmental factors, that LDs were unexpected given the child's strengths in other areas, and that children with LDs required specialized education (Lyon et al., 2003). A further belief was that by examining a child's performance on formal (e.g., ITPA) and informal assessments, an appropriate and effective intervention plan could be developed.

Formal Definition and Federal Involvement

Creation of the Term "Learning Disabilities"

Samuel Kirk is generally credited with creating the term "learning disabilities." He originally defined the condition in his1962 textbook *Educating Exceptional Children*:

> A learning disability refers to retardation, disorder, or delayed development in one or more of the processes of speech, language, reading, writing, arithmetic, or other school subjects resulting from a psychological handicap caused by a possible cerebral dysfunction and/or emotional or behavioral disturbances. It is not the result of mental retardation, sensory deprivation, or cultural or instructional factors. (cited in Hallahan & Mercer, 2002, p. 22)

It is interesting to note that emotional–behavioral factors were possible causes of LDs according to Kirk's 1962 definition. However, he excluded children who were deaf or blind, mentally retarded, or who suffered from educational or cultural disadvantages.

The term "learning disabilities" was adopted in 1963 at a meeting of groups of parents and educators of children identified with a variety of names, including minimal brain injured, perceptually handicapped, and neurologically impaired. The parents and educators met in an attempt to unify their views. Kirk suggested "learning disabilities" at that meeting as a unifying term to define the children (Shepherd, 2001). That was the beginning of the group known today as the Learning Disabilities Association of America.

Bateman, a student of Kirk, redefined "learning disabilities" in 1965:

> Children who have learning disorders are those who manifest an educationally significant discrepancy between their estimated potential and actual level of performance related to basic disorders in the learning process, which may or may not be accompanied by demonstrable central nervous system dysfunction, and which are not secondary to generalized mental retardation, educational or cultural deprivation, severe emotional disturbance, or sensory loss. (cited in Hallahan & Mercer, 2002, p. 23)

Bateman included in her definition Monroe's earlier IQ–achievement discrepancy concept as indicative of students with LDs. She also added emotional disturbance to the list of exclusionary factors. Both of Bateman's changes to

Kirk's definition were eventually incorporated into the Federal definition and regulations governing the identification of LDs, with far reaching consequences.

Federal Definition

In 1963, the U.S. government had convened three task forces to address issues related to LDs. Two of the task forces focused primarily on defining LD; they developed conflicting definitions on two controversial issues important to assessment: (1) whether or not nervous system dysfunction is a primary causal factor, and (2) whether an IQ–achievement discrepancy is a defining characteristic of LDs. As these two task forces were attempting to name and define the LD construct, the Education of the Handicapped Act was signed into law; the act did not extend Federal assistance and protection to students with LDs (Hallahan & Mock, 2003).

The United States Office of Education (USOE) asked the National Advisory Committee on Health and Disability (NACHD), headed by Samuel Kirk, to define LD. The NACHD definition was similar to that in Kirk's 1962 textbook; however, emotional disturbance was listed as an exclusionary condition in accordance with the Bateman definition (Hammill, 1990).

As a result of intense lobbying by professionals and parents with a stake in the field of LD, Federal legislation was passed to include students with LDs (Hammill, 1993). In 1969, the Elementary and Secondary Education Act of 1965 was amended to include students with LDs as a special education category.

In 1975, with the Passage of the Education for All Handicapped Children Act (Public Law No. 94-142), the Federal government mandated that school districts provide free and appropriate education to all children with handicaps, including those with LDs. During the House Subcommittee Hearing on Public Law No. 94-142, concern was expressed regarding the vagueness of the proposed definition. The Bureau of Education for the Handicapped was instructed to find a better definition that explained explicitly how children were to be identified. Consensus was not achieved, so the NACHD definition, with a few minor modifications, was adopted (Hammill, 1990).

The following definition was used in Public Law No. 94-142:

The term "specific learning disability" means a disorder in one or more of the basic psychological processes involved in understanding or using language, spoken or written, that may manifest itself in an imperfect ability to listen, read, spell, write, or to do mathematical calculations, including such conditions as perceptual handicaps, brain injury, minimal brain dysfunction, dyslexia, and developmental aphasia. The term does not include children who have learning problems that are primarily the result of visual, hearing, or motor handicaps, or mental retardation, or emotional disturbance, or of environmental, cultural, or economic disadvantage. (cited in Hallahan & Mock, 2003, p. 24)

The definition of learning disabilities that first appeared in 1975 in Public Law No. 94-142, the Education of all Handicapped Children Act, was also incorporated in revisions of that law (IDEA—1990, 1997, and 2004). The current revision of IDEA was reauthorized in December 2004.

IQ–Achievement Discrepancy

There is an operational definition in the Federal law, which first appeared in a separate set of regulations for children with LDs (USOE, 1977). These regulations, in accordance with the Bateman definition, state that a student has a specific learning disability if (1) the student does not achieve at the proper age and ability levels in one or more specific areas when provided with appropriate learning experiences, and (2) the child has a severe discrepancy between achievement and intellectual ability in one or more of seven areas (i.e., oral expression, listening comprehension, written expression, basic reading skills, reading comprehension, mathematics calculation, and mathematics reasoning). It is this operational definition that has resulted in reliance on evidence of an IQ–achievement discrepancy in LD diagnoses.

The focus in the regulations on a severe discrepancy resulted in a significant conceptual shift in LD from psychological processes to unexplained underachievement (Reschly, Hosp, & Schmied, 2003). This shift was in part a response to controversy about the psychological processing clause included in the definition (Torgesen, 2004). As discussed earlier, various programs to remediate specific processing deficits identified by assessment of processing abilities had not been proven effective for improving academic, cognitive, or even long-term perceptual–motor abilities. Although tests of specific processing abilities at that time (which often were focused on visual processing and visual–motor abilities) were ineffectual in determining appropriate intervention, they at least represented an attempt to link LD assessment to intervention. The shift to the IQ–achievement discrepancy criterion in the federal regulations abandoned this assessment goal. Discussion of psychological processes, as well as the use of the IQ–achievement discrepancy in assessment, is included later in this chapter.

In the 1976 Federal Register, the Bureau of Education for the Handicapped (USOE, 1976) suggested a formula for determining a severe discrepancy. The concept of "severe discrepancy" was defined as achievement 50% below expectations. This component, according to Hammill (1990), led to the development of state formulas for calculating a severe discrepancy between intellect and achievement. Opposition to the USOE formula approach was immediate; as a result, the formula was dropped from later regulations. However, although the USOE deleted the formula from its 1977 definition, many states seized on the idea of aptitude–achievement discrepancy, and designed and implemented their own formulas (Hammill, 1990). As of 2001, 48 of 50 states included the severe discrepancy between intellectual ability and achievement in their LD classification criteria (Reschly et al., 2003). No Federal guidance was provided regarding how the discrepancy was to be determined or what constituted a "severe" discrepancy. As a result, the definitions of and methods used to determine such a severe discrepancy vary dramatically across the states (Reschly et al., 2003).

There was another, practical rather than theoretical reason for the inclusion of discrepancy criterion in the regulations. According to Weintraub (2005), the question of whether to include students with LDs in Federal legislation was a major contention, because opponents argued that the proposed definition of LD was too vague and could possibly require services to millions of students. As a result, an amendment was agreed to on the floor of the House of Representatives, capping the number of students who could be served under the LD category at 2% (Reschly et al., 2003). This cap was subsequently lifted when the USOE adopted regulations for identification of students with

LDs, including the severe discrepancy requirement that would supposedly limit the number of students served to 1–3% of the total population (Weintraub, 2005). It is interesting to note that the current percentage of students classified as having LDs is almost double the higher limit of that estimate. Therefore, in addition to moving identification of LD away from assessment that informs instruction, the discrepancy criterion did not limit the identified population as intended. A more detailed discussion of the prevalence of LD is included later in this chapter.

The most recent edition of the *Diagnostic and Statistical Manual of Mental Disorders* (DSM-IV-TR; American Psychiatric Association, 2000) largely reflects the Federal perspective. Differences include use of the term "learning disorders" instead of learning disabilities and more emphasis on distinguishing among academic domains in diagnosis. The domains are reading, mathematics, and written expression, with an additional category for "learning disorder not otherwise specified." The similarity is the embrace of a discrepancy model. Interestingly, there is no qualification associated with use of discrepancy despite an impressive body of research that calls its validity into question.

CURRENT ISSUES IN ASSESSMENT OF LDs

Other difficulties with the diagnosis of LD are the exclusion factors maintained in the statutory definition and the likelihood that an LD co-occurs with other conditions. On the one hand, the law seemingly ignores the possibility of comorbidity via the exclusions; on the other hand, research documents comorbidity. In contrast to Federal implications, DSM-IV-TR (American Psychiatric Association, 2000) guidelines support comorbid diagnosis including not only the co-occurrence of more than one academic difficulty but also cross-classification diagnosis with mental retardation, pervasive developmental disorder, and communication disorder. We next provide a brief overview of exclusion factors in the Federal definition and the most prominent comorbid conditions.

Exclusion Factors

The exclusionary factors in the Federal definition are retained in the latest reauthorization of IDEA and include visual, hearing, or motor disabilities; mental retardation; emotional disturbance; and environmental, cultural, and economic disadvantage. Children cannot be diagnosed as having LDs if the cause of the learning problem is attributed to these sources. Fletcher and colleagues (2002) argued that the cognitive correlates of academic difficulties attributed to social, cultural, and economic disadvantage do not appear to be different from those associated with LD. Also, according to Lyon and colleagues (2001), a child's intervention needs and response to intervention do not vary according to these distinctions. The exclusion of environmental factors is problematic, because such factors interact with and exacerbate LDs (Fletcher et al., 2002). Such factors need to be considered when evaluating a student and determining treatment, rather than discounted as not being the cause of the disability.

Comorbid Conditions

Social–Emotional Problems

Accumulating evidence indicates that a significant number of children with LDs are likely to have social–emotional problems. Students with LDs evidence problems in virtually every category of social well-being, that is, affective, self-concept and attributions, and social skills (Bryan, 1998). In a meta-analysis of 152 studies, Kavale and Forness (1996) found that on average about 75% of students with LDs manifest social skills deficits that distinguished them from comparison groups. The differences were consistent across different evaluators (peers, teachers, and the students themselves) and across major dimensions of social skills.

The results of several studies comparing students with and without LDs have consistently found that students with LDs are more likely to experience feelings of depression, anxiety, and loneliness (Bryan, 1998; Bryan, Burstein, & Ergul, 2004). Wright-Strawderman and Watson (1992) investigated the prevalence of depressive symptoms in elementary school children, ages 8–11, with LDs, and found that 35.85% scored in the depressed range on the Children's Depression Inventory. Depression is not only a serious mental health issue but also an academic one. Negative affect depresses memory and produces inefficient information processing; it affects the performance of complex cognitive functions that require flexibility, integration, and utilization of cognitive material (Bryan et al., 2004). The high percentage of children with LDs who reported depressive symptoms suggests that depression should be assessed in the diagnostic process (Wright-Strawderman & Watson, 1992). Maag and Reid (2006), however, caution that although researchers have found that students with LDs obtain statistically higher scores on measures of depression than their peers, it is not known whether the degree of difference is sufficient to place them in the clinical range. The authors stated that there are not unequivocal data to indicate that students with LDs are any more likely than their peers to have clinical depression.

Children with comorbid LDs and serious emotional disturbance are underidentified and underserved in special education systems (Handwerk & Marshall, 1998). A deterrent to such comorbid diagnosis is the stipulation in the Federal regulations that an LD cannot be caused by emotional factors. The exclusion of emotional factors in the LD definition is interesting, because for a child to qualify as emotionally disturbed, the impairment must adversely affect his or her educational performance (Handwerk & Marshall, 1998). Regarding the exclusion of students with emotional disabilities, Fletcher and colleagues (2002) state that early failure to achieve may be causally related to, and often precedes, the development of behavior problems and should be considered in evaluation.

In contrast to the Federal definition, past definitions of LDs have made either a direct or indirect connection between LDs and social–emotional deficits. The Learning Disabilities Association of America (formerly the Association for Children with Learning Disabilities), the Federal Interagency Committee on Learning Disabilities, and the National Joint Committee on Learning Disabilities all defined LDs as co-occurring with social and/or emotional problems (Elksnin & Elksnin, 2004). It should be noted that Kirk's original LD definition included emotional problems as a possible causal factor. However, the current Federal definition fails to consider the social–emotional deficits of children and adolescents with LDs. No changes in the LD definition referencing the effect of social problems were included in the recent reauthorization.

Attention-Deficit/Hyperactivity Disorder

LDs are often linked to attention-deficit/hyperactivity disorder (ADHD). Although ADHD is not a category under IDEA, children with ADHD are usually included under the other health impaired category if they do not qualify under any other category, such as LD or serious emotional disturbance (SED). Estimates of comorbidity between LD and ADHD vary considerably. Tabassam and Graigner (2002) stated that for students with LD, comorbidity with ADHD ranges from 40 to 80% across studies. Voeller (2004) reported that 80% of children selected because of severe phonological awareness deficits met criteria for ADHD. Children with a primary diagnosis of ADHD often have comorbid LDs as well. Voeller (2004) stated that it is rare to encounter a child with pure ADHD, without emotional or learning problems. Mayes, Calhoun, and Crowell (2000) analyzed data for 119 children ages 8–16, evaluated in a child diagnostic clinic, and found that an LD was present in 70% of the children with ADHD. Of interest is that children with both an LD and ADHD had more severe learning problems than children with an LD alone. Also children with an LD, but not ADHD, had some attention problems, and children with ADHD, but not an LD, had some degree of learning problems. The authors stated that results of their study indicate that learning and attention problems occur on a continuum, are interrelated, and usually coexist; therefore, psychologists should take these factors into consideration when assessing either condition.

Math Disability

It is increasingly common for researchers to specify the academic domain that is the target of the LD. Thus, comorbidity among academic disabilities requires consideration. Reading disability is the most frequently studied learning disability, followed by math, and there are a few studies of their co-occurrence. Light and DeFries (1996) reported that approximately 80% of students with LDs experience reading problems, and most of these students also evidence comorbid deficits in mathematics. In contrast relatively few children with LDs have problems restricted to mathematics and quantitative reasoning. These findings are contradicted by a recent epidemiological study, wherein 35.0 to 56.7% of children with math disabilities (depending on formula used) did *not* experience a comorbid reading disability (Barbaresi, Katusic, Colligan, Weaver, & Jacobsen, 2005). They also reported that the cumulative incidence of math disability ranged from 5.9 to 13.8%, and that boys were significantly more likely to experience a problem.

Investigations indicate that children with comorbid reading and math disabilities fare worse than children with a singular diagnosis. In the elementary school years, children with math difficulties (MD) who are good readers progress faster in mathematics achievement than do children with comorbid math and reading difficulties (MD/RD), independent of other factors (Hanich, Jordan, Kaplan, & Dick, 2001; Jordan, Hanich, & Kaplan, 2003). Specifically, children with MD evidenced an advantage over those with MD/RD in areas mediated by language (e.g., word problems and verbal counting), but not in areas associated with numerical understanding or rapid retrieval of math facts. According to Hanich and colleagues (2001), children with MD should be considered separately from children with MD/RD, because children with MD may have an advantage over children with MD/RD on skills that require or are mediated by language.

Comorbid Diagnosis

Despite evidence of comorbidity between LD and other conditions, Federal regulations and state guidelines discourage comorbid diagnosis (Handwerk & Marshall, 1998). Although not explicitly prohibited, Federal reimbursements are based on number of students identified, not number of handicapping conditions identified, resulting in states' reluctance to acknowledge comorbidity (Handwerk & Marshall, 1998). This may be particularly true of comorbid conditions requiring additional treatment, such as emotional disturbance, rather than of those requiring accommodations or pharmacological interventions, such as ADHD. Furthermore, because ADHD is not listed as an exclusionary factor in the LD definition, practitioners may be more willing to consider it in assessment.

Prevalence of LDs

Since the passage of Public Law No. 94-142, there has been a steady increase in the number of students identified as having LDs. The first year the law was implemented (1977–1978) approximately 800,000 children, or 1.8% of the enrolled population, received services under the LD category. By the year 2002, the number had increased to 2.6 million, or 5.8% of the school-age population (U.S. Department of Education, 2002). State prevalence varied from a low of 2.96% in Kentucky to a high of 9.46% in Rhode Island during the 2001–2002 school year (Reschly et al., 2003). Also, 50% of all children served under IDEA are classified as learning disabled (U.S. Department of Education, 2002). Of those students classified as having an LD, 1.3% are Native American, 1.9% are Asian/Pacific Islander, 19.9% are African American (non-Hispanic), 14.5% are Hispanic, and 62.4 % are white (non-Hispanic) (U.S. Department of Education, 2002).

The disproportionate representation of certain ethnic groups in the IDEA disability categories of mental retardation and behavior disorders is an urgent issue (Hallahan & Mock, 2003). Although the degree of representation is not as great as that for other categories, African Americans are slightly overrepresented in the LD category, because they constitute 14.8% of the school-age population but 19.9% of the LD population, as are Native Americans, who constitute 1.0% of the school-age population and 1.3% of the LD population. Furthermore, the overrepresentation of these two groups in the LD category in certain states is substantial (Hallahan & Mock, 2003).

Etiology

As our discussion on history attests, LDs have long been associated with cognitive processing difficulties considered constitutional in origin. Despite the difficulty of connecting poor academic performance and brain anomalies in children with no known tissue damage, early researchers continued to draw the inference. This inference is also reflected in the Federal definition of LD through subsuming the terms "perceptual disabilities," "brain injury," and "minimal brain dysfunction." Lyon and colleagues (2003) noted that whereas early attempts to link brain and behavior in LDs were highly speculative, more recent work in neurobiology provides support for such a connection (e.g., Shaywitz et al., 2004; Simos et al., 2005; Temple et al., 2003). Lyon and colleagues are careful to point out that such linkages do not argue against environmental influences, and that the evidence is limited to reading disability associated with word decoding difficulties (dyslexia). We believe most scientists and practitioners likely agree that the locus of LDs is suboptimal cognitive processing. A primary point of disagreement is the extent to which these processes can be measured reliably with valid connections to brain activity. This issue is elaborated in our review of assessment methods that follows.

OVERVIEW OF EVALUATION OF ASSESSMENT METHODS

The next sections of the chapter evaluate the validity of psychological–cognitive processing and RTI models of LD identification. Our use of the term "validity" is based on Messick's (1989a, 1989b, 1995) broader conceptualization of test validity. In the current context the "test" to be considered includes procedures to operationalize LDs. Messick proposed that traditional methods of evaluating validity are too narrow, and that not only data associated with test scores but also consequences of applying test scores require examination. In our evaluation of LD assessment procedures, we focus on what Messick called "construct validity," which comprises traditional ideas about types of validity: reliability, content, criterion and construct validity, and relevance. Relevance reflects users' evaluations of usefulness (Good & Jefferson, 1998) and we interpret this to mean connections between assessment data and intervention. Other aspects of Messick's view of validity include examining consequences of test use. We touch briefly on consequences, as appropriate. For each method reviewed, evidence for construct validity is presented, followed by evidence for relevance.

ASSESSING PSYCHOLOGICAL PROCESSING DISORDERS

The term "psychological processes" has been retained as part of the definition of LDs in every reauthorization of IDEA. This is so despite (1) early dissatisfaction with the term that led to the 1977 Federal regulations instituting intellectual ability–achievement discrepancies as a criterion for identification rather than psychological processes (Reschly et al., 2003; Torgesen, 2004) and (2) consistent research

findings from earlier eras that the psychological processing approach to assessment and intervention were not valid (e.g., Kavale & Mattson, 1983; Klenck & Kirby, 2000).

Present-day proponents of psychological–cognitive processing assessment for LD identification argue that past attempts using discrepancy were flawed, because the measure of intelligence (primarily the Wechsler scales) lacked a theoretical base (Kavale, Holdnakc, & Mostert, 2005; Naglieri, 2003). They argue that its measurement rather than the conceptual base for IQ–achievement discrepancy is flawed. Although the number of professional writers who support this position is rather small, the number of supportive practitioners is potentially large. Machek and Nelson (in press) reported that 75% of the school psychologists they surveyed endorsed assessment of cognitive processes in diagnosing LDs and over 60% were endorsed using IQ–achievement discrepancies. We review and evaluate several processing approaches, including the Wechsler Intelligence Scale for Children–IV (Wechsler, 2003), the Woodcock–Johnson Tests of Cognitive Abilities–III (Woodcock, McGrew, & Mather, 2001), the Cognitive Assessment System (Naglieri & Das, 2005), and the Kaufman Assessment Battery for Children–II (Kaufman & Kaufman, 2004).

Wechsler Intelligence Scale for Children–IV

A method used historically by diagnosticians to identify a processing disorder is examination of subtest scores from intellectual assessments to determine patterns of cognitive strengths and weaknesses. Such an analysis determines whether the resulting pattern of subtest scores differentiates between students with LDs and other, low-achieving students (Kavale, 2002). Hale and Fiorello (2004) reported that 90% of school psychologists use factor or index scores, subtest profile analysis, or both, in interpreting IQ tests. Because intelligence tests are the basis of such assessments and the Wechsler Intelligence Scale for Children is often used, we present a description and evaluation of the latest edition developed for children.

Description

The Wechsler Intelligence Scale for Children–IV (WISC-IV), released in 2003, is the current version of Wechsler's intelligence tests for children and adolescents. It is an individually administered test for individuals ages 6 years to 16 years, 11 months. Each of the three Weschler Scales (Wechsler Adult Intelligence Scales, WAIS; Wechsler Intelligence Scales for Children, WISC; and Wechsler Preschool and Primary Scales of Intelligence, WPPSI) originally provided three IQ scores: Full Scale IQ (FSIQ), Verbal IQ, and Performance IQ. Calculation of these three IQ scores was based on performance on individual subtest scores. The WISC is a downward extension of the WAIS, and the WPPSI is a downward extension of the WISC. In 1999, in addition to the three aforementioned scales, the Psychological Corporation published the Wechsler Abbreviated Scale of Intelligence (WASI) that comprises four subtests (Similarities, Vocabulary, Block Design, and Matrix Reasoning). Also available is the WISC-IV Integrated version, which can be

ordered as an upgrade and incorporates the core and supplemental subtests of the WISC-IV, along with 12 "process approach" subtests (McCloskey & Maerlender, 2005).

The WISC-IV has more changes than any previous model (Flanagan & Kaufman, 2004; Groth-Marnat, 2003), including the elimination of the traditional Verbal and Performance IQs. In place of the performance and verbal scores, the primary scores are now derivatives of four factor-based index scores: Verbal Comprehension, Perceptual Reasoning, Processing Speed, and Working Memory (Prifitera, Weiss, Saklofske, & Rolfhus, 2005). Table 13.1 lists these indices and describes the associated subtests. A detailed description of changes is provided by Prifitera and colleagues (2005). In general, subtests and indices were updated to reflect contemporary views of cognitive processes and achievement.

TABLE 13.1. Subtests of the Wechsler Intelligence Scales for Children—4th Edition (WISC-IV) Organized by Index

Index	Subtest
Verbal Comprehension	• Comprehension: The student is required to answer orally presented questions pertaining to social rules or problems. • Similarities: The student is required to explain the similarities between oral word pairs. • Vocabulary: The student is required to name pictures or provide definitions for words. • Information (Supplemental): The student is required to answer factual questions of learned content. • Word Reasoning (Supplemental): The student is required to identify a common concept based on successive verbal clues.
Perceptual Reasoning	• Block Design: The student is required to rearrange a set of blocks to match visual patterns presented on a card (timed). • Picture Concepts: The student is required to choose pictures from rows in an array to form a group with common characteristics. • Matrix Reasoning: The student is required to draw visual analogies and respond to multiple-choice questions. • Picture Completion (Supplemental): The student is required to identify missing element of picture of common object or setting (timed).
Processing Speed	• Coding: The student is required visually to match numbers with corresponding symbols and record appropriate symbols under numbers (timed). • Symbol Search: The student is required visually to scan an array and mark target symbols (timed). • Cancellation (Supplemental): The student is required to scan both a random and a nonrandom arrangement of pictures and mark target pictures (timed).
Working Memory	• Digit Span: The student is required to repeat orally presented numbers forwards and backwards. • Letter-Number Sequencing: The student is required to recode orally presented letter–number combinations, stating the numbers in ascending order and the letters in alphabetic order. • Arithmetic (Supplemental): The student is required to solve mentally and express orally the answer to orally presented arithmetic problems.

Use and Validity

The FSIQ and index scores are generally the first scores examined by the practitioner (Zhu & Weiss, 2005). The four WISC Index scores (Verbal Comprehension, Perceptual Reasoning, Working Memory, and Processing Speed) are often compared in the diagnosis of an LD to determine an individual's pattern of cognitive strengths and weaknesses. In fact, the primary level of interpretation of the WISC-IV is at the index score level (Weiss, Prifitera, & Saklofske, 2005). The diagnostician typically compares the index scores either to the mean of the index scores or among themselves to determine an individual's relative strengths and weaknesses (Prifitera et al., 2005). However, interpretations should be made cautiously, because moderate index differences are common to the general population (Groth-Marnat, 2003), indicating little empirical support for the practice.

Another traditional practice of psychologists is to interpret the pattern of WISC subtest scores and classify the patterns of cognitive strengths and weaknesses based on subtest analysis. Often WISC subtest scores are combined to establish a profile supposedly characteristic of students with learning disabilities. Bannatyne (1968, 1974) was one of the earliest to define such a profile. Bannatyne believed that the WISC's division of subtests into Performance and Verbal IQ measures was not diagnostically helpful in identifying students with LDs (Smith & Watkins, 2004). He recategorized the WISC subtest scores into those testing spatial abilities, conceptual abilities, sequencing abilities, and acquired knowledge. Bannatyne suggested that the performance of students with LD would demonstrate spatial abilities > conceptual abilities > sequencing abilities > acquired knowledge. The theory underlying Bannatyne's recategorization was that people with LDs would be expected to do better on spatial, holistic tasks that require simultaneous processing than on learning tasks that require sequential processing (Groth-Marnat, 2003). However, although more students with LDs exhibit the Bannatyne profile than do students in general, score differences are well below significance (Kavale, 2002). Also, the majority of students with LDs do not have the profile (Groth-Marnat, 2003; Smith & Watkins, 2004).

Others have attempted to define profiles of subtests on which students with LDs score lower compared to their overall performance. Three such WISC profiles are the ACID, the ACIDS, and the SCAD. Originally developed for the WISC-R (Groth-Marnat, 2003), the ACID refers to the scores on Arithmetic, Coding, Information, and Digit Span subtests; the WISC-III's Symbol Search subtest was added to the ACID profile to create the ACIDS profile (Groth-Marnat, 2003); the SCAD profile comprises Symbol Search, Coding, Arithmetic, and Digit Span subtests. Children with LDs have been found to score poorly on the ACID, ACIDS, and SCAD subtests relative to their overall performance. Although these profiles occur more frequently in individuals with LDs than in the general population, other groups also have the same profiles, the frequency for students with LD is not that much higher, and the majority of individuals with LDs do not exhibit the profiles (D'Angiulli & Siegel, 2003; Groth-Marnat, 2003).

To investigate profile analysis and students with LDs, Mayes and colleagues (1998) compared the performance of 66 children with LDs and 51 children without LDs, ages 6–16, on the WISC-III. Analyses involving the younger children (6–7 years old) were conducted separately, because the authors determined that their age might have precluded identification as having LDs. Mayes and colleagues found that the only profile with statistically significant frequency differences between children ages 8–16 with and without LD on the WISC-III was the AD (Arithmetic, Digit Span). For children with LDs, 38% had Arithmetic and Digit Span as two of their three lowest subtest scores, whereas only 9% of students without LD exhibited that profile. It should be noted, however, that the majority of students with LD did not exhibit the AD profile. Furthermore, the authors found that for children age 6–7 years, there were no profile differences between students with and without LDs. According to Maller (2005), although the WISC-IV manuals promote the use of profile analysis for interpreting an examinee's strengths and weaknesses, practitioners should be wary that such an interpretation increases the likelihood of findings due to chance.

Another strategy frequently used in diagnosis of LDs is to determine the meaning of extremely high or low individual subtest scores. A common method of such subtest analysis is to compute ipsative deviation scores, comparing the individual's subtest scores and the mean to identify strengths and weaknesses (Robinson

& Harrison, 2005). However, according to Flanagan and Kaufman (2004), ipsative scores have poor reliability, are not stable over time, and do not add anything to predicting achievement beyond measures of general intelligence. Groth-Marnat (2003) cautions that such an analysis needs to be undertaken with care, because individual subtests are not sufficiently reliable or specific, and a high degree of subtest scatter is fairly common. Groth-Marnat recommends the following when interpreting subtest variation: (1) Statistical significance of the fluctuations should be ascertained; (2) hypotheses should be checked against performance on other subtests requiring similar skills; and (3) hypotheses should be confirmed with additional information, such as the student's motivation, school records, teacher reports, other test scores, and medical records.

The WISC is also frequently used as a measure of overall IQ (FSIQ) to identify children with IQ–achievement discrepancies that have long been considered a hallmark of LD diagnosis. This discrepancy is thought to indicate "unexpected" learning problems, presumably due to psychological or cognitive processing problems. Both logic and research have accumulated over the last 25 years, indicating that IQ–achievement discrepancies do not identify a unique group of children, they have a number of statistical and measurement problems, they require a history of failure before a discrepancy is apparent, and they do not inform instruction or prevention efforts (e.g., Fletcher et al., 1994; Share, McGee, & Silva, 1989; Stanovich & Siegel, 1994; Stuebing et al., 2002). This work is reviewed in a number of articles (e.g., Fletcher et al., 2002) and is not elaborated here. Our conclusion is that little evidence supports the use of intellectual–achievement discrepancies, and the burden is on its proponents to provide validity evidence.

Summary of Validity

The evidence supporting the construct and relevance validity of the WISC-IV is uneven. Some reviewers believe it is psychometrically sound (Groth-Marnat, 2003; Hale & Fiorello, 2004), whereas others do not (Maller, 2005). The previously mentioned review suggests that clinical practices such as profile analysis for identification of LDs are not valid. Furthermore, its usefulness in informing instruction for students with LDs is questionable. Braden and Niebling (2005) provided a detailed analysis of the valid-

ity of the WISC-IV and stated that "little or no direct evidence is provided for specific claims regarding treatment planning or links to neuropsychological foundations" (p. 620). Its usefulness as part of an index to measure discrepancy has been soundly rejected. So what conclusion should one draw then in terms of the role of the WISC-IV in the assessment of children with LDs? Should it be used under certain circumstances? In a particular way? Not at all? In summary, although the WISC has a historical role in the diagnosis of LDs, its validity or usefulness for that purpose has not been established. In our opinion its use should be reserved in LD diagnosis for measuring overall IQ to rule out the possibility of mental retardation. It should not be routinely administered as part of a diagnostic battery.

Woodcock–Johnson III Psychoeducational Battery

Description

The Woodcock–Johnson III Psychoeducational Battery (WJ-III) comprises two batteries: the Woodcock–Johnson III Tests of Cognitive Abilities (WJ-III-COG) and the Woodcock–Johnson III Tests of Achievement (WJ-III-ACH). The authors describe the WJ-III-COG as a comprehensive set of individually administered tests for measuring cognitive abilities, scholastic aptitudes, and oral language for individuals from age 24 months to 90 years, which is complemented by the WJ-III-ACH (Mather & Woodcock, 2001). The WJ-III Diagnostic Supplement to the WJ-III-COG includes additional subtests.

The WJ-III-COG is based on the Cattell–Horn–Carroll (CHC) theory of cognitive abilities, a hierarchical framework of human cognitive abilities that comprises three strata: general intelligence, broad cognitive abilities, and narrow cognitive abilities. Although the Woodcock–Johnson Achievement battery is one of the most frequently used measures of achievement, the Cognitive battery historically has not been used as frequently as the Wechsler scales. Recently there has been increased interest in the WJ-III-COG, because it is based on the CHC model of intelligence, which many believe to be the most empirically supported and theoretically sound model (Taub & McGrew, 2004). Cizek (2005) stated that the W-J-III (COG and ACH) is a comprehensive, norm-referenced, individually administered assessment of those cognitive abilities, skills, and academic knowledge most recognized as constituting human intelligence, and routinely encountered in school and other settings.

The cognitive battery contains 20 subtests, 10 of which are part of the standard battery, and 10, part of the extended battery. The subtests are organized into the following broad CHC cognitive ability clusters: Comprehension-Knowledge (Gc), Long-Term Retrieval (Glr), Visual–Spatial Thinking (Gv), Auditory Processing (Ga), Fluid Reasoning (Gf), Processing Speed (Gs), and Short-Term Memory (Gsm). The WJ-COG subtests organized by broad CHC factors are listed in Table 13.2.

TABLE 13.2. Subtests of the Woodcock–Johnson III Tests of Cognitive Abilities (WJ-III-COG) Organized by Broad Cattell–Horn–Carroll (CHC) Factor

Broad CHC factor	Subtest
Comprehension–Knowledge (Gc)	• Verbal Comprehension (Standard): The student is required to identify objects, provide antonyms and synonyms, and complete verbal analogies. • General Information (Extended): The student is required to explain where objects are found and how they are typically used.
Long-Term Retrieval (Glr)	• Visual–Auditory Learning (Standard): The student is required to learn and recall pictographic representations of words. • Visual–Auditory Learning-Delayed (Standard): The previous subtest is readministered after a time delay to measure ease of relearning. • Retrieval Fluency (Extended): The student is required to name as many examples as possible from a given category.
Visual–Spatial Thinking (Gv)	• Spatial Relations (Standard): The student is required to identify the subset of pieces required to form a target shape. • Picture Recognition (Extended): The student is required to identify a subset of previously presented pictures within a field of distracting pictures. • Planning (Extended): The student is required to trace a pattern without removing the pencil from the paper or retracing any lines.
Auditory Processing (Ga)	• Sound Blending (Standard): The student is required to listen to and blend phonemes or syllables to pronounce a word. • Incomplete Words (Standard): The student is required to identify words orally presented with missing phonemes. • Auditory Attention (Extended): The student is required to identify auditorily presented words amid increasingly intense background noise.
Fluid Reasoning (Gf)	• Concept Formation (Standard): The student is required to identify, categorize, and determine rules applied to visual information. • Analysis–Synthesis (Extended): The student is required to analyze puzzles to determine missing components. • Planning (Extended): The student is required to trace a pattern without removing the pencil from the paper or retracing any lines. (subtest also under Visual–Spatial Thinking Index)
Processing Speed (Gs)	• Visual Matching (Standard): The student is required to locate and circle two identical numbers in a row (timed). • Decision Speed (Extended): The student is required to circle the two pictures that are conceptually most similar in a row (timed). • Rapid Picture Naming (Extended): The student is required to recognize and name pictured objects (timed). • Pair Cancellation (Extended): The student is required to identify and circle a repeated pattern of pictures (timed).
Short-Term Memory (Gsm)	• Numbers Reversed (Standard): The student is required to repeat a series of numbers in reverse order. • Auditory Working Memory (Standard): The student is required to remember a set of numbers and letters and reorder them into the two corresponding sequences. • Memory for Words (Extended): The student is required to repeat lists of unrelated words in correct sequence.

Use and Validity

Mather and Woodcock (2001) stated that the goal of a learning disability assessment is to uncover the individual student's pattern of strengths and weaknesses to design an appropriate intervention and the W-J-III-COG battery provides such information. They further asserted that the use of the Cognitive battery in conjunction with the Achievement battery allows the practitioner to identify cognitive factors associated with achievement problems.

The WJ-III-COG's validity appears adequate (Salvia & Ysseldyke, 2004). Cizek (2005) stated that it is apparent that Standards for Educational and Psychological testing (Joint Committee on Standards for Educational and Psychological Testing of the AERA [American Education Research Association], American Psychological Association [APA], and National Council on Measurement in Education [NCME], 1999) informed the current revision of the WJ-III. He also reported that correlational evidence supports the validity of the WJ-III-COG, because the expected pattern of relationships among tests was observed; tests hypothesized to measure similar characteristics correlated more strongly than tests measuring dissimilar constructs, as hypothesized by CHC theory. Sandoval (2005) concluded that the WJ-III-COG has good concurrent validity overall, because the cognitive clusters intended to predict achievement correlate with the achievement clusters in the .70 range. Evans, Floyd, McGrew, and Leforgee (2002) examined relations between the WJ-III-COG and the CHC theory of cognitive abilities, and found that measures of CHC cognitive abilities obtained from the WJ-III were significantly related to components of reading achievement. They stated that the results supported the external validity for the WJ-III cognitive clusters. Other researchers have found links between the WJ-III-COG clusters and achievement in math (Floyd, Evans, & McGrew, 2003; McGrew & Hessler, 1995).

Hale and Fiorello (2004) described a model for developing and evaluating individual interventions using the CHC model. Fiorello and Primrano (2005) designed worksheets linking CHC abilities to specific achievement areas and derived programming recommendations from the cognitive processing findings. The authors recommended research or data collection to measure the effectiveness of the recommendations.

Fiorello and Primrano (2005) stated that collective research findings establish the differential diagnostic validity of the CHC-based WJ-III-COG. However, they caution that such links do not automatically lead to interventions. Braden and Niebling (2005), in a comprehensive analysis of validity evidence, stated that "no direct evidence to support claims of value for educational planning . . . is provided" (p. 626).

Summary of Validity

The WJ-III-COG has initial evidence of traditional validity (criterion related). A question to be considered is the extent to which this type of validity evidence is meaningful for an LD diagnosis. If achievement is the important validity criterion for cognitive processes, what is added by using cognitive processing scores? It would be more sensible to use the more direct measure (achievement) than a correlate (cognitive processes). This criticism applies to all processing tests in which achievement is viewed as the important criterion. Proponents of cognitive processing need to establish, at a minimum, that these scores provide more in-depth information about a child than can be derived from achievement scores. This may include identifying differential patterns of performance unique to children with LDs and connecting intervention plans with testing results.

Cognitive Assessment System

Description

Designed for youth ages 5–17 years, the Cognitive Assessment System (CAS; Naglieri & Das, 1997) is an individually administered, norm-referenced test of cognitive processing. The CAS has four components derived from the PASS theory of intelligence (planning, attention, simultaneous, and successive cognitive processes) based on the theoretical work of Luria. Specifically, PASS processes were derived from Luria's 1973 neuropsychological theory of brain functions (Joseph, McCachran, & Naglieri, 2003; Naglieri & Reardon, 1993).

According to Naglieri and Rojahn (2004) the four separate dimensions of ability were developed as a modern approach to intelligence. Naglieri (2005) claimed that the PASS theory places emphasis on cognitive processes related to performance rather than on a general intelligence model. Naglieri (2001, 2005) suggested that the CAS be used in the identification of students with LDs and that the four PASS processes represent the types of basic psychological processes described in IDEA. He claimed that the four basic psychological processes are used to design appropriate interventions to discover a child's strengths and weaknesses.

According to Naglieri and Das (1997), *planning* is the ability to formulate, execute, and judge the effectiveness of a strategy; *attention* is the ability to attend selectively to relevant versus irrelevant stimuli; *simultaneous processing* is the ability to survey and integrate elements into the whole; and *successive processing* is the ability to process information serially. Because the CAS subtests were developed specifically to operationalize the PASS theory of cognitive processing, the sole criterion for inclusion was each subtest's correspondence to the PASS the-

oretical framework (Naglieri, 2001). Table 13.3 summarizes the 12 CAS subtests organized by process. The CAS Standard Battery comprises all 12 subtests. The CAS Basic Battery comprises the first two subtests listed under each process.

Naglieri (2003, 2005) argued that all of the major intelligence tests except the CAS and the Kaufman Assessment Battery for Children (K-ABC) are biased in the assessment of minority children and children with limited English or limited academic skills, because the tests measure achievement rather than ability. Naglieri (2000) stated that removing verbal achievement from ability measures and focusing on cognitive processes increases fairness to minority populations. A study investigating the difference in performance on tests of ability by race found that the CAS test exhibited the

TABLE 13.3. Subtests of the Cognitive Assessment System (CAS) Organized by Process

Process	Subtest
Planning	• Matching Numbers: The student is required to identify and underline two identical numbers consisting of from one to seven digits (timed). • Planned Codes: The student is required to fill in code letters in accord with a legend (timed). • Planned Connections: The student is required to connect randomly ordered numbers, as well as numbers and letters, in sequential order (timed).
Attention	• Expressive Attention: The student (ages 5–7) is required to state whether a pictured animal is large or small in real life, ignoring the relative size of the picture. The student (ages 8 and older) is required to: (1) read color words, (2) name the color of a series of rectangles, and (3) name the color of ink a color word is printed in, ignoring the color word (timed). • Number Detection: The student is required to underline specific numbers printed in an outlined typeface (timed). • Receptive Attention: The student (ages 5–7) is required to (1) underline pairs of drawings that are identical in appearance, and (2) underline pairs of drawings that have the same name. The student (ages 8 and older) is required to do the same with letters (timed).
Simultaneous	• Nonverbal Matrices: The student is required to complete geometric matrices interrelated through spatial or logical organization. • Verbal–Spatial Relations: The student is required to select the appropriate spatial configuration in response to a verbal description. • Figure Memory: The student is required to identify a two- or three-dimensional figure (previously displayed for 5 seconds) embedded within a larger figure.
Successive	• Word Series: The student is required to repeat a series of single-syllable, high-frequency words. • Sentence Repetition: The student is required to repeat sentences composed of color words (e.g., *The blue is yellowing*). • Speech Rates (ages 5–7): The student is required to repeat a series of three one- and two-syllable words 10 times in a row (timed). • Sentence Questions (ages 8–17): Used instead of speech rate for older students. The student is required to respond after reading questions similar to those used in sentence repetition (e.g., *The blue is yellowing. Who is yellowing?*).

smallest difference between black and white participants (Naglieri, 2003).

Use and Validity

Naglieri and Sullivan (1998) suggested that identification of an LD begins with an examination of the PASS profile to identify intra- and interindividual weaknesses on the PASS processes. Then the student's academic achievement is evaluated for areas of low achievement. Thus, the determination of a cognitive weakness is based on dual processing criteria (a low score relative to both the child's mean and the norm group) and accompanied by a weakness in an achievement domain (Naglieri & Das, 2005). In interpreting the CAS, emphasis is placed at the PASS process level rather than at the specific subtest level (Naglieri & Das, 2005). The PASS scale scores are computed on the basis of the sum of subtest scaled scores included in each scale. These four scales, representing a child's cognitive processing in specific areas, are intended to be used diagnostically to examine cognitive strengths and weaknesses (Naglieri, 2005). Each of the 12 subtests measures the specific PASS process corresponding to the scale in which it is included; the subtests are not considered to represent specific abilities (Naglieri, 2005). Rather, subtests are intended as varying ways to measure each of the four processes and have less reliability than the composite scores for the PASS processes (Naglieri & Das, 2005).

To establish the construct validity of the CAS many researchers investigated the correlation between the CAS and achievement. Joseph and colleagues (2003) explored the relationship between the CAS performance of 62 primary grade children referred for reading problems, and their phonological processing and reading achievement. They hypothesized and found that some processes were strongly related both to phonological processes and reading performance. The strongest intercorrelation was between phonological memory and the successive processes composite on the CAS (.81). However, the best predictor of performance on word-level skills was the phonological awareness measure, not CAS scores.

Johnson, Bardos, and Tayebi (2003) explored the relationships between CAS performance and writing achievement in junior high school students with and without written expression disabilities. Ninety-six students were administered the CAS and the writing subtests

of the WIAT. Significant relationships were found between the planning and attention composites of the CAS and the WIAT writing scales in the students with writing disabilities. In contrast, simultaneous and successive composites of the CAS were significantly related to writing achievement in the students without writing disabilities.

Naglieri and Das (1997) investigated the predictive relationship between CAS performance and achievement compared to other tests of cognitive ability. The median correlation between the CAS Full Scale and the revised WJ-ACH was .70. The correlation with achievement was higher than coefficients obtained with the WISC-III (.59), the revised WJ-COG (.63), and the K-ABC (.63). Naglieri and Rojahn (2004) reported similar correlations between CAS performance and achievement. They interpreted these data as evidence of construct validity.

According to Naglieri (2001, 2003), the finding that the CAS had the highest correlation among the major intelligence tests with achievement was especially important for two reasons. First, one of the most important dimensions of validity for a test of cognitive ability is the relationship to achievement. Second, the CAS, unlike the Wechsler scales, does not include subtests that are highly reliant on acquired knowledge.

Kranzler and colleagues (Keith, Kranzler, & Flanagan, 2001; Kranzler & Keith, 1999) questioned the construct validity of the CAS, suggesting that the scales are more consistent with the CHC theory of intelligence than with the PASS theory based on the work of Luria. Therefore, they suggested that the CAS is not an appropriate tool for diagnostic or intervention purposes.

According to Salvia and Ysseldyke (2004), the validity of the CAS is problematic, because the underlying model of intelligence is so different from the models used by other tests of IQ. However, they stated that the CAS does correlate well with other tests of intelligence and does predict scores on standardized achievement tests. Thompson (2005), in a review of the CAS, stated that data presented by the authors in the interpretive handbook provide generally strong support for the construct validity. Furthermore, the criterion-related validity studies suggest that the CAS correlates highly with other measures of ability and achievement.

Naglieri (2000, 2001) believes data from CAS can inform instructional and intervention needs, therefore speaking to relevance. Two approaches designed in accord with PASS theory are the PASS Remedial Program (PREP; Das, 1999), which targets reading decoding, and the Planning Facilitation Program (Naglieri, 1999), which originally targeted math calculation but has been used in other academic areas as well.

The focus of the PREP is primarily on successive processing. The program teaches children to focus on the successive nature of a variety of tasks, each of which has two forms, global and bridging (Naglieri, 2005). The global tasks are nonacademic in content and are designed to illustrate the underlying concept. The bridging tasks contain reading content and illustrate the same concept. For example, a global task of matching the head to the appropriate rear of an animal's body is paired with the bridging task of joining the beginning letters of a word to appropriate ending letters (Naglieri, 2001). Researchers found that students with decoding difficulties who were trained in the PASS-based PREP program made significantly greater gains than controls in word reading skills (Boden & Kirby, 1995; Carlson & Das, 1997; Das, Mishra, & Pool, 1995; Parrila, Das, Kendrick, Papadopolous, & Kirby, 1999).

The Planning Facilitation Program is based on the assumption that planning processes should be facilitated rather than directly instructed, so that children discover the value of strategy use (Naglieri, 2001). The approach, which was used in a number of research studies, varied from study to study but, in general, used a verbalization technique that encouraged a well-planned and organized examination of the demands of the task. Self-reflection and discussion were facilitated in all variations of the program (Naglieri, 2001, 2003). Naglieri and his colleagues (Haddad et al., 2003; Naglieri & Gottling, 1995; Naglieri & Johnson, 2000) reported that students with low planning scores on the CAS improved more following instruction targeting planning than did students with high scores. However, a study with a larger sample failed to replicate these findings (Kroesbergen, Van Luit, & Naglieri, 2003). The results of this line of research are tempered by the need for experimental designs that interpret intervention effects and have larger samples and testable hypotheses. For example, Naglieri and Johnson (2000) conducted an intervention with nine children, only three of whom evidenced a planning weakness, to ex-amine the differential effectiveness of a version of the Planning Facilitation Program; Naglieri and Gottling (1997) conducted an intervention with eight children, with no experimental controls; and Kroesbergen and colleagues (2003) reported findings that contradicted the theoretical points made in the introduction to the study. Meikamp (2005) noted that few CAS intervention studies incorporated exceptional populations; therefore, caution should be used in prescribing PASS-based instruction for remedial students.

Summary of Validity

There appears to be general agreement on the criterion-related validity but some question regarding evidence for construct validity of the CAS. Studies of relevance are beginning to appear but have not yet met the burden of evidence required to link assessment with intervention.

Kaufman Assessment Battery for Children–II

Description

The Kaufman Assessment Battery for Children–II (K-ABC-II) is an individually administered battery of tests used to measure the IQ of children and adolescents. The first edition of the K-ABC was the first test to be influenced by Luria's cognitive processing model of human functioning (Naglieri, 2003). In developing the K-ABC, Kaufman and Kaufman departed from the common conception of intelligence as an overall global entity (Lichtenberger, 2001). Both the information processing approach of Luria and the cerebral specialization theory of Sperry, Bogen, Kinsbourne, Wada, Clarke, and Hamm provided the theoretical framework for the sequential and simultaneous process emphasis of the K-ABC (Lichtenberger, 2001).

The K-ABC-II, in contrast with the K-ABC, is based on a dual theoretical foundation: (1) Luria's processing model of human functioning, and (2) the CHC broad and narrow abilities model (Kaufman, Kaufman, Kaufman-Singer, & Kaufman, 2005). The K-ABC-II represents a substantial revision of the K-ABC, with a greatly expanded age range (3 years to 18 years, 11 months instead of 2 years, 6 months to 12 years, 6 months), the replacement of eight subtests, and the addition of a Delayed Recall scale. The K-ABC-II comprises core and supplemental subtests that are administered depending on the age of the child and the model the examiner chooses to use. Change in the complexity of the theoretical structure of the test that is dependent upon the child's age is roughly consistent with milestones of intellectual development identified by other theorists, such as Piaget (Thorndike, 2005).

The KABC-II includes four or five broad ability scales depending on the model used. The CHC model organizes subtests into Short-Term Memory (G*sm*), Visual Processing (G*v*), Long-Term Retrieval (G*lr*), Fluid Reasoning (G*f*), and Crystallized Ability (G*c*) scales, and gives a Fluid–Crystallized Index composite score. The

Luria model renames the scales into Sequential Processing (Short-Term Memory, G*sm*), Simultaneous Processing (Visual–Spatial Thinking, G*v*), Learning Ability (Long-Term Retrieval, G*lr*), and Planning Ability (Fluid Reasoning, G*f*) scales, and gives a composite Mental Processing Index score; the Crystallized Ability scale is not included in the Luria model. The test developers claim that the K-ABC-II can be interpreted using either the Luria model or the CHC model. Table 13.4 summarizes the K-ABC-II subtests organized by Fluid–Crystallized Index/Mental Processing Index.

TABLE 13.4. Subtests of the Kaufman Assessment Battery for Children—2nd Edition (K-ABC-II) Organized by Fluid–Crystallized Index/Mental Processing Index

Fluid–Crystallized Index/ Mental Processing Index	Subtest
Visual Processing (G*v*)/ Simultaneous	• Triangles: The student is required to copy designs with plastic triangles or shapes. • Face Recognition: The student is required to identify a face that was shown earlier. • Conceptual Thinking: The student is required to identify a picture that does not belong in a group. • Rover: The student is required to select the shortest path on a checkerboard-like grid to move a dog toward a bone. • Block Counting: The student is required to visualize unseen blocks to determine how many are in a stack. • Gestalt Closure: The student is required to fill in gaps to complete an inkblot picture.
Short-Term Memory (G*sm*)/Sequential	• Word Order: The student is required to touch silhouettes of common objects in correct sequence following examiner naming. • Number Recall: The student is required to repeat a series of numbers. • Hand Movements: The student is required to repeat a sequence of hand movements in response to examiner modeling.
Fluid Reasoning (G*f*)/ Planning	• Pattern Reasoning: The student is required to select a missing shape in a series to complete a pattern. • Story Completion: The student is required to select a missing picture in a series of pictures that tell a story.
Long-Term Storage and Retrieval (G*lr*)/Learning	• Atlantis: After learning nonsense names for colorful pictures, the student is required to point to the appropriate picture in response to hearing its name. • Rebus: The student is required to learn words associated with simple line drawings, then read the drawings. • Delayed Recall: The student is required to recall paired associations learned earlier during the Atlantis and Rebus subtests.
Crystallized Ability (G*c*): included in CHC model only	• Riddles: The student is required to answer riddles in response to a set of clues. • Expressive Vocabulary: The student is required verbally to identify objects represented in color drawings. • Verbal Knowledge: The student is required to point to a picture that corresponds to a vocabulary word or general information prompt.

Note. Different subtests are administered at different student ages (core or supplemental status also changes with age of student). Subtests are generally untimed for younger students, but they can be administered on a timed or untimed basis for older students.

Use and Validity

According to Kaufman and colleagues (2005), like the original K-ABC, the K-ABC-II was designed to assist in the identification of process integrities and deficits for assessment of individuals with specific LDs, among other purposes. The K-ABC-II assesses 15 of the approximately 70 CHC narrow abilities. The Broad Ability scales that comprise these narrow abilities are of primary importance for interpreting the child's cognitive profile (Kaufman et al., 2005).

The K-ABC-II also includes supplementary subtests (e.g., Delayed Recall, Hand Movements) that are not included in the computation of standard scores but are intended to allow the examiner to follow up hypotheses suggested by the profile of scores on the Core Battery (Kaufman et al., 2005). For example, Delayed Recall measures the evaluation of a child's recall of paired associations learned 20 minutes earlier.

Because the K-ABC-II utilizes a dual theoretical approach, it permits alternate interpretation of the scales based on either the examiner's orientation or the specific individual being evaluated. For example, the index containing the Word Order, Number Recall, and Hand Movements subtests may be interpreted as Sequential Processing Skill (problem solving based on linear input) under the Luria model or Short-Term Memory (ability to apprehend and briefly hold information) under the CHC model.

The CHC is ordinarily the model of choice, particularly when assessing children with known or suspected LDs (Kaufman et al., 2005). However, the Luria model is recommended when exclusion of measures of acquired knowledge from the global scale promotes fairer assessment, for example, with individuals who have a receptive or expressive language disability or come from a bilingual background (Kaufman et al., 2005). Similar to the K-ABC, the K-ABC-II also provides a Nonverbal scale, with subtests that can be administered in pantomime and require a motor response.

Braden (2005) stated that although the manual justifies why crystallized ability knowledge is omitted from the Luria model, it does not justify why the same subtest scores can be interpreted in two different ways (e.g., why the same subtest reflects sequential processing in one examinee but short-term memory in another when interpreted under a different model). Kaufman and colleagues (2005) explained that the change in the two models was in response to criticism that the K-ABC interpreted mental processing scales solely from the sequential–simultaneous perspective. Braden (2005), in his review, concluded that the absence of direct evidence to support one model over another leaves the examiner wondering what the K-ABC-II actually tests.

Braden (2005) further stated that although the K-ABC does not explicitly use the current measurement standards to organize and evaluate validity evidence, it presents substantial evidence of validity in three domains (i.e., content validity, relationships within the test, and relationships to other tests). However, there is little evidence that K-ABC-II score patterns or profiles effectively discriminate among individuals with different types of LDs or ADHD. Another criticism is that there is no evidence that derived test data are useful in designing interventions. According to Thorndike (2005), in a review of the K-ABC, an important piece of validity evidence was not presented by the test's authors. Because the CAS was explicitly designed to assess the Luria processing model and extensive work has been done to validate the CAS, Thorndike suggests that the CAS should have been used to validate the K-ABC's use of the Luria model. Also, although most of the clinical studies reported in the manual in support of the K-ABC-II reveal mean differences between groups with disabilities and the norm group, the pattern of differences for the various scales for students with LDs is relatively flat, suggesting little diagnostic utility.

Summary of Validity

The K-ABC-II has evidence of content and criterion validity. Reviewers question the strength of the evidence to support the construct of intelligence, as defined by the selected processes. Most critical to this chapter is the need for an assessment to distinguish between children with LDs and the general population, and provide information to guide intervention. Currently the K-ABC-II cannot be recommended for these purposes.

Summary of Psychological Processes

Many professionals believe in the existence of intrinsic processing weaknesses as a construct underlying LD (Torgesen, 2002). The direct diagnosis of students with LDs through analysis of processing weaknesses potentially has several advantages over the IQ discrepancy approach, including early identification, inclusion of students without discrepancy between IQ and achievement, and the potential to focus instruction in areas of greatest need.

Similar to Torgesen (2004), we conclude that whereas psychological processing differences likely underlie the condition we call LDs, current understanding of processing operations and their relationship to learning are not sufficiently developed for either diagnosis or intervention. This conclusion does not mean it will never be possible to assess cognitive processes in a meaningful way, only that the necessary evidence is not currently available. The issue of diagnostic relevance is essential when evaluating measures of cognitive processing. Two questions arise: Are measures of psychological processing effective in diagnosing students with LD, and are they helpful in designing interventions? It seems that there is not solid evidence to support their relevance in either area. Fletcher, Coulter, Reschly, and Vaughn (2004) stated that "anecdotal links between cognitive processing and instruction are at best appealing experimental hypotheses that have not been validated despite extensive efforts over the past 30 years" (p. 321).

Certainly there are those who disagree with this conclusion. Kavale and colleagues (2005) argue that the negative perceptions regarding intellectual assessment/psychological processing and the development of useful diagnostic profiles from such assessments is a result of the strong influence of the *g* factor (general intelligence) implicit in the Wechsler scales. Kavale and colleagues suggested that newer tests of cognitive abilities (e.g., CAS) that have moved away from the *g* factor and are theory based will result in better individualized interventions.

Although these authors are appropriately impressed with the importance of theory, what seems to be missing in their formulations is the realization that a theory is important because one can generate and test hypotheses based on it. Theory in and of itself does not buy much if it is not used this way. It would seem that relevant propositions could be developed and tested (Fletcher et al., 2004).

A major hurdle to overcome is the lack of consensus on the meaning of the term "processing." Are the processing abilities to be evaluated those proposed by, for example, Naglieri,

those examined by indexes of the WISC or the WJ-COG, or those at the sublexical level, as in phonological processing? The issue is more than semantic, and research comparing the hypothesized processes across measures and perspectives would be valuable as one step toward consensus. Evidence of relevance to instruction needs to follow.

RESPONSE TO INTERVENTION

Background and Definition

RTI has gained favor as an important element in Federal regulations that govern the identification of LDs. The essence of RTI models is that evidenced-based instruction is provided with fidelity, progress is monitored frequently, and the child's responsiveness is evaluated (Batsche et al., 2005; Vaughn & Fuchs, 2003). In the context of the regulations for the implementation of IDEA (2004), there is a two-pronged test for LD eligibility: (1) The child does not achieve commensurate with peers in one of eight domains despite appropriate instruction, and (2) the child fails to make sufficient progress in meeting state-approved results. One of two methods can be used to judge the latter criterion. The first, an RTI method, was clearly favored in the discussion that accompanied the *proposed* regulations (*wrightslaw.com/idea/law.htm*). The second criterion requires a pattern of strengths and weaknesses either alone or in conjunction with intellectual ability that the multidisciplinary team believes is relevant for an LD diagnosis. The approved regulations maintain the exclusionary clauses that include sensory impairments, mental retardation, and economic and cultural differences. In addition, IDEA specifically states that a child may *not* be identified as having an LD if there was a lack of appropriate instruction in reading or math, or if the child has limited English proficiency.

It was anticipated that the regulatory language specifying a severe discrepancy between achievement and intellectual ability as a defining characteristic of LD would be altered. However, the final regulations for IDEA 2004 retained both RTI and IQ–achievement discrepancies, the latter a hallmark of LD identification since the first regulations were put in place in 1977.

In any event, the new emphasis in diagnosis is clearly on instruction. Although "failure to learn despite adequate instruction" has always been part of the Federal regulations for learning disabilities, documentation of "adequate instruction" never received serious consideration as part of a diagnostic workup (Speece & Shekitka, 2002). In schools, diagnostic information may include both classroom observations and prereferral activities designed to improve teaching and learning by making changes in the general education classroom prior to an eligibility decision. However, our experience suggests that the decision largely rests on data derived from published, norm-referenced tests, and not on observation, regardless of whether the school or a private practitioner makes the diagnosis.

RTI is an umbrella term encompassing a variety of different assessment and instructional approaches (e.g., D. Fuchs, Mock, Morgan, & Young, 2003; Marston, Muyskens, Lau, & Carter, 2003) However, there is some consensus on conceptualizing RTI as three tiers of increasingly intense instruction, with ongoing monitoring of progress. Tier 1 is general education instruction in which all children are receiving instruction deemed to be effective. Prior to the new regulations, general education was assumed to be effective without any substantiation. The thrust of the new regulations is a more rigorous approach to documenting the quality of general education, emphasizing instruction and curricula that have scientific support. Another proposal for assessing quality is monitoring student progress. When most students are making progress, the instruction is presumed to be effective (L. S. Fuchs, 1995; Fuchs & Fuchs, 1998). The extent to which this will mean monitoring all children is not clear, but several authors urge universal screening at a minimum, if not regular monitoring of all children (e.g., L. S. Fuchs, 1995; Speece & Case, 2001).

Tier 2 instruction may occur in the general education classroom (e.g., Fuchs & Fuchs, 1998; O'Connor, 2000; Speece & Case, 2001) or as an extra classroom supplement (e.g., Vaughn, Linan-Thompson, & Hickman, 2003; Vellutino et al., 1996). Tier 2 often includes two learning trials for a child considered at risk for learning problems, each lasting between 8 and 10 weeks. If the first trial does not result in improved learning, instruction is further modified and a second trial is undertaken. Tier 3 is associated with assessment for eligibility as an LD diagnosis, as well as more intensive instruc-

tion and continued monitoring of progress. Tier 3 is the most poorly defined of the three tiers, with no clear consensus on what further assessment may include or how an LD will be defined.

An RTI approach to diagnosis contains many moving parts, and a lack of integrity in any one part greatly damages the validity of the system. Elements include screening, research-based instruction, fidelity of implementation, valid progress monitoring, and interpretation. The inseparable linkage between instruction (research-based, fidelity) and assessment (screening, progress monitoring, interpretation) complicates the diagnostic process. The most fully developed model of RTI was presented by Fuchs and Fuchs (1998; L. S. Fuchs, 1995; Fuchs, Fuchs, & Speece, 2002). Originally called "treatment validity," Fuchs and Fuchs (1998) credited Messick (1984) with laying the groundwork for a special education diagnostic system that would result in more accurate identification of children from minority groups. In their initial four-phase model, all children receive frequent (e.g., weekly) assessments with curriculum-based measures (e.g., reading, math) in Phase 1. Within-classroom (or grade level) progress is quantified by two indices: level of performance at the end of the measurement period and slope reflecting growth across the measurement period. Children who deviate from the class level and slope by some amount (e.g., 1 SD below classroom means) are considered at risk for academic problems and are identified at the end of Phase 1. Fuchs and Fuchs (1998) referred to deficiencies on both level and slope as "dual discrepancies." In Phases 2 and 3, the general educator, continuing with progress monitoring, provides interventions to at-risk (dually discrepant) children. If after these two phases, a child's performance has not improved to acceptable standards, he or she would then proceed to Phase 4 to receive a trial placement in special education to determine whether the placement resulted in better learning.

Several nuances in this system deserve mention (Fuchs & Fuchs, 1998). First, general education instruction is considered adequate if level and slope data indicate that most children are profiting from the instruction. Classrooms with low performance compared to others would receive intervention at the classroom level to improve the overall learning trajectory of all children before identifying an individual child as being at risk. This procedure acknowledges the potential problem of poor instruction confounding risk status. Second, Fuchs and Fuchs specify that the first round of interventions occurs in general education, not in a separate setting with a different teacher. Fuchs (2002) makes a convincing case that to do otherwise blurs the distinction between general and special education. For example, what does it mean, diagnostically, when a child responds well to small-group instruction delivered by a specialist (or a paraprofessional for that matter)? Is the child remediated and ready to return to the general education classroom? Or does it mean the child should receive special education in which reduced teacher–child ratios are common? Fuchs argues that if the instruction needed to enhance a child's response cannot be implemented reasonably in general education, then the child likely needs special education.

Third, special education placement is not automatic. The same interpretation rules that apply at other phases remain in place; that is, the child must demonstrate a positive response to special education instruction for it to be considered a valid treatment. Holding special education accountable for progress is noteworthy and an aspect that should not get lost in transition to new systems. This requirement is not without problems, many of which have been discussed with recommendations (Fuchs, Fuchs, & Speece, 2002). The major issue is, what happens if special education is not successful? Returning the child to the general education environment is not reasonable, because it was a source of initial failure. Fuchs and colleagues (2002) suggested that educators and parents consider an alternative curriculum that may be better suited to the child's needs.

Validity of RTI Frameworks

Of importance to our consideration in this chapter is the extent to which treatment validity/RTI systems have demonstrated validity. Establishing validity for complex systems is daunting but no less a requirement than for single tests. It is certainly true that there are more published opinions than published evidence about RTI, a fact that gives us some pause. Two studies indicate that both academics and practicing professionals are in favor of an RTI approach to identifying reading disabilities. These data can serve as one piece of evidence in

Messick's validity matrix (values). Speece and Shekitka (2002), in a study that predated the acceptance of the RTI term, surveyed editorial board members of LD and related journals on criteria that should be used to identify reading disabilities. Two-thirds of respondents were in favor of RTI (treatment validity) as a criterion, with 30% endorsing IQ–achievement discrepancies and almost 50% selecting cognitive processing as a criterion. Whereas only 42% of respondents would include intelligence cutoff scores, 72% believed mental retardation should be retained as an exclusionary criterion. Because IQ tests would be required to rule out mental retardation, this result suggests that there is some ambivalence about the role of IQ tests in the identification of LDs.

Machek and Nelson (in press) (reviewed earlier in the chapter) replicated the Speece and Shekitka (2002) study with practicing school psychologists. This group also was in favor of RTI as a criterion (over 80% agreed or strongly agreed). Interestingly, over 60% also endorsed IQ–achievement discrepancies, and over 75% endorsed cognitive processing. The findings from both studies suggest that whereas RTI holds considerable appeal and acceptance, it is not unanimous. Considerable work in establishing relevance that also translates to training is needed, if RTI is to replace long-held beliefs about the roles of intelligence tests, achievement discrepancies, and cognitive processes in LDs.

A handful of studies address different validity questions. They are primarily concerned with construct validity—determining whether nonresponsive children are different from other children (Fuchs, 2003; Fuchs et al., 2005; McMaster, Fuchs, Fuchs, & Compton, 2005; Speece & Case; 2001; Speece, Case, & Molloy, 2003). There also are analyses of relevance based primarily on longitudinal outcomes (Case, Speece, & Molloy, 2003; Vaughn et al., 2003; Vellutino et al., 2003), with some attention to social-consequential validity (Speece & Case, 2001; Vaughn et al., 2003). These studies are reviewed to assess the extent to which evidence for validity is obtained.

Construct Validity

Speece and Case (2001) assessed the validity of three methods of identifying reading disability: (1) curriculum-based measurement (CBM) dual discrepancy on level and slope of oral reading fluency (ORF) performance compared to classmates (RTI), (2) IQ–reading achievement discrepancy, and (3) low reading achievement. From a population screen of 694 first- and second-grade children, they identified an epidemiological sample of at-risk and not-at-risk children based on performance early in the academic year on letter–sound fluency (LSF; first grade) and ORF (second grade). In this study, responsiveness was measured in relation to peers receiving general education instruction over most of the school year. The CBM dual-discrepancy group was compared to both IQ–reading discrepancy and low achievement groups on a battery of reading, reading-related, and behavioral measures. Although there were no differences on word-level reading skills, the CBM dual-discrepancy group was younger, more impaired on reading processes (phonological awareness and rapid automatic naming [RAN]), and was rated lower by teachers on academic competence. Furthermore, the CBM dual-discrepancy group reflected the gender and ethnic/racial distributions of the population. The IQ–reading discrepancy group was disproportionately white. Differences were larger for the comparisons between the CBM dual-discrepancy and IQ–reading discrepancy groups than for the CBM dual-discrepancy and low achievement groups. These findings were interpreted as providing evidence of both construct and social consequential validity in support of one aspect of RTI (identification in general education). CBM dual-discrepancy criteria (1 *SD* below classroom means for level and slope) identified 8% of the population *before* any specialized intervention, which is close to the 5% prevalence of LDs. However, the three identification methods were not distinct. There was a 25% overlap between CBM dual discrepancy and IQ–reading discrepancy, and a 60% overlap between CBM dual discrepancy and the low achievement criterion.

Interestingly, measures administered in the beginning of the academic year were not sensitive indicators of which children would experience reading problems at the end of the year. Neither of the two CBM measures nor phonological awareness fared well in the prediction of year-end reading status. These findings held for the classification of the CBM dual-discrepancy group and the entire pool of poor readers (Speece & Case, 2001). This suggests that more time-consuming methods that incorporate growth in learning may be necessary for

valid classification. Speece, Case, and Molloy (2003) further investigated the relative merits of a static versus a growth view of identification with respect to classification accuracy. First- and second-grade children who scored above a standard score of 90 on the Basic Reading Skills cluster score (WJ-R) were examined with respect to their oral reading fluency skill and status as CBM dually discrepant to determine who might be missed if a static low achievement criterion was used to identify early reading failure. Twenty percent of first-grade children and 25% of second-grade children who scored above 90 also scored *below* the 25th percentile on ORF (15 words per minute [wpm], first grade; 51 wpm, second grade), indicative of severe reading difficulty. Thus, the Basic Reading Skills cluster score was not sensitive to poor oral reading fluency and would result in missing children who were deficient in a critical reading skill. Of the 48 first- and second-grade children who were above 90 on Basic Reading Skills but below the 25th percentile on CBM ORF, 12 were also identified as CBM dually discrepant. Not only were their levels of fluency discrepant from peers, but also their rate of growth. These and other findings support the inference that the addition of growth measures to an identification formula may assist in the identification of true-positive cases (Compton, Fuchs, Fuchs, & Bryant, 2005; Fuchs et al., 2005; Speece, 2005).

L. S. Fuchs and colleagues (Fuchs, 2003; D. Fuchs, Fuchs, & Compton, 2004; Fuchs et al., 2005) also examined the validity of different RTI identification strategies. Their general approach was to apply a variety of identification criteria to a sample and compare them on relevant measures. Methods that identify larger between-group differences on relevant measures and a reasonable number of children with problems are viewed more favorably. For example, Fuchs (2003) compared CBM level, CBM slope, and CBM dual discrepancy to see which would function as the best identification method (number of children identified, size of group differences). Second-grade children comprised the sample. Performance level and slope estimates were based on the first 10 weeks of school. Outcomes included end-of-year level and across-year slope on word identification, word attack, and comprehension. CBM dual discrepancy yielded the smallest number of nonresponsive children (5%) compared to CBM slope (15%) and CBM level (16%). Both

CBM level and CBM dual discrepancy yielded significant and large differences on the word measures but not comprehension. Although obtaining CBM dual discrepancies requires more time devoted to identification, in this analysis, it was the superior method.

Using the same approach with first-grade children, McMaster and colleagues (2005) examined nonresponsiveness to Tier 2 reading interventions. Tier 2 children were those who showed lower rates of response to a validated general education reading program. Five definitions of nonresponsiveness to Tier 2 interventions were analyzed: dual discrepancy; level on either published, norm-referenced measures or a CBM benchmark; and either no growth or limited growth on published, norm-referenced word-level measures. The percentages of nonresponders based on the total Tier 2 sample as defined by each definition were 70, 45, 100, 7, and 39, respectively. These figures illustrate how dramatic the differences may be with various criteria. Although there is no consensus on how to evaluate these Tier 2 percentages given that they do not represent population prevalence, the CBM benchmark definition (< 40 wpm) that yielded 100% nonresponders is likely too high, because no child is identified as responsive. Other researchers have reached the same conclusion regarding this criterion (D. Fuchs et al., 2004; Speece, 2005).

In a rare study of identification of math disability and response to intervention, Fuchs and colleagues (2005) compared 17 definitions that included IQ–achievement discrepancy, low achievement–average IQ, normalized achievement RTI, and slope RTI (including dual discrepancy on level and slope). The validity of each method was judged positively if it produced a prevalence rate of math disability between 4 and 7% and an effect size of 0.50 or better on one of several math outcome measures. Several approaches met the validity criteria: IQ–achievement discrepancy with untimed math concepts and applications as the achievement measure; normalized achievement on either untimed math concepts and applications or basic addition fact fluency, and CBM dual discrepancy based on math computation fluency. The authors noted that the IQ–achievement discrepancy method may produce valid findings, because the achievement measure was sensitive to performance differences at the low end of the achievement range, a fact that may not be true of published, norm-referenced mea-

sures such as the WJ-III-ACH. The study by Speece, Case, and Molloy (2003) reviewed earlier also supports this insight.

SUMMARY OF CONSTRUCT VALIDITY

The bulk of the evidence suggests that some RTI methods identify a group of children who experience serious learning problems. Methods that include slope as a criterion, in addition to level of performance, identify a reasonable number of children (i.e., 4–10%) who differ significantly, and often substantially, from children who do not have academic growth and level deficits. These studies provide evidence of construct validity. Whether these children should be labeled learning disabled is open to debate and further inquiry. The database is limited to early elementary school children and reading, with few exceptions. This limited coverage of developmental levels and academic domains is of concern given Federal initiatives to support RTI approaches to the identification of LDs. Studies are needed that incorporate larger and more diverse samples and a wider array of measures and domains. Another issue that hinders evaluation is that RTI criteria are arbitrary. For example, to identify students for further intervention, Speece and Case (2001) defined "dual discrepancy" as 1 SD below the mean level and slope of classmates who were not considered at risk for reading problems. McMaster and colleagues (2005), however, defined "dual discrepancy" as .5 SD below the mean level and slope of all average achieving students in the study. Thus, the case for RTI construct validity is positive but limited in scope to children in early elementary school and reading.

Relevance

Relevance, in terms of RTI, is interpreted as an evaluation of the extent to which the procedures produce meaningful outcomes. This criterion might include consumer satisfaction, the extent to which children were over- or underidentified, and longitudinal outcomes. As with construct validity, the data are limited but interpreted as promising.

Compton and colleagues (2005) investigated the usefulness of slope as a predictor of reading status for 206 children at risk for reading problems. The focus of their study was to identify effective screening procedures to identify which children should receive a Tier 2 intervention. Slope was based on CBM word identification fluency (WIF) across 5 weeks in first grade, signifying responsiveness to general education instruction. Other predictors included WIF level, phonemic awareness, rapid naming, and oral vocabulary. A composite measure of reading based on the end of second grade performance was used to classify children as reading disabled. Several models were evaluated for their classification sensitivity (correct identification of at-risk children with RD) and specificity (correct identification of children without RD). The first model, which included all variables except WIF level and slope, resulted in reasonable classification rates. The addition of WIF initial level, WIF slope, and WIF 5-week level resulted in much better classification accuracy, with 90% sensitivity and 83% specificity in one case, and 100% sensitivity and 93% specificity in another model. Although the classification approaches tested require statistical sophistication, the results indicate that fluency growth measures, which are often used in RTI models, provide important information to identify children in need of more intensive instruction.

Case and colleagues (2003) asked if persistent nonresponsiveness to classroom literacy instruction over time identified a unique group of poor readers. In addition to the screening procedures and classification of poor readers (CBM dual discrepancy) used by Speece and Case (2001), the investigators worked with 25 general education teachers across 3 years to develop reading interventions that the teachers then implemented in their classrooms for children classified as poor readers. Dual-discrepancy status was assessed two to three times per year. The longitudinal sample comprised 36 first- and second-grade children identified as being at risk on Fall screening measures in one school. These at-risk children were placed into one of three groups based on their responsiveness to instruction across 3 years: never dually discrepant (NDD; *n* = 12), infrequently dually discrepant (IDD, *n* = 17), and frequently dually discrepant (FDD; *n* = 7). The IDD group was identified one to three times and the FDD group was identified four or more times as dually discrepant. Case and colleagues hypothesized that the FDD group should be more impaired on reading, reading-related, behavioral, and school attention measures if responsiveness to instruction is a valid indicator of child status. School attention was the sum of extra classroom assistance (e.g., reading specialist, special educator) and services (e.g., parent meetings, IEP meetings) received by the child. There were clear and significant differences between FDD and NDD (word reading, pseudoword reading, word reading fluency, academic competence, problem behavior, school attention) and between FDD and IDD (Word Reading, Word Reading Fluency, Academic Competence, Problem Behavior, School Attention). In all cases cited, the FDD group performed less well than the comparison group. The sensitivity of these groupings was reflected by one NDD–IDD difference (Problem Behavior) and small to moderate effect sizes (ESs) on other measures (e.g., ES = 0.25 for phonological awareness, –0.60 for problem behaviors). Contextual measures (classroom observations of instruction, teachers' years of experience, classroom reading slopes) did not produce differences between the groups, but the effect size for classroom slope (NDD–FDD ES = –0.42) suggested that the FDD group might have experienced stronger instructional environments.

The Case and colleagues (2003) study spanned 3 years but RTI models in practice would identify children for more intensive instruction within one school year, as was done by Vaughn and colleagues (2003) in a study of Tier 2 interventions. They provided small groups of at-risk second-grade readers with daily supplemental reading instruction and evaluated their progress every 10 weeks. Children who met the criterion were dismissed from the instruction, whereas the others continued to receive instruction for up to 30 weeks. Regardless of status, children continued to receive assessments. Children who responded quickly to the instruction (after 10 weeks) were more likely to maintain progress in general education than were children who needed 20 weeks of supplemental instruction. This finding suggests that Tier 2 instruction defined as a pullout service may differentiate between students who need a short-term "boost" and those students who need more intensive and long-term support. However, whereas all children in the 10-week exit group continued to make good progress after 10 weeks in the general education curriculum, 30% were making *minimal* growth after 20 weeks. Thus, quick response is not synonymous with a "quick fix," and the finding emphasizes the importance of constant progress monitoring. The researchers also reported that the children who met the criterion at 10 or 20 weeks differed from children who never met the criterion on passage comprehension, passage reading fluency, and rapid naming of letters and digits measured at baseline. Thus, children who were persistently nonresponsive did experience more serious problems.

Vellutino and colleagues (1996) provided individual reading tutoring to at-risk first-grade children for one or two semesters and assessed differences between groups defined by their responsiveness to the tutoring. Participants had to be nominated by their first-grade teachers, have either a performance or verbal intelligence test score of 90 or above, and score at or below the 15th percentile on a word-level test. The study was framed to differentiate between reading problems due to educational experience and those due to within-child deficits, a basic tenet of RTI frameworks (Fuchs & Fuchs, 1998). The authors concluded that the primary difference between at-risk children who had higher and lower responsiveness rates was skill with phonological measures when compared to normal readers. Interestingly, and similar to Vaughn and colleagues (2003), phonological measures did not distinguish between the very high- and very low-growth tutored children, but rapid naming tasks did. Vellutino, Scanlon, and Jacard (2003) provided a follow-up report on the tutored children at the end of third and fourth grades. The percentage of children in the very high-growth group who scored above the 25th percentile was similar at the end of second, third, and fourth grades, 95–100%, as was the percentage of very limited-growth readers, 10–16%. The authors do not state whether the same children were in the normal range at each assessment point, an important consideration in determining if the low-growth students who did respond to the tutoring maintained their advantage. In any event, these data suggest that children who do not respond to a very structured and intensive intervention in first and second grades will likely require special education and could conceivably be considered reading disabled.

SUMMARY OF RELEVANCE VALIDITY

All four studies provide evidence that children identified by RTI approaches have meaningfully different outcomes over time. This conclusion holds whether instruction reflects usual general education instruction, modified general education instruction, or small-group or individual tutoring. The Case and colleagues (2003) study also showed that teachers across 3 years viewed the persistent nonresponders as less academically competent, and the school provided these children with more resources. The implication is that children who do not respond to instruction represent a meaningful and recognizable group to practitioners. A major methodological issue is the small sample sizes associated with these studies; thus, replication and extension are required to elaborate the case for validity.

Measuring Responsiveness

Academic Domains

CBM is by far the most frequently used measurement system to document response to intervention. CBM represents a set of measures with multiple alternate probes (test forms) in the basic academic domains of reading, math, spelling, and writing. They are designed to be brief, time-based assessments that measure fluency (accuracy and rate). Importantly, they are general outcome measures and, because of this feature, can be distinguished from other types of curriculum-based assessment (CBA) procedures such as mastery measurement (Fuchs & Deno, 1991; Hintze, Christ, & Methe, 2006). The distinction is that general outcome measures assess progress toward a goal (e.g., proficiency in end-of-year reading curriculum), whereas mastery measures assess what was taught. Mastery measurement is based on a task-analysis conceptualization of learning in which discrete skills are taught and assessed. The assumption is that the accumulation of such activities represents progress monitoring (Fuchs, 2004). In contrast, items for CBM probes are sampled randomly from the entire curriculum, or from the part of the curriculum that represents goal material (e.g., books that represent end-of-year reading). Thus, each probe is a parallel form that either represents the entire curriculum or the goal curriculum.

For example, the familiar weekly spelling test is a mastery measurement assessment. Typically each lesson contains a specific grapheme or grapheme–phoneme convention (e.g., silent *e*, double vowels, consonant blends). Children study a list of words, take a test on Friday, and begin again with a new list the following Monday. In contrast, CBM spelling begins with defining the curriculum (all words in the second-grade spelling text), randomly selecting 20 words from the pool of all words for each probe, and repeating the selection process to have enough probes for weekly assessment. The advantage of CBM for RTI is sensitivity to growth in the curriculum.

The research that supports CBM reflects the validity issues emphasized by Messick (1989, 1995): technical adequacy (construct validity), treatment validity (consequences), and feasibility (relevance) (Deno, Fuchs, Marston, & Shin, 2001; Fuchs & Fuchs, 1998). A number of reviews of this voluminous literature confirm excellent reliability and validity, the connection between growth on CBM and achievement, and usefulness for teachers (Fuchs & Fuchs, 1986; Hosp & Hosp, 2003; Madelaine & Wheldall, 1999; Shinn, 1989; Stecker, Fuchs, & Fuchs, 2005). The Research Institute on Progress Monitoring identified over 500 documents devoted to CBM, with 141 representing published studies (Espin & Wallace, 2004). Reading was the most frequent content area reflected in the articles (58%), followed by math (18%), writing (5%), and spelling (4%). A searchable database for these documents may be accessed online at *progressmonitoring.org*.

Administration of CBM is relatively easy, especially for professionals who are proficient with timing responses, and who understand the importance of standard administration and scoring. The several sources for probes include the World Wide Web (e.g., *www.aimsweb.com* and *www.dibels.uoregon.edu*) and educational publishers (e.g., *Monitoring Basic Skills Progress*; Fuchs, Hamlett, & Fuchs [1998]). The website for the National Center on Student Progress Monitoring (*www.studentprogress. org*) is recommended as the first stop for the examiner interested in training, evaluation of the available instruments, and further information on probe availability that includes no-cost options.

Examples of an examiner protocol and child copy for passage reading fluency (PRF) are shown in Figures 13.1 and 13.2, respectively. The examiner reads the directions at the top of the protocol; the child reads for 1 minute while the examiner marks errors. The measure of interest is the number of words read correctly in 1 minute. The time varies depending on measure and academic domain. Figure 13.3 illustrates first- and second-grade PRF progress

monitoring data for a child. The graphs were produced with the software available from Fuchs and colleagues (1998). The vertical lines indicate that a change of instruction occurred; "G" represents the goal established for the child, and "T" is the child's trend (average) line. In Janis's case, three interventions were attempted in her first (Reading 1) and second (Reading 2) general education classrooms, because she demonstrated a dual discrepancy relative to her classmates. There were not enough data points to establish a trend line for the last intervention, but it is evident that Janis was not making sufficient progress to meet the goal. These data illustrate a possible scenario for Tier 3 assessment and intervention when general education is not effective.

Although there are many reasons to recommend CBM as a progress monitoring tool, there are limitations. The lack of national norms makes it difficult to interpret data outside the local context. There are several sources that compile benchmarks and growth rates from the available literature (Deno et al., 2001; Fuchs & Fuchs, 2004; Hosp & Hosp, 2003), and the DIBELS website (*www.dibels. uoregon.edu*) provides benchmarks based on extensive, unpublished data. These sources provide guidelines that can be supplemented with school system norms. Another drawback is the primary focus on measures for the elementary school years. Progress monitoring measures for secondary students are in development, but the research base is in its early stages (e.g., Espin & Foegen, 1996; Espin et al., 2000). Finally, results from CBM progress monitoring data with decision rules indicate whether an instructional change is required, but not necessarily what the instructional change should be. There is some work in this area (Fuchs, Fuchs, & Hamlett, 1994) that requires elaboration. We find that analysis of several probes (e.g., PRF) provides sufficient clinical information upon which to offer instructional ideas, but systematizing an approach would be of benefit to most users.

Preacademic Skills

The strength of CBM research and practice coupled with national interest in early reading assessment, prevention, and intervention (e.g., National Reading Panel 2000; Snow, Burns, & Griffin, 1998) spawned the development of prereading and premath fluency tasks that mir-

CBM #1/Grade 1

Student:		Teacher:	
School:		Date:	
Grade:		Examiner:	
# attempted		# of errors	# read correctly

Instructions

You are going to read this story titled *Frog Feels Sick* out loud. This story is about when Toad tried to make his friend Frog feel better. (*Place the reading passage in front of the student, face down.*) Try to read each word. You can use your finger to keep your place. If you come to a word you don't know, I'll tell it to you. You will read for one minute. Be sure to do your best reading. Do you have any questions? (*Turn the passage right-side up.*) Put your finger on the first word. Begin.

Frog Feels Sick

One day in summer Frog was not feeling well.	9
Toad said, "Frog, you are looking quite green."	17
"But I always look green," said Frog. "I am a frog."	28
"Today you look very green even for a frog," said Toad.	39
"Get into bed and rest."	44
Toad made Frog a cup of hot tea. Frog drank the tea, and	57
then he said, "Tell me a story while I am resting."	68
"All right," said Toad. "Let me think of a story to tell	80
you."	81
Toad thought and thought. But he could not think of a	92
story to tell Frog.	96
"I will go out on the front porch and walk up and down,"	109
said Toad. "Perhaps that will help me think of a story."	120

FIGURE 13.1. Example of an examiner's protocol for a curriculum-based measurement probe of passage reading fluency.

Frog Feels Sick

One day in summer Frog was not feeling well.

Toad said, "Frog, you are looking quite green."

"But I always look green," said Frog. "I am a frog."

"Today you look very green even for a frog," said Toad.

"Get into bed and rest."

Toad made Frog a cup of hot tea. Frog drank the tea, and then he said, "Tell me a story while I am resting."

"All right," said Toad. "Let me think of a story to tell you."

Toad thought and thought. But he could not think of a story to tell Frog.

"I will go out on the front porch and walk up and down," said Toad. "Perhaps that will help me think of a story."

FIGURE 13.2. Example of a child's protocol for a curriculum-based measurement probe of passage reading fluency.

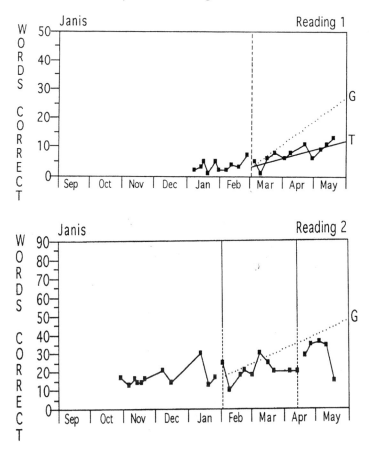

FIGURE 13.3. Graph of passage reading fluency performance for a child in first (top panel) and second grade. G, goal; T, trendline; vertical lines signal a change in instruction.

ror CBM tasks. The best known effort is the Dynamic Indicators of Early Literacy (DIBELS; 2001) system, in which fluency of sublexical skills such as letter names, initial sounds, and phonemic segmentation are measured (Good, Simmons, & Kame'enui, 2001; Kaminski & Good, 1996). This is a new area of research and as such, most of the validity data reflect that of construct validity in Messick's terms (1995). Researchers also have investigated the validity of letter–sound fluency (Ritchey & Speece, 2006; Speece, Mills, Ritchey, & Hillman, 2003; Stage, Sheppard, Davidson, & Browning, 2001) and premath skills (VanDerHeyden et al., 2004; VanDerHeyden, Witt, Naquin, & Noell, 2001).

Although these preacademic tasks are often called "CBM," there are important distinctions (Fuchs & Fuchs, 1999). Prereading fluency measures assess a single skill that does not rep-

resent the general outcome of word recognition and reading comprehension. In contrast, PRF reflects word recognition and comprehension processes (Jenkins, Fuchs, van den Broek, Espin, & Deno, 2003), the goals of reading instruction. There is concern that single-skill measurement may narrow the range of skills teachers may teach, and that the measures may not adequately model growth in the curriculum (Fuchs & Fuchs, 1999). Ritchey and Speece (2006) reported that letter–sound fluency slope predicted word reading at the end of kindergarten, suggesting some relation between sublexical growth and reading outcomes. The DIBELS website provides benchmarks that could be construed as evidence of growth. However, several research reports indicate that the benchmarks yield too many false-positive cases (Fuchs, 2003; Hintze, Ryan, & Stoner, 2003; Speece, 2005). Further work along the lines of the research program that guided CBM is required to understand the full range of validity questions. Construct validity is established for several of the measures, so they can be viewed as predictors of literacy outcomes, but their use as progress monitoring or diagnostic measures is premature.

RECOMMENDATIONS AND FUTURE DIRECTIONS

Although our own work focuses on RTI, not psychological processes, and, accordingly, we view RTI as more viable for the identification of LDs, examination of validity indicates both approaches require more work to claim the high ground. There is evidence of construct validity for each. It is true that RTI has a stronger hold on relevance given the direct tie to instruction and child outcomes (e.g., Speece & Case, 2001; Vaughn et al., 2003; Vellutino et al., 1996), but there remain a large number of questions to be examined, such as validity for older children, academic domains beyond reading and math, applicability to children in kindergarten and preschoolers, methods to ensure fidelity of treatment as RTI goes to scale in schools, and methods to reduce the cumbersome nature of the RTI enterprise. Major issues for psychological processing methods include demonstrating a contribution beyond what is learned from achievement tests and evaluating instructional relevance through tighter research designs that include experimental control and larger samples. Both methods need to be more definitive about the criteria for diagnosing a learning disability.

Obviously, clinicians and practitioners do not have the luxury of waiting for definitive answers if, indeed, any are forthcoming. Current best practice is to implement an RTI system with all the components (increasingly intensive instruction across three tiers, progress monitoring, and fidelity of instruction). In line with IDEA, Tier 3 must include a multifaceted assessment in relevant domains *as needed*, in addition to continued progress monitoring. This *may* mean an intellectual assessment, if mental retardation is suspected, but this assessment would not be routine. We advocate greater sensitivity to potential comorbid conditions, including social emotional functioning, ADHD, and academic domains other than that cited in the referral. There is a great deal of evidence that chil-

dren's attention to task predicts academic performance (e.g., McKinney, Mason, Perkerson, & Clifford, 1975; McKinney & Speece, 1983; Speece & Cooper, 1990; Stage et al., 2003; Torgesen et al., 1999). This general conclusion holds whether behavior is measured directly through observation or inferred from behavior ratings by teachers. A number of instruments are available to assess attention and should be incorporated as indicated in a comprehensive assessment. Our preference is to conduct minimalist assessments beyond the information on discrepant learning levels and rates provided by RTI. Selected measures should emphasize informing instruction and not comparisons with a norm group.

As the foregoing suggests, RTI is a school-based process. This raises the question of how private practitioners will participate in LD identification if RTI holds sway. If a state educational agency decides that an RTI process is required as part of the diagnostic process, then nonschool practitioners will need to develop additional procedures to work in schools. The proposed regulations, however, provide leeway for a business as usual approach (i.e., testing to document discrepancy and psychological processing difficulties). This flexibility will likely lead to conflict between school systems that adopt RTI and outside practitioners who base diagnosis on a different set of criteria. States will need to consider this possibility and be clear on what counts as evidence. One possible resolution may be the development of dynamic assessment procedures in which test–train–test paradigms administered in single sessions or over a brief amount of time assess responsiveness (e.g., Speece, Cooper, & Kibler, 1990; Swanson & Howard, 2005). Dynamic assessment connected to academic learning holds promise as an efficient approach to RTI and is in development (D. Fuchs, personal communication, October 2005).

Advances in the neurosciences also hold promise for informing psychological processing methods of assessment. Recent work documenting changes in brain activation patterns as a result of reading interventions may ultimately assist in linking these patterns with behavioral measures (e.g., Shaywitz et al., 2004; Simos et al., 2005; Temple et al., 2003). It will be important to expand the behavioral measures to include newer versions of intellectual assessment (i.e., CAS, K-ABC-II) to further assess construct validity.

Although it is unsettling to have such ambiguity in definition and identification for a construct with a long history, as Doris (1986) noted, the LD field actually has a short scientific past. Assessment of LD is more a clinical than a statistical enterprise. Paul Meehl (1954) urged us to put more work in the latter to achieve the validity that the LD field demands.

ACKNOWLEDGMENTS

Work on this chapter was supported by Grant No. H325D020040 from the Office of Special Education Programs, U.S. Department of Education. The opinions expressed here are not necessarily those of the funding institute. We acknowledge with appreciation the contributions of Ming-yi Cho and Caroline Walker.

REFERENCES

Adams, M. (1990). *Beginning to read*. Cambridge, MA: MIT Press.

American Psychiatric Association. (2000). *Diagnostic and statistical manual of mental disorders* (4th ed., text rev.). Washington, DC: Author.

Bannatyne, A. (1968). Diagnosing learning disabilities and writing remedial prescriptions. *Journal of Learning Disabilities*, 1, 242–249.

Bannatyne, A. (1974). Diagnosis: A note on recategorization of the WISC scaled scores. *Journal of Learning Disabilities*, 7, 272–274.

Barbaresi, W. J., Katusic, S. K., Colligan, R. C., Weaver, A. L., & Jacobsen, S. J. (2005). Math learning disorder: Incidence in a population-based birth cohort, 1976–82, Rochester, MN. *Ambulatory Pediatrics*, 5, 281–289.

Bateman, B. (2005). The play's the thing. *Learning Disabilities Quarterly*, 28, 93–95.

Batsche, G., Elliott, J., Graden, J. L., Grimes, J., Kovaleski, J. F., Prasse, D., et al. (2005). *Response to intervention: Policy considerations and implementation*. Alexandria, VA: National Association of State Directors of Special Education.

Boden, C., & Kirby, J. R. (1995). Successive processing, phonological coding and the remediation of reading. *Journal of Cognitive Education*, 4, 19–31.

Braden, J. P., & Niebling, B. C. (2005). Using the joint test standards to evaluate the validity evidence for intelligence tests. In D. P. Flanagan & P. L. Harrison (Eds.), *Contemporary intellectual assessment: Theories, tests, and issues* (2nd ed., pp. 615–641). New York: Guilford Press.

Braden, J. P., & Outzs, S. M. (2005). [Review of the test Kaufman Assessment Battery for Children Second Edition]. *Sixteenth Mental Measurements Yearbook*. Retrieved March 10, 2007, from the Mental Measurements Yearbook database, accession no. 16073158.

Bryan, T. (1998). Social competence of students with learning disabilities. In B. Wong (Ed.), *Learning about learning disabilities* (2nd ed., pp. 237–275). San Diego, CA: Academic Press.

Bryan, T., Burstein, K., & Ergul, C. (2004). The social–emotional side of learning disabilities: A science-based presentation of the state of the art. *Learning Disabilities Quarterly*, 27, 45–51.

Carlson, J., & Das, J. P. (1997). A process approach to remediating word decoding difficulties in Chapter 1 children. *Learning Disabilities Quarterly*, 20, 93–102.

Case, L. P., Speece, D. L., & Molloy, D. E. (2003). The validity of a response-to-instruction paradigm to identify reading disabilities: A longitudinal analysis of individual differences and contextual factors. *School Psychology Review*, 32, 557–582.

Cizek, G. J. (2005). [Review of the test Woodcock–Johnson(R) III]. *Sixteenth Mental Measurements Yearbook*. Retrieved March 10, 2007, from Mental Measurements Yearbook database, accession no. 15072743.

Compton, D. L., Fuchs, D., Fuchs, L. S., & Bryant, J. D. (2005). *Selecting at-risk readers in first grade for early intervention: A two-year longitudinal study of decision rules and procedures*. Unpublished manuscript, Vanderbilt University.

D'Angiulli, A., & Siegel, L. S. (2003). Cognitive functioning as measured by the WISC-R. *Journal of Learning Disabilities*, 36, 48–59.

Das, J. P. (1999). *PASS reading enhancement program*. Deal, NJ: Sacra Educational Resources.

Das, J. P., Mishra, R. K., & Pool, J. E. (1995). An experiment on cognitive remediation of word-reading difficulty. *Journal of Learning Disabilities*, 28, 66–79.

Deno, S. L., Fuchs, L. S., Marston, D., & Shin, J. (2001). Using curriculum-based measurement to establish growth standards for students with learning disabilities. *School Psychology Review*, 30, 507–524.

DIBELS. (2001). *Dynamic Indicators of Early Literacy Skills*. Retrieved September 6, 2001, from *www.dibels.uoregon.edu/measures*

Doris, J. (1986). Learning disabilities. In S. J. Cecil (Ed.), *Handbook of cognitive, social, and neuropsychological aspects of learning disabilities* (Vol. 1, pp. 3–53). Hillsdale, NJ: Erlbaum.

Elksnin, L. K., & Elksnin, N. (2004). The social–emotional side of learning disabilities. *Learning Disabilities Quarterly*, 27, 3–8.

Espin, C. A., & Foegen, A. (1996). Validity of general outcome measures for predicting secondary students' performance on content-area tasks. *Exceptional Children*, 62, 497–514.

Espin, C. A., Shin, J., Deno, S. L., Skare, S., Robinson, S., & Benner, B. (2000). Identifying indicators of written expression proficiency for middle school students. *Journal of Special Education*, 34, 140–153.

Espin, C. L., & Wallace, T. (2004, May). *CBM literature* (Working document). Minneapolis: University of

Minnesota Research Institute on Progress Monitoring.

Evans, J. J., Floyd, R. G., McGrew, K. S., & Leforgee, M. H. (2002). The relations between measures of Cattell–Horn–Carroll (CHC) Cognitive Abilities and Reading Achievement during childhood and adolescence. *School Psychology Review*, 31, 246–263.

Fiorello, C. A., & Primrano, D. (2005). Research into practice: Cattell–Horn–Carroll Cognitive Assessment in practice: Eligibility and program development issues. *Psychology in the Schools*, 42, 525–536.

Flanagan, D. P., & Kaufman, A. S. (2004). *Essentials of WISC-IV assessment.* Hoboken, NJ: Wiley.

Fletcher, J. M., Coulter, W. A., Reschly, D. J., & Vaughn, S. (2004). Alternative approaches to the definition and identification of learning disabilities: Some questions and answers. *Annals of Dyslexia*, 54, 304–331.

Fletcher, J. M., Lyon, G. R., Barnes, M., Stuebing, K. K., Francis, D. J., Olson, R., et al. (2002). Classification of learning disabilities: An evidence based evaluation. In R. Bradley, L. Danielson, & D. P. Hallahan (Eds.), *Identification of learning disabilities: Research to practice* (pp. 185–250). Mahwah, NJ: Erlbaum.

Fletcher, J. M., Morris, R. D., & Lyon, G. R. (2003). Classification and identification of learning disabilities. In H. L. Swanson, K. R. Harris, & S. Graham (Eds.), *Handbook of learning disabilities* (pp. 30–56). New York: Guilford Press.

Fletcher, J. M., Shaywitz, S. E., Shankweiler, D. P., Katz, L., Liberman, I. Y., Stuebing, K. K., et al. (1994). Cognitive profiles of reading disability: Comparisons of discrepancy and low achievement definitions. *Journal of Educational Psychology*, 86, 6–23.

Floyd, R. G., Evans, J. J., & McGrew, K. (2003). Relations between measures of Cattell–Horn–Carroll (CHC) cognitive abilities and mathematical achievement across the school age years. *Psychology in the Schools*, 40, 155–171.

Fuchs, D., Fuchs, L. S., & Compton, D. L. (2004). Identifying reading disabilities by responsiveness-to-instruction: Specifying measures and criteria. *Learning Disability Quarterly*, 27, 216–227.

Fuchs, D., Mock, D., Morgan, P. L., & Young, C. L. (2003). Responsiveness to intervention: Definitions, evidence, and implications for the learning disabilities construct. *Learning Disabilities Research and Practice*, 18, 157–171.

Fuchs, L. S. (1995, May). *Incorporating curriculum-based measurement into the eligibility decision-making process: A focus on treatment validity and student growth.* Paper presented at the Workshop on IQ Testing and Educational Decision Making, National Research Council, National Academy of Science, Washington, DC.

Fuchs, L. S. (2002). Three conceptualizations of "treatment" in a responsiveness-to-treatment framework for LD identification. In R. Bradley, L. Danielson, & D. P. Hallahan (Eds.), *Identification of learning disabilities* (pp. 521–529). Mahwah, NJ: Erlbaum.

Fuchs, L. S. (2003). Assessing intervention responsiveness: Conceptual and technical issues. *Learning Disabilities Research and Practice*, 81, 172–186.

Fuchs, L. S. (2004). The past, present, and future of curriculum-based measurement research. *School Psychology Review*, 33, 188–192.

Fuchs, L. S., Compton, D. L., Fuchs, D., Paulsen, K., Bryant, J. D., & Hamlett, C. L. (2005). The prevention, identification, and cognitive determinants of math difficulty. *Journal of Educational Psychology*, 97(3), 493–513.

Fuchs, L. S., & Deno, S. L. (1991). Paradigmatic distinctions between instructionally relevant measurement models. *Exceptional Children*, 57, 488–500.

Fuchs, L. S., & Fuchs, D. (1986). Effects of systematic formative evaluation: A meta-analysis. *Exceptional Children*, 53, 199–208.

Fuchs, L. S., & Fuchs, D. (1998). Treatment validity: A unifying concept for reconceptualizing the identification of learning disabilities. *Learning Disabilities Research and Practice*, 13, 204–219.

Fuchs, L. S., & Fuchs, D. (1999). Monitoring student progress toward the development of reading competence: A review of three forms of classroom-based assessment. *School Psychology Review*, 28, 659–671.

Fuchs, L. S., & Fuchs, D. (2004). Determining adequate yearly progress from kindergarten through grade 6 with curriculum-based measurement. *Assessment for Effective Intervention*, 29(4), 25–37.

Fuchs, L. S., Fuchs, D., & Compton, D. L. (2004). Monitoring early reading development in first grade: Word identification fluency versus nonsense word fluency. *Exceptional Children*, 71, 7–21.

Fuchs, L. S., Fuchs, D., & Hamlett, C. L. (1994). Strengthening the connection between assessment and instructional planning with expert systems. *Exceptional Children*, 61, 138–146.

Fuchs, L. S., Fuchs, D., & Speece, D. L. (2002). Treatment validity as a unifying construct for identifying learning disabilities. *Learning Disability Quarterly*, 25, 33–45.

Fuchs, L. S., Hamlett, C., & Fuchs, D. (1998). *Monitoring Basic Skills Progress.* Austin, TX: PRO-ED.

Good, R. H., & Jefferson, G. (1998). Contemporary perspectives on curriculum-based measurement validity. In M. R. Shinn (Ed.), *Advanced applications of curriculum-based measurement.* New York: Guilford Press.

Good, R. H., III, Simmons, D. C., & Kame'enui, E. J. (2001). The importance and decision-making utility of a continuum of fluency-based indicators of foundational reading skills for third-grade high-stakes outcomes. *Scientific Studies of Reading*, 5, 257–288.

Groth-Marnat, G. (2003). *Handbook of psychological assessment* (4th ed.). Hoboken, NJ: Wiley.

Haddad, F. A., Garcia, Y. E., Naglieri, J. A., Grimditch, M., McAndrews, A., & Eubanks, J. (2003). Planning facilitation and reading comprehension: Instructional relevance of the PASS theory. *Journal of Psychoeducational Assessment*, 21, 282–289.

Hale, J. B., & Fiorello, C. A. (2004). *School neuropsychology: *A practitioner's handbook*. New York: Guilford Press.

Hallahan, D. P., & Mercer, C. D. (2002). Learning disabilities: Historical perspectives. In R. Bradley, L. Danielson, & D. P. Hallahan (Eds.), *Identification of learning disabilities: Research to practice* (pp. 1–79). Mahwah, NJ: Erlbaum.

Hallahan, D. P., & Mock, D. R. (2003). A brief history of the field of learning disabilities. In H. L. Swanson, K. R. Harris, & S. Graham (Eds.), *Handbook of learning disabilities* (pp. 16–29). New York: Guilford Press.

Hammill, D. D. (1990). On defining learning disabilities: An emerging consensus. *Journal of Learning Disabilities, 23,* 74–84.

Hammill, D. D. (1993). A brief look at the learning disabilities movement in the United States. *Journal of Learning Disabilities, 26,* 295–310.

Handwerk, M. L., & Marshall, R. M. (1998). Behavioral and emotional problems of students with learning disabilities, serious emotional disturbance, or both conditions. *Journal of Learning Disabilities, 31,* 327–338.

Hanich, L., Jordan, N. C., Kaplan, D., & Dick, J. (2001). Performance across different areas of mathematical cognition in children with learning disabilities. *Journal of Educational Psychology, 93,* 615–626.

Hintze, J. M., Christ, T. J., & Methe, S. A. (2006). Curriculum-based assessment. *Psychology in the Schools, 43,* 45–56.

Hintze, J. M., Ryan, A. L., & Stoner, G. (2003). Concurrent validity and diagnostic accuracy of the Dynamic Indicators of Basic Early Literacy Skills and the Comprehensive Test of Phonological Processing. *School Psychology Review, 32,* 541–556.

Hosp, M. K., & Hosp, J. L. (2003). Curriculum-based measurement for reading, spelling, and math: How to do it and why. *Preventing School Failure, 48,* 10–17.

Individuals with Disabilities Education Improvement Act, Pub. L. No. 108-446 (2004).

Jenkins, J. R., Fuchs, L. S., van den Broek, P., Espin, C., & Deno, S. L. (2003). Sources of individual differences in reading comprehension and reading fluency. *Journal of Educational Psychology, 95,* 719–729.

Johnson, J. A., Bardos, A. N., & Tayebi, K. A. (2003, August). *Relationship between written expression achievement and the Cognitive Assessment System.* Paper presented at the annual conference of the American Psychological Association, Toronto, Canada.

Joint Committee on Standards for Educational and Psychological Testing of the AERA, APA, and NCME. (1999). *Standards for educational and psychological testing.* Washington, DC: American Educational Research Association.

Jordan, N. C., Hanich, L. B., & Kaplan, D. (2003). A longitudinal study of the mathematical competencies in children with specific mathematical difficulties

versus children with comorbid mathematics and reading difficulties. *Child Development, 74,* 834–850.

Joseph, L. M., McCachran, M. E., & Naglieri, J. A. (2003). PASS cognitive processes, phonological processes, and basic reading performance for a sample of referred primary-grade children. *Journal of Research in Reading, 26,* 304–314.

Kaminski, R. A., & Good, R. H., III (1996). Toward a technology for assessing basic early literacy skills. *School Psychology Review, 25,* 215–227.

Kaufman, A. S., & Kaufman, N. L. (2001). Assessment of specific learning disabilities in the new millennium: Issues, conflicts, and controversies. In A. S. Kaufman & N. L. Kaufman (Eds.), *Specific learning disabilities and difficulties in children and adolescents: Psychological assessment and evaluation* (pp. 433–461). Cambridge, UK: Cambridge University Press.

Kaufman, A. S., & Kaufman, N. L. (2004). *Kaufman Assessment Battery for Children—Second Edition (KABC-II).* Circle Pines, MN: American Guidance Service.

Kaufman, J. C., Kaufman, A. S., Kaufman-Singer, J., & Kaufman, N. L. (2005). The Kaufman Assessment Battery for Children—Second Edition and the Kaufman Adolescent and Adult Intelligence Test. In D. P. Flanagan & P. L. Harrison (Eds.), *Contemporary intellectual assessment: Theories, tests, and issues* (2nd ed., pp. 344–370). New York: Guilford Press.

Kavale, K. (2002). Discrepancy models in the identification of learning disabilities. In R. Bradley (Ed.), *Identification of learning disabilities: Research to practice* (pp. 369–426). Mahwah, NJ: Erlbaum.

Kavale, K. A., & Forness, S. R. (1996). Social skills deficits and learning disabilities: A meta-analysis. *Journal of Learning Disabilities, 29,* 226–244.

Kavale, K. A., Holdnack, J. A., & Mostert, M. P. (2005, Winter). Responsiveness to intervention and the identification of specific learning disability: A critique and alternate proposal. *Learning Disability Quarterly, 28,* 3–16.

Kavale, K., & Mattson, P. D. (1983). One jumped off the balance beam. *Journal of Learning Disabilities, 16,* 165–173.

Keith, T. Z., Kranzler, J. H., & Flanagan, D. P. (2001). What does the cognitive assessment system (CAS) measure?: Joint confirmatory factor analysis of the CAS and the Woodcock–Johnson Tests of Cognitive Ability (3rd edition). *School Psychology Review, 30,* 89–119.

Klenk, L., & Kirby, M. W. (2000). Re-mediating reading difficulties: Appraising the past, reconciling the present, constructing the future. In M. E. Kamil (Ed.), *Handbook of reading research* (Vol. 3, pp. 667–690). Mahwah, NJ: Erlbaum.

Kranzler, J. H., & Keith, T. Z. (1999). Independent confirmatory factor analysis of the Cognitive Assessment System (CAS): What does the CAS measure? *School Psychology Review, 28,* 117–144.

Kroesbergen, E. H., Van Luit, J. E. H., & Naglieri, J. A. (2003). Mathematical learning difficulties and PASS cognitive processes. *Journal of Learning Disabilities, 36*, 574–585.

Lichtenberger, E. O. (2001). The Kaufman tests—K-ABC and KAIT. In A. S. Kaufman & N. L. Kaufman. (Eds.), *Specific learning disabilities and difficulties in children and adolescents: Psychological assessment and evaluation* (pp. 97–140). Cambridge, UK: Cambridge University Press.

Light, J. G., & DeFries, J. C. (1996). Comorbidity of reading and mathematics disability: Genetic and environmental etiologies. *Journal of Learning Disabilities, 28*, 96–107.

Lyon, G. R., Fletcher, J. M., & Barnes, M. C. (2003). Learning disabilities. In E. J. Mash & R. A. Barkley (Eds.), *Child psychopathology* (2nd ed., pp. 520–586). New York: Guilford Press.

Lyon, G. R., Fletcher, J. M., Shaywitz, S. E., Shaywitz, B. A., Torgesen, J. K., Wood, F. B., et al. (2001). Rethinking learning disabilities. *Rethinking special education for a new century.* Washington, DC: Thomas B. Fordham Foundation and Progressive Policy Institute. Retrieved on February 2, 2006, from *www.educationnext.org/20012/22.html*

Maag, J. W., & Reid, R. (2006). Depression among students with learning disabilities: Assessing the risk. *Journal of learning Disabilities, 39*, 97–99.

Machek, G. R., & Nelsen, J. M. (in press). How should reading disabilities be operationalized? A survey of practicing school psychologists. *Learning Disabilities Research and Practice.*

Madelaine, A., & Wheldall, K. (1999). Curriculum-based measurement of reading: A critical review. *International Journal of Disability, Development, and Education, 46*, 71–85.

Maller, S. J. (2005). Wechsler Intelligence Scale for Children [Review of the test]. *Sixteenth Mental Measurement Yearbook.* Lincoln: University of Nebraska Press.

Marston, D., Muyskens, P., Lau, M., & Carter, A. (2003). Problem-solving model for decision making with high-incidence disabilities: The Minneapolis Experience. *Learning Disabilities Research and Practice, 81*, 187–200.

Mather, N., & Woodcock, R. W. (2001). The Woodcock–Johnson Tests of Cognitive Ability—Revised. In A. S. Kaufman & N. L. Kaufman (Eds.), *Specific learning disabilities and difficulties in children and adolescents: Psychological assessment and evaluation* (pp. 55–96). Cambridge, UK: Cambridge University Press.

Mayes, S. D., Calhoun, S. L., & Crowell, E. W. (1998). WISC-III profiles for children with and without learning disabilities. *Psychology in the Schools, 35*, 309–316.

Mayes, S. D., Calhoun, S. L., & Crowell, E. W. (2000). Learning disabilities and ADHD: Overlapping spectrum disorders. *Journal of Learning Disabilities, 33*, 417–424.

McCloskey, G., & Maerlender, A. (2005). The WISC-IV Integrated. In A. Prifitera, D. H. Saklofske, & L. G. Weiss (Eds.), *WISC-IV clinical use and interpretation* (pp. 101–149). Amsterdam: Elsevier.

McGrew, K. S., & Hessler, G. L. (1995). The relationship between the WJ-R Gf-Gc cognitive clusters and mathematics achievement across the life-span. *Journal of Psychoeducational Assessment, 13*, 21–38.

McKinney, J. D., Mason, J., Perkerson, K., & Clifford, M. (1975). Relationship between classroom behavior and Academic achievement. *Journal of Educational Psychology, 67*, 198–203.

McKinney, J. D., & Speece, D. L. (1983). Classroom behavior and the Academic progress of learning disabled students. *Journal of Applied Developmental Psychology, 4*, 149–161.

McMaster, K. L., Fuchs, D., Fuchs, L. S., & Compton, D. L. (2005). Responding to nonresponders: An experimental field trial of identification and intervention methods. *Exceptional Children, 71*, 445–463.

Meehl, P. E. (1954). *Clinical vs. statistical prediction.* Minneapolis: University of Minnesota Press.

Meikamp, J. (2005). Das-Naglieri Cognitive Assessment System [Review of the test]. *Sixteenth Mental Measurements Yearbook.* Lincoln: University of Nebraska Press.

Messick, S. (1984). Assessment in context: Appraising student performance in relation to instructional quality. *Educational Researcher, 13*, 3–8.

Messick, S. (1989a). Meaning and values in test validation: The science and ethics of assessment. *Educational Researcher, 18*(2), 5–11.

Messick, S. (1989b). Validity. In R. L. Linn (Ed.), *Educational measurement* (3rd ed., pp. 13–103). New York: Macmillan.

Messick, S. (1995). Validity of psychological assessment: Validation of inferences from persons' responses and performances as scientific inquiry into score meaning. *American Psychologist, 50*, 741–749.

Naglieri, J. A. (1999). *Essentials of CAS assessment.* New York: Wiley.

Naglieri, J. A. (2000). Intelligence testing in the 21st century: A look at the past and suggestions for the future. *Education and Child Psychology, 17*, 6–18.

Naglieri, J. A. (2001). Using the Cognitive Assessment System (CAS) with learning disabled children. In A. S. Kaufman & N. L. Kaufman (Eds.), *Specific learning disabilities and difficulties in children and adolescent: Psychological assessment and evaluation* (pp. 141–177). Cambridge, UK: Cambridge University Press.

Naglieri, J. A. (2003). Current advances in assessment and intervention for children with learning disabilities. *Advances in Learning and Behavioral Disabilities, 16*, 163–190.

Naglieri, J. A. (2005). The Cognitive Assessment System. In D. P. Harrison & P. L. Flanagan (Eds.), *Con-

temporary intellectual assessment: Theories, tests, and issues (2nd ed., pp. 441–460). New York: Guilford Press.

Naglieri, J. A., & Das, J. P. (1997). *Cognitive Assessment System.* Itasca, IL: Riverside.

Naglieri, J. A., & Das, J. P. (2005). Planning, attention, simultaneous, successive (PASS) theory. In D. P. Flanagan & P. L. Harrison (Eds.), *Contemporary intellectual assessment: Theories, tests, and issues* (2nd ed., pp.120–135). New York: Guilford Press.

Naglieri, J. A., & Gottling, S. H. (1997). Mathematics instruction and PASS cognitive processes: An intervention study. *Journal of Learning Disabilities, 30,* 513–520.

Naglieri, J. A., & Johnson, D. (2000). Effectiveness of a cognitive strategy intervention to improve math calculation based on the PASS theory. *Journal of Learning Disabilities, 33,* 591–597.

Naglieri, J. A., & Reardon, S. (1993). Traditional IQ is irrelevant to learning disabilities—intelligence is not. *Journal of Learning Disabilities, 26,* 127–133.

Naglieri, J. A., & Rojahn, J. (2004). Construct validity of the PASS theory and CAS: Correlations with achievement. *Journal of Educational Psychology, 96*(1), 174–181.

Naglieri, J. A., & Sullivan, L. (1998). IDEA and identification of children with specific learning disabilities. *Communique, 27,* 20–21.

National Reading Panel. (2000). *Report of National Reading Panel: Teaching children to read: An evidence-based assessment of the scientific research literature on reading and its implications for reading instruction: Report of the subgroups.* Washington, DC: National Institutes of Child Health and Human Development.

O'Connor, R. (1999). Increasing the intensity of interventions in kindergarten and first grade. *Learning Disabilities Research and Practice, 15,* 43–54.

Parrila, R. K., Das, J. P., Kendrick, M., Papadopoulos, T., & Kirby, J. (1999). Efficacy of a cognitive reading remediation program for at-risk children in grade 1. *Developmental Disabilities Bulletin, 27,* 1–31.

Prifitera, A., Weiss, L. G., Saklofske, D. H., & Rolfhus, E. (2005). The WISC-IV in the clinical assessment context. In A. Prifitera, D. H. Saklofske, & L. G. Weiss (Eds.), *WISC-IV: Clinical use and interpretation* (pp. 3–32). Amsterdam: Elsevier Academic.

Reschly, D. J., Hosp, J. L., & Schmied, C. M. (2003). *And Miles to go . . . : State SLD requirements and authoritative recommendations.* Washington, DC: U.S. Department of Education, Office of Special Education Programs.

Ritchey, K. D., & Speece, D. L. (in press). From letter names to word reading: The nascent role of sublexical fluency. *Contemporary Educational Psychology.*

Robinson, B. R., & Harrison, P. L. (2005). WISC-III core profiles for students referred or found eligible for special education and gifted programs. *School Psychology Quarterly, 20,* 51–65.

Salvia, J., & Ysseldyke, J. E. (2004). *Assessment in inclusive and special education* (9th ed.). Boston: Houghton Mifflin.

Sandoval, J. (2005). Woodcock–Johnson (R) III [Review of the test]. *Sixteenth Mental Measurements Yearbook.* Lincoln: University of Nebraska Press.

Share, D., McGee, R., & Silva, P. D. (1989). I.Q. and reading progress: A test of the capacity notion of I.Q. *Journal of the American Academy of Child and Adolescent Psychiatry, 28*(1), 97–100.

Shaywitz, B. A., Shaywitz, S. E., Blachman, B. A., Pugh, K. R., Fulbright, R. K., Skudlarski, P., et al. (2004). Development of left occipitotemporal systems for skilled reading in children after a phonologically-based intervention. *Biological Psychiatry, 55,* 926–933.

Shepherd, M. J. (2001). History lessons. In A. S. Kaufman & N. L. Kaufman (Eds.), *Specific learning disabilities and difficulties in children and adolescents: Psychological assessment and evaluation* (pp. 3–28). Cambridge, UK: Cambridge University Press.

Shinn, M. R. (Ed.). (1989). *Curriculum-based measurement: Assessing special children.* New York: Guilford Press.

Shinn, M. R. (1989). Identifying and defining Academic problems: CBM screening and eligibility procedures. In M. R. Shinn (Ed.), *Curriculum-based measurement: Assessing special children.* New York: Guilford Press.

Simos, P. G., Fletcher, J. M., Sarkari, S., Billingsley, R. L., Francis, D. J., Castillo, E. M., et al. (2005). Early development of neurophysiological processes involved in normal reading and reading disability: A magnetic source imaging study. *Neuropsychology, 19,* 787–798.

Smith, C. B., & Watkins, M. W. (2004). Diagnostic utility of the Bannatyne WISC-III pattern. *Learning Disability Practice, 19,* 49–56.

Snow, C. E., Burns, M. S., & Griffin, P. (Eds.). (1998). *Preventing reading difficulties in young children.* Washington, DC: National Academy Press.

Speece, D. L. (2005). Hitting the moving target known as reading development: Some thoughts on screening first grade children for secondary interventions. *Journal of Learning Disabilities, 38,* 487–493.

Speece, D. L., & Case, L. P. (2001). Classification in context: An alternative approach to identifying early reading disability. *Journal of Educational Psychology, 93,* 735–749.

Speece, D. L., Case, L. P., & Molloy, D. E. (2003). Responsiveness to general education instruction as the first gate to learning disabilities identification. *Learning Disabilities Research and Practice, 18,* 147–156.

Speece, D. L., & Cooper, D. H. (1990). Ontogeny of school failure: Classification of first grade children.

American Educational Research Journal, 27, 119–140.

Speece, D. L., Cooper, D. H., & Kibler, J. M. (1990). Dynamic assessment, individual differences, and academic achievement. *Learning and Individual Differences, 2,* 113–127.

Speece, D. L., Mills, C., Ritchey, K. D., & Hillman, E. (2003). Initial evidence that letter fluency tasks are valid indicators of early reading skill. *Journal of Special Education, 36,* 223–233.

Speece, D. L., & Shekitka, L. (2002). How should reading disabilities be operationalized?: A survey of experts. *Learning Disabilities Research and Practice, 17,* 118–123.

Stage, S. A., Abbott, R. D., Jenkins, J. R., & Berninger, V. W. (2003). Predicting response to early reading intervention from verbal IQ, reading-related language abilities, attention ratings, and verbal IQ-word reading discrepancy: Failure to validate discrepancy method. *Journal of Learning Disabilities, 36,* 24–33.

Stage, S. A., Sheppard, J., Davidson, M. M., & Browning, M. M. (2001). Prediction of first-graders' growth in oral reading fluency using kindergarten letter fluency. *Journal of School Psychology, 39,* 225–237.

Stanovich, K. E., & Siegel, L. S. (1994). Phenotypic performance profile of children with reading disabilities: A regression-based tests of the phonological-core variable-difference model. *Journal of Educational Psychology, 86*(1), 24–53.

Stecker, P. M., Fuchs, L. S., & Fuchs, D. (2005). Using curriculum-based measurement to improve student achievement: Review of research. *Psychology in the Schools, 42,* 795–819.

Stuebing, K. K., Fletcher, J. M., LeDoux, J. M., Lyon, G. R., Shaywitz, S. E., & Shaywitz, B. A. (2002). Validity of IQ-discrepancy classifications of reading disabilities: A meta-analysis. *American Educational Research Journal, 39,* 465–518.

Swanson, H. L., & Howard, C. B. (2005). Children with reading disabilities: Does dynamic assessment help in the classification? *Learning Disabilities Quarterly, 28,* 17–34.

Tabassam, W., & Graigner, J. (2002). Self-concept, attributional style and self-efficacy beliefs of students with learning disabilities with and without attention deficit disorder. *Learning Disabilities Quarterly, 25,* 141–151.

Taub, G. E., & McGrew, K. S. (2004). A confirmatory factor analysis of Cattell–Horn–Carroll theory of cross-age-invariance of the Woodcock–Johnson Tests of Cognitive Abilities III. *School Psychology Quarterly, 19,* 72–87.

Temple, E., Deutsch, G. K., Poldrack, R. A., Miller, S. L., Tallal, P., Merzenich, M. M., et al. (2003). Neural deficits in children with dyslexia ameliorated by behavioral remediation: Evidence from functional MRI. *Proceedings of the National Academy of Sciences of the United States of America, 100,* 2860–2865.

Thompson, D. (2005). The Das–Naglieri Cognitive Assessment System [Review of the test]. *Sixteenth Mental Measurements Yearbook.* Lincoln: University of Nebraska Press.

Thorndike, R. M. (2005). The Kaufman Assessment Battery for Children, Second Edition [Review of the test]. *Sixteenth Mental Measurements Yearbook.* Lincoln: University of Nebraska Press.

Torgesen, J. K. (1998). Learning disabilities: An historical and conceptual overview. In B. Wong (Ed.), *Learning about learning disabilities* (2nd ed., pp. 3–34). San Diego, CA: Academic Press.

Torgesen, J. K. (2002). Empirical and theoretical support for direct diagnosis of learning disabilities by assessment of intrinsic processing weaknesses. In R. Bradley, L. Danielson, & D. P. Hallahan (Eds.), *Identification of learning disabilities: Research to practice* (pp. 565–613). Mahwah, NJ: Erlbaum.

Torgesen, J. K. (2004). Learning disabilities: An historical and conceptual overview. In B. Wong (Ed.), *Learning about learning disabilities* (3rd ed., pp. 3–40). San Diego, CA: Academic Press.

Torgesen, J. K., Wagner, R. K., Rashotte, C. A., Rose, E., Lindamood, P., Conway, T., et al. (1999). Preventing reading failure in young children with phonological processing disabilities: Group and individual responses to instruction. *Journal of Educational Psychology, 91,* 579–593.

U. S. Department of Education. (2002). *Individuals with Disabilities Education Act: To assure the free appropriate education of all children with disabilities* (Twenty-Fourth Annual Report to Congress on the Implementation of the Individuals with Disabilities Education Act). Washington, DC: U.S. Government Printing Office.

U. S. Office of Education (USOE). (1976). Proposed rulemaking. *Federal Register, 41*(230), 52404–52407.

U. S. Office of Education (USOE). (1977). Assistance to states for education of handicapped children: Procedures for evaluating specific learning disabilities. *Federal Register, 42*(250), 65082–65085.

VanDerHeyden, A. M., Broussard, C., Fabre, M., Stanley, J., Legendre, J., & Creppel, R. (2004). Development and validation of curriculum-based measures of math performance for preschool children. *Journal of Early Intervention, 27,* 27–41.

VanDerHeyden, A. M., Witt, J. C., Naquin, G., & Noell, G. (2001). The reliability and validity of curriculum-based measurement readiness probes for kindergarten students. *School Psychology Review, 30,* 363–382.

Vaughn, S., & Fuchs, L. S. (2003). Redefining learning disabilities as inadequate response to instruction: The promise and potential problems. *Learning Disabilities Research and Practice, 18,* 137–146.

Vaughn, S., Levy, S., Coleman, M., & Bos, C. S. (2002). Reading instruction for students with LD and EBD: A synthesis of observation studies. *Journal of Special Education, 36,* 2–21.

Vaughn, S., Linan-Thompson, S., & Hickman, P. (2003). Response to treatment as a means of identifying students with reading/learning disabilities. *Exceptional Children*, 69, 391–409.

Vellutino, F. R., Scanlon, D. M., & Jacard, J. (2003). Toward distinguishing between cognitive and experiential deficits as primary sources of difficulty in learning to read: A two year follow-up of difficult to remediate and readily remediated poor readers. In B. R. Foorman (Ed.), *Preventing and remediating reading difficulties* (pp. 73–120). Baltimore: York.

Vellutino, F. R., Scanlon, D. M., & Lyon, G. R. (2000). Differentiating between difficult-to-remediate and readily remediated poor readers: More evidence against the IQ–achievement discrepancy definition of reading disability. *Journal of Learning Disabilities*, 323, 223–238.

Vellutino, F. R., Scanlon, D. M., Sipay, E. R., Small, S. G., Pratt, A., Chen, R. S., et al. (1996). Cognitive profiles of difficult to remediate and readily remediated poor reader: Early intervention as a vehicle for distinguishing between cognitive and experiential deficits as basic causes of specific reading disability. *Journal of Educational Psychology*, 88, 607–638.

Voeller, K. K. S. (2004). Attention-deficit hyperactivity disorder (ADHD). *Journal of Child Neurology*, 19, 798–814.

Wechsler, D. (2003). *Wechsler Intelligence Scale for Children: Fourth Edition*. San Antonio, TX: Psychological Corporation.

Weintraub, F. (2005). The evolution of LD policy and future challenges. *Learning Disabilities Quarterly*, 28, 97–99.

Weiss, L. G., Prifitera, A., & Saklofske, D. H. (2005). Interpreting the WISC-IV Index scores. In A. Prifitera, D. H. Saklofske, & L. G. Weiss (Eds.), *WISC-IV clinical use and interpretation* (pp. 71–100). Amsterdam: Elsevier.

Wiederholt, J. L. (1974). Historical perspectives on the education of the learning disabled. In L. Mann & D. A. Sabatino (Eds.), *The second review of special education* (pp. 103–152). Philadelphia: JSE Press.

Woodcock, R. W. McGrew, K. S., & Mather, N. (2001). *Woodcock–Johnson Tests of Cognitive Abilities, III*. Itasca, IL: Riverside.

Wright-Strawderman, C., & Watson, B. L. (1992). The prevalence of depressive symptoms in children with learning disabilities. *Journal of Learning Disabilities*, 25, 258–264.

Zhu, J., & Weiss, L. (2005). The Wechsler scales. In D. P. Flanagan & P. L. Harrison (Eds.), *Contemporary Intellectual assessment: Theories, tests, and issues* (2nd ed., pp. 297–324). New York: Guilford Press.

PART VI

Children at Risk

CHAPTER 14

Child Abuse and Neglect

Claire V. Crooks
David A. Wolfe

In this chapter we present a comprehensive update and review of the major findings on child abuse and neglect to formulate a multilevel framework for psychological assessment. Because of the advances in theory and research since the last edition of this volume, new information has led to considerable changes and refinements in our assessment strategy. Most notably, assessing the child is much more detailed due to the sizable number of new instruments and approaches that have been investigated; previously, the parent was the focus of the lion's share of assessment procedures, and little information was available as to either the effects on or the needs of the children. Although physical abuse continues to receive more coverage than child neglect, many recent studies' added specificity to their procedures has allowed for better discrimination among factors relevant to assessment. In particular, specific measures of neglect have been developed since the previous edition of this volume.

Child abuse and neglect occur within ongoing relationships that are expected to be protective, supportive, and nurturing. Children from abusive and neglectful families grow up in environments that fail to provide consistent and appropriate opportunities that guide development; instead, these children are placed in jeopardy of physical and emotional harm. Because their ties to their families, even to the abuser, are very important, child victims may feel torn between a sense of belonging and a sense of fear and apprehension. For this and many other reasons discussed in this chapter, the assessment of abused children, their caregivers, and their family environment is fraught with challenges.

The chapter begins with an overview of the types of child maltreatment, epidemiological findings, and developmental consequences, all of which are important for formulating an assessment strategy. This overview is followed by a comprehensive look at the state of assessment approaches for this multidimensional problem. Our assessment strategy incorporates procedures for assessing many areas of emotional and behavioral development of maltreated children; moreover, it addresses critical areas associated with parent and family functioning that affect maltreatment, such as parental history, childrearing skills, stressful events, and so on. The approach to assessment, derived from research and clinical literature, involves a multistage process that profits from advances in observational and self-report assessment strategies.

TYPES OF CHILD ABUSE AND NEGLECT

Many societies are struggling to balance parental rights (e.g., parents' rights to discipline their children) and the rights of children to be safe and free of harm. Consequently, a significant shift is underway in how child maltreatment is defined and in how its effects are studied. In the past, abuse was defined primarily by visible physical injuries. However, physical injuries are only one of many consequences; maltreatment can also damage individuals' developing relations with others and their fundamental sense of safety and self-esteem.

At its most basic level, "child maltreatment" is a generic term describing volitional or neglectful acts on the part of a child's caregiver that result in, or have the potential to result in, physical injuries and/or psychological harm. Maltreatment includes four primary acts of commission or omission: (1) *neglect* (failure to provide care in accordance with expected societal standards for food, shelter, protection, affection); (2) *emotional abuse* (verbal abuse, isolation, exposing children to violence); (3) *physical abuse* (nonaccidental bodily injury); and (4) *sexual abuse* (sexual contact, including attempts or threats). Importantly, most child maltreatment occurs in the context of the caregiver–child *relationship*, which has significance because this relationship is central to the child's ongoing sense of safety, trust, and fulfillment of needs. Although there are other forms of maltreatment that are not caregiver- or family-based (e.g., child sexual exploitation/prostitution, child labor, abuse/assault by nonfamily persons known to the child), we limit our discussion herein to physical abuse and neglect by a child's primary caregiver (interested readers on these other forms of exploitation are referred to Cooper, Estes, Giardino, Kellogg, & Vieth [2005]). Thus, from a psychological perspective, maltreatment is harmful or potentially harmful to the child's immediate and future well-being not only because of physical injuries, but also because of what it often represents in terms of interfering with the child's ongoing social, cognitive, and behavioral development (Wekerle, Miller, Wolfe, & Spindel, 2006).

Physical abuse is the deliberate application of force to any part of a child's body, which results, or may result, in a nonaccidental injury. It may involve hitting a child a single time, or it may involve a pattern of incidents. Physical abuse also includes behaviors such as shaking, choking, biting, kicking, burning, or poisoning a child, holding a child under water, or any other harmful or dangerous use of force or restraint (e.g., locking a child in a closet or tying him or her to a chair). Child physical abuse is often connected to physical punishment or may be confused with child discipline. *Neglect* occurs when a child's parents or other caregivers are not providing essential requisites for a child's emotional, psychological, and physical development. Physical neglect involves inadequate provision of a child's needs for food, clothing, shelter, cleanliness, medical care, and protection from harm. The determination of child abuse and neglect typically requires consideration of cultural values and standards of care, as well as recognition that some forms of maltreatment may be bound by poverty.

In addition to these more clearly defined forms of abuse and neglect, the definition of "child maltreatment" for purposes of assessment and intervention often includes cases of high-risk parenting practices that may fall short of documented injuries. Rather than a dichotomous definition (abusive–not abusive), such a view considers the full continuum of childrearing acts, which may range from appropriate and developmentally sensitive behaviors to physically and verbally abusive ones (Wolfe, 1999). Examples of family problems that are addressed by this assessment strategy include reliance upon high-intensity physical punishment, use of excessive criticism and verbal harassment, use of unorthodox disciplinary techniques, lack of physical or verbal affection toward the child, failure to provide developmentally appropriate stimulation or opportunities to the child, exposure to domestic violence, and similar trauma-inducing experiences caused directly or indirectly by caregivers. These and many similar instances of parental inadequacy or ineffectiveness often warrant professional involvement. Because determination of such events involves professional judgment, definitions of child abuse and neglect vary somewhat in accordance with the purpose of the assessment and intervention concerns. This ambiguity is considered necessary and acceptable in view of the current state of knowledge and the presumed advantage to the child and family in seeking assistance for wide-ranging problems (as opposed to labeling or punishing individual family members).

Legal definitions of abuse and neglect emphasize parental deviance and wrongdoing, thereby focusing on the implicit intent to harm or the parent's inability to protect the child from harm. In contrast, social science definitions allow greater recognition of the individual, family, and social context of maltreatment, because most incidents involve non-life-threatening injuries rather than major acts of assault. The social science perspective, reflected herein, places primary importance on the relational context of maltreatment, because the child's short- and long-term adjustment following incident(s) of abuse or neglect are highly dependent on the overall quality of this relationship. In other words, a parent who is abusive on some occasions may be a source of support and nurturance for the child at other times; thus, the overall psychological impact of abuse may be tempered by other aspects of the relationship (although this process does not negate the significance of the act or the parent's responsibility).

The most distinguishing aspect of parents who have been reported for abuse, compared to their socioeconomically matched counterparts, is the chronic and escalating pattern of parent–child conflict, culminating in more and more serious harm over time. Neglectful parents are usually distinguished by the chronicity and severity of their behavior rather than by single events (Hildyard & Wolfe, 2002; Slack, Holl, McDaniel, Yoo, & Bolger, 2004). Furthermore, both abuse and neglect are most detrimental when they occur in the absence of compensatory factors, such as positive interactions or a strong social support network, which are crucial to facilitating a child's social, cognitive, and emotional development. Thus, rather than being categorically distinct from other parental actions, childhood maltreatment is best understood in terms of a continuum of parenting behaviors. At one extreme on the continuum are those practices considered to be most harmful and inappropriate; at the other extreme are methods that promote the child's social, emotional, and intellectual development. From this perspective, "child abuse and neglect" can be defined in terms of the degree to which a parent uses aversive or inappropriate control strategies in an attempt to inflict physical or emotional pain upon a child, and/or fails to provide minimal standards of caregiving and nurturance (Wolfe, 1999). Furthermore, abuse and neglect often involve a negative and rejecting stance toward the child, which translates into limited opportunities for the child to re-

ceive positive attention and nurturance, or to develop a sense of trust in relationships.

INCIDENCE AND PROFILE

Every week, more than 50,000 children are reported as victims of suspected child abuse and neglect in the United States alone (U.S. Department of Health and Human Services [USDHHS], 2005). This weekly toll translates into an annual rate of about 3 million reports of *suspected* child abuse and neglect cases each year, a figure that has changed very little over the last decade (USDHHS, 2004). About one-third of these reports end up as *substantiated* cases by child protective services, yielding a rate of 12.4 per 1,000 children in the population. Child neglect (including medical neglect) continues to be the most common form of maltreatment, accounting for close to 60% of all documented cases in the United States. Almost one-fifth of the children suffered physical abuse, and nearly 10% were sexually abused. In addition, about one-fourth of these children suffered more than one type of maltreatment.

By comparison, Canada's substantiated incidence of maltreatment was 9.7 per 1,000 children based on a 1998 sample (Trocmé et al., 2001). However, Canada's incidence rate more than doubled in the more recent 2003 study (21.71/1,000 children), mostly because the latter survey included children exposed to domestic violence (as a category of neglect) (Trocmé et al., 2005). Notably, almost two-thirds of the families in the Canadian Incidence Study were known previously to child protective services, underscoring the chronicity and repetitive nature of most forms of maltreatment.

Lifetime prevalence estimates of maltreatment are derived by asking adults if they ever experienced particular forms of maltreatment as children. For example, the Ontario Health Supplement, a general population survey of nearly 10,000 residents of Ontario, Canada, asks people 15 years and older about physical and sexual abuse in childhood (MacMillan et al., 1997). A history of child physical abuse was reported more often by males (31.2%) than by females (21.1%), whereas sexual abuse during childhood was more commonly reported by females (12.8%) than by males (4.3%). Retrospective reports of childhood experiences are inexact, and it is rarely possible to corroborate episodes of maltreatment to get precise accounts (Hardt & Rutter, 2004). Nevertheless, on the whole, these incidence and prevalence data indicate a substantial problem affecting a sizable proportion of the child and adult population.

Child abuse and neglect occur in all societies, and more and more countries are committed to an ongoing surveillance of reported cases for better awareness and planning. Cross-culturally, the World Health Organization (WHO; 2002) estimates that 40 million children ages 0–14 are victims of child abuse and neglect annually around the world, confirming suspicions that child abuse is found in all societies and is almost always a highly guarded secret.

Certain child characteristics identified through incidence studies help to identify the overall probability and type of maltreatment. Incidence studies have consistently found that children's age and sex are related to risk of maltreatment but that ethnic identity is not, once other factors such as poverty and homelessness are taken into account (Trocmé et al., 2001; USDHHS, 2003). Younger children, who have the greatest need for care and supervision, are the most common victims of physical neglect. Along with young adolescents, toddlers and preschoolers are the most common victims of physical and emotional abuse, which corresponds to the emergence of greater independence and parental conflict at these developmental periods. Sexual abuse, in contrast, is relatively constant from age 3 on, which attests to children's vulnerability from early preschool years throughout childhood. Although both boys and girls are more likely to be sexually abused by someone they know and trust, boys are more likely to be abused by male *nonfamily* members (e.g., camp staff, teachers, scout leaders), whereas girls are more likely to be sexually abused by male *family* members (Berliner & Elliott, 2002; Wolfe, Jaffe, Jetté, & Poisson, 2003).

Abuse and neglect are more common among the poor and disadvantaged, although they also occur among higher income families. This socioeconomic connection is not likely accounted for by reporting bias, as it has not changed for the past 30 years despite increased awareness and reporting (USDHHS, 2003). Family structure is also connected to the probability of child maltreatment. Children living with a single parent are at significantly greater risk of both physical abuse and neglect. Those living in father-only homes are almost twice as likely to be physically abused as those living with mothers alone (Sedlak & Broadhurst, 1996; Trocmé et al., 2001). The majority of child victims are maltreated by one or both parents (85%) across all forms of maltreatment. However, there are important exceptions, as well as key sex differences in the nature of abuse or neglect. Child neglect is committed predominantly—about 90% of the time—by mothers, which fits with the fact that mothers and mother substitutes tend to be primary caretakers and are more likely to be charged with child neglect, even when a father figure is present in the family. In contrast, sexual abuse is committed more often—about 90% of the time—by males, about half of whom are the child's father or father figure. Although males are the dominant perpetrators in sexual abuse, the most common perpetrator pattern overall is a female parent acting alone, who is typically younger than 30 years of age (USDHHS, 2003). The finding that a single mother is the most frequently identified perpetrator of child abuse is to some extent a reflection of the number of single-parent families headed by mothers.

DEVELOPMENTAL CONSIDERATIONS AND IMPAIRMENTS

The development of the abused child seldom follows a predictable course, because child abuse is characterized by many other negative socialization forces, including family instability, parenting inconsistency, and socioeconomic disadvantage. Information about the developmental sequelae of abuse has gradually grown from its early beginnings (i.e., case histories, clinical interventions, comparative studies of abused and nonabused children) to include more sophisticated longitudinal investigations. These studies continue to suggest that maltreated children, as a group, do not reveal characteristic adjustment patterns or long-term developmental problems that clearly distinguish them from nonabused children. At the same time, the range and extent of problems in this population implicate abuse as a contributory factor in a wide range of child (e.g., delinquency, school problems, speech and language delays) and adult (e.g., criminal behavior, marital conflict, childrearing problems) developmental impairments (Trickett, Kurtz, &

Pizzigati, 2004). This wide range of possible developmental trajectories poses a challenge for assessment due to the number of areas that are potentially affected by child abuse and neglect. A developmental psychopathology perspective of abuse views the emergence of maladaptive behaviors, such as peer aggression, school failure, and delinquency, within a longitudinal and multidimensional framework (Cicchetti, Toth, & Maughan, 2000). This perspective facilitates an ongoing investigation of the *changes over time* observed among samples of abused children, and attempts to account for these changes on the basis of both global (e.g., socioeconomic and normative factors affecting all children) and more specific (e.g., type of maltreatment, child and family resources) intervening variables.

Because child abuse and neglect are the result of adult actions and not child disorders, it is important for assessment purposes to examine the major developmental impacts that have been linked to these phenomena. These developmental impairments show up in children from infancy through adolescence, and can have consequences throughout adulthood. Some of the effects on development lead to mental disorders in childhood or later life, such as posttraumatic stress disorder (PTSD), mood disorders, substance abuse, and so on, whereas others affect ongoing relationships, educational attainment, criminal behavior, and many other aspects of personality and adjustment. Below is a snapshot of the major developmental processes most affected by child physical abuse and various forms of child neglect, followed by discussion of major disorders often associated with longer-term outcomes. Assessment implications and approaches for these impairments follow in subsequent sections.

Episodes of child abuse and neglect, whether chronic or sporadic, can disrupt the important process of early childhood attachment, and interfere with children's ability to seek comfort and to regulate their own physiological and emotional processes. As a result, young maltreated children are more likely than other children to show an absence of an organized attachment strategy (Lyons-Ruth, Yellin, Melnick, & Atwood, 2003). Without consistent stimulation, comfort, and routine to aid in the formation of secure attachments, maltreated infants and toddlers have considerable difficulty establishing a reciprocal, consistent pattern of interaction with their caregivers. In-

stead, they may show a pattern described as *insecure–disorganized attachment*, characterized by a mixture of approach and avoidance, helplessness, apprehension, and a general disorientation (Barnett, Ganiban, & Cicchetti, 1999). The lack of a secure, consistent basis for relationships places maltreated children at greater risk of falling behind in their cognitive and social development, and can result in their having problems regulating their emotions and behavior with others (Sroufe, Carlson, Levy, & Egeland, 1999).

Parent–child attachment and the home climate also play a critical role in emotion regulation, another early developmental milestone. "Emotional regulation" refers to the ability to modulate or control the intensity and expression of feelings and impulses, especially intense ones, in an adaptive manner (Cicchetti, Ganiban, & Barnett, 1991; Maughan & Cicchetti, 2002). Because maltreated children live in a world of emotional turmoil and extremes, it is very difficult for them to understand, label, and regulate their internal states (Shipman, Zeman, Penza, & Champion, 2000). Expressions of affect, such as crying or signals of distress, may trigger disapproval, avoidance, or abuse from caregivers, so maltreated youngsters have a greater tendency to inhibit their emotional expression and regulation, and remain more fearful and hypervigilant (Klorman, Cicchetti, Thatcher, & Ison, 2003). Similarly, they show increased attention to anger- and threat-related signals, such as facial expressions, and less attention to other emotional expressions (Pollak & Tolley-Schell, 2003). Difficulties modulating emotions can be expressed as depressive reactions, as well as intense angry outbursts (Wekerle & Wolfe, 2003). Accordingly, as they grow older and are faced with new situations involving peers and other adults, poor emotional regulation becomes more and more problematic. Over time, this inability to regulate emotions is associated with both internalizing symptoms, such as depression and fearfulness, as well as externalizing symptoms, such as hostility, aggression, and various forms of acting out (Burack et al., 2006; Éthier, Lemelin, & Lacharité, 2004).

Neuroscientists have connected the behavioral signs of poor emotional regulation among maltreated children to alterations in the developing brain. Studies with maltreated children and adults with a history of childhood abuse show long-term alterations in the hypothalamic–pituitary–adrenal (HPA) axis and norepinephrine systems, which have a pronounced affect on one's responsiveness to stress (Bremner & Vermetten, 2001; Nemeroff, 2004). Brain areas implicated in the stress response include the hippocampus (involved in learning and memory) the prefrontal cortex, and the amygdala. The impact of child abuse on these areas of the brain may lead to long-term mental health problems (Bremner, 2003). In effect, acute and chronic forms of stress associated with maltreatment may cause changes in brain development, resulting in changes in structure and function. Due to prolonged and unpredictable episodes of abuse or neglect, cortisol levels become depleted, and the feedback systems that control hormone levels in the brain may become dysfunctional. As a result, the neuroendocrine system becomes highly sensitive to stress (De Bellis, Keshavan, Spencer, & Hall, 2000). These neurobiological changes that occur in response to untoward early-life stress may partially account for the psychiatric problems that emerge throughout the lifespan among individuals who were maltreated in childhood.

Maltreated children may also lack core positive beliefs about themselves and their world, because their negative experiences in relationships are carried forward to new situations (Cicchetti, Rogosch, Maughan, Toth, & Bruce, 2003). They may develop negative representational models of themselves and others based on a sense of inner "badness," self-blame, shame, or rage that further impairs their ability to regulate their affective responses (Feiring, Taska, & Lewis, 2002). The child's developing sense of personal self-efficacy can be undermined by physical and verbal abuse, as well as by physical and emotional neglect, because such maltreatment devalues the child as a person. Feelings of betrayal can also challenge an individual's sense of self, because a person on whom the individual was dependent violated that trust and confidence.

Maltreated children's relationships with their peers and teachers typically mirror the models of relationships they know best. Instead of a healthy sense of autonomy and self-respect, their models of relationships have elements of being both victim and victimizer—those who rule and those who submit—and during interactions with peers, maltreated children may alternate between being the aggressor

and being the victim (Dodge, Pettit, & Bates, 1994). Their adaptation strategies, such as hypervigilance and fear, evolve to become highly responsive to threatening or dangerous situations. These strategies conflict, however, with the new challenges of school and peer groups. As a result, children with histories of physical abuse and neglect may be more distracted by aggressive stimuli and misread the intentions of their peers and teachers as being more hostile than they actually are (Dodge et al., 1994). Given their propensity to attribute hostile intent to others and their lack of empathy and social skills, it is not surprising that abused and neglected children are rejected by their peers (Bolger & Patterson, 2001; Burack et al., 2006; Shields, Ryan, & Cicchetti, 2001), and have severe and wide-ranging problems in school and interpersonal adjustment (Egeland, Yates, Appleyard, & van Dulmen, 2002). This pattern of poor adjustment often persists, leading to higher rates of personality disorders in early adulthood, especially among neglected children (Johnson, Smailes, Cohen, Brown, & Bernstein, 2000).

LIFE COURSE

As children approach adulthood, the developmental impairments stemming from child maltreatment can lead to more pervasive and chronic psychiatric disorders, including anxiety and panic disorders, depression, eating disorders, sexual problems, and personality disturbances (Brown, Cohen, Johnson, & Smailes, 1999; Edwards, Holden, Felitti, & Anda, 2003; Felitti et al., 1998). Four of the prominent developmental outcomes of abuse and neglect discussed herein include mood and affect disturbances, substance abuse, posttraumatic stress-related problems, and antisocial or abusive behavior in relationships.

Symptoms of depression, emotional distress, and suicidal ideation are common features of individuals of all ages with histories of physical as well as sexual abuse, especially in the absence of positive relationships and opportunities to develop healthy coping strategies and social supports (Leifer, Kilbane, Jacobsen, & Grossman, 2004). Symptoms of depression and mood disturbance often increase during late adolescence and adulthood, especially among those who were abused since childhood (Brown et al., 1999; Kolko, 2002), and can lead to life-threatening suicide attempts and self-mutilating behavior (Kaplan, Pelcovitz, Salzinger, Mandel, & Weiner, 1997).

Similarly, teens with histories of maltreatment have a much greater risk of substance abuse (Kilpatrick et al., 2003), which in turn increases the risk of other adjustment problems. Perhaps as a result of chronic emotional pain, some teens and adults attempt to cope with unpleasant memories and current stressors by abusing alcohol and drugs, in a futile effort to diminish their distress. Substance abuse may also bolster self-esteem and temporarily reduce feelings of isolation (Bensley, Eenwyk, & Simmons, 2000). Thus, drug and alcohol use may function as a coping mechanism for increased stress brought on by childhood abuse. Alcohol and other illegal drug use may reduce symptoms of hyperarousal and unpleasant emotions, and produce emotional numbing and euphoria.

A significant number of men and women who have been subjected to severe physical or sexual abuse during childhood suffer long-term stress-related disorders. Between 20 and 50% of children and adolescents with histories of maltreatment involving sexual abuse or combined sexual and physical abuse meet criteria for PTSD (McCloskey & Walker, 2000; Scott, Wolfe, & Wekerle, 2003). The prevalence among adults is equally disturbing: About one-third of the childhood victims of sexual abuse, physical abuse, or neglect meet criteria for lifetime PTSD (Kilpatrick et al., 2003; Widom, 1999). Because of the emotional and physical pain of abusive experiences, children may voluntarily or involuntarily induce an altered state of consciousness known as "dissociation," which can be adaptive when neither resistance nor escape are possible (Herman, 1992). The process allows the victim to feel detached from the body or self, as if what is happening is not happening to him or her. Child abuse victims may come to rely on this form of psychological escape to the extent that profound disruptions to self and memory can occur (Macfie, Cicchetti, & Toth, 2001).

Finally, although most child victims of abuse and neglect do not grow up to be perpetrators of violence, a disturbingly high number, approximately 30%, carry the pattern into adolescence and adulthood (Kaufman & Zigler, 1987). Growing up with power-based, authoritarian methods of asserting power, even if they do not result in physical injuries or identified maltreatment, can be toxic to relationship and social patterns (Straus, 2001). For example, youth who have learned to adapt to violence and intimidation as a way of life, and who lack suitable alternative role models or experiences, are more likely to approach dating with inappropriate expectations about relationships. Youth (girls as well as boys) who grow up in violent homes report more violence, especially verbal abuse and threats, both toward and from their dating partners (Wolfe, Scott, Wekerle, & Pittman, 2001; Wolfe, Wekerle, Scott, Straatman, & Grasley, 2004). Dating violence during adolescence, combined with a past history of violence in their own family, are strong prerelationship predictors of intimate violence in early adulthood and marriage (O'Leary, Malone, & Tyree, 1994; White & Widom, 2003).

SUMMARY

The perspective on abused and neglected children presented herein has focused on knowledge of the wide range of developmental changes and deviations that have been documented in this diverse population. This developmental viewpoint embraces the subtly interacting conditions that work in combination either to attenuate the effects of powerful traumatic events or to turn a minor developmental crisis into a major impairment. Accordingly, maltreatment during infancy is strongly associated with characteristics of both anxious and disorganized attachments that may, over time, adversely affect the child's intellectual and socioemotional development. Preschool-age abused children are more difficult to manage and have more marked developmental delays in language, self-control, and peer interactions than do nonabused children. As they reach school age, these children continue to have significant learning and motivational problems at school, and higher rates of aggressive and destructive behavior with peers. Finally, as abused children reach adolescence and adulthood, they are likely to continue this pattern of altered development, manifested by elevated symptoms of mood and affect disorders, substance abuse, posttraumatic stress, and abuse and violence in their close relationships.

Despite the potential for these serious consequences, child maltreatment, like other forms of adversity and trauma during childhood, does not affect each child in a predictable or consistent fashion. To the contrary, the impact of maltreatment depends on not only the severity and chronicity of the events themselves but also how such events interact with the child's individual and family characteristics (Felitti et al., 1998). Accordingly, because of the wide-ranging causes and effects of maltreatment, a comprehensive assessment framework must be followed that includes child, parent, family, and cultural influences. We describe the global and specific aspects to such a framework for assessing these areas in the sections to follow.

ETIOLOGY

Physical abuse, in particular, may be understood as a special case of aggression in which child behavior often represents an immediate aversive stimulus that precipitates adult aggression. This perspective also recognizes the significance of contextual factors, such as crowded housing, ambient noise level, and socioeconomic disadvantages that contribute to the uncontrolled expression of aggression in the family. Although such precursors to abuse are highly relevant to our understanding of the problem, the question remains as to why only a relatively small percentage of adults exhibit such behavior in the presence of these common aversive events. To answer this question, a consideration of parent, child, and situational characteristics that may serve to accent or buffer the impact of such events is required.

Child physical abuse and neglect are often considered *relational disorders*, because they occur in the context of critical relationship roles. These relationships are particularly salient during periods of stressful role transitions for parents, such as the postnatal attachment period, the early childhood and early adolescence "oppositional" periods of testing limits, and times of family instability and disruption. Caregivers' failure to provide nurturing, sensitive, available, and supportive care, especially during critical periods, is a fundamental feature of maltreatment.

Abuse and neglect are rarely caused by a single risk factor, notwithstanding the critical role of the adult offender. In addition, even though risk signs and indicators may be present, it is still very difficult to predict who may become abusive and who will not. Because child maltreatment is an event, not a uniform disorder, it is necessary to consider multiple interactive causes. The presence of stress can convert static conditions into dynamic, chaotic patterns. For example, physical abuse and neglect occur most often in the context of social and economic family deprivation, which can transform predisposed, high-risk parents into abusive or neglectful ones. The greater degree of stress in the social environment of the abusive parent increases the probability that violence will surface as an attempt to gain control or cope with irritating, stressful events. In the case of neglect, stress may be so great that parents withdraw from their child care responsibilities.

For many parents, childrearing is a difficult and aversive event that can escalate unpredictably into a sudden abusive incident, or more gradually turn into avoidance and neglect. Lacking experience and guidance in childrearing, and faced with overwhelming stress, these parents cannot think of ways to handle a situation. Instead, they are often hypersensitive to perceived child misbehavior or have unrealistic expectations of child behavior, and respond overaggressively. Many abusive and neglectful parents have had little past or present exposure to positive parental models and supports. Their own childhoods were often full of difficult, sometimes very traumatic episodes of family violence, alcoholism, and harsh family circumstances related to frequent moves, unemployment, and poverty (Wolfe, 1999). As adults, they find daily living stressful and irritating, and they prefer to avoid potential sources of support, because it takes additional energy to maintain social relationships. Chronic physical ailments and a pervasive mood of discontentment, both common complaints, are understandable in light of the circumstances and limited coping resources.

Offender Characteristics

Because abuse and neglect usually occur in relation to childrearing demands, it is not surprising that both neglectful and abusive parents interact less often with their children than other parents during everyday activities. In general, neglectful parents actively avoid interacting with their child, even when the child appropriately seeks attention, most likely because social interaction is unfamiliar and even unpleasant. Physically abusive parents, in contrast, tend to deliver to their children a lot of threats or angry commands that exceed the demands of the situation, rather than positive forms of guidance and praise (Azar & Wolfe, 2006). Because of hostile information-processing biases, maltreating parents may misperceive or mislabel typical child behavior in ways that lead to inappropriate responses and increased aggression (Azar, 2002; Milner, 2003). They are unfamiliar with what is developmentally appropriate for a child at a given age. Some parents apply the same faulty reasoning to themselves as well, which results in lowered self-efficacy ("I'm not a good mother; other mothers can get their children to do these things") and greater interpersonal dependency (Bornstein, 2005). Unrealistic expectations and negative intent attributions can lead to greater punishment for child misbehavior and less reliance on explanation and positive teaching methods (Azar & Wolfe, 2006). Children are seen as deserving of harsh punishment, and its use is rationalized as a way to maintain control (Bugental, Blue, & Cruzcosa, 1989).

Neglectful parents have received far less research attention than physically abusive ones, perhaps because *omissions* of proper caretaking behaviors are more difficult to describe and detect than *commissions*. Although personality characteristics and lifestyle choices of abusive and neglectful parents overlap considerably, as a group, neglectful parents have more striking personality disorders and inadequate knowledge of children's needs, and they suffer more chronic patterns of social isolation than both abusive and nonabusive parents (Hildyard & Wolfe, 2002). Furthermore, neglectful caregivers typically disengage when under stress, whereas abusive parents become emotionally and behaviorally reactive (Azar, 2002). Neglectful parents try to cope with the stress of childrearing and related family matters through escape and avoidance, which can lead not only to severe consequences for the child but also to higher risk of substance abuse and similar coping failures for these parents (Crittenden & Claussen, 2002).

Child and Family Influences

Even though children might do things that are annoying, adults are fully responsible for abuse and neglect. Children's behavior or developmental limitations may increase the potential for abuse, but only if accompanied by the other critical factors noted previously. Unintentionally, however, the child may still play a role in the continuation or escalation of an abusive or neglectful relationship. For example, children with disabilities such as mental retardation or physical impairments were three times more likely to be abused than were their nondisabled peers based on a large population-based sample (Sullivan & Knutson, 2000).

Abusive incidents occur most often during difficult to manage, but not uncommon, episodes of child behavior such as disobedience, fighting and arguing, accidents, and dangerous behavior, which may produce anger and tension in some adults. Circumstances surrounding incidents of neglect, in contrast, relate more to chronic adult inadequacy, which spills over into daily family functioning (Herrenkohl, Herrenkohl, & Egolf, 1983). Neglected children's early feeding problems or irritability may place an increased strain on the parents' limited child care abilities, again setting in motion an escalation in the child's dependency needs and demandingness, accompanied by further parental withdrawal (Drotar, 1999).

Family circumstances, most notably conflict and marital violence, also have a causal connection to child maltreatment. In about half of the families in which adult partners are violent toward one another, one or both parents have also been violent toward a child at some point during the previous year (Edleson, 1999). Domestic conflicts and violence against women most often arise during disagreements over childrearing, discipline, and each partner's responsibilities in child care (Edleson, Mbilinyi, Beeman, & Hagemeister, 2003). Children may be caught in the crossfire between angry adults, or in some cases, they might instigate a marital conflict by misbehaving or demanding attention. In either case, an escalating cycle of family turmoil and violence begins, whereby children's behavioral and emotional reactions to the violence create additional stress on the marital relationship, further aggravating an already volatile situation.

Child maltreatment usually occurs in the context of multiproblem homes and neighborhoods, where poverty, social isolation, and wide acceptance of corporal punishment exert major influence on child development. Perhaps as a result of cultural and social factors, maltreating families often lack significant social connections to others in their extended families, neighborhoods, and communities, as well as to social assistance agencies (Korbin, 2003; Thompson & Flood, 2002). Unfortunately, maintaining family privacy and isolation may come at the cost of restricted access to healthier childrearing models and social supports. Neglectful families are especially prone to such isolation and insularity, which may be tied to the parents' significant interpersonal problems (Gaudin, Polansky, Kilpatrick, & Shilton, 1996).

In summary, abusive and neglectful parents may be characterized as coming from multi-problem families of origin, in which they were exposed to traumatic or negative childhood experiences, such as family violence and instability. As adults, they often are incapable of managing the levels of stress found in their environment, and tend to avoid social contacts that they may perceive as additional sources of stress. Inadequate or inappropriate exposure to positive parental models and supports (both in the present and the past), coupled with limited problem-solving skills and ability to make appropriate judgments during childrearing situations, may serve to make childrearing a difficult and aversive event. Consequently (or concomitantly), such parents may report symptoms indicative of health and coping problems that further impair their ability to function effectively as parents. As a result, strategies for assessing parents must balance between screening for a wide range of possible difficulties without being cumbersome in an attempt to be exhaustive.

ASSESSMENT OF CHILD ABUSE AND NEGLECT

The preceding overview has emphasized the interplay of a constellation of factors that involve the entire family, including the parent's childhood and early adult history, childrearing skills, recent stressful events, social relationships, and features of the child, among others. We have also seen that the causes and outcomes of abuse are entwined with general background factors that may impair child development, such as socioeconomic disadvantage, health status, and family instability. In view of the complexity of this problem, several implications for the assessment of maltreating families emerge. Whereas home and clinic observations of behavior have demonstrated their value for pinpointing specific problem areas, by themselves such observations may be insufficient to reveal the range and significance of contextual events that may be dramatically influencing

parent and child behavior. Therefore, indirect assessment methods (e.g., self-report and collateral report instruments, interviews, and standardized psychological tests) that assess such things as parental attitudes, perceived social supports, and physical and emotional health are important methods for examining low-frequency behaviors and qualitative factors that relate to parental competence and possible marital, social, or financial problems.

Another assessment issue that deserves emphasis relates to the extremely wide range of behaviors that may be shown by abused children. Typically, functional components of the abuse process, such as marital conflict, family instability, and elevated expressions of anger, are associated with an unusual pattern of child behavior. However, it is not uncommon to find maltreated children who either lack any signs of overt problems or distress or exhibit very self-defeating behavior with no obvious function. Rather than assuming that an apparent absence of distress is indicative of the benign effects of abuse, other alternatives must be carefully considered. Therefore, the ongoing assessment of abused children's development and behavior over an extended time period may be necessary both to understand the relationship of their behavior to previous and current experiences, and to determine the (possible) adaptive nature of their coping and adjustment patterns at different developmental periods.

Referral Questions

Assessing child abuse and neglect is a complex undertaking, in part because there are many different assessment purposes. Unlike assessing pathology such as depression or anxiety, in which the assessment questions tend to be more consistent, there is a range of referral reasons for an assessment evaluating child maltreatment. It is critical to have a clear understanding of the parameters and focus of the assessment at the outset, because child maltreatment assessments range on a variety of dimensions, including the likelihood of becoming part of a court proceeding. Because child maltreatment occurs within a system rather than an individual, evaluation typically includes an assessment of the parent(s), child(ren), and/or the parent–child relationship. A comprehensive assessment almost always includes all three elements. Some common referral purposes include the following.

Assessment of Risk of Abuse and/or Competence of Parenting

One of the most common purposes of referral, assessment of risk for abuse and/or parenting capacity, is often ordered to assist child protective services or the court in making placement decisions. The importance of a clear referral purpose cannot be overstated. Even within this particular type of assessment, the more focused the purpose of referral the better, because vague or global reasons for referral (e.g., "to evaluate this mother's parenting ability") are likely to lead to vague and global reports (Budd, 2001). These assessments may be very labor intensive, because they often include a review of significant amounts of collateral information and require interviews with many individuals who have been involved with the family. Assessing allegations about parenting capacity and/or abuse occurs with higher frequency in high-conflict custody cases than in the general public (see Box 14.1).

Assessment of a Family Where Child Maltreatment Has Been Identified for the Purposes of Intervention Planning

General treatment planning for various members of a family is another common purpose for assessment. In these cases, maltreatment has already been substantiated in the child protection system (or the family has been identified as high risk) and the purpose of the referral is to identify appropriate intervention(s). Although protocols related to mandatory reporting of child abuse still apply, there is less focus on whether an incident did or did not occur and more emphasis on identifying strengths and weaknesses of the family. In these assessments, recommendations typically focus more on identifying required interventions and supports than on specific placement decisions.

Assessment of the Adult Perpetrator of Child Maltreatment for the Purposes of Intervention Planning

In some cases, an adult perpetrator of child abuse is referred for an assessment to assist intervention planning. Although the focus is the adult perpetrator, an understanding of the parent–child dynamics associated with child abuse is critical for conducting these assessments. Because these assessments are more typically the domain of child protective services or

adult forensic work, and less likely to be part of general psychological practice, they are not covered in great detail in this chapter.

Assessment of Child Victim for the Purposes of Intervention Planning

Social workers and psychologists are often called upon to assess child victims of abuse to evaluate the extent of trauma and other difficulties that have arisen due to the abuse. These assessments provide a critical basis for intervention planning. The assessment may include overt symptomatology (e.g., trauma symptoms, depression and anxiety, behavioral problems), more subtle attitudinal components (e.g., attributions about blame, attitudes about acceptability of violence), and deficits in interpersonal and academic functioning.

Screening for Child Abuse in a General Clinical Setting

Sometimes a child or family that has come into contact with professionals for reasons other than child maltreatment may evidence a "red flag" for neglect or abuse. Situations in which abuse might be suspect include the following: (1) The history of the child's injury given by the parent is incompatible with the present injury; (2) the parent's account of the "accident" changes during the course of questioning; (3) repeated episodes of trauma or accidents are known to the agency, setting, or interagency records; and (4) there is an inexplicable delay in seeking treatment for the child's injury or illness. Typically, such assessment or screening is done by emergency care staff in hospitals and child protection agencies, although any professional who comes into contact with families may be called upon to offer his or her opinion about the nature and probable cause of an atypical pattern of child injuries, delays, or behavior.

Victim Impact Assessment of Adults Who Were Victims of Child Abuse

A final, highly specialized focus is assessment of the impact of historical child abuse on individuals who are now adults. These assessments, conducted for the purpose of criminal or civil litigation, document the severity and pervasiveness of the effects of the abuse. In some of these assessments there is a vocational component to highlight the gap between possi-

BOX 14.1. Legal Issue: Assessing Child Abuse Allegations in the Context of High-Conflict Custody Cases

Psychologists and social workers who conduct custody assessments for the court are often presented with competing claims of child maltreatment by divorcing parties (Jaffe, Crooks, & Bala, 2006). One California-based study of high-conflict separation cases in the family courts found that more than half involved an allegation of spousal or child abuse (Johnston, Lee, Olesen, & Walters, 2005). Allegations in the context of high-conflict divorce might be dismissed by professionals as symptoms of the parental conflict, and child protective services often want the matter settled in civil or family court. However, the results of the California study suggest that these allegations should be taken seriously and evaluated on their own merit. In this sample, about one-half of the abuse allegations were substantiated, and in about one-fourth of the cases some form of child or spousal abuse was perpetrated by both parents. Professionals may be (understandably) suspicious about the timing of child abuse allegations in the context of custodial proceedings and worry that a parent is making unfounded allegations to gain the upper hand in the civil proceedings. However, there may be other good reasons why allegations are made at the point of separation. In some cases, the child or parent feels too intimidated or guilty to disclose the abuse until after separation; in other cases, child abuse may not begin until after separation. Nonetheless, false allegations remain a weighty concern for mental health and justice system professionals.

What is the incidence of false allegations in child custody proceedings? It is impossible to say definitively, and it may be more useful to think about unfounded allegations (rather than maliciously false). Overall, in the few empirical studies that have been conducted, there is a significantly higher incidence of unfounded allegations of child abuse in the post separation context than in other situations (Bala & Schuman, 1999; Trocmé & Bala, 2005). However, it is important to note that a relatively small number of the unfounded postseparation allegations of child abuse in these studies were deemed to be due to deliberate or malicious fabrication. More common are cases of unfounded postseparation allegations, in which the accusing parent has an honestly held (albeit erroneous) belief about abuse based on numerous factors. For example, children's vague descriptions or symptoms, the parent's own abuse history, their poor view of the other parent, and lack of trust between parents may well contribute to the unfounded belief that abuse occurred.

In some cases, the accusing parent's erroneous beliefs about the other parent perpetrating child abuse are held so strongly that he or she will reject repeated independent, professional opinions refuting the allegations. In these cases, courts and community service providers have to manage their limited resources to ensure that repeated assessments and the litigation process are not harming the children. The fact that a parent continues to hold unfounded beliefs about child abuse perpetrated by the other parent in the face of clear refutation by investigating professionals may be symptomatic of serious emotional problems and require intervention.

Implication for Assessment

Regardless of the particular context, allegations of child abuse require thoughtful and thorough assessment. Custody proceedings tend to be conceptualized by the parties as having a winner and a loser, and there is an implicit assumption that at least one of the parents can provide safe and adequate parenting. In reality, both parents may have significant parenting deficits and/or engage in child abusive behaviors, requiring assessors to make a report to child protective services. Custody assessments in general tend to trigger the highest number of complaints about practitioners to licensing boards across jurisdictions. Assessors are cautioned to undertake these assessments with great care, and to ensure adequate supervision and professional development before entering into this area of practice.

ble career success and the individual's actual path. Similar to parenting capacity assessments, victim impact assessments are conducted with the understanding that the report will become part of a settlement or trial proceeding, and the assessor may be called to testify. These assessments may focus on historical familial abuse but, increasingly, they relate to historical institutional abuse (Wolfe et al., 2003).

Although the basic standards of good assessment apply to all of the preceding referral issues, there are additional considerations for assessments relating to child maltreatment. The American Psychological Association (APA) has published guidelines to assist psychologists who engage in child protection evaluations (APA Committee on Professional Practice and Standards, 1998). These guidelines address numerous areas, including orientation, preparing for a child protection evaluation, and procedures. Although not intended to be binding standards, they are highly recommended for any professional undertaking these assessments. Also, there are additional considerations specific to the broader area of child maltreatment assessments (over and above child protection evaluations). These considerations provide a critical context for the entire assessment process, and competent assessment of child maltreatment is grounded in an appreciation of these factors.

1. *Child maltreatment encompasses a range of behaviors.* As noted in the first section of this chapter, there is a wide range of patterns that span the subject of child maltreatment, from the legal definition of child abuse to a more encompassing clinical concept of maltreatment. Generally, it is recognized that officially documented cases of legal child abuse represent only the "tip of the iceberg" (Trocmé, et al., 2001). The legal definition of child abuse is predicated on whether or not a specific event occurred, but beyond these discrete incidents that have met the legal threshold, there may be ongoing toxic and coercive parent–child interactions that do not meet the legal definition. It is important for an assessor to be clear about whether he or she is documenting child abuse in the formal, legal sense or maltreatment in a broader sense. Regardless of the parameters of the referral question, inclusion of subabusive violence directed toward children in the assess-

ment process is key (Graziano, 1994). Furthermore, as difficult as it is to measure physical child maltreatment, neglect and emotional abuse are even more complicated due to differences in definitions and conceptualizations (see Straus & Kantor [2005] and Hamarman, Pope, & Czaja [2002], respectively).

2. *Families are typically seeking service involuntarily or with significant coercion.* Families undergoing assessment for child abuse and neglect often have been referred for psychological services involuntarily or under duress. This referral pattern has implications in terms of both eliciting the necessary, accurate information from the parents and establishing credibility and rapport that will increase clients' motivation to change their parenting style. In general, such clients are more reserved and defensive than self-referred clients in terms of acknowledging their need for mental health services. In addition, there are specific concerns with respect to response patterns for well-established standardized measures (Carr, Moretti, & Cue, 2005). These response patterns are discussed in more detail in the section of this chapter on assessing adults. Assessing defensiveness is an important piece of a comprehensive assessment, because readiness to change has been found to predict improvement and recidivism in a child welfare sample (Littell & Girvin, 2005). Finally, it is important to be aware that informed consent in these cases may have a coercive element.

3. *Child abuse represents an entrenched style of interaction with many barriers to change.* The task of learning unfamiliar child management procedures may appear overwhelming to parents, strengthening their desire to adhere to more familiar, aversive control methods. This "resistance to change" is also embedded in cultural and familial factors (e.g., proclivity toward physical punishment and rigid control) that may conflict with the therapist's style of assistance and intended goals for the family. In our parenting program for abusive fathers, men typically begin by saying that they are simply "not going to do it again"; however, even with the desire to change, these men face significant challenges associated with altering overlearned patterns of relating (Crooks, Scott, Francis, Kelly, & Reid, 2006).

4. *Abusive families are a heterogeneous group of multiproblem families.* Abusive families are a heterogeneous group of multiproblem families that possess unique combinations of

assets and liabilities. Recent research efforts have begun to identify profiles or types of parents who are abusive (Haskett, Scott, & Ward, 2004; Herron & Holtzworth-Munroe, 2002), but the reality remains that each family is idiosyncratic in terms of its own strengths and weaknesses. Thus, each family requires a uniquely tailored, ongoing assessment strategy that is sensitive to its particular needs. It is a widely recognized clinical principle that the likelihood of positive treatment outcomes is maximized when interventions are matched to specific targets on the basis of an appropriate assessment. A mismatch of intervention and needs is at best inefficient, and at worst dangerous, particularly in families where child maltreatment is an issue (Saunders, Berliner, & Hanson, 2003).

General Assessment Methods and Process

Assessment for all comprehensive child abuse referral questions involves assessing parents, children, and parent–child dynamics separately. The overall options for data collection are the same as for other types of assessment (i.e., interview, self-report, administered tests, and observation) and the general principles of competent assessment still apply (i.e., multimethod, multi-informant approaches). However, there are many additional considerations unique to the nature of the problem being assessed.

In the next sections we discuss assessment of parents, followed by children, and finally parent–child abuse-related dynamics. In the parent and child sections, our focus is on specific abuse assessment considerations and concerns rather than reiteration of basic assessment principles. Where specific measures have been researched more carefully with a child abuse population, we describe the findings. We highlight recent innovations and include comments on feasibility of measures and approaches throughout.

STEP 1: ASSESSING PARENTS

Issues in Assessing Maltreating Adults

The assessment of abusive parents must be tailored to the needs of the referral source, as well as those of the particular family. The complex array of factors that contribute to abuse and neglect requires an assessment approach that attends to the major problem areas in an organized and progressive fashion, without becoming overburdened by the number of potential concerns.

Because the possible consequences associated with the family's participation during assessment and issues of confidentiality are often initially unclear, parents may behave in a cautious or defensive manner. It is important that the interviewer explains his or her professional role (i.e., to assess areas in need of change) and standards concerning client confidentiality; however, it is equally important to clarify for the parents the assessor's legal obligation to report any suspicions of child maltreatment to protective services. Usually this can be done in a matter-of-fact manner as the session begins:

> "I'll be asking you to tell me a lot of detail concerning your child's behavior and your feelings and actions related to your child. My role is to find out whether the problems you are having can be lessened in any way. Please understand that I'm not here to make any judgments about your parenting ability without your agreement and understanding. I am under no obligation to report to anyone outside of this room about what we discuss unless there is a risk of your child or another child being at risk for harm. This means that if you tell me that you hurt your child or may hurt him/her I must notify your caseworker (or protective services). Beyond the immediate safety of children, I will not discuss anything with your worker unless we have both agreed to this beforehand. If you have any other concerns about your situation and my role, let's discuss them now before proceeding with the interview."

Mental health professionals who have been asked by the court to prepare a written report on parental competence and risk will have to modify this statement to clarify for the parent exactly what the court is asking, and what does and does not need to be reported.

A wide range of assessment domains may be pertinent for a particular adult, and the breadth of the assessment, of course, stems from referral concerns. There has been a move away from extensive personality testing, in part because there is not an "abusive personality" for which to assess. At the same time, a general measure of personality (e.g., the Personality Assessment Inventory, the Minnesota Multiphasic Personality Inventory—Second Edition) may be incorporated to help develop an overall pattern of strengths and weaknesses. Typically, an assessment includes a general evaluation of psychosocial functioning and possible symptomatology, emotional functioning and regulation, social support, life stress, and the marital relationship or other intimate partner relationships. Additional indicated areas, such as a more in-depth mental health or substance abuse assessment, are included on an as-needed basis.

Interview

Initial information concerning both parent and child functioning is typically obtained from a semistructured interview with the parent, as well as reports from others. To assist in organizing the material in a comprehensive fashion, a Parent Interview and Assessment Guide, presented in Table 14.1, provides an overview of the major issues that we address below.

TABLE 14.1. Parent Interview and Assessment Guide: Abuse and Neglect

The following is a selected summary of the major factors associated with child abuse and neglect, requiring further interviewing and assessment of the parent, as indicated. The framing and emphasis of each question are left up to the discretion of the interviewer.

I. Identifying general problem areas
    A. Family background
        1. Early rejection or abuse during own childhood; relationship with biological and/or psychological parents
        2. Methods of punishment and reward receiving during own childhood
        3. Family planning and effect of children on the marital relationship
        4. Preparedness for and sense of competence in childrearing
        5. Early physical, emotional, behavioral problems of child (i.e., illnesses, trauma, temperament)

    B. Marital relationship
        1. Length, stability, and quality of present relationship
        2. Examples of conflict of physical violence
        3. Support from partner in family responsibilities
        4. Substance abuse

    C. Areas of perceived stress and supports
        1. Employment history and satisfaction
        2. Family income and expenses, chronic economic problems
        3. Stability of occupation, income, and living arrangements
        4. Perceived support from within or outside of the family
        5. Daily/weekly contacts with others (e.g., neighbors, social workers)
        6. Quality of social contacts and major life events (i.e., positive vs. negative influence on the parent)

    D. Symptomatology
        1. Recent or chronic health problems; treatment; drug and alcohol use
        2. Identifiable mood and affect changes; anxiety; social dysfunction
        3. Previous psychiatric evaluations of treatment

II. Assessing parental responses to childrearing demands
    A. Emotional reactivity
        1. Perception of how particular child differs from siblings or other children known to the parent
        2. Feelings of anger and loss of control when interacting with child (describe circumstances, how the parent felt, how the parent reacted)
        3. Typical ways of coping with arousal during/following stressful episodes

    B. Childrearing methods
        1. Parental expectations of child (i.e., accuracy of expectations for child behavior and development, in reference to child's actual developmental status)
        2. Examples of recent efforts to teach new or desirable behavior to child
        3. "Preferred" and "typical" manner of controlling/disciplining child
        4. Attitudes toward learning different or unfamiliar childrearing methods
        5. Perceived effectiveness of parent's teaching and discipline approach
        6. Pattern of child behavior in response to typical discipline methods (i.e., accelerating, decelerating, manipulative, responsive)

Family Background

The importance of careful investigation of parents' previous childhood experiences that may affect current behavior cannot be overstated. Abusive parents can often relate to the examiner several significant events, such as early rejection or abuse during childhood, or strong cultural values, such as adherence to corporal punishment and disavowal of "bribery methods," that have influenced or guided their behavior within the family. Although these events and perceptions may have little to do with changing current behaviors per se, they may suggest to the examiner the type of treatment approach that might be most effective (emphasis on cognitive and attitudinal change, modeling, problem solving, etc.). Most importantly, knowledge of the parent's history enables the therapist to develop an intervention plan that is most likely to succeed in relation to the parent's expectations, abilities, and needs.

The interview should trace the origins and development of significant areas of stress within the family system, beginning with family planning and the effects of children on the marital relationship. This discussion includes, for example, whether the child was planned, the effect of the pregnancy on parental attitudes and lifestyle, support of the biological father, the mother's/father's preparedness and sense of competence in childrearing (i.e., emotional maturity, family support, peer influences), and early childhood problems (e.g., illnesses, trauma, and temperament). It is often useful to allow time for general discussion of the child throughout the interview, because the parent may have justified or rationalized his or her actions based on the child's "difficult behavior." The parent can be encouraged to describe the child's desirable and undesirable behaviors, and to discuss how he or she would like to see these changed.

Marital and Family Adjustment

Because the parent's childrearing effectiveness and appropriateness is often related to his or her interactions and experiences with other significant adults, the interviewer should be careful to assess areas of non-child-related stress within the family. In many instances of child maltreatment, the marital (or common-law) relationship is a primary source of added conflict and stress that interferes with childrearing. A discussion of the length, stability, and quality of the present relationship may provide insight into the manner in which adult conflict may influence parent–child interactions, such as tolerance for child misbehavior, noise, and interruptions. Interestingly, family functioning may be an area where there are different risk factors for men and women. In one study of military parents, depression, parental distress, and family conflict predicted child abuse potential scores for both mothers and fathers, whereas low family expressiveness was predictive only for fathers, and marital dissatisfaction, low social support, and low family cohesion were predictive only for mothers (Schaeffer, Alexander, Bethke, & Kretz, 2005).

In addition, the interviewer should be sensitive to other signs of major distress or conflict in the family system that may play a major role in the perpetration of child maltreatment, especially physical violence between partners, extramarital relationships, substance abuse, interference from relatives, and lack of spousal assistance in handling family affairs. These topics may need to be addressed during private, individual sessions with each partner as circumstances require.

Areas of Perceived Stress and Support

The major purpose of assessing the family's or individuals' degree of stress and support is to locate areas that are perceived as highly stressful and to determine what resources family members use to manage these areas of stress, either effectively or ineffectively. Assessment of highly stressful socioeconomic factors can be accomplished during the interview by discussing employment history and satisfaction, family income and expenses, housing and living arrangements, and similar circumstances that may be contributing to family problems.

Parental Emotional Regulation and Functioning

The parent's reactivity to unpleasant or aversive environmental events is an important factor believed to mediate anger and aggression (Wolfe, 1999). Because emotional reactivity involves involuntary somatic responses (e.g., changes in cardiovascular function, temperature of peripheral organs, muscle tension) that are very difficult to observe or measure under realistic conditions, self-report ratings of annoyance, anger, or unpleasant changes in affect have most commonly been used. Abusive parents are often willing to describe their feelings of anger and "loss of control" when provided with distinctive cues or examples, such as interacting with their child in a high-conflict situation or discussing a recent conflict (e.g., Koverola, Elliot-Faust, & Wolfe, 1984); that is, feelings of anger, tension, and frustration can be identified by asking parents to provide recent examples of irritating child behaviors, the circumstances in which they occurred, how they felt, and how they reacted. At the same time, the clinician can ask parents to identify fluctuations in mood (especially depression, anxiety, and agitation) that precede or follow incidences of parent–child conflict (MacMillan et al., 1991).

Throughout the interview it is important for the clinician to attend to the process as well as the content relayed by the parent's responses. By attending to *how* responses are given and looking for patterns, an understanding of the parent's worldview will begin to emerge. Do they see authority figures and helping professionals as trustworthy or do they feel hostile towards people in general? Do they feel that they have some control over events or do things just seem to happen to them? Can they link the causes and consequences of some of the events they have experienced? Listening to the phrases a parent uses to attribute intent towards their children is also helpful. For example, a parent who reports that a child really knows their "triggers" or "how to push their buttons" suggests a belief system that may predispose them to coercive and abusive parenting strategies due to the perception of malicious intent on the child's part. Although it may not be possible to record the entire interview verbatim, recording key responses in the exact language used by the parent will provide helpful material for the report.

If the clinician has concerns about significant psychopathology, a structured diagnostic interview might be indicated. For example, the Structured Clinical Interview for DSM-IV Axis I Disorders (SCID; First, Spitzer, Gibbon, & Williams, 1996) is a semistructured diagnostic interview designed to assist clinicians in making reliable DSM-IV Axis I (clinical) psychiatric diagnoses. Although the presence of a mental health disorder in and of itself does not determine whether parenting is ineffective or abusive, a diagnosis can alert the assessor to specific areas of functioning that might be impaired. For example, if a parent has been diagnosed with bipolar disorder and experiences periods of mania accompanied by poor impulse control and judgment, it would be important to assess the parent's insight into the need for parenting support during these episodes.

Self-Report Measures of Interpersonal Functioning, Adjustment, and Personality

During the interview, a history of the parent's clinical symptomatology may be addressed by discussing mood and affect changes, anxiety, recent or chronic health problems, and medical treatments. This interview procedure may be assisted by the administration of a standardized psychiatric symptom checklist or inventory to rule out particular forms of psychopathology and/or determine the extent of psychopathology. Several options are presented here that vary in length, extent to which they focus on pathology versus general functioning and personality, and ability to detect social desirability. These measures are further summarized in Table 14.2.

The Symptom Checklist–90—Revised (SCL-90-R; Derogatis, 1983), a relatively brief self-report symptom inventory designed to reflect psychological and health-related symptoms of the respondent over the past 7 days, has been shown to have strong psychometric properties. Two subscales of this 90-item questionnaire are particularly useful indicators of adult interpersonal style: (1) Interpersonal Sensitivity, which measures personal inadequacy and inferiority (e.g., self-deprecation, feelings of uneasiness); and (2) Hostility, which reflects thoughts, feelings, or actions that are characteristic of the negative affect state of anger. The SCL-90-R has demonstrated utility with at-risk parents (Ammerman & Patz, 1996; Budd, Heliman, & Kane, 2000). There is also a shorter version of the SCL-90-R, the 53-item Brief Symptom Inventory (BSI—Derogatis, 1992; Derogatis & Melisaratos, 1983). Although the efficiency of the BSI makes it an attractive alternative, little research has been conducted with the BSI in the context of assessing parenting competence or risk (Budd, 2001). More recently the BSI-18 was developed as a brief, self-report symptom inventory designed to screen for psychological distress and psychiatric disorders (Derogatis, 2000). The 18 items take approximately 4–5 minutes to complete and provide scores on So-

TABLE 14.2. General Measures of Personality, Psychopathology and Interpersonal Functioning for Assessing Parents

Measure	Description of scales	No. of items (time)	Validity scales	Comments
Symptom Checklist-90-R	9 primary symptoms scales plus 3 global indices measuring overall distress, intensity of symptoms, and number of symptoms	90 (12–15 min)	No	The SCL-90-R and shorter versions have not received much research attention with respect to utility in child abuse assessments.
Brief Symptom Inventory	9 primary symptoms scales plus 3 global indices measuring overall distress, intensity of symptoms, and number of symptoms	53 (8–10 min)	No	
Brief Symptom Inventory–18	3 scales—Anxiety, Depression, Somatization, plus an Overall Severity Index	18 (4 min)	No	
Minnesota Multiphasic Personality Inventory–2	10 clinical scales 9 restructured clinical (RC) scales 15 content scales 27 content component scales 20 supplementary scales 31 clinical subscales (Harris–Lingoes and social introversion subscales) Various special or setting-specific indices	567 (60–90 min)	Yes: 8 validity scales	Validity scales make the MMPI very useful in child abuse assessments.
Personality Assessment Inventory	11 clinical scales 5 treatment scales 2 interpersonal scales	344 (40–60 min)	Yes: 5 validity scales	Has validity scales, but there is preliminary evidence that these may not detect defensive responding patterns in child abuse assessments.

matization, Depression, and Anxiety subscales, in addition to a Global Severity Index.

One of the most commonly used but relatively time-consuming self-report options for assessing functioning and pathology is the Minnesota Multiphasic Personality Inventory—Second Edition (Butcher, Dahlstrom, Graham, Tellegen, & Kaemmer, 1989). The MMPI-2 is considered by many to be the gold standard in personality and psychopathology assessment. It has 567 true–false items and is estimated to take between 60 and 90 minutes to complete. Scores are produced on a wide range of clinical, content, and validity scales, and there are now more than 50 years of research on the original MMPI. Several translations of the MMPI-2 are available, including Spanish, Hmong, and French for Canada. Although the MMPI-2 is significantly longer than the SCL-90-R and other, similar measures, it was found to be much more useful in detecting

defensive responding in a sample of parents undergoing parenting capacity assessments (Carr et al., 2005). Based on the results of all of the measures evaluated in this study, the authors recommended that the MMPI-2 be used routinely in all assessments due to its rigorous validity scales. Furthermore, they note that self-report measures that do not have validity scales are of little use in this context (Carr et al., 2005). Although the pattern of defensive responding investigated in this study was based on clients undergoing parenting capacity assessments, it is consistent with our experience in assessing maltreating parents pre- and postintervention (Scott & Crooks, in press).

The Personality Assessment Inventory (PAI; Morey, 1991, 1996) is a 344-item measure that takes approximately 50–60 minutes to complete. It has 11 clinical scales, 5 treatment scales, and 2 interpersonal scales. In addition, the PAI has a number of validity scales, some of which correspond in concept to scales on the MMPI-2. However, in the aforementioned study evaluating social desirability in parenting capacity assessments, the PAI was found to be more conservative than the MMPI-2 in detecting positive impression management, and likely missed a number of individuals who were not completely forthcoming in their responses (Carr et al., 2005). Furthermore, the style of defensive responding that was found to be pervasive among participants in this study had a profound impact on clinical scale elevations; thus, rather than being an independent issue, defensiveness has significant implications for identifying areas of challenge for the client.

In summary, there are a number of measures and approaches for assessing general personality functioning and psychopathology, and the three discussed in this section each have their strengths and weaknesses. The SCL-90-R is relatively brief and has shown some discriminant validity for use with abusive parents; however, defensive responding patterns for adults being assessed in the context of child abuse have not been studied. The MMPI-2 has undergone extensive research and has more sophisticated validity scales, which may be more successful in identifying overt and subtle defensiveness. On the negative side, the length of the MMPI-2 is daunting. The PAI is longer than the SCL-90-R but shorter than the MMPI-2. Although the PAI has validity scales, these did not detect positive impression management reliably in a child protection context. Given these various trade-offs, clinician must base their choices on time, resources, and concerns about detecting defensiveness.

Social Support and Life Stress

As noted, social support and life stressors may be assessed during the parent interview. Clinicians may wish to include some short, standardized measures, but if they are attempting to minimize the administration of paper-and-pencil tasks, these are not areas of priority. Standardized measures of social support and life stress are highly face valid and the information is quite easily obtained during an interview. One reason *to* include standardized measures in these domains is to assess the impact of treatment, if increasing social support is a specifically articulated intervention goal.

If a standardized measure of social support is preferred, two widely used options are the So-

cial Support Questionnaire (SSQ; Sarason, Levine, Basham, & Sarason, 1983) and the Perceived Social Support from Friends and Family scales (PSS: Procidano & Heller, 1983). The SSQ, a 27-item measure, has individuals rate both availability and satisfaction with social support from specific individuals in a particular scenario. There is also a 6-item brief version of the SSQ that correlates well with the original measure (Sarason, Sarason, Shearin, & Pierce, 1987). The PSS, a 20-item scale, differs from the SSQ in that it distinguishes between the sources of perceived social support (i.e., friends vs. family), on the grounds that these sources may serve different social support functions, with different consequences. One advantage of the PSS is that it is available in the widely used third edition of the handbook *Measures for Clinical Practice: A Sourcebook* (Corcoran & Fischer, 2000). As an interesting aside, Swedish and Turkish translations of the PSS scales have been reported in the research literature (see summary on METRIC website, retrieved April 18, 2006, from *www.metric.research.med.va. gov/index.asp*).

Stress may be measured by one of two general approaches, either by evaluating the perceived experience of stress or by looking more objectively at the number of stressors experienced. One widely used instrument that takes the former approach is the Perceived Stress Scale (Cohen, Kamarck, & Mermelstein, 1983; Cohen & Williamson, 1988). The Perceived Stress Scale is a measure of the degree to which situations in one's life are appraised as stressful. Items were designed to tap how unpredictable, uncontrollable, and overloaded respondents find their lives. There are three versions of the scale, with 4 items, 10 items, or 14 items, although the 10-item scale has the best reliability.

Life stressor indices typically ask participants to indicate which of a number of events have occurred within a particular time frame. The list includes major stressful life events that occur in people's lives, such as death of a loved one, loss of a job, being divorced, moving, and going to court. In general, the idea of life events instruments is that the negative impact of major life events increases with the number of events. No life event instrument is appropriate for all populations or generally accepted in the field. There are also questions about the sensitivity (appropriateness) of any of the standard life events instruments for lower socioeconomic status (SES), or specific ethnic populations, in part because events are only counted if they are part of the scale, and these measures may not represent the breadth of negative experiences faced by a particular group. Strategies to measure parenting-related stress are discussed more specifically later in this chapter.

Intimate Relationships: Satisfaction, Conflict, and Violence

Marital conflict and satisfaction may be assessed through several methods, including interview, standardized instruments, and observation of interactions during conflict resolution tasks. For child abusive families (in which couples have not requested marital counseling and are often hesitant to discuss other issues), it may be useful to follow the previously discussed interview procedure with a brief satisfaction measure, such as the *Dyadic Adjustment Scale* (DAS; Spanier, 1976).

Violence between intimate partners should be assessed for a number of reasons. The presence of adult violence has implications for individuals' capacity to parent, role models to which children are being exposed, and is a general red flag for physical child abuse, given that the overlap between the two forms of violence is estimated to be in the range of 30–60% (Edleson, 1999). In some jurisdictions, exposure to domestic violence has been defined as a form of child maltreatment and/or risk that triggers a child protection response (see Box 14.2). The *Conflict Tactics Scales* measure (CTS—Straus, 1979, 1995; revised version [CTS2]—Straus, Hamby, Boney-McCoy, & Sugarman, 1996) was specifically designed to elicit information concerning conflict resolution tactics between adults and/or between parents and child(ren). The CTS is administered in an interview fashion, whereby each partner is asked to rate the frequency of occurrence (on a 7-point scale, ranging from *Never*, to *More than 20 times*) of tactics that he or she has used toward the partner in disputes over the past 12 months. These tactics include, for example, "Discussed the issue calmly," "Insulted or swore at the other one," "Threatened to hit or throw something at the other one," and "Kicked, bit, or hit with a fist." This instrument has been widely used in clinical and research studies to assess verbal and physical aggression in the family (see Archer [1999] for meta-analytic review on couples agreement of

aggression ratings). A shorter version has been developed; however, the authors note that the brief version may miss cases of violence and is best used as an initial screen (Straus et al., 1996). Regardless of the version of the CTS used, information obtained from this approach should be combined with other sources (e.g., interview, direct observation) to provide the best estimate of marital conflict resolution tactics (Jouriles & O'Leary, 1985; for additional procedures for assessing marital violence, see Jacobson, Gottman, Waltz, & Rushe, 1994).

Although there are many measures of general marital satisfaction, the Parenting Alliance Measure (PAM; Abidin & Konold, 1999) is unique in its evaluation of the parenting aspects of a couple's relationship. Parents' perceptions of their own cooperativeness, communicativeness, and respectfulness with regard to caring for their children are assessed. The PAM is appropriate for a variety of parenting partners and living situations.

Use of Collateral Information

Parent interviews, self-reports, and testing should be augmented with collateral information where possible. For example, child protection services, physician, police, and other service provider information help to provide a more comprehensive picture. If the assessment has a particularly forensic focus (e.g., a parenting capacity assessment), careful documentation of collateral information becomes even more critical.

Collateral information is important in two ways. The first and more obvious benefit is the additional information, which may highlight difficulties that parents did not mention or help to resolve a difference in reported versions of a particular event (e.g., when a police report of a domestic violence call clarifies parents' contradictory accounts of the events). A second way that collateral information may be useful is to review it with the parents and provide them with the opportunity to clarify or help the clinician understand the reports. This review is important, because written records sometimes contain incorrect information. Beyond the factual verification, it is informative to assess parents' understanding and/or responsibility taking for previous events. For example, reviewing police records that relay multiple charges of drinking and driving provides clinicians with an opportunity to assess whether a parent un-

---

BOX 14.2. Legal Issue: Should Exposure to Domestic Violence be Considered a Form of Legal Child Abuse?

Over the past 20 years, concern about children exposed to domestic violence (DV) has grown rapidly, as a result of an emerging awareness that these children may experience difficulties similar to those of children who are directly abused. In response, legislators and policymakers have attempted to develop laws and protocols to protect these children (Jaffe, Crooks, & Wolfe, 2003). In some jurisdictions, exposing children to DV has been defined as a form of criminal child abuse, whereas in others, it may be considered abuse if there is direct, observable harm to the children. In yet other states, none of these laws has been implemented. These legal changes have been the subject of significant debate.

Proponents of defining exposure to DV as child abuse identify benefits such as sending a clear message to perpetrators about the unacceptability of the behavior, recognizing children exposed as a vulnerable group, and providing a mechanism for accessing and offering service to children who need it. In addition, given the significant overlap between DV and physical child abuse, the presence of DV may warrant further inspection of other risks children may be facing.

At the same time, there are a number of potential problems with identifying exposure to DV as a form of child abuse. First, although children exposed to DV have more problems in general, there is considerable variability in adjustment, and many exposed children do not experience these difficulties (Wolfe, Crooks, Lee, McIntyre-Smith, & Jaffe, 2003). Second, women's advocates have noted that although these legal changes are intended to help hold perpetrators of violence more accountable, the result may be revictimization of an abused mother, who in extreme cases can be charged with failure to protect. Third, in cases where there needs to be a demonstrated link between exposure to DV and the harm experienced by children, assessments methods have lagged behind these policy changes. The concept of a demonstrated link seems to make sense, but the practicality of assessing the *cause* of particular child difficulties is a challenge, especially in multiproblem families in which partner violence may be one of a multitude of risk factors. Finally, promoting legal changes as a way to identify and provide service to more children is flawed logic, in that these services typically are not available. The end result in such cases may be more children being identified (and possibly drawn into the child protection system) but not receiving any further service (Edleson, Gassman-Pines, & Hill, 2006).

The growing consensus among experts in the field is that the best practice in such cases is a *differentiated response*, which means saving the most intensive supports and resources for the families who need it. Broad-based laws identifying all exposure to domestic violence as a form of child abuse are not consistent with a differentiated response.

Implications for Assessment

As the framework for differentiated response emerges, there will be an increasing need for assessors to help guide the process of a system that can respond appropriately to different levels of severity. Research in the area of assessing the specific impact of children's exposure to domestic violence is greatly needed.

---

derstands the severity of the behavior, takes responsibility (vs. explaining it away on external factors), and has developed a plan to avoid future similar difficulties.

At the end of the adult portion of the assessment, the evaluator should have an overall view of the parents' strengths and challenges as individuals and in relation to their parenting roles. This view will have emerged within the context of a historical understanding of parents' families of origin, as well as their relationship with each other. Significant psychological difficulties should be clear, as well as resources

and coping styles that the individuals use to mitigate the impact of these difficulties.

STEP 2: ASSESSING CHILDREN

Children may be assessed as part of a larger strategy to determine a family's overall intervention needs. In these cases they are one component of an assessment addressing the strengths and needs of the larger family system. They may also be assessed with a very narrow focus to answer a specific question about the children's intervention needs. The following three examples demonstrate this more focused, narrow type of child abuse assessment.

Brenda, an 8-year-old, was removed from her mother's care following substantiated allegations of child abuse. In foster care, she has continued to demonstrate significant trauma symptoms such as nightmares, bedwetting, and hypervigilance. Despite these difficulties, Brenda is adamant about wanting to move back home. Her mother has completed a parenting program and is also requesting reunification. An assessment has been requested to explore the possible impact on Brenda of being reunited with her mother and to identify necessary supports for this family.

Juan, a 17-year-old with a long history of chronic abuse, neglect, and disrupted living arrangements, has been seeing an individual therapist for the past year to help him with anger and stress management, as well as interpersonal functioning. His therapist has become concerned about symptoms that might be consistent with early psychotic processes. She has referred him for an assessment to determine whether his symptoms of alienation, paranoia, and hostility are indicative of emerging psychosis or more likely sequelae of his long-standing abuse and losses.

Gina, a 6-year-old currently in inpatient care at a hospital following breakdown of her foster placement and several group home placements, has a documented history of abuse, and recent computed tomographic (CT) scans show some anomalies in her brain structure. The possibility of a seizure disorder has been raised in the past but is not well documented. She is observed by the hospital staff to have tantrums that seem to appear out of nowhere and are noteworthy for their magnitude and intensity. The referring psychiatrist is wondering whether the tantrums and observed emotional dysregulation could be related to a seizure disorder, or whether they are better understood as a result of psychosocial stressors and abuse.

Some assessment components would be common for all of these referral questions, such as administering standardized measures that compare the child's behavior to others of his or her age, obtaining a history of school and academic functioning, and identifying possible strengths or protective factors through interview and/or questionnaires. Other components would vary depending on the age of the child

and the specific referral question. For Brenda, assessment strategies that measure the range and severity of PTSD symptoms would be important. In the example of Juan, measuring his reality testing would be indicated. In addition, understanding the nature of his paranoid thoughts would be important. Due to the concerns about possible neurological impairment, a more thorough assessment of memory and learning would be indicated for Gina than for Juan or Brenda. There is always a trade-off between a broad assessment strategy that addresses the widest range of functioning and a more efficient, focused strategy that addresses the specific needs of any one child in greater depth.

In formulating an assessment strategy for an individual child, the clinician must be concerned about achieving some balance among child self-report (both interview and questionnaires), report by parents (especially if he or she is suspected of maltreatment), and observation of the child with peers and/or caregivers. The assessment usually begins with reports from significant sources in the child's life (including the referral source), because generally speaking such information from these sources (i.e., teachers, parents, social workers) provides a global understanding of the child that is then useful for narrowing down the choices for additional self-report, interview, or observational procedures. Following a clinical interview, self-report and observational methods yield considerable information concerning the child's strengths and deficits, especially in terms of his or her views of self and others (social cognition), and feeling states (socioemotional development).

Interview

An individual interview with the preschooler or school-age child can assist the practitioner in understanding the child's overall functioning and provide insight as to current fears or anxiety that might be quite debilitating. The possibility that the older child (age 6 or older) has developed a distorted perspective of family life in which violence is commonplace or acceptable should be investigated by discussing his or her attitudes about interpersonal aggression, sex roles, and responsibility for aggressive behavior. For example, when asked, children who have witnessed violence toward their mothers state that men should not hit women, but more subtle questioning may reveal that these children believe violence is permissible in certain situations (e.g., if a parent has been drinking, if the wife does not do what her husband says). The child may also respond to the examiner in a very guarded manner that is not a valid reflection of his or her typical behavior, out of possible fear of reprisal or confusion over the events that have occurred. For this reason the examiner should prioritize developing a rapport with the child and establishing a sense of trust and comfort prior to discussing his or her family's problems. Seeing the child on more than one occasion might be more important in these cases than in some other assessment situations.

Due to the sensitive (and possibly litigious) nature of the material being discussed, it is imperative that clinicians have a good sense of developmentally appropriate interviewing. A highly readable book to assist both novice and experienced clinicians is *What Children Can Tell Us: Eliciting, Interpreting, and Evaluating Critical Information from Children* (Garbarino & Stott, 1989). If a practitioner seeks to become specialized in forensic interviewing, additional training and ongoing professional development are highly advisable.

A good beginning point is to use a semi-structured interview format in discussing the child's comprehension and reaction to family problems. The interview begins with a general discussion of activities and events that the child enjoys, which leads to a more specific discussion of recent crisis events. The child's "crisis adjustment" is assessed in reference to (1) his or her feelings about changes in the family (e.g., foster care, parental separation) and (2) discussion of major life events (e.g., aided by the Life Events Checklist for Children; Johnson & McCutcheon, 1980). Safety skills (e.g., "What do you do if your mom and dad are arguing?"; "How can you tell when your mom or dad is angry?"; "Who do you call in an emergency?") are also important areas to consider during the child interview. The child's comprehension of personal safety and knowledge of appropriate actions to take provides useful information in planning for the immediate needs of the child (i.e., out-of-home placement, alternative actions to avoid high-conflict situations).

The clinician can then turn the discussion to the child's attitudes and responses to interpersonal conflict and expression of anger, by encouraging the child to discuss events, for example that "make you really mad," followed by identification of his or her actions, feelings, and attitudes about such "anger situations." We find it useful to describe attitudes and reactions to anger provocation in reference to favorite television characters, to determine the child's ability to recognize the inappropriateness of aggressive behavior. For example, some abused children reveal the influence of aggressive modeling in the family or on TV through their inability to recognize nonviolent means for resolving interpersonal conflicts. Although this impaired social problem solving is by no means unique to abused children, the presence of such rigid adherence to coercive problem solving signals a need for exposure to alternative strategies.

Standardized Assessment of Behavioral, Cognitive, and Emotional Development

Assessments of children need to be abuse-informed but not abuse-specific (Saunders et al., 2003). The task of assessing all potentially relevant dimensions of child psychopathology can become unmanageable unless a systematic, problem-solving approach is used. As noted in the first part of this chapter, child abuse is a nonspecific risk factor and can lead to impaired functioning in virtually every domain of children's adjustment. Rather than attempting to address all possible outcomes, we identify strategies for assessing major domains of functioning that may be impaired by experiencing child maltreatment and more narrow, abusive-specific concerns. When widely used measures have been researched with a child maltreatment population, implications for the measure's use are discussed. Self- and other-report measures and standardized procedures are discussed in the following section under the major headings of social and behavioral functioning, cognitive and social-cognitive development, and emotional and moral development. There may be areas outside of these that have been influenced by inadequate or abusive parenting (e.g., academic performance). If there were concerns of this nature in a particular case, a standard psychoeducational assessment would be performed.

Social and Behavioral Functioning

The child's primary caregiver, usually the parent, is a critical source of information concerning the child's development and behavior. Parental report of child behavior is a useful starting point for assessment and intervention planning, because it permits the clinician to obtain a broad spectrum of information as to the parent's perception of problem areas in the child. The Child Behavior Checklist (CBCL; Achenbach, 1991) is the most widely used measure of child social, emotional, and behavioral functioning. The CBCL requires only a sixth-grade reading level, takes about 20 minutes to complete, and the results can be easily discussed with the respondent to clarify the nature and specific circumstances surrounding his or her report of child behavior problems.

Although the CBCL has excellent general psychometric properties and has been used extensively in research, in a recent study of participants undergoing parenting capacity assessments, parents' general tendency to respond in socially desirable ways extended to their ratings of their children (Carr et al., 2005). In other words, in this particular study, parents undergoing parenting capacity assessments (i.e., parents who had perpetrated abuse or neglect, or were considered high risk for perpetrating) *underreported* their children's problems compared to the reports of teachers and foster parents. This finding is somewhat surprising in that general clinical wisdom is that abusive parents tend to *overreport* child misbehavior, in part because of their attributions of having less power over their children. These concerns notwithstanding, the CBCL is an efficient way to gather information on a range of behaviors. Furthermore, the availability of a Teacher Report Form and a Youth Self Report (YSR; for children age 12 and older) create the ability to look at differences in perception among informants. As of February 2006, versions of the CBCL had been translated into 74 languages (retrieved April 20, 2006, from *www.aseba.org/ordering/translations.html*).

An alternative system for assessing child and adolescent functioning, the Behavior Assessment System for Children, Second edition (BASC-2; Reynolds & Kamphaus, 2004), comprises a set of rating scales and forms, including Teacher Rating Scales, Parent Rating Scales, Self-Report of Personality, Student Observation System, and Structured Developmental History. Taken together, these forms provide a comprehensive overview of children and adolescents' emotional and behavioral functioning. The Self-Report of Personality form can be used with both college-age students and younger adolescents. Similar to the CBCL and related forms, the BASC-2 includes a wide range of internalizing and externalizing scales, as well as other learning-related dimensions. Compared to the earlier version of the tool, the BASC-2 has several new scales, new norms, and the addition of content scales, including Anger Control, Bullying, Emotional Self-Control, Executive Functioning, Resiliency, Ego Strength, and Test Anxiety (although not all content scales are applicable for all age ranges). One of the advantages of the BASC-2 over alternative assessment measures is the inclusion of three validity indices, which are not found in the CBCL measures, that help clinicians assess the quality of the information received from each informant (i.e., adolescent, parent, and teacher).

The Eyberg Child Behavior Inventory (ECBI; Eyberg & Pincus, 1999) provides a shorter measure of child behavior (compared to the CBCL) by focusing on more common behavior problems. It comprises 36 items and is appropriate for children ages 2–16 years. Caregiver respondents rate the frequency of a particular behavior along a 7-point scale and indicate whether the behavior is considered a problem with a dichotomous rating. The ECBI generates both an intensity score and a problem score from these ratings. The reliability and validity are well established, and the ECBI has been widely used in research. The trade-off between the ECBI and the CBCL or BASC-2 is that the ECBI takes less time to complete, but the latter two provide more detailed information about the *nature* of the behavior problem and are more likely to detect unusual behaviors.

More recently, the Social Behavior Inventory (SBI; Gully, 2001) was developed specifically as a measure of children's interpersonal behavior in a child abuse population. In comparison to more general measures of children's interpersonal functioning, the SBI was designed to measure five dimensions of social behavior that are especially pertinent for children who have been maltreated—Aversive–Miscommunication, Aversive–Insensitive, Aversive–Argumentative, Prosocial–Genuine, and Prosocial–Direct. Furthermore, it was developed to be quick (30 items) and sensitive enough to monitor progress in therapy. Although there is some preliminary evidence for the reliability and validity of this measure, more research is needed.

The Brief Symptom Inventory (BSI; Derogatis, 1993), mentioned in the assessing parents section of this chapter, is also suitable for use with adolescents. As noted, it has Hostility (e.g., "Feeling easily annoyed or irritated") and Interpersonal Sensitivity (e.g., "Feeling that people are unfriendly or dislike you") scales, which may be particularly useful in capturing the perceived experience of maltreated adolescents and identifying interpersonal difficulties. Other scales include Somatization, Obsessive–Compulsive, Depression, Anxiety, Phobic Anxiety, Paranoid Ideation, and Psychoticism, and as such, the measure covers a broad spectrum of psychological difficulties. At 53 items, it is much shorter than the YSR and may create less testing fatigue. Finally, there are specific adolescent norms to which scores may be compared.

In addition to these general measures of internalizing and externalizing symptoms, and interpersonal functioning, there is a need for abuse-specific measures in an assessment, especially concerning trauma symptoms and sexual behavior problems. Table 14.3 highlights several measures designed specifically to assess abuse-related difficulties in functioning. A well-established tool for measuring trauma symptoms, the Trauma Symptom Checklist for Children (TSCC; Briere, 1996), was designed to measure the impact of child abuse (sexual, physical, and psychological) and neglect, other interpersonal violence, witnessing trauma to others, major accidents, and disasters. In addition to measuring posttraumatic stress, it evaluates other symptom clusters evident in traumatized children. Its 54 items load onto six clinical scales (Anxiety, Depression, Posttraumatic Stress, Sexual Concerns, Dissociation, and Anger). In addition there are two validity scales (Underresponse and Hyperresponse). TSCC items are explicitly written at a level thought to be understood by children age 8 years or older. The TSCC requires approxi-

TABLE 14.3. Measures of Abuse-Related Child Functioning

Measure	Purpose/scales	No. of items	Informants/versions	Comments
Social Behavior Inventory	5 scales: aversive-miscommunication, aversive-insensitive, aversive-argumentative, prosocial-genuine, prosocial-direct	30	Self-report	Developed to measure social functioning in children and adolescents who have been abused. Psychometrics are preliminary at this point.
Trauma Symptom Checklists	6 clinical scales (anxiety, depression, posttraumatic stress, sexual concerns, dissociation, and anger)	44–90 depending on version	Self-report version for ages 8–16 years Alternate version without sexual content	Has good validity scales and strong psychometric properties.
	2 validity scales		Caregiver report version for children as young as 3 (and up to 12) years	
Sexual Behavior Inventories (Child and Adolescent Clinical versions)	Measures normative and non-normative sexual behavior in 9 content areas (boundary issues, sexual interest, exhibitionism, sexual intrusiveness, gender role behavior, sexual knowledge, self-stimulation, voyeuristic behavior, sexual anxiety)	38 in Child version	Caregiver report for children Adolescent version has self-report and caregiver report forms	Only standardized measure of children's sexual behavior. Has strong psychometric properties and considerable use in research.
	Adolescent version also measures sexual risk taking, nonconforming sexual behaviors, sexual interest, and sexual avoidance	45 in Adolescent version		

mately 10–20 minutes to complete for all but the most traumatized or clinically impaired children, and can be scored and profiled in approximately 10 minutes. A 44-item Alternate version of the TSCC (the TSCC-A) that does not contain Sexual Concerns items is for use in circumstances where sexual item content must be avoided. The TSCC (and TSCC-A) have been demonstrated to have strong reliability and validity. Particular strengths include the validity scales (especially for identifying underreporting), large samples used to generate norms, and norms that are specific to different age ranges.

More recently, a version has been developed that is completed by a caregiver and can be used for children as young as age 3 (and as old as age 12). The Trauma Symptom Checklist for Young Children (TSCYC; Briere et al., 2001) is a 90-item instrument that contains two caregiver validity scales in addition to clinical scales similar to the TSCC. In a multisite sample of 219 traumatized children (Briere et al., 2001), the TSCYC clinical scales had good reliability (alpha values for the clinical scales ranged from .81 to .93) and were predictive of exposure to childhood sexual abuse, physical abuse, and witnessing domestic violence. In addition to tapping posttraumatic difficulties, the TSCC appears to be sensitive to the effects of therapy for abused children (Lanktree & Briere, 1995). The TSCC has been translated into several languages to study the effects of trauma in other cultures.

Another cluster of symptoms that deserves special attention among maltreated children is sexual behavior problems. Although a history of sexual abuse (see Wolfe, Chapter 15, this volume, for a discussion of the assessment of children who have been sexually abused) has been posited as a major predictor of sexualized behavior, empirical evidence suggests a much more complex picture. Indeed, in a study involving more than 2,300 children ages 2–12 years, sexual abuse was not found to be the predominant predictor of sexual acting out. A multidimensional model that incorporated family adversity, modeling of coercive behavior, exposure to sexuality, and child emotional and behavioral factors provided much better prediction of sexual behavior problems than did a history of sexual abuse alone (Friedrich, Davies, Feher, & Wright, 2003). Thus, sexualized behavior problems can be part of a clinical pattern for children from disorganized and vio-

lent families, even in the absence of sexual abuse. It is important to inquire explicitly about sexual behavior problems, because children and parents may not spontaneously disclose them due to embarrassment and the highly private nature of the behavior. The Child Sexual Behavior Inventory (CSBI; Friedrich, 1997), the only standardized measure available, has been used extensively in research. The CSBI is a parent- or caregiver-administered checklist that assesses the presence of a wide range of normative and nonnormative sexual behaviors in nine content areas (e.g., Intrusiveness, Gender Role Behavior, Sexual Anxiety). More recently, the Adolescent Clinical Sexual Behavior Inventory (ACSBI; Friedrich, Lysne, Sim, & Shamos, 2004) was developed to measure sexual risk taking, nonconforming sexual behaviors, sexual interest, and sexual avoidance in clinical samples. The ACSBI has both adolescent and parent report forms, and preliminary research has indicated good psychometric properties.

Although most of the measures discussed to this point emphasize deficits in functioning (with some subscales that measure prosocial functioning), it is also important to evaluate the children's or adolescents' strengths and the resources available to them. A number of measures have recently been developed to measure youth assets. These measures vary in length but tend to share certain similarities, such as being very face valid. The Youth Asset Survey (YAS; Oman et al., 2002), for example, is a 54-item measure that provides scores on eight subscales of assets: Family Communication, Peer Role Models, Future Aspirations, Responsible Choices, Community Involvement, Non-Parental Role Models, Constructive Use of Time—Groups/Sports, and Constructive Use of Time—Religious Time. The use of a measure such as the YAS provides a systematic means to assess protective factors and possible resources upon which to build intervention plans. Including a measure such as the YAS balances out the negative focus of some of the other checklists and allows youth to identify and share some of the areas of life about which they may feel more positive.

Cognitive and Social-Cognitive Development

Research with both child and adult victims of violence points to the importance of the victim's assessment of the conflict, because individual attribution may in turn influence the victim's emotional reaction. For example, the child who attributes physical maltreatment to his or her parent's mean character would be expected to fare worse than the child who sees the same behavior as caused by external circumstances (e.g., job stress). Moreover, as the severity of the maltreatment increases, attributions of blame to the perpetrator increase (Wolfe & McGee, 1991). If attributions of blame (either to self or to the perpetrator) result from the maltreatment, then emotional reactions of sadness or anger are more likely to result. Children's attributions may be measures by self-report with the Children's Attribution Style Questionnaire—Revised (CASQ-R), which is available in a 48-item version or a briefer, 24-item format (Kaslow, & Nolen-Hoeksema, 1991; Thompson, Kaslow, Weiss, Nolen-Hoeksema, 1998). The CASQ-R measures the extent to which children attribute negative events to internal, global, and stable causes (e.g., "I failed the test because I am dumb") versus external, specific, and unstable causes (e.g., "I failed the test because I stayed up late and watched TV instead of studying"). Although the CASQ-R was not specifically designed to measure attribution in abused children, its use has identified attributional style as a mediator between parental child abuse risk and children's internalizing symptoms (Rodriguez, 2006).

A more abuse-specific attributional assessment may be done with the Attribution for Maltreatment Interview (AFMI; McGee, 1990), which comprises four structured interviews, corresponding to hostile maltreatment (i.e., physical and emotional abuse), exposure to family violence, sexual abuse, and neglect (respondents only complete those interviews that pertain to their experiences). After generating a list of all possible causes for their maltreatment, they are asked to make agreement ratings (from 1, *Do not agree* to 4, *Strongly agree*) in relation to 26 statements read aloud by the interviewer. For each of the maltreatment types, the AFMI yields five subscales (derived from theory and factor analysis): Self-Blaming Cognition, Self-Blaming Affect, Self-Excusing, Perpetrator Blame, and Perpetrator Excusing. In a study involving 160 maltreated youth, Wolfe and McGee (1994) found that the majority viewed the offender as the major cause for their maltreatment; however, for physical and emotional abuse, one-third of the sample identified their own behavior as the major cause for what happened. Further research in this area has indicated that attributions about maltreatment contribute uniquely to adolescent adjustment, even after accounting for maltreatment severity (McGee, Wolfe, & Olson, 2001). In the latter study, adolescents rarely saw themselves as causing the maltreatment, but they did exhibit more nuanced self-blame cognitions (such as self-recrimination for not doing anything to *prevent* the abuse). These findings underscore the importance of assessing the youth's attributions for maltreatment, both for targeting self-blame statements and the underlying beliefs that he or she could have prevented such acts and was therefore somewhat at fault.

An alternative procedure, the Home Interview with Children (Conduct Problems Prevention Research Group, 1991), provides an assessment of the degree to which children attribute hostile intent to hypothetical peer behavior and the extent to which it manifests in their problem-solving ability. The measure comprises eight vignettes accompanied by pictures that depict problematic peer interactions in which the peer's intentions are ambiguous. Four problems relate to exclusion by peers and four relate to a physical conflict. Participants are asked to imagine that they are the protagonist child in each situation, and to tell why the antagonist child in each vignette behaved as he or she did. Responses are coded as either hostile (e.g., "He was being mean") or benign (e.g., "It was an accident"). The child is also asked what he or she would do in response to the other child's behavior, and these responses are coded as either aggressive (e.g., hitting the other child), assertive (e.g., asking the other child to fix the problem), passive (e.g., walking away), solution-focused (e.g., cleaning up the mess), or seeking information (e.g., asking the other child why he or she did that). As with the AFMI, the Home Interview with Children is likely more useful as a research tool at this point, and less practical as a clinical measure. Alternatively, the procedure might be a useful interview aid when a child is reluctant to share personal information, and it can be used to branch into discussing peer conflicts and problem solving in the child's life. Thus, attribution can be measured more generally with an easily available, quick self-report measure (i.e., the CASQ-R) or with a more involved interview procedure that requires additional experience to administer and code.

Emotional and Moral Development

Children's emotional functioning, particularly with respect to self-perception, can be profoundly shaped by experiences of maltreatment and neglect. In particular, negative perceptions of individual competence across a wide range of domains may result. Rather than measuring global self-esteem, a multidimensional measure of self-perception may be more informative and help to identify any relative strengths experienced by the child. Some of the most widely used instruments for assessing perceived self-competence are the Harter scales (Self-Perception Profile for Children [SPPC; Harter, 1982] and Self-Perception Profile for Adolescents [SPPA; Harter, 1988]). There are numerous domains, and the clinician or researcher can pick and choose the domain(s) of interest. For example, the SPPA contains eight domains of perceived competence (i.e., Scholastic Competence, Athletic Competence, Social Acceptance, Close Friendship, Romantic Appeal, Physical Appearance, Behavioral Conduct, and Job Competence), as well as a Global Self-Worth subscale. The format of both versions is similar, in that individuals are presented with two options that define opposite ends of a spectrum and asked to decide which end is more like them, for example, "Some teenagers do very well at their classwork, or other teenagers don't do very well at their classwork." After choosing which "self" is more like them, they are asked to indicate whether this is *Sort of true for me* or *Really true for me*. This structured alternative format was used specifically to decrease socially desirable responding. One of the advantages of a multidomain self-perception scale is that it allows clinicians to identify potential strengths and weaknesses to assist in treatment planning. For example, knowing that an adolescent who had been abused has high perceived competence in the area of athletics, but low perceived competence in peer and romantic relationships, would allow a therapist to build on strengths, and use the adolescent's skill and confidence in a particular area to scaffold new skills in weaker areas.

The Harter scales have several attractive feature related to their development, availability, and applicability, including the fact they have been widely used in research for more than 20 years. These scales are available for a nominal cost from the developer and involve a one-time purchase of a manual that allows for photocopying of actual items, making them very accessible both to researchers and clinicians. There have also been some promising cross-cultural studies and language translations with the Harter scales, specifically the SPPC (e.g., with African American and biracial children [Schumann et al., 1999], with Spanish-speaking children [Pereda & Forns, 2004], with Dutch schoolchildren [Muris, Meesters, & Fijen, 2003], with Mexican American schoolchildren [Hess & Petersen, 1996], and with samples from three Chinese cultures [Wang, Meredith, & Tsai, 1996]). Although there have been relatively fewer studies on cultural adaptation with the SPPA (compared to the SPPC), there are some promising studies, including published psychometrics for a sample of early-adolescent African American youth (Thomson & Zand, 2002), with French Canadian adolescents (Bouffard et al., 2002), and with a rural Mexican American sample (Dimmitt, 1996). Other ongoing initiatives include validating the measure with Native American youth, for whom the format has been changed to accommodate cultural taboos about referencing the self compared to others. The combination of cross-cultural studies with both the SPPC an SPPA indicate that perceived self-competence may have both different norms and different domains (i.e., factor structure) for different cultural groups, and highlights the importance of these measures being adapted for and normed with nonwhite populations.

Whereas the Harter scales measure a wide range of perceived self-competence, other measures have a more narrow focus. The *Adolescent Interpersonal Competence Questionnaire* (AICQ; Buhrmester, 1990), a 32-item measure, assesses domains of competence that are important in adolescent close relationships: Self-Disclosure, Providing Emotional Support to Friends, Management of Conflicts, and Negative Assertion. This measure can also be completed by another respondent, such as a dating partner, parent, and so on, who knows the person well. The respondent rates his or her own competence on a 5-point scale (1, *Poor at this; would be so uncomfortable and unable to handle this situation that it would be avoided if possible*, to 5, *Extremely good at this; would feel very comfortable and could handle this situation very well*). Reliability for the factor scores has been high, and the scales correlate with adjustment and friendship intimacy measures (Buhrmester, 1990). The *AICQ* does not cover as wide a range of competencies as the SPPA; however, it covers relationship-related competence in more detail, which may be more pertinent to difficulties faced by maltreated adolescents.

Moral reasoning and development subsequent to a history of maltreatment often reflect poor self-regulation and aggressive themes (e.g., Smetana, Kelly, & Twentyman, 1984). Although difficult to measure in a standardized way, innovative procedures that prompt the child's thinking process merit recognition. One prominent example was reported by Buchsbaum, Toth, Clyman, Cicchetti, and Emde (1992) in which a play narrative "stem technique" was used to elicit a child's internal representations of relationships and emotion regulation. The interviewer begins with a story (the "stem") using doll play, and the child is asked to complete it. In addition to recording verbal and behavioral responses, standard probes are used to challenge the child to resolve the dilemma posed by the stem and to pursue the reasons he or she chose to complete the story a particular way. The stories were developed to elicit certain themes of moral reasoning: for example, empathic or prosocial responses; ways to adhere to a rule in the face of temptation; maternal responses to stealing; parental responses to a transgression in which the transgression results in potential harm to the child; and conflict between members of the family/parents. In their study involving a sample of over 100 maltreated preschool-age children and a matched comparison sample, Buchsbaum and colleagues found that the narratives of the maltreated children tended to have more themes involving inappropriate aggression, neglect, and sexualized behavior. Their self-statements also reflected their views of themselves as "bad," and contained more punitive and abusive language. This standard form of administration of story stems serves to avoid the problem of leading questions that often plagues interviews with maltreated children, and offers considerable promise for assessing the younger child's belief system and moral reasoning. Clearly, widespread adoption of standardized measures that require this level of training in administration and coding remains a challenge.

What should emerge from an assessment of the children's current adaptive abilities and cognitive and emotional development is an understanding of their resources for coping with the level of family problems that may exist, as well as their current attitudes, beliefs, and emotional and behavioral expression vis-à-vis their role in their families. Children who have been removed from the home (or who have had their parents separate or leave the home), as well as older children who have experienced prolonged family conflict and abuse, often display the more extreme signs of adjustment difficulties (e.g., aggression, withdrawal, peer problems, anger at family members). This finding presumably reflects the relationship between child behavior and critical situational variables that must be considered throughout the interpretation of the child's needs. Information provided by the parent, child, caseworker, and through interview procedures should be integrated in a fashion that permits a comparison of how the *parent* views the child and how the child views his or her own situation, behavior, and affect that follow from the assessment procedures described herein. Furthermore, objective information on the child's cognitive development and behavioral adjustment, obtained through observational or normative assessment devices, can provide a framework for establishing treatment priorities that are consistent with the child's abilities and needs.

STEP 3: ASSESSING PARENT–CHILD RELATIONSHIP AND ABUSE–NEGLECT DYNAMICS

Assessing the parent–child relationship, particularly with respect to abuse and neglect dynamics, is perhaps the most challenging part of child abuse assessments. Due to the private and shameful nature of abuse and neglect, assessing related dynamics may be more realistic than assessing the actual maltreatment (although parents are clearly questioned specifically about abuse as well). Furthermore, developing an understanding of the underlying dynamics of abuse in a family provides important direction for changing parent behavior. Domains of interest in this area include abuse risk, neglect, parents' view of their children, and empathy. Table 14.4 highlights some of the measures most related to directly assessing child abuse and neglect in the parent–child relationship.

For practitioners seeking a semistructured interview guide, the Child Abuse and Neglect Interview Schedule—Revised (CANIS-R; Ammerman, Van Hasselt, & Hersen, 1993) assesses the presence of maltreatment behaviors

TABLE 14.4. Measuring Risk for, or Presence of, Abuse and Neglect in the Parent–Child Relationship

Measure	Purpose/description	Format	Comments
Child Abuse and Neglect Interview Schedule—Revised	Assesses presence of maltreatment behaviors and factors related to abuse and neglect. Four sections include: • Child behavior problems and disciplinary practices • Parental past and current history of family violence • Child's exposure to violence, psychological abuse, and neglect • Sexual abuse (both the child's and parent's experiences)	Semistructured interview with parent	Unpublished interview (available from author). Requires skilled administration.
Child Abuse Potential Inventory	Designed to measure areas related to increased likelihood of abuse; 160 items result in six subscales: • Distress • Rigidity • Unhappiness • Problems with child and self • Problems with family • Problems with others Has validity scales	Parent self-report	Brief version available. Has validity scales, but concerns have been raised about the validity of the measure for certain purposes. Rigidity scale may be most resistant to defensive responding. Used widely in research.
Adult–Adolescent Parenting Index—Second Edition	Designed to measure dimensions pertinent to child abuse risk patterns: • Inappropriate expectations of children • Lack of empathy towards the needs of children • Strong belief in the use of corporal punishment, • Reversing parent–child family roles • Oppressing children's power and independence	Parent self-report	Good scales in theory, but lack of validity scales makes the use of the measure questionable in abuse assessments.
Children's Experiences of Victimization Questionnaire	Measures experiences of: • Child physical abuse • Child sexual abuse • Witnessing domestic violence • Physical punishment • Peer-on-peer violence	Youth self-report	Covers a broad range of victimization experiences. Developed for research, not clinical use.

Measure	Description	Format/Informant	Comments
Mother–Child Neglect Scale	Measures mother-reported neglectful behavior toward children	Parent self-report	Developed based on interview format as part of a large research project. Developers caution against clinical use until more research is conducted.
Multidimensional Neglectful Behavioral Scale—Child Report	Measures four broad domains of neglect including: • Cognitive • Emotional • Physical • Supervisory Additional scales assess exposure to violence, alcohol-related neglect, abandonment, and children's appraisals of parenting	Child self-report Computer-assisted technology	First standardized measure of neglect for children to complete. Computer-assisted technology is a strength of the measure but also makes it expensive to obtain.
Parental Empathy Measure	Measures several components of parental empathy: • Attention to signals • Attributions • Behavior • Emotion • Overall empathy Also contains a "faking good" validity scale	Semistructured interview with parent	Promising preliminary psychometrics, but needs more research.
Parenting Stress Index	Measures parental stress related to: • The child domain (related to children's adaptability, acceptability, demandingness, mood, distractibility, and responsivity to parent) • The parent domain (i.e., stress related to depression, role restriction, sense of parental competence, social isolation, health, and relationship with spouse) • The parent–child domain An optional 19-item Life Events Stress scale is contained within the PSI. Also provides a total stress score.	Parental self-report Standard version, short-form version, and version for parents of adolescents	Has a validity index. Useful to see how parents explain source of their stress.

(e.g., corporal punishment, physical abuse), as well as factors related to abuse and neglect (e.g., parental history of maltreatment). The CANIS-R comprises over 100 questions and takes approximately 45 minutes to administer. The four sections include child behavior problems and disciplinary practices; parental past and current history of family violence; child exposure to violence, psychological abuse and neglect; and sexual abuse (both child and parental experiences). The CANIS-R is a semi-structured interview rather than a set of questions to be read verbatim; as such, the training and skill of the interviewer is an important component in administration.

Standardized Self-Report Measures and Administered Procedures

Self-report measures are used routinely with parents and children to assess components of parent–child interactions and/or child abuse risk. Although standardized measures have many attractive features, it is critical to be aware of whether a particular measure was developed for the express purpose of assessing child maltreatment. Use of measures that were developed for other purposes and normed on other groups must be undertaken with caution (Budd, 2001). Even instruments developed to measure parent–child problems are not necessarily specific to measurement of attributes of parents at risk for maltreatment (Budd & Holdsworth, 1996). Furthermore, many of the measures have been developed and used predominantly for research. In some cases, these measures may detect between-group differences well (i.e., distinguish between groups of abusive and nonabusive parents). However, between-group differences may mask important within-group differences, and concepts such as sensitivity and specificity, or clinical cutoffs (established with valid criteria) may be more important than deviation from a population mean.

Unfortunately, many of these self-report measures are used routinely, without an appreciation of the complexity of the issues. Furthermore, strong general psychometrics and the ability to differentiate among groups are important starting points for a measure, but there are additional considerations. Issues such as feasibility, sensitivity of the measure to treatment effects, and predictive validity are also important considerations. We include these

considerations in relation to the measures as they are discussed. Most of the measures that consider parent–child relationships vis-à-vis abuse risk are administered to parents, although there are also a few child-report options.

Risk for Abuse–Presence of Abuse

Attempts to develop a direct measure of child abuse dynamics in the parent–child relationship have met with limited success. The Child Abuse Potential Inventory (CAPI; Milner, 1986) is the best known and most widely used measure in this regard. The CAPI was specifically designed to measure problem areas related to parental and family background associated with an increased probability of abuse. Since its development in the late 1970s, this instrument has undergone considerable psychometric investigations by the author and others (see Milner, 1989; Ondersma, Chaffin, Mullins, & LeBreton, 2005) that have produced norms for general and abusive populations, and reliability and validity information. The Major Abuse Scale comprises six factor subscales: Distress, Rigidity, Unhappiness, Problems with Child and Self, Problems with Family, and Problems with Others. In addition, a Lie Scale indicates the degree of deceptive responding (e.g., "I love all children"). The 160 items on the scale are written at the grade 3 reading level and require only an *Agree* or *Disagree* response (e.g., "I am often mixed up"; "A child should never talk back"; "My parents did not understand me"). More recently, a brief version of the CAPI has been published, with psychometric properties similar to the original version (Ondersma et al., 2005).

Despite reasonably strong general psychometric properties, relatively easy and quick administration, and its widespread popularity, recent studies have raised concerns about some aspects of the clinical validity of the CAPI. Indeed, among parents being investigated for child abuse and neglect, a positive self-presentation bias substantially compromises the interpretation of traditional self-report measures such as the CAPI, although the Rigidity Scale did not appear to be as affected as the other scales (Carr et al., 2005). Furthermore, the validity of interpreting *changes* in CAPI scores as being indicative of change in child abuse risk is questionable. In a study utilizing data from 459 parents in 27 community-based interventions, improvements in CAPI scores following intervention did *not* predict reduced rates of official child maltreatment reports in the ensuing 2 years (Chaffin & Valle, 2003). In this study, algorithms classifying significant change produced counterintuitive and misleading results; that is, participants classified as improved were actually at similar or even high risk to perpetrate future abuse compared to those classified as unchanged or worse. In our work with abusive fathers, clients who have been referred with a documented history of child maltreatment consistently avoid detection with the clinical cutoffs of the CAPI (Scott & Crooks, 2006). Thus, despite being a measure specifically designed to assess child abuse risk, the CAPI does not detect risk reliably in many cases, nor can changes in risk, as measured by the CAPI, be considered an adequate indicator of success in the absence of corroborating information. This latter shortcoming is particularly concerning given that the CAPI is routinely used to indicate success following intervention. Ironically, the test developer (Milner) has raised many of these questions and concerns in his own research (e.g., Milner, 1989, 1994); nonetheless, other researchers and clinicians have adopted the measure wholesale and without regard for these intricacies. Thus, the CAPI is probably best used as one piece of a comprehensive assessment, with the proviso that it is not a litmus test for abuse. Similarly, it should not be the sole outcome in intervention research to judge treatment success; unfortunately, it is often used in this manner.

A second widely used measure, the Adult–Adolescent Parenting Index—Second Edition (AAPI-2; Bavolek & Keene, 1999) has even greater problems than the CAPI, due to the lack of validity scales. At a construct level, the AAPI-2 was designed to measure dimensions that are highly pertinent to measuring child abuse risk patterns: inappropriate expectations of children, parental lack of empathy toward the needs of children, strong parental belief in the use of corporal punishment, reversal of parent–child family roles, and oppression of children's power and independence. The AAPI-2 is problematic in that items are highly face valid, which is concerning given client defensiveness and the sensitivity of the topics being addressed, and because there are no validity scales to evaluate or temper the effects of socially desirable responding (Carr et al., 2005). In our work with abusive fathers, we have virtually no men endorse the Corporal Punishment scale, despite the fact that many of these same clients describe spanking as part of their parenting repertoire during the interview portion of the assessment, and harsh and frequent corporal punishment has been recorded by child protective services in many cases.

In comparison to the CAPI and AAPI-2, which are administered to parents, other measures assess children's experiences of abuse directly. The Childhood Experiences of Violence Questionnaire (CEVQ; Walsh, MacMillan, Trocmé, Boyle, & Jamieson, 2006) is one such measure that directly assesses children's experiences of a broad range of victimization. The CEVQ has 18 items that measure Child Physical Abuse, Child Sexual Abuse, Witnessing Domestic Violence, and Physical Punishment (Wekerle et al., 2006). One strength of the CEVQ is that it includes extrafamilial (peer-on-peer) violence, which may be an important area to assess and to accommodate in treatment planning with abused children. The CEVQ was developed for large, survey-based research studies and has not been used clinically to date; however, it provides a relatively efficient format for assessing a range of victimization experiences with adolescents and may be a useful adjunct to an interview.

Neglect

Although neglect is by definition difficult to measure (because it involves acts of omission rather than commission), a couple of well-designed, standardized neglect measures have emerged during the past 5 years. The Mother–Child Neglect Scale (MCNS; Lounds, Norkowski, & Whitman, 2004) was adapted from the Neglect Scale (Straus, Kinard, & Williams, 1995), a self-report measure of personal experience of neglect as a child, to assess neglectful behaviors perpetrated by a parent. The MCNS was developed as part of a longitudinal study of adolescent mothers and their firstborn children that followed mother–child dyads from the third trimester of pregnancy through the child's 14th year of life (Whitman, Borkowski, Keogh, & Weed, 2001). The questionnaire included a phone interview in which mothers were asked about their behavior toward their children when the children were 8 years of age. The questionnaire was validated with videotaped play episodes between mothers and children, and an adapted, shorter version of the CAPI (Milner, 1986), which primarily used items from the Rigidity and Unhappiness Scales. The resulting 20-item MCNS (and a briefer 8-item form) show promise in terms of reliability and validity, and may be useful as part of a multimethod approach to assessing neglect in research settings. However, the developers clearly caution against its application in clinical or child protective settings, until much more research can be undertaken (Lounds et al., 2004).

A major, recent advance in the direct measurement of neglect is the development of the Multidimensional Neglectful Behavior Scale—Child Report (MNBS-CR; Kantor et al., 2004), the first standardized measure to canvas children in a systematic way about the level of care they receive and possible neglect. The MNBS-CR taps into four broad domains of neglect, including Cognitive (e.g., parent does not talk to child a lot, does not read to child), Emotional (e.g., parent does not comfort child, does not do fun activities with child), Physical (e.g., child is improperly dressed for weather, has poor dental hygiene), and Supervisory (e.g., parent does not know where child is playing, leaves child alone in the car for lengthy periods). Additional scales assess exposure to violence, alcohol-related neglect, abandonment,

and children's appraisals of parenting. This measure has utilized computer technology in an innovative manner to gain several advantages over traditional paper-and-pencil surveys. Using audio computer-assisted self-interview (ACASI) technology, children see pictorial items, hear a voice read the item, and respond by touching the computer screen.

ACASI technology offers several benefits. The items can be tailored to the child's age (item content differs for older and younger children as threshold for neglectful behavior differs) and gender (pictorial representations are generated to match the child's gender). In addition, the audio-assisted portion means that reading level is less important, and the child experiences a more comfortable and private administration than possible in a face-to-face interview with an adult. Finally, the use of a computer program is perceived to be fun. The format of items involves showing children at two different ends of a parenting care–neglect spectrum with respect to a particular behavior, and the child indicates which is more like his or her own experience. The next computer screen has the child rate the extent to which the item represents his or her experience (see Figure 14.1 for a sample from the MNBS-CR Physical Neglect scale).

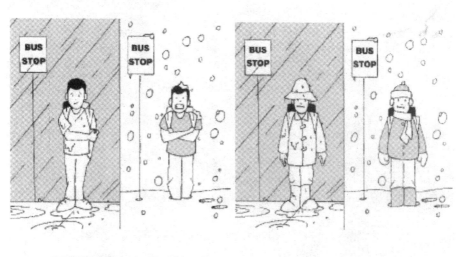

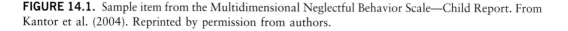

FIGURE 14.1. Sample item from the Multidimensional Neglectful Behavior Scale—Child Report. From Kantor et al. (2004). Reprinted by permission from authors.

Developing these pictorial items was a challenging undertaking. In the words of the lead developer, operationalizing neglect can be like trying to hear "one hand clapping"; nonetheless, the early psychometrics are very promising (Kantor et al., 2004). The extent to which the MNBS-CR is adopted into clinical practice remains to be seen, in part because the proprietary nature of the ACASI technology makes it a very expensive measure for the developers to make available to others. Even with the expense associated, its use in research will likely grow due to the lack of alternative child-based measures of neglect. A parent version of the MNBS is under development (G. Kantor, personal communication, April 2006).

Parenting Attitudes and Behaviors

Although identifying parent personality traits and general characteristics that predict abuse has not been very useful to date, there is emerging interest in empathy as a foundational construct that mediates risk of abuse (Donald & Jureidini, 2004; Kilpatrick, 2005; Scott & Crooks, 2004). The focus is on parents' empathy toward their own children specifically, not the more general concept of empathy as a broad characteristic. Donald and Jureidini (2004, p. 5, original emphasis) argue that it is "the parents' ability to empathetically understand and give priority to *their* children's needs" that is the critical determining factor in risk to children, *not* the broader constructs of parenting knowledge and social support, and so on. In developing the first measure of parental empathy, Kilpatrick (2005) notes that a model of parental empathy must include a number of emotional, cognitive, and behavioral elements that combine to create empathy. These factors include attending to the child's signals or emotional cues, making accurate attributions about why the child is feeling that way, and experiencing child-focused positive emotions. Furthermore, these emotions and cognitions must lead to child-focused behavior. The Parental Empathy Measure is a semi-structured interview that uses a combination of forced-choice items, scenarios, and open-ended questions to assess Parent Beliefs, Behavioral Responses (both typical responses and on a "bad day"), Emotional Responses, and Attributions (Kilpatrick, 2005). There is also a Social Desirability scale included in the measure. Although the *Parental Empathy Measure* is rel-

atively new, the initial developmental work suggests promising psychometrics in terms of good internal reliability, interrater reliability, construct validity, and concurrent validity.

Parents' Views of Children and Parenting Stress

There are a number of measures designed to assess parents' views and expectations of their children, as well as stress experienced in the parenting role. A number of these measures are discussed herein. Parental views about their influence on their children's behavior may be assessed with the Parent Attribution Test (PAT; Bugental et al., 1989). This measure grew out of research indicating that abusive parents tend to experience subjectively less power over their children and attribute more negative intent to child behavior compared to nonabusive parents. The PAT measures respondents' attributions about potential causes of caregiving success and failure on a 7-point scale. Items are grouped according to four subscales (e.g., attributed control to adults for unsuccessful outcomes, attributed control to children for unsuccessful outcomes). The construct and discriminant validity of the PAT has been established in numerous studies (Bugental & Lewis, 1999; Bugental, Lewis, Lin, Lyon, & Kopeikin, 1999).

The Parental Childrearing Cognitions Questionnaire (PCCQ; Jefferis & Oliver, 2006) was developed to measure dysfunctional cognitions that likely influence parenting behavior and the quality of the parent–child relationship negatively. Respondents are presented with six challenging but developmentally appropriate child-rearing dilemmas (i.e., noncompliance, overactive and impulsive behavior, and demanding behavior that interrupts parental activity) and asked to imagine themselves in that scenario. Next they are presented with a series of statements with which they indicate their agreement. Categories for the statements include Attribution of Child Behavior to Negative Motivations, Negative Cognitions Concerning Limit Setting, Child Perceived as Excessively Demanding or Problematic, and Behavior Perceived as Predictive of Future Problems. The PCCQ has shown promising psychometrics with respect to reliability and validity (comparing clinical and nonclinical parents; Jefferis & Oliver, 2006).

The Parent Opinion Questionnaire (POQ; Azar, Robinson, Hekimian, & Twentyman,

1984), an 80-item questionnaire that measures unrealistic parental expectations of appropriate children's behavior, has six subscales based on content areas of unrealistic expectations (i.e., Self-Care, Family Responsibility and Care of Siblings, Help and Affection to Parents, Leaving Children Alone, Proper Behavior and Feelings, and Punishment). POQ scores have been found to distinguish between maltreating and nonmaltreating parents (Azar et al., 1984), as well as between parents who are perpetrating abuse and those who are not, within the same family (Azar & Rohrbeck, 1986). More recently, POQ scores (particularly with respect to unrealistic expectations about children providing support to parents) were associated with at-risk maternal behavior in videotaped mother–child interactions among mothers with major mental illnesses who were involved with the child welfare system (Leventhal, Jacobsen, Miller, & Quintana, 2004). It has also been recommended for use as part of a clinical assessment for parenting capacity (Budd, 2001).

The Parenting Stress Index (PSI; Abidin, 1995) is a widely used measure that assesses the stress experienced by parents, as well as the perceived source of the stress. The PSI contains 120 items rated on a 5-point scale. It is grouped into the Child domain (i.e., parental report of stress related to their children's adaptability, acceptability, demandingness, mood, distractibility, and responsive to the parent); the Parent domain (i.e., stress related to depression, role restriction, sense of parental competence, social isolation, health, and relationship with spouse); and the Parent–Child domain. An optional 19-item Life Events Stress Scale is contained within the PSI. The PSI also provides a total stress score that sums across all of the domains. It has strong psychometrics and is widely used in both clinical and research settings. In addition to the full 120-item version, a 36-item PSI Short Form (PSI-SF) yields a total stress score from three subscales: Parental Distress, Parent–Child Dysfunctional Interaction, and Difficult Child. Although the PSI-SF does not capture the same richness of data as the original, longer version, it has been shown to have reasonably strong psychometric properties with a range of populations and purposes (Haskett, Ahern, Ward, & Allaire, 2006).

The PSI (both the original and short form) was developed for use with parents of children ages 3 months to 10 years, but an upward extension is also available with the Stress Index for Parents of Adolescents (SIPA; Sheras, Abidin, & Konold, 1998). The SIPA is for use with parents of children ages 11–19. It is a 90-item self-report questionnaire and, similar to the PSI, measures stress with reference to an Adolescent domain (Moodiness/Lability, Social Isolation/Withdrawal, Delinquent/Antisocial, and Failure to Achieve/Persevere), a Parent domain (Life Restrictions, Relationship with Spouse/Partner, Social Alienation, and Incompetence/Guilt), and an Adolescent–Parent Relationship domain.

The PSI and SIPA are useful in child abuse assessments, because they measure not only stress (which, in and of itself, is linked to maltreatment) but also the source of the stress. The extent to which the parent views the child as the source of all negative experience in his or her life is an important clinical consideration in assessment and treatment planning. Furthermore, PSI scores have been found to differentiate between abusive and nonabusive parents (e.g., Holden & Banez, 1996), although they may not be very effective at detecting defensive responding patterns (Milner & Crouch, 1997).

Observations

Child abuse researchers have long recognized the validity and feasibility of direct parent–child observations with this population (Wolfe, 1985). There are several ways to approach this task, each with advantages and disadvantages. For example, observing families in the home may provide the most naturalistic setting, yet the family's typical pattern of interaction may be so disrupted that little information is gained (particularly with abusive families who have *not* requested service). In terms of setting, structured clinic observations have gained wide acceptability and support as a valid assessment of parent–child interactions, and they have the potential advantage of videotaping the observed interactions. In addition to coding behavior from the tape, the scenes may be played back to have the parent retrospectively indicate his or her emotional reactions, level of arousal, and thoughts during the interaction. Another consideration for using structured clinic observations is that observations of low-frequency behaviors (yelling, grabbing, etc.) yield more relevant data in a more efficient manner when structured tasks are presented (e.g., Herrenkohl, Herrenkohl, Toedter, & Yanushefski, 1984; Oldershaw, Walters, & Hall, 1986).

Observations of child behavior in the home or clinic serve two assessment functions: They provide a measure of the child's typical behavior with his or her parent, and they also allow the examiner to view the child's range of behavior under controlled conditions. By observing the parent and child from behind an observational mirror the examiner may record selected target behaviors during contrived situations and free interaction. For very young children and infants, these situations are limited primarily to basic caregiving, such as feeding, holding, verbal and physical forms of communication, and simple compliance or instructional tasks (e.g., attending to the parent's voice commands). Preschool and older children may be given more specific instructions by the parent to engage in activities that resemble common areas of conflict at home (e.g., to complete one activity, then switch to another).

Quantitative assessment of family interactions is best approached by using an existing or modified structured procedure for coding family interactions. Since no particular behavior categories are unique to abusive families, the investigator can choose from among an expanding variety of family observation systems, and base his or her choice upon considerations such as diversity of definitional codes, ability to conduct sequential interactions, and field experience. These assessment strategies range from highly formal coding of videotaped interactions to ratings of more unstructured home observations, and an example of each is provided here. There are relative advantages and disadvantages associated with either approach.

The Dyadic Parent Interaction Coding System–III (DPICS-III; Eyberg, Nelson, Duke, & Boggs, 2005) is a well-researched behavioral coding system that measures the quality of parent–child social interactions. In the DPICS-III, behaviors are recorded, with 26 behavioral categories to measure child and parent verbalizations (i.e., the content of the verbal behavior) and physical behaviors (i.e., positive and negative touch). In addition, child vocalizations (i.e., the tone of the verbal behavior) and response behaviors (e.g., compliance to command, answer to question, no opportunity to comply) are also coded. The DPICS-III has a number of supplemental scales in addition to the standard ones. The various iterations of the DPICS have been shown to have good psychometrics. A thorough description of psychometric properties and research using the DPICS is

included in the manual, which is available online (Eyberg et al., 2005).

A less rigidly scored procedure than the DPICS-III is the Home Observation for Measurement of the Environment Inventory (HOME; Caldwell & Bradley, 1984). The HOME was designed to measure the quality and quantity of stimulation and support available to a child in the home environment. Since its original development, multiple versions have emerged to correspond to children's stages. In addition to the original Infant/Toddler version, there is an Early Childhood version for children ages 3–6, a Middle Childhood version for ages 6–10, and an Early Adolescent version for youth ages 10–15. Administration of the HOME requires an unstructured home visit, lasting typically between 45 and 90 minutes. In addition to the target child and his or her primary caregiver, other family members and even guests may be present, but their presence is not necessary. The procedure is a low-key, semistructured observation and interview aimed at minimizing intrusiveness and allowing family members to act normally.

The intent is to understand the child's opportunities and experiences; in essence, to understand what life is like for the particular child in the child's most intimate surroundings. This inventory was designed to sample certain aspects of the quantity and quality of social, emotional, and cognitive support available to a young child. The HOME is completed following visits to the family's residence, and items not obtained by direct observation (e.g., "takes the child out of home more than twice per week") are based on parental report. The original version comprised 45 yes–no ratings corresponding to 6 subscales: Emotional and Verbal Responsivity of the Mother, Avoidance of Restriction and Punishment, Organization of the Physical and Temporal Environment, Provision of Appropriate Play Materials, Maternal Involvement with the Child, and Opportunities for Variety in Daily Stimulation. Subsequent versions differ slightly in length and number of subscales. Psychometric information about all of the different versions is found in the administration manual (Caldwell & Bradley, 1984). The alpha coefficients for the total scores are all above .90; and the interobserver agreement for each measure is 90% or higher. The measure has been used throughout North and South America (including the Caribbean), in several European and Asian countries, in

Australia, and in at least two African nations. It has been used in a wide variety of clinical and research settings, and to evaluate the impact of intervention programs. Reviews of research on HOME can be found in Bradley (1994; Bradley, Corwyn, & Whiteside-Mansell, 1996).

If a formal behavioral coding system or checklist is not practical, possibly due to the logistics of the parent–child interaction (i.e., visit undertaken in an office, videotaping is not available) or impractical because of the extensive training necessary for some of the coding systems, a plan for outlining areas to assess during the observation session is still a useful adjunct to general impressions. The clinician needs to be alert to parent behaviors, child behaviors, and the interaction between these. Budd (2001) provides a useful list of questions to guide observation for a parent–child interaction assessment in the context of parenting capacity assessments (see Table 14.5). This list should not be considered exhaustive, but it highlights several key areas to which clinicians must remain vigilant. Furthermore, it underscores the importance of evaluating what is left unsaid or undone, in addition to the more obvious observations about what is being said and done. Although parents are typically on their best behavior while being observed, children's reactions to particular parental overtures will help the clinician assess whether Mom or Dad is behaving in an unusual manner. At the same time, it is important to remember that the situation itself is stressful and may elicit some negative behavior patterns from parents and/or children.

Checklists that are completed following a home visit or by a social worker who is familiar with the family can be useful assessment tools, particularly in identifying cases of neglect. Polansky, Chalmers, Butenweiser, and Williams (1978) developed the *Childhood Level of Living Scale* (CLLS) to assess the extent of positive and negative influences present in the child's home environment. This instrument is particularly well suited for assessing neglectful families, in that it lists the major areas of concern relative to children's minimal health, safety, and stimulation requirements. The CLLS has two main scales: Physical Care, containing items comprising five subscales labeled General Positive Care, State of Repair of House, Negligence, Quality of Household Maintenance, and Quality of Health Care and Grooming; and

TABLE 14.5. Potential Content Areas for Informally Observing Parent–Child Interactions

I. Parent behavior patterns

  A. How does parent structure interactions through instructions, toys, or activities?

  B. How does parent show understanding or misunderstanding of children's developmental levels?

  C. How does parent convey acceptance or approval of children's behavior (praise, descriptive feedback, physical affection)?

  D. How does parent convey disapproval of children's behavior (criticisms, negative comments, threats, physical roughness)?

  E. Does parent notice and attend to children's physical needs (e.g., hunger, need to use bathroom, safety risks)?

  F. Is parent responsive to children's initiations via verbalizations, facial expressions, and actions?

  G. Does parent accept children's right to disagree or express their own opinions?

  H. Does parent follow through with his or her instructions or rules?

  I. Does parent spread attention fairly across children, if more than one child is present?

  J. Does parent appear distracted, withdrawn, or bored during session (e.g., ignoring children or watching television instead of interacting with children)?

  K. Does parent make "troublesome" comments (e.g., asking children if they love parent, making negative comments about family members or foster parents, swearing)?

II. Child behavior patterns

  A. Are children at ease around parent (e.g., smiling, playing, and verbalizing vs. remaining distant, quiet, or fearful)?

  B. Do children initiate interactions with parent?

  C. Do children display developmental, emotional, or behavioral difficulties that require more skilful parenting strategies than the parent exhibits?

  D. Do children respond to parent's initiations by showing interest and acceptance of parent's attention?

  E. Do children disagree with parent or express their own opinions?

  F. How do children show affection and interest toward parent?

  G. What topics do children bring up in conversations with parent (e.g., activities in foster family, desire to be with parent)?

Note. Data from Budd (2001).

Emotional–Cognitive Care, with subscales labeled Encouraging Competence, Inconsistency of Discipline and Coldness, Encouraging Superego Development, and Material Giving. The 99 items are rated by home visitors as *yes* or *no*. The authors provide preliminary normative data for this instrument, with cutoff scores indicating neglectful care, adequate care, and good child care, although reliability and validity data are limited (with the exception of one report indicating discriminative validity between neglect and control families; Polansky et al., 1978). The CLLS has both rural and urban versions available, because neglect concerns vary somewhat with context; however, it has been argued that widespread adoption of the CLLS has been limited due to its length (Lounds et al., 2004) and concerns about item relevance (Gaudin, Polansky, & Kilpatrick, 1992).

Specifically designed to measure key components of the home environment that are perceived to be representative of child neglect (Trocmé, 1996), the Ontario Child Neglect Index requires social workers to make ratings of neglect in three major areas that are identified in legislation, with the assistance of behavioral anchors. These areas include supervision, physical care (rating food/nutrition, and clothing and hygiene separately), and provision of health care (evaluating physical health care, mental health care, and development and educational care separately). Although the measure was designed to match a specific jurisdiction's neglect laws, it can easily be adapted for other jurisdictions (Trocmé, 1996). Strengths include its brevity and face validity (for the social worker completing the measure).

In summary, assessment of the parent–child relationship requires special attention due to the relational nature of child abuse. This assessment is best conducted through a combination of parent and child report and observation. The domains being measured include specific abuse and neglect categories, as well as related parent–child dynamics (e.g., stress and communication).

INTEGRATING INFORMATION AND MAKING RECOMMENDATIONS

Subsequent to undertaking the assessment procedures described in this chapter, the assessor is faced with the challenge of integrating findings from parents, children, and parent–child relationships, and noting both challenges and strengths upon which to build intervention. It is important to return to the specific referral question(s) when formulating results and making recommendations; vague recommendations rarely serve either the family or the referral agent. Some additional challenges are involved with child abuse assessments compared to other areas.

First, due to the dynamics of defensiveness and minimization displayed by many abusive families, it is especially important to note the limitations and source of the data for a particular finding. For example, rather than noting that an individual does not have a police record, the assessor might note that the individual *reported* no police record, but that confirmation was not received directly from the police. Because the individuals making decisions on the basis of the report may not be familiar with particular tests or measurement theory, conveying an understanding about the meaning of validity scale scores is crucial, rather than assuming that the referral agent will make the connection between elevated validity scale scores and likely underreporting of difficulties.

A second challenge relates to the difficulty of providing feedback in a way that is respectful to clients, yet accurate and honest. All too often clients seem to be given a watered-down version of assessment findings in the verbal feedback meeting, and are then shocked when they later see the report, or conversely, never realize what has actually been written, because the report is not shared with them. Although it is challenging to convey negative feedback in a forthright yet compassionate manner, these skills are critical to develop if clinicians want to be effective in this area.

Finally, it is important to include findings that do not fit the overall conceptualization, as well as those that do. Although it may be tempting to focus on the findings that support the assessors' global view of the family, the complexity of abusive families is such that it is rarely a uniformly bleak picture. Capturing the strengths of a family, even if the resulting recommendations of the assessment are that the parents continue to pose a risk to their children, or that the children should be placed outside of the family, is a way to ensure respectful service to the most difficult families and may result in their feeling more validated in the process than they would otherwise feel.

REFERENCES

Abidin, R. R. (1995). *The Parenting Stress Index: Professional manual.* Odessa, FL: Psychological Assessment Resources.

Abidin, R. R., & Konold, T. R. (1999). *Parenting Alliance Measure: Professional manual.* Odessa, FL: Psychological Assessment Resources.

Achenbach, T. M. (1991). *Manual for the Child Behavior Checklist/4–18 and 1991 profile.* Burlington: University of Vermont, Department of Psychiatry.

American Psychological Association Committee on Professional Practice and Standards. (1998). *Guidelines for psychological evaluations in child protection matters.* Washington, DC: American Psychological Association.

Ammerman, R. T., & Patz, R. J. (1996). Determinants of child abuse potential: Contribution of parent and child factors. *Journal of Clinical Child Psychology, 25,* 300–307.

Ammerman, R. T., Van Hasselt, V., & Hersen, M. (1993). *The Child Abuse and Neglect Interview Schedule—Revised.* Pittsburgh, PA: Western Pennsylvania School for Blind Children.

Archer, J. (1999). Assessment of the reliability of the Conflict Tactics Scales: A meta-analytic review. *Journal of Interpersonal Violence, 14,* 1263–1289.

Azar, S. T. (2002). *Parenting and child maltreatment.* Mahwah, NJ: Erlbaum.

Azar, S. T., Robinson, D. R., Hekimian, E., & Twentyman, C. T. (1984). Unrealistic expectations and problem-solving ability in maltreating and comparison mothers. *Journal of Consulting and Clinical Psychology, 52,* 687–691.

Azar, S. T., & Rohrbeck, C. A. (1986). Child abuse and unrealistic expectations: Further validation of the parent opinion questionnaire. *Journal of Consulting and Clinical Psychology, 54,* 867–868.

Azar, S., & Wolfe, D. (2006). Child physical abuse and neglect. In E. J. Mash & R. A. Barkley (Eds.), *Treatment of childhood disorders* (3rd ed., pp. 595–646). New York: Guilford Press.

Bala, N., & Schuman, J. P. (1999). Allegations of sexual abuse when parents have separated. *Canadian Family Law Quarterly, 17,* 191–241.

Barnett, D., Ganiban, J., & Cicchetti, D. (1999). Maltreatment, negative expressivity, and the development of type D attachments from 12 to 24 months of age. *Monographs of the Society for Research in Child Development, 64,* 97–118.

Bavolek, S. J., & Keene, R. G. (1999). *Adult–Adolescent Parenting Inventory—Second Edition.* Park City, UT: Family Development Resources.

Bensley, L. S., Eenwyk, J. V., & Simmons, K. W. (2000). Self-reported childhood sexual and physical abuse and adult HIV-risk behaviors and heavy drinking. *American Journal of Preventive Medicine, 18,* 151–158.

Berliner, L., & Elliott, D. M. (2002). *Sexual abuse of children.* Thousand Oaks, CA: Sage.

Bolger, K. E., & Patterson, C. J. (2001). Developmental pathways from child maltreatment to peer rejection. *Child Development, 72,* 549–568.

Bornstein, R. F. (2005). Interpersonal dependency in child abuse perpetrators and victims: A meta-analytic review. *Journal of Psychopathology and Behavioral Assessment, 27,* 67–76.

Bouffard, T., Seidah, A., McIntyre, M., Boivin, M., Vezeau, C., & Cantin, S. (2002). Mesure de l'estime de soi à l'adolescence: Version canadienne-française de self-perception profile for adolescents de Harter [Measuring adolescent self-esteem: A French-Canadian version of Harter's Self-Perception Profile for Adolescents]. *Canadian Journal of Behavioural Science, 34,* 158–162.

Bradley, R. H. (1994). The HOME inventory: Review and reflections. In H. W. Reese (Ed.), *Advances in child development and behavior* (Vol. 25, pp. 241–288). San Diego, CA: Academic Press.

Bradley, R. H., Corwyn, R. F., & Whiteside-Mansell, L. (1996). Life at home: Same time, different places—an examination of the HOME inventory in different cultures. *Early Development and Parenting, 5,* 251–269.

Bremner, J. D. (2003). Long-term effects of childhood abuse on brain and neurobiology. *Child and Adolescent Psychiatric Clinics of North America, 12,* 271–292.

Bremner, J. D., & Vermetten, E. (2001). Stress and development: Behavioral and biological consequences. *Development and Psychopathology, 13,* 473–489.

Briere, J. (1996). *Trauma Symptom Checklist for Children (TSCC).* Odessa, FL: Psychological Assessment Resources.

Briere, J., Johnson, K., Bissada, A., Damon, L., Crouch, J., Gil, E., et al. (2001). The Trauma Symptom Checklist for Young Children (TSCYC): Reliability and association with abuse exposure in a multi-site study. *Child Abuse and Neglect, 25,* 1001–1014.

Brown, J., Cohen, P., Johnson, J. G., & Smailes, E. M. (1999). Childhood abuse and neglect: Specificity and effects on adolescent and young adult depression and suicidality. *Journal of the American Academy of Child and Adolescent Psychiatry, 38,* 1490–1496.

Buchsbaum, H. K., Toth, S. L., Clyman, R. B., Cicchetti, D., & Emde, R. N. (1992). The use of a narrative story stem technique with maltreated children: Implications for theory and practice. *Development and Psychopathology, 4,* 603–625.

Budd, K. S. (2001). Assessing parenting competence in child protection cases: A clinical practice model. *Clinical Child and Family Psychology Review, 4,* 1–18.

Budd, K. S., Heilman, N. E., & Kane, D. (2000). Psychosocial correlates of child abuse potential in multiply disadvantaged adolescent mothers. *Child Abuse and Neglect, 24,* 611–625.

Budd, K. S., & Holdsworth, M. J. (1996). Issues in clinical assessment of minimal parenting competence. *Journal of Clinical Child Psychology, 25,* 2–14.

Bugental, D. B., Blue, J., & Cruzcosa, M. (1989). Perceived control over caregiving outcomes: Implications for child abuse. *Developmental Psychology*, *25*, 532–539.

Bugental, D. B., & Lewis, J. C. (1999). The paradoxical misuse of power by those who see themselves as powerless: How does it happen? *Journal of Social Issues*, *55*, 51–64.

Bugental, D. B., Lewis, J. C., Lin, E., Lyon, J., & Kopeikin, H. (1999). In charge but not in control: The management of teaching relationships by adults with low perceived power. *Developmental Psychology*, *35*, 1367–1378.

Buhrmester, D. (1990). Intimacy of friendship, interpersonal competence, and adjustment during preadolescence and adolescence. *Child Development*, *61*, 1101–1111.

Burack, J. A., Flanagan, T., Peled, T., Sutton, H. M., Zygmuntowicz, C., & Manly, J. T. (2006). Social perspective-taking skills in maltreated children and adolescents. *Developmental Psychology*, *42*, 207–217.

Butcher, J., Dahlstrom, W., Graham, J., Tellegen, A., & Kaemmer, B. (1989). *MMPI-2: Manual for administration and scoring*. Minneapolis: University of Minnesota Press.

Caldwell, B., & Bradley, R. (1984). *Home Observation for Measurement of the Environment*. Little Rock: University of Arkansas.

Carr, G. D., Moretti, M. M., & Cue, B. J. H. (2005). Evaluating parenting capacity: Validity problems with the MMPI-2, PAI, CAPI, and ratings of child adjustment. *Professional Psychology: Research and Practice*, *36*, 188–196.

Chaffin, M., & Valle, L. A. (2003). Dynamic prediction characteristics of the Child Abuse Potential Inventory. *Child Abuse and Neglect*, *27*, 463–481.

Cicchetti, D., Ganiban, J., & Barnett, D. (1991). Contributions from the study of high-risk populations to understanding the development of emotion regulation. In J. Garber & K. A. Dodge (Eds.), *The development of emotion regulation and dysregulation: Cambridge studies in social and emotional development* (pp. 15–48). New York: Cambridge University Press.

Cicchetti, D., Rogosch, F. A., Maughan, A., Toth, S. L., & Bruce, J. (2003). False belief understanding in maltreated children. *Development and Psychopathology*, *15*, 1067–1091.

Cicchetti, D., Toth, S. L., & Maughan, A. (2000). An ecological–transactional model of child maltreatment. In A. J. Sameroff, M. Lewis, & S. M. Miller (Eds.), *Handbook of developmental psychopathology* (2nd ed., pp. 689–722). Dordrecht, The Netherlands: Kluwer Academic.

Cohen, S., Kamarck, T., & Mermelstein, R. (1983). A global measure of perceived stress. *Journal of Health and Social Behavior*, *24*, 385–396.

Cohen, S., & Williamson, G. (1988). Perceived stress in a probability sample of the United States. In S. Spacapan & S. Oskamp (Eds.), *The social psychology of health: Claremont Symposium on Applied Social Psychology*. Newbury Park, CA: Sage.

Conduct Problems Prevention Research Group and the Fast Track Project. (1991). *Fast Track study cumulative data files*, 1992–2003 [Computer files]. Durham, NC: Fast Track Data Center, Duke University. Retrieved June 2006 from *www.pubpol.duke.edu/centers/child/fasttrack/techrept/h/hic*

Cooper, S. W., Estes, R. J., Giardino, A. P., Kellogg, N. D., & Vieth, V. I. (Eds.). (2005). *Medical, legal, and social science aspects of child sexual exploitation: A comprehensive review of pornography, prostitution, and Internet crimes, Volumes 1 and 2*. St. Louis, MO: G. W. Medical Publishing.

Corcoran, K., & Fischer, J. (2000). *Measures for clinical practice: A sourcebook* (3rd ed.). New York: Free Press.

Crittenden, P. M., & Claussen, A. H. (2002). Developmental psychopathology perspectives on substance abuse and relationship violence. In C. Wekerle & A. Wall (Eds.), *The violence and addiction equation: Theoretical and clinical issues in substance abuse and relationship violence.* (pp. 44–63). New York: Brunner-Routledge.

Crooks, C. V., Scott, K. L., Francis, K., Kelly, T., & Reid, M. (2006). Eliciting change in maltreating fathers: Goals, processes, and desired outcomes. *Cognitive and Behavioral Practice*, *13*, 71–81.

De Bellis, M. D., Keshavan, M. S., Spencer, S., & Hall, J. (2000). N-acetylaspartate concentration in the anterior cingulate of maltreated children and adolescents with PTSD. *American Journal of Psychiatry*, *157*, 1175–1177.

Derogatis, L. R. (1983). *SCL-90-R: Administration, scoring, and procedures manual–II*. Towson, MD: Clinical Psychometric Research.

Derogatis, L. R. (1992). *The Brief Symptom Inventory (BSI): Administration, scoring, and procedures manual–II* (2nd ed.). Minneapolis, MN: National Computer Systems.

Derogatis, L. R. (2000). *The Brief Symptom Inventory 18: Administration, scoring, and procedures manual–II* (2nd ed.). Minneapolis, MN: Pearson Assessments.

Derogatis, L. R., & Melisaratos, N. (1983). The Brief Symptom Inventory: An introductory report. *Psychological Medicine*, *13*, 595–605.

Dimmitt, J. H. (1996). Translation and reassessment of the adolescent self-perception profile for a rural, Mexican-American population. *Journal of Nursing Measurement*, *4*, 5–18.

Dodge, K. A., Pettit, G. S., & Bates, J. E. (1994). Socialization mediators of the relation between socioeconomic status and child conduct problems. *Child Development*, *65*, 649–665.

Donald, T., & Jureidini, J. (2004). Parenting capacity. *Child Abuse Review*, *13*, 5–17.

Drotar, D. (1999). Child neglect in the family context: Challenges and opportunities in pediatric settings. *Children's Health Care*, *29*, 109–121.

Edleson, J. E., Gassman-Pines, J., & Hill, M. B. (2006). Defining child exposure to domestic violence as neglect: Minnesota's difficult experience. *Social Work*, 5,167–174.

Edleson, J. L. (1999). The overlap between child maltreatment and woman battering. *Violence Against Women*, 5, 134–154.

Edleson, J. L., Mbilinyi, L. F., Beeman, S. K., & Hagemeister, A. K. (2003). How children are involved in adult domestic violence: Results from a four-city telephone survey. *Journal of Interpersonal Violence*, 18, 18–32.

Edwards, V. J., Holden, G. W., Felitti, V. J., & Anda, R. F. (2003). Relationship between multiple forms of childhood maltreatment and adult mental health in community respondents: Results from the Adverse Childhood Experiences Study. *American Journal of Psychiatry*, 160, 1453–1460.

Egeland, B., Yates, T., Appleyard, K., & van Dulmen, M. (2002). The long-term consequences of maltreatment in the early years: A developmental pathway model to antisocial behavior. *Children's Services: Social Policy, Research, and Practice*, 5, 249–260.

Éthier, L. S., Lemelin, J., & Lacharité, C. (2004). A longitudinal study of the effects of chronic maltreatment on children's behavioral and emotional problems. *Child Abuse and Neglect*, 28, 1265–1278.

Eyberg, S. M., Nelson, M. M., Duke, M., & Boggs, S. R. (2005). *Manual for the Dyadic Parent–Child Interaction Coding System* (3rd ed.). Retrieved June 30, 2006, from *phhp.ufl.edu/~seyberg/pcitweb2004/dpicsfiles/dpics%20draft%203.03.pdf*

Eyberg, S., & Pincus, D. (1999). *ECBI and SESBI-R: Eyberg Child Behavior Inventory and Sutter–Eyberg Student Behavior Inventory—Revised, professional manual*. Odessa, FL: Psychological Assessment Resources.

Feiring, C., Taska, L., & Lewis, M. (2002). Adjustment following sexual abuse discovery: The role of shame and attributional style. *Developmental Psychology*, 38, 79–92.

Felitti, V. J., Anda, R. F., Nordenberg, D., Williamson, D. F., Spitz, A. M., & Edwards, V., et al. (1998). Relationship of childhood abuse and household dysfunction to many of the leading causes of death in adults: The Adverse Childhood Experiences (ACE) study. *American Journal of Preventive Medicine*, 14, 245–258.

First, M. B., Spitzer, R. L., Gibbon, M., & Williams, J. B. W. (1996). *Structured Clinical Interview for DSM-IV Axis I Disorders, Clinician Version* (SCID-CV). Washington, DC: American Psychiatric Press.

Friedrich, W. N. (1997). *Child Sexual Behavior Inventory: Professional manual*. Odessa, FL: Psychological Assessment Resources.

Friedrich, W. N., Davies, W. H., Feher, E., & Wright, J. (2003). Sexual behaviour problems in preteen children: Developmental, ecological, and behavioural correlates. *Annals of the New York Academy of Sciences*, 989, 95–104.

Friedrich, W. N., Lysne, M., Sim, L., & Shamos, S. (2004). Assessing sexual behavior in high-risk adolescents with the Adolescent Clinical Sexual Behavior Inventory (ACSBI). *Child Maltreatment*, 9, 239–250.

Garbarino, J., & Stott, F. M. (1989). *What children can tell us: Eliciting, interpreting, and evaluating information from children*. San Francisco: Jossey-Bass.

Gaudin, J. M., Polansky, N. A., & Kilpatrick, A. C. (1992). The Child Well-Being Scales: A field trial. *Child Welfare*, 71, 319–328.

Gaudin, J. M., Polansky, N. A., Kilpatrick, A. C., & Shilton, P. (1996). Family functioning in neglectful families. *Child Abuse and Neglect*, 20, 363–377.

Graziano, A. M. (1994). Why we should study subabusive violence against children. *Journal of Interpersonal Violence*, 9, 412–419.

Gully, K. J. (2001). The Social Behavior Inventory for children in a child abuse treatment program: Development of a tool to measure interpersonal behavior. *Child Maltreatment*, 6, 260–270.

Hamarman, S., Pope, K. H., & Czaja, S. J. (2002). Emotional abuse in children: Variations in legal definitions and rates across the United States. *Child Maltreatment*, 7, 303–311.

Hardt, J., & Rutter, M. (2004). Validity of adult retrospective reports of adverse childhood experiences: Review of the evidence. *Journal of Child Psychology and Psychiatry*, 45, 260–273.

Harter, S. (1982). The Perceived Competence Scale for Children. *Child Development*, 53, 87–97.

Harter, S. (1988). *Manual for the Self-Perception Profile for Adolescents*. Denver, CO: University of Denver.

Haskett, M. E., Ahern, L. S., Ward, C. S., & Allaire, J. C. (2006). Factor structure and validity of the Parenting Stress Index—Short Form. *Journal of Clinical Child and Adolescent Psychology*, 35, 302–312.

Haskett, M. E., Scott, S., & Ward, C. (2004). Subgroups of physically abusive parents based on cluster analysis of parenting behavior and affect. *American Journal of Orthopsychiatry*, 74, 436–447.

Herman, J. L. (1992). Complex PTSD: A syndrome in survivors of prolonged and repeated trauma. *Journal of Traumatic Stress*, 5, 377–391.

Herrenkohl, E. C., Herrenkohl, R. C., Toedter, L., & Yanushefski, A. M. (1984). Parent–child interactions in abusive and nonabusive families. *Journal of the American Academy of Child Psychiatry*, 23, 641–648.

Herrenkohl, R. C., Herrenkohl, E. C., & Egolf, B. P. (1983). Circumstances surrounding the occurrence of child maltreatment. *Journal of Consulting and Clinical Psychology*, 51, 424–431.

Herron, K., & Holtzworth-Munroe, A. (2002). Child abuse potential: A comparison of subtypes of martially violent and nonviolent men. *Journal of Family Violence*, 17, 1–21.

Hess, R. S., & Petersen, S. J. (1996). Reliability and validity of the Self-Perception Profile for children with Mexican American elementary-age children. *Journal of Psychoeducational Assessment*, 14, 229–239.

Hildyard, K. L., & Wolfe, D. A. (2002). Child neglect: Developmental issues and outcomes. *Child Abuse and Neglect, 26,* 679–695.

Holden, E. W., & Banez, G. A. (1996). Child abuse potential and parenting stress within maltreating families. *Journal of Family Violence, 11,* 1–12.

Jacobson, N. S., Gottman, J. M., Waltz, J., & Rushe, R. (1994). Affect, verbal content, and psychophysiology in the arguments of couples with a violent husband. *Journal of Consulting and Clinical Psychology, 62,* 982–988.

Jaffe, P. G., Crooks, C. V., & Bala, N. (2005). *Making appropriate parenting arrangements in family violence cases: Applying the literature to identify promising practices* [Family, Children and Youth Section Research Report No. 2005-FCY-3E]. Ottawa: Department of Justice, Canada.

Jaffe, P. G., Crooks, C. V., & Wolfe, D. A. (2003). Legal and policy responses to children exposed to domestic violence: The need to evaluate intended and unintended consequences. *Clinical Child and Family Psychology Review, 6,* 205–213.

Jefferis, P. G., & Oliver, C. (2006). Associations between maternal childrearing cognitions and conduct problems in young children. *Clinical Child Psychology and Psychiatry, 11,* 83–102.

Johnson, J., & McCutcheon, S. (1980). Assessing life stress in older children and adolescents: Preliminary findings with the Life Events Checklist. In I. Sarason & C. Spielberger (Eds.), *Stress and anxiety* (Vol. 7, pp. 111–125). Washington, DC: Hemisphere.

Johnson, J. J., Smailes, E. M., Cohen, P., Brown, J., & Bernstein, D. P. (2000). Associations between four types of childhood neglect and personality disorder symptoms during adolescence and early adulthood: Findings of a community-based longitudinal study. *Journal of Personality Disorders, 14,* 171–187.

Johnston, J. R., Lee, S., Olesen, N. W., & Walters, M. G. (2005). Allegations and substantiations of abuse in custody-disputing families. *Family Court Review, 43,* 283–294.

Jouriles, E. N., & O'Leary, K. D. (1985). Interspousal reliability of reports of marital violence. *Journal of Consulting and Clinical Psychology, 53,* 419–421.

Kantor, G. K., Holt, M. K., Mebert, C. J., Straus, M. A., Drach, K. M., & Ricci, L. R., et al. (2004). Development and preliminary psychometric properties of the Multidimensional Neglectful Behavior Scale—Child Report. *Child Maltreatment, 9,* 409–428.

Kaplan, S. J., Pelcovitz, D., Salzinger, S., Mandel, F., & Weiner, M. (1997). Adolescent physical abuse and suicide attempts. *Journal of the American Academy of Child and Adolescent Psychiatry, 36,* 799–808.

Kaslow, N. J., & Nolen-Hoeksema, S. (1991). *Children's Attributional Style Questionnaire—Revised.* Unpublished manuscript, Emory University, Atlanta, GA.

Kaufman, J., & Zigler, E. F. (1987). Do abused children become abusive parents? *American Journal of Orthopsychiatry, 7,* 186–192.

Kilpatrick, D. G., Ruggiero, K. J., Acierno, R., Saunders, B. E., Resnick, H. S., & Best, C. L. (2003). Violence and risk of PTSD, major depression, substance abuse/dependence, and comorbidity: Results from the National Survey of Adolescents. *Journal of Consulting and Clinical Psychology, 71,* 692–700.

Kilpatrick, K. L. (2005). The Parental Empathy Measure: A new approach to assessing child maltreatment risk. *American Journal of Orthopsychiatry, 75,* 608–620.

Klorman, R., Cicchetti, D., Thatcher, J. E., & Ison, J. R. (2003). Acoustic startle in maltreated children. *Journal of Abnormal Child Psychology, 31,* 359–370.

Kolko, D. J. (2002). *Child physical abuse.* Thousand Oaks, CA: Sage.

Korbin, J. E. (2003). Neighborhood and community connectedness in child maltreatment research. *Child Abuse and Neglect, 27,* 137–140.

Koverola, C., Elliot-Faust, D., & Wolfe, D. A. (1984). Clinical issues in the behavioral treatment of a child abusive mother experiencing multiple life stresses. *Journal of Clinical Child Psychology, 13,* 187–191.

Lanktree, C. B., & Briere, J. (1995). Outcome of therapy for sexually abused children: A repeated measures study. *Child Abuse and Neglect, 19,* 1145–1155.

Leifer, M., Kilbane, T., Jacobsen, T., & Grossman, G. (2004). A three-generational study of transmission of risk for sexual abuse. *Journal of Clinical Child and Adolescent Psychology, 33,* 662–672.

Leventhal, A., Jacobsen, T., Miller, L., & Quintana, E. (2004). Caregiving attitudes and at-risk maternal behavior among mothers with major mental illness. *Psychiatric Services, 55,* 1431–1433.

Littell, J. H., & Girvin, H. (2005). Caregivers' readiness for change: Predictive validity in a child welfare sample. *Child Abuse and Neglect, 29,* 59–80.

Lounds, J. J., Norkowski, J. G., & Whitman, T. L. (2004). Reliability and validity of the mother–child neglect scale. *Child Maltreatment, 9,* 371–381.

Lyons-Ruth, K., Yellin, C., Melnick, S., & Atwood, G. (2003). Childhood experiences of trauma and loss have different relations to maternal unresolved and hostile–helpless states of mind on the AAI. *Attachment and Human Development, 5,* 330–352.

Macfie, J., Cicchetti, D., & Toth, S. L. (2001). Dissociation in maltreated versus nonmaltreated preschool-aged children. *Child Abuse and Neglect, 25,* 1253–1267.

MacMillan, H. L., Fleming, J. E., Trocmé, N., Boyle, M. H., Wong, M., Racine, Y. A., et al. (1997). Prevalence of child physical and sexual abuse in the community: Results from the Ontario Health Supplement. *Journal of the American Medical Association, 278,* 131–135.

Maughan, A., & Cicchetti, D. (2002). Impact of child maltreatment and interadult violence on children's emotion regulation abilities and socioemotional adjustment. *Child Development, 73,* 1525–1542.

McCloskey, L. A., & Walker, M. (2000). Posttraumatic

stress in children exposed to family violence and single-event trauma. *Journal of the American Academy of Child and Adolescent Psychiatry, 39,* 108–115.

McGee, R. A. (1990). *The Attribution for Maltreatment Interview.* Unpublished manuscript, University of Western Ontario, London, Ontario, Canada.

McGee, R., Wolfe, D. A., & Olson, J. (2001). Multiple maltreatment, attribution of blame, and adjustment among adolescents. *Development and Psychopathology, 13,* 827–846.

Milner, J. S. (1986). *The Child Abuse Potential Inventory manual—second edition.* DeKalb, IL: Psytec.

Milner, J. S. (1989). Applications and limitations of the Child Abuse Potential Inventory. *Early Child Development and Care, 42,* 85–97.

Milner, J. S. (1994). Assessing physical child abuse risk: The Child Abuse Potential Inventory. *Clinical Psychology Review, 14,* 547–583.

Milner, J. S. (2003). Social information processing in high-risk and physically abusive parents. *Child Abuse and Neglect, 27,* 7–20.

Milner, J. S., & Crouch, J. L. (1997). Impact and detection of response distortions on parenting measures used to assess risk for child physical abuse. *Journal of Personality Assessment, 69,* 633–650.

Morey, L. C. (1991). *The Personality Assessment Inventory: Professional manual.* Odessa, FL: Psychological Assessment Resources.

Morey, L. C. (1996). *An interpretive guide to the Personality Assessment Inventory.* Odessa, FL: Psychological Assessment Resources.

Muris, P., Meesters, C., & Fijen, P. (2003). The Self-Perception Profile for Children: Further evidence for its factor structure, reliability, and validity. *Personality and Individual Differences, 35,* 1791–1802.

Nemeroff, C. B. (2004). Neurobiological consequences of childhood trauma. *Journal of Clinical Psychiatry, 65*(Suppl. 1), 18–28.

Oldershaw, L., Walters, G. C., & Hall, D. K. (1986). Control strategies and noncompliance in abusive mother–child dyads: An observational study. *Child Development, 57,* 722–732.

O'Leary, K. D., Malone, J., & Tyree, A. (1994). Physical aggression in early marriage: Prerelationship and relationship effects. *Journal of Consulting and Clinical Psychology, 62,* 594–602.

Oman, R. F., Vesely, S. K., McLeroy, K. R., Harris-Wyatt, V., Aspy, C. B., Rodine, S., et al. (2002). Reliability and validity of the Youth Asset Survey (YAS). *Journal of Adolescent Health, 31,* 247–255.

Ondersma, S. J., Chaffin, M. J., Mullins, S. M., & LeBreton, J. M. (2005). A brief form of the Child Abuse Potential Inventory: Development and validation. *Journal of Clinical and Consulting Psychology, 34,* 301–311.

Pereda, N., & Forns, M. (2004). Psychometric properties of the Spanish version of the Self-Perception Profile for Children. *Perceptual and Motor Skills, 98,* 685–699.

Polansky, N. A., Chalmers, M. A., Butenweiser, E., & Williams, D. (1978). Assessing adequacy of child caring: An urban scale. *Child Welfare, 7,* 439–449.

Pollak, S. D., & Tolley-Schell, S. A. (2003). Selective attention to facial emotion in physically abused children. *Journal of Abnormal Psychology, 112,* 323–338.

Procidano, M., & Heller, K. (1983). Measures of perceived social support from friends and from family: Three validational studies. *American Journal of Community Psychology, 11,* 1–24.

Reynolds, C. R., & Kamphaus, R. W. (2004). *Behavioral Assessment Scale for Children, Second Edition (BASC-2).* Bloomington, MN: Pearson Assessments.

Rodriguez, C. M. (2006). Attributional style as a mediator between parental abuse risk and child internalizing symptomatology. *Child Maltreatment, 11,* 121–130.

Sarason, I. G., Levine, H. M., Basham, R. B., & Sarason, B. R. (1983). Assessing social support: The Social Support Questionnaire. *Journal of Personality and Social Psychology, 44,* 127–139.

Sarason, I. G., Sarason, B. R., Shearin, E. N., & Pierce, G. R. (1987). A brief measure of social support: Practical and theoretical implications. *Journal of Social and Personal Relationships, 4,* 497–510.

Saunders, B. E., Berliner, L., & Hanson, R. F. (Eds.). (2003). *Child physical and sexual abuse: Guidelines for treatment.* Charlston, SC: National Crime Victims Research and Treatment Center.

Schaeffer, C. M., Alexander, P. C., Bethke, K., & Kretz, L. S. (2005). Predictors of child abuse potential among military parents: Comparing mothers and fathers. *Journal of Family Violence, 20,* 123–129.

Schumann, B. C., Striegel-Moore, R. H., McMahon, R. P., Waclawiw, M. A., Morrison, J. A., & Schreiber, G. B. (1999). Psychometric properties of the Self-Perception Profile for Children in a biracial cohort of adolescent girls: The NHLBI Growth and Health Study. *Journal of Personality Assessment, 73,* 260–275.

Scott, K. L., & Crooks, C. V. (2004). Effecting change in maltreating fathers: Critical principles for intervention planning. *Clinical Psychology: Science and Practice, 11,* 95–111.

Scott, K. L., & Crooks, C. V. (in press). Preliminary evaluation of an intervention program for maltreating fathers. *Brief Treatment and Crisis Intervention.*

Scott, K. L., Wolfe, D. A., & Wekerle, C. (2003). Maltreatment and trauma: Tracking the connections in adolescence. *Child and Adolescent Psychiatric Clinics of North America, 12,* 211–230.

Sedlak, A. J., & Broadhurst, D. D. (1996, September). *Third National Incidence Study of Child Abuse and Neglect: Final report.* Washington, DC: U.S. Department of Health and Human Services.

Sheras, P. L., Abidin, R. R., & Konold, T. R. (1998). *SIPA: Stress Index for Parents of Adolescents.* Odessa, FL: Psychological Assessment Resources.

Shields, A., Ryan, R. M., & Cicchetti, D. (2001). Narrative representations of caregivers and emotion dys-regulation as predictors of maltreated children's rejection by peers. *Developmental Psychology*, *37*, 321–337.

Shipman, K., Zeman, J., Penza, S., & Champion, K. (2000). Emotion management skills in sexually maltreated and nonmaltreated girls: A developmental psychopathology perspective. *Development and Psychopathology*, *12*, 47–62.

Slack, K. S., Holl, J. L., McDaniel, M., Yoo, J., & Bolger, K. (2004). Understanding the risks of child neglect: An exploration of poverty and parenting characteristics. *Child Maltreatment*, *9*, 395–408.

Smetana, J. G., Kelly, M., & Twentyman, C. T. (1984). Abused, neglected, and nonmaltreated children's conceptions of moral and social-conventional transgressions. *Child Development*, *55*, 277–287.

Spanier, G. B. (1976). Measuring dyadic adjustment: New scales for assessing the quality of marriage and similar dyads. *Journal of Marriage and the Family*, *38*, 15–28.

Sroufe, L. A., Carlson, E. A., Levy, A. K., & Egeland, B. (1999). Implications of attachment theory for developmental psychopathology. *Development and Psychopathology*, *11*, 1–13.

Straus, M. A. (1979). Measuring intrafamily conflict and violence: The Conflicts Tactics (CTS) Scales. *Journal of Marriage and the Family*, *41*, 75–88.

Straus, M. A. (1995). *Manual for the Conflict Tactics Scales*. Durham: Family Research Laboratory, University of New Hampshire.

Straus, M. A. (2001). *Beating the devil out of them: Corporal punishment in American families and its effects on children*. New Brunswick, NJ: Transaction.

Straus, M. A., Hamby, S. L., Boney-McCoy, S., & Sugarman, D. B. (1996). The revised Conflict Tactics Scales (CTS2): Development and preliminary psychometric data. *Journal of Family Issues*, *17*, 283–316.

Straus, M. A., & Kantor, G. K. (2005). Definition and measurement of neglectful behavior: Some principles and guidelines. *Child Abuse and Neglect*, *29*, 19–29.

Straus, M. A., Kinard, E. M., & Williams, L. M. (1995, July). *The Neglect Scale, Form A: Adolescent and Adult-Recall version*. Paper presented at the Fourth International Conference on Family Violence Research, Durham, NH.

Sullivan, P., & Knutson, J. (2000). Maltreatment and disabilities: A population-based epidemiological study. *Child Abuse and Neglect*, *24*(10), 1257–1273.

Thompson, M., Kaslow, N. J., Weiss, B., & Nolen-Hoeksema, S. (1998). Children's Attributional Style Questionnaire—Revised: Psychometric examination. *Psychological Assessment*, *10*, 166–170.

Thompson, R. A., & Flood, M. F. (2002). Toward a child-oriented child protection system. In G. B. Melton, R. A. Thompson, & M. A. Small (Eds.), *Toward a child-centered, neighborhood-based child protection system: A report of the Consortium on Children, Families, and the Law* (pp. 155–194). Westport, CT: Praeger.

Thomson, N. R., & Zand, D. H. (2002). The Harter Self-Perception Profile for Adolescents: Psychometrics for an early adolescent, African American sample. *International Journal of Testing*, *2*, 297–310.

Trickett, P. K., Kurtz, D. A., & Pizzigati, K. (2004). Resilient outcomes in abused and neglected children: Bases for strengths-based intervention and prevention policies. In K. I. Maton, C. J. Schellenbach, B. J. Leadbeater, & A. L. Solarz (Eds.), *Investing in children, youth, families, and communities: Strengths-based research and policy* (pp. 73–95). Washington, DC: American Psychological Association.

Trocmé, N. (1996). Development and preliminary evaluation of the Ontario Child Neglect Index. *Child Maltreatment*, *1*, 145–155.

Trocmé, N., & Bala, N. (2005). False allegations of abuse and neglect when parents separate. *Child Abuse and Neglect*, *29*, 1333–1345.

Trocmé, N., MacLaurin, B., Fallon, B., Daciuk, J., Billingsley, D. A., & Tourigny, M., et al. (2001). *Canadian Incidence Study of Reported Child Abuse and Neglect: Final report*. Ottawa: Minister of Public Works and Government Services Canada.

Trocmé, N. B., Fallon, B., MacLaurin, J., Daciuk, C., Felstiner, T., Black, L., et al. (2005). *Canadian Incidence Study of Reported Child Abuse and Neglect–2003: Major findings*. Ottawa: Minister of Public Works and Government Services Canada.

U.S. Department of Health and Human Services. (2004). *Child maltreatment 2002: Reports from the states to the National Center on Child Abuse and Neglect*. Washington, DC: U.S. Government Printing Office.

U.S. Department of Health and Human Services. (2003). *Child welfare outcomes 2000: Annual report*. Washington, DC: U.S. Government Printing Office.

U.S. Department of Health and Human Services, Administration on Children, Youth, and Families. (2005). *Child Maltreatment 2003*. Washington, DC: U.S. Government Printing Office.

Walsh, C. A., MacMillan, H. L., Trocmé, N., Jamieson, E., & Boyle, M. (2006). *Measurement of victimization in adolescence: Development and validation of the Childhood Experience of Violence Questionnaire*. Manuscript submitted for publication.

Wang, A., Meredith, W. H., & Tsai, R. (1996). Comparison in three Chinese cultures of scores on the Self-Perception Profile for Children. *Perceptual and Motor Skills*, *82*, 1087–1095.

Wekerle, C., Miller, A., Wolfe, D. A., & Spindel, C. B. (2006). *Childhood maltreatment*. Cambridge, MA: Hogrefe & Huber.

Wekerle, C., & Wolfe, D. A. (2003). Child maltreatment. In E. J. Mash & R. A. Barkley (Eds.), *Child psychopathology* (2nd ed., pp. 632–684). New York: Guilford Press.

White, H. R., & Widom, C. S. (2003). Intimate partner violence among abused and neglected children in young adulthood: The mediating effects of early aggression, antisocial personality, hostility and alcohol problems. *Aggressive Behavior*, *29*, 332–345.

Whitman, T. L., Borkowski, J. G., Keogh, D. A., & Weed, K. (2001). *Interwoven lives: Adolescent mothers and their children.* Mahwah, NJ: Erlbaum.

Widom, C. S. (1999). Posttraumatic stress disorder in abused and neglected children grown up. *American Journal of Psychiatry, 156,* 1223–1229.

Wolfe, D. A. (1985). Child-abusive parents: An empirical review and analysis. *Psychological Bulletin, 97,* 462–482.

Wolfe, D. A. (1999). *Child abuse: Implications for children development and psychopathology* (2nd ed.). Thousand Oaks, CA: Sage.

Wolfe, D. A., Crooks, C. V., Lee, V., McIntyre-Smith, A., & Jaffe, P. G. (2003). The effects of children's exposure to domestic violence: A meta-analysis and critique. *Clinical Child and Family Psychology Review, 6,* 171–187.

Wolfe, D. A., Jaffe, P. G., Jetté, J. L., & Poisson, S. E. (2003). The impact of child abuse in community institutions and organizations: Advancing professional and scientific understanding. *Clinical Psychology: Science and Practice, 10,* 179–191.

Wolfe, D. A., & McGee, R. (1991). Assessment of emotional status among maltreated children. In R. H. Starr, Jr. & D. A. Wolfe (Eds.), *The effects of child abuse and neglect: Issues and research* (pp. 257–277). New York: Guilford Press.

Wolfe, D. A., & McGee, R. A. (1994). Dimensions of child maltreatment and their relationship to adolescent adjustment. *Development and Psychopathology, 6,* 165–181.

Wolfe, D. A., Scott, K., Wekerle, C., & Pittman, A. (2001). Child maltreatment: Risk of adjustment problems and dating violence in adolescence. *Journal of the American Academy of Child and Adolescent Psychiatry, 40,* 282–298.

Wolfe, D. A., Wekerle, C., Scott, K., Straatman, A., & Grasley, C. (2004). Predicting abuse in adolescent dating relationships over one year: The role of child maltreatment and trauma. *Journal of Abnormal Psychology, 113,* 406–415.

World Health Organization. (2002). *World report on violence and health: Summary.* Geneva, Switzerland: Author.

CHAPTER 15

Child Sexual Abuse

Vicky Veitch Wolfe

The study of childhood sexual abuse (CSA) began in earnest in the 1970s, a relative latecomer in the field of childhood psychopathology. However, since that time, tremendous gains have been made in our understanding of this serious problem. The growing recognition of the extent of CSA, and concern about its lifelong effects, led to significant changes in law, social work, education, and mental health. Indeed, there is even evidence that our increased knowledge and efforts toward recognition, prevention, and intervention have led to overall reductions in the prevalence of sexual abuse (Finkelhor & Jones, 2004). The professions of psychology and the behavioral sciences have made enormous contributions toward the understanding of the effects of sexual abuse and have led to great improvements in assessment, prevention, and treatment of sexually abused children and adolescents, and their families. These advancements have moved the field forward from the initial need to document and describe sexual abuse, to advancements in understanding the specific ways that sexual abuse affects children and results in psychological processes that often lead to lifelong adjustment difficulties.

This chapter reviews current issues related to child sexual abuse, with the general assumption that from our core bases of knowledge, assessment methodology will grow. The chapter consists of three main parts: (1) an epidemio-logical overview of the problem of sexual abuse, including prevalence and incidence, characteristics of the abuse and perpetrators, child victims, their families and communities, and the types of stress they encounter subsequent to abuse disclosures; (2) an overview of the impact of sexual abuse on children and adolescents, and factors that attenuate and exacerbate those effects; and (3) an overview of assessment strategies and tools that have been developed especially for CSA victims and their families. Drawing from extant evidence-based methods, practical suggestions are made for clinical assessments.

EPIDEMIOLOGICAL OVERVIEW OF THE PROBLEM

Epidemiological studies of CSA have varied considerably in methodology, yielding large discrepancies in sexual abuse estimates, ranging from 2 to 62% for women and from 3 to 16% for men among U.S. studies, and from 3 to 20% for women and from 7 to 36% for men among international studies (Finkelhor, 1994b). Prevalence rates vary considerably depending on how sexual abuse is defined. For instance, studies that include noncontact forms of abuse and abuse by peers tend to yield high abuse estimates (Goldman & Padayachi, 2000). Due to the complicating factor of adolescent consensual sexual activity, definitions for adolescents tend to vary regarding the upper age limited considered as abuse, the age difference required between the victim and offender for noncoercive sexual contacts (typically increased to 10 years), and the ways that coercion and abuse of authority are defined. Survey questions about sexual abuse also vary across studies. Some studies use a general question about sexual abuse history as a gate to asking more detailed questions, sometimes using vague terms such as "unwanted sexual touching," whereas other studies ask about history of a number of specific acts without necessarily defining the acts as sexual abuse. The latter method tends to yield higher estimates of abuse, because some respondents may not consider their experiences as abusive (e.g., young males abused by older females). Research suggests that more inclusive definitions have an advantage when studying the impact of abuse, because more victims who are affected by abuse are included (Long & Jackson, 1990).

Based on a review of 19 studies of adult retrospective reports of childhood experiences, Finkelhor (1994a) concluded that approximately 20% of women and 5–10% of men had at least one episode of sexual abuse during their childhood. More recent studies yield similar estimates. A large-scale study of 17,337 adult members of a managed care program in California revealed that 25% of women and 16% of men reported at least one episode of abuse during childhood (Dong, Anda, Dube, Giles, & Felitti, 2003). In another large-scale population-based study (N = 3,958), Fleming, Mullen, and Bammer (1997) found that 20% of women reported CSA. Although some have suggested that epidemiological studies overestimate prevalence, most studies indicate that even in anonymous studies, individuals tend to underreport CSA by at least 16–50% (Fergusson, Horwood, & Woodward, 2000; Goodman et al., 2003; Greenhoot, McCloskey, & Gisky, 2005; Widom & Morris, 1997; Williams, 1994). Overall, these statistics reveal that sexual victimization is higher among youth compared to adults. Indeed, Hashimi and Finkelhor (1999) reported that rates of abuse of adolescents ages 12–17 were 2.0 to 3.3 times higher than rates for young adults ages 18–24.

Incidence data reflect the number of cases made known to public agencies during a specified period of time. Incidence data grossly underestimate true rates of sexual abuse, because most cases are never reported to official agencies. However, in addition to providing information about agency-reported abuse, incidence data may be used to detect epidemiological trends, including rates of disclosure to official agencies. Recent retrospective surveys estimate that between 8.7 and 12.0% of CSA was reported to police or other authorities (MacMillan et al., 1997; MacMillan, Jamieson, & Walsh, 2003; Saunders, Villeponteaux, Lipovsky, Kilpatrick, & Veronon, 1993). However, Finkelhor (1994a), combining prevalence and incidence estimates, calculated that approximately 30% of sexual abuse is currently disclosed to official agencies during childhood. In some cases, abuse is disclosed to parents and peers, but not to official agencies. Data from the National Survey of Adolescents, which included 1,958 girls ages 12–17 years, revealed that 48% of sexual abuse victims had disclosed their abuse to an adult, and an additional 25% had disclosed to a peer (Kogan, 2004). Hanson, Resnick, Saunders, Kilpatrick, and Best (1999), also reporting data from the National Survey of Adolescents, found that only half of those who disclosed their abuse to a relative, friend, or other confidant had also made a disclosure to an official agency.

Based on both incidence and prevalence data, evidence suggests a decrease in sexual abuse during the past two decades. Adult retrospective surveys from Australia and Ireland have demonstrated trends toward less abuse reported by younger, compared to older, cohorts (Dunne, Purdie, Cook, Boyle, & Najman, 2003; McGee, Garavan de Barra, Byrne, & Conroy, 2002). Surveys of adolescents have also demonstrated decreases in rates of sexual abuse and sexual assaults from 1992 to 2001 that range from 22 to 56% (Finkelhor & Jones, 2004). Reports of sexual abuse to official agencies have also decreased since the mid-1990s, with a 39% decrease in the United States (Jones, Finkelhor, & Kopiec, 2001) and a 49% decrease in Ontario, Canada (Trocmé, Fallon, MacLaurin, & Neves, 2003). Indeed, 1990 U.S. statistics indicated that sexual abuse cases comprised 17% of all confirmed or validated reports of maltreatment, whereas in 2004, CSA accounted for only 9.7% of reported maltreatment cases (Sedlak & Broadhurst, 1996; U.S. Department of Health and Human Services, 2004). In Ontario, the decrease in sexual abuse substantiation occurred at the same time that reports of other forms of maltreatment were on the rise (Trocmé et al., 2003). However, in the United States, these declines coincided with similar declines in physical abuse, crime, teen pregnancies, runaway youth, and teen suicides (Finkelhor & Jones, 2004). Although there is some evidence that declines in incidence rates were in part due to changes in child protective service procedures, verification, and recording methods, other evidence indicates that the trend appears to reflect actual declines in sexual abuse. Positive effects of prevention programs, public awareness campaigns, and increased prosecution likely contribute to the decline (Jones et al., 2001). Finkelhor and Jones (2004) argued that societal deterrents against sexual abuse have been particularly effective. Between 1986 and 1997, the number of persons incarcerated for sex crimes against children doubled (Finkelhor & Ormrod, 2001), and this data did not include the increased number of offenders who received nonincarceration penalties following sexual abuse charges (e.g., probation). Citing data collected in Illinois and Pennsylvania, Finkelhor and Jones highlighted significant declines in sexual abuse cases involving fathers. They argued that biological fathers, who may be the least compulsive of CSA offender types, may be particularly deterred by the possibility of detection and prosecution.

Abuse Characteristics

Perpetrators

Sexual abuse varies on a number of dimensions, including the child's relationship to the perpetrator, the sexual acts involved, the use of coercion or force, and the duration and frequency of abuse. For female sexual abuse victims, 92% report abuse by males, 2% report abuse by females, and 4% report abuse by both males and females; for male sexual abuse victims, 51% report abuse by males, 21% report abuse by females, and 18%, by both males and females (Dube et al., 2005). Researchers have historically distinguished intrafamilial or incestuous abuse from extrafamilial abuse. Roughly 33–50% of female victims and 10–20% of male victims are abused by family members; 10–30% are abused by strangers, and approximately 40% are abused by someone known but not related to them (Fergusson, Lynskey, & Horwood, 1996; Finkelhor, 1994b; Vogeltanz et al., 1999). From 4.5 to 6.0% of girls are

abused by a father figure (Bagley & Mallick, 2000; Hanson et al., 2003; Russell, 1984). Although biological fathers account for more sexual abuse than do stepfathers (more children live with fathers than stepfathers), stepfathers are up to seven times more likely to abuse their stepdaughters and are more likely to commit more serious forms of abuse (Russell, 1983, 1984). Indeed, males in surrogate father roles (e.g., stepfathers, adoptive father, the mother's boyfriends) account for 18% of reported sexual abuse, whereas biological fathers account for 14% of reported sexual abuse (U.S. Department of Health and Human Services, 2004). Sexual abuse by family members tends to be more severe and repeated. Fergusson and colleagues (1996) reported that 61% of CSA episodes involving family members involved attempted or completed intercourse, and more than one incident occurred in 71% of cases.

Despite considerable focus on abuse by father figures, sibling abuse is the most prevalent form of incest, with between 7 and 15% of women and 10% of males reporting abuse by a sibling during childhood (Finkelhor, 1980; Hardy, 2001; Romero, Wyatt, Loeb, Carmona, & Solis, 1999). Sibling abuse occurs at least five times more often than does parent–child abuse (Finkelhor, 1980; Smith & Israel, 1987) and accounts for between 16 and 50% of incest cases (Laurence, 2000; Romero et al., 1999). In most cases, sibling incest is perpetrated by boys between the ages of 10 and 14, and their victims are typically at least 5 years younger (Laurence, 2000). Although some might consider sibling incest to be within the realm of sexual exploration, there is growing awareness that sibling incest can lead to serious emotional sequelae for victims (Adler & Schultz, 1995). Clinic-based studies of sibling incest reveal that 46–89% of cases involve attempted or completed vaginal or anal penetration, with most victims at least 5 years younger than the offenders. Russell (1986) found that 44% of brothers who committed sibling incest used physical force, such as pushing and pinning down the victim.

In their review of the literature, Pithers and Gray (1998) estimated that 40% of CSA was perpetrated by youth under the age of 20, and that 13–18% of offenses were committed by children ages 6–12. Likewise, in their study of sexual abuse among U.S. Latinos, Romero and colleagues (1999) found that 51% of offenders against females were younger than age 20 years. From a United Kingdom study, 32% of offenders were younger than age 18 (Oaksford & Frude, 2001). In the United States, individuals under age 18 account for 17% of all arrests for sexual crimes (Federal Bureau of Investigation, 1999) and roughly 33% of all arrests for sexual offenses against children (Snyder & Sickmund, 1999). Well over half (57%) of identified adolescent offenders had multiple victims prior to being caught (Fehrenbach, Smith, Monastersky, & Deisher, 1986). Furthermore, Sperry and Gilbert (2005) found that 8% of females and 4% of males reported sexual abuse prior to the age 12 by a peer who was 12 years old or younger.

During recent years, Internet-initiated sexual abuse has become a serious concern. A recent national survey documented that 20% of children and adolescents report at least one episode of Internet-initiated sexual solicitation within a 1-year period (Mitchell, Finkelhor, & Wolak, 2003). Case-based evidence suggests that Internet predators operate in ways similar to other perpetrators (Dombrowski, LeMasney, Ahia, & Dickson, 2004; Walsh & Wolak, 2005); that is, they select children and adolescents who show some level of vulnerability—either through the use of sexually suggestive nicknames on the Internet or by presenting themselves as isolated, lonely, passive, or emotionally vulnerable. Internet perpetrators may at first present themselves as peers. Like other perpetrators, they may engage in grooming behaviors in the forms of exchanging pictures, and providing pornography and gifts. Once a relationship is established, online predators may progress to requesting personal information, phone numbers, and face-to-face meetings. Adolescents, more than children, tend to be more common targets of online predators because they have greater autonomy, mobility, and sexual curiosity.

Walsh and Wolak (2005) studied Internet-initiated, nonforcible sex crimes against youth that resulted in felony charges. The majority of victims were adolescents (81%), 61% female and 39% male. In most cases, the abuse was discovered by a parent or guardian and reported directly to police. Investigation by police revealed that 45% of perpetrators were in possession of child pornography, 39% had given pornography to the victim, and 27% had taken pornographic pictures of their victims. Fifty percent of cases involved sexual penetra-

tion, and in 34% of cases, the victims were supplied drugs or alcohol. Of great concern, many offenders (30%) volunteered or had jobs that put them in positions of trust with minors. Nine percent had prior sexual offense arrests. Because Internet predators typically leave computer-based evidence of their crimes, prosecution of these types of offenses tends to be successful. Of the 77 arrests reviewed for the study, the conviction rate was 91%, with 59 individuals incarcerated, 59 placed on a sexual offender registry, and half ordered into mental health treatment.

Abusive Acts

Sexually abusive acts vary along a number of dimensions, ranging from inappropriate sexual overtures to fondling, and to oral, vaginal, and anal intercourse. Most epidemiological studies make a distinction between abuse that involves some form of penetration and other forms of abuse, and estimates have varied considerably. Several studies of adult retrospective reports reveal that approximately 25% of male and female abuse includes sexual intercourse (Coxell, King, Mezey, & Kell, 2000; Dube et al., 2005; Sachs-Ericsson, Blazer, Plant, & Arnow, 2005; Ullman & Filipas, 2005; Vogeltanz et al., 1999). Studies of adolescents and young adults suggest that younger generations experience more severe forms of abuse that include sexual intercourse. Data from the National Survey of Adolescents revealed that roughly 33% of victims reported sexual intercourse (Hanson et al., 2003). Tubman, Gil, and Wagner (2004) found that 42% of 18- to 23-year-old males and females who experienced sexual abuse prior to age 16 reported that their abuse had included sexual intercourse.

A *Los Angeles Times* poll (Timnick, 1985), which defined "coercion" as abuse that involved a weapon or forcible physical restraint, found that 15% of male victims and 19% of female victims experienced coercion. In more recent studies, Vogeltanz and colleagues (1999) reported that 38% of female victims reported some form of physical coercion, 15% thought their lives were in danger, and 3% sustained physical injury. Hanson and colleagues (2003) found that 27% of adolescents felt that their life was in jeopardy as a result of the sexual abuse.

Adult and adolescent retrospective studies indicate that 60–71% of abuse occurs only once (Finkelhor, 1979; Stevens, Ruggiero, Kilpatrick, Resnick, & Saunders, 2005; Wyatt, Loeb, Solis, Carmona, & Romero, 1999). Boys tend to be abused less frequently and over shorter durations compared to girls (Kendall-Tackett & Simon, 1992), with 11% of girls and 8% of boys abused repeatedly over at least 1 year (Timnick, 1985). Bagley and Mallick (2000) noted differences in onset between those who experienced one-time versus multiple abuse episodes. Among those who experienced one-time abuse, onset during preschool years was rare (3%), whereas one-time episodes were more common among girls age 11 and older (12–19%). In contrast, among those who reported multiple episodes of abuse, onset during preschool years was not uncommon (14%), but it was uncommon after age 11 (5%). Not surprisingly, those who experience multiple episodes of abuse are more likely to report more serious forms of maltreatment. Bagley and Mallick found that only 3% of one-episode abuse cases include vaginal or anal penetration; for those who experienced multiple abuse episodes, 48% experienced vaginal penetration, and 19% experienced anal penetration.

Sexual abuse often occurs amid other forms of maltreatment and adversity. In addition to the cumulative effects of these events and circumstances, multiple forms of abuse and adversity suggest serious familial and social inadequacies that fail to protect and nurture the child (Fleming, Mullen, Sibthorpe, & Bammer, 1999). In a large-scale epidemiological study, Dong and colleagues (2003) found that CSA was associated with a history of physical abuse (45.5% of women, 42.7% of men), emotional maltreatment (26.1% of women, 17.3% of men), emotional neglect (29.6% of women, 19.9% of men), exposure to domestic violence (23.6% of women, 20.5% of men), and parental substance abuse (43.3% of women, 34.4% of men). Only 22% of sexual abuse victims reported no other form of maltreatment, and 29% had four or more forms of maltreatment and adversity. Finkelhor and his colleagues conducted two nationwide surveys of children and adolescents (ages 10 and older) that revealed high prevalences of nonsexual victimizations among sexually abused children (Boney-McCoy & Finkelhor, 1995; Finkelhor, Ormrod, Turner, & Hamby, 2005): 43% experienced another form of maltreatment (physical abuse, emotional abuse, neglect, family abduction, custodial interference); 70% experienced property victimization (e.g., vandalism, theft), and 84% witnessed violence or indirect victimization (e.g., witnessed domestic violence, saw a violent crime). Children who present for clinical services are even more likely to have multiple victimization experiences. For example, two clinic-based studies of CSA victims reported that more than 50% had witnessed spousal violence (Bowen, 2000; Kellogg & Menard, 2003), with 77% reporting that the spousal violence and sexual abuse occurred within the same time period. Bowen (2000) found that 41% of victims reported delaying disclosure out of fear of violence by the perpetrator.

Children who experience CSA are also particularly likely to experience subsequent, distinct sexual victimizations in later childhood, adolescence, and as adults (Classen, Palesh, & Aggarwal, 2005). Stevens and colleagues (2005), drawing from the National Survey of Adolescents, found that children who are abused at a young age and those who experienced more severe forms of abuse are particularly likely to be revictimized. In their survey of children and adolescents, Boney-McCoy and Finkelhor (1996) found that those with a history of sexual abuse were 11.7 times more likely to report a different sexual victimization within the next year. Indeed, a number of studies have identified that history of sexual abuse was related to revictimization during adolescent years. For example, Small and Kerns (1993) found that roughly 33% of adolescents who experienced a sexual assault reported prior childhood sexual abuse. Fergusson, Horwood, and Lynsky (1996), in their longitudinal sample of adolescents, found that among those who reported contact forms of CSA, 10% experienced rape or attempted rape between the ages of 16 and 18, five times the risk of their nonabused peers. An additional 13% experienced other forms of sexual assault during that period, three times the risk of their nonabused peers. In a long-term follow-up of a sample of sexual abuse victims in Australia, Swanston and colleagues (2002) found that 17% had official reports reflecting subsequent sexual victimizations. In turn, adolescent sexual victimization is a powerful predictor of subsequent sexual victimization of young women (Gidycz, Coble, Latham, & Layman, 1993; Humphrey & White, 2000).

Victim Risk and Resiliency Factors

Three child factors have received attention as risk factors for CSA: age, gender, and disabilities. Approximately 10% of sexually abused children are under age 6, with a slight increase in onset at age 6–7 years, and a dramatic increase around age 10 (33%; Bagley & Mallick, 2000; Finkelhor & Baron, 1986; Vogeltanz et al., 1999). Indeed, data from the National Survey of Adolescents (Hanson et al., 2003) revealed that 60% of sexual abuse occurred between the ages of 11 and 16. Because of the large age span considered under the umbrella of sexual abuse, the nature, impact, and etiology of sexual victimization vary at different developmental points (Black, Heyman, & Slep, 2001).

Not surprisingly, girls are at higher risk for sexual abuse than boys, and are victims 3 to 5 times more often than boys (Boney-McCoy & Finkelhor, 1995; Fergusson, Lynskey, & Horwood, 1996; Sachs-Ericcson et al., 2005; Sedlak & Broadhurst, 1996). Sexual abuse experiences differ for boys and girls (Gordon, 1990; Watkins & Bentovim, 1992), with girls generally describing their experiences more negatively (Fischer, 1991). This may be because girls tend to be younger at the onset of their abuse (Dong et al., 2003) and their perpetrators tend to be older (Romano & DeLuca, 2001). Girls are abused by family members more often, and abuse perpetrated by family members tends to be more serious. Fergusson, Lynskey, and Horwood (1996) reported that 61.3% of abuse perpetrated by family members included some form of intercourse, and that 71% of familial abuse involved more than one episode. Boys are more likely to be abused by adolescent males and by females (Dube et al., 2005; Finkelhor, 1990). They may perceive abuse by adolescent males as a form of sexual experimentation (Romano & De Luca, 2001), and up to 20% of males describe sexual abuse by older females as either nonthreatening or pleasurable (Bagley & Thurston, 1996).

Children with developmental disabilities are at heightened risk for sexual abuse, with prevalence estimates two to three times greater than those of children without disabilities (Crosse, Kaye, & Ratnofsky, 1993; Sullivan & Knutson, 1998). Four factors have been linked to increased risk among children with disabilities (Westcott & Jones, 1999): (1) greater physical and social isolation; (2) increased dependence and lack of control over their lives and bodies (e.g., need for assistance when bathing, dressing, and toileting, often by individuals other than parents, such as residential and disability care providers); (3) institutional care, with concerns raised about the level of staff training and qualifications, and insufficient efforts to ensure patient safety; and (4) communication impairments that may increase risk of being selected by perpetrators, prevent reporting, and impede validation of abuse allegations. Much of the increased vulnerability in this population is among boys, particularly those between ages 6 and 11 (Randall, Parrila, & Sobsey, 2000; Sobsey, Randall, & Parrila, 1997; Sullivan, Brookhouser, Scanlan, Knutson, & Schulte, 1991). Sobsey and Doe (1991) found that increased contact with disability service providers accounted for 78% of the increased risk to children with disabilities. Indeed, Sobsey and colleagues (1997) queried whether the disproportionate representation of boys among sexually abused children with disabilities is related to a tendency for their nonfamilial caregivers to be male, whereas nonfamilial caregivers of girls tend to be female.

Family Risk and Resiliency Factors

Several interrelated family factors have been linked with risk of sexual abuse: unplanned pregnancy, low maternal education, parental alcohol and drug abuse, parental mental illness, harsh discipline, parent–child relationship problems, maternal death, living with only one or with no natural parent, marital discord, separation, divorce, and maternal remarriage (Bagley & Mallick, 2000; Boney-McCoy & Finkelhor, 1995; Brown, Cohen, Johnson, & Salzinger, 1998; Dong et al., 2003; Fergusson, Lynskey, & Horwood, 1996; Finkelhor, Moore, Hamby, & Straus, 1997; Hanson et al., 2006; Mullen, Martin, Anderson, Romans, & Herbison, 1993; Walsh, MacMillan, & Jamieson, 2003). Increasing levels of family-related adversity correspond to increasing risk of child sexual victimization, and family-based risk factors are relevant to both intrafamilial and extrafamilial sexual abuse of boys and girls (Fergusson, Lynskey, & Horwood, 1996). Indeed, in a longitudinal study of 267 low socioeconomic status (SES) primiparous women and their children, Pianta, Egeland, and Erickson (1989) found that children identified as having experienced sexual abuse ($n = 11$) had mothers who previously had reported more stressful life events and less social support at every prior assessment point, which occurred at 6- to 12-month intervals when the children were between the ages of 2 and 5 years. Compared to the other mothers in the study, mothers whose children were sexually abused had described themselves as more tense, depressed, angry, confused, restless, skeptical, and calculating.

Factors that negatively affect parental ability to monitor child safety appear to be particularly potent in predicting risk for sexual abuse. Drawing from the National Survey of Adolescents, Hanson and colleagues (2006) found that not living with a biological parent increased the odds of sexual abuse by 1.8. As well, parental alcohol abuse, which affects parental availability and child monitoring, increased the odds of adolescent reports of extrafamilial sexual abuse by 1.7 and doubled the odds of multiple victimization (Hanson et al., 2006; Stevens et al., 2005). Finkelhor and colleagues (1997) found that leaving a child at home alone without adequate supervision increased the odds of child sexual victimization by 3.4. Likewise, Fergusson, Lynskey, and Horwood (1996) found that poor parental supervision, lack of knowledge about sexual abuse risk factors, and child exposure to risky social environments increased odds of sexual abuse.

In line with intergenerational theories of child abuse, maternal history of childhood sexual abuse has been linked with increased risk of problematic parenting, child adjustment problems, and risk of sexual abuse and other forms of child maltreatment. Parenting issues are apparent even during pregnancy. Smith, Poschman, Cavaleri, Howell, and Yonkers (2006) reported greater alcohol use during pregnancy among women with posttraumatic stress disorder (PTSD); although the sample experienced different forms of traumas, CSA was the most commonly identified trauma. A number of studies have found that mothers with sexual abuse histories tend to lack confidence and competence in their parenting skills and abilities (Banyard, 1997; DiLillo & Damashek, 2003; Ruscio, 2001; Zuravin & Fontanella, 1999). Maternal mental health, particularly PTSD and depression, along with low levels of maternal social support and high levels of stress, appear to mediate the links between maternal CSA history and their children's adjustment problems, including both internalizing and externalizing behavior problems and child

social competence (Banyard, Williams, & Siegel, 2003; Koverola et al., 2005; Pianta et al., 1989; Wright, Fopma-Loy, & Fischer, 2005). In their national survey of children and adolescents, Finkelhor and colleagues (1997) found that parents with a history of childhood sexual victimization were 10 times more likely to have a child who experienced sexual abuse compared to parents without such a history. Zuravin and Fontanella (1999) also found that adolescent mothers with a sexual abuse history, compared to other adolescent mothers, were more likely to neglect their children.

Community/Social Risk Factors

Studies that have examined race, culture, and ethnicity as risk factors for sexual abuse have been inconclusive (Kenny & McEachern, 2000). However, there is some evidence that sexual abuse is more common among lower SES families (Costello, Erkanli, Fairbank, & Angold, 2002; Finkelhor et al., 1997; Sedlak, 1997; Manion et al., 1996). Living in high-risk communities also appears to increase CSA risk. Drake and Pandey (1996) found that communities with higher percentages of families in poverty (> 41%) had significantly higher rates of child sexual victimization compared to other communities. As well, Boney-McCoy and Finkelhor (1995) found that children from dangerous communities were at increased risk for child sexual victimization (odds ratio [OR] = 1.5) compared to other communities.

Postdisclosure Stressors

Who Discloses Abuse?

Despite widespread efforts to encourage early disclosure (Finkelhor & Dziuba-Leatherman, 1995; Wurtele, 2002), 50–70% of children and adolescent sexual abuse victims do not disclose their abuse to anyone during childhood (Arata, 1998; Finkelhor, 1990; Usher & Dewberry, 1995). As noted earlier, even fewer cases are reported to official agencies (Arata, 1998; Fergusson, Lynskey, & Horwood, 1996; Hanson et al., 2003; Smith et al., 2000; Usher & Dewberry, 1995). Among those who disclose their abuse during childhood, less than 33% disclose shortly after the incident (Arata, 1998; Smith et al., 2000) and another 33% within 6 months (Smith et al., 2000), with 42% disclosing within 1 year (Finkelhor, 1990). For those who disclose during childhood, delays average at least 1.5 to 3.0 years (Goodman et al., 1992; Henry, 1997; Oxman-Martinez, Rowe, Straka, & Thibault, 1997; Sas, Cunningham, Hurley, Dick, & Farnsworth, 1995).

Failure to disclose and delays in disclosure pose serious problems for victims and society. The most serious outcome of delayed disclosure is the risk of further abuse. Sas and colleagues (1995) reported that among those who did not immediately report their abuse, 44% were abused again by the same perpetrator. Failure to disclose also places other children at risk, because many offenders have multiple victims, including incestuous offenders (Abel, Becker, Cunningham-Rathner, Mittelman, & Rouleau, 1988). Delays in disclosure diminish prospects for prosecution when the abuse is eventually disclosed (Goodman-Brown, Edelstein, Goodman, Jones, & Gordon, 2003; Myers, 1992). As well, disclosures delayed by 1 month or more are associated with increased risk of developing PTSD and major depressive disorder (MDD) (Ruggiero et al., 2003), and delay access to mental health services that can address early-onset symptoms.

Children's decisions to disclose sexual abuse should be viewed within a developmental framework, influenced by issues relevant to the abuse itself, the perpetrator, the family, and personal characteristics of the child. Older children are more likely to disclose their abuse in a planned and purposeful way (Mian, Wehrspann, Klajner-Diamond, LeBaron, & Winder, 1986), whereas younger children are often prompted to disclose after an adult suspects abuse, often due to inappropriate sexualized behaviors, changes in personality, detection of a sexually transmitted disease, or learns that a child spent time with someone suspected of abusing others (Kelley, Brant, & Waterman, 1993; Sorenson & Snow, 1991). Even after an initial disclosure, young children are less likely than older children to disclose in the context of formal investigations (DiPietro, Runyan, & Frederick, 1997), though additional interviews may aid the disclosure process (Gries, Goh, & Cavanaugh, 1996). School-age children tend to confide their abuse experiences to a parent or primary caregiver (Arata, 1998; Lamb & Edgar-Smith, 1994), but adolescents are more likely to confide in a peer (Everill & Waller, 1995; Henry, 1997; Kellogg & Huston, 1995; Lamb & Edgar-Smith, 1994).

There are many reasons why children avoid disclosure; they may fear retaliation from the perpetrator or others, may wish to avoid the stigma and family turmoil that might ensue, or may worry that they will be blamed or punished. Unfortunately, these fears are often justified, in that disclosures are often met with disbelief, do not lead to protection, and result in significant family upheaval and victim blaming (Sauzier, 1989; Sorenson & Snow, 1991). Although children sometimes deny abuse even when faced with compelling evidence (DiPietro et al., 1997; Lawson & Chaffin, 1994), in cases with strong corroborating evidence, 84% of children disclose abuse when interviewed or shortly thereafter (London, Bruck, Ceci, & Shuman, 2005). Stressors associated with disclosure increase the possibility of recantation, including disbelief by mothers (Elliott & Briere, 1994) and court proceedings (Gonzalez, Waterman, Kelly, McCord, & Oliveri, 1993). As well, abuse-related PTSD avoidance symptoms may serve as a catalyst to recant abuse allegations, particularly when children are faced with situations that require them to remember and talk about what happened (Gonzalez et al., 1993; Koverola & Foy, 1993).

Several additional predictors of disclosure in childhood have been identified. Boys are less likely to disclose their sexual abuse than girls (Hanson et al., 2002; Lynch, Stern, Oates, & O'Toole, 1993; Stroud, Martens, & Barker, 2000; Violatao & Genius, 1993), in part due to the stigmatization of male-perpetrated abuse, and also because some boys may not define sexual acts by older girls or women as abuse (Hecht & Hansen, 1999). Disclosures are more common when the perpetrator is a stranger rather than a family member (Hanson et al., 2003; Smith et al., 2000), and delays in disclosure tend to be longer for intrafamilial than for extrafamilial abuse (Sas et al., 1995; Usher & Dewberry, 1995). Despite higher prevalence of sexual abuse among children with disabilities, disclosure rates are disproportionately small, and disclosures are often not reported to child protective service agencies (Kvam, 2000).

Some victims report that school-based personal safety programs or conversations with their parents influenced their decisions to disclose. Children's motivations also influence disclosure, including need for protection and emotional support, and feelings of anger and desire for revenge (Lamb & Edgar-Smith, 1994; Sas et al., 1995; Sorenson & Snow, 1991). Children who experience severe forms of maltreatment (e.g., sexual penetration), physical coercion, and threats tend to have one of two reactions (Gomes-Schwartz, Horowitz, & Cardarelli, 1990). For some, the severity of the abuse facilitates disclosure, because the children may fear for their lives. However, other children may delay their disclosure until they feel safe from retribution. Paine and Hansen (2002) reported that delays in disclosure were twice as lengthy when perpetrators were violent with either the children themselves or with members of their families. Kogan (2004) found that children were most likely to delay disclosures when family members had been threatened.

The Justice System for Juvenile Victims

INVESTIGATIONS

Finkelhor, Cross, and Cantor (2005) coined the term "justice system for juvenile victims" in reference to the complex set of agencies and institutions that serve child victims and their families, which includes police, prosecutors, child protection agencies, mental health services, and criminal, civil, and family courts. Collaboration among professionals and agencies facilitates thorough investigations, protects children from unnecessarily redundant interviews, and helps to ensure child safety. Among the system-induced stressors associated with children's disclosures, having to endure multiple investigative interviews by various interviewers with different agencies has repeatedly been demonstrated to have negative effects on children (Berliner & Conte, 1995; Goodman et al., 1992; Henry, 1997). To avoid the problems associated with multiple interviews and to encourage interagency cooperation, many communities conduct joint police–child protective service investigations, whereas other communities pool resources to create child abuse multidisciplinary teams. Some multidisciplinary teams have a designated workspace such as a child advocacy center (CAC) or a child abuse assessment center (CAAC), whereas others meet informally to plan investigation strategies and review evidence. The National Child Advocacy Center in Huntsville, Alabama, serves as a prototype for multiagency cooperation. It provides office space for professionals involved in investigations and treatment, comfortable interviewing rooms for children, and a Court Prep Group (Pence & Wilson, 1994; Whitcomb, 2003). There are now at least 724 such centers in all 50 states and the District of Columbia (National Children's Alliance, 2006). Programs typically have multidisciplinary teams and case review procedures that include law enforcement, child protective services, prosecutors, health care, mental health care, and victim advocates. Most have trained interviewers on site and provide ongoing staff training. Emerging evidence indicates that these programs are rated more positively by children, and require fewer child interviews by fewer interviewers in fewer locations (Saywitz, Goodman, & Lyon, 2002). Multidisciplinary teams also tend to facilitate access to investigative and treatment services, enhance the efficacy of court-related decision making and substantiation of allegations, promote more confessions and guilty pleas by perpetrators, and increase criminal charges and conviction rates (Joa & Edelson, 2004; Smith, Witte, & Fricker-Elhai, 2006).

In the United States, approximately 30% of reported maltreatment cases are substantiated, with 12% of those involving sexual abuse (Golden, 2000). From the Canadian Incidence Study, which surveyed child protective service agencies across Canada, 38% of sexual abuse allegations were substantiated, 20% were suspected (evidence that allegations are true, but insufficient to substantiate), 36% were unsubstantiated, and 6% were considered intentionally false (Trocmé & Bala, 2005). These findings are similar to earlier studies that found that half of allegations tend to be substantiated or suspected (Everson & Boat, 1989; Jones & McGraw, 1987). Studies indicate that only about 2.5% of allegations are deliberately false (Oates et al., 2000; Trocmé, McPhee, & Tam, 1995). The Canadian Incidence Study found that false reports of sexual abuse by children were very rare (none were identified); otherwise, false reports tended to come from custodial parents (19%), noncustodial parents (16%), relatives, neighbors, and acquaintances (14%), and anonymous reporters (16%). When maltreatment allegations were made in the context of custody and access allegations, 12% of allegations were deemed false, mostly by anonymous reports and noncustodial fathers. However, evidence suggests that only a small percentage (0.3%) of custody and access disputes involve allegations of sexual abuse (Thoennes & Tjaden, 1990; Trocmé & Bala, 2005).

CRIMINAL PROSECUTION AND COURTROOM TESTIMONY

Compared to other forms of maltreatment, sexual abuse is more likely to result in criminal charges (Sedlak et al., 2005), and sexual abuse cases are the most common type of trial that involves child witnesses (Goodman, Quas, Bulkley, & Shapiro, 1999). However, only about half of substantiated cases of sexual abuse result in criminal charges, and up to half of those are dropped or dismissed following preliminary hearings (Cross, Whitcomb, & De Vos, 1995; Martone, Jaudes, & Cavins, 1996; Stroud et al., 2000). Cases that involve latency-age female victims, older male perpetrators, and multiple victims are more likely to be prosecuted. On the other hand, prosecution is less likely when a child is preschool age or male, when the mother does not support prosecution, and when the accused individual is a family member (Cross, De Vos, & Whitcomb, 1994; Cross et al., 1995; Stroud et al., 2000).

Of those cases that remain viable following preliminary hearings, most take at least 1 year to resolve. To address the problem of excessive delays, 12 states and the District of Columbia have statutes mandating speedy trials that involve children as victims and/or witnesses (American Prosecutors Research Institute, National District Attorneys Association, 2007). On the whole, cases slated for trial are successful for the prosecution. Fifty to 85% of defendants plead guilty prior to trail, and of the small number of cases proceeding to trial, roughly 67% result in guilty verdicts (Cross et al., 1995; DeJong & Rose, 1991; Faller & Henry, 2000; Martone et al., 1996; Stroud et al., 2000). Sentencing varies considerably across jurisdictions. For example, Stroud and colleagues (2000) reported that convicted perpetrators (guilty pleas and guilty verdicts) averaged 11-year jail terms, but most sentences were suspended. Parole sentences averaged just less than 4 years. On the other hand, Martone and colleagues (1996) found that most perpetrators served time, with average sentences of 6.8 years. Cross and colleagues (1995) reported that 38% were incarcerated more than 1 year, 40% were incarcerated less than 1 year, and 22% were placed on probation.

Approximately 50% of cases referred for prosecution require that children testify at some legal proceeding, such as a preliminary hearing (Goodman et al., 1992); if cases proceed to trial, at least 80% of child victims testify (Cross et al., 1995). However, because of the small number of cases that proceed to trial, this accounts for only 1–4% of sexually abused children known to official agencies (Saunders, Kilpatrick, Resnick, Hanson, & Lipovsky, 1992; Stroud et al., 2000). Most children find testifying in court to be very stressful (Lipovsky, Tidwell, Kilpatrick, Saunders, & Dawson, 1991; Sas et al., 1995). Prior to testifying, children identify a number of fears, including fears of the testimony itself, of the defense attorney, and of seeing the defendant; after testifying, children report that the most distressing aspects were seeing the defendant and not having their parents in the courtroom (Goodman et al., 1992). Children also fear that the defendant will retaliate and that they will not be believed.

INVOLVEMENT WITH CHILD PROTECTIVE SERVICES

Child protective services (CPS) tend to limit their continued involvement to cases in which parents or caregivers are implicated in the abuse, or when concerns are raised that parents cannot protect the children from further harm by the perpetrators or other potential offenders. In most cases, CPS monitor "at-risk" children in their home through voluntary agreements or through court-imposed supervision orders. However, approximately 17% of sexually abused children go into foster care (Finkelhor, 1983), often because of concerns about the mother's ability to protect the child from further abuse (Ryan, Warren, & Weincek, 1991). Indeed, sexually abused children who go into foster care are more likely to come from low-SES families, to have experienced multiple abuse episodes, and to have mothers who did not support their allegations (Hunter, Coulter, Runyan, & Everson, 1990; Leifer, Shapiro, & Kassem, 1993). Placement outside the home following sexual abuse allegations is associated with greater mental health concerns, particularly when children experience multiple placements (Gomes-Schwartz et al., 1990; Melton et al., 1995); however, because of the close connection between foster placement, poor maternal support, and preexisting behavioral and emotional problems, it is difficult to determine whether foster placement has an additive effect on adjustment problems. Compared to other reasons for foster placement (e.g., neglect, physical abuse), sexually abused children tend to remain in foster care for shorter durations (approximately 8 months shorter; Lie & McMurtry, 1991). Thus, because reintegration with families is highly likely for CSA victims in foster care, efforts to resolve family problems and facilitate successful reunification are very important.

Family Reactions

FAMILY SUPPORT REGARDING ABUSE ALLEGATIONS

Drawing from the Adolescent Health Survey, Chandy, Blum, and Resnick (1997) found that one of the strongest predictors of resilience subsequent to sexual abuse was children's perception that their parents cared about them. Although maternal support has received considerable attention, supportive reactions from other family members have also been identified as a resilience factor (Garbarino, Dubrowi, Kostelney, & Pardo, 1992). Several studies have investigated mothers' reactions to their children's abuse allegations. Gomes-Schwartz and colleagues (1990) described four types of maternal responses: (1) a decisive, nonambiguous, protective response, with responsibility attributed to the accused; (2) ambivalent loyalties between child and perpetrator, requiring support from CPS to ensure adequate protection; (3) an immobilization response, resulting in a failure to protect the child, but moderate support and no overt blame of the child; and (4) rejection of the child, alignment with the perpetrator, and no child protective action. However, Elliott and Carnes (2001) note that maternal reactions of belief and support tend to be fluid and change over time with different circumstances. Nonetheless, evidence suggests that parental support and protection subsequent to abuse allegations are a function of the quality of the preexisting parent–child bond (Bolen & Lamb, 2002). Although most mothers are decisive, supportive, and protective in response to their children's allegations, 16–50% of mothers do not support their children's allegations (Pierce & Pierce, 1985; Sas et al., 1995; Tufts New England Medical Center, 1984). Belief in a child's allegations does not

necessarily result in protective action, however. Pintello and Zuravin (2001) found that, on the one hand, 20% of mothers who believed their children's allegations failed to take protective actions. On the other hand, they also found that 52% of mothers who were ambivalent about their children's allegations nonetheless took protective action. Although one might anticipate that previous involvement with CPS might sensitize parents to concerns about abuse and neglect, this does not appear to be the case. Previous involvement with CPS has been found to have either no relationship to parental belief and protection (Pintello & Zuravin, 2001) or a negative relationship (Bolen & Lamb, 2002).

The more seriously the abuse allegations affect a mother's lifestyle and sense of self, the less likely the mother is to believe the allegations (Elliott & Briere, 1994; Gomes-Schwartz et al., 1990; Lawson & Chaffin, 1992; Sirles & Franke, 1989). Mothers tend to have more difficulty believing allegations against their current partners, particularly when allegations are against stepfathers and common-law partners with whom the mother has either a new, intense, or financially reliant relationship (Elliott & Briere, 1994; Everson, Hunter, Runyan, Edelsohn, & Coutler, 1989; Faller, 1984; Gomes-Schwartz et al., 1990; Leifer, Kilbane, & Grossman, 2001). Alaggia and Turon (2005) examined the impact of spousal abuse on responses to child sexual abuse allegations. Interestingly, mothers who were abused in nonphysical, psychological, or emotional ways were less supportive of their child's sexual abuse allegations compared to those who experienced physical spousal violence. When mothers are faced with the difficult choice between their spouses and their children, approximately one-fourth of them opt to stay with their spouses (Everson et al., 1989; Gomes-Schwartz et al., 1990). In contrast, mothers are often quite supportive when allegations occur in the midst of preexisting spousal problems or when the spouses have already separated (Faller, 1984; Sirles & Franke, 1989).

Mothers are also less likely to believe their children's allegations when alternative explanations are available (Sirles & Franke, 1989). Young children are perceived as having little sexual knowledge and little motive for making false allegations, and are therefore most often believed. As children grow older, allegations are less likely to be believed, particularly when the allegations include very serious forms of abuse or when a child's story indicates that the mother was home when the abuse occurred. Sadly, children with unsupportive mothers tend to suffer more episodes of abuse and are ultimately more likely to recant their allegations (Elliott & Briere, 1994; Leifer et al., 1993). Mothers also tend to have more difficulty believing their children when their partners have substance use problems or when their partners also physically abuse the children. Apparently, in these circumstances, mothers are more likely to find a reason for the children to lie about the abuse (e.g., retaliation for the physical abuse), or are more accustomed to making excuses for the partners' inappropriate behavior (Elliott & Briere, 1994).

ONGOING CONTACT WITH THE OFFENDER AFTER ABUSE ALLEGATIONS

In paternal and sibling abuse cases, many children continue to have contact with their incestuous relative following disclosure, although this contact is usually supervised by a CPS agency, a supervised access program, or a family member (Hamilton, 1997). Supervised access with an incestuous relative can serve several positive functions (Straus, 1995): It can (1) help the child gain a realistic assessment of the person and their relationship; (2) serve as a stepping-stone to less restricted access; and (3) allow the child to maintain a relationship with the family member in a safe situation. On the negative side, a child may fear this relative, and visits may stimulate PTSD symptoms. When legal proceedings are in progress, a child's access may introduce divided loyalties between wanting to please the perpetrator and following through with prosecution. Tebbutt, Swanston, Oates, and O'Toole (1997), in their longitudinal study of abuse-related sequelae, found that contact between intrafamilial perpetrators and victims between the 18-month and the 5-year follow-up period was predictive of long-term depressive symptoms. In an exploratory study, Hamilton (1997) reviewed 40 CPS files to examine factors associated with father–child access and with positive adjustment to access. Access supervisors were more likely to note positive adjustment to access when the father (1) had admitted to the abuse, (2) emotionally supported the child, (3) abided by supervision rules, (4) was highly involved in treatment services, and (5) demonstrated positive parenting behaviors during access visits.

IMPACT OF ABUSE ALLEGATIONS ON MATERNAL MENTAL HEALTH

Mothers of sexual abuse victims tend to have relatively high rates of psychopathology. As noted earlier, in some cases the mothers may have had mental health problems prior to their child's sexual abuse; however, for many, their child's disclosure of sexual abuse can lead to great psychological distress, increasing the odds of mothers' developing their own posttraumatic stress symptoms and/or depression (Davies, 1995; Deblinger, Hathaway, Lippman, & Steer, 1993; Elliott & Carnes, 2001; Hooper, 1992; Manion et al., 1996). In many cases, mothers of sexual abuse victims are victims of domestic violence by the same offender (Bowen, 2000; Kellogg & Menard, 2003). In addition to concerns about their child's well-being, many mothers often feel guilt and self-blame after learning about their child's sexual abuse. As well, the aftermath of the disclosure can lead to serious financial, occupational, and residential setbacks (Hooper, 1992; Massat & Lundy, 1998). Parental psychopathology tends to interfere with parenting in general, and may interfere with caregivers' ability to provide the nurturance needed to support children following sexual abuse (Kelly, Faust, Runyon, & Kenny, 2002). Indeed, the level of distress shown by sexually abused children often mirrors their parents' level of distress (Avery, Massat, & Marta, 1998; Lipton, 1997; Newberger, Gremy, Waternaux, & Newberger, 1993). Research indicates that depressed mothers tend to be less responsive and more helpless, hostile, critical, disorganized, and inconsistent in their parenting compared to nondepressed mothers (Gelfand & Teti, 1990; Goodman, 1992). Parental depression increases the odds of a number of child mental health problems, including depression, anxiety, somatic complaints, and behavior problems (Downey & Coyne, 1990; Gelfand & Teti, 1990). Depressed mothers of sexual abuse victims, compared to nondepressed mothers of sexual abuse victims, are more likely to describe their children as having externalizing behavior problems, attentional problems, and as being immature and showing extreme forms of pathology, such as delusions and hallucinations (Kelly et al., 2002).

To complicate matters, mothers of sexually abused children often have their own history of childhood sexual abuse and/or other forms of maltreatment (Collin-Vézina & Cyr, 2003). Preliminary evidence indicates mothers who experienced childhood maltreatment find parenting more stressful, report less effective parenting styles, find parenting less rewarding, and report less spousal support than mothers without abuse histories (Cole, Woolger, Power, & Smith, 1992; DeOliveira, Bailey, Wolfe, & Evans, 2006; DiLillo & Damashek, 2003; Douglas, 2000; Fitzgerald, Shipman, Jackson, McMahon, & Hanley, 2005; Ruscio, 2001). Although the literature is quite underdeveloped at this point, different types of childhood maltreatment appear to have different effects on subsequent parenting. Lyons-Ruth and Block (1996), in one of the few studies to examine the impact of childhood maltreatment on parenting behaviors, found that a history of physical abuse was associated with mothers' increased hostile–intrusive behavior toward their infants, whereas a history of sexual abuse was associated with decreased involvement and restricted maternal affect. Mental health issues such as depression, dissociative tendencies, and avoidant coping likely mediate the relationship between maternal history of childhood maltreatment and parenting outcomes (Banyard et al., 2003; Koverola et al., 2005; Schuetz & Eiden, 2005; Wright et al., 2005). DeOliveira et al. (2006) found that maternal history of maltreatment affected parenting in different ways based on the child's gender. Mothers with trauma-related intrusive symptoms were less likely to engage in emotion-focused dialogues with their sons, whereas mothers who experienced either emotional neglect or physical abuse showed more hostility in their interactions with girls.

Implications of Epidemiological Findings on Clinical Assessment

Epidemiological findings provide an important framework for identifying the types of background and contextual information relevant to clinical assessment. Most importantly, however, extant epidemiological data highlight the broad extent of CSA and other life adversities, and relatively low rates of disclosures. Although considerable attention has been given to false CSA reports, underreporting of CSA is more common and its detection is essential for proper diagnosis and treatment. Thus, all clinicians working with children and youth, not just those who specialize in CSA and childhood trauma, should be mindful that many children who are identified for mental health service have undisclosed histories of CSA and life adversities. Underreporting of CSA is most common among males, children with disabilities, and children who perceive either negative or ineffectual consequences to their disclosures. Adolescents tend to disclose to their peers rather than to adults. In many cases, CSA is reported to caregivers, but caregivers do not inform official agencies. At the very least, it is important to screen for known histories of CSA, other forms of maltreatment, and other negative life events and adversities, through CPS records and/or caregiver reports. Consideration should also be given to routinely asking children about maltreatment experiences. Recent large-scale surveys with children and youth have demonstrated the feasibility of collecting such information from children. Research demonstrates that most children do not disclose CSA unless prompted, so well planned, nonsuggestive interviews can provide a catalyst for disclosures that might not otherwise occur.

When screening for CSA, clinicians need to discard some common myths. Although most consider sexual abuse to be perpetrated by adults, particularly parents and caregivers, abuse by siblings, older youth, and peers is quite common. For disabled youth, attention should be paid to institutional caregivers and to whether institutional policies are in place to protect and monitor children. The way questions are asked about history of CSA is also important. Simply asking about CSA may not be sufficient, because some children and parents may have a limited understanding of what CSA includes. Thus, more detailed questions without reference to "abuse" likely prompt more accurate information.

Epidemiological studies have also revealed the sad fact that for many CSA victims, *when it rains, it pours.* CSA often occurs in the midst of dysfunctional and inadequate caregiving that falls short in monitoring and protecting children, lacks the emotional sensitivity needed to detect child problems, and fails to nurture adequate communication needed to promote early disclosures. CSA victims often experience other forms of childhood maltreatment, witness domestic violence, live in violent and impoverished communities, and experience other life adversities. They are also at increased risk of subsequent sexual victimization during their childhood, adolescence, and adult years. Thus, in addition to documenting CSA and other adversities, it is important to obtain historical and current information about parenting, with the goal of identifying past and current risk factors. Given the high risk of revictimization, assessment strategies must identify current child, family, and community risks risk factors.

Disclosure of CSA exposes children and youth to a host of family and system stressors. Family reactions to the disclosure are among the most potent predictors of child adjustment subsequent to CSA. Caretakers' inability to provide protection from further maltreatment leads to children's placement outside of the home with relatives or in foster or group homes. Alternative care can be stressful for youth, who may perceive these protective actions as punishment for their disclosure. Even when in alternate care, most youth continue to have contact with their families, and in some cases have ongoing contact with the accused. Furthermore, most CSA victims in CPS care eventually return home. In many cases, CSA leads to a number of criminal and child protection legal proceedings. Although most children do not testify in criminal or child welfare proceedings, those who do often find the experience very stressful. Even when the child is not directly involve in the process, criminal and child protection legal proceedings create stress for those involved in the child's care, which is often communicated to the child. Thus, the assessment process should include an examination of how family, alternative care, and system stressors have affected the child, and how the family, child, and system adapt to these stressors.

IMPACT OF SEXUAL ABUSE ON CHILD VICTIMS

Sexual abuse is not a disorder with a clearly delineated list of symptoms. Rather, sexual abuse is best considered a negative life event that poses significant risk for the development of a broad spectrum of behavioral and emotional problems. Because of the magnitude of problems that often result from sexual abuse, and because of the associated familial and social contexts, sexual abuse has the potential to affect a number of developmental processes negatively, setting the stage for a lifetime of sequelae. In some cases, the sexual abuse was a defining event that led to abuse-related mental health concerns. However, many sexual abuse victims had behavioral, emotional, and developmental problems before the abuse occurred, or live within familial and/or community contexts that likely would have led to mental health problems even if the sexual abuse had not occurred. Thus, evaluating the impact of sexual abuse per se can be quite complex, particularly given developmental issues that affect manifestation of symptoms for preschoolers, latency-age children, and adolescents.

For the purposes of this chapter, sexual abuse effects are conceptualized at three levels. *Abuse-specific* symptoms are specifically linked with sexual abuse experiences, characterize a significant proportion of sexual abuse victims, and differentiate between sexual abuse victims and their nonabused peers, and other clinic-referred children. *Abuse-related* symptoms are linked with the sexual abuse experience, characterize a significant proportion of sexual abuse victims, and differentiate between sexual abuse victims and their nonabused peers, but either do not differentiate between sexual abuse victims and other, clinic-referred children or are likely not caused by the sexual abuse, but rather by individual, family, and community risk factors associated with sexual abuse (e.g., family dysfunction, increased negative affect). *Pathological changes in psychological processes* refer to changes resulting from exposure to sexual abuse that have implications for adjustment problems in general, such as changes in affect regulation ability, cognitive style, or coping reactions.

In the past, it was difficult to assess the impact of sexual abuse during childhood and adolescence due to ethical and methodological difficulties associated with surveying large populations of children and adolescents on the topic. As a result, up until the past decade, most studies that investigated the impact of CSA on children and adolescents relied upon assessment of sexual abuse victims identified through CPS agencies or clinical services, and were thus based on small, nonrepresentative samples. Several large-scale representative surveys of children and adolescents that are now available provide evidence of the impact of sexual abuse in the general population of children, particularly for those 10 years of age and older. These include the National Youth Victimization Prevention Study (*n* = 2,000; Boney-McCoy & Finkelhor, 1996), the Developmental Victimization Survey (*n* = 2,030; Turner, Finkelhor, & Ormrod, 2006); the National Survey of Adolescents (*n* = 4,023; Danielson, de Arellano, Kilpatrick, Saunders, & Resnick, 2005; Kilpatrick et al., 2003), the Youth Risk Behavior Survey (*n* = 13,601; Howard & Wang, 2005), and a large survey of U.S. high school students in the Midwest (*n* = 17,465; Luster, Small, & Lower, 2002). As well, several large-scale longitudinal studies have surveyed children and adolescents over time and linked mental health adjustment with history of sexual abuse and other forms of maltreatment. These include a New Zealand high school sample (*n* = 1,019; Fergusson, Horwood, & Lynsky, 1996), a South Carolina high school sample (*n* = 3,283; Cuffe et al., 1998), and a New York sample followed from age 5 through adulthood (*n* = 776; Brown, Cohen, Johnson, & Smailes, 1999). One additional study surveyed a large, multisite sample of clinic-referred children and adolescents (*n* = 3,479; Walrath et al., 2003).

Abuse-Specific Symptoms

Posttraumatic Stress Disorder

The literature on posttraumatic stress disorder (PTSD) (see Fletcher, Chapter 9, this volume) provides an important research and clinical framework for conceptualizing sexual abuse sequelae. The fourth, text revision edition of the *Diagnostic and Statistical Manual of Mental Disorders* (DSM-IV-TR; American Psychiatric Association [APA], 2000) supports consideration of PTSD as a possible diagnosis for CSA victims; in fact, in defining trauma, it includes "developmentally inappropriate sexual experiences with or without threatened or actual violence or injury" (p. 464). A diagnosis of PTSD requires four conditions: (1) experience of an event posing serious threat, to which the individual responds with great helplessness, fear, or horror (criteria A1 and A2, respectively); (2) three sets of symptoms—reexperiencing aspects of the trauma (criterion B), avoidance strategies that serve as a means to escape from trauma-related stimuli (criterion C), and increased autonomic arousal (criterion D); (3) duration of symptoms for at least a 1-month period beyond the initial 3-month

posttrauma period (criterion E); and (4) significant interference with the ability to function effectively at home, with friends, and/or at work or school (criterion F). DSM-IV-TR notes that young children may differ from older children and adults in the manifestation of PTSD symptoms. Young children may express intrusive thoughts through thematic, repetitive play. They may complain of frightening dreams but be unable to describe or recognize the content as trauma-related. Finally, rather than describing flashbacks, young children may reenact their trauma through play or art (APA, 2000).

In a prevalence study with a community sample of older adolescents, experiencing rape or CSA increased the odds of developing PTSD by 49% (Cuffe et al., 1998). Several additional studies with large, representative samples of older children and adolescents have also demonstrated relatively high levels of PTSD symptoms among sexually abused boys and girls compared to their nonabused peers (Bal, Van Oost, de Bourdeaudhuij, & Crombez, 2003; Boney-McCoy & Finkelhor, 1995, 1996; Danielson et al., 2005; Kilpatrick et al., 2003). Other studies of identified sexual abuse victims indicate that between 36 and 60% meet diagnostic criteria for PTSD (Bal, de Bourdeaudhuij, Crombez, & van Oost, 2004; Dubner & Motta, 1999; Kendall-Tackett, Williams, & Finkelhor, 1993; McLeer et al., 1998; Wolfe & Birt, 2005a; Wolfe, Sas, & Wekerle, 1994). Research with clinical and CPS samples have demonstrated relatively high rates of PTSD compared to nonabused controls via a number of assessment strategies, including parent reports (e.g., Wells, McCann, Adams, Voris, & Ensign, 1995); child reports (e.g., Dubner & Motta, 1999; Friedrich, Jaworski, Hexschl, & Bengston, 1997; Wolfe & Birt, 2005a), social worker checklists (e.g., Mennen & Meadow, 1993), chart reviews (e.g., Kiser, Heston, Millsap, & Pruitt, 1991), and diagnostic interviews (e.g., McLeer, Deblinger, Henry, & Orvaschel, 1992; McLeer et al., 1998). Compared with other negative life events in childhood and adolescence, such as serious accidents, natural and man-made disasters, and even physical abuse, sexual abuse is particularly potent in provoking PTSD symptomatology (Bal, Crombez, Van Oost, & Debourdeaudhuij, 2003; Bal et al., 2003; Boney-McCoy & Finkelhor, 1996; Cuffe et al., 1998; Dubner & Motta, 1999). Despite relatively high rates of negative life events among clinic-referred children, PTSD is more prevalent among CSA victims than among other clinic-referred children and adolescents (McLeer et al., 1998; Wolfe & Birt, 2005a) and as compared to those who experience other types of maltreatment (Runyon & Kenny, 2002). Even when prior mental health and quality of parent–child relationships were controlled, Boney-McCoy and Finkelhor (1996) found that sexually abused youth reported more PTSD symptoms than their nonabused peers, revealing a medium effect size.

A number of factors have been related to the development of PTSD among sexually abused children and adolescents. Younger children and girls appear to be at increased risk of developing PTSD subsequent to sexual abuse (Dubner & Motta, 1999; Feiring, Taska, & Lewis, 1999, 2002; Kaplow, Dodge, Amaya-Jackson, & Saxe, 2005; Wolfe & Birt, 2005a; Wolfe, Gentile, & Wolfe, 1989). Young children may have limited ability to cope effectively with stressors and may be more negatively affected than older youth by sexually abusive acts, the aftermath of disclosure, and involvement in the legal system (Quas et al., 2005). Because of developmental issues, young children may experience more system-induced stressors associated with abuse verification, pretestimony interviews, and court-related adverse experiences, such as continuances, lack of corroborative evidence, defendant acquittal, case being dropped, and having to testify repeatedly (Quas et al., 2005).

Surprisingly, despite considerable variability in individual experiences considered under the umbrella of sexual abuse, most studies have found that these variations add little to the prediction of PTSD symptoms (e.g., Bal et al., 2004, 2005; Feiring, Taska, & Lewis, 2002; Kaplow et al., 2005; Naar-King, Silvern, Ryan, & Sebring, 2002; Spaccarelli, 1995; Wolfe & Birt, 2005a). Indeed, although some studies have identified some aspects of sexual abuse as predictors of PTSD (e.g., age at onset, sexual abuse frequency and duration, and relationship to perpetrator; Ruggiero, McLeer, & Dixon, 2000), no single abuse characteristic, or set of characteristics, has shown a consistent pattern of predicting PTSD across studies. Instead, experiencing other negative life events appears to increase the risk of developing PTSD subsequent to sexual abuse (Cuffe et al., 1998). This is particularly true for youth who experience both sexual and physical abuse (Kiser et al.,

1991; Wolfe & Birt, 2005a). As noted earlier, multiple forms of maltreatment are indicative of serious family dysfunction (Fleming et al., 1999). Indeed, experiencing both sexual and physical abuse has been linked with family alcohol and other problems, and more severe forms of abuse (Stevens et al., 2005).

Goodman and colleagues (1992) and Quas and colleagues (2005), studying a large sample of sexually abused children slated for courtroom testimony, found that the strongest predictor of PTSD-related symptoms in both the short run (subsequent to disclosure and legal proceedings) and the long run (on average 10 years later) was testifying in multiple court proceedings, particularly when victims had to testify repeatedly about very serious forms of sexual abuse. In addition, testifying only once and waiting in court to testify (but not actually testifying) were also associated with long-term PTSD symptoms. Quas and colleagues speculated that such events are not only traumatic but also promote self-perceptions of being a victim. Not testifying in court can be detrimental as well, particularly when offenders do not plead guilty or when they receive a lenient sentence, leading to perceptions that the legal system is unfair.

One reason that abuse-specific factors do not add to the prediction of PTSD may be that even within specific researcher-defined categorizations there may be considerable untapped variation in abuse severity. For example, intrafamilial abuse typically includes abuse by resident father figures, but also often includes family members who have limited contact with the victims (e.g., estranged father figures), and individuals who are not emotionally close with the victim (e.g., nonresident uncle). In some studies the severity of the abuse is captured by penetration, which sometimes includes penile–vaginal penetration, as well as fellatio and digital penetration. However, even fine gradations of trauma dimensions do not necessarily enhance the predictive power of abuse variables (Spaccarelli, 1995; Wolfe & Birt, 2005a), a finding that is mirrored in research with other types of violence exposure (Jaycox, Marshall, & Orlando, 2003).

It is possible that subjectively reported peritraumatic reactions and retrospective cognitive appraisals more accurately reflect the stress associated with negative life events such as sexual abuse, and are thus more closely linked with the development of PTSD. However, appraisals of events may reflect not only the stressfulness of the trauma but also individual differences in cognitive and coping styles, and trauma-related sequelae. Peritraumatic reactions are the thoughts, emotions, and behaviors experienced at the time of the trauma. DSM-IV-TR PTSD criterion A2 refers to the peritraumatic reactions of feeling great horror, fear, and helplessness at the time of the traumatic event, and dissociative peritraumatic reactions are part of the diagnostic criteria for acute stress disorder. Nonetheless, peritraumatic reactions have generally not been formally assessed until recently, and even when assessed, only a limited range of peritraumatic response options, such as peritraumatic dissociation, has been tapped. For sexual abuse, studies have thus far only assessed peritraumatic reactions retrospectively; as such, recollections of past peritraumatic reactions may be affected by current cognitive style and abuse-related symptomatology. Even so, with nonabusive traumatic events such as vehicle accidents and disasters, evidence suggests that peritraumatic reactions are more potent predictors of PTSD than specific trauma factors (Ehler, Mayou, & Bryant, 2003; Shannon, Lonigan, Finch, & Taylor, 1994; Stallard, Velleman, & Baldwin, 1998). Likewise, Wolfe and Birt (2005b) found that children's retrospective recollections of their peritraumatic reactions to their sexual abuse experiences were more powerful predictors of PTSD than specific abuse characteristics, such as abuse severity, force, frequency, duration, and relationship to the perpetrator. Interestingly, peritraumatic reactions were not predicted by abuse characteristics. Negative cognitive appraisals of stressors can have implications for long-term adjustments. In the Quas and colleagues (2005) 10-year follow-up of child victims–witnesses, emotional reactions to the courtroom experience predicted later PTSD, greater internalizing symptoms, and more negative attitudes toward the legal system.

In addition to event appraisals and peritraumatic reactions, PTSD has been linked with both general and abuse-specific attributions and coping. Two studies have linked general attributional style for negative events with PTSD (Feiring, Taska, & Lewis, 2002; Runyon & Kenny, 2002). Specifically, the risk of developing PTSD has been linked with general tendencies to attribute negative life events to factors that are internal, global, and stable. Abuse-specific attributions of self-blame, guilt,

and shame have also been linked with PTSD (Feiring, Taska, & Chen, 2002; Feiring, Taska, & Lewis, 2002; Negrao, Bonanno, Noll, Putnam, & Trickett, 2005; Spaccarelli & Fuchs, 1997; Wolfe et al., 1994; Wolfe, Gentile, Michienzi, Sas, & Wolfe, 1991). Furthermore, positive changes in abuse-related attributions have been linked with improvements in PTSD symptoms (Feiring, Taska, & Lewis, 2002).

Attributional style may affect adjustment in part by affecting the ways that individuals cope with stressors (Muris, Schmidt, Lambrichs, & Meesters, 2001). Several studies have demonstrated links among sexual abuse trauma, emotional distress, and ineffective coping strategies, such as wishful thinking, inappropriate tension reduction strategies (eating, drinking, drug use, sex), emotion-focused coping, and avoidant coping (Bal, Crombez, et al., 2003; Bal, Van Oost, et al., 2003; Chaffin, Wherry, & Dykman, 1997; Tremblay, Hebert, & Piche, 1999). Furthermore, Bal, Crombez, and colleagues (2003) found that avoidant coping mediated the relationship between sexual abuse and psychological distress. Similar mediating effects have been demonstrated with adult CSA survivors (Merrill, Thomsen, Sinclair, Gold, & Milner, 2001; Runtz & Schallow, 1997). Browne, Cloitre, and Linehan (2002) found that perhaps as a reflection of interpersonal trust issues adolescents in foster care with sexual and/or physical abuse histories were more likely to cope with stressful situations independently (without seeking social support or assistance from others), whereas their nonabused peers in foster care were more likely to seek support from peers.

As noted earlier, family support is one of the strongest predictors of resilience subsequent to sexual abuse (Chandy et al., 1997; Garbarino et al., 1992). For both intrafamilial and extrafamilial abuse, both preabuse and concurrent family functioning, particularly family cohesiveness, have been linked with PTSD symptoms (Bal et al., 2004; Boney-McCoy & Finkelhor, 1995, 1996).

COMPLEX TRAUMA AND COMPLEX OR TYPE II PTSD

Early efforts to conceptualize sexual abuse sequelae as PTSD were criticized for failing to account for the full range of symptoms described for sexually abused children (Finkelhor, 1990) and for adult survivors of abuse (Herman, 1992). Terr (1987) recognized that

CSA differs from many forms of trauma, in that it is often repeated over long periods in secret, thereby requiring victims to adapt to their abusive situation via strategies that are either developmentally or psychologically inappropriate or damaging, particularly when these strategies are generalized beyond the abusive situation. Terr described these adaptations as psychogenic numbing, dissociation, distrust, relationship problems, suicidal ideation, rage, and "unremitting sadness." Terr (1987, 1991) proposed a dual classification for trauma-related disorders: Type I disorders follow exposure to a single traumatic event, whereas Type II disorders result from multiple or long-standing experiences with extreme stress (e.g., sexual abuse). Although patients with both types of PTSD are thought to experience core PTSD symptoms (reexperiencing, avoidance, and hyperarousal), those with Type II PTSD also develop atypical coping patterns and psychological symptoms that eventually become integrated into their personalities. Similar dual conceptualizations of PTSD emerged simultaneously within the adult literature (e.g., Herman, 1992).

Over the years, the term "complex trauma" has been used to describe the experience of multiple, chronic, and prolonged traumatic circumstances, typically within the realm of childhood maltreatment. As such, these events are often interpersonal in nature, begin in early life, and have the potential to disrupt normal developmental pathways (van der Kolk, 2005). The complex and intertwined combination of early life traumas, and emotional maltreatment and neglect, has been linked with multiple adverse outcomes. Indeed, Cook and colleagues (2005) identified seven areas of impairment linked with childhood complex trauma: attachment problems, psychophysiological concerns (e.g., medication problems, somatization), affect regulation, dissociation, and poor behavioral control, cognition, and self-concept. Given the unique characteristics and outcomes of complex trauma, van der Kolk (2005) suggested a new diagnostic classification, developmental trauma disorder.

Nonetheless, the idea of an alternative diagnostic classification requires considerable study. Currently, symptom variations are often treated diagnostically and therapeutically as comorbid conditions; some patients with PTSD have concurrent diagnoses such as MDD, dissociative identity disorder, and/or borderline personality disorder (Shalev, Friedman, Foa, & Keane, 2000). This approach has considerable validity, because several of the common comorbid diagnoses have well developed conceptual underpinnings and empirically supported treatment strategies that inform the study and treatment of trauma effects. Some symptoms identified for developmental trauma disorder may be conceptualized as extreme manifestations of PTSD, and may simply require the addition of refinements to the description of symptom criteria. For example, affect dysregulation and somatization symptoms might be considered part of the PTSD hyperarousal domain, and some dissociative symptoms might be considered extreme manifestations of the avoidance domain. Some symptoms of complex PTSD may be associated with conditions other than trauma, such as dysfunctional family backgrounds and premorbid propensities to cope with life stressors in ineffective ways.

Dissociation

Dissociation is an ephemeral phenomenon that has been difficult to study. Because it is an intrapsychic event that affects one's ability to self-monitor internal states, dissociation is difficult to document by self-report, particularly by children, and only the behavioral manifestations of dissociation are observable by others. In the face of trauma, dissociation can be considered a defensive process that enables a child to avoid mentally the ongoing trauma that he or she cannot avoid physically (Terr, 1991; van der Kolk, van der Hart, & Marmar, 1996). If traumatic events and dissociative reactions occur repeatedly or continuously, dissociation can become a habit-like, unconscious and automatic response triggered by less severe day-to-day stressors, thereby affecting everyday information processing and functioning (Liotti, 1999; Post et al., 1998).

Dissociation is thought to have its roots in early childhood trauma, particularly sexual abuse, physical abuse, and neglect (Briere & Runtz, 1989; Chu & Dill, 1990; Hornstein & Putnam, 1992; Ogawa, Sroufe, Weinfield, Carlson, & Egeland, 1997; Sanders & Giolas, 1991; Yeager & Lewis, 1996). In fact, one meta-analytic study demonstrated a strong relationship between sexual trauma and dissociative symptoms, with an effect size of 0.42 (van IJzendoorn & Schuengel, 1996). Family factors such as parental dissociation and lack of family cohesion appear to contribute to the development of childhood dissociation (Bal et al., 2004; Coons, 1985), perhaps due to psychological unavailability of the parent or because the parent and child experienced simultaneous traumas (e.g., child and spouse abuse). Alternatively, parental dissociation has been linked with increased probability of child maltreatment (Egeland & Sussman-Stillman, 1996). Research into possible genetic contributions are limited, though it is possible that genetic predispositions (e.g., autohypnotic tendencies) define the boundaries of dissociative states available to a particular individual (Putnam, 1997).

Early childhood trauma may set the stage for dissociative disorders because of the extreme vulnerability of young children, who are more likely to experience extreme distress under frightening circumstances, or because young children appear to have innate dissociative abilities that dissipate as more effective coping strategies develop. For instance, Perry, Pollard, Blakley, Baker, and Vigilante (1995) described infantile dissociation as occurring when a caregiver is not available to rescue an infant from a fear-producing situation. If crying fails to summon support, the infant moves from a hyperaroused condition to dissociation, reflecting either a "freeze" or "surrender" response.

The perpetuation and exacerbation of early dissociative processes disrupt normal processes that integrate different aspects of experience, resulting in the three main components of dissociation: memory disturbance, distortion of perceptions, and failure to develop a consistent and integrated sense of "self" and "identity" (Macfie, Cicchetti, & Toth, 2001; Waller, Putnam, & Carlson, 1996; Zayed, Wolfe, & Birt, 2006). Dissociative individuals often experience lapses in memory for personally experienced events, become so engrossed in an intrapsychic activity that awareness of ongoing events and surroundings is lost, and show variations in personality and behavior patterns across time and situation, as well as failure to integrate thoughts, sensations, and feelings associated with experiences. Dissociation is generally considered to fall along a continuum from typical everyday occurrences (e.g., intense thought absorption, lapses in memory when driving) to the most extreme form of dissociation, dissociative identity disorder (Ross & Joshi, 1992). In contrast, Waller and colleagues (1996) proposed that some dissociative symptoms are inherently pathological. Based on taxometric analyses of the Dissociative Experiences Scale with adults (Bernstein & Putnam, 1986), eight items were identified as pathological dissociation: finding oneself in a place and not knowing how one got there; finding new things among one's belongings that cannot be accounted for; feeling as if one is standing next to oneself; not recognizing friends or family members; other people and objects not feeling real; feeling that one's body does not belong to oneself; acting differently in different situations; and hearing voices.

Although the onset is believed to occur in early childhood, dissociative disorders are rarely diagnosed in children, perhaps because our current nosologies are based more on the adult than on the child literature. Indeed, Putnam, Hornstein, and Peterson (1996) noted that young children with dissociative symptoms typically do not meet diagnostic criteria for disorders such as dissociative identify disorder; they are more often given the diagnosis of dissociative disorder not otherwise specified. Children's dissociative symptoms are often attributed to other causes. For instance, trancelike behaviors may be misdiagnosed as truancy, conduct problems, or moodiness (McElroy, 1992). Some dissociative symptoms, such as imaginary friends, may be interpreted as typical (McElroy, 1992). Often dissociation goes undiagnosed, because either symptoms are not evident at the time of assessment (Kluft, 1985) or other diagnoses are given, such as PTSD, MDD, schizophrenia, or borderline personality disorder (Coons, Bowman, & Milstein, 1988). Because children's sense of self evolves and becomes more cohesive with age, the self aspect of dissociation may not be evident until adolescence or young adulthood. Perhaps with the development of more reliable and valid tools for defining and assessing dissociation in children, diagnostic practices will improve as well.

Depression, Learned Helplessness, and Cognitive Style

The most commonly investigated mental health problem subsequent to sexual abuse is depression. Because history of negative life events has long been linked with increased risk of depression (e.g., Ge, Lorenz, Conger, Edler, & Simmons, 1994; Nolen-Hoeksema, Girgus, & Seligman, 1992), it is not surprising that research has demonstrated increased risk of depression for sexual abuse victims. Numerous studies have found higher prevalences of depressive symptoms and mood disorders among sexually abused youth compared to nonabused community controls (Boney-McCoy & Finkelhor, 1996; Brant, King, Olson, Ghaziuddin, & Naylor, 1996; Bryant & Range, 1996; Fergusson, Horwood, & Lynskey, 1996; Garnefski & Diekstra, 1997; Howard & Wang, 2005; Kilpatrick et al., 2003; Kiser et al., 1991; Koverola, Pound, Heger, & Lytle, 1993; Ligiezinska et al., 1996; Luster et al., 2002; Mannarino & Cohen, 1996b; Runyon, Faust, & Orvaschel, 2002). Even after controlling for prior adjustment and parent-child relationship, sexual abuse victims show a four-fold increase in risk for depression subsequent to sexual abuse (Boney-McCoy & Finkelhor, 1996). As well, even when controlling for other types of adversities, including physical abuse, history of sexual abuse is linked with increased risk for depression (Fergusson, Horwood, & Lynskey, 1996; Luster et al., 2002). Indeed, like PTSD, history of child sexual abuse puts individuals at risk for depression more so than other negative life events, including history of neglect and physical abuse (Brown et al., 1999). In their longitudinal study of child sexual abuse victims, Brown and colleagues (1999) reported that one-third of sexual abuse victims met criteria for a depressive disorder in either adolescence or adulthood or both. One-third also had a suicide attempt. ORs for dysthymia and MDD for CSA victims were 9.74 and 3.17, respectively, whereas ORs were 5.71 for suicide attempt and 15.78 for repeated suicide attempts. Furthermore, compared to other clinic-referred youth, CSA victims are more likely to have a diagnosis of depression (Deblinger, McLeer, Atkins, Ralphe, & Foa, 1989; Kolko, Moser, & Weldy, 1988; Walrath et al., 2003).

PTSD subsequent to sexual abuse tends to be comorbid with other disorders, particularly major depressive episodes (Kilpatrick et al., 2003). Having experienced multiple forms of maltreatment increases the odds of having comorbid depression and PTSD. Using data from the National Survey of Adolescents, Danielson and colleagues (2005) found that 11% of depressed youth who had experienced sexual abuse had a comorbid diagnosis of PTSD, whereas among youth who experienced both sexual and physical abuse, comorbidity with PTSD was 34%. Comorbidity of PTSD and depression appears to be particularly common for girls and is characterized by the depressive symptoms of anhedonia, worrying, loneliness, sleep and appetite disturbance, and difficulty making decisions, and by the PTSD symptoms of flashbacks and sleep disturbance (Runyon et al., 2002).

A number of factors have been linked to increased risk of depression among sexually abused youth. Unlike children, adolescents tend to have more depressive symptoms than PTSD symptoms (Feiring, Taska, & Lewis, 2002; Tebbutt et al., 1997). However, as in PTSD, girls show more symptoms of depression than do boys (Danielson et al., 2005; Feiring et al., 1999; Feiring, Taska, & Lewis, 2002; Runyon et al., 2002). A number of abuse-related factors have been linked to increased risk of depression, including abuse severity, physical coercion and assault during the sexual abuse, repeated episodes, and abuse by a family member (Danielson et al., 2005; Feiring, Taska, & Lewis, 2002; Garnefski & Diekstra, 1997). Having experienced other negative life events and/or additional forms of maltreatment, particularly physical abuse, has also been linked with increased depressive symptoms and suicidal ideation (Boney-McCoy & Finkelhor, 1995; Danielson et al., 2005; Garnefski & Diekstra, 1997; Naar-King et al., 2002). Furthermore, continued contact with the offender, which is more common with intrafamilial cases, is associated with long-term problems with depression and self-esteem (Tebbutt et al., 1997).

As with other populations, research with sexual abuse victims has demonstrated a link between depression and attributional style (Feiring, Taska, & Chen, 2002). Abuse-specific appraisals, including shame, have also been linked with depression (Danielson et al., 2005; Feiring, Taska, & Lewis, 2002; Spaccarelli & Fuchs, 1997). Family dysfunction, particularly maternal depression, has been linked with risk of depression and low self-esteem, in both the short and long run (Bal et al., 2004; Kelly et al., 2002; Meyerson, Long, Miranda, & Marx, 2002; Swanston et al., 2003; Tebbutt et al., 1997).

Sexual abuse victims show elevated risks for suicidal ideation and gestures, as well as completed suicides (Fergusson et al., 2000). Sexually abused boys are twice as likely as sexually abused girls to report suicidal ideation (Garnefski & Diekstra, 1997). Risk factors for suicidal ideation and behaviors among sexual abuse victims include family dysfunction and socioeconomic adversity (Fergusson et al.,

2000). Danielson and colleagues (2005) found that 70% of depressed youth with a history of both sexual and physical abuse experienced suicidal ideation.

Sexual Problems

Unlike most of the other problems associated with CSA, childhood sexuality problems have not been identified by DSM-IV-TR as constituting a specific disorder, possibly because there was relatively little research on the topic prior to the 1990s. However, considerable research has since documented the frequencies of various sexual behaviors across childhood and adolescence that now serve to help delineate between typical and atypical and problematic childhood sexual interests and behaviors. For children age 12 years and younger, sexual problems can be sorted into several categories (Friedrich et al., 1992): personal boundary deviations, exhibitionism, general role diversions, self-stimulation, sexual anxiety, excessive or precocious sexual interest, sexual intrusiveness, sexual knowledge, and voyeuristic behavior. For adolescents age 13 and older, other issues emerge (Friedrich, Lysne, Sim, & Shamos, 2004): excessive sexual interest and preoccupation, early onset of sexual activity, multiple sexual partners, sexual anxiety, excessive concern about appearance, divergent sexual interests, prostitution, sexual aggression, and behaviors that place them at risk for pregnancy, sexually transmitted diseases, including HIV infection, and victimization.

SEXUAL PROBLEMS DURING CHILDHOOD

Childhood is typically considered a period of relatively little sexual interest or sexual activities. However, surveys in the United States, Sweden, and Finland reveal that some sexual behaviors are fairly common in children, though the frequencies of various sexual behaviors vary with age (Friedrich, Fisher, Broughton, Houston, & Shafran, 1998). For example, among preschoolers, 44% of girls and 60% of boys engage in genital self-touching, up to 44% of boys and girls touch women's breasts, and 27% of boys and girls try to look at people when they are nude. Among children ages 6–9, it is still fairly common for boys and girls to engage in genital self-touching (40% and 21%, respectively) and to try to look at people when they are nude (20% for both

genders). From ages 10–12, common sexual behaviors include interest in looking at nudity in pictures or on TV (8.5% to 15% for boys and girls, respectively), and both genders show increased interest in the opposite sex (24–29%). Most sexual behaviors decrease across the span of childhood, including genital self-touching, attempts to look at people when they are nude, and touching women's breasts; however, interest in looking at nudity in media (TV, pictures) and interest in the opposite sex tend to increase with age. Several behaviors are unusual regardless of age, particularly overt sexual acts that involve others, such as invitations to engage in sexual acts, French kissing, oral–genital contact, touching animal genitalia, undressing playmates, making sexual sounds, pretend sexual play, and trying to have sexual intercourse. Other unusual sexual behaviors across all childhood ages are drawings that include sex parts, pretending that toys are having sex, and inserting objects in the vagina or rectum.

Chaffin, Letourneau, and Silovsky (2002) defined child sexual problem behaviors by the following conditions: (1) occur at greater frequency than developmentally expected; (2) interfere with child's development; (3) occur with coercion, intimidation, or force; (4) occur in association with emotional distress; (5) occur between children of divergent ages or developmental abilities; and (6) repeatedly recur in secrecy after intervention by caregivers. Research has clearly linked child sexual behavior problems to a history of child sexual abuse. Kendall-Tackett and colleagues (1993) estimated that approximately one-fourth of sexually abused children display such problems. However, the link between sexual behavior problems and CSA appears to be strongest among preschool-age children. Johnson (1988) reported that 72% of 4- to 6-year-olds with sexual behavior problems had a history of being sexually abused, compared with 42% of 7- to 10-year-olds and 35% of 11- to 12-year-olds. Numerous studies have documented sexual behavior differences between sexually abused children and their nonabused peers (see Friedrich [1993] for a review). More recently, Friedrich and colleagues (2001) demonstrated differences on the Child Sexual Behavior Inventory between sexually abused children and both normative and psychiatric controls.

In the Friedrich and colleagues (2001) study, sexual behavior problems were related to several sexual abuse characteristics: penetration abuse by a family member, multiple perpetrators, and frequent and longer-term abuse. Family sexuality and child life stress (e.g., events such as parental separations, illnesses, and foster care) also contributed to predictions of sexual behavior problems. Others have linked child sexual problems to child characteristics such as impulsivity, aggression, poor interpersonal skills, and lack of empathy for others (Johnson & Felmeth, 1993; Rasmussen, Burton, & Christopherson, 1992). Several parental characteristics have also been identified: poor monitoring, family violence, life stress, and poor parent–child attachment (Pithers, Gray, Busconi, & Houchens, 1998; Rasmussen et al., 1992). Friedrich and colleagues (2005) found significant continuity of problematic sexualized behaviors over a 1-year period, which was most pronounced for children living in residential treatment centers (perhaps because these were the most disturbed children in the study).

Pithers and colleagues (1998), using cluster analyses with a sample of 6- to 12-year-old children with sexual behavior problems, identified five types of childhood sexual problems. *Sexually aggressive* children were characterized by being male, having conduct disorders, using aggression to gain victim submission, and perpetrating serious sexual offenses that included sexual penetration. Compared to other types of children with sexual behavior problems, sexually aggressive children were less likely to have been sexually or physically abused and, if they had been abused, had fewer abuse episodes. *Abuse reactive* children were also characterized by being male and as not only having high levels of externalizing problems but also parent-reported internalizing problems. They often had a high level of sexual and physical maltreatment, often displaying sexual problems soon after their own abuse. Abuse reactive children were distinguished by the frequency of their sexually abusive acts against others, which often included penetration and aggression to gain compliance. The *highly traumatized* group included both boys and girls who experienced extensive sexual and physical maltreatment. In many cases their first victimization occurred at a young age, and several children were abused by multiple perpetrators. Compared to the other groups, this group had the highest number of psychiatric diagnoses, including PTSD. Children in the highly traumatized group did not penetrate their victims. The

two remaining groups were overrepresented by girls, *rule breakers* and *nonsymptomatic*. Rule breakers tended to have high levels of externalizing behavior problems, but parents also reported high levels of internalizing symptoms. Although their histories reflected moderate levels of sexual and physical victimization, this group had a high proportion of extended families members identified as being a sexual offender. Although they often used aggression to gain victim submission, penetration was not common. For the nonsymptomatic group, most did not have psychiatric diagnoses, though one-fourth of children had attention-deficit/hyperactivity disorder (ADHD). Most did not have a history of physical abuse, though the group was mixed in terms of sexual abuse history. Half were reported to have additional sexual offenders within their extended families. Their sexual behavior problems typically did not include aggressive behavior or penetration, and they tended to have relatively few victims. Nonsymptomatic, highly traumatized, and abuse reactive children were the most responsive to a modified relapse prevention program, and rule breakers were responsive to a combination of modified relapse prevention and expressive therapy. However, the sexually aggressive children did not show benefits from either type of treatment approach.

SEXUAL PROBLEMS DURING ADOLESCENCE

Sexual Offending. Unfortunately, adolescent sexual offending is not uncommon. Adolescent offenders under age 18 are responsible for up to 41% of sexual assaults against children under age 12 (Finkelhor & Dziuba-Letherman, 1995; Snyder & Sickmund, 1999;), with the peak rate of offending between the ages 13 and 14 years (Canadian Centre for Justice Statistics, 1999; Snyder, 2000). Juvenile arrest records indicate that in a 1-year period, 0.19% of males between the ages 11 and 18 are arrested for a sexual offense (Federal Bureau of Investigation, 2000). Even in community samples, up to 2.6% of adolescent males report having used some form of physical force or threat in a sexual act (Ageton, 1983). The most frequently identified risk factors for adolescent and adult sexual offenses are being male and having been a victim of sexual abuse in childhood (Salter et al., 2003). Very little is known about adolescent female sexual offenders, primarily because they comprise only 5% of adolescent offenders (Fehrenbach et al., 1986). Although sexual abuse is common among adolescent offenders, many have experienced other forms of maltreatment as well. Way, Satwah, and Drake (1999) found that 35% of adolescents who were reported to child welfare agencies for sexually abusing a child had documented histories of themselves being the victim of CSA, physical abuse, or neglect. Among those involved in a specialized treatment for adolescent offenders, 67.7% reported a history of sexual abuse, 72.3% reported physical abuse, and 39.6%, neglect (Way et al., 1999).

It should be noted, however, that only a small percentage of sexually abused children go on to engage in sexually abusive behavior. Salter and colleagues (2003) identified the following risk factors, evident at a postdisclosure sexual abuse assessment, that predicted subsequent sexual offenses: female perpetrator (OR = 3.03), witnessed to severe forms of domestic violence (OR = 3.1), physical and supervisory neglect (ORs = 3.4 and 2.0, respectively), history of cruelty to animals (OR = 7.9), and history of encopresis (OR = 2.8). These results replicate those of other researchers, who also identified witnessing domestic violence, neglect, and abuse by a female relative as risk factors for sexual offending among sexually abused boys (Butler & Seto, 2002; Glasser et al., 2001; Widom & Ames, 1994). The pathway between CSA and later offenses as adolescents and adults may in part be a history of childhood sexual behavior problems. Burton (2000) found that among adolescents with an admitted history of sexual offending, 47% reported a history of childhood sexual problems. Those with offenses spanning childhood and adolescence had more extensive sexual abuse histories. Once adolescents are identified as sexual offenders, between 9 and 26% of them will have another sexual offense charge before age 18 (Caldwell, 2002; Hagan & Gust-Brey, 1999; Nisbet, Wilson, & Smallbone, 2004). Studies that have examined risk factors for reoffending have produced mixed results, but the evidence in general suggests that sexual recidivism is linked with evidence of sexual deviancy (e.g., phallometrically measured preference for prepubescent stimuli) and is more common among those who committed high-frequency and/or violent offenses (Caldwell, 2002).

Risky Sexual Behaviors. Both longitudinal and cross-sectional studies of sexual abuse victims indicate that sexual abuse prematurely sets in motion a series of sexual experiences that have serious lifelong consequences. Sexual abuse victims tend to be younger both when they begin consensual sexual activities and when they have their first consensual sexual intercourse experience (Fergusson, Horwood, & Lynskey, 1997; Miller, Monson, & Norton, 1995; Noll, Trickett, & Putnam, 2000; Wyatt, 1985), which places them at risk for early pregnancy (Woodward, Fergusson, & Horwood, 2001). Indeed, up to 66% of pregnant teens report a history of childhood sexual abuse (Boyer & Fine, 1991; Gershenson et al., 1989). Early teenage pregnancy has important implications of intergenerational transmission of child maltreatment. Teenage mothers tend to leave school early, to have fewer social and economic opportunities in life, to suffer greater social disadvantage, to be less competent and more punitive as parents, to suffer more depression, and to be more often the victims of spousal violence (Bardone, Moffitt, Caspi, & Dickson, 1996; Brooks-Gunn & Chase-Landsale, 1995; Woodward et al., 2001).

CSA victims are at increased risk for a number of sexually transmitted infections including chlamydia, gonnorhea, human papillomavirus (HPV), and HIV infection, as a result of both the abuse (Beck-Sague & Solomon, 1999; Gutman, St. Claire, Herman-Giddens, Johnston, & Phelps, 1992; Lindegren et al., 1998), and risky sexual behaviors (Saewyc et al., 2006; Steel & Herlitz, 2005). Adolescents who report a history of CSA and/or family violence are four times more likely than their peers to engage in sex without condoms, to have sex after drug use, and to have sex with multiple partners (Voisin, 2005). Furthermore, these risky behaviors are twice as prevalent among those who perceive that their peers engage in similar, risky sexual practices. Girls with a history of sexual abuse may find it particularly difficult to assert themselves in sexual situations, either to resist sexual advances or to ensure safe sexual practices (Brown, Kessel, Lourie, Ford, & Lipsitt, 1997; Johnsen & Harlow, 1996).

Sexual risk taking tends to occur within a broader constellation of risky adolescent behaviors that includes smoking, substance use, and involvement with a deviant peer culture (Breitenbecher, 2001; Donovan & Jessor, 1985; Willoughby, Chalmers, & Busseri, 2004). Drug dependence increases the risk of engaging in risky sexual practices, due to both impaired decision-making and issues such as running away, homelessness, and prostitution associated with both substance use and sexual victimization. In a study of women engaged in prostitution, approximately 60% reported a history of CSA prior to entering prostitution, and 73% indicated that they began prostituting while they were still minors (Fraser, 1985). In a longitudinal investigation of sexual abuse victims, both childhood sexual abuse and neglect were linked with subsequent prostitution (Widom & Kuhns, 1996).

Noll and colleagues (2000) identified three trajectories for sexual development among adolescents/young women with prior histories of sexual abuse. Those who had been abused by their biological fathers, compared to other sexual abuse survivors, tended to be more preoccupied with sex, felt more pressure to have sex, were less effective in their birth control practices, and were more likely to have given birth at least once. These young women reported more male friends and fewer female friends, fewer nonpeer male relationships (father, grandfathers, etc.), and low satisfaction with male nonpeers. Concerns were raised that girls who were abused by their fathers were predisposed to be overly sexual in their relationships with boys, perhaps due to socialization within the father–daughter relationship. In contrast, those who were abused by multiple, nonparental family members and who experienced physical coercion showed less sexual preoccupation, had more negative attitudes toward sex, felt little pressure to engage in sex, and reported more responsible birth control use. Young women who had experienced abuse by one nonparental family member were no different than the comparison group in sexual attitudes and behaviors.

Sexual Revictimization. As noted previously, several literature reviews have highlighted the link between childhood and adolescent sexual abuse, and sexual assaults and subsequent assaults during adult years (Classen et al., 2005; Muehlenhard, Highby, Lee, Bryan, & Dodrill, 1998; Roodman & Clum, 2001). In addition to the invasiveness of the sexual acts, a number of other abuse and trauma variables have been linked with increased risk of subsequent victimization, including closer relationship to the perpetrator, abuse that was more frequent and of longer duration, use of force,

and experiencing other childhood traumas, particularly childhood physical abuse (Classen et al., 2005). Several family variables have also been linked with revictimization, including parent–child conflict, spousal violence, changes in caregivers, and drug and alcohol problems (Classen et al., 2005). Fergusson et al. (1997) found that family-related factors such as disadvantaged home environments, family dysfunction, and parental drug and alcohol problems partially mediated the link between child sexual abuse and subsequent victimization during late adolescence. Lifestyle factors appear to place sexual abuse victims at risk for revictimization (Breitenbecher, 2001). Consensual sexual intercourse at an early age, drug and alcohol problems, and depression also increase risk for revictimization during later adolescence (Breitenbecher, 2001; Fergusson et al., 1997). Wilson, Calhoun, and Bernat (1999) provided experimental evidence that risk of revictimization may be due in part to diminished perception of threat in high-risk situations.

Abuse-Related Symptoms

Externalizing Problems

Across childhood and adolescence, sexual abuse has been linked with increased risk of anger, aggression, and conduct problems. During the preschool and early primary school years, sexually abused children show increased anger and aggression, particularly among children who were very young when the abuse first occurred, and among those who experienced multiple types of maltreatment (English, Graham, Litrownik, Everson, & Bangdiwala, 2005; Lau et al., 2005). Externalizing behavior problems exhibited by sexually abused children can be quite serious. For example, Martin, Bergen, Richardson, Roeger, and Allison (2004) reported that history of sexual abuse is a significant risk factor for firesetting. It is unclear, however, whether these externalizing problems arise specifically from the abuse experiences or from the types of family stressors typical of children who show externalizing problems in general. In their nationally representative survey of children ages 2–11, Turner, Finkelhor, and Ormrod (2006) documented relatively high rates of externalizing problems for sexual abuse victims. However, the increase in externalizing problems was accounted for by family dysfunction and other types of negative life events and adversities. Furthermore, Tebbutt and colleagues (1997), in their 5-year follow-up of sexual abuse victims, found that increased externalizing problems were primarily linked with family dysfunction.

During adolescence, the externalizing problems displayed by sexual abuse victims graduate to more serious conduct problems in the form of increased aggression, criminal behavior, and addiction-risk behaviors (Bagley & Mallick, 2000; Dube et al., 2006; Fergusson, Horwood, & Lynskey, 1996; Garnefski & Diekstra, 1997; Howard & Wang, 2005; Kilpatrick et al., 2003; Luster & Small, 1997; Luster et al., 2002; Turner et al., 2006). Garnefski and Diekstra (1997) found that history of sexual abuse increased the odds of these externalizing problems for girls 2.5 and 2.3 times, respectively, and for boys, 1.7 and 1.6. Sexually abused boys were particularly likely to report a combination of aggressive/criminal behavior and addiction-risk behavior compared to nonabused boys (OR = 20). Unlike children under age 11, increased problems with anger and aggression among adolescents appear to have direct links with the sexual abuse itself, even when family dysfunction and other life adversities are controlled (Quas et al., 2005; Spaccarelli & Fuchs, 1997; Turner et al., 2006).

Adolescent Substance Use

The link between substance use problems and history of sexual abuse is most pronounced for girls. As a whole, studies do not show elevated substance use problems for sexually abused boys compared to boys in the general population. In their review of this issue, Simpson and Miller (2002) found that adolescent girls who were victims of sexual abuse were overrepresented among females with alcohol and drug problems, regardless of whether the research was conducted with treatment seekers, medical clinic attenders, elementary or high school students, or general community dwellers. Even when other childhood adversities and family dysfunction were considered, history of sexual abuse continued to be a significant predictor of substance use problems for girls.

Eating Disorders

Despite some inconsistent findings across studies, both a literature review (Jacobi, Hayward, de Zwaan, Kraemer, & Agras, 2004) and a meta-analysis of 53 studies (Smolak & Murnen, 2002) confirmed that CSA is a significant risk factor for both subclinical and clinical eating disorder symptomatology. However, it appears that eating disorder symptoms are not an abuse-specific outcome, but the relationship is mediated through abuse-related negative affect (depression, PTSD) and ineffective coping mechanisms (Hund & Espelage, 2005; Thompson & Wonderlich, 2004). Hund and Espelage (2005) found that both emotional distress and alexithymia mediated the relationship between history of sexual abuse and eating disorder symptoms in a sample of university women. Alexithymia reflects deficits in identifying, verbalizing, and understanding emotions, and inabilities in identifying emotional and physical sensations.

Self-Harm Behaviors

Self-harm behaviors refer to intentional self-injury without the direct intention to commit suicide (Briere & Gil, 1998) and often include repetitive behaviors that inflict superficial wounds, such as making cuts on the arms and other body parts. Superficial self-harm appears to have increased over the past decade (Boyce, Oakley, Brown, & Hatcher, 2001), with up to 15% of adolescents (Laye-Gindhu & Schonert-Reichl, 2005; Ross & Heath, 2002), 12% of university students (Favazza, DeRosear, & Conterio, 1989), and 4% of the general adult populations reporting a history of self-mutilating behavior (Briere & Gil, 1998). Research with adults has demonstrated a link between history of sexual and physical abuse and intentional self-harm behaviors (Low, Jones, MacLeod, Power, & Duggan, 2000; van der Kolk, Perry, & Herman, 1991; Yates & Carleson, 2003), relationships that continue to be apparent even after other negative childhood life events are controlled. However, at this point, the connection between intentional self-harm and history of child sexual or physical abuse has not been demonstrated with child or adolescent populations. With adults, intentional self-harm is often comorbid with a number of mental health problems, including borderline personality disorder, PTSD, depression, and dissociation, which in turn are all linked with histories of child sexual abuse. Surveys of self mutilators reveal that the most common reason for intentional self-harm behavior is to gain emotional relief and to regulate emotions (Browne et al., 2002), which may be maintained through the negative reinforcement associated with the subsequent reduction or termination of unwanted emotional states (Chapman, Gratz, & Brown, 2006; Nock & Prinstein, 2004).

Pathological Changes in Psychological Processes

Affect Dysregulation and Emotional Competence

Ford (2005) described childhood maltreatment as a "developmentally adverse interpersonal trauma," noting that maltreatment may not only be traumatic but also may have the potential to alter biological, psychological, and interpersonal regulatory capacities that contribute to a host of child and adolescent problems. Psychophysiological research indicates that childhood maltreatment may negatively affect central nervous system development and functioning, impacting the ability to regulate emotional states (Glasser, 2000; Teicher, Yutaka, Glod, & Anderson, 1997)). Affect regulation requires competence in coordinating responses across three systems—physiological, cognitive, and behavioral. Three components of emotional competence have been identified: (1) the ability to recognize emotions and communicate emotional states effectively; (2) the ability to understand the causes and consequences of emotional expressions, and the ability to respond effectively to one's own emotions, as well as the emotional displays of others; and (3) the ability to regulate emotional expression and emotional experience within differing social and cultural contexts. Within the realm of typical social development, these skills have been linked to children's social competence and psychological adjustment (Garber, Braafladt, & Weiss, 1995; Rubin, Coplan, Fox, & Calkins, 1995).

Concerns have been raised that child sexual maltreatment, particularly abuse that occurs within the context of family relationships, may disrupt children's emotional development, as a function of not only the trauma associated with the abuse but also the family context in which abuse occurs (Cole & Putnam, 1992). From a functionalist perspective, atypical social contexts such as sexually abusive relationships and family environments associated with risk for sexual abuse result in atypical emotion management skills (Campos, Mumme, Kermoian,

& Campos, 1994); that is, emotion management strategies that effectively modulate affect in the abusive environment (e.g., decreased emotional awareness, suppression of emotional expression), may subsequently interfere with successful adaptations in other, nonabusive contexts. Research indicates that physically abused children are less able than their nonabused peers to encode and decode facial expressions, understand the dynamics behind emotionally arousing situations, or regulate emotions within the context of peer relationships (Camras et al., 1988; Rogosch, Cicchei, & Aber, 1995). Shields, Ryan, and Cicchetti (2001) studied a group of children who had experienced mixed forms of maltreatment (sexual abuse, physical abuse, and/or neglect) and a comparison sample during a summer camp experience. Camp counselors rated the maltreated children as more emotionally dysregulated, and peers rated them as less cooperative, and more disruptive and aggressive. The relationship between maltreatment and social adjustment was partially mediated by the children's negative representations of caregivers and by their emotion regulation abilities.

One study specifically examined emotion management skills among intrafamilially abused girls in comparison to a nonabused control group (Shipman, Zeman, Penza, & Champion, 2000). Sexually maltreated girls had poorer understanding of emotions, more difficulty accurately appraising the causes and consequences of emotionally arousing situations, and more negative expectations about reactions to their own emotional expressions. They were less aware of their own emotions, showed more emotion dysregulation, and failed to respond to others' emotional displays in a culturally appropriate manner. The results suggested that sexually maltreated girls may fail to attend to, process, and interpret emotional information, and that this failure then interferes with their ability to establish and maintain positive interpersonal relationships. For example, in response to questions about how to respond to negative emotional displays in others, maltreated girls were more likely to say that they would ignore the emotional displays or leave the situation. In contrast, their nonmaltreated peers were more likely to indicate that they would provide assistance or support. Thus, although avoidance strategies may protect an intrafamilially maltreated girl in the course of conflict with her parents (i.e., it might be unsafe for her to confront either the perpetrator or the nonabusing parent), similar avoidance patterns with peers may interfere with her ability to establish relationships outside the maltreatment context.

Cognitive Style

As noted earlier, cognitive style has important implications for the development of a number of mental health problems, including PTSD and depression (Joiner & Wagner, 1995). Cognitive style appears to develop during the latency years and is influenced by the experience of both high- and low-magnitude negative life events (Compas, Ey, & Grant, 1993; Garber & Flynn, 2001; Gibb et al., 2001; Gibb, Alloy, Abramson, & Marx, 2003; Hankin, Abramson, & Siler, 2001; McGinn, Cukor, & Sanderson, 2005), and parenting style (Garber & Flynn, 2001; Stuewig & McCloskey, 2005). Even over the course of adolescence, negative life events continue to mold cognitive style (Garber & Flynn, 2001; Spence, Sheffield, & Donovan, 2002). Research with adults indicates that a history of childhood abuse, including sexual abuse, is particularly linked to negative cognitive style and risk for depression (Rose, Abramson, Hodulik, Halberstadt, & Leff, 1994).

Coping

Coping has been defined as "any and all responses made by an individual who encounters a potentially harmful outcome" (Silver & Wortman, 1980, p. 281). Causey and DeBow (1992) identified six coping factors. Two factors are considered effective (problem solving and seeking social support), and three are considered ineffective (distancing, internalizing, and externalizing). The sixth factor assesses perception of the event as controllable or uncontrollable. Causey and DeBow also highlight that coping is situation-specific, and that no single coping strategy is appropriate for every situation. For example, when a stressor is moderate and controllable, strategies intended to alter the situation are associated with lower levels of distress and fewer negative emotions (Hubert, Jay, Saltoun, & Hayes, 1988; Hyson, 1983). However, when a person is faced with high-stress, uncontrollable stressors, coping

strategies that reduce emotional distress or enable the person to avoid the stressors appear to be most effective (Altshuler & Ruble, 1989; Band & Weisz, 1988; Spirito, Stark, & Williams, 1988). For instance, distraction is a commonly used coping strategy when stressors are perceived as uncontrollable (David & Suls, 1999). Coping may also differ depending on the magnitude of the stressor. High-magnitude stressors, compared to low-magnitude stressors, tend to evoke more negative coping reactions (internalizing and externalizing) and fewer problem-solving reactions (Fair et al., 2006; Wolfe & Birt, 2003). Evidence also suggests that changes in coping over time, particularly utilization of social supports, are related to interim levels of adversity (Fair et al., 2006). Leitenberg, Gibson, and Novy (2004) examined differences in coping among undergraduate women as a function of childhood maltreatment. Women who reported more extensive childhood adversity (sexual abuse, physical abuse, witnessing domestic violence, having an alcoholic parent, and/or parental rejection) reported an increased reliance on disengagement methods of coping (wishful thinking, problem avoidance, social withdrawal, and self-criticism).

Implications for Clinical Assessment

As is evident from this review, CSA has numerous affects throughout the lifespan. Thus the assessment of CSA must be developmentally informed, multidimensional, and integrate historical and current contextual information with an array of emotional and behavioral symptoms and psychological processes. CSA sets in motion a number of negative mental health processes that have the capacity cumulatively to affect a broad range of adjustment concerns. Compared to other serious negative life events, CSA is strongly linked to the development of depression and PTSD, and early childhood abuse appears to sow the seeds of dissociative processes and disorders. CSA is linked with a number of sexuality problems, ranging from increased risk of sexual victimization to age-inappropriate interest in sexual activities, to sexual offending. These problems are exacerbated by disturbances in a number of psychological processes, including affect regulation skills, cognitive style, and coping strategies. In the following section, assessment strategies are reviewed for each of these issues, with the goal of identifying important assessment strategies, methods, and tools.

ASSESSING SEXUAL ABUSE AND OTHER FORMS OF MALTREATMENT AND ADVERSITY

Inherent in conducting an assessment of a child who has been sexually abused is obtaining accurate background information relevant not only to the sexual abuse but also to other forms of maltreatment, trauma, and adverse childhood events, along with other types of family-based adversities. Given that many sexual abuse victims experience multiple types of maltreatment and adversity, broad-based assessment of negative life events is important to gain an understanding of factors that might contribute to child adjustment problems and have bearing on service delivery. Although there is growing awareness of the need to assess multiple forms of adversity, little attention has been paid to the development of psychometrically sound assessment tools for these purposes, particularly tools that are appropriate and feasible for clinical settings (Hanson, Smith, Saunders, Swenson, & Conrad, 1995). Indeed, given the complexity of child maltreatment and adversity, and the difficulty in obtaining such sensitive information on a large sample of children and youth, the task of developing these tools has been quite daunting, particularly because large sample sizes are required to address the many relevant issues adequately.

Due to unique risk factors and psychological outcomes, types of maltreatment need to be considered separately for both research and clinical purposes (Egeland & Sroufe, 1981; Higgins & McCabe, 2000); however, the reality is that many maltreated children experience multiple forms of abuse and adversity, and various combinations of different forms of abuse and adversity appear to have unique outcomes that are not accounted for by simply summing forms of maltreatment. Thus, when assessing the effects of a specific form of maltreatment, it is necessary to assess and consider the impact other forms of maltreatment and adversity. As well, it is important to assess the specific aspects of that particular form of maltreatment, and to consider how that form of maltreatment interacts with other forms of adversity to predict unique outcomes. Broad-based assessment strategies typically assess five types of maltreat-

ment: sexual abuse, physical abuse, emotional abuse, exposure to family violence, and neglect (see Crooks & Wolfe, Chapter 14, this volume). For each type of maltreatment, important details include the acts involved, the offender, the age when the events occurred and ended, the frequency and duration of the events, and whether there were any injuries and health, or developmental consequences directly linked with the maltreatment (Barnett, Manly, & Cicchetti, 1993; Hanson et al., 1995; Wolfe & Birt, 1997).

Developmental issues should also be considered, such as age of first abusive episode and continuity of abuse across the preschool, latency, and adolescent years. For sexual abuse, details about the disclosure process are important, including how the abuse was discovered, to whom the child disclosed (if at all), and whether any CPS, family, and/or criminal legal matters have occurred, are planned, or are in progress. To assess and control comprehensively for other forms of adversity, exposure to nonmaltreatment negative life events should be assessed, as well as family-based risk factors. Many sexually abused children have complex and chaotic backgrounds that necessitate careful history taking; details about biological parents and stepparents, parental separations, past and current living arrangements, and school placements should all be assessed. As noted earlier, caregiver mental health, substance abuse problems, and history of maltreatment have important implications for the adjustment of sexual abuse victims and should also be assessed.

Whenever possible, it is wise to solicit historical data, and maltreatment and adversity information, from multiple sources. In most cases, abuse-related information reported by parents, medical personnel, CPS, and children themselves is consistent and reliable (Kaufman, Jones, Stielglitz, Vitulano, & Mannarino, 1994; McGee, Wolfe, Yuen, Wilson, & Carnochan, 1995). However, Kaufman and colleagues (1994) found that medical records and parent reports often yielded information about abuse severity and other forms of abuse that was not available in CPS files. For example, CPS files revealed that 77% of their sample of sexually abused children and adolescents had experienced emotional maltreatment; when medical, parent, and CPS records were all surveyed for each case, 98% of cases revealed evidence of emotional maltreatment.

Broad-Based Assessment of Child Maltreatment

Chart Reviews

The History of Victimization Form (HVF; Wolfe, Gentile, & Bourdeau, 1986) was designed for completion through CPS chart reviews, supplemented with information from other sources, such as parents, mental health agencies, and children and adolescents, as appropriate. The format was designed to provide the greatest level of detail possible about history of maltreatment, with the idea that users can identify dimensions of abuse relevant for particular purposes. The HVF assesses six sexual abuse dimensions: Severity of Sexual Acts, Use of Coercion or Force, Relationship to the Perpetrator, Number of Perpetrators, and Estimates of Frequency and Duration. Severity of Sexual Abuse, Use of Coercion or Force, and Relationship to the Perpetrator are rated on a Gutman-type scale, with the most serious level of abuse recorded. The number of perpetrators is recorded, along with estimates of the duration and frequency. Frequency of abuse is particularly difficult to ascertain from chart reviews, so estimates are gathered by determining the duration of abuse multiplied by an estimate of frequency within a time period. For example, a child may have said it occurred for a 3-month period when her mother went to play bingo once a week, so the estimate for frequency would be 12. Physical abuse, neglect, emotional maltreatment, and exposure to family violence are also assessed in a similar fashion, with some slight variations relevant to the type of maltreatment considered. In addition to detailed information about each form of maltreatment, the HVF also solicits background information about the child's disclosure and legal status, and the family's involvement with CPS.

Complex measurement systems such as the HVF yield a lot of information, but reduction of variables into meaningful constructs has been a challenge. The majority of research using the HVF has focused on sexual abuse victims, as have psychometric analyses. Based on two separate samples, principal component analyses have yielded two theoretically meaningful factors (Birt, 1996; Gentile, 1988): Severity (a combination of severity, coercion, and number of perpetrators) and Course (a combination of duration, frequency, and relationship to perpetrator). Relationship to perpetrator appears to link with duration and frequency, because familial abuse tends to occur more frequently over longer durations. These two dimensions have important theoretical relevance, since PTSD and other abuse-related sequelae appear to be related to both the intensity of the trauma and the duration and course of the abuse. Although detailed background information is important for clinical purposes, concerns have been raised about the efficiency of detailed chart reviews to gather abuse information systems for research purposes. Relative to the extensive time required to review files, the incremental predictive power of fine-grain details appears to be limited. Indeed, research with the Record of Maltreatment Experiences (ROME; McGee, Wolfe, & Wilson, 1990), an abbreviated version of the HVF, found that simple ratings of maltreatment severity were as predictive of outcomes as the detailed ROME recordings (McGee et al., 1995).

The most researched maltreatment assessment tool for children under 12 is the Maltreatment Classification Scheme (MCS; Barnett et al., 1993), which has been adapted for use by LONGSCAN, a consortium of five longitudinal studies of child abuse and neglect conducted at several sites across the United States (Runyan et al., 1998). At all sites, assessments are planned for ages 4, 6, 8, 12, 14, 16, and 20 years; for the most recent publications, the sample totaled 1,435 children and their families (English et al., 2005). The MCS was originally developed to collect information from CPS records; LONGSCAN's adapted version is referred to as the Modified Maltreatment Classification Scheme (MMCS). The MCS assesses severity of incidents within each subtype of maltreatment, frequency and chronicity, length of CPS involvement, developmental period during which the events occurred, type and number of placements outside the home, and the perpetrators of the incident. Within the major forms of maltreatment, different subtypes are recorded. For example, the Neglect scale is subdivided into Lack of Supervision, Moral/Legal/Educational Maltreatment, and Failure to Provide subscales; within Failure to Provide, details are provided as to whether the concern is related to food, clothing, or shelter. At each level of maltreatment, severity is rated on a 5-point, Gutman-like scale based on a combination of caretaker actions (or lack thereof) and impact on child (e.g., weight loss for neglect). The Sexual Abuse subscale has the following hierarchical designations: (1) Child is exposed to explicit sexual stimuli or activities but not directly involved (e.g., child is exposed to pornography, sexual activity, sexual talk in his or her presence); (2) child is invited to engage in sexual activity and/or exposed to caretaker's genitals; (3) offender fondles the child or has the child sexually touch him or her; (4) attempts and actual penetration of child, including coitus, oral sex, anal sex, or any other form of sodomy; and (5) intercourse involving restraint, weapons, brutality, or physical force; prostitution of child. The MCS is available in Barnett and colleagues (1993), and the MMCS LONGSCAN version is available at *www.iprc. unc.edu/longscan.*

As noted earlier, these complex systems are difficult to reduce to parsimonious, meaningful constructs. In a special issue of *Child Abuse and Neglect* (English, Bangdiwala, & Runyon, 2005), several articles addressed questions related to calculation of abuse type, severity, and chronicity using LONGSCAN data for assessment of children at ages 4 and 8. Overall, despite concerns to the contrary (e.g., McGee et al., 1995), findings supported the importance of preserving fine gradations in abuse information when examining the links between maltreatment and outcome. Lau and colleagues (2005) found that differentiation among multiple maltreatment type combinations was particularly effective in predicting multiple child outcomes (e.g., Child Behavior Checklist [CBCL] total, Internalizing, and Externalizing scores [Achenbach & Rescorla, 2001]; Trauma Symptom Checklist for Children [TSCC; Briere, 1996, 2006a] Posttraumatic Stress and Anger scores). Specifically, the co-occurrence of multiple types of maltreatment was robustly related to multiple outcomes, particularly when sexual abuse was involved. Furthermore, Litrownik and colleagues (2005) found that preserving severity ratings within different types of maltreatment was the most effective strategy for predicting a broad range of outcomes (e.g., CBCL broad-band scores, Vineland Adaptive Behavior Scales [Sparrow, Balla, & Cicchetti, 1985] Socialization scores; TSCC Anger scale]) compared to both an amalgamated score that combined severity rating across maltreatment types or the highest rating received across different maltreatment types. The maximum severity by type strategy yielded five maltreatment severity scores, based on the highest severity rating of reports within the five maltreatment domains during a specified period of time. This strategy has a conceptual advantage, because different forms of maltreatment are likely to have different types of outcomes (e.g., the ultimate effect of physical abuse is death, whereas the ultimate effect of emotional maltreatment is psychological trauma; Manly, 2005).

In contrast, it appears that chronicity of maltreatment is best considered by combining different abuse subtypes to form one chronicity variable. English and colleagues (2005) identified five progressively detrimental levels of chronicity: situational, limited episodic, limited continuous, extended episodic, and extended continuous). They found that the more developmental periods with any form of maltreatment reported, the more child externalizing behavior problems. Likewise, anxiety and anger were less pronounced for children with developmental periods that were free from maltreatment. These findings mirror those of Bolger, Patterson, and Kupersmidt (1998; Bolger & Patterson, 2001), who found that chronically maltreated children are less popular with peers, regardless of subtype or severity. Evidence also links chronic maltreatment to aggression, and aggression mediated the link between chronic maltreatment and peer rejection (Bolger & Patterson, 2001; Manly, Cicchetti, & Barnett, 1994).

Parent Reports

The Abuse Dimensions Inventory (ADI; Chaffin, Wherry, Newlin, Crutchfield, & Dykman, 1997) was designed to be completed by caregivers in a semistructured interview format, though it has subsequently been used to gather information from CPS workers (Silovsky & Niec, 2002). The ADI has six sections: physical abuse (12 items), sexual abuse (13 items), force or coercion used to gain submission to sexual abuse (9 items), force or coercion used to gain secrecy about either physical or sexual abuse (6 items), role relationships between child and abuser (9 relationships identified), and postdisclosure reactions abusers might express regarding admission and blame (5 items). Rank ordering of items for severity was based on a survey of mental health professionals with specialization in child abuse, with the following rank order from least to most serious for sexual abuse: (1) sexually suggestive talk, hugs, or kisses; (2) exposure to pornography, exposure of genitals, or voyeurism; (3)

fondling of child over clothes; (4) fondling of child under clothes; (5) simulated intercourse over clothes; (6) simulated intercourse under clothes with no penetration, having child masturbate abuser; (7) abuser oral contact with child genitals; (8) child required to have oral contact with abuser's genitals; (9) digital or object penetration; (10) vaginal or anal intercourse, including unsuccessful attempts; (11) paraphilic sex (e.g., urine, feces, bondage) or prostitution; and (12) ritual or satanic abuse or sexualized torture. Interrater agreement was calculated based on 25 interviews that were audiotaped for coding by four independent raters. The overall mean kappa was .80, ranging across scales from .65 to 1.00. Factor analyses of 136 ADIs yielded four factors: Sexual Abuse Severity and Coercion, Sexual Abuse Duration and Number of Events, Physical Abuse Severity and Coercion, and Physical Abuse Duration and Number of Events. Role relationship and abuser's reaction did not load heavily on any factor. In a subsequent study, ADI sexual abuse severity ratings correlated with child-reported PTSD symptoms (Chaffin & Shultz, 2001).

Child and Adolescent Self-Reports

Large-scale epidemiological studies have necessitated the development of assessment tools for children and adolescents to determine prevalence of maltreatment, victimization, and adversity. The Juvenile Victimization Questionnaire (JVQ; Finkelhor et al., 2005; Hamby & Finkelhor, 2001, 2004) has been used as a self-report measure for children and youth age 8 years and older. A caregiver version uses similar wording, so that it is directly comparable to the youth report version, and can be used for children under the age of 8. The JVQ assesses 34 offenses against youth in five areas: Conventional Crime (assaults, property crimes), Child Maltreatment (physical, sexual, and emotional abuse, neglect, family abduction/custodial interference), Peer and Sibling Victimization (assaults and property offenses), Sexual Assault (rape and sexual assaults attempted or completed, flashing, sexual harassment, and statutory sexual offenses), and Witnessing and Indirect Victimization (domestic violence, abuse of a sibling, community violence, civil disturbances and riots, and warzone violence). Thus far, the JVQ has only been used to assess 1-year incidence data, so it is un-

clear how it would work assessing lifetime maltreatment experiences. The JVQ takes 20–30 minutes to complete, depending on the number of victimizations reported. Following screener questions, more in-depth information is obtained, including perpetrator characteristics, use of a weapon, injuries, and co-occurrence of the event with another reported event (in case one event falls into more than one category).

The Child Trauma Questionnaire (CTQ), perhaps the most commonly used self-report measure of childhood victimization, is a 70-item, Likert-like self-report inventory (Bernstein & Fink, 1998; Bernstein et al., 1994) that yields five subscales: Emotional Abuse, Physical Abuse, Emotional Neglect, Sexual Abuse, and Physical Neglect. Although originally developed for adults, it has been used with youth as young as 12 years. The five subscales are based on two factor analyses, one with adults and a second with adolescents. For the adolescent study, the CTQ demonstrated good sensitivity and specificity with known maltreatment information (Bernstein, Ahluvalia, Pogge, & Handelsman, 1997). Bernstein and colleagues (2003) created a shortened, 28-item version of the CTQ. Using confirmatory factor analyses, results revealed that the five scales were a good fit for the data, which was true with several samples, including adolescent inpatients, adult substance users, and a community sample that provided normative data. As well, the shortened version demonstrated good convergent and discriminant validity, with clinician ratings based on known information about patients.

The Traumatic Events Questionnaire— Adolescents (TEQ-A; Lipschitz, Bernstein, Winegar, & Southwick, 1999), a 46-item self-report questionnaire, uses a multiple-choice format to elicit details about six forms of traumatic experiences: Witnessing Home Violence, Witnessing or Being the Victim of Community Violence, Accidental Physical Injuries, Physical Abuse, and Sexual Abuse. The TEQ-A defines "sexual abuse" as sexual contact between a minor and an adult 5 years older or a peer 2 years older. A two-level gating system is used, with two initial sexual abuse questions: "When you were growing up, did anyone try to have some kind of sexual contact with you in a way that made you feel uncomfortable?" and "If so, how old was the person who did this?" Details of each sexual incident are then obtained, including the age of onset, duration, identity of perpetrators, use of force, and exact nature of each traumatic experience. When adolescents' responses on the TEQ-A were compared to a best-estimate source (based on information from therapist interviews, chart reviews, and child welfare agencies), the agreement for sexual abuse was 88% (kappa = .75) and physical abuse was 84% (kappa = .66). Comparisons between the TEQ-A and the CTQ revealed that 71% of respondents who reported sexual abuse on the CTQ also reported sexual abuse on the TEQ-A; however, 35% of those above the clinical cutoff on the CTQ did not report sexual abuse on the TEQ-A (kappa = −.41). Discrepancies between the two measures in reports of sexual abuse were more common among males, who reported less severe abuse experiences and fewer mental health problems. Thus, the CTQ is more sensitive than the TEQ-A in detecting sexual abuse of lesser severity. Lipschitz and colleagues (1999) suggested that the differences in format might account for the differences in reporting, in that the Likert-like format might facilitate reporting of less frequent and less distressing events, possibly including events that technically meet criteria for sexual abuse but are not considered by the respondent to have been abusive (e.g., sexual "initiation" of adolescent boys by an older female).

Several available life events checklists include items reflecting childhood maltreatment, as well as other types of negative life events and adversities. The Child and Adolescent Psychiatric Assessment (CAPA) Life Events Module (Costello, Angold, March, & Fairbank, 1998) was developed for use with the Great Smoky Mountain Epidemiological Study. Both high- and low-magnitude negative life events are assessed. The 15 high-magnitude events are death of close relative or friend; witnessing a traumatic event; natural disaster; diagnoses of a life-threatening or disabling physical illness; serious accident, fire, or exposure to a toxic agent; learning of a traumatic event affecting a close family member or friend; war, terrorism, or death or serious harm to someone else; physical violence by someone other than a family member; physical abuse by a family member; being kidnapped or held hostage; and sexual abuse, rape, and sexual abuse with coercion. Low-magnitude events include new child in home (if unwelcome); pregnancy (own or partner's—learned of, premature termination, childbirth, placement of child); parental sepa-

ration; parental divorce; new parental figure; moving recently or repeatedly; change of school other than normal promotion; loss of best friend through move; breakup with best friend; breakup with boyfriend or girlfriend; parental arrest; serious reduction in standard of living; forced separation from home; other event. Comparisons of parent and child completed versions yielded good intraclass correlations (.72 [child] and .83 [parent] for high-magnitude events, and .62 [child] and .58 [parent] for low-magnitude events). Kappa coefficients ranged from high for violence and sexual abuse to low for child reports of serous accidents and natural disasters. This format has been adapted as a preface for the Children's Impact of Traumatic Events Scale–II (CITES-II; Wolfe, 2002), which is used to identify negative life events, past (greater than 2 years) and current (within the past 2 years), and has been used in gathering normative data as a tool for participants to identify a negative life event, for which they then complete the event-related questions of the various CITES-II sections.

Unidimensional Detailed Assessment of Specific Traumatic Events

In some cases, a researcher or clinician may prefer to assess the details of a specific identified event rather than survey the full range of negative life events that occurred for a particular individual. The Dimensions of Stressful Events (DOSE; Fletcher, 1996) rating scale is applicable to a broad-range of specified negative life events. The DOSE includes 25 general trauma items and 24 items specific to sexual abuse. A scoring template available for the initial 25 items yields a total DOSE score, and a recommended procedure is provided for obtaining a total score for sexual abuse victims. Fletcher (Chapter 9, this volume) reports a number of studies with diverse populations linking DOSE scores to PTSD symptoms.

Measures That Tap Abuse-Related Stressors

Quas and colleagues (2005) described a long-term follow-up (10 years) of child and adolescent victims of CSA involved in the legal system. They developed a system for quantifying four types of adversity: sexual abuse, family, legal, and other traumas. For the CSA Index, three abuse characteristics were identified from a literature search for those that were robustly associated with mental health outcomes: severity of the sexual acts (penetration vs. no penetration), closeness in relationship to the perpetrator (parent vs. not a parent), and duration of the abuse (1 day vs. more than 1 day). The CSA Index was the average of the three items. A Trauma Risk Index included additional adverse experiences at long-term follow-up: victim of a crime (with each type of crime coded separately—physical assault, burglary, physical abuse, other crime), death of loved one, foster or group home care, changes in foster/group homes, serious accident, school failure, unwanted pregnancy, rape as a adult, and sexual assault. Again, each was dichotomized and the index was the average of the items. The Legal Risk Index included the following: trial being canceled and rescheduled at least once, case lasting at least 1 year, lack of maternal support following disclosure or during legal trial, case lacking corroborating evidence, child testified in trial, and defendant not serving prison/jail term.

Spaccarelli developed two questionnaires that specifically assess aspects of the sexual abuse experience. The Abusive Sexual Exposure Scale (ASES; Spaccarelli, 1993), developed for use with girls ages 11–18, includes 28 questions about the occurrence of 14 types of sexual abuse and identity by relationship of all perpetrators for each type of abuse. In addition to two noncontact forms of abuse (peeped at, photographed when nude), six other contact forms of abuse are assessed: breast or genital fondling of victim, or victim required to fondle perpetrator; oral copulation of victim, or victim doing same to perpetrator; digital penetration of victim's anus or vagina, and genital penetration of victim's anus or vagina. The Checklist of Sexual Abuse and Related Stressors (C-SARS; Spaccarelli, 1995) includes 70 items designed to assess stressors commonly associated with sexual abuse experiences, falling into three theoretically devised scales: abuse-specific stressors, abuse-related events, and public disclosure events, such as repeated interviews. Abuse-specific stressors included several subscales: Negative Coercion, Inducements in the Form of Bribes or Rewards, Misrepresentation of Issues Related to the Sexual Abuse, Seduction, Violation of Trust, Stigmatizing Messages, and Victim Denigration. Abuse-related events included three subscales: Increased Family Conflict/Dysfunction, Loss of Social Contacts, and Nonsupportive Reactions.

As evidence of convergent validity, C-SARS scales correlated significantly with therapists' ratings of abuse-specific and abuse-related stressors. Internal consistency for the entire scale was .93, and the three scales ranged from .66 to .91.

Subjective Appraisals of Sexual Abuse

The *Children's Impact of Traumatic Events Scale–II: Peritraumatic Reactions Scales* (CITES-II) is a self-report measure that assesses negative life events, peritraumatic reactions, PTSD symptoms, attributions, perceptions of social reactions following abuse discovery/disclosure, and sexuality. It is appropriate for children and adolescents ages 8–16, and depending on reading level, can be administered as a structured interview or as an independently completed questionnaire. A number of psychometric evaluations have been completed with the CITES. A factor analysis of the initial 54-item version of the CITES (Wolfe et al., 1991) supported a two-tiered scale structure of four broad-band categories (PTSD, Attributions, Social Reactions, and Sexuality) and 11 narrow-band scales associated with the broader domains. A multitrait–multimethod analysis supported the convergent and divergent validity of the CITES scales. The original CITES was designed to assess PTSD symptoms and related constructs for sexual abuse victims (Wolfe et al., 1991; Wolfe & Birt, 2004a). The CITES-II has been reworded so that it can now be used to assess PTSD-related constructs with any negative life event. As well, previous versions of the CITES randomly interspersed PTSD, Attributional, and Social Support items throughout the questionnaire. The CITES-II now comprises five sections: Negative Life Event Checklist, Peritraumatic Reactions, PTSD, Attributions/Social Reactions, and two experimental sections, Posttraumatic Growth and Sexuality Issues (divided into child and adolescent sections). Thus, clinicians can administer the entire questionnaire or select particular sections as appropriate for an individual clinical case or research need. The diverse constructs assessed by the CITES-II are discussed within the various sections of the chapter that address different assessment issues relevant to sexual abuse victims (i.e., peritraumatic reactions [PR], PTSD symptoms, abuse-specific attributions, abuse-specific social support, and sexuality issues).

The CITES-II PR scales were developed in the absence of other measures to assess peritraumatic experiences with children. The items were originally a separate questionnaire called the Children's Peritraumatic Reactions Questionnaire (Wolfe & Birt, 2005b). The CITES-II PR includes 38 items and forms five scales based on a principal component analysis: Extreme Reactions (8 items; e.g., *Like I might die*; *Like I might faint*; *Like I wanted to kill the person who did this*); Fear and Anxiety (5 items; e.g., *Scared*; *Shaky*; *Worried*); Dissociation (9 items, e.g., *Like I left my body*; *Like I wasn't there*; *Like I lost sense of time*); Anger and Negative Affect (10 items; e.g., *Mad*; *Disgusted*; *Upset*); and Guilt/Self-Blame (5 items; e.g., *Like I caused it*; *Guilt*; *Like it was my fault*). Respondents are asked to consider their thoughts and feelings at the time of sexual abuse (or another identified negative life event) and identify their reactions on a 3-point scale of *None*, *Some*, or *A lot*. All of the scales have good internal consistency alphas (> .80), with the exception of the three-item Guilt scale (alpha = .54), which has since been expanded to include five items. With the exception of the Guilt scale, youth who completed the CITES-II PR scales with regard to sexual abuse experiences reported more intense peritraumatic reactions on all scales compared to youth who responded with regard to other negative life events. For the five scales, Extreme Reactions showed the strongest relationships with PTSD symptoms, whether reported by the child or the parent (Wolfe & Birt, 2005b).

Abuse-Related Attributions

The *CITES-II Attributional Scales* were originally developed to reflect the three attributional dimensions associated with the revised learned helpless model of depression (internal, global, and specific attributions for negative events), as well as the traumagenic factors (guilt, betrayal, sexualization, and stigmatization) identified by Finkelhor and Browne (1985). Two principal component analyses of two datasets have shaped the content and focus of the Attributional Scales, yielding the following four subscales: Guilt/Self-Blame (7 items; alpha = .81; e.g., "I feel guilty about what happened"), Empowerment (3 items; alpha = .78; e.g., "I know enough about sexual abuse now that I can protect myself in the future"), Dan-

gerous World (7 items; alpha = .67; e.g., "People often take advantage of children"), and Distrust (4 items; alpha = .65; e.g., "Something like this might happen to me again"). A recent psychometric analysis of the revised CITES (CITES-R; Wolfe & Birt, 2005a) resulted in some minor changes to a previous subscale, Personal Vulnerability, with a name change to Distrust. The three more negatively valenced scales correlated moderately (Guilt/Self-Blame, Dangerous World, Distrust; r's = .26–.29), but Empowerment did not correlate with the other Attributional Scales. Guilt/Self-Blame, Distrust, and Dangerous World correlated with PTSD Reexperiencing and Hyperarousal scales (r's = .28–.52), and Distrust also correlated with PTSD Avoidance (r = .32). As well, Guilt/Self-Blame and Distrust correlated with PTSD Sexual Anxiety (r's = .62 and .25, respectively). Empowerment did not correlate with any of the PTSD scales. However, Empowerment correlated significantly with both of the Social Reaction scales (r's = .37 for Social Support and –.22 for Negative Reactions). Of the four attributional scales, only Distrust distinguished between sexual abuse victims and both community controls and other clinic-referred youth. As well, both Distrust and Dangerous World had higher scores among sexual abuse victims with PTSD compared to those without PTSD.

Research from other studies has also supported the psychometric properties of the CITES Attributional Scales. Crouch, Smith, Ezzell, and Saunders (1999) found that Guilt/Self-Blame, Personal Vulnerability, and Empowerment all correlated with the TSCC (Briere, 1996) PTSD scale (r's = .47, .65, and –.53, respectively). Chaffin and Shultz (2001) found that Guilt/Self-Blame was sensitive to treatment-related changes. Taska and Feiring (1995) found that all four attributional scales correlated with both abuse-related and general measures of shame.

The Children's Attributions and Perceptions Scale (CAPS; Mannarino, Cohen, & Berman, 1994), an 18-item, self-report questionnaire for children ages 7 to 12, was designed for administration in an interview format that uses a 5-point Likert-like scale ranging from *Never* (1) to *Always* (5). The CAPS yields four conceptually derived scales: Feeling Different from Peers (4 items; alpha = .68; e.g., "Do you feel different than other girls your age?"); Personal Attributions for Negative Events (4 items; alpha = .65; e.g., "Do you blame yourself when things go wrong?"); Perceived Credibility (5 items; alpha = .73; e.g., "Do you think people believe you when you tell them something?"); and Interpersonal Trust (5 items; alpha = .64; e.g., "Do you ever feel that people whom you trust do things to hurt you?"). Test–retest reliabilities after 2 weeks were .82, .70, .62, .60 for the individual scales, respectively, and .75 for the total scale. The items do not refer specifically to sexual abuse, so the CAPS can be used with normal comparison samples. Mannarino and colleagues (1994) found that sexually abused children endorsed more items for the total CAPS score and three of the four scales compared to nonabused controls (Feeling Different from Peers, Personal Attributions for Negative Events, and Interpersonal Trust. CAPS scales correlated with measures of depression, anxiety, and PTSD (Cohen & Mannarino, 2000; Mannarino et al., 1994). As well, scores from the CAPS predicted treatment outcome for sexually abused children (Cohen & Mannarino, 2000).

The Negative Appraisals of Sexual Abuse Scale (NASAS; Spaccarelli, 1995; Spaccarelli & Fuchs, 1997) is a 56-item self-report of perceptions of threat or harm related to sexual victimization. The scale yields a total score, as well as eight theoretically based subscales: Physical Pain/Damage, Negative Self-Evaluation–Global, Negative Self-Evaluation–Sexuality, Negative Evaluation by Others, Loss of Desired Resources, Harm to Relationships/Security, Harm to Others, and Criticism of Others. Each item begins with the stem "Because of what happened with (offender's name), did it make you think or feel. . . . " Responses are rated on a 4-point scale, from *Not at all* to *A lot*. Spaccerelli (1995) recommended using the full scale rather than individual scales because of high intercorrelations among the individual scales. The total score also had a strong internal consistency alpha value of .93. Scores from the NASAS correlated significantly with higher numbers of sexual acts, as assessed by the ASES, and with scores from the C-SARS. Whereas abuse resulting from stress accounted for only 2% of the variance in PTSD scores, negative appraisals significant predicted PTSD and accounted for 25% of the variance. Negative appraisals also significantly predicted depression scores, accounting for 29% of the variance.

Measures of Shame

The concepts *guilt/self-blame* and *shame* differ primarily in the focus of the emotional attribution, with guilt/self-blame focusing on the event and actions taken or not taken, and shame focusing on the negative emotions oriented toward oneself in relation to an event (Berliner, 2005). Shame is considered an important emotional reaction to abuse because of its implication for PTSD; that is, shame is thought to motivate avoidance of self-exposure (Barrett, Zahn-Waxler, & Cole, 1993; Feiring & Taska, 2005; Tangney, 1995; Zupanic & Kreidler, 1998), thus inhibiting the healing processes needed to adjust following negative life events. As an example, Bonanno and colleagues (2002) asked CSA victims to talk about their most negative life event as part of an assessment procedure. Victims who selected an event other than their sexual abuse (presumably indicating avoidance of talking about their sexual abuse), showed more nonverbal indicators of shame while discussing their event. Shame also has implications for depression. Concerns have been raised that shame engenders a wide array of negative self-representations that are consistent with the negative thinking characteristics of depression, and that shame interferes with the development of positive self-traits such as self-agency and self-affectivity (Alessandri & Lewis, 1996).

Feiring, Taska, and Lewis (2002) followed sexual abuse victims from disclosure across several years. At each assessment point, abuse-related shame was linked with PTSD symptoms, demonstrating that shame has significant predictive power for PTSD even years after disclosure. In fact, changes in shame over time were linked with concomitant changes in PTSD. Feiring and colleagues have used several different strategies to assess shame. For two studies, they used four items: I feel ashamed because I think that people can tell from looking at me what happened; When I think about what happened I want to go away by myself and hide; I am ashamed because I feel I am the only one in my school who this has happened to; and What happened to me makes me feel dirty. Each item was rated on a 3-point scale (*Not true* to *Very true*). Despite the small number of items, internal consistency of the scale was good (alpha = .85). As well, test–retest reliability with a small sample of 10 over a 2-week period was good (r = .78). At the third assessment, four more items were added to the scale: *When I think about what happened, I feel like covering my body; When I think about what happened, I wish I were invisible; When I think about what happened, I feel disgusted with myself;* and *When I think about what happened, I feel exposed.* For the eight items, internal consistency continued to be good (alpha = .86).

Feiring, Taska, and Lewis (2002) also developed a nonverbal assessment tool with line drawings that depicted various postures associated with shame. Participants were asked to rate each drawing for the extent to which it described how they felt when thinking about their sexual abuse, using the same 3-point scale used for the verbal shame scale described previously. The internal consistency for the drawing measure was also high (alpha = .92), and the measure correlated with the concurrently administered verbal items described earlier. As well, the drawing measure results were predicted by prior administrations of the verbal items.

Negrao and colleagues (2005) used facial expressions to examine shame, which were coded from videotapes of CSA victims as they described their most negative life event. The Emotional Facial Action Coding System (EMFACS), which is based on the Facial Action Coding System (FACS; Ekman & Friesen, 1976, 1978), assessed only emotionally relevant facial muscle movements identified in previous research with the FACS. Using the EMFACS, anger, shame, and embarrassment were coded with a 5-point scale, ranging from *Minimum intensity* to *Extreme intensity.* Interrater agreement averaged .80. Interestingly, whereas facial expressions tended to be congruent with verbal content for a nonabused sample, for CSA victims, facial expressions were not necessarily congruent with verbal content. Victims who chose to discuss their sexual abuse tended to express shame and humiliation through words but not facial expressions. However, those who chose not to disclose their abuse history did not display verbal evidence of shame, but instead displayed nonverbal evidence of shame (Bonanno et al., 2002; Negrao et al., 2005).

Other studies have focused more on a general attribute of shame proneness rather than shame that is specific to sexual abuse or maltreatment. The Adolescent Shame Measure (ASM; Reimer, 1995) assesses shame proneness

by presenting 13 brief scenarios (e.g., *You say something mean about a friend. Your friend overhears you*), to which respondents rate the likeliness of four reactions that reflect Shame, Guilt, Anger/Blame, and Detachment (e.g., the shame statement is "I would feel totally awful about myself"; the guilt statement is "I would be sorry that I hurt their feelings"). Internal consistency for Shame ranged from .77 to .81, and for Guilt, .72 to .78 (Reimer, 1995; Stuewig & McCloskey, 2005). Reimer (1996) linked these concepts with self-esteem, self-consciousness, and depressed mood in adolescents. With a mixed sample of adolescents who experienced various forms of maltreatment, shame proneness was linked with parental criticism and depression. Interestingly, guilt was negatively associated with delinquent behavior. Some evidence has linked the experience of guilt with empathetic abilities (Tangney, 1991), perhaps enhancing one's ability to see the harmful consequence of behavioral offenses (Stuewig & McCloskey, 2005).

Bennett, Sullivan, and Lewis (2005) assessed shame proneness with a sample of physically abused and neglected preschool children using success–failure tasks. Conditions were manipulated so that the child experienced either success or failure on timed color-matching and puzzle completion tasks. Facial, body, and vocal behaviors were used to code shame, anger, and sadness from videotapes. "Shame" was defined as collapsed body, turned down corners of mouth, tucked up lower lip, eyes lowered or askance, withdrawal from the task, and negative self-evaluations, such as "I'm too slow." Average interrater reliability across the three emotions' codes was 93%, ranging from 85–97%, with kappas averaging .73, ranging from .62 to .82. Physical abuse, but not neglect, was related to increased shame responses, and shame was linked with anger.

Social and Family Supports and Stressors

The *CITES-II Social Reactions Scales* are two factor-derived scales that tap reactions to the disclosure and postdisclosure support: Social Support (Cronbach's alpha = .72) and Negative Reactions (Cronbach's alpha = .81). The modest negative correlation between the two scales (–.31) suggests that these scales are not opposite ends of one construct, but rather tap different aspects of postdisclosure social reactions. Negative Reactions items include concerns that people disbelieve the allegations, blame the victim, or no longer care about the child. Social Support items reflect a perception that people believed the allegations, protected the victim from further maltreatment, and were helpful and supportive. The Negative Reactions scale appears to tap an important construct related to postabuse adjustment problems. Negative Reactions correlates positively with CITES-II PTSD Reexperiencing ($r = .36$) and Hyperarousal scales ($r = .53$), and differentiates between those who meet PTSD symptom criteria from those who do not (Wolfe & Birt, 2005a). As well, Crouch and colleagues (1999) found significant correlations between the Negative Reactions scale and several TSCC scales, including Posttraumatic Stress ($r = .50$), Anxiety ($r = .38$), Depression ($r = .62$), Anger ($r = .42$), Dissociation ($r = .38$), and Sexual Concerns ($r = .49$). As evidence of convergent validity, Chaffin and Shultz (2001) found that the Negative Reactions scale correlated significantly with a therapists' ratings of parental support using the Parental Response to Abuse Disclosure Scale (PRADS; Runyan, Hunter, Everson, & De Vos, 1992).

Mannarino and Cohen (1996a) developed two parent report measures to assess parental reactions to their child's sexual abuse. The Parent Emotional Reaction Questionnaire (PERQ) is a 15-item, Likert-like 5-point scale (*Never* to *Always*) that assesses parental emotional reactions to their child's sexual abuse, including fear, sadness, guilt, anger, embarrassment, shame, and emotional preoccupation (Mannarino & Cohen, 1996a, 1996b). Psychometric properties include good internal consistency for the scale (alpha = .87) and test–retest reliability at a 2-week interval ($r = .90$). Two studies have demonstrated a positive relationship between the intensity of the parent's emotional reaction and child adjustment problems, both before and after treatment, with preschool- and latency-age children (Cohen & Mannarino, 1998; Mannarino & Cohen, 1996b).

The Parental Support Questionnaire (PSQ) includes 19 items and yields two scales, Support (Cronbach's alpha = .73) and Blame (Cronbach's alpha = .70). The PSQ was designed to assess parental perceptions of their own behaviors in response to their child's sexual abuse experience. The Support scale includes items such as parents encouraging the child to express feelings associated with the abuse, efforts to enhance the child's sense of security, and communication of support to the child. The Blame scale includes items such as parental belief that the child could have stopped the abuse if he or she had wanted to and criticism and/or punishment of the child over issues related to the abuse. Like the PERQ, the PSQ had good test–retest reliability over a 2-week period (.79 and .83, respectively). Although it did not predict baseline adjustment with preschoolers (perhaps because most of the sample reported strong support for the children; Mannarino & Cohen, 1996b), Cohen and Mannarino (1998) found that the PSQ was a significant predictor of adjustment at 6- and 12-month posttreatment follow-up points.

The Parental Reaction to Incest Disclosure Scale (PRIDS; Everson et al., 1989) is a three-item scale designed to document parental reactions and support following disclosure of intrafamilial sexual abuse. Professionals rate three issues along a continuum from +5 (*Most supportive*) to –5 (*Least supportive*), based on interviews with the family members and reports from agency staff members involved with the family. The three items are Emotional Support (e.g., from *Committed to child and provides meaningful support*, to *Is threatening or hostile; has abandoned the child psychologically*); Belief of the Child (e.g., from *Makes clear, public statement of belief* to *Totally denies that abuse occurred*); and Action toward Perpetrator (e.g., from *Actively demonstrates disapproval of perpetrator's abusive behavior* to *Chooses perpetrator over child at child's expense*). In Everson and colleagues' (1989) sample of 88 families, interrater agreement was quite high (.95), with 44% of mothers classified as "supportive" (+3 or greater), 32% as "ambivalent" (+2 to –2), and 24% as "unsupportive" (at or below –3). Maternal support on the PRIDS was significantly related to child distress and psychological adjustment, accounting for more variance than any abuse-related variable. Interestingly, supportive mothers and their children had similar reports of child behavioral and emotional adjustment. However, CBCL scores from ambivalent and unsupportive mothers did not correspond to information obtained in clinical interviews with their children.

Measures of General Family Functioning

In addition to assessing abuse-specific aspects of family support, many studies have examined overall family functioning in terms of how families of sexual abuse victims differ from other families, and how family adjustment affects child psychopathology. Two questionnaires have been used by several researchers, the *Family Environment Scale* (FES; Moos & Moos, 1986) and the *Family Adaptability and Cohesion Scales* (FACES; versions II and III; Olson, Portner, & Bell, 1982; Olson, Portner, & Lavee, 1985). The FES yields seven scales, but research with sexual abuse victims has focused on two scales, Conflict and Cohesion. Families of sexual abuse victims tend to have low levels of Cohesion (Bal et al., 2004; Cecil & Matson, 2005; Dadds, Smith, Webber, & Robinson, 1991; Hanson, Saunders, & Lipovsky, 1992), and two studies have revealed high levels of Conflict, but only for families of girls (Cecil & Matson, 2005; Meyerson et al., 2002). The FACES-II and III both yielded two scores, Adaptability and Cohesion. Mannarino and Cohen (1996b) found relatively low Cohesion for families of sexual abuse victims and linked low levels of Adaptability to higher rates of child behavior problems (Mannarino & Cohen, 1996b). The FACES-IV (Olson & Gorall, 2006), an expansion of the original form, now comprises 62 items. The original Cohesion and Adaptability scales were preserved, but the Adaptability scale was renamed Flexibility. The Cohesion and Flexibility scales are considered balanced, in that higher scores reflect better family functioning. Four new scales were added, labeled unbalanced scales, which assess the low and high extremes of Cohesion (i.e., Disengaged and Enmeshed), and the lows and highs of Flexibility (i.e., Rigid and Chaotic). The circumplex model is used to interpret the scales, which are plotted to yield profile types (Olson & Gorall, 2006). The circumplex model examines different combinations of high and low extremes for Cohesion and Adaptability, and how the variations reflect different forms of familial dysfunction.

Assessing PTSD

Over the past decade, there have been tremendous strides in the assessment of PTSD with children and adolescents (Ohan, Myers, & Collett, 2002; Strand, Sarmiento, & Pasquale, 2005). Fletcher (Chapter 9, this volume) provides a review of these measures as a whole. In this chapter, the discussion is limited to measures that have been used extensively to assess PTSD with sexually abused children.

The Trauma Symptom Checklist for Children (TSCC; Briere, 1996, 2006a) is a 54-item self-report measure designed to assess children's reactions to trauma across several symptom areas: Anxiety, Depression, Anger, Posttraumatic Stress, Dissociation, and Sexual Concerns (Sexual Preoccupation and Sexual Distress). A 44-item alternative version does not include the Sexual Concerns items. The TSCC also yields two validity scales, Underresponse and Hyperresponse, that have demonstrated usefulness in detecting response biases (Davies & Flannery, 1998). Norms are available for males and females ages 6–17, representing over 3,000 youth from various locations across the United States. Each scale has good internal consistency, with alphas in the mid to high .80's; however, the Sexual Concerns scale is somewhat less reliable, with alphas in the .60's to .70's. Several studies have demonstrated the reliability and convergent, divergent, discriminant, and construct validity of the TSCC (Briere, 1996; Elliott & Briere, 1994; Friedrich et al., 1997; Lanktree & Briere, 1995; Sadowski & Friedrich, 2000; Singer, Anglin, Song, & Lunghofer, 1995). As well, the TSCC appears to be sensitive to change following mental health interventions (Henry, 1997; Lanktree & Briere, 1995). The TSCC has been translated into several languages, and the French Canadian version has demonstrated positive psychometric properties (Wright et al., 1998).

The Trauma Symptom Checklist for Young Children (TSCYC; Briere, 2006b; Briere et al., 2001) is a caregiver report measure designed to assess trauma-related symptoms in children ages 3–12. The 90-item measure, written at a grade 6 reading level, yields eight clinical scales: Posttraumatic Stress–Intrusion, Posttraumatic Stress–Avoidance, Posttraumatic Stress–Arousal, Sexual Concerns, Dissociation, Anxiety, Depression, and Anger or Aggression. The three Posttraumatic Stress scales can be amalgamated to form a summary PTSD score. As well, item responses can be used to determine DSM-IV PTSD diagnostic status for children age 5 and older, with a sensitivity of .72 and specificity of .75 (Briere, 2006b). Norms are based on a stratified sample of 750 children. Alpha values for the norm sample averaged .86 per scale, ranging from .78 to .92;

similar alphas have been reported for clinical and child abuse samples. Test–retest reliability ranges between .68 and .96, averaging .88 across scales. Overall, the scales have demonstrated good discriminant, predictive, and construct validity.

Like the other CITES-II scales, the *CITES-II PTSD scale* (Wolfe, 2002) has been shaped by two previous psychometric evaluations. The original PTSD items were influenced by the Impact of Event Scale (IES; Horowitz, Wilner, & Alvarez, 1979), and additional items have been added to tap issues relevant to children and adolescents, and to cover all the symptoms identified in DSM-IV-TR. The CITES-II PTSD scales contain 46 items, reflecting four scales: Reexperiencing, Avoidance, Hyperarousal, and Sexual Anxiety. Past studies have indicated that the CITES-R PTSD scales have good internal consistency (Chaffin & Shultz, 2001; Crouch et al., 1999). As well, the CITES-R PTSD scales have good convergent validity with the TSCC PTSD scales (Crouch et al., 1999; $r = .72$) and with Diagnostic Interview for Children and Adolescents—Revised (DICA-R) PTSD Child Report scale (Reexperiencing, $r = .50$; Avoidance, $r = .38$; Hyperarousal, $r = .45$; and Sexual Anxiety, $r = .25$—Chaffin & Shultz, 2001). As well, the CITES-R was sensitive in detecting pre- to posttreatment changes (Berliner & Saunders, 1996; Chaffin & Shultz, 2001). Collin-Vézina and Hébert (2005), using a French translation of the CITES-R PTSD scales, reported good internal consistency for the total PTSD score (alpha = .81), and found that history of sexual abuse increased the odds of CITES-R-based PTSD diagnoses fourfold. They also found that sexual penetration was associated with higher PTSD scores.

Wolfe and Birt (2005a) conducted a psychometric analysis of the CITES-R with a sample of sexual abuse victims, clinic-referred youth without a sexual abuse history, and community controls without a history of maltreatment or mental health problems. A principal component analysis of the CITES-R supported the existing factor structure. Alpha values for the PTSD scales follow: Reexperiencing (12 items; .88); Sexual Anxiety (.84); Avoidance (18 items, .78); and Hyperarousal (13 items; .63). Sexual abuse victims reported more total PTSD symptoms than did the comparison samples, with the Reexperiencing, Sexual Anxiety, and Avoidance scales also discriminating among the groups. The CITES-R covers all the DSM-IV-TR diagnostic criteria; thus, diagnostic status can be calculated for the symptom criteria. Wolfe and Birt found higher rates of PTSD for sexual abuse victims using the CITES-R compared to both clinic-referred and community youth. Depending on the level of symptoms required for a diagnosis, 55% of CSA victims met the low PTSD criterion (sufficient symptoms endorsed, each at least rated as *Somewhat or sometimes true*), and 24% met the high PTSD criterion (sufficient symptoms endorsed, all rates as *Very or often true*).

Thus far, my colleagues and I have created two CITES-II databases, a clinical trauma sample ($n = 60$) and a representative sample of high school girls ($n = 151$). For the clinical trauma sample, Cronbach alpha values for the scales are Reexperiencing (.87); Avoidance, (.76); and Hyperarousal (.89). For the high school girls sample, alpha values are Reexperiencing (.86); Avoidance (.91); and Hyperarousal (.90). In addition to including all symptom criteria for a DSM-IV-TR PTSD diagnosis, the CITES-II PTSD items are followed by three items designed to assess perceived functional impairment of relationships with family and friends, and school performance.

The CITES-II—Parent Report version (CITES-II-PR; Wolfe, 2000) comprises the CITES-II PTSD and Social Reactions items. The CITES-PR has 24 PTSD items, 6 Social Support items, and 8 Negative Reactions items. Based on a sample of children and adolescents referred to a trauma-focused mental health clinic ($n = 122$), internal consistency alpha values were .91, .80, and .81, respectively. Based on 52 individuals administered both the CITES-II and the CITES-PR, the total PTSD scores correlated significantly ($r = .47$). As expected, parent-reported PTSD symptoms correlated significantly with the Negative Reactions ($r = .30$) scale. Unexpectedly, parent-reported PTSD symptoms also correlated positively with the Social Support scale ($r = .28$). Perhaps children who experience PTSD subsequent to negative life events are more likely to provide and to recall social support given to themselves and to others.

The Child Behavior Checklist (CBCL; Achenbach & Rescorla, 2001) is a commonly used parent report questionnaire that assesses a broad spectrum of child adjustment problems. Although the CBCL was not designed to assess PTSD, many of the items reflect PTSD symptoms. In an effort to document PTSD symptoms via parent report, Wolfe and colleagues (1989) selected 20 CBCL items that matched PTSD diagnostic criteria. Compared to the standardization sample, parents of sexually abused children endorsed PTSD items five times more frequently. Wolfe and Birt (1997) compared individual CBCL items across three samples: sexually abused, clinic-referred (but not sexually abused), and the CBCL standardization sample. Nineteen of the 20 items were more common in the sexually abused sample compared to the standardization group, and 11 of the 20 items differentiated between the sexually abused and the clinic-referred groups. Ruggiero and colleagues (2000) investigated the psychometric properties of the 20 CBCL PTSD items. The CBCL PTSD scale significantly discriminated between PTSD and no PTSD sexual abuse cases. CBCL PTSD scale scores were higher among sexually abused victims compared to a general school sample but did not differentiate between the sexual abuse sample and outpatient psychiatric controls. Fourteen items either correlated significantly with the number of PTSD symptoms reported during diagnostic interviews or significantly differentiated between sexually abused victims who either met or did not meet PTSD diagnostic criteria. Wolfe and Birt (2005a) modified the CBCL PTSD scale to include the 14 items identified by Ruggiero and colleagues. Thus, the CBCL PTSD scale now comprises the following items: Argues a lot, difficulty concentrating, obsessive thoughts, clings to adults, too guilty, secretive, moody, unhappy, withdrawn, fears doing something bad, feels persecuted, nervous, nightmares, and too fearful. Based on a mixed sample of sexual abuse victims, agency referred youth, and community controls, Cronbach's alpha value for the 14 items was .86. For the sexual abuse sample, the correlation between the CITES-R PTSD scale and the CBCL PTSD scale was .28 ($p <$ .001). To examine the discriminative validity of the PTSD CBCL scale, the CITES-R was used to determine PTSD status for the sexual abuse sample. For the sexual abuse sample, CBCL PTSD scores were higher among those with PTSD compared to those who scored low on PTSD symptoms. Furthermore, CBCL PTSD scores among sexual abuse victims

were predicted by factors that tend to predict PTSD via other assessment strategies, including having experienced physical abuse in addition to the sexual abuse, and reports of extreme peritraumatic reactions at the time of the sexual abuse.

Assessing Dissociation

Current assessment strategies for childhood dissociation are limited (Silberg, 2000). Regardless of age, dissociative symptoms are very difficult to identify through typical psychological assessment strategies, because dissociated individuals are required to self-report on phenomena that affect their own continuity of consciousness, thus impairing their capacities for self-awareness and self-monitoring. In addition to these general difficulties, the assessment of dissociation in childhood is further complicated by several factors (Friedrich, 2002; McElroy, 1992; Ogata, Silk, & Goodrich, 1990; Putnam, 1997): (1) Relative to adults, children have a limited capacity to report on behavioral, cognitive, and emotional states; (2) relative to adults, they have a poorer sense of continuity in their experience, behavior, and the flow of time; (3) child dissociation presents subtly in childhood relative to adulthood, perhaps due to its diagnostically confounded nature with normative childhood dissociative experiences and other childhood disorders (such as oppositional problems, PTSD, MDD, or schizophrenia); and (4) given that one's sense of self and identity are not formed until late adolescence, dissociative disorders that are more directly related to identity and self (e.g., dissociative identity disorder [DID]) may manifest only subtly and progressively during later childhood and adolescence.

Parent/Caregiver Report

The Child Dissociation Checklist (CDC; Putnam, 1990; Sidran Traumatic Foundation, 2000b) was developed for use with children and adolescents ages 5–14. Parents report dissociative symptoms displayed by their child over the past 12 months, with the response options *Very true*, *Somewhat or sometimes true*, and *Not true*. Several dissociative symptoms are assessed, including imaginary friends, different identities, moodiness, forgetfulness, thought absorption, and "spaciness." Based on an initial psychometric evaluation of the CDC, the 20-item scale yielded one score, with a Cronbach's alpha of .91 (Putnam, Helmers, & Trickett, 1993), and a 1-year test–retest reliability of .84 for sexually abused children and .79 for controls. The CDC total score discriminates between maltreated and nonmaltreated children, and between children with DID and those with other dissociative disorders and normal controls (Macfie et al., 2001; Putnam et al., 1993). Collin-Vézina and Hébert (2005) found that a history of sexual abuse increased eightfold the odds of pathological levels of dissociation on the CDC. As well, higher scores have been associated with more extensive abuse history (Putnam & Peterson, 1994). Norms are available based on modest samples for sexually abused, dissociative, and community youth ages 6–14 years. High CDC total scores have been linked with younger age, family dysfunction, and hypnotizability (Ohan et al., 2002).

Because of the breadth of the symptoms included on the CDC, clinical interpretation of the total CDC score can to be difficult. Six conceptually defined domains have been identified (Feindler, Rathus, & Silver, 2003; Putnam & Peterson, 1994): Dissociative Amnesia, Rapid Shifts in Demeanor and Abilities, Spontaneous Trance States, Hallucinations, Identity Alterations, and Aggressive or Sexualized Behavior. Psychometric properties and norms for the individual scales are not available. To aid in the clinical interpretation of the CDC, Zayed and colleagues (2006) conducted a series of psychometric analyses to examine scale content and structure. Based on group comparisons (sexually abused, clinic-referred/nonabused, and community control boys and girls) and a principal component analysis, the scale content was reduced to 14 items that produced three scales: Forgetful/Confused (Cronbach's alpha = .67; e.g., Child is unusually forgetful or confused about things that he or she should know), Absorption/Fantasy Proneness (alpha = .74; e.g., Child has vivid imaginary companion or companions; child may insist that the imaginary companion is responsible for things that he or she has done), and Identity/Self-Disturbance (Cronbach's alpha = .79; e.g., Child refers to him- or herself in the third person when talking about self, or at time insists on being called by a different name). Group comparisons revealed that all three scales differentiate between sex-

ual abuse victims and community controls, but not between sexual abuse victims and other agency-referred youth.

Self-Report of Dissociation

MEASURES SUITABLE FOR CHILDREN

The Child Dissociation Checklist—Child (CDC-C; Wolfe & Birt, 2002) was developed as a self-report version of the CDC, with language appropriate for children as young as 8 years. Zayed and colleagues (2006) conducted a series of psychometric analyses that resulted in a 17-item version that yields three scales: Forgetful/Confused (Cronbach's alpha = .67), Spaciness/Daydreaming/Fantasy (Cronbach's alpha = .74), and Identity/Self (Cronbach's alpha = .79). The Identify/Self scale was psychometrically sound only for the adolescent sample, suggesting that these personality dimensions are less well formulated or less often self-identified by children. As with the parent report version, although the scales differentiated between sexually abused and the community comparison samples, the sexually abused group did not differ from other agency-referred youth.

The Children's Perceptual Alteration Scale (CPAS; Evers-Szostak, 2002; Evers-Szostak & Sanders, 1992), drawn from the adult self-report Perceptual Alteration Scale (Sanders, 1986), is another self-report scale for children ages 8–12 years. Although the scale yields one total score, the items reflect six aspects of dissociation: Automatic Experiences, Imaginary Playmates, Amnesia, Loss of Time, Heightened Monitoring, and Loss of Control over Behaviors and Emotions. Internal consistency was reported to be good for a clinical sample but moderate for a nonclinical sample (Ohan et al., 2002). Rhue, Lynn, and Sandberg (1995) compared CPAS results for sexually abused, physically abused, and nonabused children. Although the total score distinguished between physically abused and nonabused children, it did not identify sexual abuse victims. The scale differentiated between children with and without mental health problems, and also correlated positively with measures of fantasy and imagination. Ohan and colleagues (2002) noted that some of the CPAS items are general and not specific to dissociation (e.g., I am hungry; I cannot sit still; I don't like going to school), and recommended caution in interpreting individual items.

MEASURES SUITABLE FOR ADOLESCENTS

The *Adolescent Dissociative Experiences Scale* (A-DES; Armstrong, Putnam, Carlson, Libero, & Smith, 1997; Sidran Traumatic Stress Foundation, 2002a; Smith & Carlson, 1996) is an adolescent version (ages 11–21 years) of the adult Dissociative Experiences Scale (DES; Bernstein & Putnam, 1986; Van IJzendoorn & Schuengel, 1996). The 28-item A-DES yields a total score, as well as four conceptually derived subscale scores: Dissociative Amnesia, Absorption and Imaginative Involvement, Passive Influence, and Depersonalization/Derealization. However, a principal component analysis with a community sample failed to support a four-factor structure (Farrington, Waller, Smerden, & Faupel, 2001). Internal consistency for the total score was .91, and the subscale alpha values ranged from .64 to .83. Test–retest reliability at a 2-week interval was .77. Norms are available based on a diverse but modest-size sample (Ohan et al., 2002), and a French Canadian version is available. The A-DES discriminates between clinically referred traumatized youth, including samples of physically and sexually abused youth, and nontraumatized youth (Armstrong et al., 1997; Farrington et al., 2001; Svedin, Nilsson, & Lindell, 2004). As well, the A-DES has good sensitivity (80%) and specificity (74%) in detecting dissociative disorders with both clinic-referred and nonclinical samples. Interestingly, Prohl, Resch, Parzer, and Brunner (2001) found that A-DES scores correlated with declarative memory scores.

Direct Observation for Preschool-Age Children

The Attachment Story Completion Task (ASCT; Bretherton, Ridgeway, & Cassidy, 1990) was designed to elicit responses reflecting the attachment relationship between child and parent. Children are told the beginning of stories, with the aid of dolls and props, and are asked to complete the story. Five story-stems are used: (1) parent as an authority figure (story depicts a child that spilled his or her juice); (2) parent as comforter (child falls off a rock and hurts his or her knee); (3) parent as protector (child calls for parents at night thinking he or she has seen a monster); (4) separation of the child from his or her parents (par-

ents leave for a trip, leaving the children with their grandmother); and (5) the reunion (child and parents reunite the next day). The ASCT takes about 25 minutes to administer and is videotaped for later coding. Macfie and colleagues (2001) developed 15 codes within six domains designed to capture dissociation in children's narrative story-stem completions. The six domains include Disruptions in Memory, Disruptions in Perception, Disruptions in Identity, Inconsistent Parents, Difficulty with Loss, and Controllingness. Kappas ranged from .65 to 1.00, with a mean kappa of .86. Twelve of the 15 codes correlated significantly with the CDC total score, and were used to form a total narrative dissociation score. With a sample of 79 preschool children (ages 3–5), narrative dissociation correlated significantly with the parent-completed CDC (r = .68) and with a CBCL Dissociation scale (r = .46) (Ogawa et al., 1997). Cronbach's alpha was .79. As evidence of discriminant validity, and to address concerns that measures of dissociation simply assess proneness toward behavior problems, the narrative dissociation scores correlated significantly more strongly with the CDC than with the majority of the CBCL scales. As well, physically and sexually maltreated children demonstrated more dissociation than did the nonmaltreated group. Maltreated and community control children were tested twice, with a 1-year interval. Whereas sexually and physically abused children showed an increase in dissociative behaviors over time, neglected and nonmaltreated children showed no changes.

Assessing Sexual Problems in Children

Sexual behavior is generally private and not readily reported by children. Thus, assessment of children's sexual behavior has typically relied on parent report (Kendall-Tackett et al., 1993). However, as children grow older, parents know less about their children's sexual behaviors. Thus, parent reports of children's sexual behaviors typically yields the most accurate information, whereas adolescent reports are more reliable and valid.

The Child Sexual Behavior Inventory (CSBI; Friedrich, 1997), a 38-item, parent report measure, is designed to assess child sexual behaviors such as self-stimulation, sexual aggression, gender role discrepancies, and personal boundary violations. The CSBI, appropriate for children ages 2–12 years, is rated on a 4-point scale for the previous 6-month period. In addition to a total CSBI score, two other scale scores are provided: Development-Related Sexual Behavior and Sexual Abuse Specific Items (Feindler et al., 2003). Norms for age and gender are provided, and the CSBI is available in French, Spanish, German, and Swedish, in addition to English. Internal consistencies for the total score ranged from .82 for a nonclinical sample and .93 for a clinical sample. Test–retest reliability was .85 for both 1-month and 3-month intervals. In the normative sample, young children were rated as displaying more sexual behaviors than older children (Friedrich et al., 1992). In fact, less sexual behavior is typically reported for each year after age 5 (Friedrich, 1997). Another study found that 26 of the 35 items were endorsed significantly more often for sexually abused children than for the normative sample (Friedrich et al., 1992). The CSBI discriminates between sexually abused and nonabused children more reliably than the CBCL Sexual Problems scale and is more strongly related to sexual abuse characteristics (including type of abuse, number of perpetrators, and use of force).

The Adolescent Clinical Sexual Behavior Inventory (ACSBI; Friedrich et al., 2004) was designed for clinical use to assess sexual risk taking, nonconforming sexual behaviors, sexual interest, and sexual avoidance/discomfort. Items were created to assess high-risk behaviors pertinent to adolescent physical and mental health concerns such as early-onset sexual behavior, unprotected intercourse, sexual victimization, multiple partners, running away from home, heightened sexual interest, sexual avoidance, fear or discomfort around the opposite sex, sexual aggression, and prostitution (Friedrich et al., 2004). The 45-item checklist has three response options (*Not true*, *Somewhat true*, and *Very true*) with consideration of the previous 12 months. A parent report version (ACSBI-P) that mirrors the adolescent self-report version (ACSBI-S) was also developed. Based on principal component analyses, the ACSBI yields five scores: Divergent Sexual Interest (5 items; alpha = .65; e.g., owns pornography); Sexual Knowledge/Interest (10 items; alpha = .84; e.g., is very interested in the opposite sex); Sexual Risk/ Misuse (10 items; alpha = .77; e.g., gets used sexually by others); Concerns about Appearance (4 items; alpha = .68; e.g., is unhappy with looks); and Fear/Discomfort (5 items; alpha = .45; e.g., has no friends of

the opposite sex). The ACSBI-P also yields the same five scores with some variation in item content: Divergent Sexual Interest (9 items; alpha = .81; e.g., has been accused of sexually abusing another person); Sexual Knowledge/ Interest (13 items; alpha = .76; e.g., flirts with other teens or adults); Sexual Risk/Misuse (8 items; alpha = .79; e.g., has unprotected sex); Concerns about Appearance (4 items; alpha = .65; e.g., is concerned about looking just right); and Fear (7 items; alpha = .39; e.g., does not like to shower or bathe). Internal consistencies were .86 for the self-report total score and .84 for the parent total score. One-week test–retest reliability for the ACSBI-S with a sample of adolescent inpatients was .74. The parent and self-report versions of the ACSBI correlated .50 for the total scores. Both versions significantly correlated with the Adolescent Sexual Concerns Questionnaire (Hussey & Singer, 1993) and the TSCC Sexual Concerns scales (Briere, 1996). With some slight variations in prediction patterns across the five scales, both the parent- and self-report versions were linked with histories of physical and sexual abuse, family problems, and negative life events.

BEST PRACTICES FOR ASSESSING SEXUALLY ABUSED YOUTH

Reason for Referral

The first consideration when assessing CSA victims is to determine the purpose of the assessment and the questions to be asked. In many cases, CSA victims are referred to identify how the abuse affected them and to provide direction for the types of interventions needed to help them recover. This typically occurs in the context of mental health services, but it can also occur in the context of legal proceedings, such as child welfare matters, custody and access disputes, civil litigation, and victim compensation applications. In most cases, adjustment problems have instigated the referral, but in some cases, caregivers and social workers want a "checkup" to determine the impact of the abuse and explore ways to prevent future adjustment problems. In some cases, youth are referred for assessment because of other problems, such as conduct problems or intentional self-harm. Because of the child's CSA history, questions arise as to whether the abuse contributed to the development or exacerbation of the problem. Thus, assessments for CSA may focus specifically on the effects of the abuse or be part of a broader assessment that addresses a number of adjustment concerns.

Even if the original assessment was not intended for legal purposes, assessment reports are often requested or subpoenaed for such proceedings. Prior to initiating an assessment, all parties should be informed of limits of confidentiality, particularly the possibility that the report might be subpoenaed by a judge. Other limits of confidentiality, including report of the abuse, should also be reviewed. Issues relevant to legal proceedings should be considered. For instance, if new details about maltreatment were reported by the youth during the course of the assessment, then care should be taken to document both the context of the disclosure and the youth's verbatim statements, and subsequent reports to CPS. This is important to avoid potential allegations that the disclosures were in some way "led" by assessment questions, misinterpreted by the assessor, or in some way mishandled in terms of child protection mandates. Care should also be taken to document all sources of information, and to interpret assessment information in line with knowledge of CSA-related research.

Start with Standard Good Assessment Strategies

Psychological assessment of children and youth require some basic components. Positive rapport is essential to all assessments, but is particularly important for CSA victims and their families. Families who have undergone CPS and justice system investigations are often wary of mental health services, and children may fear yet another interview about the abuse. Exploration of child and family concerns, and their goals at the outset of the assessment, may be helpful, and assessors should take time to explain the assessment process and how assessment information is used to assist with planning services. To understand the impact of CSA on children, it is best to assess the "whole child," not just the sexual abuse; that is, take time to learn about the children's interests, strengths, friends, and family. Although much of the focus of assessment is on mental health problems, the goals of mental health interventions include positive adjustment and personal growth. Knowing the child's strengths and interests identifies areas on which to build resilience and competence, and helps the child and family feel hopeful and balanced about mental

health services. This chapter has focused on CSA-specific types of information. However, other basic information is required, including child developmental history, academic adjustment, and family and social relationships. Past efforts toward resolving problems should be explored, both within the family and through mental health services, including methods that have been successful and unsuccessful, and perceptions of the reasons behind these outcomes.

Build an Assessment Protocol

Individual assessors tend to establish preferred assessment methods and strategies. The purpose of this chapter is not to recommend specific assessment tools, but to provide information about the assessment methods available for establishing an assessment protocol. Given the breadth and complexity of issues inherent in assessing CSA victims, an assessment approach is recommended that is multi-gating, multivariate, multi-informant, and multimethod. Multi-gating refers to using broadband assessment tools to guide more specific areas of inquiry. Broad-band assessments include interviews, questionnaires, and personality measures that span multiple factors. For instance, the CBCL (Achenbach & Rescorla, 2001) provides an excellent overview of both child competencies and behavioral and emotional problems. As well, diagnostic interviews, such as the Diagnostic Interview for Children and Adolescents–IV (Reich, Welner, & Herjanic; 1997) and the Diagnostic Interview Schedule for Children (Shaffer et al., 1996), provide a thorough investigation of common mental health problems. Available computer-administered versions of these interviews for parent and adolescent completion enhance feasibility within clinical settings. Once specific mental health issues are identified from these broad-band assessments, more narrow-band evaluations can be conducted. That said, these broad-band assessment tools are often not sensitive to some of the specific effects of CSA. Thus, it is recommended that for identifying symptoms and for diagnostic purposes, broad-band assessment tools be supplemented with measures that independently assess PTSD and sexual problems.

The multivariate aspects of assessment protocols refer to four domains: (1) background, (2) symptoms, (3) psychological processes, and (4) family and other social supports and stressors. By assessing these four domains, the child's problems may be conceptualized in terms of antecedents and consequences of the maltreatment and adversity, and identified child and family factors may serve as objectives and goals for interventions. The multi-informant and multi-method aspects of an assessment protocol provide a layered strategy for ensuring a thorough evaluation and guard against biases stemming from different informants or methods. Assessment strategies should include the child and the child's primary caregivers, and when possible and relevant, information from social workers, therapists, and teachers. For background information, it is often helpful to gather information from multiple sources (charts, CPS workers, parents, and sometimes the children themselves), because it is unlikely that any single source presents a full account of all relevant information. As well, inconsistencies from different sources are not uncommon and may call for clarification. Whenever CPS is involved in a case, it is often helpful to invite the primary worker to participate in the assessment process. CPS workers can clarify custodial status and the provisions of supervisory orders, and provide information about past and ongoing child welfare concerns, often with detail that is not readily available from CPS reports, which may not reflect the most recent events relevant to the case.

Although parents generally provide a good assessment of externalizing types of problems, parents with mental health problems sometimes overreport child problems and may underreport symptoms in other circumstances (e.g., during custody and access or child welfare proceedings (Friedrich, 2002; Sourander et al., 2006). Teacher reports can provide an unbiased alternative assessment of adjustment problems and provide additional information about the child's academic and social adjustment. For sexual problems, parents are typically the best informants for sexualized behaviors of children (who often deny anything sexual), but adolescents are typically the better informants for themselves, because parents are often unaware of their sexual activities, and adolescents are less hesitant than children to report sexual issues. PTSD symptoms are best reported by the child or adolescent, because many symptoms are cognitive in nature. However, some youth may wish to avoid having their PTSD symptoms detected (as part of the avoidance aspect of PTSD); thus, parental re-

ports provide an alternative source of information, particularly about the more observable aspects of PTSD. Likewise, youth tend to be the best informants of other internalizing symptoms, but some children may under- or overreport their symptoms (Friedrich, 2002). Varying assessment methods can help to ensure that information drawn from children is consistent and reliable. Whereas self-report measures are very helpful, supplementing the assessment protocol with projective and observational tools may provide checks against method biases.

Assessing PTSD and Event-Related Issues with CSA Victims

One of the three symptoms domains of PTSD is avoidance, and avoidance of thoughts and conversations related to an identified trauma is a commonly endorsed symptom within that domain (Wolfe & Birt, 2005a). Thus, it is important to establish rapport before delving into these sensitive issues. As well, it is often helpful in the beginning to schedule assessment tasks with less sensitive measures (e.g., ways of coping) before moving to more sensitive measures (abuse-related PTSD). Open-ended questions about CSA-related issues typically do not yield detailed responses, because youth are often reluctant to discuss CSA, and they generally do not have a framework to conceptualize their behavioral and emotional thoughts, feelings, and symptoms in relationship to their abuse experiences. Therefore, abuse-specific questionnaires can be very helpful. The CITES-II asks respondents to remember their abuse experiences (but they are not asked to retell what happened) and to answer the questions with that set of events in mind. Children and adolescents appear to tolerate the questions well, though because of the different sections, completion of the full CITES-II sometimes takes more than one session. Because the CITES-II identifies the specific trauma and includes items that cover all DSM-IV-TR PTSD diagnostic criteria, the diagnostic process is facilitated (a diagnostic algorithm is provided). Detailed information about abuse-related attribution, social reactions, and coping is relevant to intervention. In some cases, children may not have fully disclosed their abuse, may have recanted their allegations, or the suspected abuse has not yet been disclosed. Questionnaires such as the TSCC (Briere, 2006a) can help to identify trauma-related symptoms, because a designation of a specific event is not required. The TSCC also provides a broad overview of additional symptoms often associated with CSA and other traumatic events, and may serve as a screening tool for more in-depth assessments.

Assessment throughout the Intervention Process

Like the assessment process, interventions for CSA victims tend to be multidimensional, to address multiple problems, and often require long-term involvement (see Wolfe [2006] for an overview of interventions with CSA victims). Assessment information is essential in developing an effective treatment and intervention plan, and can help the clinician triage and prioritize treatment objectives. Once a treatment plan is in place, it is important to monitor progress of specific objectives on an ongoing basis, through tailored methods such as parent or child daily monitoring of symptoms and clinician sessional ratings of progress toward goals. Once a specific set of goals is met, new goals and objectives may be set and monitored, with a continuation of the process until the child's mental health difficulties are addressed in full. For example, for a sexually abused child with sexual behavior problems, a treatment priority might be decreasing inappropriate sexual behaviors with other children. Multiple sessions are required to address those problems, and tailored monitoring strategies may be put in place until the sexualized problems are under control. At that point, other problems may be considered as a second stage of intervention, such as addressing the child's PTSD symptoms, which also may be monitored until symptoms are resolved.

SUMMARY AND CONCLUSIONS

This chapter provides an overview of issues related to CSA, including epidemiological findings, situational correlates of sexual abuse, and the impact of sexual abuse on victims. The findings reviewed provide a framework for assessing sexually abused children for both clinical and research purposes. The research indicates that sexual abuse is a serious negative life event that has great potential to set in motion a lifetime of adjustment problems. A number of mental health problems are clearly linked with sexual abuse, including PTSD, dissociation, depression, sexuality problems, and risk for subsequent revictimization. Additional problems are likely not only influenced by the sexual abuse experience but also linked with the emotional, familial, and social contexts associated with sexual abuse. For example, eating disorders and intentional self-harm appear to be disproportionately represented among sexual abuse victims, but the link with these disorders is the negative emotional states and dysphoria associated with the abuse. As well, behavioral and conduct problems have links with the sexual abuse, but the links are likely through depression and PTSD symptoms such as hyperarousal, as well as a dysfunctional family and social contexts that often accompany sexual abuse.

There are clearly great individual differences in risk for developing mental problems subsequent to sexual victimization. Understanding the effects of sexual abuse requires consideration of many layers of contributing factors that are interrelated in complex ways. Sexual abuse itself constitutes a heterogeneous set of circumstances, including different acts, perpetrators, types of coercion, and frequencies and durations. Although these factors are related to sexual abuse sequelae, research suggests that children's perceptions of abuse severity have much more to do with subsequent impact than specific abuse factors. Furthermore, children's perceptions of abuse severity do not necessarily correspond to the severity dimensions typically assessed by researchers (i.e., abusive acts, coercion, relationship to perpetrator). This suggests that either researchers have not yet found a way to define abuse severity that reflects children's experiences, or that individual differences in the ways children experience negative life events such as sexual abuse have much to do with the child's resilience. It is possible that children's perceptions of their sexual abuse are influenced by factors other than the abuse itself, such as postdisclosure stressors related to family reactions, involvement with CPS and the legal system, and the experience of other forms of maltreatment and subsequent sexual victimization. It is also possible that children's ways of coping with sexual abuse reflect premorbid coping tendencies; that is, well-adjusted children who have good coping skills and good family support may cope more effectively at the time of the abuse, perceive less threat and helplessness, act in effective ways to minimize the probability of further abuse or negative impact, and subsequently experience fewer negative mental health outcomes. But children with poor self-esteem, who rely on avoidant, internalizing, or externalizing forms of coping and have distant, nonsupportive familial relationships may react at the time of the sexual abuse with great horror and helplessness, may fail to disclose their abuse, and may therefore experience repeated episodes of abuse. Further longitudinal research is needed with large representative samples to investigate how premorbid adjustment and coping factors affect the impact of sexual abuse. The good news on this front is the success of several large-scale research projects that have assessed both mental health and histories of negative life events, including sexual abuse, thus providing methodological templates for future prospective longitudinal studies. These findings have important implications for developing prevention programs that promote healthy coping when children face serious, negative life events, including but not limited to sexual abuse.

Over the past decade, the field has been enhanced by the development and refinement of a number of tools to assess CSA victims. In particular, we now have a number of tools that assess PTSD, dissociation, and sexuality problems at different developmental points. As well, numerous tools that are now available assess both details about sexual abuse and details of other childhood maltreatment, adversities, and family-related problems. Our tool kit now also includes measures that assess children's perceptions and attributions about their abuse and their family situation. Clinically, these tools may be used as part of a more comprehensive assessment of victim adjustment that is multigating, multitrait, multimethod, multi-informant, ensuring that all appropriate symptoms are assessed, that results do not just reflect method variance, and that the perspectives of multiple people involved in a child's life are considered.

REFERENCES

Abel, G. G., Becker, J., Cunningham-Rathner, J., Mittelman, M. S., & Rouleau, J. L. (1988). Multiple paraphilic diagnoses among sex offenders. *Bulletin of the American Academy of Psychiatry and the Law, 16*, 153–168.

Achenbach, T. M., & Rescorla, L. A. (2001). *Mental health practitioners' guide to the Achenbach System of Empirically Based Assessment (ASEBA)* (2nd ed.). Burlington: University of Vermont, Research Center for Children, Youth, and Families.

Adler, N. A., & Schultz, J. (1995). Sibling incest offenders. *Child Abuse and Neglect, 19*, 811–820.

Ageton, S. S. (1983). The dynamics of female delinquency, 1976–1980. *Criminology: An Interdisciplinary Journal, 21*, 555–584.

Alaggia, R., & Turon, J.V. (2005). Against the odds: The impact of woman abuse on maternal response to child sexual abuse. *Journal of Child Sexual Abuse, 14*, 95–113.

Alessandri, S. M., & Lewis, M. (1996). Differences in pride and shame in maltreated and nonmaltreated preschoolers. *Child Development, 67*, 1857–1869.

Altshuler, J., & Ruble, D. (1989). Developmental changes in children's awareness of strategies of coping with uncontrollable events. *Child Development, 60*, 1337–1349.

American Prosecutors Research Institute—National District Attorneys Association. (2007). *"Speedy trial" statutes for allegations involving children.* Retrieved March 2, 2007, from *www.ndaa.org/pdf/ncpca_statute_trial_statutes_chart.pdf*

American Psychiatric Association (APA). (2000). *Diagnostic and statistical manual of mental disorders* (4th ed., text revision). Washington, DC: Author.

Arata, C. M. (1998). To tell or nor to tell: Current functioning of child sexual abuse survivors who disclosed their victimization. *Child Maltreatment, 3*, 63–71.

Armstrong, J. G., Putnam, F. W., Carlson, E. B., Libero, D. Z., & Smith, S. R. (1997). Development and validation of a measure of adolescent dissociation: The Adolescent Dissociative Experiences Scale. *Journal of Nervous and Mental Disease, 185*, 491–497.

Avery, L., Massat, C. R., & Marta, L. (1998). The relationship between parent and child reports of parental supportiveness and psychopathology of sexually abused children. *Child and Adolescent Social Work Journal, 15*, 187–205.

Bagley, C., & Thurston, W. E. (1996). *Understanding and preventing child sexual abuse: Vol. 2. Male victims, adolescents, adult outcomes and offender treatment.* Hampshire, UK: Ashgate.

Bagley, C. C., & Mallick, K. (2000). Prediction of sexual, emotional, and physical maltreatment and mental health outcomes in a longitudinal cohort of 290 adolescent women. *Child Maltreatment, 5*, 218–226.

Bal, S., Crombez, G., Van Oost, P., & Debourdeaudhuij, I. (2003). The role of social support in well-being and coping with self-reported stressful events in adolescents. *Child Abuse and Neglect, 27*, 1377–1395.

Bal, S., DeBourdeaudhuij, I., Crombez, G., & Van Oost, P. (2004). Differences in trauma symptoms and family functioning in intra- and extrafamilial sexually abused adolescents. *Journal of Interpersonal Violence, 19*, 108–123.

Bal, S., Debourdeaudhuij, I., Crombez, G., & Van Oost, P. (2005). Predictors of trauma symptomatology in sexually abused adolescents: A 6-month follow-up study. *Journal of Interpersonal Violence, 20,* 1390–1405.

Bal, S., Van Oost, P., De Bourdeaudhuij, I., & Crombez, G. (2003). Avoidant coping as a mediator between self-reported sexual abuse and stress-related symptoms in adolescents. *Child Abuse and Neglect, 27,* 883–897.

Band, E., & Weisz, J. (1988). How to feel better when it feels bad: Children's perspectives on coping with everyday stress. *Developmental Psychology, 24,* 247–253.

Banyard, V. L. (1997). Childhood maltreatment and the mental health of low-income women. *American Journal of Orthopsychiatry, 69,* 1095–1107.

Banyard, V. L., Williams, L. M., & Siegel, J. A. (2003). The impact of complex trauma and depression on parenting: An exploration of mediating risk and protective factors. *Child Maltreatment, 8,* 334–349.

Bardone, A. M., Moffitt, T., Caspi, A., & Dickson, N. (1996). Adult mental health and social outcomes of adolescent girls with depression and conduct disorder. *Development and Psychopathology, 8,* 811–829.

Barnett, D., Manly, J. T., & Cicchetti, D. (1993). Defining child maltreatment: The interface between policy and research. In D. Cicchetti & S. Toth (Eds.), *Child abuse, child development, and social policy* (pp. 7–73). Norwood, NJ: Ablex.

Barrett, K. C., Zahn-Waxler, C., & Cole, P. M. (1993). Avoiders vs. amenders: Implications for the investigation of guilt and shame during toddlerhood? *Cognition and Emotion, 7,* 481–505.

Beck-Sague, C. M., & Solomon, F. (1999). Sexually transmitted diseases in children and adolescent and adult victims of rape: Research of selected literature. *Clinical Infectious Diseases, 28,* S74–S83.

Bennett, D. S., Sullivan, M. W., & Lewis, M. (2005). Young children's adjustment as a function of maltreatment, shame, and anger. *Child Maltreatment, 10,* 311–323.

Berliner, L. (2005). Shame in child maltreatment: Contribution and caveats. *Child Maltreatment, 10,* 387–390.

Berliner, L., & Conte, J. (1995). The process of victimization: The victims' perspective. *Child Abuse and Neglect, 14,* 29–40.

Berliner, L., & Saunders, B. E. (1996). Treating fear and anxiety in sexually abused children: Results of a controlled 2-year follow-up study. *Child Maltreatment, 1,* 294–309.

Bernstein, D. P., Ahluvalia, T., Pogge, D., & Handelsman, L. (1997). Validity of the Childhood Trauma Questionnaire in an adolescent psychiatric population. *Journal of the American Academy of Child and Adolescent Psychiatry, 36,* 340–348.

Bernstein, D. P., & Fink, L. (1998). *Childhood Trauma Questionnaire: A retrospective self-report.* San Antonio, TX: Psychological Corporation.

Bernstein, D. P., Fink, L., Handelsman, L., Foote, J., Lovejoy, M., Wenzel, K., et al. (1994). Initial reliability and validity of a new retrospective measure of child abuse and neglect. *American Journal of Psychiatry, 15,* 1132–1136.

Bernstein, D. P., & Putnam, F. W. (1986). Development, reliability, and validity of a dissociation scale. *Journal of Nervous and Mental Disease, 174,* 727–735.

Bernstein, D. P., Stein, J. A., Newcomb, M. D., Walker, E., Pogge, D., Ahluvalia, T., et al. (2003). Development and validation of a brief screening version of the Childhood Trauma Questionnaire. *Child Abuse and Neglect, 27,* 169–190.

Birt, J. H. (1996). *Abuse-related variables, attributions, coping, and negative sequelae of sexually abused girls.* Unpublished doctoral dissertation, University of Windsor, Ontario, Canada.

Black, D. A., Heyman, R. E., & Slep, A. M. S. (2001). Risk factors for child sexual abuse. *Aggression and Violent Behavior, 6,* 203–229.

Bolen, R. M., & Lamb, L. J. (2002). Guardian support of sexually abused children: A study of its predictors *Child Maltreatment, 7,* 265–276.

Bolger, K. E., & Patterson, C. J. (2001). Developmental pathways from child maltreatment to peer rejection. *Child Development, 72,* 549–568.

Bolger, K. E., Patterson, C. J., & Kupersmidt, J. B. (1998). Peer relationships and self-esteem among children who have been maltreated. *Child Development, 69,* 1171–1197.

Bonanno, G. A., Keltner, D., Noll, J. G., Putnam, F. W., Trickett, P. K., LeJune, J., et al. (2002). When the face reveals what words do not: Facial expressions of emotion, smiling, and the willingness to disclose childhood sexual abuse. *Journal of Personality and Social Psychology, 83,* 94–110.

Boney-McCoy, S., & Finkelhor, D. (1995). Prior victimization: A risk factor for child sexual abuse and for PTSD-related symptomatology among sexually abused youth. *Child Abuse and Neglect, 19,* 1401–1421.

Boney-McCoy, S., & Finkelhor, D. (1996). Is youth victimization related to trauma symptoms and depression after controlling for prior symptoms and family relationships?: A longitudinal, prospective study. *Journal of Consulting and Clinical Psychology, 64,* 1406–1416.

Bowen, K. (2000). Child abuse and domestic violence in families of children seen for suspected sexual abuse. *Clinical Pediatrics, 39*(1), 33–40.

Boyce, P., Oakley-Browne, M. A., & Hatcher, S. (2001). The problem of deliberate self-harm. *Current Opinion in Psychiatry, 14,* 107–111.

Boyer, D., & Fine, D. (1991). Sexual abuse as a factor in adolescent pregnancy and child maltreatment. *Family Planning Perspectives, 24,* 4–11.

Brant, E. F., King, C. A., Olson, E., Ghaziuddin, N., & Naylor, M. (1996). Depressed adolescents with a history of sexual abuse: Diagnostic comorbidity and suicidality. *Journal of the American Academy of Child and Adolescent Psychiatry, 34,* 34–41.

Breitenbecher, K. H. (2001). Sexual revictimization among women:. A review of the literature focusing on empirical investigations. *Aggression and Violent Behavior, 6,* 415–432.

Bretherton, I., Ridgeway, D., & Cassidy, J. (1990). Assessing internal working models of the attachment relationship: An attachment story completion task for 3-year-olds. In D. Cicchetti, M. Greenberg, & E. M. Cummings (Eds.), *Attachment during the preschool years: Theory, research and intervention* (pp. 272–308). Chicago: University of Chicago Press.

Briere, J. (1996). *Trauma Symptom Checklist for Children (TSCC): Professional manual.* Lutz, FL: Psychological Assessment Resources.

Briere, J. (2006a). *Trauma Symptom Checklist for Children (TSCC).* Retrieved on August 23, 2006, from *johnbriere.com/psych_tests.htm*

Briere, J. (2006b). *Trauma Symptom Checklist for Young Children (TSCYC).* Retrieved on August 23, 2006, from *johnbriere.com/psych_tests.htm*

Briere, J., & Gil, E. (1998). Self-mutilation in clinical and general population samples: Prevalence, correlates, and functions. *Journal of Orthopsychiatry, 68,* 609–620.

Briere, J., Johnson, K., Bissada, A., Damon, L., Crouch, J., Gil, E., et al. (2001). The Trauma Symptom Checklist for Young Children (TSCYC): Reliability and association with abuse exposure in a multi-site study. *Child Abuse and Neglect, 25,* 1001–1014.

Briere, J., & Runtz, M. (1989). University males' sexual interest in children: Predicting potential indices of "pedophilia" in a nonforensic sample. *Child Abuse and Neglect, 13,* 65–75.

Brooks-Gunn, J., & Chase-Lansdale, P. L. (1995). Adolescent parenthood In M. H. Bornstein (Ed.), *Handbook of parenting: Vol. 3. Status and social conditions of parenting* (pp. 113–149). Hillsdale, NJ: Erlbaum.

Brown, J., Cohen, P., Johnson, J. G., & Salzinger, S. (1998). A longitudinal analysis of risk factors for child maltreatment: Findings of a 17-year prospective study of officially recorded and self-reported child abuse and neglect. *Child Abuse and Neglect, 22,* 1065–1978.

Brown, J., Cohen, P., Johnson, J. G., & Smailes, E. M. (1999). Childhood abuse and neglect: Specificity and effects on adolescent and young adult depression and suicidality. *Journal of the American Academy of Child and Adolescent Psychiatry, 38,* 1490–1496.

Brown, L. K., Kessel, S. M., Lourie, K. J., Ford, H., & Lipsitt, L. (1997). Influence of sexual abuse on HIV-related attitudes and behaviors in adolescent psychiatric inpatients. *Journal of the American Academy of Child and Adolescent Psychiatry, 36,* 316–322.

Browne, M. Z., Cloitre, K. A., & Linehan, M. M. (2002). Reasons for suicide attempts and nonsuicidal self-injury in women with borderline personality disorder. *Journal of Abnormal Psychology, 111,* 198–202.

Bryant, S. L., & Range, L. M. (1996). Suicidality in college women who report multiple versus single types

of maltreatment by parents: A brief report. *Journal of Child Sexual Abuse, 4,* 87–94.

Burton, D. L. (2000). Were adolescent sexual offenders children with sexual problems? *Sexual Abuse: A Journal of Research and Treatment, 12,* 37–48.

Butler, S. M., & Seto, M. C. (2002). Distinguishing two types of adolescent sex offenders. *Journal of the American Academy of Child and Adolescent Psychiatry, 41,* 83–90.

Caldwell, M. F. (2002). What we do not know about juvenile sexual reoffense risk? *Child Maltreatment, 7,* 291–302.

Campos, J., Mumme, D., Kermoian, R., & Campos, R. (1994). A functionalist perspective on the nature of emotion. In N. A. Fox (Ed.), The development of emotion regulation: Biological and behavioral considerations. *Monographs of the Society for Research in Child Development, 59*(2–3, Serial No. 240), 284–303.

Camras, L. A., Ribordy, S., Hill, J., Martino, S., Sachs, V., & Spaccarelli, S. (1988). Recognition and posing of emotional expressions by abused children and their mothers. *Developmental Psychology, 24,* 776–781.

Canadian Centre for Justice Statistics. (1999). *Sex offenders* (Juristat Catalogue No. 85-002-XIE, Vol. 19, Issue 3). Ottawa: Statistics Canada.

Causey, D. L., & DeBow, E. F. (1992). Development of a self-report coping measure for elementary school children. *Journal of Clinical Child Psychology, 21,* 47–59.

Cecil, H., & Matson, S. C. (2005). Differences in psychological health and family dysfunction by sexual victimization type in a clinical sample of African American adolescent women. *Journal of Sex Research, 42,* 203–214.

Chaffin, M., Letourneau, E., & Silovsky, J. (2002). Adults, adolescents, and child who sexually abuse children: A developmental perspective. In J. Meyers (Ed.), *The APSAC handbook on child abuse and neglect.* Thousand Oaks, CA: Sage.

Chaffin, M., & Shultz, S. K. (2001). Psychometric evaluation of the Children's Impact of Traumatic Events Scale—Revised. *Child Abuse and Neglect, 25,* 401–411.

Chaffin, M., Wherry, J. N., & Dykman, R. (1997). School-age children's coping with sexual abuse: Abuse stresses and symptoms associated with four coping strategies. *Child Abuse and Neglect, 21,* 227–240.

Chaffin, M., Wherry, J. N., Newlin, C., Crutchfield, A., & Dykman, R. (1997). The Abuse Dimensions Inventory: Initial data on a research measure of abuse severity. *Journal of Interpersonal Violence, 12,* 569–589.

Chandy, J. M., Blum, R. W., & Resnick, M. D. (1997). Sexually abused male adolescents: How vulnerable are they? *Journal of Child Sexual Abuse, 6*(2), 1–16.

Chapman, A. L., Gratz, K. L., & Brown, M. Z. (2006). Solving the puzzle of deliberate self-harm: The experiential avoidance model. *Behavior Research and Therapy, 44,* 371–394.

Chu, J. A., & Dill, D. L. (1990). Dissociative symptoms in relation to childhood physical and sexual abuse. *American Journal of Psychiatry, 147,* 887–892.

Classen, C. C., Palesh, O. G., & Aggarwal, R. (2005). Sexual victimization: A review of the empirical literature. *Trauma, Violence, and Abuse, 2,* 103–129.

Cohen, J. A., & Mannarino, A. P. (1998). Factors that mediate treatment outcome of sexually abused preschool children: Six- and 12-month follow-up. *Journal of the American Academy of Child and Adolescent Psychiatry, 37,* 44–51.

Cohen, J. A., & Mannarino, A. P. (2000). Predictors of treatment outcome in sexually abused children. *Child Abuse and Neglect, 24,* 983–994.

Cole, P., & Putnam, F. (1992). Effect of incest on self and self functioning: A developmental psychopathology perspective. *Journal of Consulting and Clinical Psychology, 60,* 174–184.

Cole, P. M., Woolger, C., Power, T. G., & Smith, K. D. (1992). Parenting difficulties among adult survivors of father–daughter incest. *Child Abuse and Neglect, 16,* 239–249.

Collin-Vézina, D., & Cyr, M. (2003). La transmission de la violence sexuelle: Description du phénomene et pistes de comprehension [Transmission of sexual violence: Description of the phenomenon and current understanding]. *Child Abuse and Neglect, 27,* 489–507.

Collin-Vézina, D., & Hébert, M. (2005). Comparing dissociation and PTSD in sexually abused school-age girls. *Journal of Nervous and Mental Disease, 193,* 47–52.

Compas, B. E., Ey, S., & Grant, K. E. (1993). Taxonomy, assessment, and diagnosis of depression during adolescence. *Psychological Bulletin, 114,* 323–344.

Cook, A., Spinazzola, J., Ford, J., Lanktree, C., Blaustein, M., Cloitre, M., et al. (2005). Complex trauma in children and adolescents. *Psychiatric Annals, 35,* 390–398.

Coons, P. M. (1985). Children of parents with multiple personality disorder. In R. P. Kluft (Ed.), *Childhood antecedents of multiple personality disorder* (pp. 151–165). Washington, DC: American Psychiatric Press.

Coons, P. M., Bowman, E. S., & Milstein, V. (1988). Multiple personality disorder: A clinical investigation of 50 cases. *Journal of Nervous and Mental Disease, 176,* 519–527.

Costello, E. J., Angold, A., March, J., & Fairbank, J. (1998). Life events and post-traumatic stress: The development of a new measure for children and adolescents. *Psychological Medicine, 28,* 1275–1288.

Costello, E. J., Erkanli, A., Fairbank, J., & Angold, A. (2002). The prevalence of potentially traumatic events in childhood and adolescence. *Journal of Traumatic Stress, 15,* 99–112.

Coxell, A. W., King, M. B., Mezey, G. C., & Kell, P. (2000). Sexual molestation of men: Interviews with 224 men attending a genitourinary medicine service. *International Journal of STD and AIDS, 11,* 574–578.

Cross, T. P., De Vos, E., & Whitcomb, D. (1994). Prosecution of child sexual abuse: Which cases are accepted? *Child Abuse and Neglect, 18,* 663–677.

Cross, T. P., Whitcomb, D., & De Vos, E. (1995). Criminal justice outcomes of prosecution of child sexual abuse: A case flow analysis. *Child Abuse and Neglect, 19,* 1431–1442.

Crosse, S. B., Kaye, E., & Ratnofsky, A. C. (1993). *A Report on the Maltreatment of Children with Disabilities* (National Centre on Child Abuse and Neglect, Contract No. 105-89-11639). Washington, DC: Westat.

Crouch, J., Smith, D., Ezzell, C., & Saunders, B. (1999). Measuring reactions to sexual trauma among children: Comparing the Children's Impact of Traumatic Events Scale and the Trauma Symptom Checklist for Children. *Child Maltreatment, 4,* 255–263.

Cuffe, S. P., Addy, C. L., Garrison, C. Z., Waller, J. L., Jackson, K. L., McKeown, R. E., et al. (1998). Prevalence of PTSD in a community sample of older adolescents. *Journal of the American Academy of Child and Adolescent Psychiatry, 37,* 147–154.

Dadds, M., Smith, M., Webber, Y., & Robinson, A. (1991). An exploration of family and individual profiles following father–daughter incest. *Child Abuse and Neglect, 15,* 575–586.

Danielson, C. K., de Arellano, M. A., Kilpatrick, D. G., Saunders, B. E., & Resnick, H. S. (2005). Child maltreatment in depressed adolescents: Differences in symptomatology based on history of abuse. *Child Maltreatment, 10,* 37–48.

David, J., & Suls, J. (1999). Coping efforts in daily life: Role of Big Five traits and problem appraisals. *Journal of Personality, 67,* 265–294.

Davies, M. (1995). Parental distress and ability to cope following disclosure of extra-familial sexual abuse. *Child Abuse and Neglect, 19,* 399–408.

Davies, W. H., & Flannery, D. J. (1998). Post-traumatic stress disorder in children and adolescents exposed to violence. *Pediatric Clinics of North America, 45,* 341–353.

Deblinger, E., Hathaway, C. R., Lippmann, J., & Steer, R. (1993). Psychosocial characteristics and correlates of symptom distress in non-offending mothers of sexually abused children. *Journal of Interpersonal Violence, 8,* 155–168.

Deblinger, E., McLeer, S., Atkins, M. S., Ralphe, D., & Foa, E. (1989). Posttraumatic stress in sexually abused, physically abused, and nonabused children. *Child Abuse and Neglect, 13,* 403–408.

DeJong, A. R., & Rose, M. (1991). Legal proof of child sexual abuse in the absence of physical evidence. *Pediatrics, 88,* 506–511.

DeOliveira, C. A., Bailey, H. N., Wolfe, V. V., & Evans, E. (2006, April). *The moderating effects of gender on the impact of maternal trauma and adjustment on child emotion socialization.* Paper presented at the annual meeting of the International Society for Traumatic Stress Studies, Hollywood, CA.

DiLillo, D., & Damashek, A. (2003). Parenting characteristics of women reporting a history of childhood sexual abuse. *Child Maltreatment, 8,* 319–333.

DiPietro, E. K., Runyan, D. K., & Frederick, D. D. (1997). Predictors of disclosure during medical evaluation for suspected sexual abuse. *Journal of Child Sexual Abuse, 6,* 133–142.

Dombrowski, S. C., LeMasney, J. W., Ahia, C. E., & Dickson, S. A. (2004). Protecting children from on-line sexual predators: Technological, psychoeducational, and legal considerations. *Professional Psychology: Research and Practice, 35,* 65–73.

Dong, M., Anda, R. F., Dube, S. R., Giles, W. H., & Felitti, V. J. (2003). The relationship of exposure to childhood sexual abuse to other forms of abuse, neglect, and household dysfunction during childhood. *Child Abuse and Neglect, 27,* 625–639.

Donovan, J. E., & Jessor, R. (1985). Structure of problem behavior in adolescence and young adulthood. *Journal of Consulting and Clinical Psychology, 53,* 890–904.

Douglas, A. R. (2000). Reported anxieties concerning intimate parenting in women sexually abused as children. *Child Abuse and Neglect, 24,* 425–434.

Downey, G., & Coyne, J. C. (1990). Children of depressed parents: An integrative review. *Psychological Bulletin, 108,* 50–76.

Drake, B., & Pandey, S. (1996). Understanding the relationship between neighborhood poverty and specific types of child maltreatment. *Child Abuse and Neglect, 20,* 1003–1018.

Dube, S. R., Anda, R. F., Whitfield, C. L., Brown, D. W., Felitti, V. J., Dong, M., et al. (2005). Long-term consequences of childhood sexual abuse by gender of victim. *American Journal of Preventive Medicine, 28,* 430–438.

Dube, S. R., Miller, J. W., Brown, D. W., Giles, W. H., Felitti, V. J., Dong, M., et al. (2006). Adverse childhood experiences and the association with ever using alcohol and initiating alcohol use during adolescence. *Journal of Adolescent Health, 38,* e-1–e-10.

Dubner, A. E., & Motta, R. W. (1999). Sexually and physically abused foster children and posttraumatic stress disorder. *Journal of Consulting and Clinical Psychology, 67,* 367–373.

Dunne, M. P., Purdie, D. M., Cook, M. D., Boyle, F. M., & Najman, J. M. (2003). Is child sexual abuse declining?: Evidence from a population-based survey of men and women in Australia. *Child Abuse and Neglect, 27,* 141–152.

Egeland, B., & Sroufe, A. (1981). Attachment and early maltreatment. *Child Development, 52,* 44–52.

Egeland, B., & Sussman-Stillman, A. (1996). Dissociation as a mediator of child abuse across generations. *Child Abuse and Neglect, 20,* 1123–1132.

Ehlers, A., Mayou, R. A., & Bryant, B. (2003). Cognitive predictors of posttraumatic stress disorder in children: Results of a prospective longitudinal study. *Behaviour Research and Therapy, 41,* 1–10.

Ekman, P., & Friesen, W. V. (1976). Measuring facial movement. *Journal of Environmental Psychology and Nonverbal Behavior, 1,* 56–75.

Ekman, P., & Friesen, W. V. (1978). *Facial action coding system: A technique for the measurement of facial movement.* Palo Alto, CA: Consulting Psychologists Press.

Elliott, A. N., & Carnes, C. N. (2001). Reactions of non-offending parents to the sexual abuse of their child: A review of the literature. *Child Maltreatment, 6,* 314–331.

Elliott, D. M., & Briere, J. (1994). Forensic sexual abuse evaluations of older children: Disclosures and symptomotogy. *Behavioral Sciences and the Law, 12,* 261–277.

English, D. J., Bangdiwala, S. I., & Runyan, D. K. (2005). The dimensions of maltreatment: Introduction [Special issue: Longitudinal Studies of Child Abuse and Neglect (LONGSCAN). *Child Abuse and Neglect, 29,* 441–460.

English, D. J., Graham, J. C., Litrownik, A. J., Everson, M., & Bangdiwala, S. I. (2005). Defining maltreatment chronicity: Are there differences in child outcomes? *Child Abuse and Neglect, 29,* 575–595.

Everill, J. T., & Waller, G. (1995). Disclosure of sexual abuse and psychological adjustment in female undergraduates. *Child Abuse and Neglect, 19,* 93–100.

Everson, M. D., & Boat, B. W. (1989). False allegations of sexual abuse of children and adolescents. *Journal of the American Academy of Child and Adolescent Psychiatry, 28,* 230–235.

Everson, M. D., Hunter, W. M., Runyan, D. K., Edelsohn, G. A., & Coulter, M. L. (1989). Maternal support following disclosure of incest. *American Journal of Orthopsychiatry, 59,* 197–207.

Evers-Szostak, M. (2002). *The Children's Perceptual Alteration Scale (CPAS).* Available from Mary Evers-Szostak, PhD, Department of Psychology, University of North Carolina, Chapel Hill, NC.

Evers-Szostak, M., & Sanders, S. (1992). The Children's Perceptual Alteration Scale (CPAS): A measure of children's dissociation. *Dissociation, 5,* 91–97.

Fair, J., Wolfe, V. V., Zayed, R., Farbstein, J., Lewis, A., & Nickels, A. (2006, November). *How do I cope?: The effects of negative life events on coping styles for adolescent girls.* Poster presented at the annual meeting of the International Society for Traumatic Stress Studies, Hollywood, CA.

Faller, K. (1984). Is the child victims of sexual abuse telling the truth? *Child Abuse and Neglect, 8,* 473–481.

Faller, K., & Henry, J. (2000). Child sexual abuse: A case study in community collaboration. *Child Abuse and Neglect, 24,* 1215–1225.

Farrington, A., Waller, G., Smerden, J., & Faupel, A. W. (2001). The Adolescent Dissociative Experience Scale: Psychometric properties and differences in scores across age groups. *Journal of Nervous and Mental Disorders, 189,* 722–727.

Favazza, A. R., DeRosear, L., & Conterio, K. (1989). Self-mutilation and eating disorders. *Suicide and Life-Threatening Behavior, 19,* 352–362.

Federal Bureau of Investigation. (1999). *Crime in the United States: Uniform crime reports 1998.* Washington, DC: U.S. Government Printing Office.

Federal Bureau of Investigation. (2000). *Crime in the United States, 1999.* Washington, DC: U.S. Government Printing Office.

Fehrenbach, P. A., Smith, W., Monastersky, C., & Deisher, R. (1986). Adolescent sexual offenders: Offender and offense characteristics. *American Journal of Orthopsychiatry, 56,* 225–233.

Feindler, E., Rathus, J., & Silver, L. (2003). *Assessment of family violence: A handbook for research and practitioners.* Washington, DC: American Psychiatric Association.

Feiring, C., & Taska, L. S. (2005). The persistence of shame following sexual abuse: A longitudinal look at risk and recovery. *Child Maltreatment, 10,* 337–349.

Feiring, C., Taska, L. S., & Chen, K. (2002). Trying to understand why horrible things happen: Attribution, shame and symptom development following sexual abuse. *Child Maltreatment, 7,* 26–41.

Feiring, C., Taska, L., & Lewis, M. (1999). Age and gender differences in children and adolescents adaptation to sexual abuse. *Child Abuse and Neglect, 23,* 115–128.

Feiring, C., Taska, L., & Lewis, M. (2002). Adjustment following sexual abuse discovery: The role of shame and attributional style. *Developmental Psychology, 38,* 79–92.

Fergusson, D. M., Horwood, J., & Lynskey, M. (1996). Childhood sexual abuse and psychiatric disorder in young adulthood: II. Psychiatric outcomes of childhood sexual abuse. *Journal of the American Academy of Child and Adolescent Psychiatry, 35,* 1365–1374.

Fergusson, D. M., Horwood, J., & Lynskey, M. (1997). Childhood sexual abuse, adolescent sexual behaviors and sexual revictimization. *Child Abuse and Neglect, 21,* 789–803.

Fergusson, D. M., Horwood, J., & Woodward, (2000). Risk factors and life processes associated with the onset of suicidal behavior during adolescence and early adulthood. *Psychological Medicine, 30,* 23–39.

Fergusson, D. M., Lynskey, M., & Horwood, J. (1996). Childhood sexual abuse and psychiatric disorder in young adulthood: I. Prevalence of sexual abuse and factors associated with sexual abuse. *Journal of the American Academy of Child and Adolescent Psychiatry, 34,* 1355–1364.

Finkelhor, D. (1979). *Sexually victimized children.* New York: Free Press.

Finkelhor, D. (1980). Sex among siblings. *Archives of Sexual Behavior, 9,* 171–194.

Finkelhor, D. (1983). Removing the child–prosecuting the offender in cases of sexual abuse: Evidence from the National Reporting System for Child Abuse and Neglect. *Child Abuse and Neglect, 7,* 195–205.

Finkelhor, D. (1990). Early and long term effects of child sexual abuse: An update. *Professional Psychology: Research and Practice, 21,* 325–330.

Finkelhor, D. (1994a). Current information on the scope and nature of child sexual abuse. *The Future of Children, 4,* 31–53.

Finkelhor, D. (1994b). The international epidemiology of child sexual abuse. *Child Abuse and Neglect, 18,* 409–417.

Finkelhor, D., & Baron, L. (1986). High risk children. In D. Finkelhor, S. Araji, L. Baron, A. Browne, S. Peters, & G. Wyatt (Eds.), *A sourcebook on child sexual abuse* (pp. 60–88). Beverly Hills, CA: Sage.

Finkelhor, D., Cross, T. P., & Cantor, E. N. (2005). The justice system for juvenile victims: A comprehensive model of case flow. *Trauma, Violence and Abuse, 6,* 83–102.

Finkelhor, D., & Dziuba-Leatherman, J. (1995). Victimization prevention programs: A national survey of children's exposure and reactions. *Child Abuse and Neglect, 19,* 129–139.

Finkelhor, D., Hotaling, G., Lewis, I. A., & Smith, C. (1990). Sexual abuse in a national survey of adult men and women: Prevalence, characteristics, and risk factors. *Child Abuse and Neglect, 14,* 19–28.

Finkelhor, D., & Jones, L. M. (2004, January). Explanations for the decline in child sexual abuse cases. *Juvenile Justice Bulletin.* Retrieved April 26, 2006, from *www.ojp.usdoj.gov/ojjdp*

Finkelhor, D., Moore, D., Hamby, S. L., & Straus, M. A. (1997). Sexually abused children in a national survey of parents: Methodological issues. *Child Abuse and Neglect, 21,* 1–9.

Finkelhor, D., & Ormrod, R. K. (2001). *Offenders incarcerated for crimes against juveniles* (Bulletin). Washington, DC: U.S. Department of Justice, Office of Justice Programs, Office of Juvenile Justice and Delinquency Prevention.

Finkelhor, D., Ormrod, R., Turner, H., & Hamby, S. L. (2005). The victimization of children and youth: A comprehensive, national survey. *Child Maltreatment, 10,* 5–25.

Finkelhor, D., Williams, L. M., Burns, N., & Kalinowski, M. (1988). *Nursery crimes: Sexual abuse in day care.* Thousand Oaks, CA: Sage.

Fischer, G. J. (1991). Is lesser severity of child sexual abuse a reason more males report having liked it? *Annals of Sex Research, 4,* 131–139.

Fitzgerald, M. M., Shipman, K. L., Jackson, J. L., McMahon, R. J., & Hanley, H. M. (2005). Perceptions of parenting versus parent–child interactions among incest survivors. *Child Abuse and Neglect, 29,* 661–681.

Fleming, J., Mullen, P., & Bammer, G. (1997). A study of potential risk factors for sexual abuse in childhood. *Child Abuse and Neglect, 21,* 49–58.

Fleming, J., Mullen, P., Sibthorpe, B., & Bammer, G. (1999). The long-term impact of childhood sexual abuse in Australian women. *Child Abuse and Neglect, 23,* 145–159.

Fletcher, K. E. (1996). Psychometric review of Dimensions of Stressful Events (DOSE) rating scale. In B. H. Stamm (Ed.), *Measurement of stress, trauma, and adaptation* (pp. 144–150). Lutherville, MD: Sidran Press.

Ford, J. D. (2005). Treatment implications of altered affect regulation and information processing following child maltreatment. *Psychiatric Annals, 35,* 410–419.

Fraser, P. (1985). *Pornography and prostitution in Canada.* Ottawa: Government of Canada.

Friedrich, W. N. (1993). Sexual victimization and sexual behavior in children: A review of recent literature. *Child Abuse and Neglect, 17,* 59–66.

Friedrich, W. N. (1997). *Child Sexual Behavior Inventory professional manual.* Odessa, FL: Psychological Assessment Resources.

Friedrich, W. N. (2002). *Psychological assessment of sexually abused children and their families.* Thousand Oaks, CA: Sage.

Friedrich, W. N., Baker, A. J. L., Parker, R., Schneiderman, M., Gries, L., & Archer, M. (2005). Youth with problematic sexualized behaviors in the child welfare system: A one-year longitudinal study. *Sexual Abuse: Journal of Research and Treatment, 17,* 391–406.

Friedrich, W. N., Fisher, J., Broughton, D., Houston, M., & Shafran, C. R. (1998). Normative sexual behavior in children: A contemporary sample. *Pediatrics, 101*(4), E9. Retrieved March 4, 2007, from *www.Pediatrics.org/cgi/content/full/.101/4/e9*

Friedrich, W. N., Fisher, J. L., Dittner, C. A., Acton, R., Berliner, L., Butler, J., et al. (2001). Child Sexual Behavior Inventory: Normative, psychiatric, and sexual abuse comparisons. *Child Maltreatment, 6,* 37–49.

Friedrich, W. N., Grambsch, P., Damon, L., Hewitt, S. K., Koverola, C., Lang, R. A., et al. (1992). Child Sexual Behavior Inventory: Normative and clinical comparisons. *Psychological Assessment, 4,* 303–311.

Friedrich, W. N., Jaworski, T. M., Hexschl, J. E., & Bengston, B. S. (1997). Dissociative and sexual behaviors in children and adolescents with sexual abuse and psychiatric histories. *Journal of Interpersonal Violence, 12,* 155–171.

Friedrich, W. N., Lysne, M., Sim, L., & Shamos, S. (2004). Assessing sexual behavior in high-risk adolescents with the Adolescent Clinical Sexual Behavior Inventory (ACSBI). *Child Maltreatment, 9,* 239–250.

Garbarino, J., Dubrowi, N., Kostelney, K., & Pardo, C. (1992). *Children in danger: Coping with the consequences of community violence.* San Francisco: Jossey-Bass.

Garber, J., Braafladt, N., & Weiss, B. (1995). Affect regulation in depressed and nondepressed children and young adolescents. *Development and Psychopathology, 7,* 93–115.

Garber, J., & Flynn, C. (2001). Predictors of depressive cognitions in young adolescents. *Cognitive Therapy and Research, 25,* 353–376.

Garnefski, N., & Diekstra, R. F. W. (1997). Child sexual abuse and emotional and behavioral problems in adolescence: Gender differences. *Journal of the American Academy of Child and Adolescent Psychiatry, 36,* 323–329.

Ge, X., Lorenz, F., Conger, R., Edler, C., & Simmons, R. (1994). Trajectories of stressful life events and depressive symptoms during adolescence. *Developmental Psychology, 30,* 467–483.

Gelfand, D. M., & Teti, D. M. (1990). The effects of maternal depression on children. *Clinical Psychology Review, 10,* 329–353.

Gentile, C. (1988). *Factors mediating the impact of child sexual abuse: Learned helplessness and severity of abuse.* Unpublished master's thesis, University of Western Ontario, London, Ontario, Canada.

Gershenson, H., Musick, J., Ruch-Ross, H., Magee, V., Rubino, K., & Rosenberg, D. (1989). The prevalence of coercive sexual experience among teenage mothers. *Journal of Interpersonal Violence, 4,* 204–219.

Gibb, B. E., Alloy, L. B., Abramson, L. Y., & Marx, B. P. (2003). Childhood maltreatment and maltreatment-specific inferences: A test of Rose and Abramson's (1992) extension of the hopelessness theory. *Cognition and Emotion, 17,* 917–931.

Gibb, B., Alloy, L., Abramson, L., Rose, D., Whitehouse, W., Donovan, P., et al. (2001). History of childhood maltreatment, negative cognitive styles, and episodes of depression in adulthood. *Cognitive Therapy and Research, 25,* 425–446.

Gidycz, C. A., Coble, C. N., Latham, L., & Layman, M. J. (1993). Sexual assault experience in adulthood and prior victimization experiences: A prospective analysis. *Psychology of Women Quarterly, 17,* 151–168.

Glasser, D. (2000). Child abuse and neglect and the brain: A review. *Journal of Child Psychology and Psychiatry, 41,* 97–116.

Glasser, M., Kolvin, I., Campbell, D., Glasser, A., Leitch, I., & Farrelly, S. (2001). Cycle of child sexual abuse: Links between being a victim and becoming a perpetrator. *British Journal of Psychiatry, 179,* 482–494.

Golden, O. (2000). The federal response to child abuse and neglect. *American Psychologist, 55,* 1050–1053.

Goldman, J. D. G., & Padayachi, U. K. (2000). Some methodological problems in estimating incidence and prevalence in child sexual abuse research. *Journal of Sex Research, 37,* 305–314.

Gomes-Schwartz, B., Horowitz, J. M., & Cardarelli, A. P. (1990). *Child sexual abuse: The initial effects.* Newbury Park, CA: Sage.

Gonzalez, L. S., Waterman, J., Kelly, R., McCord, J., & Oliveri, M. K. (1993). Children's patterns of disclosures and recantations of sexual and ritualistic abuse allegations in psychotherapy. *Child Abuse and Neglect, 17,* 281–289.

Goodman, G. S., Ghetti, S., Quas, J. A., Edelstein, R. S., Alexander, K. W., Redlich, A. D., et al. (2003). A prospective study of memory for child sexual abuse: New findings relevant to the repressed memory controversy. *Psychological Science, 14,* 113–118.

Goodman, G. S., Pyle-Taub, E. P., Jones, D. P. H., England, P., Port, L. K., Rudy, L., et al. (1992). The effects of court testimony on child assault victims. *Monographs of the Society for Research in Child Development*, 57, 1–163.

Goodman, G. S., Quas, J. A., Bulkley, J., & Shapiro, C. (1999). Innovations for child witnesses: A national survey. *Psychology, Public Policy, and Law*, 5, 255–281.

Goodman, S. (1992). Understanding the effects of depressed mothers on their children. *Progress in Experimental Personality and Psychopathology Research*, 47–109.

Goodman-Brown, T. B., Edelstein, R. S., Goodman, G. S., Jones, D. P. H., & Gordon, D. S. (2003). Why children tell: A model of children's disclosure of sexual abuse. *Child Abuse and Neglect*, 27, 525–540.

Gordon, M. (1990). The family environment of sexual abuse: An examination of the gender effect. *Journal of Family Violence*, 5, 321–332.

Greenhoot, A. F., McCloskey, L. A., & Gisky, E. (2005). A longitudinal study of adolescents' recollections of family violence. *Applied Cognitive Psychology*, 19, 719–743.

Gries, L. T., Goh, D. S. & Cavanaugh, J. (1996). Factors associated with disclosure during child sexual abuse assessment. *Journal of Child Sexual Abuse*, 5, 1–18.

Gutman, L. T., St. Claire, K., Herman-Giddens, M. E., Johnston, W. W., & Phelps, W. C. (1992). Evaluation of sex abused and nonabused young girls for intravaginal human papillomavirus infection. *American Journal of Diseases of Children*, 146, 694–699.

Hagan, M. P., & Gust-Brey, K. L. (1999). A ten-year longitudinal study of adolescent rapists upon return to the community. *International Journal of Offender Therapy and Comparative Criminology*, 43, 448–458.

Hamby, S. L., & Finkelhor, D. (2001). *Choosing and using child victimization questionnaires* (NCJ186027). Washington, DC: U.S. Department of Justice, Office of Juvenile Delinquency and Prevention.

Hamby, S. L., & Finkelhor, D. (2004). *The Comprehensive Juvenile Victimization Questionnaire*. Durham: University of New Hampshire.

Hamilton, L. (1997). *Contact between sexually abused children and their incestuous fathers: Implications for child post-disclosure adjustment*. Unpublished senior honors thesis, University of Western Ontario, London, Ontario, Canada.

Hankin, B. L., Abramson, L. Y., & Siler, M. (2001). A prospective test of the hopelessness theory of depression in adolescence. *Cognitive Therapy and Research*, 5, 607–632.

Hanson, R., Smith, D., Saunders, B., Swenson, C., & Conrad, L. (1995). Measurement in child abuse research: A survey of researchers. *APSAC Advisor*, 8, 7–10.

Hanson, R. F., Kievit, L. W., Saunders, B. E., Smith, D. W., Kilpatrick, D. G., Resnick, H. S., et al. (2003). Correlates of adolescent reports of sexual assault: Findings from the National Survey of Adolescents. *Child Maltreatment*, 8, 261–272.

Hanson, R. F., Resnick, H. S., Saunders, B. E., Kilpatrick, D. G., & Best, C. (1999). Factors related to the reporting of childhood rape. *Child Abuse and Neglect*, 23, 559–569.

Hanson, R. F., Saunders, B. E., & Lipovsky, J. A. (1992). The relationship between self-reported levels of distress in parents and victims in incest families. *Journal of Child Sexual Abuse*, 1, 49–61.

Hanson, R. F., Seer-Brown, S., Fricker-Elhai, A. E., Kilpatrick, D. G., Saunders, B. E., & Resnick, H. S. (2006). The relations between family environment violence exposure among youth: Findings from the national survey of adolescents. *Child Maltreatment*, 11, 3–15.

Hanson, R. K., Gordon, A., Harris, A. J., Marques, J. K., Murphy, W., Quinsey, V. L., et al. (2002). First report of the Collaborative Outcome Data Project on the effectiveness of psychological treatment for sex offenders. *Sexual Abuse: A Journal of Research and Treatment*, 14, 169–194.

Hardy, M. S. (2001). Physical aggression and sexual behavior among siblings: A retrospective study. *Journal of Family Violence*, 16, 255–268.

Hashimi, P. Y., & Finkelhor, D. (1999). Violent victimization of youth versus adults in the National Crime Victimization Survey. *Journal of Interpersonal Violence*, 14, 799–820.

Hecht, D., & Hansen, D. (1999). Adolescent victims and intergenerational issues in sexual abuse. In V. Van Hasselt & M. Hersen (Eds.), *Handbook of psychological approaches with violent criminal offenders: Contemporary strategies and issues* (pp. 303–328). New York: Plenum Press.

Henry, J. (1997). System intervention trauma to child sexual abuse victims following disclosure. *Journal of Interpersonal Violence*, 12, 499–512.

Herman, J. L. (1992). Complex PTSD: A syndrome in survivors of prolonged and repeated trauma. *Journal of Traumatic Stress*, 5, 377–391.

Higgins, D. J., & McCabe, M. P. (2000). Relationships between different types of maltreatment during childhood and adjustment in adulthood. *Child Maltreatment*, 5, 261–272.

Hooper, C. (1992). *Mothers surviving child sexual abuse*. London: Rutledge.

Hornstein, N. L., & Putnam, F. W. (1992). Clinical phenomenology of child and adolescent dissociative disorders. *Journal of the American Academy of Child and Adolescent Psychiatry*, 31, 1077–1085.

Horowitz, M. J., Wilner, N., & Alvarez, W. (1979). Impact of Event Scale: A measure of psychosomatic stress. *Archives of General Psychiatry*, 32, 85–92.

Howard, D. E., & Wang, M. Q. (2005). Psychosocial correlates of U.S. adolescents who report a history of forced sexual intercourse. *Journal of Adolescent Health*, 36, 372–379.

Hubert, N., Jay, S., Saltoun, M., & Hayes, M. (1988). Approach–avoidance and distress in children undergoing preparation for painful medical procedures. *Journal of Clinical Child Psychology, 17*, 194–202.

Humphrey, J. A., & White, J. W. (2000). Women's vulnerability to sexual assault from adolescence to young adulthood. *Journal of Adolescent Health, 27*, 419–424.

Hund, A. R., & Espelage, D. L. (2005). Childhood sexual abuse, disordered eating, alexithymia, and general distress: A mediation model. *Journal of Counseling Psychology, 52*, 559–573.

Hunter, W. M., Coulter, M. L., Runyan, D. K., & Everson, M. D. (1990). Determinants of placement for sexually abused children. *Child Abuse and Neglect, 14*, 407–417.

Hussey, D., & Singer, M. I. (1993). Psychological distress, problem behaviors, and family functioning of sexually abused adolescent inpatients. *Journal of the American Academy of Child and Adolescent Psychiatry, 32*, 954–961.

Hyson, M. (1983). Going to the doctor: A developmental study of stress and coping. *Journal of Child Psychology and Psychiatry and Allied Disciplines, 24*, 247–259.

Jacobi, C., Hayward, C., de Zwaan, M., Kraemer, H. C., & Agras, W. S. (2004). Coming to terms with risk factors for eating disorders: Application of risk terminology and suggestions for a general taxonomy. *Psychological Bulletin, 130*, 19–65.

Jaycox, L., Marshall, G. N., & Orlando, M. (2003). Predictors of acute distress among young adults injured by community violence. *Journal of Traumatic Stress, 16*, 237–245.

Joa, D., & Edelson, M. G. (2004). Legal outcomes for children who have been sexually abused: The impact of child abuse assessment center evaluations. *Child Maltreatment, 9*, 263–276.

Johnsen, L. W., & Harlow, L. L. (1996). Childhood sexual abuse linked with adult substance use, victimization, and AIDS-risk. *AIDS Education and Prevention, 8*, 44–57.

Johnson, T. C. (1988). Child perpetrators–children who molest other children: Preliminary findings. *Child Abuse and Neglect, 13*, 571–585.

Johnson, T. C., & Feldmeth, J. R. (1993). Sexual behaviors: A continuum. In E. Gil & T. C. Johnson (Eds.), *Sexualized children: Assessment and treatment of sexualized children and children who molest* (pp. 41–52). Rockville, MD: Launch Press.

Joiner, T. E., & Wagner, K. D. (1995). Attributional style and depression in children and adolescents: A meta-analytic review. *Clinical Psychology Review, 15*, 777–798.

Jones, D. P. H., & McGraw, J. M. (1987). Reliable and fictitious accounts of sexual abuse of children. *Journal of Interpersonal Violence, 2*, 27–45.

Jones, L. M., Finkelhor, D., & Kopiec, K. (2001). Why is sexual abuse declining?: A survey of state child protection administrators. *Child Abuse and Neglect, 25*, 1139–1158.

Kaplow, J., Dodge, K. A., Amaya-Jackson, L., & Saxe, G. N. (2005). Pathways to PTSD: Part II. Sexually abused children. *American Journal of Psychiatry, 162*, 1305–1310.

Kaufman, J., Jones, B., Stieglitz, E., Vitulano, L., & Mannarino, A. P. (1994). The use of multiple informants to assess children's maltreatment experiences. *Journal of Family Violence, 9*, 227–248.

Kelley, S. J., Brant, R., & Waterman, J. (1993). Sexual abuse of children in day care centers. *Child Abuse and Neglect, 17*, 71–89.

Kellogg, N. D., & Huston, R. L. (1995). Unwanted sexual experiences in adolescence: Patterns of disclosure. *Clinical Pediatrics, 34*, 306–312.

Kellogg, N. D., & Menard, S. W. (2003). Violence among family members of children and adolescents evaluated for sexual abuse. *Child Abuse and Neglect, 27*, 1367–1376.

Kelly, D., Faust, J., Runyon, M. K., & Kenny, M. C. (2002). Behavior problems in sexually abused children of depressed versus nondepressed mothers. *Journal of Family Violence, 17*, 107–116.

Kendall-Tackett, K., & Simon, A. F. (1992). Perpetrators and their acts: Data from 365 adults molested as children. *Child Abuse and Neglect, 11*, 237–245.

Kendall-Tackett, K. A., Williams, L. M., & Finkelhor, D. (1993). Impact of sexual abuse on children: A review and synthesis of recent empirical studies. *Psychological Bulletin, 113*, 164–180.

Kenny, M. C., & McEachern, A. G. (2000). Racial, ethnic, and cultural factors of childhood sexual abuse: A selected review of the literature. *Clinical Psychology Review, 20*, 905–922.

Kilpatrick, D. G., Ruggiero, K. J., Acierno, R., Saunders, D. E., Resnick, H. S., & Best, C. L. (2003). Violence and risk of PTSD, major depression, substance abuse/dependence, and comorbidity: Results from the National Survey of Adolescents. *Journal of Consulting and Clinical Psychology, 71*, 692–700.

Kiser, L. J., Heston, J., Millsap, P. A., & Pruitt, D. B. (1991). Physical and sexual abuse in childhood: Relationship with post-traumatic stress disorder. *Journal of the American Academy of Child and Adolescent Psychiatry, 30*, 776–783.

Kluft, R. P. (1985). Introduction: Multiple personality disorder in the 1980's: In R. P. Kluft (Ed.), *Childhood antecedents of multiple personality disorder* (pp. xiii–xiv). Washington, DC: American Psychiatric Press.

Kogan, S. M. (2004). Disclosing unwanted sexual experiences: Results from a national sample of adolescent women. *Child Abuse and Neglect, 28*, 1–19.

Kolko, D. J., Moser, J. T., & Weldy, S. R. (1988). Medical/health histories and physical evaluation of physically and sexually abused child psychiatric patients: A controlled study. *Journal of Family Violence, 5*, 249–267.

Koverola, C., & Foy, D. (1993). Post traumatic stress disorder symptomatology in sexually abused children: Implications for legal proceedings. *Journal of Child Sexual Abuse, 2*, 21–35.

Koverola, C., Papas, M. A., Pitts, S., Murtaugh, C., Black, M. M., & Dubowitz, H. (2005). Longitudinal investigation of the relationship among maternal victimization, depressive symptoms, social support, and children's behavior and development. *Journal of Interpersonal Violence, 20,* 1523–1546.

Koverola, C., Pound, J., Heger, A., & Lytle, C. (1993). Relationship of child sexual abuse to depression. *Child Abuse and Neglect, 17, 390–400.*

Kvam, M. H. (2000). Is sexual abuse of children with disabilities disclosed?: A retrospective analysis of child disability and the likelihood of sexual abuse among those attending Norwegian hospitals. *Child Abuse and Neglect, 24,* 1073–1084.

Lamb, S., & Edgar-Smith, S. (1994). Aspects of disclosure: Mediators of outcome of childhood sexual abuse. *Child Abuse and Neglect, 17,* 515–526.

Lanktree, C., & Briere, J. (1995). Outcome of therapy for sexually abused children: A repeated measures study. *Child Abuse and Neglect, 19,* 1145–1156.

Lau, A. S., Leeb, R. T., English, D., Graham, J. C., Briggs, E. C., Brody, K. E., et al. (2005). What's in a name?: A comparison of methods for classifying predominant type of maltreatment. *Child Abuse and Neglect, 29,* 533–551.

Laurence, J. (2000, November 19). Revealed: The truth about child sex abuse in Britain's families. *The Independent News.* Retrieved from *www.ipce.info/piceweb/Library/oonov19d_new_report.htm*

Lawson, L., & Chaffin, M. (1994). False negatives in sexual abuse disclosure interviews: Incidence and influence of caretaker's belief in abuse in cases of accidental abuse discovery by diagnosis of STD. *Journal of Interpersonal Violence, 7,* 532–542.

Laye-Gindhu, A., & Schonert-Reichl, K. A. (2005). Nonsuicidal self-harm among community adolescents: Understanding the "whats" and "whys" of self harm. *Journal of Youth and Adolescence, 34,* 447–457.

Leifer, M., Kilbane, T., & Grossman, G. (2001). A three-generational study comparing the families of supportive and unsupportive mothers of sexually abused children. *Child Maltreatment, 6,* 353–364.

Leifer, M., Shapiro, J. P., & Kassem, L. (1993). The impact of maternal history and behavior upon foster placement and adjustment in sexually abused girls. *Child Abuse and Neglect, 17,* 755–766.

Leitenberg., H., Gibson, L. E., & Novy, P. L. (2004). Individual differences among undergraduate women in methods of coping with stressful events: The impact of cumulative childhood stressors and abuse. *Child Abuse and Neglect, 28,* 181–192.

Lie, G., & McMurtry, S. L. (1991). Foster care for sexually abused children: A comparative study. *Child Abuse and Neglect, 15,* 111–121.

Ligezinska, M., Firestone, P., Manion, I. G., McIntyre, J., Ensom, R., & Wells, G. (1996). Children's emotional and behavioral reactions following disclosures of extrafamilial sexual abuse: Initial effects. *Child Abuse and Neglect, 20,* 111–125.

Lindegren, M. L., Hanson, I. C., Hammett, T. A., Beil, J., Fleming, P. L., Ward, J. W., et al. (1998). Sexual abuse of children: Intersection with the HIV epidemic. *Pediatrics, 102,* p. e46. Retrieved from *www.pediatrics.org/cgi/content/full/102/4/e46*

Liotti, G. (1999). Disorganization of attachment as a model for understanding dissociative psychopathology. In J. Solomon & C. George (Eds.), *Attachment disorganization* (pp. 291–317). New York: Guilford Press.

Lipovsky, J., Tidwell, R., Kilpatrick, D., Saunders, B., & Dawson, V. (1991, November). *Children as witnesses in criminal court: Is the process harmful?* Paper presented at the 25th Annual Meeting of the Advancement of Behavior Therapy, New York.

Lipschitz, D. S., Bernstein, D. P., Winegar, R. K., & Southwick, S. M. (1999). Hospitalized adolescents' reports of sexual and physical abuse: A comparison of two self-report measures. *Journal of Traumatic Stress, 12,* 641–654.

Lipton, M. (1997). The effect of the primary caregiver's distress on the sexually abused child: A comparison of biological and foster parents. *Child and Adolescent Social Work Journal, 14,* 115–127.

Litrownik, A. J., Lau, A., English, D. J., Briggs, E., Newton, R. R., Romney, S., et al. (2005). Measuring the severity of child maltreatment. *Child Abuse and Neglect, 29,* 553–573.

London, K., Bruck, M., Ceci, S. J., & Shuman, D. W. (2005). Disclosure of child sexual abuse: What does the research tell us about the ways that children tell? *Psychology, Public Policy, and Law, 11,* 194–226.

Long, P. J., & Jackson, J. L. (1990, November). *Defining childhood sexual abuse.* Poster presented at the annual meeting of the Association for Advancement of Behavior Therapy, San Francisco.

Low, G., Jones, D., MacLeod, A., Power, M., & Duggan, C. (2000). Childhood trauma, dissociation and self-harming behaviour: A pilot study. *British Journal of Medical Psychology, 73,* 269–278.

Luster, T., & Small, S. A. (1997). Sexual abuse history and problems in adolescence: Exploring the effects of moderating variables. *Journal of Marriage and the Family, 59,* 131–142.

Luster, T., Small, S. A., & Lower, R. (2002). The correlates of abuse and witnessing abuse among adolescents. *Journal of Interpersonal Violence, 17,* 1323–1340.

Lynch, D. L., Stern, A. E., Oates, K., & O'Toole, B. I. (1993). Who participates in child sexual abuse research? *Journal of Child Psychology and Psychiatry, 34,* 935–944.

Lyons-Ruth, K., & Block, D. (1996). The disturbed caregiving system: Relations among childhood trauma, maternal caregiving, and infant affect and attachment. *Infant Mental Health Journal, 17,* 257–275.

Macfie, J., Cicchetti, D., & Toth, S. L. (2001). The development of dissociation in maltreated preschool-age children. *Development and Psychopathology, 13*, 233–254.

MacMillan, H. L., Fleming, J. E., Trocmé, N., Boyle, M. H., Wong, M., Racine, Y. A., et al. (1997). Prevalence of child physical and sexual abuse in the community: Results from the Ontario Health Supplement. *Journal of the American Medical Association, 278*, 131–135.

MacMillian, H. L., Jamieson, E., & Walsh, C. A. (2003). Reported contact with child protection services among those reporting child physical and sexual abuse: Results from a community survey. *Child Abuse and Neglect, 27*, 1397–1408.

Manion, I. G., McIntyre, J., Firestone, P., Ligezinska, M., Ensom, R., & Wells, G. (1996). Secondary traumatization in parents following the disclosure of extrafamilial child sexual abuse: Initial effects. *Child Abuse and Neglect, 20*, 1095–1109.

Manly, J. T. (2005). Advances in research definitions of child maltreatment. *Child Abuse and Neglect, 29*, 425–439.

Manly, J. T., Cicchetti, D., & Barnett, D. (1994). The impact of subtype, frequency, chronicity, and severity of child maltreatment on social competence and behavior problems. *Development and Psychopathology, 6*, 121–143.

Mannarino, A., & Cohen, J. (1996a). Abuse-related attributions and perceptions, general attributions, and locus of control in sexually abused girls. *Journal of Interpersonal Violence, 11*, 162–180.

Mannarino, A., & Cohen, J. (1996b). Family-related variables and psychological symptom formation in sexually abused girls. *Journal of Child Sexual Abuse, 5*, 105–120.

Mannarino, A., Cohen, J., & Berman, S. (1994). The Children's Attributions and Perceptions Scale: A new measure of sexual abuse related factors. *Journal of Clinical Child Psychology, 23*, 204–211.

Martin, G., Bergen, H. A., Richardson, A. S., Roeger, L., & Allison, S. (2004). Correlates of firesetting in a community sample of young adolescents. *Australian and New Zealand Journal of Psychiatry, 38*, 148–154.

Martone, M., Jaudes, P. K., & Cavins, M. K. (1996). Criminal prosecution of child sexual abuse cases. *Child Abuse and Neglect, 20*, 457–464.

Massat, C. R., & Lundy, M. (1998). Reporting costs to nonoffending parents in cases of intrafamilial child sexual abuse. *Child Welfare, 77*, 371–388.

McElroy, L. P. (1992). Early indicators of pathological dissociation in sexually abused children. *Child Abuse and Neglect, 16*, 833–846.

McGee, H., Garavan de Barra, M., Byrne, J., & Conroy, R. (2002). *The SAVI Report: Sexual abuse and violence in Ireland: A national study of Irish experiences, beliefs, and attitudes concerning sexual violence*. Dublin: Liffey.

McGee, R. A., Wolfe, D. A., & Wilson, S. K. (1990). *A record of maltreatment experiences*. Unpublished manuscript, University of Western Ontario, London, Ontario, Canada.

McGee, R. A., Wolfe, D. A., Yuen, S. A., Wilson, S. K., & Carnochan, J. (1995). The measurement of maltreatment: A comparison of approaches. *Child Abuse and Neglect, 19*, 233–249.

McGinn, L. K., Cukor, D., & Sanderson, W. C. (2005). The relationship between parenting style, cognitive style, and anxiety and depression: Does increased early adversity influence symptom severity through the mediating role of cognitive style? *Cognitive Therapy and Research, 29*, 219–242.

McLeer, S. V., Deblinger, E., Henry, D., & Orvaschel, H. (1992). Sexually abused children at high risk for post-traumatic stress disorder. *Journal of the American Academy of Child and Adolescent Psychiatry, 31*, 875–879.

McLeer, S., Dixon, J. F., Henry, D., Ruggiero, K., Escovitz, K., Niedda, T., et al. (1998). Psychopathology in non-clinically referred sexually abused children. *Journal of the American Academy of Child and Adolescent Psychiatry, 37*, 1326–1333.

Mennen, F. E., & Meadow, D. (1993). The relationship of sexual abuse to symptom levels in emotionally disturbed girls. *Child and Adolescent Social Work Journal, 10*, 319–328.

Melton, G., Goodman, G. S., Kalichman, S. C., Levine, M., Saywitz, K., & Koocher, G. P. (1995). Empirical research on child maltreatment and the law. *Journal of Clinical Child Psychology, 24*, 47–77.

Merrill, L. L., Thomsen, C. J., Sinclair, B. B., Gold, S. R., & Milner, J. S. (2001). Predicting the impact of child sexual abuse on women: The role of abuse severity, parental support, and coping strategies. *Journal of Consulting and Clinical Psychology, 69*, 992–1006.

Meyerson, L. A., Long, P. L., Miranda, R., & Marx, B. P. (2002). The influence of childhood sexual abuse, physical abuse, family environment, and gender on the psychological adjustment of adolescents. *Child Abuse and Neglect, 26*, 387–405.

Mian, M., Wehrspann, W., Klajner-Diamond, H., LaBaron, D., & Winder, C. (1986). Review of 125 children 6 years of age and under who were sexually abused. *Child Abuse and Neglect, 4*, 223–229.

Miller, B. C., Monson, B. H., & Norton, M. C. (1995). The effects of forced sexual intercourse on white female adolescents. *Child Abuse and Neglect, 19*, 1289–1303.

Mitchell, K. J., Finkelhor, D., & Wolak, J. (2003). The exposure of youth to unwanted sexual material on the Internet: A national survey of risk, impact, and prevention. *Youth and Society, 34*, 330–358.

Moos, R. H., & Moos, B. S. (1986). *Family Environment Scale manual*. Palo Alto, CA: Consulting Psychologists Press.

Muehlenhard, C. L., Highby, B. J., Lee, R. S., Bryan, T.

S., & Dodrill, W. A. (1998). The sexual revictimization of women and men sexually abused as children: A review of the literature. *Annual Review of Sex Research, 9,* 1–47.

Mullen, P. E., Martin, J. L., Anderson, J. C., Romans, S. E., & Herbison, G. P. (1993). Childhood sexual abuse and mental health in adult life. *British Journal of Psychiatry, 163,* 721–732.

Muris, P., Schmidt, H., Lambrichs, R., & Meesters, C. (2001). Protective and vulnerability factors of depression in normal adolescents. *Behaviour Research and Therapy, 39,* 555–565.

Myers, J. E. B. (1992). *Legal issues in child abuse and neglect.* Newbury Park, CA: Sage.

Naar-King, S., Silvern, L., Ryan, V., & Sebring, D. (2002). Type and severity of abuse as predictors of psychiatric symptoms in adolescence. *Journal of Family Violence, 17,* 133–149.

National Children's Alliance. (2006). *Children's advocacy centers.* Retrieved August 26, 2006, from *www.nca-online.org*

Negrao, C., Bonanno, G. A., Noll, J. G., Putnam, F. W., & Trickett, P. K. (2005). Shame, humiliation, and childhood sexual abuse: Distinct contributions and emotional coherence. *Child Maltreatment, 10,* 350–363.

Newberger, C. M., Gremy, I. M., Waternaux, C. M., & Newberger, E. H. (1993). Mothers of sexually abused children: Trauma and repair in longitudinal perspective. *American Journal of Orthopsychiatry, 63,* 92–102.

Nisbit, I. A., Wilson, P. H., & Smallbone, S. W. (2004). A prospective longitudinal study of sexual recidivism among adolescent sex offenders. *Sexual Abuse: A Journal of Research and Treatment, 16,* 223–234.

Nock, M. K., & Prinstein, M. J. (2004). A functional approach to the assessment of self-mutilative behavior. *Journal of Consulting and Clinical Psychology, 72,* 885–890.

Nolen-Hoeksema, S., Girgus, J., & Seligman, M. E. (1992). Predictors and consequences of childhood depressive symptoms: A 5-year longitudinal study. *Journal of Abnormal Psychology, 101,* 405–422.

Noll, J. G., Trickett, P. K., & Putnam, F. W. (2000). Social network constellation and sexuality of sexually abused and comparison girls in childhood and adolescence. *Child Maltreatment, 5,* 323–337.

Oaksford, K. L., & Frude, N. (2001). The prevalence and nature of child sexual abuse: Evidence from a female university sample in the UK. *Child Abuse Review, 10,* 49–59.

Oates, R. K., Jones, D. P. H., Denson, D., Sirotnak, A., Gary, N., & Krugman, R. D. (2000). Erroneous concerns about child sexual abuse. *Child Abuse and Neglect, 24,* 149–157

Ogata, S., Silk, K., & Goodrich, S. (1990). The childhood experience of the borderline patients. In P. Links (Ed.), *Family environment and borderline personality disorder* (pp. 87–103). Washington, DC: American Psychiatric Association.

Ogawa, J. R., Sroufe, L. A., Weinfield, N. S., Carlson, E. A., & Egeland, B. (1997). Development and the fragmented self: Longitudinal study of dissociative symptomatology in a nonclinical sample. *Development and Psychopathology, 9,* 855–879.

Ohan, J. L., Myers, K., & Collett, B. R. (2002). Ten-year review of rating scales. IV: Scales assessing trauma and its effects. *Journal of the American Academy of Child and Adolescent Psychiatry, 41,* 1401–1422.

Olson, D. H., & Gorall, D. M. (2006). *FACES-IV and the circumplex model.* Retrieved August 25, 2006, from *www.facesiv.com/pdf/3.innovations/pdf*

Olson, D. H., Portner, J., & Bell, R. (1982). *Family Adaptability and Cohesion Evaluation Scales (FACES II).* Manual published by the University of Minnesota, Family Social Science Department, 290 McNeal Hall, 1985 Buford Avenue, St. Paul, MN 55108.

Olson, D. H., Portner, J., & Lavee, Y. (1985). *FACES III manual.* Manual published by the University of Minnesota, Family Social Science Department, 290 McNeal Hall, 1985 Buford Avenue, St. Paul, MN 55108.

Oxman-Martinez, J., Rowe, W. S., Straka, S. M., & Thibault, Y. (1997). La baisse d'abuse sexuels [The decline in the reported incidence of child sexual abuse cases and their delayed disclosure]. *Revue Québecoise de Psychologie, 18,* 77–90.

Paine, M. L., & Hansen, D. J. (2002). Factors influencing children to disclose sexual abuse. *Clinical Psychology Review, 22,* 271–295.

Pence, D., & Wilson, C. (1994). Reporting and investigating child sexual abuse. *The Future of Children, 4,* 70–83.

Perry, B. D., Pollard, R. A., Blakley, T. L., Baker, W. L., & Vigilante, D. (1995). Child trauma, the neurobiology of adaptation, and use dependent development of the brain: How states become traits. *Infant Mental Health Journal, 16,* 271–291.

Pianta, R., Egeland, B., & Erickson, M. (1989). The antecedents of maltreatment: Results of the Mother–Child Interaction Research Project. In D. Cicchetti & V. Carlson (Eds.), *Child maltreatment: Theory and research on the causes and consequences of child abuse and neglect* (pp. 203–253). New York: Cambridge University Press.

Pierce, R., & Pierce, L. H. (1985). The sexually abused child: A comparison of male and female victims. *Child Abuse and Neglect, 9,* 191–199.

Pintello, D., & Zuravin, S. (2001). Intrafamilial child sexual abuse: Predictors of postdisclosure maternal belief and protective action. *Child Maltreatment, 6,* 344–352.

Pithers, W., & Gray, A. (1998). The other half of the story: Children with sexual behaviour problems. *Psychology, Public Policy, and Law, 4,* 200–217.

Pithers, W., Gray, A., Busconmi, A., & Houchens, P. (1998). Children with sexual behavior problems: Identification of five distinct child types and related treatment considerations. *Child Maltreatment, 3,* 384–406.

Post, R. M., Weiss, S. R. B., Li, H., Smith, M. A., Zhang, E. X., Xing, G., et al. (1998). Neural plasticity and emotional memory. *Development and Psychopathology, 10,* 829–856.

Prohl, J., Resch, F., Parzer, P., & Brunner, R. (2001). Relationship between dissociative symptomatology and declarative procedural memory in adolescent psychiatric patients. *Journal of Nervous and Mental Disease, 189,* 602–607.

Putnam, F. W. (1990). *Child Dissociation Checklist (CBCL).* Unpublished manuscript, National Institute of Mental Health, Bethesda, MD.

Putnam, F. W. (1997). *Dissociation in children and adolescents.* New York: Guilford Press.

Putman, F. W., Helmers, K., & Trickett, P. K. (1993). Development, reliability, and validity of a child dissociation scale. *Child Abuse and Neglect, 19,* 645–656.

Putnam, F. W., Hornstein, N., & Peterson, G. (1996). Clinical phenomenology of child and adolescent dissociative disorders: Gender and age effects. *Child and Adolescent Psychiatric Clinics of North America, 5,* 351–360.

Putnam, F. W., & Peterson, G. (1994). Further validation of the Child Dissociation Checklist. *Dissociation, 7,* 204–211.

Quas, J. A., Goodman, G. S., Ghetti, S., Alexander, K. W., Edelstein, R., Redlich, A. D., et al. (2005). Childhood sexual assault victims: Long-term outcomes after testifying in criminal court. *Monographs of the Society for Research in Child Development, 70,* 1–145.

Randall, W., Parrila, R., & Sobsey, D. (2000). Gender, disability status, and risk for sexual abuse in children. *Journal of Developmental Disabilities, 7,* 1–15.

Rasmussen, L. A., Burton, J. E., & Christopherson, B. J. (1992). Precursors to offending and the trauma outcome process in sexually reactive children. *Journal of Child Sexual Abuse, 1,* 33–48.

Reimer, M. (1995). *The Adolescent Shame Measure (ASM).* Philadelphia: Temple University Press.

Reimer, M. S. (1996). "Sinking into the ground": The development and consequences of shame in adolescence. *Developmental Review, 16,* 321–363.

Rhue, J. W., Lynn, S. J., & Sandberg, D. (1995). Dissociation, fantasy, and imagination in childhood: A comparison of physically abused, sexually abused, and non-abused children. *Contemporary Hypnosis, 12,* 131–136.

Rogosch, F. A., Cicchetti, D., & Aber, J. L. (1995). The role of child maltreatment in early deviations in cognitive and affective processing abilities and later peer relationship problems [Special issue: Developmental Processes in Peer Relationships and Psychopathology]. *Development and Psychopathology, 7,* 591–609.

Romano, E., & De Luca, R. V. (2001). Male sexual abuse: A review of effects, abuse characteristics, and links with latter psychological functioning. *Aggression and Violent Behavior, 6,* 55–78.

Romero, G. J., Wyatt, G. E., Loeb, T. B., Carmona, J. V., & Solis, B. M. (1999). The psychology of Latina women [Special issue]. *Hispanic Journal of Behavioral Sciences, 21,* 351–365.

Roodman, A. A., & Clum, G. A. (2001). Revictimization rates and method variance: A meta-analysis. *Clinical Psychology Review, 21,* 183–204.

Rose, D. T., Abramson, L. Y., Hodulik, C. J., Halberstadt, L., & Leff, G. (1994). Heterogeneity of cognitive style among depressed inpatients. *Journal of Abnormal Psychology, 103,* 419–429.

Ross, C., & Joshi, S. (1992). Schneiderian symptoms and childhood trauma in the general population. *Comprehensive Psychiatry, 33,* 269–273.

Ross, S., & Heath, N. (2002). A study of the frequency of self-mutilation in a community sample of adolescents. *Journal of Youth and Adolescence, 31,* 67–77.

Rubin, K. H., Coplan, R. J., Fox, N. A., & Calkins, S. (1995). Emotionality, emotion regulation, and preschoolers' social adaptation. *Development and Psychopathology, 7,* 49–62.

Ruggiero, K. J., McLeer, S. V., & Dixon, J. F. (2000). Sexual abuse characteristics associated with survivor psychopathology. *Child Abuse and Neglect, 24,* 951–964.

Ruggiero, K. J., Smith, D. W., Hanson, R. F., Resnick, H. S., Saunders, B. E., Kilpatrick, D. G., et al. (2003). Is disclosure of childhood rape associated with mental health outcome?: Results from the National Women's Study. *Child Maltreatment, 9,* 62–77.

Runtz, M. G., & Schallow, J. R. (1997). Social support and coping strategies as mediators of adult adjustment following childhood maltreatment. *Child Abuse and Neglect, 21,* 211–226.

Runyan, D. K., Curtis, P., Hunter, W., Black, M., Kotch, J., Bangdiwala, K., et al. (1998). LONGSCAN: A consortium for longitudinal studies of maltreatment and the life course of children. *Aggression and Violent Behavior, 3,* 275–285.

Runyan, D. K., Hunter, W. M., Everson, M. D., & De Vos, E. (1992). *Maternal support for child victims of sexual abuse: Determinants and implications (final report).* Washington, DC: National Clearinghouse on Child Abuse and Neglect.

Runyon, M. K., Faust, J., & Orvaschel, H. (2002). Differential symptom patterns of post-traumatic stress disorder (PTSD) in maltreated children with and without concurrent depression. *Child Abuse and Neglect, 26,* 39–53.

Runyon, M. K., & Kenny, M. C. (2002). Relationship of attributional style, depression, and posttrauma distress among children who suffered physical or sexual abuse. *Child Maltreatment, 7,* 254–264.

Ruscio, A. M. (2001). Predicting the child-rearing practices of mothers sexually abused in childhood. *Child Abuse and Neglect, 25,* 369–387.

Russell, D. E. H. (1983). The incidence and prevalence of intrafamilial sexual abuse of female children. *Child Abuse and Neglect, 7,* 133–146.

Russell, D. E. H. (1984). The prevalence and seriousness

of incestuous abuse: Stepfathers versus biological fathers. *Child Abuse and Neglect, 8*, 15–22.

Russell, D. E. H. (1986). *The secret trauma: Incest in the lives of girls and women.* New York: Basic Books.

Ryan, P., Warren, B. L., & Weincek, P. (1991). Removal of the perpetrator versus removal of the victim in cases of intrafamilial child sexual abuse. In D. D. Knutson & J. L. Miller (Eds.), *Abused and battered: Social and legal responses of family violence* (pp. 123–133). Hawthorne, NY: Aldine de Gruyter.

Sachs-Ericsson, N., Blazer, D., Plant, E. A., & Arnow, B. (2005). Childhood sexual and physical abuse and the 1-year prevalence of medical problems in the National Comorbidity Survey. *Health Psychology, 24*, 32–40.

Sadowski, C. M., & Friedrich, W. N. (2000). Psychometric properties of the Trauma Symptom Checklist for Children (TSCC) with psychiatrically hospitalized adolescents. *Child Maltreatment, 5*, 354–372.

Saewyc, E., Skay, C., Richens, K., Reis, E., Poon, C., & Murphy, A. (2006). Sexual orientation, sexual abuse, and HIV-risk behaviors among adolescents in the Pacific Northwest. *American Journal of Public Health, 96*, 1104–1110.

Salter, D., McMillan, D., Richards, M., Talbot, T., Hodges, J., Bentovim, A., et al. (2003). Development of sexually abusive behaviour in sexually victimised males: A longitudinal study. *Lancet, 361*, 471–476.

Sanders, B., & Giolas, M. H. (1991). Dissociation and childhood trauma in psychologically disturbed adolescents. *American Journal of Psychiatry, 148*, 50–54.

Sanders, S. (1986). The Perceptual Alteration Scale: A scale measuring dissociation. *American Journal of Clinical Hypnosis, 29*, 95–102.

Sas, L. D., Cunningham, A. H., Hurley, P., Dick, T., & Farnsworth, A. (1995). *Tipping the balance to tell the secret: Public discovery of child sexual abuse.* London, Ontario, Canada: Family Court Clinic.

Saunders, B., Villeponteaux, L., Lipovsky, J., Kilpatrick, D., & Veronen, L. (1993). Child sexual abuse as a risk factor for mental disorders among women: A community survey. *Journal of Interpersonal Violence, 7*, 189–204.

Saunders, B. E., Kilpatrick, D. G., Resnick, H. S., Hanson, R., & Lipovsky, J. (1992). *Epidemiological characteristics of child sexual abuse: Results from Wave II of the National Women's Study.* Paper presented at the sixth annual San Diego Conference on Responding to Child Maltreatment, San Diego, CA.

Sauzier, M. (1989). Disclosure of child sexual abuse: For better or for worse? *Psychiatric Clinics of North America, 12*, 455–569.

Saywitz, K. J., Goodman, G., & Lyon, T. (2002). Interviewing children in and out of court: Current research and practice implications. In J. E. B. Myers, L. Berliner, J. Briere, C. T. Hendrix, C. Jenny, & T. A. Reid (Eds.), *The APSAC handbook on child maltreatment* (2nd ed., pp. 349–377). Thousand Oaks, CA: Sage.

Schuetz, P., & Eiden, R. D. (2005). The relationship between sexual abuse during childhood and parenting outcomes: Modeling direct and indirect pathways. *Child Abuse and Neglect 29*, 645–659.

Sedlak, A. J. (1997). Risk factors for the occurrence of child abuse and neglect. *Journal of Aggression, Maltreatment, and Trauma, 1*, 149–187.

Sedlak, A. J., & Broadhurst, D. D. (1996). *The Third National Incidence Survey of Child Abuse and Neglect.* Washington, DC: U.S. Department of Health and Human Services.

Sedlak, A. J., Doueck, H. J., Lyons, P., Wells, S. J., Schultz, D., & Gragg, F. (2005). Child maltreatment and the justice system: Predictors of Court involvement. *Research on Social Work Practice, 15*, 389–403.

Shaffer, D., Fisher, P., Dulkan, M. K., & Davies, M. (1996). The NIMH Diagnostic Interview Schedule for Children: Description, acceptability, prevalence rates and performance in the MECA study. *Journal of the American Academy of Child and Adolescent Psychiatry, 35*, 865–877.

Shalev, A. Y., Friedman, M. J., Foa, E. B., & Keane, T. M. (2000). Integration and summary. In E. B. Foa, T. M. Keane, & M. J. Friedman (Eds.), *Effective treatments for PTSD: Practice guidelines from the International Society for Traumatic Stress Studies* (pp. 359–379). New York: Guilford Press.

Shannon, M. P., Lonigan, C. J., Finch, A. J., & Taylor, C. M. (1994). Children exposed to disaster: I. Epidemiology of post-traumatic symptoms and symptom profiles. *Journal of the American Academy of Child and Adolescent Psychiatry, 33*, 80–93.

Shields, A., Ryan, R. M., & Cicchetti, D. (2001). Narrative representations of caregivers and emotion dysregulation as predictors of maltreated children's rejection by peers. *Developmental Psychology, 37*, 321–337.

Shipman, K., Zeman, J., Penza, S., & Champion, K. (2000). Emotion management skills in sexually maltreated and nonmaltreated girls: A developmental psychopathology perspective. *Development and Psychopathology, 12*, 47–62.

Sidran Traumatic Stress Foundation. (2000a). *The Adolescent Dissociative Experiences Scale.* Available from the Sidran Traumatic Stress Foundation, 200 East Joppa Road, Suite 207, Baltimore, MD 21286.

Sidran Traumatic Stress Foundation. (2000b). *The Child Dissociation Checklist.* Available from the Sidran Traumatic Stress Foundation, 200 East Joppa Road, Suite 207, Baltimore, MD 21286.

Silberg, J. (2000). Fifteen years of dissociation in maltreated children: Where do we go from here? *Child Maltreatment, 5*, 119–136.

Silver, R. L., & Wortman, C. (1980). Coping with undesirable events. In J. Garber & M. Seligman (Eds.), *Human helplessness: Theory and applications* (pp. 279–340). New York: Academic Press.

Silovsky, J. F., & Niec, L. (2002). Characteristics of

young children with sexual behavior problems: A pilot study. *Child Maltreatment, 7,* 187–197.

Simpson, T. L., & Miller, W. R. (2002). Concomitance between childhood sexual and physical abuse and substance use problems: A review. *Clinical Psychology Review, 22,* 27–77.

Singer, M. I., Anglin, T. M., Song, L. Y., & Lunghofer, L. (1995). Adolescents' exposure to violence and associated symptoms of psychological trauma. *Journal of the American Medical Association, 273,* 477–482.

Sirles, E. A., & Franke, P. J. (1989). Factors influencing mothers' reactions to intrafamilial sexual abuse. *Child Abuse and Neglect, 13,* 131–139.

Small, S. A., & Kerns, D. (1993). Unwanted sexual activity among peers during early and middle adolescence: Incidence and risk factors. *Journal of Marriage and the Family, 55,* 941–952.

Smith, D. W., Letourneau, E. J., Saunders, B. E., Kilpatrick, D. G., Resnick, H. S., & Best, C. L. (2000). Delay in disclosure of childhood rape: Results from a national survey. *Child Abuse and Neglect, 24*(2), 273–287.

Smith, D. W., Witte, T. H., & Fricker-Elhai, A. E. (2006). Service outcomes in physical and sexual abuse cases: A comparison of child advocacy center-based and standard services. *Child Maltreatment, 11,* 354–360.

Smith, H., & Israel, E. (1987). Sibling incest: A study of the dynamics of 25 cases. *Child Abuse and Neglect, 11,* 101–108.

Smith, M. V., Poschman, K., Cavaleri, M. A., Howell, H. B., & Yonkers, K. A. (2006). Symptoms of posttraumatic stress disorder in a community sample of low-income pregnant women. *American Journal of Psychiatry, 163,* 881–884.

Smith, S. R., & Carlson, E. B. (1996). Reliability and validity of the Adolescent Dissociative Experiences Scale. *Dissociation, 9,* 125–129.

Smolak, L., & Murnen, S. K. (2002). A meta-analytic examination of the relationship between child sexual abuse and eating disorders. *International Journal of Eating Disorders, 31,* 136–150.

Snyder, H. N. (2000). *Juvenile arrests 1999.* Washington, DC: U.S. Department of Justice, Office of Juvenile Justice and Delinquency Prevention.

Snyder, H. N., & Sickmund, M. (1999). *Juvenile Offenders and Victims: 1999 National Report.* Washington, DC: Office of Juvenile Justice and Delinquency Prevention.

Sobsey, D., & Doe, T. (1991). Patterns of sexual abuse and assault. *Sexuality and Disability, 9,* 243–259.

Sobsey, D., Randall, W., & Parrila, R. K. (1997). Gender differences in abused children with and without disabilities. *Child Abuse and Neglect, 21,* 707–720.

Sorenson, T., & Snow, B. (1991). How children tell: The process of disclosure in child sexual abuse. *Child Welfare, 70,* 3–15.

Sourander, A., Pihlakoshi, L., Aromaa, M., Rautara, P., Helenius, H., & Sillanpää, M. (2006). Early predictors of parent- and self-reported global psychological difficulties among adolescents: A prospective cohort study from age 3 to age 15. *Social Psychiatry and Psychiatric Epidemiology, 41,* 173–182.

Spaccarelli, S. (1993). *Documentation of scales for the study of stress and coping in child sex abuse.* Unpublished manuscript, Arizona State University, Tempe.

Spaccarelli, S. (1995). Measuring abuse stress and negative cognitive appraisals in child sexual abuse: Validity data on two new scales. *Journal of Abnormal Child Psychology, 23,* 703–724.

Spaccarelli, S., & Fuchs, C. (1997). Variability in symptom expression among sexually abused girls: Developing multivariate models. *Journal of Clinical Child Psychology, 26,* 24–35.

Sparrow, S. S., Balla, D. A., & Cicchetti, D. V. (1985). *Vineland Adaptive Behavior Scales.* Circle Pines, MN: American Guidance Service.

Spence, S. H., Sheffield, J., & Donovan, C. (2002). Problem-solving orientation and attributional style: Moderators of the impact of negative life events on the development of depression in adolescence? *Journal of Clinical Child Psychology, 31,* 219–229.

Sperry, D. M., & Gilbert, B. O. (2005). Child peer sexual abuse: Preliminary data on outcomes and disclosure experiences. *Child Abuse and Neglect, 29,* 889–904.

Spirito, A., Stark, L., & Williams, C. (1988). Development of a brief coping checklist for use with pediatric populations. *Journal of Pediatric Psychology, 13,* 555–574.

Stallard, P., Valleman, R., & Baldwin, S. (1998). Prospective study of posttraumatic stress disorder in children involved in road traffic accidents. *British Medical Journal, 317,* 1619–1623.

Steel, J. L., & Herlitz, C. A. (2005). The association between childhood and adolescent sexual abuse and proxies for sexual risk behavior: A random sample of the general population of Sweden. *Child Abuse and Neglect, 29,* 1141–1153.

Stevens, T. N., Ruggiero, K. J., Kilpatrick, D. G., Resnick, H. S., & Saunders, B. E. (2005). Variables differentiating singly and multiply victimized youth: Results from the National Survey of Adolescents and implications for secondary prevention. *Child Maltreatment, 10,* 211–223.

Strand, V. C., Sarmiento, T., & Pasquale, L. E. (2005). Assessment and screening tools for trauma in children and adolescents: A review. *Trauma, Violence, and Abuse, 6,* 55–78.

Straus, M. (1995). Corporal punishment of children and adult depression and suicidal ideation. In J. McCord (Ed.), *Coercion and punishment in long-term perspectives* (pp. 59–77). New York: Cambridge University Press.

Stroud, D. D., Martens, S., & Barker, J. (2000). Criminal investigation of child sexual abuse: A comparison of cases referred to the prosecutor to those not referred. *Child Abuse and Neglect, 24,* 689–700.

Stuewig, J., & McCloskey, L. A. (2005). The relation of child maltreatment to shame and guilt among adolescents: Psychological routes to depression and delinquency. *Child Maltreatment, 10,* 324–336.

Sullivan, P. M., Brookhouser, P. E., Scanlan, J. M., Knutson, J. F., & Schulte, L. E. (1991). Patterns of physical and sexual abuse of communicatively handicapped children. *Annals of Otology, Rhinology, and Laryngology, 100,* 188–194.

Sullivan, P. M., & Knutson, J. F. (1998). The association between child maltreatment and disabilities in a hospital-based epidemiological study. *Child Abuse and Neglect, 22,* 271–288.

Svedin, C. G., Nilsson, D., & Lindell, C. (2004). Traumatic experiences and dissociative symptoms among Swedish adolescents: A pilot study using Dis-Q-Sweden. *Nordic Journal of Psychiatry, 58,* 349–/355.

Swanston, H. Y., Parkinson, P. N., Oates, R. K., O'Toole, B. I., Plunkett, A. M., & Shrimpton, S. (2002). Further abuse of sexually abused children. *Child Abuse and Neglect, 26,* 115–127.

Swanston, H. Y., Plunkett, A. M., O'Toole, B. I., Shrimpton, S., Parkinson, P. N., & Oates, R. K. (2003). Nine years after child sexual abuse. *Child Abuse and Neglect, 27,* 967–984.

Tangney, J. P. (1991). Moral affect: The good, the bad, and the ugly. *Journal of Personality and Social Psychology, 61,* 598–607.

Tangney, J. P. (1995). Recent advances in the empirical study of shame and guilt. *American Behavioral Scientist, 38,* 1132–1145.

Taska, L., & Feiring, C. (1995, November). *Children's adaptation to sexual abuse: The role of shame and attribution.* Poster presented at the annual meeting of the Association for Advancement of Behavior Therapy, Washington, DC.

Tebbutt, J., Swanston, H., Oates, R. K., & O'Toole, B. I. (1997). Five years after child sexual abuse: Persisting dysfunction and problems of prediction. *Journal of the American Academy of Child and Adolescent Psychiatry, 35,* 330–339.

Teicher, M., Yutaka, I., Glod, C. A., & Anderson, S. (1997). Preliminary evidence of abnormal cortical development in physically and sexually abused children using EEG coherence and MRI. *Annals of the New York Academy of Sciences, 821,* 160–175.

Terr, L. C. (1987, May). *Severe stress and sudden shock: The connection.* Lecture presented at the annual convention of the American Psychiatric Association, Chicago.

Terr, L. C. (1991). Childhood traumas: An outline and overview. *American Journal of Psychiatry, 148,* 10–20.

Thoennes, N., & Tjaden, P. (1990). The extent, nature, and validity of sexual abuse allegations in custody and visitation disputes. *Child Abuse and Neglect, 14,* 151–163.

Thompson, K., & Wonderlich, S. (2004). Child sexual abuse and eating disorders. In K. Thompson (Ed.), *Handbook of eating disorders and obesity* (pp. 679–694). Hoboken, NJ: Wiley.

Timnick, L. (1985, August 25). 22% in survey were child abuse victims. *Los Angeles Times,* pp. 1, 34.

Tremblay, C., Hebert, M., & Piche, C. (1999). Coping strategies and social support as mediators of consequence in child sexual abuse victims. *Child Abuse and Neglect, 23,* 929–945.

Trocmé, N., & Bala, N. (2005). False allegations of abuse and neglect when parents separate. *Child Abuse and Neglect, 29,* 1333–1345.

Trocmé, N., Fallon, B., MacLaurin, B., & Neves, T. (2003). What is driving increasing child welfare caseloads in Ontario?: Analysis of the 1993 and 1998 Ontario Incidence Studies. *Child Welfare, 84,* 341–362.

Trocmé, N. McPhee, D., & Tam, K. K. (1995). Child abuse and neglect in Ontario: Incidence and characteristics. Changing the child welfare agenda: Contributions from Canada [Special issue]. *Child Welfare Journal, 74,* 563–586.

Tubman, J. G., Gil, A. G., & Wagner, E. (2004). Co-occurring substance use and delinquent behavior during early adolescence: Emerging relations and implications for intervention strategies. *Criminal Justice and Behavior, 31,* 463–488.

Tufts New England Medical Center, Division of Child Psychiatry. (1984). *Sexually exploited children: Service and research project* (Final report for the Office of Juvenile Justice and Delinquency Prevention). Washington, DC: U.S. Department of Justice.

Turner, H. A., Finkelhor, D., & Ormrod, R. (2006). The effect of lifetime victimization on the mental health of children and adolescents. *Social Sciences and Medicine, 62,* 13–27.

Ullman, S. E., & Filipas, H. H. (2005). Gender differences in social reactions to abuse disclosures, postabuse coping, and PTSD of child sexual abuse survivors. *Child Abuse and Neglect, 29,* 767–782.

U.S. Department of Health and Human Services. (2004). *Child Maltreatment 2002: Reports from the States to the National Child Abuse and Neglect Data Systems—National Statistics on Child Abuse and Neglect.* Washington, DC: Author.

Usher, J. M., & Dewberry, C. (1995). The nature and long-term effects of childhood sexual abuse: A survey of adult women survivors in Britain. *British Journal of Clinical Psychology, 34,* 177–192.

van der Kolk, B. (2005). Developmental trauma disorder: Toward a rational diagnosis for children with complex trauma histories. *Psychiatric Annals, 35,* 401–408.

van der Kolk, B. A., Perry, J. C., & Herman, J. L. (1991). Childhood origins of self destructive behaviour. *American Journal of Psychiatry, 148,* 1665–1676.

van der Kolk, B. A., van der Hart, O. V., & Marmar, C. R. (1996). Dissociation and information processing in posttraumatic stress disorder. In B. A. van der Kolk, A. C. McFarlane, & L. Weisaeth (Eds.), *Traumatic stress: The effects of overwhelming experience* on mind, body, and society (pp. 303–327). New York: Guilford Press.

van IJzendoorn, M. H., & Schuengel, C. (1996). The measurement of dissociation in normal and clinical populations: Meta-analytic validation of the Dissociative Experiences Scale (DES). *Clinical Psychology Review, 16*, 365–382.

Violatao, C., & Genius, M. (1993). Problems of research in male child sexual abuse: A review. *Journal of Child Sexual Abuse, 2*, 33–54.

Vogeltanz, N. D., Wilsnack, S. C., Harris, T. R., Wilsnack, R. W., Wonderlich, S. A., & Kristjanson, A. F. (1999). Prevalence and risk factors for childhood sexual abuse in women: National survey findings. *Child Abuse and Neglect, 23*, 579–592.

Voisin, D. R. (2005). The relationship between violence exposure and HIV sexual risk behavior: Does gender matter? *American Journal of Orthopsychiatry, 75*, 497–506.

Waller, N., Putnam, F. W., & Carlson, E. B. (1996). Types of dissociation and dissociative types: A taxometric analysis of dissociative experiences. *Psychological Methods, 1*, 300–321.

Walrath, C., Ybarra, M., Holden, W., Liao, Q., Santiago, R., & Leaf, P. (2003). Children with reported histories of sexual abuse: Utilizing multiple perspectives to understand clinical and psychosocial profiles. *Child Abuse and Neglect, 27*, 509–524.

Walsh, C., MacMillan, H. L., & Jamieson, E. (2003). The relationship between parental substance abuse and child maltreatment: Findings from the Ontario Health Supplement. *Child Abuse and Neglect, 27*, 1409–1425.

Walsh, W., & Wolak, J. (2005). Nonforcible Internet-related sex crimes with adolescent victims: Prosecution issues and outcomes. *Child Maltreatment, 10*, 260–271.

Watkins, B., & Bentovim, A. (1992). The sexual abuse of male children and adolescents: A review of current research. *Journal of the American Academy of Child and Adolescent Psychiatry, 33*, 197–248.

Way, I., Satwah, R., & Drake, B. (1999, January). *Adolescent sexual offenders: A comparison of maltreated and nonmaltreated youths.* Poster presented at the annual meeting of the Society for Social Work and Research, Austin, TX.

Wells, R. D., McCann, J., Adams, J., Voris, J., & Ensign, J. (1995). Emotional, behavioral, and physical symptoms reported by parents of sexually abused, nonabused, and allegedly abused prepubescent females. *Child Abuse and Neglect, 19*, 155–164.

Westcott, H. L., & Jones, D. P. H. (1999). Annotation: The abuse of disabled children. *Journal of Child Psychology and Psychiatry, 40*, 497–506.

Whitcomb, D. (2003). Legal interventions for child victims. *Journal of Traumatic Stress, 16*, 149–157.

Widom, C. S., & Ames, M. A. (1994). Criminal consequences of childhood sexual victimization. *Child Abuse and Neglect, 18*, 303–318.

Widom, C. S., & Kuhns, J. B. (1996). Childhood victimization and subsequent risk for promiscuity, prostitution, and teenage pregnancy: A prospective study. *American Journal of Public Health, 86*, 1607–1612.

Widom, C. S., & Morris, S. (1997). Accuracy of adult recollections of childhood victimization: Part 2. Childhood sexual abuse. *Psychological Assessment, 9*, 34–46.

Williams, L. M. (1994). Recall of childhood trauma: A prospective study of women's memories of child sexual abuse. *Journal of Consulting and Clinical Psychology, 62*, 1167–1176.

Willoughby, T., Chalmers, H., & Busseri, M. A. (2004). Where is the syndrome?: Examining co-occurrence among multiple problem behaviors in adolescence. *Journal of Consulting and Clinical Psychology, 72*, 1022–1037.

Wilson, A. E., Calhoun, K. S., & Bernat, J. A. (1999). Risk recognition and trauma-related symptoms among sexually revictimized women. *Journal of Consulting and Clinical Psychology, 67*, 705–710.

Wolfe, D. A., Sas, L., & Wekerle, C. (1994). Factors associated with the development of post-traumatic stress disorder among child victims of sexual abuse. *Child Abuse and Neglect, 18*, 37–50.

Wolfe, V. V. (2000). *Children's Impact of Traumatic Events Scale—Parent Report Version.* Unpublished assessment instrument. (Available from V. V. Wolfe, Child and Adolescent Centre, London Health Sciences Centre, 346 South St., London, Ontario N6A 4G5, Canada.)

Wolfe, V. V. (2002). *The Children's Impact of Traumatic Events Scale II (CITES-II).* Unpublished assessment instrument. (Available from V. V. Wolfe, Child and Adolescent Centre, London Health Sciences Centre, 346 South St., London, Ontario N6A 4G5, Canada.)

Wolfe, V. V. (2006). Child sexual abuse. In E. Mash & R. Barkley (Eds.), *Treatment of childhood disorders, third edition* (pp. 569–623). New York: Guilford Press.

Wolfe, V. V., & Birt, J. (1997). Child sexual abuse. In E. Mash & L. Terdal (Eds.), *Assessment of childhood disorders* (3rd ed., pp. 569–623). New York: Guilford Press.

Wolfe, V. V., & Birt, J. (2003, April). *Depressive symptoms, attributional styles, and coping strategies among sexual abuse victims and clinical and nonclinical controls.* Poster presented at the biennial meeting of the Society for Research in Child Development, Tampa, FL.

Wolfe, V. V., & Birt, J. H. (2005a). *The Children's Impact of Traumatic Events Scale—Revised (CITES-R): Scale structure, internal consistency, discriminant validity, and PTSD diagnostic patterns.* Unpublished manuscript. (Available from V. V. Wolfe, London Health Sciences Centre, 346 South St., London ON N6A 4G5 or vicky.wolfe@lhsc.on.ca.)

Wolfe, V. V., & Birt, J. H. (2005b). *The Peritraumatic Experiences Scale of the Children's Impact of Trau-*

matic Events Scale–II: A measure to assess DSM-IV-TR PTSD criterion A2. Unpublished manuscript. (Available from V. V. Wolfe, London Health Sciences Centre, 346 South St., London ON N6A 4G5 or *vicky.wolfe@lhsc.on.ca.*)

Wolfe, V. V., Gentile, C., & Bourdeau, P. (1987). *History of Victimization Questionnaire.* (Available from Vicky V. Wolfe, PhD, 346 South Street, London Health Sciences Centre, London, Ontario, N6A 4G5 Canada.)

Wolfe, V. V., Gentile, C., Michienzi, T., Sas, L., & Wolfe, D. A. (1991). The Children's Impact of Traumatic Events Scale: A measure of post–sexual abuse PTSD symptoms. *Behavioral Assessment, 13,* 359–383.

Wolfe, V. V., Gentile, C., & Wolfe, D. A. (1989). The impact of sexual abuse on children: A PTSD formulation. *Behavior Therapy, 20,* 215–228.

Woodward, L., Fergusson, D. M., & Horwood, L. J. (2001). Risk factors and life processes associated with teen pregnancy: Results of a prospective study from birth to 20 years. *Journal of Marriage and the Family, 63,* 1170–1184.

Wright, J., Friedrich, W. N., Cyr, M., Thériault, C., Perron, A., Lussier, Y., et al. (1998). The evaluation of Franco-Quebec victims of child sexual abuse and their mothers: The implementation of a standard assessment protocol. *Child Abuse and Neglect, 22,* 9–23.

Wright, M. O., Fopma-Loy, J., & Fischer, S. (2005). Multidimensional assessment of resilience in mothers who are child sexual abuse survivors. *Child Abuse and Neglect, 29,* 1173–1193.

Wurtele, S. K. (2002). School-based child sexual abuse prevention, In P. A. Schewe (Ed.), *Preventing violence in relationships: Interventions across the life span* (pp. 9–54). Washington, DC: American Psychological Association.

Wyatt, G. E. (1985). The sexual abuse of Afro-American and White-American women in childhood. *Child Abuse and Neglect, 9,* 507–519.

Wyatt, G. E., Loeb, T. B., Solis, B., Carmona, J. V., & Romero, G. (1999). The prevalence and circumstances of child sexual abuse: Change across a decade. *Child Abuse and Neglect, 23,* 45–60.

Yates, T. M., & Carlson, E. A. (2003, April). *Fragile foundations: The developmental antecedents of self-injurious behavior.* Paper presented at the annual meeting of the Society for Research in Child Development, Tampa, FL.

Yeager, C. A., & Lewis, D. O. (1996). The intergenerational transmission of violence and dissociation. *Child and Adolescent Psychiatric Clinics of North America, 5,* 393–430.

Zayed, R., Wolfe, V. V., & Birt, J. (2006). *Child Dissociation Checklist: Psychometric properties of parent- and child-report versions.* Unpublished manuscript. (Available from V. V. Wolfe, Ph.D., London Health Sciences Centre, 346 South Street, London, Ontario, N6A 2L2 Canada.)

Zupanic, M. K., & Kreidler, M. C. (1998). Shame and the fear of feeling. *Perspectives in Psychiatric Care, 34,* 29–34.

Zuravin, S. J., & Fontanella, C. (1999). Parenting behaviors and perceived parenting competence of child sexual abuse survivors. *Child Abuse and Neglect, 23,* 623–632.

PART VII

Problems of Adolescence

CHAPTER 16

Eating Disorders

Eric Stice
Carol B. Peterson

Eating disorders are psychiatric disturbances involving abnormal eating behaviors, maladaptive efforts to control shape and weight, and disturbances in perceived body shape. Three eating disorder syndromes are recognized in the literature: anorexia nervosa, bulimia nervosa, and binge-eating disorder. These eating disorders commonly emerge during adolescence and can result in severe subjective distress, functional impairment, morbidity, and mortality.

We first define these eating disorders, with a focus on diagnostic criteria, associated clinical features, descriptive epidemiology, psychiatric comorbidity, etiology, and young adult outcomes. Next, we discuss the assessment and diagnoses of eating disorders, including general assessment considerations, critical assessment domains, and methods for selecting measurement instruments and integrating assessment data. Finally, we review questionnaire measures and diagnostic interviews that we believe are most feasible and ecologically useful in most assessment and clinical settings, as well as those supported by reliability and validity data.

DEFINITIONS OF THE DISORDERS

Anorexia Nervosa

Diagnostic Criteria

The diagnostic criteria for anorexia nervosa include extreme emaciation (less than 85% of expected weight for height and age), intense fear of gaining weight or becoming fat despite a low body weight, disturbed perception of weight and shape, undue influence of weight or shape on self-evaluation or denial of the seriousness of the low body weight, and amenorrhea in postmenarcheal females (American Psychiatric Association [APA], 1994). Table 16.1 provides a more detailed operationalization of the diagnostic symptoms for anorexia nervosa from the fourth edition of the *Diagnostic and Statistical Manual of Mental Disorders* (DSM-IV). A distinction is made between a restricting type of anorexia nervosa, in which the person does not regularly engage in binge eating or purging (self-induced vomiting or laxative–diuretic use), and a binge eating–purging type of anorexia nervosa, in which the person does engage in these behaviors. This distinction is

TABLE 16.1. DSM-IV-TR Criteria for Anorexia Nervosa

A. Refusal to maintain body weight at or above a minimally normal weight for age and height (e.g., weight loss leading to maintenance of body weight less than 85% of that expected; or failure to make expected weight gain during period of growth, leading to body weight less than 85% of that expected).

B. Intense fear of gaining weight or becoming fat, even though underweight.

C. Disturbance in the way one's body weight or shape is experienced, undue influence of body weight or shape on self-evaluation, or denial of the seriousness of the current low body weight.

D. In postmenarcheal females, amenorrhea, i.e., the absence of at least three consecutive menstrual cycles. (A woman is considered to have amenorrhea if her periods occur only following hormone, e.g., estrogen, administration.)

Specify type:

Restricting Type: during the current episode of Anorexia Nervosa, the person has not regularly engaged in binge-eating or purging behavior (i.e., self-induced vomiting or the misuse of laxatives, diuretics, or enemas)

Binge-Eating/Purging Type: during the current episode of Anorexia Nervosa, the person has regularly engaged in binge-eating or purging behavior (i.e., self-induced vomiting or the misuse of laxatives, diuretics, or enemas)

Note. From American Psychiatric Association (2000). Copyright 2000 by the American Psychiatric Association. Reprinted by permission.

based on the observation that individuals with the binge–purge type of anorexia nervosa have elevated personal and family histories of obesity and higher rates of impulsive behaviors, including stealing, drug abuse, self-harm, and mood lability, than individuals with the restricting type of anorexia nervosa (Garner, Vitousek, & Pike, 1993).

Although the diagnostic criteria for anorexia nervosa appear straightforward, they can be challenging to implement (Commission on Adolescent Eating Disorders, 2005). With regard to criterion A, because children and adolescents are undergoing physical maturation, it can be difficult to determine whether a particular individual is actually at or below the 85th percentile for body weight. The most logical solution is to use age- and sex-adjusted norms to determine the weight percentile, but these

can be rather challenging to locate. Complicating matters is the necessity to adjust for height when considering weight, which is most typically done by focusing on the body mass index (BMI = kg/m^2). In addition, the weight and height norms are continuously changing as the prevalence of overweight and obesity increase in the general population. With regard to criterion B, younger individuals and those who are not motivated for treatment may deny that they fear weight gain, despite engaging in behaviors clearly designed to prevent weight gain and that clearly suggest a fear of gaining weight. One possible solution to this difficulty would be to reformulate this diagnostic criterion in terms of typical weight control behaviors, so that it would not be necessary to rely on unobservable cognitions for making diagnoses. Criterion D is somewhat controversial, because several studies have found that individuals who meet all of the diagnostic criteria for anorexia nervosa except amenorrhea do not differ from those who meet all of the diagnostic criteria (e.g., Garfinkel et al., 1996). In addition, the fact that certain forms of birth control produce seemingly regular menstrual cycles in those who would not otherwise experience them, whereas other forms of birth control can cause functional amenorrhea complicates matters further. These considerations suggest that this may be a less useful criterion for anorexia nervosa.

Associated Clinical Features

There are several common clinical features associated with anorexia nervosa, including a relentless pursuit of thinness and overvaluation of body shape that usually result in extreme dietary restriction and high levels of physical activity (Fairburn & Harrison, 2003). Consequent to this state of semistarvation, individuals experience mood disturbances, preoccupation with food, and ritualistic and stereotyped eating (Wilson, Becker, & Heffernan, 2003). Anorexia nervosa is also associated with the highest rates of suicidal ideation and mortality of any psychiatric condition (Herzog et al., 2000; Newman et al., 1996). According to the clinical literature (Slade, 1982), anorexia nervosa is also commonly associated with a need for control and dysfunctional relationships with family members, although it is unclear whether this is a cause or consequence of this eating disorder. Because of the extreme pursuit of thinness that characterizes individuals with anorexia nervosa, the eating disorder is often perceived as a personal accomplishment rather than a psychiatric disorder in need of treatment. Thus, individuals with anorexia nervosa are often brought to treatment by concerned family members or friends and are typically very resistant to treatment, which invariably involves weight restoration.

Common physical presenting symptoms include yellowish skin (due to hypercarotenemia), lanugo (fine, downy hair), hypersensitivity to cold, hypotension, bradycardia, and other cardiovascular problems (Wilson et al., 2003). Purging behaviors may cause enlargement of salivary glands and erosion of dental enamel. Most importantly, dehydration and electrolyte imbalance resulting from chronic purging may lead to serum potassium depletion and consequent hypokalemia, which increases risk of renal failure and cardiac arrhythmia. Osteopenia may also result from malnutrition and decreased estrogen secretion.

Epidemiology, Course, and Periodicity

Epidemiological studies that primarily have relied on diagnostic interviews suggest that between 1.4 and 2.0% of girls and women experience anorexia nervosa, and that between 0.1 and 0.2% of boys or men experience this condition during their lifetime (Favaro, Ferrara, & Santonastaso, 2003; Lewinsohn, Hops, Roberts, Seeley, & Andrews, 1993; Lewinsohn, Striegel-Moore, & Seeley, 2000; Woodside et al., 2001). Community-recruited samples indicate that the rates of subthreshold or partial-syndrome anorexia nervosa range between 1.1 and 3.0% for adolescent girls (Lewinsohn et al., 2000; Stice, Presnell, & Bearman, 2007). Point prevalence rates range between 0.3 and 0.7% for full-threshold anorexia nervosa and between 0.0 and 0.4% for subthreshold anorexia nervosa among adolescent females, but the rates for males were too low to detect in epidemiological samples (Commission on Adolescent Eating Disorders, 2005).

Retrospective data suggest two peak periods of risk for onset of anorexia nervosa: age 14 and age 18 (APA, 1994). The fact that these two peak periods of risk correspond to the developmental transitions from grade school to high school and from high school to post–high school roles (e.g., going to college or assuming full-time jobs) suggests that developmental

stressors may precipitate onset of this condition among at-risk individuals. In addition, the fact that eating disorders more broadly tend to emerge after pubertal development suggests that there may be something about physical maturation of secondary sexual characteristics or concomitant increases in the female gender role internalization that increases risk for eating pathology, though the precise mechanisms that underlie this effect are unclear.

The course and outcome of this condition are highly variable (Wilson et al., 2003). Some afflicted individuals stage a complete and lasting recovery after only one episode of anorexia nervosa. Other individuals oscillate between marked weight loss and hospitalization, and periods of restoration of normal weight. Still others show weight restoration but experience bulimia nervosa or some other eating disorder not otherwise specified (ED NOS). Finally, a sizable proportion of afflicted individuals never recover from this eating disorder.

Although much attention has focused on ethnic differences in eating disorders, to date there is little evidence of ethnic differences in the rates of eating disorder symptoms and only limited evidence of ethnic differences in risk factors for eating disorders (Shaw, Ramirez, Trost, Randall, & Stice, 2004; Striegel-Moore, Wilfley, Pike, Dohm, & Fairburn, 2000). The one consistent ethnic difference that has emerged is that African Americans report less body dissatisfaction than their European American counterparts (Smolak & Striegel-Moore, 2001).

Psychiatric Comorbidity

Very few studies have examined the rates of comorbid psychiatric disorders among children and adolescents with anorexia nervosa relative to those without this eating disorder. In addition, virtually nothing is known about comorbidity in males, because the rates of eating disorders are extremely low. However, one study that collapsed across the various eating disorders suggested that men with eating disorders show very similar psychiatric comorbidity to that of women with eating disorders (Woodside et al., 2001). Moreover, many studies examining comorbidity in any age group use treatment-seeking samples, which are typically biased toward finding elevated comorbidity relative to population levels, because each psychiatric condition that an individual has increases the odds of treatment seeking (Berkson, 1946). Another limitation of our knowledge base is that many studies have reported lifetime comorbidity, rather than concurrent comorbidity, and it is not clear that the former really should be conceptualized as comorbidity. From a clinical perspective, greater weight should be given to studies reporting concurrent comorbidity because these are the comorbid conditions that should be assessed with the greatest care among individuals with anorexia nervosa presenting for assessment or treatment.

Lewinsohn, Hops, Roberts, Seeley and Andrews (1993), one of the few groups to have collected psychiatric diagnostic data from a large cohort of community-recruited adolescents, provided detailed information about the rates of comorbid conditions among individuals with anorexia nervosa (personal communication with J. Seeley, January 2006). Relative to the base rates observed in the larger sample of female adolescents, those with anorexia nervosa had elevated rates of dysthymia (5 vs. 44%), bipolar disorder (3 vs. 33%), and oppositional defiant disorder (3 vs. 22%). However, individuals with anorexia nervosa did not show elevated rates of bulimia nervosa, major depression, conduct disorder, attention-deficit/ hyperactivity disorder, substance use disorders, social phobia, simple phobia, agoraphobia, posttraumatic stress disorder, panic disorder, obsessive–compulsive disorder, separation anxiety, generalized anxiety disorder, or borderline personality disorder. Newman and colleagues (1996), another group that has collected psychiatric diagnostic data from a large cohort of community-recruited adolescents, also provided detailed information about the rates of comorbid conditions in the past year among individuals with anorexia nervosa (T. Moffitt, personal communication, October 2001). Relative to the base rates observed in the larger sample of female adolescents, those with anorexia nervosa had elevated rates of agoraphobia (50 vs. 5%), simple phobia (25 vs. 13%), dysthymia (25 vs. 4%), marijuana dependence (50 vs. 4%), and antisocial personality disorder (1 vs. 25%). In comparison to the base rates observed in the larger sample of female adolescents, those with anorexia nervosa had lower rates of obsessive–compulsive disorder (0 vs. 7%), social phobia (0 vs. 12%), and alcohol dependence (0 vs. 5%). It was noteworthy that the rates of major depression were similar among the large sample of adolescents relative

to those with anorexia nervosa (21 vs. 25%). However, these estimates should be interpreted with care, because there were only four individuals with anorexia nervosa in the past year from the Newman sample and only nine from the Lewinsohn sample.

We were able to locate a study on a community-recruited sample of individuals with anorexia nervosa that examined the rates of personality disorders. Although it lacked a weight-matched control group, there was evidence that adult females with anorexia nervosa showed elevated rates of narcissistic, dependent, avoidant, and obsessive–compulsive personality disorders, but did not show particularly elevated rates of paranoid, schizoid, schizotypal, antisocial, borderline, or histrionic personality disorders (Gillberg, Rastam, & Gillberg, 1995).

Although there appear to be no comparable data from treatment-seeking samples of adolescents with anorexia nervosa, one large study of adults seeking treatment for anorexia nervosa likewise suggested that the current rates of several disorders were elevated relative to current prevalence data available from epidemiological studies of similar-age participants (e.g., Garfinkel et al., 1995). Herzog, Keller, Sacks, Yeh, and Lavori (1992) found that the rates of current major depression (37%), obsessive–compulsive disorder (5%), panic disorder (7%), and phobic disorder (15%) were substantially higher than the lifetime prevalence rates observed in epidemiological studies. However, Herzog and associates found that the rates of alcohol and drug use disorders (both were 0% in this sample) among treatment-seeking adults were lower than the lifetime prevalence rates observed in epidemiological studies.

Collectively, results suggest that individuals with anorexia nervosa often show elevated rates of mood, anxiety, and substance use disorders. However, the inconsistencies across studies suggest that caution should be used when interpreting these findings, particularly because of the low base rate of anorexia nervosa in the population and the limited data available from adolescent samples.

Etiology

Although there are numerous theories regarding the etiological processes that promote the development of anorexia nervosa, almost no prospective studies have investigated factors that predict subsequent onset of anorexic pathology or increases in anorexic symptoms, and there have been no prospective tests of multivariate etiological models. Thus, surprisingly little is currently known about the risk factors for anorexic pathology or how they work together to promote this pernicious eating disturbance. Prospective studies are essential to determining whether a putative risk factor is a precursor, concomitant, or a consequence of eating pathology.

Theorists have suggested a wide variety of risk factors for anorexia nervosa, including norepinephrine abnormalities, serotonergic abnormalities, childhood sexual abuse, negative life events, low self-esteem, perfectionism, need for control, disturbed family dynamics, internalization of the thin ideal, dietary restraint, and mood disturbances (Fairburn & Harrison, 2003; Kaye, Klump, Frank, & Strober, 2000; Wilson et al., 2003). These findings are largely based on cross-sectional studies that have compared individuals with and without anorexia nervosa (Commission on Adolescent Eating Disorders, 2005). However, because of the cross-sectional design of most of the studies in this literature, it is not possible to confirm whether they temporally preceded the development of anorexia nervosa, or whether they might have been a result of experiencing this pernicious eating disturbance.

Nonetheless, we were able to locate two prospective studies that examined risk factors for anorexia nervosa. In one study, which used the Swedish psychiatric inpatient registry, girls who were born prematurely (particularly those who were small for gestational age) and those born with cephalhematoma (a collection of blood under the scalp of a newborn) were at elevated risk for developing anorexia nervosa (Cnattingius, Hultman, Dahl, & Sparen, 1999). These particular obstetrical complications appear to be relatively specific to anorexia nervosa, given that they do not predict onset of schizophrenia or onset of affective or reactive psychosis (Cnattingius et al., 1999). The authors suggested that subtle brain injury at birth might result in feeding difficulties that increase risk for the onset of anorexia nervosa. Another possibility is that eating pathology in the mothers resulted in a premature birth and small gestational size of the infants because of malnourishment (Commission on Adolescent Eating Disorders, 2005). A second prospective study that tested predictors of subsequent onset of threshold or subthreshold anorexia nervosa

found that girls with the lowest relative weight and those with extremely low scores on a dietary restraint scale at baseline, when they averaged 13 years of age, were at increased risk for future onset of anorexic pathology over a 5-year period (Stice, Presnell, & Bearman, 2007). In contrast to expectancies, early puberty, perceived pressure to be thin, thin-ideal internalization, body dissatisfaction, depressive symptoms, and deficits in parental and peer support did not predict onset of anorexic pathology; however, these null findings should be interpreted with care because of the low base rate of this outcome. Unfortunately, we were unable to locate any additional prospective studies that focused on predicting onset of anorexic pathology or increases in anorexia nervosa symptoms: All of the other studies that focused on this eating disorder collapsed across anorexic and bulimic pathology (e.g., McKnight Investigators, 2003; Patton, Johnson-Sabine, Wood, Mann, & Wakeling, 1990; Santonastaso, Friederici, & Favaro, 1999), rendering it difficult to determine whether these risk factors are specific to each of these two eating disorders.

It is probable that genetic factors contribute to the development of anorexia nervosa, but twin studies have produced conflicting results, with heritability estimates ranging from 0 to 70% for anorexia nervosa and from 0 to 83% for bulimia nervosa (Fairburn, Cowen, & Harrison, 1999; Kaye et al., 2000). Other genetic findings are likewise conflicting. For example, in one study the concordance rate for monozygotic twins was greater than that for dizygotic twins (Treasure & Holland, 1989), but another observed findings in the opposite direction (Walters & Kendler, 1995). Similarly, studies that have tried to identify specific receptor genes associated with anorexia nervosa have produced highly inconsistent results that have not been replicated (e.g., Hinney et al., 1998). The large range in parameter estimates suggests fundamental problems with sampling error, resulting from small samples, the reliability of diagnostic procedures, or statistical models used to estimate genetic effects. It therefore appears premature to draw conclusions regarding the degree of genetic heritability of anorexia nervosa at this time.

Young Adult Outcomes

Research suggests that among adolescents with anorexia nervosa, 50–70% will recover, 20%

will show improvement but continue to exhibit residual symptoms, and 10–20% will not recover from this eating disorder (Commission on Adolescent Eating Disorders, 2005). Although these recovery figures appear promising, it is not uncommon for recovery to take up to 10 years (Strober, Freeman, & Morrell, 1997). In addition, those showing residual symptoms often exhibit abnormalities in weight, eating behaviors, body image, and menstrual functioning, and disturbances in psychosocial functioning. Furthermore, relapse is common after discharge from inpatient treatment, occurring in approximately 30% of the cases (Strober et al., 1997). There is also evidence that many patients with anorexia nervosa, particularly of the restricting subtype, develop binge eating and eventually satisfy criteria for bulimia nervosa after sufficient weight gain (Eddy et al., 2002). (Few individuals with bulimia nervosa show subsequent onset of anorexia nervosa.)

Anorexia nervosa also has one of the highest mortality rates of any psychiatric disturbance; approximately 6% of patients diagnosed with this disorder die per decade of illness, and anorexia nervosa patients are 12 times more likely to die than women of similar age in the population (Keel et al., 2003; Sullivan, 1995). The most common causes of death are acute starvation and suicide. The suicide rate for anorexia nervosa is 57 times greater than that for the general population (Keel, Fulkerson, & Leon, 1997).

Bulimia Nervosa

Diagnostic Criteria

The diagnostic criteria for bulimia nervosa include recurrent episodes (at least two episodes per week for the previous 3 months) of uncontrollable consumption of large amounts of food, recurrent use (at least twice weekly for the previous 3 months) of compensatory behavior to prevent consequent weight gain (e.g., self-induced vomiting, laxative abuse, diuretic abuse, fasting, or excessive exercise), and undue influence of weight and shape on self-evaluation (APA, 1994). Table 16.2 provides a more detailed operationalization of DSM-IV diagnostic symptoms for bulimia nervosa. If these symptoms occur exclusively during a period of time in which the individual satisfies diagnostic criteria for anorexia nervosa, the lat-

---

TABLE 16.2. DSM-IV-TR Criteria for Bulimia Nervosa

A. Recurrent episodes of binge eating. An episode of binge eating is characterized by both of the following:
  (1) eating, in a discrete period of time (e.g., within any 2-hour period), an amount of food that is definitely larger than most people would eat during a similar period of time and under similar circumstances
  (2) a sense of lack of control over eating during the episode (e.g., a feeling that one cannot stop eating or control what or how much one is eating)

B. Recurrent inappropriate compensatory behavior in order to prevent weight gain, such as self-induced vomiting; misuse of laxatives, diuretics, enemas, or other medications; fasting; or excessive exercise.

C. The binge eating and inappropriate compensatory behaviors both occur, on average, at least twice a week for 3 months.

D. Self-evaluation is unduly influenced by body shape and weight.

E. The disturbance does not occur exclusively during episodes of Anorexia Nervosa.

Specify type:

  Purging Type: during the current episode of Bulimia Nervosa, the person has regularly engaged in self-induced vomiting or the misuse of laxatives, diuretics, or enemas

  Nonpurging Type: during the current episode of Bulimia Nervosa, the person has used other inappropriate compensatory behaviors, such as fasting or excessive exercise, but has not regularly engaged in self-induced vomiting or the misuse of laxatives, diuretics, or enemas

Note. From American Psychiatric Association (2000). Copyright 2000 by the American Psychiatric Association. Reprinted by permission.

---

ter diagnosis is given precedence because of the treatment implications; for those with anorexia nervosa, weight restoration is a key clinical goal. During binge episodes, individuals with bulimia nervosa (and binge-eating disorder) typically consume between 1,000 and 2,000 calories, which usually involve foods with high fat and sugar content (Walsh, 1993; Yanovski et al., 1992). Bulimia nervosa is typically associated with marked feelings of guilt and shame regarding eating behaviors, which are often kept secret from friends and family (Wilson et al., 2003). One benefit is that this shame makes it easier to engage individuals with bulimia nervosa in treatment than is the case for individuals with anorexia nervosa, although the average patient has bulimia nervosa for 6 years before seeking treatment (Fairburn & Harrison, 2003). Similar to individuals with anorexia nervosa, those with bulimia nervosa often present with rigid rules regarding eating and an overvaluation of thinness.

The diagnostic criteria for bulimia nervosa may also be somewhat difficult to interpret (Commission on Adolescent Eating Disorders, 2005). The diagnostic criteria for binge eating, criterion A, has specific requirements regarding the amount of food typically consumed during a binge episode (larger than most people would eat), the duration of the binge episode (in a discrete period of time), and subjective experience of the episode (a sense of a lack of control over eating). It can be difficult to determine with certainty whether each of these conditions is satisfied for a particular individual. For example, certain clients may endorse uncontrollable binge eating in a discrete period of time but report eating a quantity of food that is not larger than what most people eat (e.g., two medium bowls of cereal). Because many clients exhibit a relatively chaotic eating pattern, it is often difficult to determine whether the reported eating episodes simply represent meals of a typical content at atypical times, or whether they truly represent clinically significant binge eating. Other clients, particularly males, may endorse eating an amount of food that is clearly larger than what most people eat (e.g., two large pizzas) but may deny that they experienced a lack of control over their eating. Criterion B requires that individuals endorse recurrent and inappropriate compensatory behaviors used to prevent weight gain. Although certain of these behaviors are discrete and easy to quantify, such as self-induced vomiting, others can be very difficult to operationalize, such as fasting and excessive exercise. A large proportion of adolescent girls endorse excessive exercise for weight control purposes, but on further probing it becomes clear that the exercise is not particularly excessive (e.g., doing 50 sit-ups or taking a 15-minute walk). It can also be difficult to determine whether the exercise is specifically used to compensate for overeating or simply part of a healthy lifestyle. It can also be challenging to determine when use of laxatives or diuretics becomes "misuse." Criterion C requires that individuals report engaging in binge eating and compensatory behaviors an average

of twice weekly for 3 months, but there is evidence that individuals slightly below this frequency and duration threshold report similar impairment and comorbidity to that of persons above this threshold (Garfinkel et al., 1995). Last, criterion D stipulates that self-evaluation be unduly influenced by weight and shape, but this criterion is endorsed by a large portion of adolescent girls and may be difficult to separate from body dissatisfaction. These ambiguities suggest that it might be beneficial to use more behavioral criteria for bulimia nervosa, or that clear decision algorithms should be developed for widescale use.

Clinical Features

There are several common clinical features of bulimia nervosa. This eating disorder is typified by rigid rules regarding eating and by dysfunctional cognitions about body shape and weight, as is the case with anorexia nervosa. Individuals with bulimia nervosa are also often secretive about their eating disturbances because of shame and guilt over these behaviors. It is not uncommon for parents and peers to be unaware of the disordered eating. In contrast to anorexia nervosa, individuals with bulimia nervosa are typically distressed about their eating behavior and are receptive to treatment, although approximately one-third of these individuals are fearful about giving up these behaviors and show a limited response to treatment. In addition, individuals with bulimia nervosa are typically in the average weight range. Laboratory-based investigations have revealed that during binge-eating episodes, individuals with bulimia nervosa primarily consume carbohydrates and fats (47 and 40% respectively; Walsh, 1993). Community-recruited samples indicate that bulimia nervosa is also associated with an increased risk for suicide attempt (Newman et al., 1996).

Bulimia nervosa may be associated with physical complaints, including fatigue, headaches, and enlarged salivary glands secondary to recurrent vomiting, and erosion of dental enamel from gastric fluids (Wilson et al., 2003). Electrolyte abnormalities (hypokalemia and hypochloremia) from frequent purging can result in cardiac arrhythmias and arrest. Regular use of laxatives may also result in dependence and withdrawal upon discontinuation, and also cause colon damage.

Epidemiology, Course, and Periodicity

Epidemiological studies suggest that between 1.1 and 4.6% of girls and women experience bulimia nervosa, and between 0.1 and 0.2% of boys or men experience this condition during their lifetime (Favaro et al., 2003; Garfinkel et al., 1995; Lewinsohn et al., 1993, 2000; Woodside et al., 2001). Community-recruited samples indicate that for adolescent females, the rates of subthreshold or partial-syndrome bulimia nervosa range between 2.0 and 5.4% (Lewinsohn et al., 2000; Stice et al., 2007). Point prevalence rates range between 0.7 and 1.5% for full-threshold bulimia nervosa, and between 0.0 and 1.2% for subthreshold bulimia nervosa among adolescent females, but the rates for males were too low to detect in epidemiological samples (Commission on Adolescent Eating Disorders, 2005). Although eating disorders such as bulimia nervosa are much more rare in males, some evidence suggests that male athletes may be at elevated risk for eating disorders (Wilson et al., 2003). Prospective epidemiological studies indicate that the peak period of risk for onset of full- and subthreshold bulimia nervosa is between 14 and 19 years of age for females (Lewinsohn et al., 2000; Stice et al., 2007).

Results in community-recruited samples suggest that bulimia nervosa typically shows a chronic course characterized by periods of recovery and relapse, whereas subthreshold bulimic pathology shows less chronicity (Bohon, Muscatell, Burton, & Stice, 2005; Fairburn, Cooper, Doll, Norman, & O'Connor, 2000). One large study followed a community-recruited cohort of 102 adolescent girls and young women with full-threshold bulimia nervosa for 5 years (Fairburn et al., 2000). Results indicated that afflicted individuals often showed marked initial improvement, followed by gradual improvement. By the end of this 5-year study, 15% of the participants still met diagnostic criteria for full-threshold bulimia nervosa, 2% met criteria for anorexia nervosa, and 34% met criteria for ED NOS. Findings also indicated instability in the course shown by this cohort; each year approximately 33% showed symptom remission, and 33% showed relapse. A second study that followed 101 community-recruited adolescent girls with full- or subthreshold bulimia nervosa indicated that 54% of the participants with bulimia

nervosa recovered over the 1-year follow-up, and that 45% of the participants with subthreshold bulimia nervosa recovered over this follow-up period (Bohon et al., 2005). In another community-recruited study, 40% of women with bulimia nervosa showed recovery over a 1-year follow-up (Grilo et al., 2003).

Psychiatric Comorbidity

As described previously, limited data are available regarding psychiatric comorbidity among adolescents with eating disorders, including bulimia nervosa. Lewinsohn and colleagues (1993), one of the few groups with comorbidity data from a large cohort of community-recruited adolescents, provided information about the rates of comorbid conditions among individuals with bulimia nervosa (J. Seeley, personal communication, January 2006). Compared to the base rates observed in the larger sample of female adolescents, those with bulimia nervosa showed elevated rates of major depression (60 vs. 89%), dysthymia (6 vs. 17%), bipolar disorder (3 vs. 11%), and conduct disorder (2 vs. 11%). However, individuals with bulimia nervosa did not show elevated rates of simple phobia, social phobia, agoraphobia, overanxious disorder, panic disorder, posttraumatic stress disorder, generalized anxiety disorder, separation anxiety, obsessive–compulsive disorder, oppositional defiant disorder, attention-deficit/hyperactivity disorder, substance use disorders, or borderline personality disorder. Moffit and associates (Newman et al., 1996) also provided detailed information about the past-year prevalence of comorbid conditions among individuals with bulimia nervosa from a community-recruited sample of adolescents (T. Moffitt, personal communication, October 2001). Relative to the base rates observed in the larger sample of female adolescents, those with bulimia nervosa had elevated rates of agoraphobia (22 vs. 5%), social phobia (22 vs. 12%), major depression (66 vs. 22%), dysthymia (22 vs. 4%), alcohol dependence (33 vs. 5%), marijuana dependence (22 vs. 4%), and antisocial personality disorder (11 vs. 1%). The rates of the remaining major psychiatric diagnoses were roughly equivalent in young women with and without bulimia nervosa. These estimates should be interpreted with care, because there were only nine individuals with bulimia nervosa in the past year from the

Newman sample, and only 18 from the Lewinsohn sample.

It is noteworthy that in one large, community-recruited sample of adolescents and adults (Garfinkel et al., 1995) relative to comparison participants without bulimia nervosa, those with current bulimia nervosa had much higher current prevalence rates of major depression (2 vs. 20%), any anxiety disorder (8 vs. 33%), social phobia (4 vs. 29%), simple phobia (4 vs. 18%), agoraphobia (2 vs. 13%), panic disorder (1 vs. 11%), generalized anxiety disorder (1 vs. 4%), and alcohol dependence (1 vs. 4%). More confidence may be placed in these estimates, because there were 55 individuals with bulimia nervosa in the Garfinkel and colleagues sample. Although there appear to be no comparable data from treatment-seeking samples of adolescents with bulimia nervosa, one large study of adults seeking treatment for this eating disorder likewise suggested that current rates of several disorders were elevated relative to current prevalence data available from epidemiological studies of similar-age participants (e.g., Garfinkel et al., 1995). Specifically, Herzog and associates (1992) found that the rates of current major depression (32%) and substance use disorders (5%) were substantially higher than the lifetime prevalence rates observed in epidemiological studies. However, the rates of obsessive–compulsive disorder (1%), panic disorder (0%), and phobic disorder (9%) were generally similar to the rates of these conditions found in epidemiological studies.

Thus, findings from both community-recruited and treatment-seeking samples suggest that individuals with bulimia nervosa often show elevated rates of mood disorders, anxiety disorders, and substance use disorders. However, the inconsistency in the findings across studies suggests that these results should be interpreted with care.

Etiology

According to the general sociocultural model of bulimia nervosa, an internalization of the socially sanctioned thin ideal for females combines with direct pressures for females thinness (e.g., weight-related teasing) to promote body dissatisfaction, which in turn is thought to increase the risk for the initiation of dieting and for negative affect and conse-

quent bulimic pathology (Cattarin & Thompson, 1994; Garner, Olmsted, & Polivy, 1983; Polivy & Herman, 1985; Stice, 2001). This body dissatisfaction is thought to lead females to engage in dietary restraint in an effort to conform to this thin ideal, which paradoxically increases the likelihood of the initiation of binge eating. Dieting also entails a shift from a reliance on physiological cues to cognitive control over eating behaviors, which leaves the individual vulnerable to overeating when these cognitive processes are disrupted. Body dissatisfaction is also theorized to contribute to negative affect, which increases the risk that these individuals will turn to binge eating to provide comfort and distraction from negative emotional states.

Consistent with the sociocultural model, thin-ideal internalization, perceived pressure to be thin, body dissatisfaction, dietary restraint, and negative affect have been consistently found to increase the risk for future onset of bulimic symptoms and bulimic pathology in prospective studies (Field, Camargo, Taylor, Berkey, & Colditz, 1999; Killen et al., 1994, 1996; Stice, Killen, Hayward, & Taylor, 1998). Experiments have confirmed that a reduction in thin-ideal internalization, body dissatisfaction, and negative affect have produced the expected decreases in bulimic symptoms but have failed to provide support for dietary restraint (for a review, see Stice, 2002). For example, randomized trials have found that assignment to a weight loss diet results in decreases in binge eating and bulimic symptoms (Klem, Wing, Simkin-Silverman, & Kuller, 1997; Presnell & Stice, 2003). A number of other risk factors have received support in a few prospective studies, such as deficits in social support, substance abuse, and elevated body mass, but other hypothesized risk factors for bulimic pathology have not received support in prospective studies, including early menarche and temperamental impulsivity (Stice, 2002).

There is also some evidence that early feeding problems may increase the risk for future binge eating and bulimic symptoms. Marchi and Cohen (1990) found that digestive problems and pica in early childhood were associated with subsequent bulimic symptoms during adolescence. Another study found that initial elevations in body mass and longer duration of infant sucking in the first year of life predicted emergence of overeating and vomiting during middle childhood (Stice, Agras, & Hammer, 1999), although these variables have not been shown to predict onset of DSM-IV binge eating or bulimia nervosa.

A variety of hypotheses have been offered regarding biological variables that may increase risk for onset or persistence of bulimia nervosa (Kaye et al., 2000). However, we were unable to locate any prospective or experimental tests of these hypotheses. In addition, it is almost certain that genetic factors contribute to the development of bulimia nervosa, but twin studies have produced conflicting results, with heritability estimates ranging from 0 to 83% for bulimia nervosa (Bulik, Sullivan, & Kendler, 1998; Fairburn et al., 1999; Kaye et al., 2000). Furthermore, studies of specific receptor genes associated with bulimia nervosa have produced inconsistent results that have not been replicated (e.g., Hinney et al., 1998). Thus, it appears premature to draw conclusions regarding the degree of genetic heritability of bulimia nervosa at this time.

Young Adult Outcomes

Approximately 40–75% of adolescents and adults with bulimia nervosa recover within a 5-year period and the remaining patients often show improvements in their symptoms (Commission on Adolescent Eating Disorders, 2005). However, the relapse rates are very high, with about one-third of patients relapsing within 1 year of recovery. In addition, many patients with bulimia nervosa exhibit residual symptoms after they no longer meet full diagnostic criteria for this eating disorder and show continued impairments in physical and psychosocial functioning (Fairburn et al., 2000). The mortality rate for bulimia nervosa is less than 1% (Keel, Mitchell, Miller, Davis, & Crow, 1999).

Furthermore, prospective studies have found that threshold and subthreshold bulimia nervosa increase the risk for future onset of depression, suicide attempts, anxiety disorders, substance abuse, obesity, and health problems (Johnson, Cohen, Kasen, & Brook, 2002; Stice, Cameron, Killen, Hayward, & Taylor, 1999; Stice, Hayward, Cameron, Killen, & Taylor, 2000; Striegel-Moore, Seeley, & Lewinsohn, 2003). For example, approximately 40% of individuals with bulimia nervosa will eventually meet diagnostic criteria for major depression,

even if they recover from their eating disorder (Fairburn et al., 2000).

Binge-Eating Disorder

Diagnostic Criteria

Binge-eating disorder is listed in DSM-IV (APA, 1994) as a provisional eating disorder diagnosis that requires further study, and as an example of eating disorder not otherwise specified. This eating disorder involves (1) repeated episodes (at least 2 days per week for previous 6 months) of uncontrollable binge eating characterized by certain features (e.g., rapid eating, eating until uncomfortably full, eating large amounts of food when not physically hungry, eating alone because of embarrassment, and feeling guilty or depressed after overeating), (2) marked distress regarding binge eating, and (3) the absence of regular compensatory behaviors (APA, 1994). Table 16.3 provides a more detailed operationalization of the provisional diagnostic symptoms for binge-eating disorder from DSM-IV. If these symptoms occur exclusively during a period of time in which the individual satisfies diagnostic criteria for anorexia nervosa or bulimia nervosa, these latter diagnoses are given precedence.

The diagnostic criteria for binge-eating disorder may also be difficult to apply. As with the criteria for bulimia nervosa, it can be challenging to determine whether purported binge episodes truly involve the consumption of an objectively large amount of food and truly involve a subjective loss of control over eating. Also, similar to bulimia nervosa, certain individuals, particularly males, may not endorse the features that reflect subjective distress regarding the binge eating, even though the binge eating may be severe. Also, few data demonstrate that the particular cutoff points regarding the frequency (twice weekly) or duration (for 6 months) optimally differentiate between individuals with and without clinically meaningful binge-eating disorder. In addition, it is often difficult for individuals to provide an accurate frequency of binge-eating episodes, because they are not punctuated by discrete compensatory behaviors (self-induced vomiting). Individuals with binge-eating disorder often report overeating continuously throughout the day (i.e., grazing), which is why it is necessary to focus on the frequency of binge-eating days

TABLE 16.3. DSM-IV-TR Research Criteria for Binge-Eating Disorder

A. Recurrent episodes of binge eating. An episode of binge eating is characterized by both of the following:
 (1) eating, in a discrete period of time (e.g., within any 2-hour period), an amount of food that is definitely larger than most people would eat during a similar period of time and under similar circumstances
 (2) a sense of lack of control over eating during the episode (e.g., a feeling that one cannot stop eating or control what or how much one is eating)

B. The binge episodes are associated with three (or more) of the following:
 (1) eating much more rapidly than normal
 (2) eating until feeling uncomfortably full
 (3) eating large amounts of food when not feeling physically hungry
 (4) eating alone because of being embarrassed by how much one is eating
 (5) feeling disgusted with oneself, depressed, or very guilty after overeating

C. Marked distress regarding binge eating is present.

D. The binge eating occurs, on average, at least 2 days a week for 6 months.
 Note: The method of determining frequency differs from that used for Bulimia Nervosa; future research should address whether the preferred method of setting a frequency threshold is counting the number of days on which binges occur or counting the number of episodes of binge eating.

E. The binge eating is not associated with the regular use of inappropriate compensatory behaviors (e.g., purging, fasting, excessive exercise) and does not occur exclusively during the course of Anorexia Nervosa or Bulimia Nervosa.

Note. From American Psychiatric Association (2000). Copyright 2000 by the American Psychiatric Association. Reprinted by permission.

rather than binge-eating episodes for diagnostic purposes.

Clinical Features

Relatively little is known about the common clinical features of binge-eating disorder, particularly during childhood and adolescence. However, studies of adults suggest that this condition often results in marked weight gain and onset of obesity (Fairburn et al., 2000).

Thus, binge-eating disorder is often associated with medical complications related to obesity, including high blood pressure, adverse lipoprotein profiles, diabetes mellitus, atherosclerotic cerebrovascular disease, coronary heart disease, colorectal cancer, reduced lifespan, and death from all causes (Dietz, 1998; Fontaine, Redden, Wang, Westfall, & Allison, 2003). In addition, individuals with binge-eating disorder often present with marked shame and guilt about their eating behaviors, which is associated with significant psychological distress.

Epidemiology, Course, and Periodicity

Epidemiological studies suggest that between 0.2 and 1.5% of girls and women experience binge-eating disorder, and between 0.9 to 1.0% of boys and men experience this condition during their lifetime (Cotrufo, Barretta, Monteleone, & Maj, 1998; Favaro et al., 2003; Hoek & van Hoeken, 2003; Kjelsas, Bjornstrom, & Gotestam, 2004). Community-recruited samples indicate that for adolescent females, the rate of subthreshold binge-eating disorder is 1.6% (Lewinsohn et al., 2000; Stice et al., 2007). Point prevalence rates range between 0.6 and 0.7% for full-threshold binge-eating disorder, but the rates for males were too low to detect in epidemiological samples (Commission on Adolescent Eating Disorders, 2005). To the best of our knowledge, there are no prospective data on the higher risk periods for onset of binge-eating disorder, although prospective studies have found that the peak period of risk for onset of DSM-IV–defined binge-eating episodes tends to occur between ages 16 and 18 years (Stice et al., 1998, 2007). However, retrospective data from clinical samples suggest that binge-eating disorder often shows a somewhat later age of onset relative to both anorexia nervosa and bulimia nervosa (Commission on Adolescent Eating Disorders, 2005).

Community-recruited natural history studies suggest that binge-eating disorder often shows a high remission rate over time, with nearly 50% of cases showing recovery by 6-month follow-up (Cachelin et al., 1999) and approximately 80% of cases showing recovery by 3- to 5-year follow-up (Fairburn et al., 2000; Wilson et al., 2003). However, some studies revealed that many of these individuals developed ED NOS or continued to show some residual symptoms, as is the case with other eating disorders. In addition, Fairburn et al. (2000) found that the rate of obesity increased from 20 to 39% over this 5-year study.

Psychiatric Comorbidity

To the best of our knowledge, no studies have examined the rates of psychiatric disorders among children and adolescents with and without binge-eating disorder, which is perhaps not surprising given that this most recently recognized eating disorder has a relatively later age of onset. In the only study of non-treatment-seeking adult individuals that used a control group, Telch and Stice (1998) found that women with binge-eating disorder did not show significantly higher rates of major depression, bipolar disorder, dysthymia, substance abuse or dependence, panic disorder, agoraphobia, social phobia, or obsessive–compulsive disorder than weight-matched comparison women (although participants with binge-eating disorder did report elevated lifetime rates of major depression). Telch and Stice also found that individuals with binge-eating disorder did not show significantly elevated rates of avoidant, dependent, obsessive–compulsive, passive–aggressive, self-defeating, paranoid, schizotypic, schizoid, histrionic, narcissistic, borderline, or antisocial personality disorders relative to weight-matched controls. In a parallel study of individuals seeking weight loss treatment, women with binge-eating disorder reported significantly higher rates of current major depression (25%) relative to weight-matched comparison participants (6%), but the two groups did not differ in terms of current bipolar disorder, dysthymic disorder, posttraumatic stress disorder, agoraphobia, panic disorder, social phobia, specific phobia, or generalized anxiety disorder (Fontenelle et al., 2003). The most likely explanation for the evidence of elevated rates of comorbid current major depression in the treatment-seeking sample, but not in the non-treatment-seeking sample, is that treatment-seeking samples are biased toward finding elevated comorbidity (Berkson, 1946). Consistent with this interpretation, the rate of current major depression was 16% in another sample (Wilfley et al., 2000) of treatment-seeking individuals with binge-eating disorder, relative to the 5% rate observed in the non-treatment-seeking sample examined by Telch and Stice (1998).

Thus, it appears that individuals with binge-eating disorder do not typically show the elevated rates of mood, anxiety, and substance use disorders documented for anorexia nervosa and bulimia nervosa, although there is evidence that individuals with binge-eating disorder may show elevated rates of depression in treatment-seeking populations. However, these findings should be generalized to adolescents with caution, because all of these estimates are from samples of adults.

Etiology

To date there have been relatively few theories regarding the etiological processes that promote binge-eating disorder, but those that have been proposed conceptually overlapped with etiological theories put forth for bulimic pathology (Vogeltanz-Holm et al., 2000). Prospective studies have provided evidence that initial elevations in body mass, body dissatisfaction, dietary restraint, negative affect, and emotional eating increase the risk for future onset of binge eating (Stice, Presnell, & Spangler, 2002; Stice et al., 1998; Vogeltanz-Holm et al., 2000).

Young Adult Outcomes

Little is known about the young adult outcome associated with binge-eating disorder. However, in one community-recruited natural history study, individuals with binge-eating disorder often manifested onset of obesity (Fairburn et al., 2000). These findings converge with evidence indicating that binge eating is a risk factor for obesity onset (Stice et al., 2002). Furthermore, low self-confidence, diminished energy level, and discrimination from teachers and peers have been found to present significant obstacles to achievement in school and other pursuits among overweight adolescents (Gortmaker, Must, Perrin, & Sobol, 1993; Morrill, Leach, Shreeve, Puhl, & Brownell, 2001).

Eating Disorder Not Otherwise Specified

In addition to the three widely recognized eating disorders noted earlier, DSM-IV also allows for the diagnosis of eating disorder not otherwise specified (ED NOS; APA, 1994). This category includes subdiagnostic levels of anorexia nervosa, bulimia nervosa, and binge-eating disorder (Fairburn & Harrison, 2003). For example, an individual who only uses compensatory behaviors an average of one time per week (versus two times per week) but meets all other diagnostic criteria for bulimia nervosa probably warrants a diagnosis of ED NOS. The ED NOS category also includes partial-syndrome eating disorders. For instance, an individual who does not evidence uncontrollable binge eating but nonetheless engages in weekly compensatory behaviors may warrant a diagnosis of ED NOS. Finally, the ED NOS category includes other atypical eating disorders, such as food avoidance or refusal, rumination (chewing food and then spitting it out), or pica (eating nonfood items) exhibited during adolescence and adulthood.

ED NOS is particularly important during childhood and adolescence, because nearly half of individuals in this developmental period who seek treatment for eating pathology do not meet full diagnostic criteria for anorexia nervosa or bulimia nervosa (Fisher, Schneider, Burns, Symons, & Mandel, 2001; Williamson, Gleaves, & Savin, 1992). The clinical features vary greatly for ED NOS.

Relatively little is known about the prevalence, course, or periodicity of ED NOS. In one study a community-recruited sample of individuals with ED NOS showed a recovery rate of 59% over a 1-year follow-up (Grilo et al., 2003), suggesting that the course may be shorter than is the case for anorexia or bulimia nervosa. Little research has been conducted on psychiatric comorbidity in samples of individuals with ED NOS, or on etiological processes and young adult outcomes within the general eating disorder category.

There are certain concerns with the current criteria for ED NOS in DSM-IV (APA, 1994). First, nearly half of adolescents seeking treatment for eating pathology do not meet full diagnostic criteria for anorexia or bulimia nervosa (Fisher et al., 2001; Herzog, Hopkins, & Burns, 1993; Williamson et al., 1992). The fact that the diagnostic net is missing nearly half of adolescents who present for treatment clearly suggests that frequency criteria for certain symptoms are overly high and that diagnostic criteria for certain syndromes are overly narrow. With regard to the former, a large portion of individuals presenting for treatment do not satisfy the frequency criteria for binge eating and compensatory behaviors for bulimia nervosa and binge-eating disorder diagnoses.

With regard to the latter, the fact that many individuals presenting for treatment have symptom compositions that fall outside the diagnostic criteria for anorexia nervosa, bulimia nervosa, and binge-eating disorder suggests the need to recognize the diversity of symptom presentation for these eating disturbances. For example, many adolescent males endorse recurrent, uncontrollable eating binges but do not satisfy criteria for binge-eating disorder, because they do not report distress and guilt over their eating behavior. Although ED NOS can be applied to these cases, because the patients, their parents, and reimbursement parties often do not consider these disturbances as serious as a full-threshold diagnosis, treatment or proper case management is often hampered.

Another limitation of the current diagnostic criteria is that there is no requirement that the eating disturbances cause clinically significant distress or impairment in social, occupational, or other important areas of functioning, as is the case for other psychiatric disorders, such as major depression. It is our understanding that this criterion was not originally included because many patients with clinically significant anorexia nervosa and bulimia nervosa deny distress or impairment. However, this criterion would be particularly useful for determining whether a diagnosis of ED NOS is warranted for individuals who do not quite meet full diagnostic criteria for another eating disorder. Such an amendment to the diagnostic criteria would also be potentially useful if a decision were made to relax the frequency requirements or symptom combination requirements we discussed previously. However, it might not be prudent to include the requirement of clinically significant distress or impairment in the diagnostic criteria for anorexia nervosa given that many patients with this condition minimize their eating disturbance.

ASSESSMENT AND DIAGNOSIS OF EATING DISORDERS

General Assessment Considerations

The assessment of youth with eating disorder symptoms poses a number of challenges for the clinician. Adolescents with eating disorders are usually referred because of concerns about weight loss or symptoms that include binge eating, purging, fasting, extreme dietary restriction, and excessive exercise. At times, relatives and school personnel express greater concern about these symptoms than do adolescents. Because individuals with eating disorders usually conceal their symptoms from others, many adolescents are symptomatic for lengthy periods of time before they seek treatment or are brought to treatment by their parents. Significant weight loss is usually apparent and tends to prompt parents' decision to pursue an evaluation. Occasionally, adolescents successfully hide their weight loss by wearing loose clothing. Some parents are aware of their child's weight loss but do not pursue treatment. Adolescents with eating disorders who are not underweight are often referred to treatment because they have been "caught" (e.g., self-induced vomiting, binge eating) or have admitted they are symptomatic. In most cases, parents are worried about their child's health and safety, and this concern is typically the main parental priority. Older adolescents may seek treatment on their own, without the family's knowledge.

One of the most difficult aspects of conducting these assessments is that many individuals with eating disorders are ambivalent about seeking treatment or refuse treatment altogether. Although treatment refusal is common among patients of all ages with eating disorders, it complicates the assessment of youth who are brought unwillingly to the evaluation by their parents. The accuracy of self-report in eating disorder assessment is compromised by a number of factors, including patients' minimization of symptoms to avoid treatment, lack of self-awareness or understanding, and cognitive biases that may affect accurate information recall (Anderson & Paulosky, 2004; Schacter, 1999; Vitousek, Daly, & Heiser, 1991). Malnourishment and nutritional deprivation may also impair concentration and memory (Keys, Brozek, Henschel, Mickelson, & Taylor, 1950).

The clinician should consider a number of factors in conducting the initial assessment and may choose to discuss some of these issues with parents by phone before the appointment. The issue of confidentiality is particularly problematic, because some youth are unwilling to disclose information to the clinician in front of the parents, or to share any information about themselves that they know will be revealed by the clinician to the parents. Parents often recognize this process and may be willing to relinquish their right to be told details about the content of the interactions between the clinician and adolescent, as long as they are assured that the clinician will inform them of any information pertinent to their child's safety (e.g., medical instability, suicidal thoughts, self-injurious behaviors, substance abuse).

In general, one of the most crucial assessment and therapeutic strategies is establishment of a solid rapport that provides a foundation for treatment and facilitates the collection of more accurate assessment data (Peterson, 2005). For this reason, the clinician should attempt to devote at least part of the initial intake to meeting alone with the adolescent to understand his or her perspective and needs. Although some youth with eating disorders deny that they have problems with eating and weight, most are willing to admit that they are struggling with interpersonal problems, academic concerns, and even depressive symptoms. In contrast, some youth are readily willing to discuss their eating disorder symptoms in detail.

As described below, a number of empirically supported instruments may be used in the assessment of eating disorder symptoms. When administered carefully, these instruments may actually enhance rapport and improve the comprehensiveness and quality of assessment data. Many adolescents with eating disorders experience significant interpersonal isolation and are ashamed of at least some of their symptoms, particularly binge eating. The use of well-articulated questions during the intake, along with appropriate assessment measures, provides for adolescents a sense that the clinician understands them and their symptoms.

When conducting an eating disorder assessment interview, semistructured or unstructured, it is most effective to convey a combination of empathy, curiosity, and patience (Miller & Rollnick, 2002; Peterson, 2005). This stance may be challenging in the face of open hostility, withdrawal, or acute medical instability, but it is nonetheless essential to building a sense of trust. When the clinician encounters anger and resistance, it is helpful to consider the source of these feelings, and to express empathy and curiosity to the adolescent. Fear is often the driving force behind this type of hostility, because most adolescents with eating disorders are terrified that they will be forced to change their eating and gain weight. The clinician can explore these possibilities with the adolescent during the initial interview (e.g., "I sense that you don't want to be here talking with me. Before I start asking you questions, let's start with your feelings about coming here today") to gradually begin the process of building rapport.

Eating disorder assessment interviews should be characterized by detailed questioning and frequent clarification (Fairburn & Cooper, 1993). Probing in detail is especially helpful to elicit accurate data and to communicate the clinician's knowledge of eating disorder patterns. For example, if an adolescent reports eating an apple for lunch, the clinician can express interest in the size of the apple, whether the apple was peeled, and how much of the apple was actually consumed. When obtaining information about the types and amounts of food eaten during a binge-eating episode, the clinician can ask, "What else did you eat?"—even after the adolescent has described the consumption of an unusually large amount of food. Once again, such a question serves to elicit accurate data, as well as convey to the adolescent that the clinician understands the nature of binge eating and is not shocked or negatively judgmental about how much food has been eaten.

In summary, the clinical assessment of eating disorders may be challenging for a number of reasons, including the need to address concerns of all family members, the importance of conducting a detailed evaluation, and the high likelihood of encountering inaccurate self-reported data. The goal of the clinician is to express empathy, patience, and curiosity regardless of hostility, anxiety, or denial that may be conveyed by adolescents or their family members. The importance of rapport in eating disorder assessment and treatment cannot be overemphasized, and the assessment phase provides a critical opportunity for the gradual development of trust and honesty.

Assessment Domains

The clinical assessment of eating disorders is multidimensional, incorporating medical, psychological and behavioral, nutritional, interpersonal, and psychosocial factors. Careful assessment in each of these domains is essential for establishing an accurate diagnosis, ensuring medical stability, and devising an effective treatment plan. Eating disorder assessment and treatment often involve a multidisciplinary team, including a psychologist, a psychiatrist, a pediatrician, and a dietician. If different professionals conduct various components of the assessment, then it is crucial that they communicate with each other and are in agreement about the assessment information and treatment plan.

Medical Evaluation

Youth with eating disorders may experience a wide range of medical problems, some of which can be both acutely and chronically dangerous (Roerig, Mitchell, Myers, & Glass, 2002). A thorough medical evaluation should be conducted as soon as possible after the initial assessment (for detailed reviews, see Pomeroy, 2004; Society for Adolescent Medicine, 1995), especially for individuals who are significantly underweight and/or purging. Blood testing for hypokalemia is particularly crucial. The medical evaluation typically informs the most immediate question of medical stability and whether the adolescent requires hospitalization.

One aspect of the medical condition that is often assessed by the mental health clinician is height and weight, because this information is needed to determine the percentage of ideal body weight as well as the BMI (kg/m^2; see the National Institutes of Health BMI website, *nhlbisupport.com/bmi/*, for calculating BMI values). These data are often required immediately to make an eating disorder diagnosis, as well as to provide preliminary information about the degree of emaciation in underweight adolescents. Self-reported height and weight should be confirmed by actual measurement, and if possible the adolescent should be weighed in a gown. Some adolescents deliberately provide misinformation about their height and weight to avoid treatment, as a way of insisting that they are "fine"; others give inaccurate information unintentionally.

Although obtaining height and weight is an important component of the initial assessment, many individuals with eating disorders find this aspect of the evaluation highly distressing. The clinician should be aware of adolescents' concerns and be as sensitive as possible about the weighing procedure. Individuals with eating disorders typically weigh themselves frequently or avoid weighing themselves out of fear or distress (Fairburn & Cooper, 1993). Asking explicitly how the adolescent feels about being weighed may help this process, as well as providing the option of a "blind weight," in which the adolescent neither sees nor hears the actual number. As important as it is to be sensitive to the adolescent's needs in the weighing process, the clinician must also be vigilant about the possibility of deception (e.g., adding weights to the pocket of the gown, drinking large amounts of fluid prior to weighing).

Psychological and Behavioral Variables

Assessment of psychological and behavioral variables is necessary to determine eating disorder and comorbid psychopathology diagnoses. This domain includes core eating disorder symptoms, comorbid Axis I and Axis II symptoms, developmental history, and other aspects of psychological functioning. In addition to establishing diagnosis, evaluating each of these factors is necessary to determine the treatment plan and intervention priorities.

Psychological and behavioral variables may be assessed with a combination of interviews and self-report instruments. In clinical settings, the interview is typically unstructured; however, the use of interviews such as the Eating Disorder Examination (EDE; Fairburn & Cooper, 1993; described below) provides a number of advantages to the clinician, yields more comprehensive and higher quality assessment data, and potentially enhances rapport (Peterson, 2005).

COMPENSATORY BEHAVIORS

The adolescent should be asked about the current and past frequency and duration of compensatory behaviors, including self-induced vomiting, fasting, excessive exercise, and abuse of laxatives and diuretics. Determining type and amount of laxatives and diuretics is also important. The clinician should also ask about the use of syrup of ipecac to induce vomiting, because it is particularly dangerous and can cause cardiomyopathy and organ dysfunction (Pomeroy, 2004). Other types of compensatory behaviors are less common but can occur, including manipulation of insulin in individuals with diabetes and the abuse of thyroid medication (APA, 1994). Although not part of the criteria, diet pill use and caffeine abuse are also important behaviors to assess and may impact the adolescent's medical status.

BINGE EATING

Among the eating disorder symptoms, binge eating is perhaps one of the most difficult to assess accurately (Wilson, 1993). Because DSM-IV requires that an episode comprise both an unusually large amount of food and a subjective sense of lack of control to be considered a binge, both of these constructs must be evaluated to determine the presence and frequency of binge eating. A number of researchers have observed that whereas the correlation between questionnaire and interview-based estimates of compensatory behaviors are generally high (e.g., Peterson & Miller, 2005), the concordance between these types of assessments for binge eating is more modest. The main source of inconsistency between self-reported and interview-based estimates of binge eating appears to be clinician raters' higher threshold for what is considered objectively or unusually large compared to individuals with eating disorders, who place more emphasis on the subjective experience of loss of control in labeling their eating as a binge (Beglin & Fairburn, 1992; Telch, Pratt, & Niego, 1998).

Because of limitations in the accuracy of written self-report data in assessing binge eating, interviews are generally essential to determine the presence and frequency of this symptom. The EDE (Fairburn & Cooper, 1993), a particularly effective method of assessing binge eating (Wilson, 1993), may be used by the clinician to determine the frequency of different types of binge eating. The EDE distinguishes between objective bulimic episodes, in which the amount of food consumed is large according to a clinical rater and the individual experiences a sense of loss of control, and subjective bulimic episodes, in which the individual experiences a sense of loss of control and feels that he or she has overeaten, but does not consume an objectively large amount of food. Although the clinical significance of the size distinction in binge-eating episodes is unclear and a topic of debate (Keel, Mayer, & Harnden-Fischer, 2001; Niego, Pratt, & Agras, 1997; Pratt, Niego, & Agras, 1998), it is nonetheless crucial to determine the size of the binge-eating episodes to make an accurate DSM-IV diagnosis.

As described earlier, careful and detailed probing is especially important when asking about binge-eating episodes. The clinician should ask for several examples of the types and amounts of food consumed during binge-eating episodes and never express shock or dismay about the amount of food consumed. Careful questioning about the subjective sense of loss or lack of control is also important and potentially challenging. Translating this construct into more concrete terms may be helpful, for example, by asking adolescents if they felt they could not resist eating food that was available, felt unable to stop eating once they started, or experienced a sense of being driven or compelled to eat (Fairburn & Cooper, 1993).

BODY IMAGE

Body image is a multidimensional construct that includes a number of different components, both perceptual and cognitive (Thompson, 2004). Effective assessment often integrates questionnaire and interview data to establish a comprehensive evaluation of body image (for detailed reviews, see Thompson & Gardener, 2002; Thompson, Roehrig, Cafri, & Heinberg, 2005). Aspects of body image include dissatisfaction with weight and/or shape; overvaluation of shape and/or weight in self-evaluation; body image distortion (i.e., misperception of body size or body parts); preoccupation with weight and shape, ideal weight and shape; and behavioral phenomena, including checking, rituals, and avoidance.

Because of the complexity of body image, the clinician should attempt to prioritize which aspects are most relevant and important to assess, particularly aspects of body image that are essential to establish a DSM-IV diagnosis: fear of weight gain, body image distortion, and overvaluation of shape and weight in self-evaluation. Fear of weight gain is generally straightforward to assess through direct questioning, although it should be noted that some individuals with anorexia nervosa fear becoming fat, whereas others fear any type of weight gain. Body image distortion is particularly difficult to measure (Thompson & Gardener, 2002). A number of devices have been used in research studies to assess the perceptual accuracy of individuals with eating disorders, and a meta-analysis suggests that, on average, samples of participants with eating disorders do overestimate their size and shape to a greater extent than do those without eating disorders (Cash & Deagle, 1997). However, these measures are generally impractical for clinical use, and questionnaire methods are not generally

effective for assessing body image distortion. Fortunately, many individuals with eating disorders are able to describe this phenomenon and admit that their perception of their bodies shifts dramatically depending on their mood, stress level, and recent food consumption. Some adolescents will agree that others perceive their bodies as thinner than they do. Body image distortion can also be inferred when an emaciated individual insists that he or she is obese (Peterson, 2005).

Although the overvaluation of shape and weight in determining self-evaluation is included in the criteria for both anorexia nervosa and bulimia nervosa, this abstract construct is challenging to assess, particularly in adolescents. Self-evaluation may be assessed using questionnaires, although the complexity of understanding self-definition and the self-awareness required to respond to these questions may result in inaccurate self-report data among adolescents. Whether using the EDE or an unstructured interview, the clinician can attempt to make self-evaluation more concrete by asking the adolescent to construct a list or pie chart to depict different components (e.g., school, relationships, work) and their importance (Fairburn & Cooper, 1993).

Other aspects of body image, although not included in the diagnostic criteria, are nonetheless core features of eating disorders and are important to address during assessment and treatment. In addition to interviews, a number of questionnaires assess body dissatisfaction and distress. Preoccupations, rituals, checking, and avoidance may also be evaluated using questionnaires or interviews. The Body Shape Questionnaire (Cooper, Taylor, Cooper, & Fairburn, 1987) and the Multidimensional Body–Self Relations Questionnaire (Brown, Cash, & Mikulka, 1990) are two measures with considerable psychometric support and clinical utility.

COMORBID PSYCHOPATHOLOGY

As described earlier, the high rates of comorbid psychopathology in eating disorders make this an important focus of assessment, especially symptoms of mood, anxiety, substance use, and personality disorders. Semistructured instruments such as the Structured Clinical Interview for DSM-IV (SCID; Spitzer, Williams, Gibbon, & First, 1990) and the Schedule for Affective Disorders and Schizophrenia for School-Age

Children (K-SADS; Puig-Antich & Chambers, 1983) can provide a thorough and comprehensive method of evaluating comorbidity. Written questionnaires that measure these types of symptoms are also clinically useful, although the clinician should be aware of potential "false positives" that can arise in the context of eating disorder symptoms. On mood disorder questionnaires, for example, adolescents with eating disorders typically endorse disturbances in eating and weight that may or may not be symptoms of depression. Semistarvation symptoms may also mimic clinical depression (Keys et al., 1950). On measures of anxiety, scores are often elevated due to anxiety that is specifically focused on weight, shape, and eating. For these reasons, data assessing comorbid psychopathology may need to be interpreted with caution for individuals with eating disorders.

PERSONALITY

Assessing personality in adolescents with eating disorders is important in several respects. First, the high rates of comorbid personality disorders make them crucial to assess, although assigning accurate Axis II diagnoses in younger adolescents can be quite difficult and may need to be provisional (see Shiner, Chapter 17, this volume). Other than accurate assignment of Axis II symptoms, assessment of personality dimensions provides important information for understanding aspects of the eating disorder (e.g., perfectionism, impulsivity) and formulating a treatment plan. Although less is known about personality and adolescents with eating disorders, individuals with restricting anorexia nervosa have been found to have elevations on measures of constraint, anxiety, and perfectionism; individuals with bulimia nervosa and the bulimic subtype of anorexia nervosa have elevated scores of impulsivity and affective instability (Cassin & von Ranson, 2005; Vitousek & Manke, 1994). Instruments that measure personality may be useful components to assess eating disorders and guide treatment plans, although they generally provide limited information about eating disorder diagnoses.

Nutrition

Collaborating with a dietician who has experience with adolescents with eating disorders is often beneficial to the mental health professional. As part of the assessment and treatment team, the dietician can focus on obtaining a careful dietary assessment (Rock, 2005) and devising meal plans. If such collaboration is not possible because of limited personnel or financial resources, the mental health clinician may include a nutritional evaluation as part of the comprehensive assessment (Brunzell & Hendrickson-Nelson, 2001; Rock, 2005).

Regardless of whether a dietician is included on the assessment team, the clinician should nonetheless ask detailed questions about current and past eating patterns, including the frequency and contents of meals and snacks, "rules" about eating (avoiding certain types of foods, calorie limits, etc.), and attempts at dietary restriction. Several methods may be used to evaluate eating habits, including unstructured interviews; standard interviews, including the EDE; dietary recalls (e.g., asking the adolescent to describe in detail types and amounts of food eaten during the past 24 hours); and written food records. Unfortunately, self-reported food intake is highly inaccurate regardless of the eating disorder diagnosis (Bandini, Schoeller, Dyr, & Dietz, 1990), and the clinician should be aware of this limitation in interpreting these types of data.

Interpersonal and Psychosocial Functioning

Assessing interpersonal and psychosocial functioning is an important aspect of assessment, because these factors are potentially causal and are also negatively affected by eating disorder symptoms. The level of detail of data collected within this assessment domain depends on several factors, including the age of the adolescent, whether the adolescent is living with the family, and the degree and scope of psychosocial impairment. Decisions about interpersonal and psychosocial assessment also depend on the treatment. For example, in interpersonal psychotherapy (IPT; Fairburn, 1997), the first phase of treatment involves a detailed assessment of interpersonal relationships in the context of eating disorder symptoms and developmental history. Family-based psychotherapy (e.g., Lock, le Grange, Agras, & Dare, 2001) requires a greater emphasis on family assessment during the initial phase.

Regardless of the type of treatment implemented, the clinician should obtain information about the adolescent's developmental history, including significant events, academic functioning, trauma experiences, and social relationships. Family history, especially of obesity and eating, mood, substance use, and anxiety disorders is also important to determine. Asking the adolescent to describe friendships and dating experiences is helpful for establishing rapport, assessing the developmental level of psychosocial functioning, evaluating the degree of impairment, determining social support resources, and formulating treatment goals. Specific questions relevant to eating disorder symptoms and peer relationships include whether the adolescent has been teased (especially about weight and shape), participation in activities in which weight and shape are emphasized (e.g., dance, gymnastics, wrestling), and the extent to which other members of the adolescent's peer group have had eating disorder symptoms.

Family assessment may be conducted with both unstructured interviews and self-report questionnaires (for a review, see le Grange, 2005). For family-based assessments, it is crucial to include all members of the cohabitating family in the assessment phase, as well as during treatment (Lock et al., 2001). Research investigations often rely on observational methods for family assessments, but these approaches are generally impractical in clinical settings.

Selecting Instruments and Integration of Assessment Data

Decisions about instrument selection depend on a number of variables, including the type of clinical setting (e.g., hospital-based vs. outpatient), the treatment orientation (e.g., family-based therapy vs. individual psychotherapy), and the age of the adolescent, because some assessment instruments are not appropriate for younger adolescents. The clinician should also consider the cost of administering and scoring, as well as the potential time burden on the adolescent and family members (Peterson & Mitchell, 2005). An important consideration in instrument selection is the extent to which an assessment measure increases the comprehensiveness and quality of the data, without creating undue time or financial burden. Self-report questionnaires may also provide more in-depth information about eating disorder symptoms, including body image, compensatory behaviors, and cognitions related to eating. The reliability and validity of each instrument is a primary concern, and the clinician should be

especially careful about selecting assessment measures that have been validated with adolescent samples.

Because of the multidimensional nature of eating disorders assessment, the clinician must often integrate various sources of information at the conclusion of the evaluation, including data from interviews, questionnaires, charts, and food records, as well as reports from other professionals. In integrating these data, the clinician should examine them for inconsistencies (e.g., discrepant information between the parents and the adolescent) and consider potential limitations in the accuracy of the data, including social desirability, inaccurate recall, and minimization of symptoms to avoid treatment. Because of the difficulty in obtaining accurate information in the initial phase (Vitousek, Daly, & Heiser, 2001), the clinician continues to gather and revise assessment data throughout the course of treatment.

ASSESSMENT INSTRUMENTS

A wide variety of self-report questionnaires and diagnostic interviews have been developed to assess eating pathology. For our purposes in this chapter, we focus on assessment devices that we believe are the most feasible and ecologically useful in most assessment and clinical settings, as well as those supported by reliability and validity data. It should be clearly noted, however, that most of the psychometric data for these scales are from samples of adolescents or young adults; very few data are available from samples of children. Although eating disorders are rare among preadolescent children, many of the measures reviewed below are probably too complex for administration to children, particularly the self-report questionnaire measures.

Questionnaire Measures

Two broad types of questionnaires assess eating pathology: one assesses general psychological disturbances often associated with eating disorders, and the other directly assesses eating disorder symptoms from DSM-IV. Both types of questionnaires have their uses in assessment and treatment settings. However, research suggests that questionnaires may provide inaccurate assessments of eating disorder symptoms relative to diagnostic interviews (Fairburn & Beglin,

1994; Wilfley, Schwartz, Spurrell, & Fairburn, 1997), presumably because interviews provide an opportunity for assessors to clarify the meaning of terms (e.g., "binge eating" and "excessive exercise"). Accordingly, unless it is unfeasible to conduct a diagnostic interview, we recommend that questionnaires be used as screening devices or to provide adjunctive information to data gathered through interviews (particularly for children). In addition, we have found that questionnaires yield the most accurate data when an office staff or research assistant is available while individuals complete the measures and when the questionnaires are immediately checked for completeness and errors (again, particularly for children).

Eating Disorder Examination–Questionnaire

The Eating Disorder Examination–Questionnaire (EDE-Q; Fairburn & Beglin, 1994), a 36-item questionnaire version of the EDE interview (Fairburn & Cooper, 1993), assesses the diagnostic symptoms of anorexia nervosa and bulimia nervosa, but not binge-eating disorder. The EDE-Q also contains subscales that assess features commonly associated with eating disorders: Restraint, Eating Concern, Shape Concern, and Weight Concern. Other investigators have created a continuous bulimic symptom composite score by averaging across the diagnostic items from this scale (e.g., Stice, 2001).

With regard to reliability, Luce and Crowther (1999) found that the Restraint, Shape Concern, Weight Concern, and Eating Concern subscales showed adequate internal consistency in a sample of late adolescent girls (mean alpha = .86). The 2-week test–retest reliability coefficient for items assessing the frequency of eating disorder behaviors were $r = .68$ for binge eating, $r = .92$ for vomiting, $r = .65$ for laxative misuse, and $r = .54$ for diuretic misuse, and the 2-week test–retest coefficients for the subscales were $r = .81$ for Restraint, $r = .94$ for Shape Concern, $r = .92$ for Weight Concern, and $r = .87$ for Eating Concern (Luce & Crowther, 1999). The bulimic symptom composite has been found to possess adequate internal consistency (mean alpha = .85) and 3-week test–retest reliability ($r = .89$) in several samples of adolescent girls (Stice, 2001; Stice, Mazotti, Weibel, & Agras, 2000; Stice, Trost, & Chase, 2003).

With regard to validity, agreement across the EDE-Q and EDE versions of the Restraint, Shape Concern, Weight Concern, and Eating Concern subscales for adult women was moderately high (mean $r = .76$; Black & Wilson, 1996; Fairburn & Beglin, 1994). Although the EDE-Q assesses symptoms of anorexia nervosa and bulimia nervosa, few studies have examined agreement between diagnoses with this scale and those with validated structured interviews, and we could not locate any that reported the kappa agreement between the two methods. Agreement between the EDE-Q and the EDE is generally good for the presence of vomiting and laxative misuse (mean Kendall's tau-b = .87), but lower for the presence of binge eating (mean Kendall's tau-b = .42; kappa = .47) across community and clinical samples of adults (Black & Wilson, 1996; Fairburn & Beglin, 1994; Mond, Hay, Rodgers, Owen, & Beumont, 2004; Wilfley et al., 1997). Studies have suggested that the concordance between the EDE and EDE-Q in terms of the frequency of bulimic symptoms tended to be higher, ranging from a high of .98 to a low of .35 (mean $r = .62$; Sysko, Walsh, & Fairburn, 2005). The agreement between the EDE and EDE-Q in terms of the frequency of binge eating was higher when more detailed instructions were provided relative to those given in the basic EDE-Q (Celio, Wilfley, Crow, Mitchell, & Walsh, 2004). There is evidence that the Restraint, Shape Concern, Weight Concern, and Eating Concern subscales of the EDE-Q are also sufficiently sensitive to detect effects of prevention interventions (Celio et al., 2000; Stewart, Carter, Drinkwater, Hainsworth, & Fairburn, 2001). The bulimic symptom composite from the EDE-Q has also been found to be sensitive to detecting change in bulimic symptoms in response to prevention programs (Stice, Mazotti, et al., 2000; Stice et al., 2003). In contrast, results in one study suggested that the EDE-Q may not provide accurate estimates of symptom change among individuals receiving treatment (Sysko, Walsh, & Fairburn, 2005). The EDE-Q has also been found to distinguish between women with and without eating disorders, with a sensitivity of .83 and a specificity of .96 (Mond et al., 2004). However, the EDE-Q Restraint scale has not shown a significant inverse correlation with objectively measured caloric intake in community and patient samples (Stice, Fisher, & Lowe, 2004; Sysko, Walsh, Schebendach, & Wilson, 2005), which suggests that it is not a valid measure of actual dietary restriction.

In summary, there is reasonable evidence regarding the internal consistency, test–retest reliability, and sensitivity of the EDE-Q for use with adolescents. However, there is relatively limited evidence of criterion validity for this scale, and most of these data were from adult samples. Normative data for adolescent girls are available for this scale, which should facilitate the use of the EDE-Q in clinical settings (Carter, Stewart, & Fairburn, 2001). Because the EDE-Q is easy to administer and score, it may be useful clinically to provide more detailed information about eating disorder symptoms, although it should not be used in lieu of a diagnostic interview.

Eating Disorder Diagnostic Scale

The Eating Disorder Diagnostic Scale (EDDS; Stice, Telch, & Rizvi, 2000) is a 1-page, 22-item self-report screening measure that assesses DSM-IV diagnostic criteria for anorexia nervosa, bulimia nervosa, and binge-eating disorder. This scale yields provisional diagnoses of these three eating disorders. In addition, the items can be averaged to form a continuous eating disorder symptom composite score.

In terms of reliability, the internal consistency for the overall symptom composite was adequate (mean alpha = .87; Stice, Fisher, & Martinez, 2004; Stice, Orjada, & Tristan, 2006; Stice & Ragan, 2002; Stice, Telch, et al., 2000). The 1-week test–retest kappa coefficient was .95 for anorexia nervosa, .71 for bulimia nervosa, and .75 for binge-eating disorder diagnoses; the 1-week test–retest correlation for the symptom composite was .87 (Stice, Telch, et al., 2000).

In terms of validity, the EDDS evidenced acceptable agreement with EDE diagnoses for anorexia nervosa (kappa = .93), bulimia nervosa (kappa = .81), and binge-eating disorder (kappa = .74) in a sample of adolescent girls and women (Stice, Telch, et al., 2000). Reasonable diagnostic agreement was also observed in a sample of primarily adolescent girls (kappa = .78; Stice, Fisher, et al., 2004). The EDDS symptom composite has also been found to detect preventive intervention effects in three independent controlled trials (Stice, Fisher, et al., 2004; Stice, Orjada, et al., 2006; Stice & Ragan, 2002). With regard to predictive validity, elevated scores on the EDDS symptom composite were found to moderate the pre- to postintervention effects of an eating disorder

prevention program (Stice, Fisher, et al., 2004). In addition, elevated scores on this symptom composite were found to predict future onset of binge eating, compensatory behaviors, and depression among initially nonafflicted individuals (Stice, Fisher, et al., 2004).

In summary, the EDDS shows promise as a brief survey designed solely to assess eating disorder symptoms and render provisional diagnoses. This scale is easy to administer and score, and takes less than 10 minutes to complete, which suggests that it might be useful for screening patients in clinical settings and monitoring change in response to preventive and treatment interventions. However, a disadvantage is that relatively less psychometric evidence has accumulated for the reliability and validity of this questionnaire. As with other survey measures, it should not be used in lieu of a diagnostic interview.

Eating Disorder Inventory–2

The Eating Disorder Inventory–2 (EDI-2; Garner, 1991) is a 91-item scale that assesses features commonly associated with anorexia nervosa and bulimia nervosa but does not provide diagnoses for eating disorders. This measure has 11 subscales including Bulimia, Body Dissatisfaction, Drive for Thinness, Perfectionism, and Impulse Regulation. Eight of these subscales remained unchanged from the previous version of this measure, and three new subscales have been added.

The EDI-2 has been found to have adequate internal consistency for women (range, .69–.92) and men (range, .57–.82) from community samples (McCarthy, Simmons, Smith, Tomlinson, & Hill, 2002; Spillane, Boerner, Anderson, & Smith, 2004). However, there is evidence that the new subscales have somewhat lower internal consistency coefficients among clinical samples of women (Eberenz & Gleaves, 1994). Research suggests that the eight subscales from the original EDI, which are also included in the EDI-2, possess adequate internal consistency and test–retest reliability (Anderson & Paulosky, 2004).

The EDI-2 has been found to discriminate significantly between individuals with and without eating disorders (Garner, 1991; Nevonen & Broberg, 2001; Schoemaker, Verbraak, Breteler, & van der Staak, 1997). For instance, in one study, the Bulimia subscale correctly classified 97% of individuals with bulimia nervosa from general psychiatric controls (Schoemaker et al., 1997). Certain EDI-2 subscales have also been found to predict dropout from eating disorder treatment (Fassino, Daga, Piero, & Rovera, 2002).

The EDI-2 is widely used clinically and may be helpful for assessing personality features, as well as a full range of eating disorder symptoms, both at intake and in assessing change over the course of treatment. Because this scale does not provide a direct assessment of the frequency of eating disorder symptoms or provide DSM-IV eating disorder diagnoses, it may be most useful as an adjunct to a diagnostic interview such as the EDE.

Diagnostic Interviews

There are several structured psychiatric interviews that generate DSM-IV (APA, 1994) diagnoses of anorexia nervosa, bulimia nervosa, and binge-eating disorder among adults, but few have been evaluated with children and adolescents.

Eating Disorder Examination

The EDE (Fairburn & Cooper, 1993), a 34-item, semistructured psychiatric interview that assesses the diagnostic criteria for anorexia nervosa and bulimia nervosa, also contains subscales that assess features commonly associated with eating disorders—Restraint, Eating Concern, Shape Concern, and Weight Concern—as well as behavioral and eating patterns.

The EDE subscales have consistently been found to have moderately high internal consistency among community and clinical samples of adult women (range, .68–.83; Fairburn & Cooper, 1993; Mond et al., 2004). The diagnostic items assessing eating behaviors have been found to have high test–retest reliability over a 2- to 7-day period (range, .82–.97) in women with eating disorders, although the agreement for subjective binge eating was much lower (number of binge days = .40; number of binge episodes = .33; Rizvi, Peterson, Crow, & Agras, 2000). This study also found that the subscales showed adequate 2- to 7-day test–retest reliability (range, .71–.76; Rizvi et al., 2000). The interrater agreement (as assessed by coding audiotapes of interviews) was high for the diagnostic items assessing eating behaviors (range, .90–.99) and for the subscales (range, .92–1.00; Rizvi et al., 2000). A

Spanish-language version of the EDE has been found to have similar test–retest and interrater reliability coefficients with Hispanic women recruited from the community, with the exception of the test–retest and interrater reliability for objective binge-eating episodes (kappas = .37 and .56, respectively; Grilo, Lozano, & Elder, 2005).

The EDE has been found to discriminate reliably between individuals with and without eating disorders, and between individuals with anorexia nervosa and those with bulimia nervosa (Fairburn & Cooper, 1993). The EDE is also sufficiently sensitive to detect intervention effects among women treated for anorexia nervosa (Pike, Walsh, Vitousek, Wilson, & Bauer, 2003), bulimia nervosa (Agras, Walsh, Fairburn, Wilson, & Kraemer, 2000; Walsh et al., 1997), and binge-eating disorder (Wilfley et al., 2002). However, Sysko, Walsh, Schebendach, & Wilson (2005) found that the EDE Restraint subscale was not significantly correlated with observed caloric intake of a yogurt shake in a laboratory setting by young women with anorexia nervosa or nondisordered control women of normal weight during two separate sessions, suggesting that this measure is not a valid measure of actual dietary restriction.

Emerging evidence supports the reliability and validity of a Child Adaptation of the EDE (ChEDE; Watkins, Frampton, Lask, & Bryant-Waugh, 2005). The subscales of the ChEDE evidenced satisfactory internal consistency (range, .80–.91), and interrater consistency was also excellent in a sample of 8- to 14-year-old girls (range, .91–1.0; Watkins et al., 2005). With regard to validity, the subscales were able to distinguish among children with anorexia nervosa, children with bulimia nervosa, and those without eating disorders. They were not able to distinguish between children with bulimia nervosa and control children, however (Watkins et al., 2005).

Another group has developed a semistructured interview, loosely adapted from the EDE, for diagnosing eating disorders among adolescents (Stice, Burton, & Shaw, 2004). This 39-item interview, the Eating Disorders Diagnostic Interview (EDDI), focuses solely on diagnosing anorexia nervosa, bulimia nervosa, and binge-eating disorder over the past year and also provides an overall eating disorder symptom composite. Research with adolescents has indicated that the symptom composite shows adequate internal consistency (mean alpha = .91) and 1-month test–retest reliability (*r* = .88; Stice, Burton, et al., 2004; Stice, Presnell, Groesz, & Shaw, 2005; Stice, Shaw, Burton, & Wade, 2006). This scale also has acceptable interrater agreement (kappa = .86), as assessed by completely independent interviews (rather than ratings of recorded interviews), and 3- to 5-day test–retest reliability in an adolescent sample (kappa = .96; Stice, Shaw, et al., 2006). This scale has shown predictive validity for future onset of obesity, depression, and substance abuse (Stice, Burton, et al., 2004; Stice, Presnell, Shaw, & Rohde, 2005), as well as sufficient sensitivity to detect intervention effects from randomized prevention and treatment trials with adolescents and young adults (Burton & Stice, 2006; Stice, Presnell, Shaw, et al., 2005; Stice, Shaw et al., 2006).

In summary, the EDE is a useful clinical interview for assessing eating disorder behaviors and associated features. The instrument has extensive reliability and validity data supporting its use among adult women, and there are adaptations that appear to be reliable and valid for use with children and adolescents. Although it has primarily been used in research settings, it may be beneficial for assessment in clinical settings as well.

Other Measures for Diagnosing Eating Disorders

Two other diagnostic interviews deserve mention that also appear to be reliable and valid, although relatively less psychometric research has investigated these measures, particularly with child and adolescent samples. First, the Structured Interview for Anorexic and Bulimic Disorders (SIAB-EX) has been found to have impressive internal consistency, interrater reliability, criterion validity with the EDE, and discriminant validity (Fichter, Herpertz, Quadflieg, & Herpertz-Dahlmann, 1998; Fichter & Quadflieg, 2001b). The SIAB-EX has also shown good agreement with a self-report version of this instrument (Fichter & Quadflieg, 2001a). The Interview for Diagnosis of Eating Disorders–IV (IDED-IV) has also shown excellent internal consistency, interrater reliability, and concurrent validity (Kutlesic, Williamson, Gleaves, Barbin, & Murphy-Eberenz, 1998). A unique feature of the IDED is that it was specifically devised to provide diagnoses of binge-eating disorder and it also provides broad coverage of ED NOS symptoms.

It is noteworthy that all of the questionnaires and interviews with adequate evidence of reliability and validity in assessing eating pathology have collected data solely from children or adolescents. In contrast, the Children's Eating Behavior Inventory (CEBI; Archer, Rosenbaum, & Streiner, 1991) was designed to be completed by parents. This questionnaire measures eating and mealtime problems in children ages 2–12 years. It contains 40 items that gather information regarding the child's food preferences, food refusal, behavioral compliance during meals, and feeding skills. The CEBI has shown satisfactory internal consistency, test–retest reliability, discriminant validity, and sensitivity to treatment interventions (Archer et al., 1991).

USE OF ASSESSMENT IN THE CONTEXT OF TREATMENT

The primary aim of assessment at the initial evaluation is to establish an accurate diagnosis and to determine the scope and severity of eating disorder and associated symptoms to formulate a detailed treatment plan. For example, if the clinician determines that the appropriate diagnosis for a particular patient is the binge–purge subtype of anorexia nervosa, then the treatment will target binge eating and compensatory behaviors, in addition to dietary restriction, excessive exercise, and body image disturbance (which would more likely be the primary focus for an individual with the restricting subtype of anorexia nervosa). If scores on a body dissatisfaction questionnaire are extremely high, the clinician may choose to focus on this type of distress early in treatment. If co-occurring symptoms of mood or anxiety are severe, the therapist may consider an adjunctive intervention including medication. Thus, the priorities of treatment are strongly influenced by the initial assessment and diagnostic information.

The selection of assessment instruments in the context of treatment depends on the type of treatment to be implemented. As described earlier, family-based and interpersonal treatments require a greater assessment focus on interpersonal variables and family patterns. Assessment in cognitive-behavioral therapy (Fairburn et al., 1993; Garner, Vitousek, & Pike, 1997) is influenced by the intervention itself, which incorporates the active assessment of behaviors and cognitions as a focus of treatment. In cognitive-behavioral therapy, the patient is asked to keep a written food log or diary. Early in treatment, in the context of nutritional rehabilitation, the main emphasis of this type of self-monitoring is the frequency and content of food consumed, as well as precipitants of problematic eating patterns. For example, review of the food diaries during the therapy sessions may reveal that purging episodes usually occur in certain places or at certain times of day. These data then influence the implementation of behavioral strategies to alter symptoms. Later in treatment, an increasing focus is placed on monitoring cognitions and thought patterns, along with eating patterns. Thus, the content of the self-monitoring varies in the course of treatment. Although many patients are at first skeptical about the use of food diaries, this type of written self-monitoring is a powerful component of treatment. It provides valuable data to review in the psychotherapy session, develops the adolescent's self-awareness as he or she monitors patterns and antecedents, and it has been found to be a therapeutic intervention for altering eating disorder symptoms, independent of psychotherapy (Agras, Schneider, Arnow, Raeburn, & Telch, 1989).

Regardless of the type of treatment, repeatedly administering assessment instruments throughout the course of treatment may be useful for ongoing planning, monitoring progress, and maintaining motivation. For example, a short battery of questionnaires to assess eating disorder and associated symptoms, including depression, may be administered on a weekly or monthly basis and reviewed by the therapist and adolescent patient together to evaluate progress. Adolescent patients often find the process of comparing current questionnaire responses to previous ones quite compelling, and they are often unaware of their progress until they observe this type of concrete change in assessment scores. Similarly, reviewing earlier food diary information may be helpful to both the therapist and the adolescent as treatment progresses.

In addition to monitoring progress, assessment data obtained throughout treatment may also highlight areas of continued struggle that require increased therapeutic focus. For example, if the adolescent patient reports that weight and shape continue to be a primary source of self-evaluation, or that he or she frequently engages in body checking rituals during the second stage of cognitive-behavioral therapy, then the therapist may modify the treatment to target these body image problems (Fairburn et al., 1993). Assessment measures, in addition to less structured interview questions, may be used to obtain a more comprehensive evaluation of symptoms and to prioritize treatment goals appropriately. Recent data also suggest that adult individuals with bulimia nervosa who ultimately respond to cognitive-behavioral therapy abstain from or significantly reduce purging by the fourth week of treatment (Agras, Crow, et al., 2000; Fairburn, Agras, Walsh, Wilson, & Stice, 2004). Although these rapid response data are based on adult samples and have not been replicated in adolescents, the clinician should nonetheless consider supplementing or altering treatment for patients who report limited reductions in purging symptoms on food logs, recall, or questionnaires by the fourth week of cognitive-behavioral treatment.

In addition to treatment planning and modification, assessment data may be useful to the clinician for documentation. Reviewing questionnaires that have been administered repeatedly may be helpful in the context of consultation or supervision. In addition, questionnaire data may be used in certain cases to document the need for ongoing treatment to third-party payors.

In summary, although assessment data are used initially to determine diagnosis and treatment goals, they are valuable to the clinician throughout the course of treatment. Repeated administration of a standard set of questionnaires provides quantitative data for both the clinician and the adolescent to monitor change. In addition, the ongoing use of assessment instruments may not only help the clinician to modify treatment appropriately but may also be useful for documentation purposes.

SUMMARY

Eating disorders in youth are serious conditions complicated by medical and psychiatric comorbidity. Accurate diagnosis of eating disorders is important for appropriate referrals and treatment planning, but this can be challenging with children and adolescents because of the complexity of the criteria and limitations in the accuracy of self-reported data. We recommend a multidimensional approach to eating disorder assessment, with a focus on medical, psychological, behavioral, nutritional, interpersonal, and psychosocial components. Assessment and treatment of adolescents with eating disorders often involve multidisciplinary team members who communicate regularly. In the initial evaluation, the clinician uses interview-based methods (both unstructured and semistructured) with the adolescent and, if appropriate, with his or her family members. The primary concern initially is to ensure that the adolescent is medically stable, and this question often informs the first phase of treatment. Self-report questionnaires are valuable for the assessment of eating disorder and comorbid symptoms, although they may not yield accurate data for certain symptoms that require clinical ratings, including binge eating. In addition to providing initial information for diagnosis and treatment planning, assessment instruments may be clinically useful for measuring quantitative change in symptoms over the course of treatment.

REFERENCES

Agras, W. S., Crow, S. J., Halmi, K. A., Mitchell, J. E., Wilson, G. T., & Kraemer, H. C. (2000). Outcome predictors for the cognitive behavior treatment of bulimia nervosa: Data from a multisite study. *American Journal of Psychiatry, 157*, 1302–1308.

Agras, W. S., Schneider, J. A., Arnow, B., Raeburn, S. D., & Telch, C. F. (1989). Cognitive-behavioral and response-prevention treatments for bulimia nervosa. *Journal of Consulting and Clinical Psychology, 57*, 215–221.

Agras, W. S., Walsh, B. T., Fairburn, C. G., Wilson, G. T., & Kraemer, H. C. (2000). A multicenter comparison of cognitive-behavioral therapy and interpersonal psychotherapy for bulimia nervosa. *Archives of General Psychiatry, 57*, 459–466.

American Psychiatric Association (APA). (2000). *Diagnostic and statistical manual of mental disorders* (4th ed., text rev.). Washington, DC: Author.

Anderson, D. A., & Paulosky, C. A. (2004). Psychological assessment of eating disorders and related features. In J. K. Thompson (Ed.), *Handbook of eating disorders and obesity* (pp. 112–129). Hoboken, NJ: Wiley.

Archer, L. A., Rosenbaum, P. L., & Streiner, D. L. (1991). The Children's Eating Behavior Inventory: Reliability and validity results. *Journal of Pediatric Psychology, 16*, 629–642.

Bandini, L. G., Schoeller, D. A., Dyr, H. N., & Dietz, W. H. (1990). Validity of reported energy intake in obese and nonobese adolescents. *American Journal of Clinical Nutrition, 52*, 421–425.

Beglin, S. J., & Fairburn, C. G. (1992). What is meant by the term "binge"? *American Journal of Psychiatry, 149*, 123–124.

Berkson, J. (1946). Limitations of the application of fourfold table analysis to hospital data. *Biometrics Bulletin, 2*, 47–53.

Black, C. M., & Wilson, G. T. (1996). Assessment of eating disorders: Interview versus questionnaire. *International Journal of Eating Disorders, 20*, 43–50.

Bohon, E., Muscatell, K., Burton, E., & Stice, E. (2005, November). *Maintenance factors for persistence of bulimic pathology: A community-based natural history study*. Poster presented at the annual meeting of the Eating Disorder Research Society, Toronto, Canada.

Brown, T. A., Cash, T. F., & Mikulka, P. J. (1990). Attitudinal body-image assessment: Factor analysis of the Body–Self Relations Questionnaire. *Journal of Personality Assessment, 55*, 135–144.

Brunzell, C., & Hendrickson-Nelson, M. (2001). An overview of nutrition. In J. E. Mitchell (Ed.), *The outpatient treatment of eating disorders: A guide for therapists, dietitians, and physicians* (pp. 216–241). Minneapolis: University of Minnesota Press.

Bulik, C. M., Sullivan, P. F., & Kendler, K. S. (1998). Heritability of binge-eating and broadly defined bulimia nervosa. *Biological Psychiatry, 44*, 1210–1218.

Burton, E. M., & Stice, E. (2006). Evaluation of a healthy-weight treatment program for bulimia nervosa: A preliminary randomized trial. *Behaviour Research and Therapy, 44*, 1727–1738.

Cachelin, F. M., Striegel-Moore, R. H., Elder, K. A., Pike, K. M., Wilfley, D. E., & Fairburn, C. G. (1999). Natural course of a community sample of women with binge eating disorder. *International Journal of Eating Disorders, 25*, 45–54.

Carter, J. C., Stewart, D. A., & Fairburn, C. G. (2001). Eating disorder examination questionnaire: Norms for young adolescent girls. *Behavior Research and Therapy, 39*, 625–632.

Cash, T. F., & Deagle, E. A. (1997). The nature and extent of body-image disturbances in anorexia nervosa and bulimia nervosa: A meta-analysis. *International Journal of Eating Disorders, 22*, 107–125.

Cassin, S. E., & von Ranson, K. M. (2005). Personality and eating disorders: A decade in review. *Clinical Psychology Review, 25*, 895–526.

Cattarin, J. A., & Thompson, J. K. (1994). A 3-year longitudinal study of body image, eating disturbance, and general psychological functioning in adolescent females. *Eating Disorders, 2*, 114–125.

Celio, A. A., Wilfley, D. E., Crow, S. J., Mitchell, J., & Walsh, B. T. (2004). A comparison of the Binge Eating Scale, Questionnaire for Eating and Weight Patterns-Revised, and Eating Disorder Examination Questionnaire with instructions with the Eating Disorder Examination in the assessment of binge eating disorder symptoms. *International Journal of Eating Disorders, 36*, 434–444.

Celio, A. A., Winzelberg, A. J., Wilfley, D. E., Eppstein-Herald, D., Springer, E. A., Dev, P., et al. (2000). Reducing risk factors for eating disorders: Comparison of an Internet- and classroom-delivered psychoeducational program. *Journal of Consulting and Clinical Psychology, 68,* 650–657.

Cnattingius, S., Hultman, C., Dahl, M., & Sparen, P. (1999). Very preterm birth, birth trauma, and the risk of anorexia nervosa among girls. *Archives of General Psychiatry, 56,* 634–638.

Commission on Adolescent Eating Disorders. (2005). Defining eating disorders. In D. L. Evans, E. B. Foa, R. E. Gur, H. Hendin, C. P. O'Brien, M. E. P. Seligman, et al. (Eds.), *Treating and preventing adolescent mental health disorders: What we know and what we don't know* (pp. 257–332). New York: Oxford University Press, the Annenberg Foundation Trust at Sunnylands, and the Annenberg Public Policy Center of the University of Pennsylvania.

Cooper, P. J., Taylor, M. J., Cooper, Z., & Fairburn, C. G. (1987). The development and validation of the Body Shape Questionnaire. *International Journal of Eating Disorders, 6,* 485–494.

Cotrufo, P., Barretta, V., Monteleone, P., & Maj, M. (1998). Full-syndrome, partial-syndrome and subclinical eating disorders: An epidemiological study of female students in southern Italy. *Acta Psychiatrica Scandinavica, 98,* 112–115.

Dietz, W. H. (1998). Childhood weight affects adult morbidity and mortality. *Journal of Nutrition, 128,* 411S–414S.

Eberenz, K. P., & Gleaves, D. H. (1994). An examination of the internal consistency and factor structure of the Eating Disorder Inventory–2 in a clinical sample. *International Journal of Eating Disorders, 16,* 371–379.

Eddy, K. T., Keel, P. K., Dorer, D. J., Delinsky, S. S., Franko, D. L., & Herzog, D. B. (2002). Longitudinal comparison of anorexia nervosa subtypes. *International Journal of Eating Disorders, 31,* 191–201.

Fairburn, C. G. (1997). Interpersonal psychotherapy for bulimia nervosa. In D. M. Garner & P. E. Garfinkel (Eds.), *Handbook of treatment for eating disorders* (2nd ed., pp. 278–294). New York: Guilford Press.

Fairburn, C. G., Agras, W. S., Walsh, B. T., Wilson, G. T., & Stice, E. (2004). Prediction of outcome in bulimia nervosa by early change in treatment. *American Journal of Psychiatry, 161,* 2322–2324.

Fairburn, C. G., & Beglin, S. J. (1994). Assessment of eating disorders: Interview or self-report questionnaire? *International Journal of Eating Disorders, 16,* 363–370.

Fairburn, C. G., & Cooper, Z. (1993). The Eating Disorder Examination (12th edition). In C. Fairburn & G. Wilson (Eds.), *Binge eating: Nature, assessment, and treatment* (pp. 317–360). New York: Guilford Press.

Fairburn, C. G., Cooper, Z., Doll, H. A., Norman, P. A., & O'Connor, M. E. (2000). The natural course of bulimia nervosa and binge eating disorder in young women. *Archives of General Psychiatry, 57,* 659–665.

Fairburn, C. G., Cowen, P. J., & Harrison, P. J. (1999). Twin studies and the etiology of eating disorders. *International Journal of Eating Disorders, 26,* 349–358.

Fairburn, C. G., & Harrison, P. J. (2003). Eating disorders. *Lancet, 361,* 407–416.

Fairburn, C. G., Marcus, M. D., & Wilson, G. T. (1993). Cognitive-behavioral therapy for binge eating and bulimia nervosa: A comprehensive treatment manual. In C. Fairburn & G. Wilson (Eds.), *Binge eating: Nature, assessment, and treatment* (pp. 361–404). New York: Guilford Press.

Fassino, S., Daga, G. A., & Piero, A., & Rovera, G. G. (2002). Dropout from brief psychotherapy in anorexia nervosa. *Psychotherapy and Psychosomatics, 71,* 200–206.

Favaro, A., Ferrara, S., & Santonastaso, P. (2003). The spectrum of eating disorders in young women: A prevalence study in a general population. *Psychosomatic Medicine, 65,* 701–708.

Fichter, M. M., Herpertz, S., Quadflieg, N., & Herpertz-Dahlmann, B. (1998). Structured Interview for Anorexic and Bulimic Disorders for DSM-IV and ICD-10: Updated (third) revision. *International Journal of Eating Disorders, 24,* 227–249.

Fichter, M. M., & Quadflieg, N. (2001a). Comparing self- and expert rating: A self-report screening version (SIAB-S) for the Structured Interview for Anorexic and Bulimic Syndromes for DSM-IV and ICD-10 (SIAB-EX). *European Archives of Psychiatry and Clinical Neuroscience, 250,* 175–185.

Fichter, M. M., & Quadflieg, N. (2001b). The structured interview for anorexic and bulimic disorders for DSM-IV and ICD-10 (SIAB-EX): Reliability and validity. *European Psychiatry, 16,* 38–48.

Field, A. E., Camargo, C. A., Taylor, C. B., Berkey, C. S., & Colditz, G. A. (1999). Relation of peer and media influences to the development of purging behaviors among preadolescent and adolescent girls. *Archives of Pediatric Adolescent Medicine, 153,* 1184–1189.

Fisher, M., Schneider, M., Burns, J., Symons, H., & Mandel, F. S. (2001). Differences between adolescents and young adults at presentation to an eating disorder program. *Journal of Adolescent Health, 28,* 222–227.

Fontaine, K. R., Redden, D. T., Wang, C., Westfall, A. O., & Allison, D. B. (2003). Years of life lost due to obesity. *Journal of the American Medical Association, 289,* 187–193.

Fontenelle, L. F., Mendlowicz, M. V., Menezes, G. B., Papelbaum, M., Freitas, W. R., Godoy-Matos, et al. (2003). Psychiatric comorbidity in a Brazilian sample of patients with binge eating disorder. *Psychiatric Research, 119,* 189–194.

Garfinkel, P. E., Lin, E., Goering, P., Spegg, C., Goldbloom, D. S., Kennedy, S., et al. (1995). Bulimia nervosa in a Canadian community sample: Prevalence and comparison of subgroups. *American Journal of Psychiatry, 152,* 1052–1058.

Garfinkel, P. E., Lin, E., Goering, P., Spegg, C., Goldbloom, D., Kennedy, S., et al. (1996). Should amenorrhea be necessary for the diagnosis of anorexia nervosa? *British Journal of Psychiatry, 168,* 500–506.

Garner, D. M. (1991). *Eating Disorder Inventory–2 manual.* Odessa FL: Psychological Assessment Resources.

Garner, D. M., Olmstead, M. P., & Polivy, J. (1983). Development and validation of a multidimensional eating disorder inventory for anorexia nervosa and bulimia. *International Journal of Eating Disorders, 2,* 15–34.

Garner, D. M., Vitousek, K. M., & Pike, K. M. (1993). Cognitive-behavioral therapy for anorexia nervosa. In D. M. Garner & P. E. Garfinkel (Eds.), *Handbook of treatment for eating disorders* (2nd ed., pp. 94–144). New York: Guilford Press.

Garner, D. M., Vitousek, K. M., & Pike, K. M. (1997). Cognitive-behavioral therapy for anorexia nervosa. In D. M. Garner & P. E. Garfinkel (Ed.), *Handbook of treatment for eating disorders* (2nd ed., pp. 94–144). New York: Guilford Press.

Gillberg, I. C., Rastam, M., & Gillberg, C. (1995). Anorexia nervosa 6 years after onset: Part 1. Personality disorders. *Comprehensive Psychiatry, 36,* 61–69.

Gortmaker, S. L., Must, A., Perrin, J., & Sobol, A. (1993). Social and economic consequences of overweight in adolescence and young adulthood. *New England Journal of Medicine, 329,* 1008–1012.

Grilo, C. M., Lozano, C., & Elder, K. A. (2005). Interrater and test–retest reliability of the Spanish language version of the Eating Disorder Examination Interview: Clinical and research implications. *Journal of Psychiatric Practice, 11,* 231–240.

Grilo, C. M., Sanislow, C. A., Shea, M. T., Skodol, A. E., Stout, R. L., Pagano, M. E., et al. (2003). The natural course of bulimia nervosa and eating disorder not otherwise specified is not influenced by personality disorders. *International Journal of Eating Disorders, 34,* 319–330.

Herzog, D. B., Greenwood, D. N., Dorer, D. J., Flores, A. T., Ekeblad, E. R., Richards, A., et al. (2000). Mortality in eating disorders: A descriptive study. *International Journal of Eating Disorders, 28,* 20–26.

Herzog, D. B., Hopkins, J., & Burns, C. D. (1993). A follow-up study of 33 subdiagnostic eating disordered women. *International Journal of Eating Disorders, 14,* 261–267.

Herzog, D. B., Keller, M. B., Sacks, N. R., Yeh, C. J., & Lavori, P. W. (1992). Psychiatric comorbidity in treatment-seeking anorexics and bulimics. *Journal of the American Academy of Child and Adolescent Psychiatry, 31,* 810–818.

Hinney, A., Bornscheuer, A., Depenbusch, M., Mierke, B., Tolle, A., Middeke, K., et al. (1998). No evidence for involvement of the leptin gene in anorexia nervosa, bulimia nervosa, underweight or early onset extreme obesity: Identification of two novel mutations in the coding sequence and a novel polymorphism in the leptin gene linked upstream region. *Molecular Psychiatry, 3,* 539–543.

Hoek, H. W., & van Hoeken, D. (2003). Review of the prevalence and incidence of eating disorders. *International Journal of Eating Disorders, 34,* 383–396.

Johnson, J. G., Cohen, P., Kasen, S., & Brook, J. S. (2002). Eating disorders during adolescence and the risk for physical and mental disorders during early adulthood. *Archives of General Psychiatry, 59,* 545–552.

Kaye, W. H., Klump, K. L., Frank, G. K., & Strober, M. (2000). Anorexia and bulimia nervosa. *Annual Review of Medicine, 51,* 299–313.

Keel, P. K., Dorer, D. J., Eddy, K. T., Franko, D., Charatan, D. L., & Herzog, D. B. (2003). Predictors of mortality in eating disorders. *Archives of General Psychiatry, 60,* 179–183.

Keel, P. K., Fulkerson, J. A., & Leon, G. R. (1997). Disordered eating precursors in pre- and early adolescent girls and boys. *Journal of Youth and Adolescence, 26,* 203–216.

Keel, P. K., Mayer, S. A., & Harnden-Fischer, J. H. (2001). Importance of size in defining binge eating episodes in bulimia nervosa. *International Journal of Eating Disorders, 29,* 294–301.

Keel, P. K., Mitchell, J. E., Miller, K. B., Davis, T. L., & Crow, S. J. (1999). Long-term outcome of bulimia nervosa. *Archives of General Psychiatry, 56,* 63–69.

Keys, A., Brozek, J., Henschel, A., Mickelsen, O., & Taylor, H. L. (1950). *The biology of human starvation.* Minneapolis: University of Minnesota Press.

Killen, J. D., Taylor, C. B., Hayward, C., Haydel, K. F., Wilson, D. M., Hammer, L., et al. (1996). Weight concerns influence the development of eating disorders: A 4-year prospective study. *Journal of Consulting and Clinical Psychology, 64,* 936–940.

Killen, J. D., Taylor, C. B., Hayward, C., Wilson, D., Haydel, K., Hammer, L., et al. (1994). Pursuit of thinness and onset of eating disorder symptoms in a community sample of adolescent girls: A three-year prospective analysis. *International Journal of Eating Disorders, 16,* 227–238.

Kjelsas, E., Bjornstrom, C., & Gotestam, K. G. (2004). Prevalence of eating disorders in female and male adolescents (14–15 years). *Eating Behaviors, 5,* 13–25.

Klem, M. L., Wing, R. R., Simkin-Silverman, L., & Kuller, L. H. (1997). The psychological consequences of weight gain prevention in healthy, premenopausal women. *International Journal of Eating Disorders, 21,* 167–174.

Kutlesic, V., Williamson, D. A., Gleaves, D. H., Barbin, J. M., & Murphy-Eberenz, K. P. (1998). The Interview for Diagnosis of Eating Disorders IV: Application to DSM-IV diagnostic criteria. *Psychological Assessment, 10,* 866–869.

le Grange, D. (2005). Family assessment. In J. E. Mitchell & C. B. Peterson (Eds.), *Assessment of eating disorders* (pp. 148–174). New York: Guilford Press.

Lewinsohn, P. M., Hops, H., Roberts, R. E., Seeley, J. R., & Andrews, J. A. (1993). Adolescent psychopathology: I. Prevalence and incidence of depression and other DSM-II-R disorders in high school students. *Journal of Abnormal Psychology, 102,* 133–144.

Lewinsohn, P. M., Striegel-Moore, R. H., & Seeley, J. R. (2000). Epidemiology and natural course of eating disorders in young women from adolescence to young adulthood. *Journal of the American Academy of Child and Adolescent Psychiatry, 39,* 1284–1292.

Lock, J., le Grange, D., Agras, W. S., & Dare, C. (2001). *Treatment manual for anorexia nervosa: A family-based approach.* New York: Guilford Press.

Luce, K. H., & Crowther, J. H. (1999). The reliability of the Eating Disorder Examination—Self-Report Questionnaire Version (EDE-Q). *International Journal of Eating Disorders, 25,* 349–351.

Marchi, M., & Cohen, P. (1990). Early childhood eating behavior and adolescent eating disorders. *Journal of the American Academy of Child and Adolescent Psychiatry, 29,* 112–117.

McCarthy, D. M., Simmons, J. R., Smith, G. T., Tomlinson, K. L., & Hill, K. K. (2002). Reliability, stability, and factor structure of the Bulimia Test—Revised and Eating Disorder Inventory-2 scales in adolescence. *Assessment, 9,* 382–389.

McKnight Investigators. (2003). Risk factors for the onset of eating disorders in adolescent girls: Results of the McKnight Longitudinal Risk Factor Study. *American Journal of Psychiatry, 160,* 248–254.

Miller, W. R., & Rollnick, S. (2002). *Motivational interviewing: Preparing people for change* (2nd ed.). New York: Guilford Press.

Mond, J. M., Hay, P. J., Rodgers, B., Owen, C., & Beumont, P. J. (2004). Validity of the Eating Disorder Examination—Questionnaire (EDE-Q) in screening for eating disorders in community samples. *Behaviour Research and Therapy, 42,* 551–567.

Morrill, C. M., Leach, J. N., Shreeve, W. C., Radebaugh, M. R., & Muriel, R. (1991). Teenage obesity: An academic issue. *International Journal of Adolescence and Youth, 2,* 245–250.

Niego, S. H., Pratt, E., & Agras, W. S. (1997). Subjective or objective binge: Is the distinction valid? *International Journal of Eating Disorders, 22,* 291–298.

Nevonen, L., & Broberg, A. G. (2001). Validating the Eating Disorder Inventory-2 (EDI-2) in Sweden. *Eating and Weight Disorders, 6,* 59–67.

Newman, D. L., Moffitt, T. E., Caspi, A., Magdol, L., Silva, P. A., & Stanton, W. R. (1996). Psychiatric disorder in a birth cohort of young adults: Prevalence, comorbidity, clinical significance, and new case incidence from ages 11 to 21. *Journal of Consulting and Clinical Psychology, 64,* 552–562.

Patton, G. C., Johnson-Sabine, E., Wood, K., Mann, A. H., & Wakeling, A. (1990). Abnormal eating attitudes in London schoolgirls—a prospective epidemiological study: Outcome at twelve month follow-up. *Psychological Medicine, 20,* 383–394.

Peterson, C. B. (2005). Conducting the diagnostic interview. In J. E. Mitchell & C. B. Peterson (Eds.), *Assessment of eating disorders* (pp. 32–58). New York: Guilford Press.

Peterson, C. B., & Miller, K. B. (2005). Assessment of eating disorders. In S. Wonderlich, J. E. Mitchell, M. de Zwaan, & H. Steiger (Eds.), *Eating disorders review, part I* (pp. 105–126). Oxford, UK: Radcliffe.

Peterson, C. B., & Mitchell, J. E. (2005). Self-report measures. In J. E. Mitchell & C. B. Peterson (Eds.), *Assessment of eating disorders* (pp. 98–119). New York: Guilford Press.

Pike, K. M., Walsh, B. T., Vitousek, K., Wilson, G. T., & Bauer, J. (2003). Cognitive behavior therapy in the posthospitalization treatment of anorexia nervosa. *American Journal of Psychiatry, 160,* 2046–2049.

Polivy, J., & Herman, C. P. (1985). Dieting and binge eating: A causal analysis. *American Psychologist, 40,* 193–204.

Pomeroy, C. (2004). Assessment of medical status and physical factors. In J. K. Thompson (Ed.), *Handbook of eating disorders and obesity* (pp. 81–111). New York: Wiley.

Pratt, E. M., Niego, S. H., & Agras, W. S. (1998). Does the size of a binge matter? *International Journal of Eating Disorders, 24,* 307–312.

Presnell, K., & Stice, E. (2003). An experimental test of the effect of weight-loss dieting on bulimic pathology: Tipping the scales in a different direction. *Journal of Abnormal Psychology, 112,* 166–170.

Rizvi, S. L., Peterson, C. B., Crow, S. J., & Agras, W. S. (2000). Test–retest reliability of the eating disorder examination. *International Journal of Eating Disorders, 28,* 311–316.

Rock, C. (2005). Nutritional assessment. In J. E. Mitchell & C. B. Peterson (Eds.), *Assessment of eating disorders* (pp. 129–147). New York: Guilford Press.

Roerig, J. L., Mitchell, J. E., Myers, T. C., & Glass, J. B. (2002). Pharmacotherapy and medical complications of eating disorders in children and adolescents. *Child and Adolescent Psychiatric Clinics of North America, 11,* 365–385.

Puig-Antich, J., & Chambers, W. J. (1983). *Schedule for Affective Disorders and Schizophrenia for School-Age Children (6–18 years).* Pittsburgh, PA: Western Psychiatric Institute.

Santonastaso, P., Friederici, S., & Favaro, A. (1999). Full and partial syndromes in eating disorders: A 1-year prospective study of risk factors among female students. *Psychopathology, 32,* 50–56.

Schacter, D. L. (1999). The seven sins of memory: Insights from psychology and cognitive neuroscience. *American Psychologist, 54,* 182–203.

Schoemaker, C., Verbraak, M., Breteler, R., & van der Staak, C. (1997). The discriminant validity of the Eating Disorder Inventory-2. *British Journal of Clinical Psychology, 36,* 627–629.

Shaw, H., Ramirez, L., Trost, A., Randall, P., & Stice, E. (2004). Body image and eating disturbances across ethnic groups: More similarities than differences. *Psychology of Addictive Behaviors, 18,* 12–18.

Slade, P. (1982). Towards a functional analysis of anorexia nervosa and bulimia nervosa. *British Journal of Clinical Psychology*, 14, 167–179.

Smolak, L., & Striegel-Moore, R. H. (2001). Challenging the myth of the golden girl: Ethnicity and eating disorders. In R. H. Striegel-Moore & L. Smolak (Eds.), *Eating disorders* (pp. 111–132). Washington, DC: American Psychological Association.

Society for Adolescent Medicine. (1995). Eating disorders in adolescents: A position paper of the Society for Adolescent Medicine. *Journal of Adolescent Health*, 16, 476–480.

Spillane, N. S., Boerner, L. M., Anderson, K. G., & Smith, G. T. (2004). Comparability of the Eating Disorder Inventory-2 between women and men. *Assessment*, 11, 85–93.

Spitzer, R. L., Williams, J. B., Gibbon, M., & First, M. B. (1990). *Structured Clinical Interview for DSM-III-R (SCID)*. Washington, DC: American Psychiatric Press.

Stewart, D. A., Carter, J. C., Drinkwater, J., Hainsworth, J., & Fairburn, C. G. (2001). Modification of eating attitudes and behavior in adolescent girls: A controlled study. *International Journal of Eating Disorders*, 29, 107–118.

Stice, E. (2001). A prospective test of the dual pathway model of bulimic pathology: Mediating effects of dieting and negative affect. *Journal of Abnormal Psychology*, 110, 124–135.

Stice, E. (2002). Risk and maintenance factors for eating pathology: A meta-analytic review. *Psychological Bulletin*, 128, 825–848.

Stice, E., Agras, W. S., & Hammer, L. (1999). Risk factors for the emergence of childhood eating disturbances: A five-year prospective study. *International Journal of Eating Disorders*, 25, 375–387.

Stice, E., Burton, E. M., Bohon, C., & Shaw, H. (2007). *Maintenance factors for persistence of bulimic pathology: A community-based natural history study.* Manuscript in preparation.

Stice, E., Burton, E. M., & Shaw, H. (2004). Prospective relations between bulimic pathology, depression, and substance abuse: Unpacking comorbidity in adolescent girls. *Journal of Consulting and Clinical Psychology*, 72, 62–71.

Stice, E., Cameron, R., Killen, J. D., Hayward, C., & Taylor, C. B. (1999). Naturalistic weight reduction efforts prospectively predict growth in relative weight and onset of obesity among female adolescents. *Journal of Consulting and Clinical Psychology*, 67, 967–974.

Stice, E., Fisher, M., & Lowe, M. R. (2004). Are dietary restraint scales valid measures of acute dietary restriction?: Unobtrusive observational data suggest not. *Psychological Assessment*, 16, 51–59.

Stice, E., Fisher, M., & Martinez, E. (2004). Eating Disorder Diagnostic Scale: Additional evidence of reliability and validity. *Psychological Assessment*, 16, 60–71.

Stice, E., Hayward, C., Cameron, R., Killen, J. D., &

Taylor, C. B. (2000). Body image and eating related factors predict onset of depression in female adolescents: A longitudinal study. *Journal of Abnormal Psychology*, 109, 438–444.

Stice, E., Killen, J. D., Hayward, C., & Taylor, C. B. (1998). Age of onset for binge eating and purging during adolescence: A four-year survival analysis. *Journal of Abnormal Psychology*, 107, 671–675.

Stice, E., Mazotti, L., Weibel, D., & Agras, W. S. (2000). Dissonance prevention program decreases thin-ideal internalization, body dissatisfaction, dieting, negative affect, and bulimic symptoms: A preliminary experiment. *International Journal of Eating Disorders*, 27, 206–217.

Stice, E., Orjada, K., & Tristan, J. (2006). Trial of a psychoeducational eating disturbance intervention for college women: A replication and extension. *International Journal of Eating Disorders*, 39, 233–239.

Stice, E., Presnell, K., & Bearman, S. K. (2007). *Risk factors for onset of threshold and subthreshold bulimia nervosa: A 5-year prospective study of adolescent girls.* Manuscript submitted for publication.

Stice, E., Presnell, K., Groesz, L., & Shaw, H. (2005). Effects of a weight maintenance diet on bulimic pathology: An experimental test of the dietary restraint theory. *Health Psychology*, 24, 402–412.

Stice, E., Presnell, K., Shaw, H., & Rohde, P. (2005). Psychological and behavioral risk factors for onset of obesity in adolescent girls: A prospective study. *Journal of Consulting and Clinical Psychology*, 73, 195–202.

Stice, E., Presnell, K., & Spangler, D. (2002). Risk factors for binge eating onset: A prospective investigation. *Health Psychology*, 21, 131–138.

Stice, E., & Ragan, J. (2002). A controlled evaluation of an eating disturbance psychoeducational intervention. *International Journal of Eating Disorders*, 31, 159–171.

Stice, E., Shaw, H., Burton, E., & Wade, E. (2006). Dissonance and healthy weight eating disorder prevention programs: A randomized efficacy trial. *Journal of Consulting and Clinical Psychology*, 74, 263–275.

Stice, E., Telch, C. F., & Rizvi, S. L. (2000). A psychometric evaluation of the Eating Disorder Diagnostic Screen: A brief self-report measure for anorexia, bulimia, and binge eating disorder. *Psychological Assessment*, 12, 123–131.

Stice, E., Trost, A., & Chase, A. (2003). Healthy weight control and dissonance-based eating disorder prevention programs: Results from a controlled trial. *International Journal of Eating Disorders*, 33, 10–21.

Striegel-Moore, R. H., Seeley, J. R., & Lewinsohn, P. M. (2003). Psychosocial adjustment in young adulthood of women who experience an eating disorder during adolescence. *American Academy of Child and Adolescent Psychiatry*, 42, 587–593.

Striegel-Moore, R. H., Wilfley, D. E., Pike, K. M., Dohm, F. A., & Fairburn, C. G. (2000). Recurrent binge eating in black American women. *Archives of Family Medicine*, 9, 83–87.

Strober, M., Freeman, R., & Morrell, W. (1997). The long-term course of severe anorexia nervosa in adolescents: Survival analysis of recovery, relapse, and outcome predictors over 10–15 years in a prospective study. *International Journal of Eating Disorders, 22,* 339–360.

Sullivan, P. F. (1995). Mortality in anorexia nervosa. *American Journal of Psychiatry, 152,* 1073–1074.

Sysko, R., Walsh, B. T., & Fairburn, C. G. (2005). Eating Disorder Examination—Questionnaire as a measure of change in patients with bulimia nervosa. *International Journal of Eating Disorders, 37,* 100–106.

Sysko, R., Walsh, T. B., Schebendach, J., & Wilson, G. T. (2005). Eating behaviors among women with anorexia nervosa. *American Journal of Clinical Nutrition, 82,* 296–301.

Telch, C. F., Pratt, E. M., & Niego, S. H. (1998). Obese women with binge eating disorder define the term binge. *International Journal of Eating Disorders, 24,* 313–317.

Telch, C., & Stice, E. (1998). Psychiatric comorbidity in a non-clinical sample of women with binge eating disorder. *Journal of Consulting and Clinical Psychology, 66,* 768–776.

Thompson, J. K. (2004). The (mis)measurement of body image: Ten strategies to improve assessment for applied and research purposes. *Body Image, 1,* 7–14.

Thompson, J. K., & Gardner, R. M. (2002). Measuring perceptual body image among adolescents and adults. In T. F. Cash & T. Pruzinsky (Eds.), *Body image: A handbook of theory, research, and clinical practice* (pp. 135–141). New York: Guilford Press.

Thompson, J. K., Roehrig, M., Cafri, G., & Heinberg, L. (2005). Assessment of body image disturbance. In J. E. Mitchell & C. B. Peterson (Eds.), *Assessment of eating disorders* (pp. 175–202). New York: Guilford Press.

Treasure, J., & Holland, A. (1989). Genetic vulnerability to eating disorders: Evidence from twin and family studies. In H. Remschmidt & M. H. Schmidt (Eds.), *Child and youth psychiatry: European perspectives* (pp. 59–68). New York: Hogrefe & Huber.

Vitousek, K. B., Daly, J., & Heiser, C. (1991). Reconstructing the internal world of the eating disordered individual: Overcoming denial and distortion in self-report. *International Journal of Eating Disorders, 10,* 647–666.

Vitousek, K., & Manke, F. (1994). Personality variables and disorders in anorexia nervosa and bulimia nervosa. *Journal of Abnormal Psychology, 103,* 137–147.

Vogeltanz-Holm, N. D., Wonderlich, S. A., Lewis, B. A., Wilsnack, S. C., Harris, T. R., Wilsnack, R. W., et al. (2000). Longitudinal predictors of binge eating, intense dieting, and weight concerns in a national sample of women. *Behavior Therapy, 31,* 221–235.

Walsh, B. T. (1993). Binge eating in bulimia nervosa. In C. G. Fairburn & G. T. Wilson (Eds.), *Binge eating: Nature, assessment, and treatment* (pp. 37–49). New York: Guilford Press.

Walsh, B. T., Wilson, G. T., Loeb, K. L., Devlin, M. J., Pike, K. M., Roose, S. P., et al. (1997). Medication and psychotherapy in the treatment of bulimia nervosa. *American Journal of Psychiatry, 154,* 523–531.

Walters, E. E., & Kendler, K. S. (1995). Anorexia nervosa and anorexia-like syndromes in a population-based female twin sample. *American Journal of Psychiatry, 152,* 64–71.

Watkins, B., Frampton, I., Lask, B., & Bryant-Waugh, R. (2005). Reliability and validity of the child version of the eating disorder examination: A preliminary investigation. *International Journal of Eating Disorders, 38,* 183–187.

Wilfley, D. E., Friedman, M. A., Dounchis, J. Z., Stein, R. I., Welch, R. R., & Ball, S. A. (2000). Comorbid psychopathology in binge eating disorder: Relation to eating disorder severity at baseline and following treatment. *Journal of Consulting and Clinical Psychology, 68,* 641–649.

Wilfley, D. E., Schwartz, M. B., Spurrell, E. B., & Fairburn, C. G. (1997). Assessing the specific psychopathology of binge eating disorder patients: Interview or self-report? *Behaviour Research and Therapy, 35,* 1151–1159.

Wilfley, D. E., Welch, R., Stein, R., Borman Spurrell, E., Cohen, L. R., Saelens, B. E., et al. (2002). A randomized comparison of group cognitive-behavioral therapy and group interpersonal psychotherapy for the treatment of overweight individuals with binge-eating disorder. *Archives of General Psychiatry, 59,* 713–721.

Williamson, D. A., Gleaves, D. H., & Savin, S. S. (1992). Empirical classification of eating disorder not otherwise specified: Support for DSM-IV changes. *Journal of Psychopathology and Behavioral Assessment, 14,* 201–216.

Wilson, G. T. (1993). Assessment of binge eating. In C. G. Fairburn & G. T. Wilson (Eds.), *Binge eating: Nature, assessment, and treatment* (pp. 227–249). New York: Guilford Press.

Wilson, G. T., Becker, C. B., & Heffernan, K. (2003). Eating disorders. In E. J. Mash & R. A. Barkley (Eds.), *Child psychopathology* (2nd ed., pp. 687–715). New York: Guilford Press.

Woodside, D. B., Garfinkel, P. E., Lin, E., Goering, P., Kaplan, A. S., Goldbloom, D. S., et al. (2001). Comparison of men with full or partial eating disorders, men without eating disorders, and women with eating disorders in the community. *American Journal of Psychiatry, 158,* 570–574.

Yanovski, S. Z., Leet, M., Yanovski, J. A., Flood, M., Gold, P. W., Kissileff, H. R., et al. (1992). Food selection and intake of obese women with binge eating disorder. *American Journal of Clinical Nutrition, 56,* 975–980.

CHAPTER 17

Personality Disorders

Rebecca L. Shiner

At times, individuals' personalities significantly interfere with their day-to-day functioning and generate internal distress and misery; this is true for youths, as well as for adults. Child psychologists and psychiatrists who routinely treat such personality difficulties need a means of conceptualizing and assessing them. Personality difficulties may be a primary focus in treating some youth, but in nearly all cases, clinicians must be attentive to patients' individual differences in emotional, cognitive, and interpersonal functioning. The fourth edition of the *Diagnostic and Statistical Manual of Mental Disorders* (DSM-IV, American Psychiatric Association [APA], 1994) acknowledges the central importance of personality by including a set of personality disorder diagnoses on Axis II. Each personality disorder in the diagnostic manual is seen as "an enduring pattern of inner experience and behavior that deviates markedly from the expectations of the individual's culture, is pervasive and inflexible, has an onset in adolescence or early adulthood, is stable over time, and leads to distress or impairment" (p. 629). This chapter elaborates the processes through which clinicians may best assess such personality disturbances in youth.

THE CASE FOR ASSESSING PERSONALITY PATHOLOGY IN ADOLESCENT PATIENTS

In assessing youth, it is essential for clinicians to consider the possibility of personality pathology; this is the most important take-home message of this chapter! In other words, it is important to consider the possibility of a personality disorder in all youth who are assessed, not just in those cases in which the youth has prototypical and obvious features of a personality disorder.

At present there is ambivalence about diagnosing personality disorders in youth, both in the DSM-IV and in the psychiatric and psychological fields at large. DSM-IV cautions clinicians to be careful about diagnosing children and adolescents with a personality disorder except in "those relatively unusual instances in which the individual's particular maladaptive personality traits appear to be pervasive, persistent, and unlikely to be limited to a particular developmental stage or an episode of an Axis I disorder" (APA, 1994, p. 631). This explicit hesitation to diagnose personality disorders in youth may arise from several sources (Freeman & Rigby, 2003; Westen & Chang, 2000). At the time when DSM-IV was written, there was a notable lack of data on early manifestations of personality disorders. There are also ongoing concerns about diagnosing youth with potentially stigmatizing disorders that are viewed as long-lasting, difficult to treat, and severe. Finally, personalities of youth are often seen as being "under construction" during childhood and adolescence, and therefore too unstable to have lasting significance. Clinicians may avoid assigning an Axis II diagnosis to their adolescent patients. In a study by Westen, Shedler, Durrett, Glass, and Martens (2003), practicing psychologists and psychiatrists were asked to report on a particular adolescent patient in their practices. Although only 28.4% of patients were assigned an Axis II diagnosis, 75.3% of the patients met criteria for an Axis II diagnosis based on their clinicians' reports of Axis II symptoms.

Over the last decade, a number of researchers have marshaled evidence that personality pathology does, indeed, occur in youth and that the pathways leading to adult personality disorders sometimes begin in childhood (Bleiberg, 2001; Cohen & Crawford, 2005; Johnson, Bromley, Bornstein, & Sneed, 2006; Johnson, Bromley, & McGeoch, 2005; Kernberg, Weiner, & Bardenstein, 2000; Westen & Chang, 2000). There has been an upsurge of empirical research on the adolescent manifestations of personality disorders in particular and on personality in adolescence more generally. This new research (reviewed in the next section of this chapter) points to several compelling reasons clinicians ought to assess personality disorders in their adolescent patients. First, personality pathology in adolescents is not rare and often poses considerable risks for development, including potential high-risk behaviors, emergence of Axis I disorders, and impairment in important life domains (e.g., academic achievement, relationships, work). Second, personality difficulties are not necessarily transient phenomena in adolescence given that pathological personality traits are already moderately stable by adolescence. Third, in light of more recent knowledge about personality change and the treatment of personality disorders in adults, a diagnosis of a personality disorder in adolescence need not be seen as consigning a youth to a permanent life of difficulty. Fourth, careful personality assessment may point to strengths youth possess that can be tremendous assets in treatment. Fifth, treatment ultimately may need to focus on personality change, even if a personality disorder is not the primary diagnosis. Many Axis I disorders likely represent varying manifestations of underlying personality pathology (Westen & Bradley, 2005). Thus, effective treatment may need to target personality change or, in the case of some newer cognitive-behavioral therapies (e.g., Hayes, Follette, & Linehan, 2004), may need to enhance patients' strategies for coping effectively with personality tendencies that may be difficult to change.

A final important reason to assess personality pathology is perhaps less obvious: the potentially large costs of misdiagnosing youth with other disorders, when a personality disorder diagnosis would be more appropriate. In some cases, well-meaning clinicians may search for another disorder to explain a youth's difficulties because of intentional or unrecognized attempts to avoid labeling the youth with a personality disorder. McClellan and Hamilton (2006) recently presented such a composite case of a 15-year-old girl, Abigail. In this illustrative case, Abigail had exhibited a range of serious symptoms for many years, including self-mutilation, explosive outbursts, alcohol and substance abuse, and self-reports of hearing voices. Her psychosocial history was characterized by maltreatment and repeated foster placements. Abigail had received a range of diagnoses, including "bipolar disorder, schizoaffective disorder, major depression with psychotic features, PTSD [posttraumatic stress disorder], conduct disorder, and substance abuse" (p. 490) and had subsequently been prescribed a wide range of psychotropic medications. Finally, she was more appropriately diagnosed with borderline personality disorder and treated with dialectical behavior therapy (DBT; Linehan, 1993a, 1993b). This case illustrates well the problem of incorrectly diagnosing a youth with a mood, anxiety, or psychotic disorder when a personality disorder diagnosis may be more accurate; incorrect diagnosis can lead to improper prescription of medications and the absence of treatment that appropriately targets the key symptoms. Certainly, it is important for clinicians to continue to be cautious about diagnosing youth with a personality disorder, because of the potential cost of stigmatization, but it is important also to recognize the costs of not diagnosing a personality disorder when it is present.

OVERVIEW OF THE CHAPTER

This chapter proceeds in five sections, the first of which articulates the two different means of conceptualizing personality pathology—as diagnostic categories and as pathological personality dimensions. The second section reviews recent research on personality disorders in youth, including prevalence, course, comorbidity, impairment, and etiology. The third section provides a set of basic underlying principles for assessing personality disorders. The fourth section outlines a set of procedures for conducting an assessment of personality disorders, including types of measures to use, information to gather, use of assessment for treatment planning and monitoring, and presentation of assessment information to patients and families. The fifth section describes and evaluates measures that can be used to assess personality pathology in youth and provides recommendations for specific measures to use. The chapter concludes with suggestions for future research on assessment of personality pathology.

MANIFESTATIONS OF PERSONALITY PATHOLOGY: DIAGNOSTIC CATEGORIES AND PERSONALITY TRAIT DIMENSIONS

DSM-IV Diagnoses

The DSM-IV provides an overarching framework for what constitutes a personality disorder. According to this general framework, personality disorders comprise deviant patterns of inner experience and behavior in at least two of the following four areas: "(1) cognition (i.e., ways of perceiving and interpreting self, other people, and events); (2) affectivity (i.e., the range, intensity, lability, and appropriateness of emotional response); (3) interpersonal functioning; (4) impulse control" (APA, 1994, p. 633). Skodol (2005) has fleshed out what these four areas often include. *Cognition* typically manifests as disturbances in how patients view themselves and others, for example, over-inflated self-views or unduly negative views of the self, profound mistrust or alienation toward others, or tendencies to idealize or devalue others. Cognition also includes deviant thinking about the world, such as expectations for perfectionism or odd, delusional beliefs. *Affectivity* involves a wide range of disturbances in patients' typical emotions, including

both restricted emotional experience and excessively intense and labile emotions. The emotions that are disturbed include the full gamut of human emotions—sadness, anxiety, anger and irritation, joy and pleasure, and love and affection. Difficulties in *interpersonal functioning* typically involve problems with one or both of the two main dimensions of interpersonal behavior: agency (ranging from dominance and self-assuredness to submission) and communion (ranging from affiliation and warmth to detachment and coldheartedness) (Wiggins & Trobst, 1999). Finally, several personality disorders involve problems with *impulse control*—either deficits in self-control (poor planning, thinking without acting, poor self-regulation of behavior and emotions) or excessive levels of self-restraint and inhibition of healthy impulses.

These deviant personality patterns are further defined by DSM-IV in several ways (APA, 1994, pp. 630–631). In making a personality disorder diagnosis, clinicians must evaluate personality difficulties in the context of the person's culture; a personality disorder diagnosis is warranted only in cases in which the patterns deviate from what is typically expected in that cultural context. Furthermore, the patterns must be enduring, inflexible, and pervasive across many contexts in the person's life. The patterns are expected to have started at least by adolescence or early adulthood. Like many other DSM-IV disorders, the personality patterns must be distressing to the person or cause impairment in important areas of daily life, such as social relationships, school, or work. Finally, the pattern must not be better accounted for as a consequence of an Axis I condition, a medical condition, or the use of some substance.

In addition to this general framework for defining the presence of a personality disorder (PD), DSM-IV outlines diagnostic criteria for 10 specific PDs, grouped into three clusters: *Cluster A*, odd or eccentric—paranoid PD, schizoid PD, and schizotypal PD; *Cluster B*, dramatic, emotional, or erratic—antisocial PD, borderline PD, histrionic PD, and narcissistic PD; and *Cluster C*, anxious or fearful—avoidant PD, dependent PD, and obsessive–compulsive PD (APA, 1994, pp. 629–630). Two additional PD diagnoses are included in the DSM-IV appendix for further study: depressive PD and passive–aggressive or negativistic PD. The primary features of the 12 personality disorders are described in Table 17.1. DSM-IV also provides the option of diagnosing personality disorder not otherwise specified (PD NOS), for those cases in which the general PD criteria are met and PD symptoms are present, but the person does not fulfill the criteria for any specific PD in the manual. The three clusters into which the diagnoses are grouped were not derived empirically; rather, they were created to help clinicians mentally group the disorders into those that share some descriptive features.

DSM-IV offers some cautions that are specific to diagnosing PDs in children and adolescents under the age of 18, who are diagnosed with personality disorders by the same set of criteria as adults; for youth under age 18, the patterns must have been present at least a year (APA, 1994, p. 631). Youth under 18 may not be diagnosed with antisocial PD, however (p. 647). Typically, youth with antisocial behavior are diagnosed with conduct disorder instead, and conduct disorder with onset before age 15 is required for an adult diagnosis of antisocial PD (p. 650). Although youth under age 18 cannot be formally diagnosed with antisocial PD, there is robust evidence that they can still exhibit the psychopathic personality traits and behaviors associated with this diagnosis, such as manipulativeness, lack of empathy, and impulsiveness (Kotler & McMahon, 2005; Lynam & Gudonis, 2005; Salekin & Frick, 2005). Because the presence of psychopathic tendencies in youth has implications for treatment, the assessment of psychopathy is discussed later in this chapter.

Alternative Dimensional Models of Personality Pathology

A key issue in conceptualizing personality pathology is whether it is most validly described as categorical patterns or variations on dimensional traits. This issue is discussed in some detail here, because it has important ramifications for the assessment of personality pathology in youth.

The model of PDs adopted in DSM-IV is a categorical one; the PDs are each seen as distinct patterns that differ qualitatively from both normal personality functioning and each other. The validity of this categorical system has been challenged on a number of fronts (reviewed in Oldham & Skodol, 2000; Trull

& Durrett, 2005; Widiger & Mullins-Sweatt, 2005). The PDs co-occur within patients at a rate that is much higher than would be expected if the disorders were truly distinct, categorical entities with distinct etiologies. The existing PD diagnoses also do not provide adequate coverage of the range of personality pathology that patients exhibit. As a result, PD NOS turns out to be the most common PD diagnosis used in actual practice with adults (Verheul & Widiger, 2004), and it may be the most prevalent PD in both adolescents and adults (Johnson, First, et al., 2005).

Rather than defining personality pathology as categorical disorders, personality pathology may be more validly conceptualized within a dimensional framework. In a dimensional taxonomy, it is recognized that psychopathology involves variation in underlying dimensions of cognition, affect, and behavior. Implicit in such a model is the recognition that there is no clear-cut boundary between normal and abnormal functioning; in other words, in a dimensional model, PDs differ from normal-range personality quantitatively rather than qualitatively. A critical issue in the upcoming development of DSM-V is whether dimensional models of psychopathology should be included (Krueger, Watson, & Barlow, 2005; Rounsaville et al., 2002). In the specific case of PDs, a dimensional model would suggest that personality pathology represents maladaptive variants of personality traits that exist in the population as a whole.

A dizzying array of dimensional models has been proposed to describe personality pathology. In fact, one recent review of such models listed 18 alternative proposals (Widiger & Simonsen, 2005)! Fortunately, there is considerable overlap among many of these models, and it is possible to integrate many of them into an overarching taxonomy of personality pathology. In one model that is particularly well supported empirically (Markon, Krueger, & Watson, 2005; Trull & Durrett, 2005; Widiger & Mullins-Sweatt, 2005; Widiger & Simonsen, 2005), personality pathology can be defined along four overarching or higher-order dimensions. First, *Extraversion versus Introversion* measures the degree to which a person is outgoing, active and energetic, expressive, and emotionally positive. At the pathological extremes, this dimension taps exhibitionism (high end) and detachment, social avoidance, and excessive shyness (low end). Second, *Antagonism*

TABLE 17.1. DSM-IV-TR Personality Disorder Diagnoses: Essential Features and Links with Big Five Personality Traits

Diagnosis	Essential features[a]	Associated Big Five traits and facets[b]
Paranoid	Distrust and suspiciousness such that others' motives are interpreted as malevolent	N—Angry–Hostility (high); E—Warmth, Gregariousness (all low); O—Actions, Ideas (all low); A—Trust, Straightforwardness, Altruism, Compliance, Tender Mindedness (all low)
Schizoid	Detachment from social relationships and a restricted range of emotional expression	E—Warmth, Gregariousness, Assertiveness, Activity, Excitement seeking, Positive Emotions (all low); O—Feelings, Actions (all low)
Schizotypal	Acute discomfort in close relationships, cognitive or perceptual distortions, and eccentricities of behavior	N—Anxiety, Self-Consciousness (all high); E—Warmth, Gregariousness, Positive Emotions (all low); O—Ideas (high); C—Order (low)
Antisocial	Disregard for, and violation of, the rights of others	N—Angry–Hostility, Impulsivity (all high) and Anxiety, Self-consciousness (all low); E—Assertiveness, Activity, Excitement Seeking (all high); O—Actions (high); A—Trust, Straightforwardness, Altruism, Compliance, Modesty, Tender Mindedness (all low); C—Dutifulness, Self-Discipline, Deliberation (all low)
Borderline	Instability in interpersonal relationships, self-image, and affects, and marked impulsivity	N—Anxiety, Angry–Hostility, Depression, Impulsiveness, Vulnerability (all high); O—Feelings, Actions (all high); C—Deliberation (low)
Histrionic	Excessive emotionality and attention seeking	N—Self-Consciousness (low) and Impulsiveness (high); E—Gregariousness, Activity, Excitement Seeking, Positive Emotions (all high); O—Fantasy, Feelings, Actions (all high); A—Trust (high); C—Self-Discipline, Deliberation (all low)
Narcissistic	Grandiosity, need for admiration, and lack of empathy	N—Angry–Hostility (high) and Self-Consciousness (low); E—Warmth (low) and Assertiveness and Excitement Seeking (all high); O—Feelings (low) and Actions (high); A—Trust, Straightforwardness, Altruism, Compliance, Modesty, Tender Mindedness (all low)
Avoidant	Social inhibition, feelings of inadequacy, and hypersensitivity to negative evaluation	N—Anxiety, Self-consciousness, Vulnerability (all high) and Impulsiveness (low); E—Gregariousness, Assertiveness, Excitement Seeking, Positive Emotions (all low); O—Actions (low); A—Modesty (high)
Dependent	Submissive and clinging behavior related to an excessive need to be taken care of	N—Anxiety, Self-Consciousness, Vulnerability (all high); E—Assertiveness (low); A—Trust, Compliance, Modesty (all high)
Obsessive–compulsive	Preoccupation with orderliness, perfectionism, and control	N—Anxiety (high) and Impulsiveness (low); E—Excitement Seeking (low); O—Feelings, Actions, Ideas, Values (all low); C—Competence, Order, Dutifulness, Achievement Striving, Self-Discipline, Deliberation (all high)
Depressive (Appendix)	Depressive cognitions and behaviors	None provided
Passive–aggressive (negativistic; Appendix)	Negativistic attitudes and passive resistance to demands for adequate performance in social and occupational situations	None provided

[a] From American Psychiatric Association (2000). Copyright 2000 by the American Psychiatric Association. Adapted by permission.
[b] N, Neuroticism; E, Extraversion; O, Openness to Experience; A, Agreeableness; C, Conscientiousness. The facets listed are those included in the NEO-PI-R (Costa & McCrae, 1992). The Big Five traits and facets associated with each personality disorder diagnosis are adapted from Lynam and Widiger (2001). Copyright 2001 by the American Psychological Association. Adapted by permission.

versus Compliance measures tendencies toward being hostile and cynical versus kind, modest, empathetic, honest, and trusting. At the pathological high end, this dimension taps mistrust and alienation, aggression, entitlement, and callousness. Third, *Constraint versus Impulsivity* measures tendencies to be responsible, attentive, persistent, orderly, high-achieving, and planful versus irresponsible, unreliable, careless, and to quit easily. At the pathological extremes, this dimension taps compulsivity and workaholism (high end), and impulsiveness, irresponsibility, and excessive risk taking (low end). Fourth, *Emotional Dysregulation versus Emotional Stability* measures individual differences in the experience of negative emotions. At the pathological high end, this dimension taps anxiousness, insecure attachment, identity problems, affective lability, feelings of worthlessness, and poor ability to cope with stress. It is not clear whether there is a pathological low end, but it may possibly involve an excessive lack of fear and anxiety (as in psychopathy). Each of these broad, higher-order dimensions in the proposed model includes a number of more narrow, lower-order dimensions that are sometimes called "facets" (e.g., Extraversion involves components such as activity level, gregariousness, and positive emotions). The lower-order components tend to covary, which is why they cohere to form a higher-order trait, but they differ enough that each lower-order component provides useful information about personality functioning.

Evidence for the proposed taxonomic framework comes from two primary sources: research linking normal-range personality traits, such as the Big Five, with personality disorders, and research delineating the structure of pathological personality trait dimensions. DSM-IV PD diagnoses may be described in terms of variation of normal-range personality traits, such as the Big Five (Costa & Widiger, 2002), which is a taxonomy of normal-range personality traits that has robust empirical support (John & Srivastava, 1999) and includes the following traits: Neuroticism, Extraversion, Openness to Experience, Agreeableness, and Conscientiousness. Support for the proposed model of personality pathology also comes from research undertaken to determine the structure of pathological personality traits. Both Livesley (Livesley & Jackson, in press) and Clark (1993) created questionnaires designed to measure the full range of personality

pathology in adults. These personality pathology measures included a greater proportion and a broader range of negative personality descriptors than normal-range personality inventories, such as those measuring the Big Five. The higher-order structure obtained in these questionnaires is generally consistent with the proposed taxonomic framework, although some differences do emerge. Normal-range personality traits and pathological personality traits in adults appear to share a common structure of higher-order traits (Markon et al., 2005). Table 17.1 presents the Big Five traits and facets that experts rated as likely to be associated with each of the DSM PDs (Lynam & Widiger, 2001).

Thus, there is compelling support for a dimensional model of personality pathology as an alternative to the categorical system now in place. This work raises an important question for the assessment of personality difficulties in children and adolescents: Can youths' personalities likewise be described validly with the proposed taxonomy of four higher-order traits? It is possible to give a tentative "yes" to this question. Children and adolescents manifest a set of Big Five traits similar to that of adults (Caspi & Shiner, 2006; Shiner, 2006); therefore, it is possible to use the Big Five traits to characterize youths' personalities in a clinical setting. As with adults, there is some evidence that PDs in adolescence may be described using Big Five personality measures (De Clercq & De Fruyt, 2003; De Clercq, De Fruyt, & Van Leeuwen, 2004). Furthermore, De Clercq, De Fruyt, Van Leeuwen, and Mervielde (2006) have created a new questionnaire measure of pathological personality in youth (similar to those created by Livesley and Clark for adults) and have found that, as with adults, four higher-order traits emerge: Introversion, Disagreeableness, Compulsivity, and Emotional Instability. Thus, clinicians who assess PDs in youth have the option of assessing personality traits, as well as determining the presence of DSM-IV PD diagnoses.

OVERVIEW OF RECENT RESEARCH ON PERSONALITY DISORDERS IN YOUTH

Prior to the mid-1990s, there was very little empirical research on the nature and development of PDs in children and adolescents. Although there is still far less known about PDs than about other disorders in youth, the last decade has seen a surge of interest. Consequently, some basic information is now available about personality pathology in adolescents, including data on prevalence, stability and course, comorbidity, life impairment, and etiology. This basic information has important implications for the assessment of PDs, because it points to crucial areas to assess. The recent research also overturns many incorrect assumptions about the nature of PDs and makes clear why it is essential that clinicians consider the possible presence of personality pathology in the youth they treat.

Prevalence and Gender

It is difficult to estimate the prevalence of PDs in both adolescents and adults, because there are not yet adequate epidemiological studies addressing this issue. Although epidemiological studies have determined prevalence rates for Axis I disorders, Axis II disorders have been excluded from these studies, with the exception of antisocial PD (Mattia & Zimmerman, 2001). For adolescents, the best available estimates of DSM-III-R and DSM-IV PDs derive from representative community or primary care samples. Prevalence estimates for having at least one PD have ranged from 6 to 17% in adolescents, with a median prevalence of 11% (Johnson, Bromley, Bornstein, & Sneed, 2006). Comparable large-scale studies with adults suggest prevalence rates of approximately 10–15% for at least one PD, and 1–2% for each specific PD diagnosis (Mattia & Zimmerman, 2001; Torgersen, 2005). Thus, there is good evidence that PDs are as prevalent in adolescence as in adulthood. In fact, PD traits and diagnoses may actually be more prevalent earlier in adolescence than during later adolescence, at which point prevalence appears to be quite comparable to that seen in adulthood (Johnson, Bromley, et al., 2006). PD rates in individuals presenting for treatment are, of course, likely to be higher.

As with general prevalence rates for PDs, epidemiological data on gender differences are lacking for both adolescents and adults. However, there is some evidence from adult community samples that although the overall prevalence rates for PDs appear to be roughly equal for males and females, some specific PDs may be more prevalent in one gender or the other (Morey, Alexander, & Boggs, 2005; Torgersen,

2005). Empirical findings are not entirely consistent with the information on gender in DSM-IV. Specifically, in adult community samples, schizoid PD, antisocial PD, and obsessive–compulsive PD may be more common in males, and histrionic and dependent PD may be more common in females (Morey et al., 2005; Torgersen, 2005). Consistent gender differences are not found in community samples for the other PDs, including borderline PD. Furthermore, findings of gender differences are often inconsistent across studies or modest in size. Very little is known about gender differences in community samples of adolescents, other than the consistent finding that conduct problems are more prevalent in samples of males (Moffitt, Caspi, Rutter, & Silva, 2001). In short, gender differences in PDs are not as common or as large in community samples as often assumed. Furthermore, even in the case of a disorder such as antisocial PD, where there is a clear male preponderance, many adolescent females still meet criteria for the diagnosis. Thus, it is important for clinicians to be vigilant about preventing preconceived ideas about gender differences from influencing their assessment of PDs and traits.

Course of Personality Disorders

DSM-IV makes a number of explicit assumptions about the stability and course of PDs. Specifically, DSM-IV describes PDs as *enduring* patterns, and these patterns need to have existed for at least a year to warrant diagnosis in youth under age 18. A number of recent longitudinal studies have examined the stability and course of PD diagnoses and symptoms in both youth and adults, and have found that the picture regarding stability is more complex than assumed. Furthermore, the results for PD diagnoses and symptoms may be understood in light of recent research on the stability of normal-range personality traits over time. Taken together, the findings for both PDs and normal-range personality traits are forcing a reanalysis of the picture of PDs presented in the DSM-IV.

Personality stability is itself a complex notion, because there are many different kinds of continuity and change. First, *rank-order stability* refers to the degree to which the relative order of individuals on a given trait or symptom is maintained over time, and it is typically measured through test–retest correlations on dimensional scores of some trait across two points in time. PD symptoms in adolescents and young adults display moderate levels of rank-order stability across time, often in the range of .40 to .65 (Cohen, Crawford, Johnson, & Kasen, 2005; Johnson, Bromley, et al., 2006), similar to the moderate levels of stability observed in adulthood (Grilo & McGlashan, 2005). These findings of moderate rank-order stability for personality disorder symptoms in adolescence are quite comparable to those found for normal-range personality traits in childhood and adolescence (Roberts & DelVecchio, 2000). The findings for personality pathology and normal personality converge on the conclusion that there is nothing transformative about the age of 18 with regard to stability of personality disorder symptoms; moderate stability is already apparent by adolescence.

Second, it is important to consider the *stability of PD diagnoses* over time. In other words, if a person meets criteria for a particular PD, is it likely that he or she will still warrant that diagnosis over time? Contrary to what might be expected from the DSM-IV, the stability of particular PD diagnoses appears to be relatively modest in both adolescent and adult samples (Cohen et al., 2005; Grilo & McGlashan, 2005; Johnson, Bromley, et al., 2006; Skodol, Gunderson, et al., 2005; Zanarini, Frankenburg, Hennen, Reich, & Silk, 2005). The relatively modest stability of PD diagnoses is due in part to the categorical system used; patients can shed a diagnosis because of crossing the arbitrary threshold set for the diagnosis. But the surprising remission rates seem to reflect more substantive processes as well. Recent longitudinal research with adults suggests that there are less stable and more stable aspects to PDs (Skodol, Gunderson, et al., 2005; Zanarini et al., 2005). The less stable aspects typically involve more acute behaviors, such as odd behavior or self-harm; in contrast, the more stable aspects involve personality traits underlying the condition (McGlashan et al., 2005). Finally, although rates of continuity may be low for specific PD diagnoses, there is some evidence that adolescent patients with a PD diagnosis may still be at higher risk of having *any* PD diagnosis over time (Chanen et al., 2004).

Third, *mean-level change* refers to increases or decreases in the average trait level of a population as a whole. In terms of mean-level

change, levels of PD symptoms appear to peak in early adolescence, then decline across the years of later adolescence and early adulthood (Cohen et al., 2005; Johnson, Bromley, et al., 2006). These findings are consistent with results for mean-level stability of normal personality traits. On average, Neuroticism decreases in young adulthood, and Agreeableness and Conscientiousness increase in young adulthood and middle age (Roberts, Walton, & Viechtbauer, 2006). Given that many PDs are characterized by high Neuroticism and low Agreeableness and Conscientiousness, it is not surprising that PD symptoms peak in adolescence and later improve. Thus, across the late adolescent and early adult years, there is on average a movement toward greater personality maturity.

The findings for mean-level changes may also help to account for why PD diagnoses are relatively unstable; individuals with PDs may experience the same maturing normative changes that occur in personality traits across the population. Despite the general improvements that typically occur in personality functioning, there may be some individuals whose PD symptoms worsen in adolescence and adulthood (Johnson, Cohen, Kasen, et al., 2000). These individuals particularly may be in need of treatment.

Comorbidity: Concurrent and Prospective Links with Axis I and Axis II Disorders

Comorbidity appears to be the rule rather than the exception for personality disorders. As noted previously, there tends to be a high level of comorbidity among the PDs in adults (Skodol, 2005). The same is true for adolescents: Comorbidity among PDs in adolescents is common (Cohen et al., 2005). There is also a high level of comorbidity between Axis I and Axis II disorders in both adults (Dolan-Sewell, Krueger, & Shea, 2001) and adolescents. All three clusters of PDs in adolescence show high rates of comorbidity with Axis I disorders, including depressive, anxiety, substance use, and disruptive behavior disorders (Cohen et al., 2005). Furthermore, earlier Axis I disorders predict heightened risk for later emergence and continuation of Axis II disorders into adulthood (Cohen et al., 2005; Lewinsohn, Rohde, Seeley, & Klein, 1997). The reverse is true as well: Earlier Axis II disorders predict greater risk for early adult Axis I disorders, even after taking into account the presence of earlier Axis I and II disorders (Cohen et al., 2005; Daley et al., 1999). It appears that there is often a transaction between Axis I and Axis II disorders across the years from adolescence to adulthood, with Axis I disorders contributing to the expression of Axis II disorders and vice versa.

PD traits in childhood are similarly linked with Axis I symptoms (Mervielde, De Clercq, De Fruyt, & Van Leeuwen, 2005): Antagonism and low Constraint with externalizing symptoms and Emotional Dysregulation and low Extraversion with internalizing symptoms. These high rates of overlap between Axis I and Axis II conditions suggest that the two axes are not nearly as distinct as originally conceived. Furthermore, it is increasingly recognized that comorbidity may often be caused by something meaningful, namely, personality dimensions that underlie both Axis I and Axis II disorders (Clark, 2005).

Impairment Associated with Personality Disorders

Personality disorders cause youth to be vulnerable to the development of a variety of risky and harmful behaviors. PDs from clusters A and B in adolescence predict risks for adolescent and adult violence, including acts such as "arson, assault, breaking and entering, initiating physical fights, robbery, and threats to injure others" (Johnson, Cohen, Smailes, et al., 2000, p. 1406) even when possible confounding variables are taken into account. Adolescent PDs from all three clusters and those in the DSM appendix are also predictive of heightened risk of suicidal ideation or attempts in early adulthood (Johnson, Cohen, et al., 1999). Self-mutilation may also be present in youth with PDs, in the form of cutting, burning, or punching oneself. In a recent study of adult patients with borderline PD approximately one-third of the patients who had engaged in self-mutilation reported that they started harming themselves as children, and another one-third reported having started as adolescents (Zanarini et al., 2006). Finally, adolescents with PDs are at heightened risk for having a high number of sexual partners and high-risk sexual behaviors more generally (Lavan & Johnson, 2002).

Beyond the effects of PDs on symptomatology and risky behaviors, there is evidence that adolescent PDs are associated with risks for problems with adaptation, both concurrently and into adulthood. Adolescent PDs and traits pose heightened risks for later conflicts with family members, as well as problems with romantic relationships, including stressful relationships, conflicts, low partner satisfaction, abuse, and unwanted pregnancy (Johnson, Bromley, et al., 2006). Adolescents with PDs also have heightened rates of problems in other domains of life, including difficulties in friendships, few social activities, poor educational achievement, and work difficulties (Bernstein et al., 1993; Johnson, First, et al., 2005). All of these findings for PDs are consistent with research on personality in childhood and adolescence more generally; youths' personalities are predictive of many important life outcomes, including peer relationships, formation of romantic relationships, academic attainment, effectiveness at work, and health (Caspi & Shiner, 2006; Shiner, 2006). It should be emphasized that although adolescent PDs are associated with risks for impairment, not all youth with PDs in the community have clearcut impairment (Cohen et al., 2005; Johnson, First, et al., 2005). Furthermore, the functioning in some youth with PDs improves as they age (Cohen et al., 2005).

In short, adolescent PDs are associated with risks for concurrent and future difficulties in many areas—Axis I disorders, high-risk behaviors (violence, suicide, risky sexual behavior), and life impairment. All of these same co-occurring problems are associated with PD NOS in adolescents as well (Johnson, First, et al., 2005). Although PD symptoms do appear to improve with age for some adolescents, the outcomes associated with these disorders can be quite serious for many youth.

The Etiology of Personality Disorders

Much of the early clinical interest in PDs in the 20th century arose from rich, complex psychodynamic theories about the origins of such disorders. Most of these etiological theories were based on clinicians' discussions with patients about their early histories. Although these theories have spurred interest in PDs and have provided a basis for interventions, relatively little is known empirically about the developmental pathways leading to PDs (with the exception of antisocial PD). Nonetheless, there are several promising leads for potential causes of PDs, including early temperament and personality traits based in part on genetics and adverse environmental experiences, particularly in the family.

Children's emerging temperaments and personalities are likely to play an important role in the emergence of personality pathology over time. Both temperament in early childhood and personality in later childhood and adolescence significantly overlap with the kinds of personality traits observed in adults (Caspi & Shiner, 2006; Rothbart & Bates, 2006; Shiner & Caspi, 2003). In early childhood, children manifest traits that tap differences in extraversion or surgency (positive emotions/pleasure), negative emotionality (fear/inhibition, irritability), and effortful control or constraint (attention); they also manifest temperament traits of activity level and soothability/adaptability (Caspi & Shiner, 2006). Thus, early in life children manifest individual differences in both their experiences of positive and negative emotions, and their ability to regulate their emotions and behavior. As children age, they display a wider range of traits, and by middle childhood these traits are structured like the Big Five traits observed in adults (Caspi & Shiner, 2006). In other words, by middle childhood, children continue to manifest individual differences in emotions (Extraversion and Neuroticism) and self-regulation (Conscientiousness), but they also manifest clear, individual differences in their prosocial versus antisocial orientation toward others (Agreeableness), and in their creativity and curiosity (Openness to Experience). There is some longitudinal evidence that childhood personality traits are predictive of later general PD symptoms; predictive childhood personality traits include introversion, low self-esteem, high emotionality, abrasiveness, immaturity, and not being goal-directed (Bernstein, Cohen, Skodol, Bezirganian, & Brook, 1996; Cohen, 1996).

Children's early personalities shape their experiences of the environment through a number of important processes (Caspi & Shiner, 2006): the ways children are conditioned by their environments, the responses children evoke from the people in their lives, the ways children interpret their experiences, the ways children evaluate themselves and form a sense of identity, the environments that children "select" for themselves, and the ways children modify and manipulate their environments.

Youths' personalities can help explain why children exposed to relatively similar environments do not have the same outcomes—a phenomenon known as "multifinality." For example, a child who is intensely anxious and irritable and lacks good self-control is going to have a very different experience of parental divorce than a child who is emotionally stable and behaviorally restrained; these differences in the experience of divorce could then lead to differing outcomes for the children.

What are the origins of individual differences in personality? Behavior genetic research on normal-range temperament and personality traits has established that individual differences in these traits are moderately heritable; estimates of heritability are in the range of .50 ± .10 in twin studies and somewhat lower (around .30) in adoption studies (Caspi & Shiner, 2006). It is interesting to note that temperament in infancy and early childhood is influenced by environmental experiences, not just by heredity (Emde & Hewitt, 2001); this research corrects common misconceptions that temperament is solely influenced by genes in infancy, and that the environment only becomes important later in life. Estimates of heritability for PD traits in adults are roughly similar in magnitude to those found for normal-range traits (Cloninger, 2005; Livesley, 2005). There is preliminary evidence for moderate heritability of PD features in a small study of children and adolescents (Coolidge, Thede, & Jang, 2001). Behavior genetic research also highlights the importance of environmental experiences as a determinant of personality differences (Caspi, Roberts, & Shiner, 2005); in nearly all behavior genetic studies, environmental differences account for a substantial portion of the variation in personality and temperament. One surprise emerging from this research, however, is that environmental experiences tend to create differences between children growing up in the same family rather than making siblings more alike (Caspi et al., 2005).

Although theories about the family origins of PDs abound, relatively few data addressed this issue until recently. There is now strong longitudinal evidence that childhood abuse (including sexual, physical, and verbal abuse) and neglect predict heightened risk for the later development of PDs (Johnson, Bromley, et al., 2005, 2006). In addition, maladaptive parenting more generally poses risks for the development of PDs; such maladaptive parenting includes low parental affection or nurturing and aversive parental behavior (e.g., harsh punishment; Johnson, Cohen, Chen, Kasen, & Brook, 2006). Abuse, neglect, and poor parenting behavior may shape children's emerging personality pathology through a number of processes. Children who face these adverse experiences lack the socialization experiences that normally help children learn how to cultivate relationships, follow societal rules, and regulate emotions and behavior (Johnson, Bromley, et al., 2005, 2006). Many children who experience family adversity also develop insecure attachments and do not learn how to trust and engage appropriately with close others (Johnson, Bromley, et al., 2005, 2006). Beyond the family environment, sociocultural factors are also likely to influence the development of PDs; for example, personality pathology characterized by poor constraint may be fostered in social contexts that do not provide structure or firm limits on the expression of impulsivity (Paris, 2005a).

Early family adversity poses significant risks for the development of personality pathology, but it is crucial to recognize that early trauma and abuse may not be present in the histories of all youth with PDs. In fact, in the best longitudinal study of personality disorders to date, the Children in the Community Study, early trauma and/or abuse "do not account for all, or even most cases of PD observed in our longitudinal cohort" (Cohen et al., 2005, p. 482). Furthermore, even in cases of maltreatment, different children are affected differently. In one study, maltreated children whose genotype conferred low levels of monoamine oxidase A (MAOA) expression more often developed conduct disorder, antisocial personality, or violence than children with a high-activity MAOA genotype (Caspi et al., 2002). Temperament may also play a more central role in some pathways, whereas trauma may be more central in other ones (Nigg, Silk, Stavro, & Miller, 2005). Research has begun to yield some clues as to the origins of personality pathology, but the task remains for future research to lay out more clearly the varied pathways through which temperament is transformed through experience into PDs (Clark, 2005; Paris, 2003). Behavior genetic designs will be particularly helpful in elucidating the roles of both genetic and environmental contributors to personality pathology.

BASIC PRINCIPLES FOR ASSESSING PERSONALITY DISORDERS

This section reviews some basic recommendations or principles for assessing PDs in youth; most of these principles should be applicable to the assessment of PDs in adults as well. Many of these principles derive from current research on the nature of PDs in youth and adults; readers are referred the earlier section of this chapter for citations of studies that document these findings.

1. *Be careful to avoid unwarranted assumptions about the manifestations or causes of PDs.* This first principle, of course, applies to assessment of all psychological conditions, but it may be especially important in the diagnosis of PDs, in which the knowledge base is relatively shallower and untested theories may sometimes hold sway. Three examples serve to illustrate the kinds of faulty assumptions to avoid. First, although childhood abuse and neglect occur at higher-than-average rates in adolescents with PDs, longitudinal data show that not all youth with PDs have been maltreated in their past. Thus, although a history of abuse or neglect should be assessed, it should not be assumed. Second, although some PDs occur at higher rates in one gender than the other, all PDs can occur in both genders (e.g., a boy with borderline PD, or a girl with early signs of antisocial PD). Third, although many youth with PDs are highly impaired in multiple areas of adaptive functioning, not all youth with PDs are severely impaired. Thus, it is important to consider the possible presence of a PD even in youth who have some areas of competent functioning.

2. *Evaluate personality pathology comprehensively to ascertain the possible presence of more than one PD diagnosis.* In evaluating PDs through unstructured methods, clinicians may sometimes settle on a PD diagnosis, then fail to adequately evaluate the presence of other PD symptoms or disorders (Westen et al., 2003; Widiger & Samuel, 2005). This tendency is particularly problematic, because comorbid PDs are common in both youth and adults. Thus, by settling on one PD diagnosis without considering others, clinicians may overlook central aspects of a patient's personality that should be addressed in treatment. Regardless of what assessment methods they use, it is important that clinicians at

least screen for a comprehensive range of personality pathology.

3. *Consider the possibility of a personality disorder not otherwise specified (NOS) diagnosis.* The DSM-IV specifies that a PD NOS diagnosis is warranted when a patient exhibits the general features of a PD and has a number of PD symptoms but does not meet criteria for any specific PD. It would be easy to overlook the possibility of this diagnosis in conducting an assessment, yet PD NOS may be the most prevalent PD in youth. Furthermore, as described previously, PD NOS is as predictive of impairment and high-risk behavior as any of the other PD diagnoses; therefore, it needs to be treated on an equal basis. Because a PD NOS diagnosis is vague and provides little guidance for treatment, clinicians need to assess and specify which personality patterns are present and particularly troubling when assigning this diagnosis.

4. *Evaluate whether personality traits and behaviors are impairing and pathological patterns versus more normative manifestations of adolescence.* Although PD symptoms may peak in adolescence and be prevalent in patients, clinicians still need to carefully discriminate between pathological patterns and more typical adolescent personality tendencies. For example, a certain amount of insecurity about relationships, confusion about one's identity, and shifting of moods and emotions is common during adolescence. Clinicians need to draw on their knowledge of adolescent behavior to determine whether particularly patterns are nonnormative. Questionnaire measures that are scored based on normative, national data are useful in this regard, as are the reports of informants who have experience with a range of adolescents (e.g., teachers).

5. *Be attentive to both acute symptoms and underlying personality patterns.* Newer models of PDs in adults indicate that PDs involve a mixture of both more acute, short-term problematic behaviors and more stable, long-term personality patterns (Skodol, Gunderson, et al., 2005; Zanarini et al., 2005). The acute behaviors may be brought on by current stress and may often be the reason for referral; for example, the patient may exhibit odd (e.g., paranoid ideation) or risky behaviors (e.g., suicidal ideation or behavior, violence, self-mutilation). In contrast, the more stable aspects involve more enduring personality patterns. The acute behaviors may be the most attention-grabbing

during an initial assessment, but it is essential to evaluate the enduring personality patterns carefully as well. The more enduring patterns are likely to provide clues to the causes of the more acute behaviors, and need to be addressed in treatment. It is also possible that the acute symptoms might be viewed as manifestations of an Axis I disorder, when they actually point to a more enduring personality pattern.

6. *Gather information from both the adolescents and others who know them well.* As with all child and adolescent disorders, it is critical for clinicians to obtain assessment information from other informants in addition to reports from the adolescent patients themselves. This is generally true when assessing children and adolescents, because different informants provide different information about them, and reports from different informants converge only modestly to moderately (Kamphaus & Frick, 1996). The need for varied informants may be especially acute in assessing PDs, however, because the disorders themselves may make it difficult for some patients to report on their functioning accurately (Klonsky, Oltmanns, & Turkheimer, 2002). Individuals with PDs may lack insight into their personality patterns, may not realize the effects of their behaviors, or may intentionally try to conceal some of their behaviors. Among adults, targets and informants agree only modestly about targets' personality disorders (Klonsky et al., 2002), and both self- and informant reports of PD symptoms provide incremental prediction of important outcomes (Klein, 2003; Ready, Watson, & Clark, 2002). Thus, informants and adolescents may have quite different perspectives on the adolescents' functioning, and these varied perspectives need to inform the assessment.

7. *Assess personality strengths as well as areas of difficulty.* In assessing PDs, it would be easy to focus entirely on areas of deficit—those aspects of youths' personalities that are causing difficulties and lead them to need treatment. Yet it is essential to assess areas of personality strengths as well; even the most troubled youth have areas of relative health in their personalities. These strengths are resources on which to draw in treatment, and a better appreciation of adolescents' individual strengths can sustain a sense of optimism in the adolescents themselves, in their caregivers, and in their treatment providers (Henggeler, Schoenwald, Borduin, Rowland, & Cunningham, 1998).

This sense of encouragement and optimism may be especially important in treating youth with PDs, who may become discouraged when treatment is difficult. Recent work in positive psychology suggests that focusing on and amplifying patients' character strengths may be a powerful complement to more traditional therapy focused on correcting deficits (Duckworth, Steen, & Seligman, 2005). One advantage to assessing personality traits rather than just PDs is that it yields information about both positive and negative traits.

RECOMMENDED PROCEDURES FOR ASSESSING PERSONALITY DISORDERS IN YOUTH

This section presents an overview of recommended procedures to follow in assessing PDs in youth. The purposes of assessment are varied; among the most important reasons are to establish a diagnosis, to formulate a case in order to plan for treatment, and to monitor treatment outcomes (Mash & Hunsley, 2005). This section considers these various purposes and recommends procedures for five aspects of assessment: (1) evaluating personality pathology, (2) obtaining other relevant information, (3) developing an effective treatment plan, (4) monitoring treatment outcomes, and (5) presenting results to adolescents and their families.

Evaluating Personality Pathology

Clinicians who assess PDs in adolescents face a formidable task, because the criteria for PDs are so wide-ranging and encompass so many different aspects of the adolescent's life. Two different types of measures are likely to be particularly helpful in gathering the information necessary to make a diagnosis: questionnaire measures and semistructured interviews. Questionnaire measures can first be administered to the adolescents and their parents to screen for the possible presence of personality pathology and to narrow down the range of personality difficulties that will require further assessment. The adolescents and their parents can then be interviewed (preferably through a semistructured interview) to determine more clearly what personality patterns are problematic. My discussion of the use of these two types of measures draws heavily on recommendations by Widiger and colleagues for assessing PDs in adults (Widiger, 2002; Widiger & Coker, 2002;

Widiger, Costa, & Samuel, 2006; Widiger & Samuel, 2005). A detailed discussion of specific questionnaires and semistructured interviews is presented in the next section.

Questionnaires

A very useful first step involves administering a self-report questionnaire to the adolescent and a separate questionnaire to his or her parent. Three different kinds of self-report omnibus questionnaires may be given to adolescents to assess personality pathology. First are measures that assess DSM-IV PD criteria in a fairly straightforward manner. Most of these are essentially screening measures that help to pinpoint which PDs require further assessment. Second are questionnaires that assess pathological personality traits that are related to but lack a clear one-to-one correspondence with the DSM-IV PDs. Third are questionnaires that assess normal personality traits that have clear relevance for the assessment of PDs. For parents, the first type of questionnaire—those that assess the DSM-IV criteria—is most appropriate, because it can be used without scoring according to norms. The latter two types of questionnaires require norms for scoring, and norms for parent reports are not available.

These different types of questionnaires vary in the information they provide. All three types of measures may potentially serve as useful screens to help determine whether to assess further for personality pathology, which PDs potentially may be skipped in a later interview, and which PDs will require more careful assessment. Although the questionnaires that assess DSM-IV PD symptoms serve most directly as screeners, the other types of questionnaires provide this sort of preliminary assessment as well. The pathological and normal-range personality trait measures serve an additional purpose: These questionnaires can help to flesh out personality patterns that are related to but not fully encompassed by the DSM-IV criteria. This is an important feature, because some clinically important aspects of personality pathology are not adequately covered by DSM-IV (Westen, 1997). These two types of questionnaires also have norms for scoring, which may be helpful in comparing the youth to adolescents in general. Finally, the normal-range personality questionnaires have the additional purpose of helping to highlight youths' personality strengths.

The questionnaires yield a rich picture of personality functioning, but they cannot be used to diagnose PDs for several reasons, the most obvious of which is that most of the recommended self-report questionnaires do not correspond exactly with DSM-IV Axis II criteria. Questionnaire measures agree only modestly with interview measures of personality (Zimmerman, 1994), in part because questionnaire measures typically overdiagnose personality pathology (Clark & Harrison, 2001; McDermut & Zimmerman, 2005). Finally, although questionnaires can pinpoint problematic personality patterns, they cannot determine the other important features of these patterns: their duration, onset, pervasiveness, and effects on patients' lives. Interviews are needed to investigate these other aspects of personality functioning.

Interviews

As noted earlier, the administration of questionnaires should be followed by interviews with adolescents and their parents. Two types of interviews may be used to assess personality disorders: unstructured and semistructured. In unstructured interviews, clinicians ask questions in the order that seems most appropriate, and the questions are typically not planned in advance (though it is likely that many clinicians typically follow a general order). In contrast, in a semistructured interview, clinicians ask a standard set of questions in a planned sequence. These questions are often followed up for clarification and elaboration. The responses to questions are scored in a structured manner. Clinicians are also usually required to score some aspects of the interview based on observations of the patient during the interview itself. Practicing clinicians tend to use unstructured interviews to assess PDs (Westen, 1997), whereas semistructured interviews are more often used in research. Semistructured interviews possess a number of advantages over unstructured interviews in assessing PDs (reviewed in Kaye & Shea, 2000; Rogers, 2003; Widiger et al., 2006): They result in more reliable diagnoses and ensure that the full range of personality pathology is considered and assessed carefully. Practicing clinicians may be hesitant to use semistructured interviews for a number of reasons, including the length of time involved, the potential formality and interference with rapport building, and the concern that patients

may have difficulty describing their personality patterns accurately and honestly. These concerns can potentially be addressed. Questionnaire measures help cut down the interview time by ruling out disorders that need not be assessed. An unstructured interview may be used initially to build rapport. Clinicians who are concerned about maintaining rapport or overcoming patients' reluctance to report problems may use one of the topically organized interviews. These topical interviews assess various areas of a patient's life (e.g., relationships, school) in a natural manner and may potentially help guarded patients be more forthcoming. Clinicians who are hesitant to use a semistructured interview are encouraged to read one nonetheless, because these interviews can help clinicians formulate questions to gather information on PDs.

As noted previously, parents should be interviewed about their children's personality patterns. The use of a PD screening questionnaire with parents helps to focus the parent interview on the relevant diagnoses. Particular attention should be paid to the parent report on Axis II diagnoses for which his or her adolescent may be a poor reporter. Some of the semistructured interviews have specific instructions for the use of informants, but all of these interviews may potentially be adapted for use with informants. The optimal way to combine informant and patient information to formulate adolescent PD diagnoses is unclear; the same is true for child and adolescent assessment more generally (Mash & Hunsley, 2005). Clinicians need to exercise considerable judgment in discerning which information yields the most valid picture of their adolescent patients' personality functioning.

Obtaining Other Relevant Information

A number of areas other than the adolescent's personality functioning are particularly important to assess in light of current research and theory on personality disorders in adolescence. These areas include the following:

Risky Behaviors

PDs in adolescence are associated concurrently and longitudinally with a number of risky behaviors: suicidality, violence, self-mutilation, and risky sexual behaviors. These troubling behaviors are likely to be the presenting problems for many youth with PDs, but clinicians should assess for these behaviors even if they are not part of the presenting picture.

Childhood Temperament

Given that childhood temperament is likely to be an important contributor to later personality pathology (Shiner, 2005), it is important to assess adolescents' early-emerging personalities. Parents may be asked about their child's early behaviors—positive emotions, willingness to approach new situations, shyness, anxiety, irritability, sensitivity to sensory stimulation, ability to maintain attention, self-control, kindness, and aggression (Caspi & Shiner, 2006). The clinician may also ask parents about responses the child's temperament evoked in them and in others, to ascertain whether the child's temperament and parents' own needs and emotional responses set in motion a problematic pattern of interaction. Adolescents themselves may be asked about their early personalities. They may have insight into internal experiences of which their parents may be unaware. Even if adolescents' recollections are not veridical, their self-descriptions are likely to illuminate their early self-concepts.

Current and Past Context

It is important to evaluate the adolescent's context carefully, because it is possible that contextual factors contributed to the development of a PD, and it is quite likely that such contextual factors may be maintaining the problematic patterns. The context should be evaluated broadly, but particular attention should be given to the adolescent's relationships with family and with peers. Recent research has substantiated that child maltreatment and poor family functioning predict heightened risk for PDs in adolescence and adulthood, so it is important that these factors be evaluated. Relationships with peers, both in childhood and concurrently, should also be assessed. Relationships with parents and peers are likely to be especially powerful contributors to internalized views of the self and of the self in relation to others.

Cyclical Patterns

A careful assessment of personality pathology can pinpoint adolescents' interpersonal behaviors that may be problematic; these behaviors include aggressiveness and hostility, lack of assertiveness, excessive social avoidance and anxiety, too much openness and trust, lack of interpersonal connectedness, or excessive interpersonal sensitivity (Gude, Moum, Kaldestad, & Friis, 2000). Adolescents may be engaging in interpersonal behaviors that perpetuate their psychological difficulties. A vicious cycle may emerge in which an individual's interpersonal behaviors evoke reactions from others that inadvertently reinforce his or her maladaptive personality tendencies (Wachtel, 1994). For example, a narcissistic individual's desperate attempt to impress others could evoke rejection from others who find the person to be a braggart, which in turn reinforces his or her underlying sense of inadequacy (that may have fueled the bravado in the first place).

Developing an Effective Treatment Plan

After determining that an adolescent patient meets criteria for a PD or has significant PD features, clinicians face a daunting task—the development of an effective treatment plan. This task is complex for a number of reasons. A key reason is that there are not yet empirically supported treatments for treating adolescent PDs. Another challenge in treating adolescents with PDs is that they are often "complex cases" that involve some combination of significant comorbidity, risk for self-harm or harm to others, substance abuse, low motivation or lack of compliance with treatment, or a stressful social environment (Ruscio & Holohan, 2006). Despite the complexities of developing a treatment plan for this population of youth, two promising routes may be followed. The first is to adapt empirically supported treatments developed for adults with PDs. The second is to define clearly youths' pathological personality patterns and use treatments that have been effective for similar problems. These two methods are discussed in turn.

Empirically supported treatments for adults with PDs may be modified for use with adolescents. Several reviews have addressed the empirical evidence of effective treatments for adult PDs (Crits-Christoph & Barber, 2004; Fonagy, Roth, & Higgitt, 2005; Leichsenring & Leibling, 2003; Perry, Banon, & Ianni, 1999). According to these reviews, there are empirically supported treatments for several specific PDs and for mixed PDs. For adult borderline PD, several treatment models have some support: schema-focused therapy (an integrative cognitive therapy; Giesen-Bloo et al., 2006); dialectical behavior therapy (DBT; an integration of cognitive-behavioral therapy and Zen mindfulness practices; see preceding reviews and Linehan et al., 2006); and psychodynamic treatment in a partial hospital program and outpatient setting (see reviews and Giesen-Bloo et al., 2006). Of these treatments, DBT has been adapted for use with adolescents (Miller, Rathus, & Linehan, 2006), and there is some preliminary empirical evidence that this treatment model may be effective with youth (Katz, Cox, Gunasekara, & Miller, 2004; Rathus & Miller, 2002). For avoidant PD, a number of behavioral treatments have proved effective in adults, including graded exposure and social skills training (see preceding reviews). Cluster C personality disorders have been treated effectively with both cognitive therapy and short-term psychodynamic therapy (see reviews and Svartberg, Stiles, & Seltzer, 2004). Finally, several forms of psychodynamic therapy have demonstrated effectiveness in treating adults with any PD diagnosis (see preceding reviews and Vinnars, Barber, Noren, Gallop, & Weinryb, 2005). In short, a number of psychodynamic, cognitive, behavioral, and integrative treatments may be adapted for use with adolescents.

Another option for devising a treatment plan is to define clearly the adolescent's pathological personality patterns and use empirically supported treatments that address similar problems in youth. Thus, in this case, the clinician is crafting a plan tailored to the needs of each individual adolescent patient. As Kazdin (2005) recently noted, "Knowing the symptoms and patterns that an individual has, working on and with these in treatment, and evaluating the impact of treatment is facilitated by leaving aside the term *disorder* and working on this child's characteristics" (p. 550). This means of developing a treatment plan may be particularly appropriate for PDs, given that the specific diagnoses possess questionable validity as discrete categories. Particular personality patterns, understood in the context of the youth's life, may be the best targets for treatment.

If clinicians conduct the sort of comprehensive personality assessment described in this chapter, then they will have a thorough understanding of their adolescent patients' problematic personality patterns to address in treatment. By the end of the assessment, they should have a good understanding of youths' difficulties in the four areas included in the PD diagnoses: *cognitions*, *affectivity*, *interpersonal functioning*, and *impulse control*. Treatments that have demonstrated efficacy for these patterns in other disorders may then be tailored to the needs of a particular youth (for a discussion of how to adapt empirically supported treatments to complex cases, see Ruscio & Holohan, 2006). For example, cognitive-behavioral therapy developed to treat depression in youth might be adapted to address an adolescent's tendencies to misinterpret others' ambiguous behaviors as malevolent. Behavioral and family treatments developed to treat conduct disorder might be adapted to address an adolescent's difficulties with controlling his or her impulses. Clinicians need to be very thoughtful in adapting treatments in this way; behavior patterns that appear similar in Axis I and Axis II conditions could, in fact, arise from quite different sources. In other words, it is essential to attend to the motivations underlying adolescents' behaviors to ensure that the selected treatments are appropriate.

Monitoring Treatment Outcomes

Research on the course of PDs has implications for which behaviors to measure at baseline to track treatment effectiveness over time. This research suggests that clinicians should measure three different kinds of targeted behaviors at the start of treatment to track adolescents' treatment outcomes; these targets include (1) disturbed personality patterns, (2) any acute problematic behaviors (e.g., suicidality, violence, or self-mutilation), and (3) life impairment.

In light of the research distinguishing between acute and stable behaviors in PDs, it may be useful to measure the more acute behaviors separately from the more stable personality patterns. Support for this idea also derives from "third-wave" cognitive-behavioral treatments (Hayes et al., 2004), including DBT for borderline PD. These third-wave therapies often focus on helping patients learn new skills for coping with painful emotions and difficult personality tendencies, while also helping patients develop a sense of acceptance of their experiences. Although the therapies do not always explicitly address the issue of personality change, they implicitly acknowledge that some personality tendencies may be relatively resistant to change, and they help patients to focus on changing their maladaptive responses to these personality tendencies. Thus, it may be helpful to measure separately the acute behaviors that may respond more quickly to treatment, and the personality patterns that may require longer bouts of treatment. By measuring these targets separately, it is possible for clinicians to document different aspects of treatment effectiveness over time.

In addition to measuring personality-relevant behaviors, it is useful to measure patients' levels of impairment at baseline and over time to determine whether treatment has helped adolescent patients achieve better life adaptation. For children and adolescents with PDs, measuring impairment includes documenting adaptation in terms of academic achievement, peer relationships, and relationships with parents or other caregivers, as well as law-breaking behavior. One of the most troubling outcomes of PDs in youth is impairment in these domains, so it is important to assess whether treatment has helped youth achieve better adaptation in their day-to-day lives.

To measure these three different targets for treatment, several kinds of measures are recommended. To assess treatment impact on PD symptoms, clinicians might use one of the questionnaire measures of PDs (perhaps one of the shorter screening measures). To assess treatment impact on the more acute PD symptoms and impairment, other measures are needed. A prototypical example of such a measure is the Youth Outcome Questionnaire (Y-OQ; Burlingame, Wells, Lambert, & Cox, 2004), a brief parent report questionnaire that assesses child and adolescent functioning in a number of areas relevant to PD treatment: intrapersonal distress, somatic, interpersonal relations, social problems, behavioral dysfunction, and critical items (paranoid ideation, obsessive–compulsive behaviors, hallucinations, delusions, suicidal feelings, mania, and eating disorder issues). A measure such as the Y-OQ might be used to complement a measure more clearly focused on PD symptoms for treatment monitoring, because it assesses both acute symptoms (e.g., suicidal feelings, paranoid ideation, distress) and life adaptation/impairment

(e.g., interpersonal relations, social problems). Other measures that serve a similar purpose include the Adolescent Treatment Outcomes Module (ATOM; Kramer & Robbins, 2004), the Child and Adolescent Functional Assessment Scale (CAFAS; Hodges, 2004), and the Child Health Questionnaire (CHQ; Landgraf, 2004). The use of such measures permits a more comprehensive evaluation of treatment impact on adolescents' acute problems and day-to-day adaptation.

Presenting Results to Adolescents and Their Families

In presenting feedback about the assessment to youth and their parents, it is important to convey the main points of the case formulation, including the key problematic personality patterns, their potential causes, and the motivations underlying them. Adolescents and their parents are likely to find little of value in being given a specific PD diagnosis. In fact, there might be some potential harm in labeling adolescents with a specific PD when providing feedback to families. There is a great deal of misinformation about the nature of PDs, and youth and their parents might easily misinterpret diagnostic information. However, there is much to be gained by conveying to adolescents and their parents the basic points of the case formulation, particularly if the information is presented in a way that conveys an empathetic understanding of the adolescents' experience of the world. The results should be presented in a manner than minimizes defensiveness on the part of both adolescents and their parents. Presenting the case formulation gives adolescents and their parents an opportunity to suggest corrections to the formulation and to begin planning for treatment.

ASSESSMENT MEASURES

This section reviews a wide range of measures used to assess PDs, maladaptive personality traits, and normal-range personality traits in youth. Four general categories of instruments are presented: (1) questionnaire measures of PDs, maladaptive personality, and normal-range personality; (2) comprehensive semistructured interviews for personality disorders; (3) measures for assessing single PDs and traits (borderline PD, narcissistic PD, and psychopathy); and (4) measures that are difficult to classify. Specific recommendations are offered for choosing among the omnibus questionnaires and semistructured interviews.

Many of the measures are the same as those used with adults (e.g., all of the semistructured interviews), and others have already been adapted from adult measures for use with adolescents. Readers are referred to several excellent general reviews of PD assessment in adults for more details on the adult-based measures: Clark and Harrison (2001); Kaye and Shea (2000); McDermut and Zimmerman (2005); Widiger and Coker (2002); Widiger, Costa, and Samuel (2006); Widiger and Samuel (2005). These reviews include some very useful adult assessment measures that are not discussed here but that may be modified for use with adolescents, such as the Dimensional Assessment of Personality Pathology—Basic Questionnaire (DAPP-BQ; Livesley & Jackson, in press), the Inventory of Interpersonal Problems—Personality Disorder scales (IIP-PD; Pilkonis, Kim, Proietti, & Barkham, 1996), and the Structured Interview for the Five-Factor Model of Personality (Trull & Widiger, 1997). Another measure not reviewed here, the Structural Analysis of Social Behavior (SASB; Benjamin, 1996; Benjamin, Rothweiler, & Critchfield, 2006), may be used to examine PDs in terms of patients' views of themselves, others, and their relationships with others. The SASB has received some use with adolescents.

Given the relatively limited amount of research on PDs in youth, it should not be surprising that information about the reliability and validity of many of these measures in youth is less than optimal. Ideally, wider knowledge of measures for assessing PDs in adolescents will spur more research in this area. When available, information on reliability and validity of the measures in adults is provided.

Omnibus Questionnaire Measures of Personality Disorders, Personality Pathology, and Normal-Range Personality Traits

As described previously, the recommended assessment procedure involves the administration of at least one questionnaire or screening measure prior to completing an interview. Table 17.2 presents the full names of the questionnaires reviewed in this section and outlines differences in the number of items and scales, informants (self or parent), age range, rating format, and material covered (DSM-IV PD criteria, pathological personality traits, or normal-range personality traits). The table also includes information about whether the questionnaires assess conditions other than PDs and where to obtain the measures.

Nearly all of the measures described have already demonstrated adequate reliability (at least in terms of internal consistency). However, most of the measures have received relatively little scrutiny in terms of whether they validly assess PDs in adolescents. Although there may be valuable validity information examining the correlations of these measures with other relevant questionnaires, many measures lack validity data demonstrating their ability to predict life outcomes, treatment effectiveness, or interview-based diagnoses of personality disorders. A number of the questionnaires are derived wholly or in part from adult instruments that have demonstrated validity for assessing personality pathology. Because of the scant validity data for most of these measures, it is especially important that clinicians consider the questionnaire results to be preliminary and to follow up on these measures with careful interviewing.

Clinicians and researchers must do a bit of work to obtain relevant materials for using and scoring some of these measures, because many of the measures lack computerized scoring systems. In other cases, it is necessary to use norms obtained for older populations. It is to be hoped that this extra bit of upfront work will not deter researchers and clinicians from using some of the less easily accessible questionnaires.

The *Adolescent Psychopathology Scale* (APS; Reynolds, 1998) self-report measure assesses five DSM-IV PDs with items that are fairly close in content to DSM criteria: avoidant, obsessive–compulsive, borderline, schizotypal, and paranoid. The APS also assesses 20 Axis I disorders (including conduct disorder) and 11 psychosocial problems (e.g., problems with anger, interpersonal relationships, suicide, self-concept), and it includes four response style scales. The items are written at a third-grade level, and computer scoring is available. The manual presents data on reliability and validity in a large school-based norming sample and a clinical sample. These data indicated

TABLE 17.2. Omnibus Questionnaire Measures Assessing Personality Disorder Diagnoses, Personality Pathology, and Normal-Range Personality Traits

Instrument	No. of items/ scales	Informants	Age range	Rating format	Material covered[a]	Non-PD scales[b]	Availability[c]
Adolescent Psychopathology Scale (APS; Reynolds, 1998)	346/40	Self	12 to 19	Varies	PD Dx and Path Pers	Yes	PAR
Assessment of DSM-IV Personality Disorders (ADP-IV; Schotte & Doncker, 1996)	94/12	Self or parent	Not stated	7-point scale	PD Dx	No	Author
Coolidge Personality and Neuropsychological Inventory for Children (CPNI; Coolidge, 1998)	200/50	Parent or guardian	5 to 17	4-point scale	PD Dx	Yes	Author
Dimensional Personality Symptom Item Pool (DIPSI; De Clerq et al., 2006)	256/ varies	Self or parent	Self: 11 to 17 Parent: 5 to 17	True–false	Path Pers	No	Author
Millon Adolescent Clinical Inventory (MACI; Millon et al., 1994)	160/31	Self	13 to 19	True–false	Path Pers	Yes	PA
Minnesota Multiphasic Personality Inventory—Adolescent (MMPI-A; Butcher et al., 1992)	478/43	Self	14 to 18	True–false	Path Pers	Yes	PA
NEO Personality Inventory—Revised (NEO-PI-R; Costa & McCrae, 1992) and NEO Personality Inventory–3 (NEO-PI-3; McCrae et al., 2005)	240/5 (plus facets)	Self	NEO-PI-R: 14+ NEO-PI-3: 12+	5-point scale	Normal Pers	No	PAR
Personality Diagnostic Questionnaire–4 (PDQ-4+; Hyler, 1994)	99/14	Self or parent	Not stated	True–false	PD Dx	No	NiJo Software *www.pdq4. com*
Schedule for Nonadaptive and Adaptive Personality—Youth version (SNAP-Y; Clark et al., 2003)	375/20	Self or parent	12 to 18	True–false	PD Dx and Path Pers	No	Author

[a] Normal Pers, Normal-range personality traits; Path Pers, pathological personality traits; PD Dx, personality disorder diagnoses based on DSM-IV criteria.

[b] Includes scales measuring constructs outside of personality disorders, pathological personality traits, or normal-range personality traits (e.g., Axis I disorders, impairment).

[c] PAR, Psychological Assessment Resources; PA, Pearson Assessments.

good internal consistency and test–retest reliability for most of the scales, and preliminary validation in terms of content and convergent and discriminant validity with other measures. The APS has received relatively little empirical attention outside the initial studies presented in the manual. The measure appears initially promising, however, and warrants further empirical evaluation, particularly with regard to its validity for assessing PD diagnoses.

The *Assessment of DSM-IV Personality Disorders Questionnaire* (ADP-IV; Schotte & De Doncker, 1996) is a brief screening measure for PDs, with items created to assess each of the DSM-IV criteria for the 10 PD and 2 appendix diagnoses. Test takers rate themselves on a 7-point scale for each item in terms of how typical the described trait is for them; when they rate themselves as a "4" or higher on the trait, they then complete a follow-up rating on a 3-point Distress scale to describe how distressing and impairing the trait is. In approximately three out of four cases, test takers do not rate the traits as distressing even when significantly present (Schotte et al., 2004). The measure yields both dimensional scores and categorical assessments of the PDs, and is scored with an Internet application, which also produces a narrative description of the results. The ADP-IV has demonstrated good reliability, convergent validity with other PD questionnaire measures, and preliminary validity in terms of predicting any Axis II diagnosis on the Structured Clinical Interview for DSM-IV Axis II Disorders (SCID-II) in adult samples (reviewed in Schotte et al., 2004). The ADP-IV was used successfully in two studies of adolescents (De Clercq & De Fruyt, 2003; De Clercq et al., 2004); thus, it seems promising as a somewhat more detailed screening measure for PDs in adolescents.

The *Coolidge Personality and Neuropsychological Inventory for Children* (CPNI; Coolidge, 1998) was developed as a straightforward parent report measure of DSM-IV PDs (including the appendix diagnoses). The measure includes at least one item to assess each of the PD criteria, and the number of items per diagnosis ranges from 7 to 10. The CPNI also includes scales assessing a number of Axis I disorders, neuropsychological conditions, personality change due to a medical condition, hostility scales, other clinical scales, and critical items. In preliminary research, most PD scales were found to have adequate internal consis-

tency and test–retest reliability, but validation of the scales is very limited (Coolidge, Thede, Stewart, & Segal, 2002). Although there are norms for calculating *T*-scores, cutoff scores should not be used given the lack of validation research. However, given how closely the items are tied to the DSM criteria, it may be possible to use this measure to ascertain parent perceptions of which PDs should be assessed further.

The *Dimensional Personality Symptom Item Pool* (DIPSI; De Clercq et al., 2006) is a newly developed parent and self-report inventory to assess personality pathology in children and adolescents. The DIPSI was developed to explore the dimensional structure of personality pathology in youth, as has been done with adults (e.g., with the Schedule of Nonadaptive and Adaptive Personality, described below). As described in the section on dimensional models of personality pathology, in preliminary research on community and clinical youth samples, a number of lower-order scales were created, and four higher-order traits emerged: Introversion, Disagreeableness, Compulsivity, and Emotional Instability. The DIPSI is not suitable at this point for clinical use, but it is a very promising instrument for research on the development of personality pathology in childhood and adolescence.

The *Millon Adolescent Clinical Inventory* (MACI; Millon, Millon, Davis, & Grossman, 1994) is a widely used omnibus self-report measure that yields scores relevant to the 12 DSM-IV PDs, as well as facet scales for these. The MACI is based on Millon's personality theory, which is strongly influenced by evolutionary theory (Millon & Davis, 1996). Although the theory relates to DSM PDs, it is not perfectly commensurate with the DSM system. The MACI yields several other types of scales as well: 8 for expressed concerns, 7 for clinical syndromes, and 3 modifying indices and 1 validity scale. A sixth-grade reading level is required. Computerized administration and scoring are available, as are interpretative reports and profiles. The measure has been found to be reliable, and preliminary validity data are available (Meagher, Grossman, & Millon, 2004). Further information on interpretation can be found in McCann (1999).

The MACI possesses both strengths and weaknesses. It is relatively efficient and easy for adolescents to complete and has the potential to yield a rich personality portrait that may provide useful targets for treatment. However, because the instrument is based on both Millon's theories and DSM criteria, the instrument may yield diagnostic information that is not as closely tied to DSM-IV as that obtained through other instruments. To obtain maximum benefit from the measure, users need to have a full understanding of Millon's personality theory and the specific content of each scale; it is important to not rely simply on the names of the scales for interpretation. There may be problems with Millon's personality theory (Widiger, 1999) and with the scoring system used. Scores adjust for age and gender differences, and also take into account estimated base rates for psychopathology; these unusual scoring procedures may yield unsupported gender differences in scores and are questionable in light of the lack of firm epidemiological data on the prevalence of PDs in adolescents.

The *Minnesota Multiphasic Personality Inventory—Adolescent* (MMPI-A; Butcher et al., 1992) is a widely used omnibus self-report measure that yields a wide range of clinically relevant scales. The MMPI-A is based in large part on the MMPI adult measures. The MMPI-A has 10 clinical scales, 15 content scales (which have more homogeneous content that the clinical scales), 11 supplemental scales, and 7 validity scales. None of the scales corresponds directly to DSM-IV PD diagnoses, but they do provide information on a wide range of topics highly pertinent to personality pathology. A sample of potentially informative scales includes the following: Depression, Hysteria, Psychopathic Deviate, Paranoia, Schizophrenia, Social Introversion, Obsessiveness, Alienation, Anger, Cynicism, Conduct Problems, Low Self-Esteem, Social Discomfort, and Family Problems. In addition, the MMPI-A may be scored to yield the Personality Psychopathology Five (PSY-5; McNulty, Harkness, Ben-Porath, & Williams, 1997), a set of scales that describe personality pathology along five dimensions: Aggressiveness, Psychoticism, Constraint, Negative Emotionality/Neuroticism, and Positive Emotionality/Extraversion.

For most items, a sixth-grade reading level is required, but some items may require more advanced reading skills (Archer, 2004). Computerized administration and scoring are available, as are interpretative reports. The measure has been found to be reliable, and preliminary validity data are available (Archer, 2004, 2005), although much of the interpretation of the instrument is based on validity research on the adult instruments. The biggest limitation of this instrument for assessing adolescent PDs is that, although the instrument assesses personality-relevant material, the scales do not specifically measure DSM-IV PDs, so clinicians would need to make links between the patterns observed on the MMPI-A and the diagnostic categories.

The *NEO-Personality Inventory—Revised* (NEO-PI-R; Costa & McCrae, 1992) is a widely used omnibus adult self-report measure of personality that assesses the Big Five higher-order traits (Neuroticism, Extraversion, Openness to Experience, Agreeableness, and Conscientiousness), as well as 30 facets (six per Big Five trait). The NEO-PI-R is reliable (Costa & McCrae, 1992), and the Big Five model and this instrument have accumulated a vast literature demonstrating their predictive validity for individuals' adaptation and day-to-day behavior (Caspi et al., 2005). The NEO-PI-R may be computer scored, and interpretive reports are available. It has been used in a number of studies with adolescents as young as age 14 and with bright youth ages 12 and 13 (reviewed in Caspi & Shiner, 2006). The NEO-PI-R may be scored for use with adolescents by using the college-age norms. A new version of the NEO has been developed, the *NEO-Personality Inventory–3* (NEO-PI-3). This new measure is a more readable version of the NEO-PI-R and has replaced some of the more difficult items with simplified versions (McCrae, Costa, & Martin, 2005). Preliminary research with the NEO-PI-3 in a large sample of adolescents demonstrated that the measure is reliable in this sample for the Big Five traits and most of the facets (McCrae, Martin, & Costa, 2005); the measure also demonstrated a valid factor structure, and convergent and discriminant validity. A new study has found that the NEO-PI-3 may also be used with middle school–age students (Costa, McCrae, & Martin, in press). The NEO-PI-3 items can be obtained from Psychological Assessment Resources, and the new instrument may be scored for use with adolescents by using either the norms in McCrae, Martin and colleagues (2005) or NEO-PI-R college student norms.

As described in the section on dimensional models of personality pathology, the NEO-PI-R has been found to predict DSM-IV PDs (Costa & Widiger, 2002). The five higher-order traits measured in the NEO-PI-R map onto the higher-order pathological personality traits in dimensional research on PDs. The facets of the NEO instruments provide particularly good coverage of variation in most PDs (Bagby, Costa, Widiger, Ryder, & Marshall, 2005; De Clercq & De Fruyt, 2003; De Fruyt, De Clercq, van de Wiele, & Van Heeringen, 2006; Miller, Reynolds, & Pilkonis, 2004), although there may be aspects of PDs not fully captured by the Big Five model (Skodol, Oldham, et al., 2005). The NEO-PI-R higher-order traits and facets provide a rich picture of a patient's personality functioning, including areas of difficulty and strength. An excellent example of the use of the NEO-PI-R (as well as other normal-range personality measures) in a clinical setting may be found in Singer (2005). The NEO-PI-R can also be scored using a prototype-matching procedure (Miller, Pilkonis, & Morse, 2004) or a simple summing procedure (Miller, Bagby, Pilkonis, Reynolds, & Lynam, 2005) to yield scores for DSM-IV personality diagnoses.

The *Personality Diagnostic Questionnaire–4+* (PDQ-4+; Hyler, 1994) is a version of two earlier measures (the PDQ and PDQ-R), which has been updated for DSM-IV. This brief screening measure assesses self-reports on each of the diagnostic criteria for DSM-IV PDs and those in the appendix. Scores for each PD are for the most part obtained by simply summing the number of criteria endorsed. The PDQ-4+ also includes two validity scales and an optional Clinical Significance scale, which is scored by having the administering clinician check on the duration, nonoverlap with Axis I conditions, and impairment and distress for each of the criteria endorsed. There is no manual for the instrument; however, a computer-assisted version is available. A substantial literature on earlier versions of this instrument suggests that it can be useful as a brief screening measure for PDs in adults; it tends to over-diagnose PDs, but it does not generally appear to miss "true" cases (Bagby & Farvolden, 2004). There is not yet enough research on the new version of the instrument to be able to establish cutoff scores for use as a screening measure (Bagby & Farvolden, 2004). The PDQ-4+ and its earlier versions have been used in a small number of studies with adolescents (e.g., Daley et al., 1999; Vito, Ladame, & Orlandini, 1999). In light of current evidence, the PDQ-4+ may potentially be used with adolescents as a brief screening measure for a later diagnostic interview.

The *Schedule of Nonadaptive and Adaptive Personality—Youth version* (SNAP-Y; Clark, Linde, & Simms, 2003) is an omnibus self-report measure of personality pathology adapted for youth from the Schedule of Nonadaptive and Adaptive Personality (SNAP; Clark, 1993) for adults. The SNAP was developed to assess criteria from DSM PD diagnoses, important aspects of other models of PDs, and some Axis I disorders that overlap potentially with PDs. Through empirical and rational means, the SNAP items were sorted to yield 12 scales that describe pathological personality traits (Mistrust, Manipulativeness, Aggression, Self-Harm, Eccentric Perceptions, Dependency, Exhibitionism, Entitlement, Detachment, Impulsivity, Propriety, and Workaholism) and three overarching temperament traits (Negative Temperament, Positive Temperament, and Disinhibition). The SNAP also includes five validity scales and can be scored to yield DSM-IV PD diagnostic information. The SNAP has strong psychometric characteristics and increasing support in terms of its validity as a measure of personality pathology (e.g., Melley, Oltmanns, & Turkheimer, 2002; Morey et al., 2003). In preliminary research with adolescents ages 12–18, the SNAP-Y has demonstrated evidence of good reliability, as well as structural validity and convergent–discriminant validity with the MMPI-A (Linde, 2002). The SNAP-Y may be scored using either the SNAP college student norms or the descriptive statistics presented in Linde (2002). Although the SNAP-Y requires further validation with adolescent samples, it appears to be a useful measure for obtaining both a more fine-grained look at adolescents' problematic and healthy personality patterns, and screening information for DSM-IV PDs.

Recommendations for Selecting Questionnaires

Assessors have a number of options in terms of youth self-report questionnaires to obtain information about problems in personality functioning. However, it is crucial to emphasize that all of these measures have received very little (if any) validation in terms of predicting interview-based PDs in adolescents; thus, all questionnaire-based findings are highly preliminary.

The selection of measures depends in part on other disorders that are being assessed and the measures that are being administered to assess those other conditions. In most clinical contexts, it is unlikely that clinicians would be assessing only PDs given the high rates of comorbidity between Axis I and Axis II conditions. If clinicians are looking for measures that assess other conditions, as well as PD features, options include the APS and the MACI (recognizing, however, that the APS does not assess all PDs and the MACI scales do not correspond exactly to DSM disorders). Clinicians with extensive experience with the MMPI-A may use this instrument to generate hypotheses about relevant personality patterns, but this measure does not assess DSM PDs directly. In contrast, when more time can be devoted specifically to PD assessment, a number of self-report measures assess DSM PDs: the SNAP-Y, the ADP-IV, the PDQ-4+, and the Structured Clinical Interview for DSM-IV Axis II Personality Disorders—Screening Questionnaire (SCID-II-Q; First, Spitzer, Williams, & Gibbon, 1997; described in the next section under the SCID-II). The SNAP-Y has the advantage of providing a rich description of personality pathology more generally rather than DSM diagnoses only. Finally, when clinicians want a more complete picture of youths' personality difficulties and strengths, the NEO-PI-R and NEO-PI-3 are recommended; new scoring procedures may be used with these instruments to generate hypotheses about DSM PD diagnoses as well.

To obtain parent report on youths' personality disorder symptoms, the SNAP-Y, ADP-IV, PDQ-4+, and SCID-II-Q are recommended; these questionnaires may be used to pinpoint which PDs should be evaluated more carefully with diagnostic interviews.

Comprehensive Semistructured Interviews for Personality Disorders

For accurate diagnosis of personality disorders, semistructured interviews are the measure of choice in research. Such measures allow assessors to determine the duration, clinical significance, and pervasiveness of particular personality patterns. As noted previously, although semistructured interviews often are not used in clinical practice, they possess many strengths that make them preferable to unstructured interviews. A thorough review of all of the semistructured interviews is provided by Rogers (2001), and readers are referred to Rogers's

(2003) practical suggestions for choosing among the PD interviews for research and clinical practice.

Five semistructured interviews allow for diagnosis of the full set of PD diagnoses found in DSM-IV. All of these interviews may be used to assess PDs in youth; however, assessors need to determine whether aspects of the interviews need to be modified for use with a younger population. For example, it is essential to ensure that the questions apply to the life context of adolescents (e.g., questions about school, friendships, romantic relationships). It is also important to ensure that the language is comprehensible to adolescents. Furthermore, assessors need to determine the expected duration of the behaviors or patterns in question. DSM-IV stipulates that the personality patterns need to have persisted for at least 1 year, but the semistructured interviews vary in terms of the required time frame for the patterns (e.g., 2 years preceding the interview, or since early adulthood). Thus, the expected duration of symptoms for adolescents may differ from that expected for adults.

The five semistructured interviews vary along a number of dimensions that need to be considered when selecting an instrument (Clark & Harrison, 2001; Rogers, 2001). First, the interviews vary according to whether they are organized by diagnosis, with all of the questions for each diagnosis clustered together, or by topic (e.g., interests and activities, work, interpersonal relationships), or whether there are two versions—one by diagnosis and the other by topic. Each organization method has potential strengths and weaknesses (reviewed in Clark & Harrison, 2001; Rogers, 2001). Second, the semistructured interviews vary according to whether they have screeners that help determine which questions and diagnoses to pursue in greater detail with the longer interview. Third, as noted, the interviews vary in the time frame during which the symptoms are expected to have persisted. Fourth, the interviews vary in number of questions and length. Fifth, some of the interviews have been used in research with adolescents, whereas others have received little or no published use in research with this population.

The *Diagnostic Interview for DSM-IV Personality Disorders* (DIPD-IV; Zanarini, Frankenburg, Sickel, & Yong, 1996) is an interview organized by diagnoses and takes approximately 90 minutes to administer. Symptoms are assessed for their presence over the 2 years preceding the assessment. The measure had received little research attention until recently; thus, there is less empirical research on this interview than on some others. However, the DIPD-IV has been used in the Collaborative Longitudinal Personality Disorders Study of (CLPS; Skodol, Gunderson, et al., 2005), a longitudinal, multisite adult study. In this study, most disorders were found to have fair to good test–retest reliability and median interrater reliability; however, test–retest reliabilities for the dimensional disorder measures were considerably higher (generally > .75) (Zanarini et al., 2000). The CLPS has provided a rich set of validity data for the four primary diagnoses assessed: schizotypal PD, borderline PD, avoidant PD, and obsessive–compulsive PD (Skodol, Gunderson, et al., 2005). I found no published clinical studies in which this interview was used with adolescents; however, the measure has been used in PD research with adolescents (M. Zanarini, personal communication, July 5, 2006). The measure may be obtained by contacting the author.

The *International Personality Disorder Examination* (IPDE; Loranger, 1995, 1999) is an interview organized by topics. It is unique in that it has two separate modules, one designed to assess DSM-IV PDs and the other designed to assess the International Classification of Diseases (ICD-10) PDs. The DSM-IV module is highly similar to an earlier, thoroughly researched version designed to assess DSM-III-R PDs. Both modules take up to 3 hours to administer, which is far too long for routine clinical use. However, the DSM-IV module takes only 60–90 minutes, and this module alone should be adequate for most clinical and research purposes. The personality patterns are assessed by determining the age of onset, and at least one trait from each disorder must have been present before the age of 25. Informant reports are optional but recommended. There is a screening measure, but Rogers (2001) raised some possible concerns about its use. Rogers noted the strengths and weaknesses of this interview. As for strengths, the instrument has demonstrated good reliability and validity (with the possible exception of poor validity for cluster A diagnoses). The instrument was also designed with international research in mind and may be especially suitable for cross-cultural settings. As for weaknesses, the instrument may not be as valid with patients with more severe Axis I diagnoses (psychotic disorders, severe depression).

The earlier version of the IPDE, the Personality Disorder Examination (PDE; Loranger, Susman, Oldham, & Russakoff, 1988), has been used in a number of studies with adolescents (see citations in Levy et al., 1999), thus providing some evidence for the validity of the measure with youth. The IPDE and PDE specify that the traits need to have been present for at least 3 years in adolescents to qualify for diagnosis; thus, the standards for duration are higher than those in DSM-IV. In at least one sample of adolescents (Becker et al., 1999), the measure demonstrated good interrater reliability, but this study also found evidence for lower internal consistency for the diagnoses and less discriminant validity than is often found in adult assessment. It is possible that these problems were due to the application of adult criteria from DSM-IV to adolescents, not problems with the interview per se. Nonetheless, this interview also has shown some promise for use with adolescents. The measure may be obtained by contacting Psychological Assessment Resources or the World Health Organization.

The *Personality Disorders Interview–IV* (PDI-IV; Widiger, Mangine, Corbitt, Ellis, & Thomas, 1995) can be administered either by diagnosis or by topic. The interview takes 90–120 minutes to administer and requires the trait to have been present at least since age 18 and for much of adulthood. However, the interview may be used with adolescents if modified to fit with the stipulations of DSM-IV. Rogers (2001) noted that some preliminary data demonstrate adequate interrater reliability, but validity data are limited, because of little empirical use of the instrument. Rogers described the instrument's strengths as its extensive and thoughtful manual, and its questions that "closely reflect that diagnostic criteria" (p. 250). Rogers noted that the instrument includes some questions that are relatively complicated and sophisticated in language; this could potentially be a problem for use with adolescents, so some questions may need to be modified. Because the PDI-IV manual provides such helpful information about PDs, the manual may be read in conjunction with other semistructured interviews that lack a detailed manual.

The *Structured Clinical Interview for DSM-IV Axis II Personality Disorders* (SCID-II; First et al., 1997) is an interview organized by diagnosis. The questions follow the order of the symptoms and diagnoses in DSM-IV. It is the shortest of all the semistructured interviews and can be completed in 30–45 minutes. Traits are assessed to determine whether they have been present for the last 5 years (clearly this time frame would need to be modified with adolescents). A self-administered screener, called the SCID-II-Q, may be used to determine which diagnoses to assess more thoroughly and cut down on administration time for the SCID-II (Piedmont, Sherman, Sherman, & Williams, 2003). There is also a computer-administered version of the SCID-II that still requires the active involvement of the interviewing clinician. The SCID-II has demonstrated good reliability and validity in adult samples (First & Gibbon, 2004; Rogers, 2001). The SCID-II has the advantages of being relatively short, straightforward, and easy to administer; drawbacks are that it may miss some important traits and be less suitable for patients who are uncomfortable acknowledging personality difficulties (Rogers, 2001, 2003).

The SCID-II requires an eighth-grade reading level and may be adapted for use with adolescents. In fact, the SCID-II and its previous DSM-III-R version appear to be the semistructured interviews that have received the most widespread use in studies of personality disorders in adolescents (Asarnow et al., 2001; Brent, Johnson, Perper, & Connolly, 1994; Chanen et al., 2004; Daley et al., 1999; Lavan & Johnson, 2002; Mittal et al., 2006; Neumann & Walker, 2003). The SCID interviews have been used in research on the full spectrum of personality disorders in adolescents. In one study of adolescents that used the SCID-II, PD features had to have persisted for at least 2 years to meet threshold criteria (Chanen et al., 2004). The adolescent PD studies have begun to establish the SCID-II's adequate reliability in adolescents. The SCID can be obtained from the American Psychiatric Press or at *www.scid4.org*.

The *Structured Interview for DSM-IV Personality* (SIDP-IV; Pfohl, Blum, & Zimmerman, 1997) is the most recent version of the earliest omnibus semistructured interview for Axis II disorders. The SIDP-IV has both diagnostic and topical versions of the interview (the diagnostic format is available only for the DSM-IV version of the SIDP). The interview takes 60–90 minutes to administer, although the interview may be shortened by omission of DSM appendix diagnoses. The informant interview, which contains some questions not found in the patient interview, may potentially be quite useful in assessing adolescents. As with the SCID-II, traits are assessed to determine whether they have been present for the last 5 years, which necessitates modification of the SIDP-IV for use with adolescents. A brief interview screener is available. The SIDP-IV and its predecessors have demonstrated good interrater reliability and validity (Rogers, 2001). Rogers (2001, 2003) has commented on a number of strengths of this interview. The topically organized version includes natural questions that make the interview flow well and that may be especially useful with defensive or guarded patients. The interview may be used with patients with a wide range of Axis I pathology (including psychotic and mood disorders). In addition, relative to other semistructured interviews, the SIDP-IV appears to yield fewer cases of comorbid PDs. The SIDP-IV interviews appear to have been used rarely with adolescents in published studies (Brent et al. [1990] and Mittal et al. [2006] are exceptions), but given the strengths of the instrument, wider use may be warranted.

Recommendations for Selecting a Semistructured Interview

All five semistructured interviews are potentially good means of assessing PDs in adolescents. Three of the interviews or their earlier versions have been used in published research with adolescents: the IPDE, the SCID-II, and the SIDP-IV; thus, these three interviews have already proved useful with this population. Deciding among these three interviews depends on several considerations. If a topical format is preferred (because of a defensive or guarded interviewee, or a need for a more conversational interview structure), then the IPDE and SIDP-IV can be used. If a diagnostic format is preferred (because of a desire to keep the interview short by omitting unlikely diagnoses based on questionnaire information), then the SCID-II or SIDP-IV can be used. Other considerations may include the need for a cross-culturally sensitive interview (the IPDE), a relatively shorter interview (the SCID-II), an interview that may be used with patients with significant Axis I disorders (the SIDP-IV), or an interview with an informant version (the SIDP-IV).

Measures of Single Personality Disorders and Traits

In addition to the omnibus questionnaire instruments and semistructured interviews described previously, a number of instruments have been used to assess single personality disorders or traits in isolation, including borderline PD (or borderline features), narcissistic PD (or narcissism), and psychopathy. The single-trait measures of borderline and narcissistic PD are not recommended generally for clinical use because of the frequent comorbidity of personality disorders. At the very least, if these measures are used in clinical practice, then it is important to screen for possible comorbid personality pathology. However, the measures may be useful in some research contexts or in selected clinical contexts; again, though, even in research, it would be useful in many cases to include an additional omnibus measure of personality pathology.

Borderline Personality Disorder Measures

There are at least three semistructured interviews and two questionnaires for assessing borderline PD or pathology in youth. The *Diagnostic Interview for Borderlines* (DIB; Gunderson, Kolb, & Austin, 1981), a 132-item, semistructured interview, yields scores for five domains of functioning: Social Adaptation, Affect, Cognition, Impulsivity, and Interpersonal Relationships. The interview was later revised, resulting in the *Diagnostic Interview for Borderlines—Revised* (DIB-R; Zanarini, Gunderson, Frankenburg, & Chauncey, 1989), which dropped the Social Adaptation section. Both the DIB and the DIB-R have been used in research with adolescents (e.g., Ludolph, Westen, Misle, & Jackson, 1990; Pinto, Grapentine, Francis, & Picariello, 1996). The interviews are based on Gunderson's conception of borderline PD, which is related to the DSM diagnostic view but does not entirely overlap (Kaye & Shea, 2000). Another variation of the DIB is the *Child Version of the Retrospective Diagnostic Interview for Borderlines* (C-DIB; Greenman, Gunderson, Cane, & Saltzman, 1986), a structured process for chart review. The C-DIB was developed to assess a condition described as "borderline pathology of childhood," which was observed in highly impaired children who exhibited the impulsivity, mood lability, and cognitive symptoms seen in adults with borderline PD. The C-DIB has been used effectively in a longitudinal study of such pathology (Guzder, Paris, Zelkowitz, & Feldman, 1999; Paris, 2005b). The *Borderline Personality Inventory* (BPI; Leichsenring, 1999), a 53-item self-report instrument developed to assess Kernberg's concept of borderline PD, appears to have good reliability and convergent validity with other borderline PD questionnaire measures. The BPI has received some preliminary research use with adolescents (Chabrol et al., 2004). Finally, the *Borderline Personality Features Scale for Children* (BPFS-C; Crick, Murray-Close, & Woods, 2005), a newly developed self-report measure for children age 9 and older, is based on the BOR (Borderline) scale of the *Personality Assessment Inventory* (PAI; Morey, 1991) for adults and was created by modifying the BOR scale to make it developmentally appropriate for children. It taps affective instability, identity problems, negative relationships, and self-harm. Based on an initial longitudinal study, the measure appears to be reliable, moderately stable over 1 year, and valid in terms of predicting other measures of borderline pathology.

Narcissistic Personality Disorder Measures

At least one semistructured interview and two modified versions of a questionnaire assess narcissistic PD or narcissism in youth. The *Diagnostic Interview for Narcissism* (DIN; Gunderson, Ronningstam, & Bodkin, 1990), a semistructured interview, includes 33 statements and results in five scores: Grandiosity, Interpersonal Relations, Reactiveness, Affects and Mood States, and Social and Moral Judgments. The DIN was developed based on Gunderson's conception of narcissism and appears to measure a broader construct than the DSM disorder. The DIN was modified for a retrospective chart review study of adolescent inpatients (Kernberg, Hajal, & Normandin, 1998). A parent version has also been developed to assess younger children ages 8–13—the *Parent Diagnostic Interview for Narcissism* (P-DIN; Guilé et al., 2004). The primary questionnaire measure of narcissism in adults, the Narcissistic Personality Inventory (NPI; Raskin & Terry, 1988), is a 40-item questionnaire. The NPI has been modified in two different versions for youth: the *Narcissistic Personality Inventory—Children* (NPIC; Barry, Frick, & Killian, 2003) and the *Narcissistic Personality*

Inventory—Junior Offender (NPI-JO; Calhoun, Glaser, & Stefurak, 2000). Hilsenroth, Handler, and Blais (1996) reviewed other adult measures of narcissism that potentially could be adapted for use with youth.

Psychopathy Measures

Psychopathy is a construct that has received a great deal of research attention over the last decade as researchers have begun to explore the nature and manifestations of this trait in youth. Psychopathy includes a number of behavioral and personality tendencies: risk-taking and impulsivity, grandiosity, manipulativeness, lack of empathy and remorse, and shallow relationships (Lynam & Gudonis, 2005). Aspects of psychopathy are included in DSM-IV diagnostic criteria for antisocial PD. However, antisocial PD cannot be diagnosed in youth under age 18, and the developmental precursor diagnosis is conduct disorder. The DSM-IV diagnosis of conduct disorder does not adequately capture aspects of psychopathy. Thus, there is no real place in DSM-IV for classifying psychopathic tendencies in youth. Yet recent research has revealed that psychopathy can be measured reliably in youth, that it is stable during the adolescent years, and that it predicts a number of important associated features and outcomes, including more severe and stable conduct problems (Kotler & McMahon, 2005; Lynam & Gudonis, 2005; Salekin & Frick, 2005). Childhood psychopathy appears to be at least partially heritable, and these inherited characteristics are likely to result in impaired socialization across development (Blair, Peschardt, Budhani, Mitchell, & Pine, 2006).

Three recent articles provide a thorough and careful review of the measures developed thus far to assess psychopathy in youth (Kotler & McMahon, 2005; Lynam & Gudonis, 2005; Vaughn & Howard, 2005). Consequently, the measures are described only briefly here; readers are referred to those reviews for more details. Presently at least four measures have been used to assess psychopathy in youth; three of these are questionnaires, and one is an interview/chart review checklist. All four measures are based in part on the most prominent adult measure of psychopathy, *Hare's Psychopathy Checklist—Revised* (PCL-R; Hare, 1991, 2003). To use the PCL-R, the clinician conducts a semistructured interview and chart review, then rates the individual on 20 items.

In the modified youth versions, inappropriate PCL-R items have been dropped (e.g., items about unstable marriages), and new, developmentally appropriate items have been added (e.g., teases others, keeps same friends). All four measures have shown good reliability at the total scale level and preliminary evidence of validity (Kotler & McMahon, 2005; Lynam & Gudonis, 2005).

The *Antisocial Process Screening Device* (ASPD; Frick & Hare, 2001) is a 20-item rating scale with self-report, parent, and teacher versions; it can be used with youth ages 6–18. It is modeled closely after the PCL-R and is the measure that has received the greatest research use thus far. The *Child Psychopathy Scale* (CPS; Lynam, 1997; revised version is in Lynam et al., 2005) is likewise based on the PCL-R but consists of 13 miniscales, each comprising two to seven items drawn from the Child Behavior Checklist (CBCL; Achenbach, 1981) and the California Child Q-set (CCQ; Block & Block, 1980). The CPS has parent, teacher, and youth versions. The *Youth Psychopathic Traits Inventory* (YPI; Andershed, Gustafson, Kerr, & Stattin, 2002), a 50-item self-report inventory for adolescents, is designed to minimize reluctance to acknowledge psychopathic traits and focuses on the affective and interpersonal features of psychopathy. The final measure is *Hare's Psychopathy Checklist—Youth Version* (PCL-YV; Forth, Hart, & Hare, 1990; Forth, Kosson, & Hare, 2003), which, like the PCL-R, comprises a 20-item rating scale completed on the basis of a thorough semistructured interview and chart review. The PCL-YV is essentially a version of the PCL-R adapted for youth. Although the questionnaire measures serve as rapid screening devices, the PCL-YV is a more time-consuming diagnostic instrument. Although all four of these psychopathy measures require further validation (including clarification about their factor structures), all show considerable potential for the measurement of this important pathological trait.

Two Personality Disorder Measures That Are Difficult to Classify

The *Children in the Community* (CIC) measures (Cohen & Crawford, 2005; Cohen et al., 2005) were developed for use in what is currently the only longitudinal epidemiological sample study of PDs. At each time point of the study, the CIC PD measure items were selected and modified from existing PD measures, and new items were added to provide developmentally appropriate coverage of the current DSM system. The CIC measures thus took different forms at different assessment points (e.g., parent and child interviews, self-report questionnaire). Although these measures are not suitable for clinical use, they could potentially be adapted for use in research studies. The authors can be contacted for more information on these measures.

The *Shedler–Westen Assessment Procedure–200 for Adolescents* (SWAP-200-A) is an assessment procedure that helps to structure clinicians' perceptions of adolescents' personality functioning. The SWAP-200-A and its adult counterpart, the *Shedler–Westen Assessment Procedure–200* (SWAP-200; Westen & Shedler, 1999), were designed in part as alternatives to the semistructured interviews and questionnaires that are typical in PD research. Westen and Shedler have argued that semistructured interviews and questionnaires are problematic for PD assessment because of their reliance on direct questioning of the patient about personality patterns. In contrast, in typical practice, clinicians look to patients' narratives about their daily lives and relationships, and to the patients' observed behavior in interaction with the clinician (Westen, 1997), presumably because clinicians implicitly view these methods as more valid.

To use the SWAP-200 or the SWAP-200-A, clinicians must first conduct a thorough systematic clinical interview with an adolescent patient and his or her parents (e.g., see the Clinical Diagnostic Interview; Westen, 2004) or obtain a thorough understanding of an adolescent through repeated clinical contact over time. The SWAP systems may then be used by the clinician to quantify clinical judgments about the patient. The SWAP-200 and SWAP-200-A both comprise 200 statements describing a fairly comprehensive set of behaviors and personality tendencies related to personality pathology, as well as statements about defense mechanisms, coping, relevant Axis I characteristics, and healthy psychological functioning (Westen & Shedler, 1999; Westen et al., 2003). Clinicians use a Q-sort procedure to quantify the appropriateness of the SWAP statements for the patient. In the Q-sort, the informant sorts a set of cards (with one SWAP statement on each) into a forced distribution based on how well each item describes the adolescent. Thus far, the SWAP-200-A has been used to explore the structure of personality pathology in adolescents (Westen et al., 2003; Westen, Dutra, & Shedler, 2005). In addition, it is possible to calculate dimensional scores for DSM-IV PD diagnoses by comparing patients' scores on the SWAP-200-A with prototype descriptions for the PD diagnoses (Westen et al., 2003). The SWAP-200-A and SWAP-200 have already proved that they can yield useful information in research on personality pathology in adolescents and adults, and the statements included in the measure seem to capture aspects of patient functioning that may be helpful for clinicians as they conceptualize cases, plan treatment, and measure treatment outcomes. Future research will help clarify the role that the SWAP systems may play in clinical practice. The SWAP-200-A is available at *www.psychsystems.net/lab*.

CONCLUSIONS AND RECOMMENDATIONS FOR FUTURE RESEARCH

This chapter has reviewed evidence demonstrating that it is possible for youth to have PDs, and that it is both important and possible to assess such patterns. Given the relative newness of research in this area, much work remains to better refine assessment procedures for adolescents with PDs. Several directions for future research are suggested. First, many of the available assessment measures for adolescents are the same instruments created for adults, adapted in various ways for use with adolescents. But, it is possible that more thorough modifications are necessary to make some of the measures (e.g., the semistructured interviews) developmentally appropriate. Some of the adult measures (e.g., the screening measures) need to be studied for use in adolescents to clarify whether they function similarly with adolescents and adults. Second, much more work is needed to determine whether the existing instruments are psychometrically sound. Although there is evidence for the reliability of many of the measures and some preliminary evidence of construct validity, many aspects of validity are unexamined. Other important aspects of validity to establish include predictive validity, discriminant validity, diagnostic utility, and treatment utility (Mash & Hunsley, 2005). Third, although it is clear that assessment information must be gathered from more than source, the relative usefulness of information from various informants is unknown. Fourth, the lack of empirically supported treatments for adolescents with PDs is a glaring and serious problem that needs to be addressed. I hope that the recent surge of interest in understanding adolescents with PDs will continue and that it will ultimately point to effective treatments for such youth.

ACKNOWLEDGMENT

Work on this chapter was supported by grants from the Colgate Research Council.

REFERENCES

Achenbach, T. M. (1981). *Manual for the Child Behavior Checklist/4–18 and 1991 profile.* Burlington: University of Vermont Department of Psychiatry.

American Psychiatric Association (APA). (1994). *Diagnostic and statistical manual of mental disorders* (4th ed.). Washington, DC: Author.

American Psychiatric Association (APA). (2000). *Diagnostic and statistical manual of mental disorders* (4th ed., text rev.). Washington, DC: Author.

Andershed, H. A., Kerr, M., & Stattin, H. (2002). The usefulness of self-reported psychopathy-like traits in the study of antisocial behaviour among non-referred adolescents. *European Journal of Personality, 16,* 383–402.

Archer, R. P. (2004). Overview and update on the Minnesota Multiphasic Personality Inventory—Adolescent (MMPI-A). In M. E. Maruish (Ed.), *The use of psychological testing for treatment planning and outcomes assessment: Vol. 2. Instruments for children and adolescents* (3rd ed., pp. 81–122). Mahwah, NJ: Erlbaum.

Archer, R. P. (2005). *MMPI-A: Assessing adolescent psychopathology* . Mahwah, NJ: Erlbaum.

Asarnow, R. F., Nuechterlein, K. H., Fogelson, D., Subotnik, K. L., Payne, D. A., Russell, A. T., et al. (2001). Schizophrenia and schizophrenia-spectrum personality disorders in the first-degree relatives of children with schizophrenia: The UCLA family study. *Archives of General Psychiatry, 58,* 581–588.

Bagby, R. M., Costa, P. T., Widiger, T. A., Ryder, A. G., & Marshall, M. (2005). DSM-IV personality disorders and the five-factor model of personality: A multi-method examination of domain and facet-level predictions. *European Journal of Personality, 19,* 307–324.

Bagby, R. M., & Farvolden, P. (2004). The Personality Diagnostic Questionnaire–4 (PDQ-4). In M. J. Hilsenroth & D. L. Segal (Eds.), *Comprehensive handbook of psychological assessment: Vol. 2. Personality assessment* (pp. 122–133). New York: Wiley.

Barry, C. T., Frick, P. J., & Killian, A. L. (2003). The relation of narcissism and self-esteem to conduct problems in children: A preliminary investigation. *Journal of Clinical Child and Adolescent Psychology, 32,* 139–152.

Becker, D. F., Grilo, C. M., Morey, L. C., Walker, M. L., Edell, W. S., & McGlashan, T. H. (1999). Applicability of personality disorder criteria to hospitalized adolescents: Evaluation of internal consistency and criterion overlap. *Journal of the American Academy of Child and Adolescent Psychiatry, 38,* 200–205.

Benjamin, L. S. (1996). *Interpersonal diagnosis and treatment of personality disorders* (2nd ed.). New York: Guilford Press.

Benjamin, L. S., Rothweiler, J. C., & Critchfield, K. L. (2006). The use of structural analysis of social behavior (SASB) as an assessment tool. *Annual Review of Clinical Psychology, 2,* 83–109.

Bernstein, D. P., Cohen, P., Skodol, A., Bezirganian, S., & Brook, J. S. (1996). Childhood antecedents of adolescent personality disorders. *American Journal of Psychiatry, 153,* 907–913.

Bernstein, D. P., Cohen, P., Velez, C. N., Schwab-Stone, M., Siever, L. J., & Shinsato, L. (1993). Prevalence and stability of the DSM-III-R personality disorders in a community-based survey of adolescents. *American Journal of Psychiatry, 150,* 1237–1243.

Blair, R. J. R., Peschardt, K. S., Budhani, S., Mitchell, D. G. V., & Pine, D. S. (2006). The development of psychopathy. *Journal of Child Psychology and Psychiatry, 47,* 262–275.

Bleiberg, E. (2001). *Treating personality disorders in children and adolescents: A relational approach.* New York: Guilford Press.

Block, J., & Block, J. H. (1980). *The California Child Q-Set.* Palo Alto, CA: Consulting Psychologists Press.

Brent, D. A., Johnson, B. A., Perper, J., & Connolly, J. (1994). Personality disorder, personality traits, impulsive violence, and completed suicide in adolescents. *Journal of the American Academy of Child and Adolescent Psychiatry, 33,* 1080–1086.

Brent, D. A., Zelenak, J. P., Bukstein, O., & Brown, R. V. (1990). Reliability and validity of the structured interview for personality disorders in adolescents. *Journal of the American Academy of Child and Adolescent Psychiatry, 29,* 349–354.

Burlingame, G. M., Wells, M. G., Lambert, M. J., & Cox, J. C. (2004). Youth Outcome Questionnaire (Y-OQ). In M. E. Maruish (Ed.), *The use of psychological testing for treatment planning and outcomes assessment: Vol. 2. Instruments for children and adolescents* (3rd ed., pp. 235–273). Mahwah, NJ: Erlbaum.

Butcher, J. N., Williams, C. L., Graham, J. R., Archer, R. P., Tellegen, A., & Ben-Porath, Y. W. (1992). *MMPI-A (Minnesota Multiphasic Personality Inventory—Adolescent): Manual for administration, scoring, and interpretation.* Minneapolis: University of Minnesota Press.

Calhoun, G. B., Glaser, B. A., & Stefurak, T. (2000). Preliminary validation of the Narcissistic Personality Inventory—Juvenile Offender. *International Journal of Offender Therapy and Comparative Criminology, 44*, 564–580.

Caspi, A., McClay, J., Moffitt, T., Mill, J., Martin, J., Craig, I. W., et al. (2002). Role of genotype in the cycle of violence in maltreated children. *Science, 297*, 851–854.

Caspi, A., Roberts, B. W., & Shiner, R. L. (2005). Personality development: Stability and change. *Annual Review of Psychology, 56*, 453–484.

Caspi, A., & Shiner, R. L. (2006). Personality development. In W. Damon & R. Lerner (Series Eds.) & N. Eisenberg (Vol. Ed.), *Handbook of child psychology: Vol. 3. Social, emotional, and personality development* (6th ed., pp. 300–365). New York: Wiley.

Chabrol, H., Montovany, A., Ducongé, E., Kallmeyer, A., Mullet, E., & Leichsenring, F. (2004). Factor structure of the borderline personality inventory in adolescents. *European Journal of Psychological Assessment, 20*, 59–65.

Chanen, A. M., Jackson, H. J., McGorry, P. D., Allot, K. A., Clarkson, V., & Yuen, H. P. (2004). Two-year stability of personality disorder in older adolescent outpatients. *Journal of Personality Disorders, 18*, 526–541.

Clark, L. A. (1993). *Manual for the Schedule for Nonadaptive and Adaptive Personality*. Minneapolis: University of Minnesota Press.

Clark, L. A. (2005). Temperament as a unifying basis for personality and psychopathology. *Journal of Abnormal Psychology, 114*, 505–521.

Clark, L. A., & Harrison, J. A. (2001). Assessment instruments. In W. J. Livesley (Ed.), *Handbook of personality disorders: Theory, research, and treatment* (pp. 277–306). New York: Guilford Press.

Clark, L. A., Linde, J. A., & Simms, L. J. (2003). *Schedule for Nonadaptive and Adaptive Personality—Youth version (SNAP-Y)*. Unpublished manuscript, University of Iowa, Iowa City.

Cloninger, C. R. (2005). Genetics. In J. M. Oldham, A. E. Skodol, & D. S. Bender (Eds.), *The American Psychiatric Publishing textbook of personality disorders* (pp. 143–154). Washington, DC: American Psychiatric Publishing.

Cohen, P. (1996). Childhood risks for young adult symptoms of personality disorder: Method and substance. *Multivariate Behavioral Research, 31*, 121–148.

Cohen, P., & Crawford, T. (2005). Developmental issues. In J. M. Oldham, A. E. Skodol, & D. S. Bender (Eds.), *The American Psychiatric Publishing textbook of personality disorders* (pp. 171–185). Washington, DC: American Psychiatric Publishing.

Cohen, P., Crawford, T. N., Johnson, J. G., & Kasen, S. (2005). The children in the community study of developmental course of personality disorder. *Journal of Personality Disorders, 19*, 466–486.

Coolidge, F. L. (1998). *Coolidge Personality and Neuro-psychological Inventory for Children manual: CPNI*. Colorado Springs, CO: Author.

Coolidge, F. L., Thede, L. L., & Jang, K. L. (2001). Heritability of personality disorders in childhood: A preliminary investigation. *Journal of Personality Disorders, 15*, 33–40.

Coolidge, F. L., Thede, L. L., Stewart, S. E., & Segal, D. L. (2002). The Coolidge Personality and Neuropsychological Inventory for Children (CPNI): Preliminary psychometric characteristics. *Behavior Modification, 26*, 550–566.

Costa, P. T., Jr., & McCrae, R. R. (1992). *Revised NEO Personality Inventory (NEO-PI-R) and NEO Five-Factor Inventory (NEO-FFI) professional manual*. Odessa, FL: Psychological Assessment Resources.

Costa, P. T., Jr., McCrae, R. R., & Martin, T. A. (in press). Incipient adult personality: The NEO-PI-3 in middle school-aged children. *British Journal of Developmental Psychology*.

Costa, P. T., Jr., & Widiger, T. A. (2002). *Personality disorders and the five-factor model of personality* (2nd ed.). Washington, DC: American Psychological Association.

Crick, N. R., Murray-Close, D., & Woods, K. (2005). Borderline personality features in childhood: A short-term longitudinal study. *Development and Psychopathology, 17*, 1051–1070.

Crits-Christoph, P., & Barber, J. P. (2004). Empirical research on the treatment of personality disorders. In J. J. Magnavita (Ed.), *Handbook of personality disorders: Theory and practice* (pp. 513–527). New York: Wiley.

Daley, S. E., Hammen, C., Burge, D., Davila, J., Paley, B., Lindberg, N., et al. (1999). Depression and Axis II symptomatology in an adolescent community sample: Concurrent and longitudinal associations. *Journal of Personality Disorders, 13*, 47–59.

De Clercq, B., & De Fruyt, F. (2003). Personality disorder symptoms in adolescence: A five-factor model perspective. *Journal of Personality Disorders, 17*, 269–292.

De Clercq, B., De Fruyt, F., & Van Leeuwen, K. (2004). A "Little Five" lexically based perspective on personality disorder symptoms in adolescence. *Journal of Personality Disorders, 18*, 479–499.

De Clercq, B., De Fruyt, F., Van Leeuwen, K., & Mervielde, I. (2006). The structure of maladaptive personality traits in childhood: A step toward an integrative developmental perspective for DSM-V. *Journal of Abnormal Psychology, 115*, 639–657.

De Fruyt, F., De Clercq, B. J., van de Wiele, L., & Van Heeringen, K. (2006). The validity of Cloninger's psychobiological model versus the five-factor model to predict DSM-IV personality disorders in a heterogeneous psychiatric sample: Domain facet and residualized facet descriptions. *Journal of Personality, 74*, 479–510.

Dolan-Sewell, R. T., Krueger, R. F., & Shea, M. T. (2001). Co-occurrence with syndrome disorders. In W. J. Livesley (Ed.), *Handbook of personality disor-*

ders: Theory, research, and treatment (pp. 84–104). New York: Guilford Press.

Duckworth, A. L., Steen, T. A., & Seligman, M. E. P. (2005). Positive psychology in clinical practice. *Annual Review of Clinical Psychology, 1,* 629–651.

Emde, R. N., & Hewitt, J. K. (2001). *Infancy to early childhood: Genetic and environmental influences on developmental change.* New York: Oxford University Press.

First, M. B., & Gibbon, M. (2004). The Structured Clinical Interview for DSM-IV Axis I Disorders (SCID-I) and the Structured Clinical Interview for DSM-IV Axis II disorders (SCID-II). In M. J. Hilsenroth & D. L. Segal (Eds.), *Comprehensive handbook of psychological assessment: Vol. 2. Personality assessment* (pp. 134–143). New York: Wiley.

First, M., Spitzer, R. L., Williams, J. B. W., & Gibbon, M. (1997). *Structured Clinical Interview for DSM-IV Axis II Personality Disorders (SCID-II) user's guide and interview.* Washington, DC: American Psychiatric Press.

Fonagy, P., Roth, A., & Higgitt, A. (2005). Psychodynamic psychotherapies: Evidence-based practice and clinical wisdom. *Bulletin of the Menninger Clinic, 69,* 1–58.

Forth, A. E., Hart, S. D., & Hare, R. D. (1990). Assessment of psychopathy in male young offenders. *Psychological Assessment, 2,* 342–344.

Forth, A. E., Kosson, D. S., & Hare, R. D. (2003). *The Psychopathy Checklist: Youth Version.* Toronto: Multi-Health Systems.

Freeman, A., & Rigby, A. (2003). Personality disorders among children and adolescents: Is it an unlikely diagnosis? In M. A. Reinecke, F. M. Dattilio, & A. Freeman (Eds.), *Cognitive therapy with children and adolescents: A casebook for clinical practice* (2nd ed., pp. 434–464). New York: Guilford Press.

Frick, P. H., & Hare, R. D. (2001). *The Antisocial Process Screening Device (ASPD).* Toronto: Multi-Health Systems.

Giesen-Bloo, van Dyck, R., Spinhoven, P., van Tilburg, W., Dirksen, C., van Asselt, T., et al. (2006). Outpatient psychotherapy for borderline personality disorder. *Archives of General Psychiatry, 63,* 649–658.

Greenman, D. A., Gunderson, J. G., Cane, M., & Saltzman, P. R. (1986). An examination of the borderline diagnosis in children. *American Journal of Psychiatry, 143,* 998–1003.

Grilo, C. M., & McGlashan, T. H. (2005). Course and outcome of personality disorders. In J. M. Oldham, A. E. Skodol, & D. S. Bender (Eds.), *The American Psychiatric Publishing textbook of personality disorders* (pp. 103–115). Washington, DC: American Psychiatric Publishing.

Gude, T., Moum, T., Kaldestad, E., & Friis, S. (2000). Inventory of Interpersonal Problems: A three-dimensional balanced and scalable 48-item version. *Journal of Personality Assessment, 74,* 296–310.

Guilé, J., Sayegh, L., Bergeron, L., Fortier, H., Goldberg, D., & Gunderson, J. (2004). Initial reliability of the Diagnostic Interview for Narcissism Adapted for Preadolescents: Parent version (P-DIN). *Canadian Child and Adolescent Psychiatry Review, 13,* 74–80.

Gunderson, J. G., Kolb, J. E., & Austin, V. (1981). The Diagnostic Interview for Borderline Patients. *American Journal of Psychiatry, 138,* 896–903.

Gunderson, J. G., Ronningstam, E., & Bodkin, A. (1990). The Diagnostic Interview for Narcissistic Patients. *Archives of General Psychiatry, 47,* 676–680.

Guzder, J., Paris, J., Zelkowitz, P., & Feldman, R. (1999). Psychological risk factors for borderline pathology in school-age children. *Journal of the American Academy of Child and Adolescent Psychiatry, 38,* 206–212.

Hare, R. D. (1991). *The Hare Psychopathy Checklist—Revised.* Toronto: Multi-Health Systems.

Hare, R. D. (2003). *The Hare Psychopathy Checklist—Revised, second edition.* Toronto: Multi-Health Systems.

Hayes, S. C., Follette, V. M., & Linehan, M. M. (2004). *Mindfulness and acceptance: Expanding the cognitive-behavioral tradition.* New York: Guilford Press.

Henggeler, S. W., Schoenwald, S. K., Borduin, C. M., Rowland, M. D., & Cunningham, P. B. (1998). *Multisystemic treatment of antisocial behavior in children and adolescents.* New York: Guilford Press.

Hilsenroth, M. J., Handler, L., & Blais, M. A. (1996). Assessment of narcissistic personality disorder: A multi-method review. *Clinical Psychology Review, 16,* 655–683.

Hodges, K. (2004). The Child and Adolescent Functional Assessment Scale (CAFAS). In M. E. Maruish (Ed.), *The use of psychological testing for treatment planning and outcomes assessment: Vol. 2. Instruments for children and adolescents* (3rd ed., pp. 405–441). Mahwah, NJ: Erlbaum.

Hyler, S. E. (1994). *Personality Disorder Questionnaire IV (PDQ-IV).* New York: New York State Psychiatric Institute.

John, O. P., & Srivastava, S. (1999). The Big Five trait taxonomy: History, measurement, and theoretical perspectives. In L. A. Pervin & O. P. John (Eds.), *Handbook of personality: Theory and research* (2nd ed., pp. 102–138). New York: Guilford Press.

Johnson, J. G., Bromley, E., Bornstein, R. F., & Sneed, J. R. (2006). Adolescent personality disorders. In D. A. Wolfe & E. J. Mash (Eds.), *Behavioral and emotional disorders in children and adolescents: Nature, assessment, and treatment* (pp. 463–484). New York: Guilford Press.

Johnson, J. G., Bromley, E., & McGeoch, P. G. (2005). Role of childhood experiences in the development of maladaptive and adaptive personality traits. In J. M. Oldham, A. E. Skodol, & D. S. Bender (Eds.), *The American Psychiatric Publishing textbook of personality disorders* (pp. 209–221). Washington, DC: American Psychiatric Publishing.

Johnson, J. G., Cohen, P., Chen, H., Kasen, S., & Brook, J. S. (2006). Parenting behaviors associated with risk for offspring personality disorder during adulthood. *Archives of General Psychiatry, 63,* 579–587.

Johnson, J. G., Cohen, P., Kasen, S., Skodol, A. E., Hamagami, F., & Brook, J. S. (2000). Age-related change in personality disorder trait levels between early adolescence and adulthood: A community-based longitudinal investigation. *Acta Psychiatrica Scandinavica, 102,* 265–275.

Johnson, J. G., Cohen, P., Skodol, A. E., Oldham, J. M., Kasen, S., & Brook, J. S. (1999). Personality disorders in adolescence and risk of major mental disorders and suicidality during adulthood. *Archives of General Psychiatry, 56,* 805–811.

Johnson, J. G., Cohen, P., Smailes, E., Kasen, S., Oldham, J. M., & Skodol, A. E. (2000). Adolescent personality disorders associated with violence and criminal behavior during adolescence and early adulthood. *American Journal of Psychiatry, 157,* 1406–1412.

Johnson, J. G., First, M. B., Cohen, P., Skodol, A. E., Kasen, S., & Brook, J. S. (2005). Adverse outcomes associated with personality disorder not otherwise specified in a community sample. *American Journal of Psychiatry, 162,* 1926–1932.

Kamphaus, R. W., & Frick, P. J. (1996). *Clinical assessment of child and adolescent personality and behavior.* Boston: Allyn & Bacon.

Katz, L. Y, Cox, B. J., Gunasekara, S., & Miller, A. L. (2004). Feasibility of dialectical behavior therapy for suicidal adolescent inpatients. *Journal of the American Academy of Child and Adolescent Psychiatry, 43,* 276–282.

Kaye, A. L., & Shea, T. M. (2000). Personality disorders, personality traits, and defense mechanisms. In A. J. Rush, H. A. Pincus, & M. B. First (Eds.), *Handbook of psychiatric measures* (pp. 713–749). Washington, DC: American Psychiatric Publishing.

Kazdin, A. E. (2005). Evidence-based assessment for children and adolescents: Issues in measurement development and clinical application. *Journal of Clinical Child and Adolescent Psychology, 34,* 548–558.

Kernberg, P. F., Hajal, F., & Normandin, L. (1998). Narcissistic personality disorder in adolescent inpatients: A retrospective record review study of descriptive characteristics. In E. F. Ronningstam (Ed.), *Disorders of narcissism: Diagnostic, clinical, and empirical implications* (pp. 437–456). Washington, DC: American Psychiatric Publishing.

Kernberg, P. F., Weiner, A. S., & Bardenstein, K. K. (2000). *Personality disorders in children and adolescents.* New York: Basic Books.

Klein, D. N. (2003). Patients' versus informants' reports of personality disorders in predicting 7½-year outcome in outpatients with depressive disorders. *Psychological Assessment, 15,* 216–222.

Klonsky, E. D., Oltmanns, T. F., & Turkheimer, E. (2002). Informant-reports of personality disorder: Relation to self-reports and future research directions. *Clinical Psychology: Science and Practice, 9,* 300–311.

Kotler, J. S., & McMahon, R. J. (2005). Child psychopathy: Theories, measurement, and relations with the development and persistence of conduct problems. *Clinical Child and Family Psychology Review, 8,* 291–325.

Kramer, T. L., & Robbins, J. M. (2004). The Adolescent Treatment Outcomes Module (ATOM). In M. E. Maruish (Ed.), *The use of psychological testing for treatment planning and outcomes assessment: Vol. 2. Instruments for children and adolescents* (3rd ed., pp. 355–370). Mahwah, NJ: Erlbaum.

Krueger, R. F., Watson, D., & Barlow, D. H. (2005). Introduction to the special section: Toward a dimensionally based taxonomy of psychopathology. *Journal of Abnormal Psychology, 114,* 491–493.

Landgraf, J. M. (2004). The Child Health Questionnaire (CHQ) and psychological assessments: A brief update. In M. E. Maruish (Ed.), *The use of psychological testing for treatment planning and outcomes assessment: Vol. 2. Instruments for children and adolescents* (3rd ed., pp. 443–460). Mahwah, NJ: Erlbaum.

Lavan, H., & Johnson, J. G. (2002). The association between Axis I and II psychiatric symptoms and high-risk sexual behavior during adolescence. *Journal of Personality Disorders, 16,* 73–94.

Leichsenring, F. (1999). Development and first results of the Borderline Personality Inventory: A self-report instrument for assessing borderline personality organization. *Journal of Personality Assessment, 73,* 45–63.

Leichsenring, R., & Leibling, E. (2003). The effectiveness of psychodynamic therapy and cognitive-behavioral therapy in the treatment of personality disorders: A meta-analysis. *American Journal of Psychiatry, 160,* 1223–1232.

Levy, K. N., Becker, D. F., Grilo, C. M., Mattanah, J. J. F., Garnet, K. E., Quinlan, D. M., et al. (1999). Concurrent and predictive validity of the personality disorder diagnosis in adolescent patients. *American Journal of Psychiatry, 156,* 1522–1528.

Lewinsohn, P. M., Rohde, P., Seeley, J. R., & Klein, D. N. (1997). Axis II psychopathology as a function of Axis I disorders in childhood and adolescence. *Journal of the American Academy of Child and Adolescent Psychiatry, 36,* 1752–1759.

Linde, J. A. (2002). Validation of the Schedule for Nonadaptive and Adaptive Personality—Youth Version (SNAP-Y): Self and parent ratings of adolescent personality (Doctoral dissertation, University of Iowa, Iowa City). *Dissertation Abstracts International, 62,* AAI3034123.

Linehan, M. M. (1993a). *Cognitive-behavioral treatment of borderline personality disorder.* New York: Guilford Press.

Linehan, M. M. (1993b). *Skills training manual for treating borderline personality disorder.* New York: Guilford Press.

Linehan, M. M., Comtois, K. A., Murray, A. M., Brown, M. Z., Gallop, R. J., Heard, H. L., et al.

(2006). Two-year randomized controlled trial and follow-up of dialectical behavior therapy vs. therapy by experts for suicidal behaviors and borderline personality disorder. *Archives of General Psychiatry, 63,* 757–766.

Livesley, W. J. (2005). Behavioral and molecular genetic contributions to a dimensional classification of personality disorder. *Journal of Personality Disorders, 19,* 131–155.

Livesley, W. J., & Jackson, D. (in press). *Manual for the Dimensional Assessment of Personality Pathology—Basic Questionnaire.* London, Ontario: Research Psychologists Press.

Loranger, A. W. (1995). *International Personality Disorder Examination Manual: ICD-10 Module.* Geneva, Switzerland: World Health Organization.

Loranger, A. W. (1999). *International Personality Disorder Examination Manual: DSM-IV module.* Washington, DC: American Psychiatric Publishing.

Loranger, A. W., Susman, V. L., Oldham, J. M., & Russakoff, M. (1998). *The Personality Disorder Examination (PDE) manual.* Yonkers, NY: DV Communications.

Ludolph, P. S., Westen, D., Misle, B., & Jackson, A. (1990). The borderline diagnosis in adolescents: Symptoms and developmental history. *American Journal of Psychiatry, 147,* 470–476.

Lynam, D. R. (1997). Pursuing the psychopath: Capturing the fledgling psychopath in a nomological net. *Journal of Abnormal Psychology, 106,* 425–438.

Lynam, D. R., Caspi, A., Moffitt, T. E., Raine, A., Loeber, R., & Stouthamer-Loeber, M. (2005). Adolescent psychopathy and the Big Five: Results from two samples. *Journal of Abnormal Child Psychology, 33,* 431–443.

Lynam, D. R., & Gudonis, L. (2005). The development of psychopathy. *Annual Review of Clinical Psychology, 1,* 381–407.

Lynam, D. R., & Widiger, T. A. (2001). Using the five-factor model to represent the DSM-IV personality disorders: An expert consensus approach. *Journal of Abnormal Psychology, 110,* 401–412.

Markon, K. E., Krueger, R. F., & Watson, D. (2005). Delineating the structure of normal and abnormal personality: An integrative hierarchical approach. *Journal of Personality and Social Psychology, 88,* 139–157.

Mash, E. J., & Hunsley, J. (2005). Evidence-based assessment of child and adolescent disorders: Issues and challenges. *Journal of Clinical Child and Adolescent Psychology, 34,* 362–379.

Mattia, J. I., & Zimmerman, M. (2001). Epidemiology. In W. J. Livesley (Ed.), *Handbook of personality disorders: Theory, research, and treatment* (pp. 107–123). New York: Guilford Press.

McCann, J. T. (1999). *Assessing adolescents with the MACI: Using the Millon Adolescent Clinical Inventory.* New York: Wiley.

McClellan, J. M., & Hamilton, J. D. (2006). An evidence-based approach to an adolescent with emotional and behavioral dysregulation. *Journal of the American Academy of Child and Adolescent Psychiatry, 45,* 489–493.

McCrae, R. R., Costa, P. T. J., & Martin, T. A. (2005). The NEO-PI-3: A more readable revised NEO Personality Inventory. *Journal of Personality Assessment, 84,* 261–270.

McCrae, R. R., Martin, T. A., & Costa, P. T. J. (2005). Age trends and age norms for the NEO Personality Inventory–3 in adolescents and adults. *Assessment, 12,* 363–373.

McDermut, W., & Zimmerman, M. (2005). Assessment instruments and standardized evaluation. In J. M. Oldham, A. E. Skodol, & D. S. Bender (Eds.), *The American Psychiatric Publishing textbook of personality disorders* (pp. 89–101). Washington, DC: American Psychiatric Publishing.

McGlashan, T. H., Grilo, C. M., Sanislow, C. A., Ralevski, E., Morey, L. C., Gunderson, J. G., et al. (2005). Two-year prevalence and stability of individual DSM-IV criteria for schizotypal, borderline, avoidant, and obsessive–compulsive personality disorders: Toward a hybrid model of Axis II disorders. *American Journal of Psychiatry, 162,* 883–889.

McNulty, J. L., Harkness, A. R., Ben-Porath, Y. S., & Williams, C. L. (1997). Assessing the Personality Psychopathology Five (PSY-5) in adolescents: New MMPI-A scales. *Psychological Assessment, 9,* 250–259.

Meagher, S. E., Grossman, S. D., & Millon, T. (2004). Studying outcomes in adolescents: The Millon Adolescent Clinical Inventory (MACI) and Millon Adolescent Personality Inventory (MAPI). In M. E. Maruish (Ed.), *The use of psychological testing for treatment planning and outcomes assessment: Vol. 2. Instruments for children and adolescents* (3rd ed., pp. 123–140). Mahwah, NJ: Erlbaum.

Melley, A. H., Oltmanns, T. F., & Turkheimer, E. (2002). The Schedule for Nonadaptive and Adaptive Personality (SNAP): Temporal stability and predictive validity of the diagnostic scales. *Assessment, 9,* 181–187.

Mervielde, I., De Clercq, B., De Fruyt, F., & van Leeuwen, K. (2005). Temperament, personality, and developmental psychopathology as childhood antecedents of personality disorders. *Journal of Personality Disorders, 19,* 171–201.

Miller, A. L., Rathus, J. H., & Linehan, M. M. (2006). *Dialectical behavior therapy with suicidal adolescents.* New York: Guilford Press.

Miller, J. D., Bagby, R. M., Pilkonis, P. A., Reynolds, S. K., & Lynam, D. R. (2005). A simplified technique for scoring DSM-IV personality disorders with the five-factor model. *Assessment, 12,* 404–415.

Miller, J. D., Pilkonis, P. A., & Morse, J. Q. (2004). Five-factor model prototypes for personality disorders: The utility of self-reports and observer ratings. *Assessment, 11,* 127–138.

Miller, J. D., Reynolds, S. K., & Pilkonis, P. A. (2004). The validity of the Five-Factor Model prototypes for personality disorders in two clinical samples. *Psychological Assessment*, 16, 310–322.

Millon, T., & Davis, R. O. (1996). *Disorders of personality: DSM-IV and beyond* (2nd ed.). New York: Wiley.

Millon, T., Millon, C., Davis, R., & Grossman, S. (1994). *The Millon Adolescent Clinical Inventory (MACI)*. Minneapolis, MN: National Computer Systems.

Mittal, V. A., Tessner, K. D., McMillan, A. L., Delawalla, Z., Trotman, H. D., & Walker, E. F. (2006). Gesture behavior in unmedicated schizotypal adolescents. *Journal of Abnormal Psychology, 115*, 351–358.

Moffitt, T. E., Caspi, A., Rutter, M., & Silva, P. A. (2001). *Sex differences in antisocial behaviour: Conduct disorder, delinquency, and violence in the Dunedin Longitudinal Study*. New York: Cambridge University Press.

Morey, L. (1991). *Personality Assessment Inventory*. Odessa, FL: Psychological Assessment Resources.

Morey, L. C., Alexander, G. M., & Boggs, C. (2005). Gender. In J. M. Oldham, A. E. Skodol, & D. S. Bender (Eds.), *The American Psychiatric Publishing textbook of personality disorders* (pp. 541–559). Washington, DC: American Psychiatric Publishing.

Morey, L. C., Warner, M. B., Shea, M. T., Gunderson, J. G., Sanislow, C. A., Grilo, C., et al. (2003). The representation of four personality disorders by the Schedule for Nonadaptive and Adaptive Personality dimensional model of personality. *Psychological Assessment, 15*, 326–332.

Neumann, C. S., & Walker, E. F. (2003). Neuromotor functioning in adolescents with schizotypal personality disorder: Associations with symptoms and neurocognition. *Schizophrenia Bulletin, 29*, 285–298.

Nigg, J. T., Silk, K. R., Stavro, G., & Miller, T. (2005). Disinhibition and borderline personality disorder. *Development and Psychopathology, 17*, 1129–1149.

Oldham, J. M., & Skodol, A. E. (2000). Charting the future of Axis II. *Journal of Personality Disorders, 14*, 17–29.

Paris, J. (2003). *Personality disorders over time: Precursors, course, and outcome*. Washington, DC: American Psychiatric Publishing.

Paris, J. (2005a). A current integrative perspective on personality disorders. In J. M. Oldham, A. E. Skodol, & D. S. Bender (Eds.), *The American Psychiatric Publishing textbook of personality disorders* (pp. 119–128). Washington, DC: American Psychiatric Publishing.

Paris, J. (2005b). The development of impulsivity and suicidality in borderline personality disorder. *Development and Psychopathology, 17*, 1091–1104.

Perry, J. C., Banon, E., & Ianni, F. (1999). Effectiveness of psychotherapy for personality disorders. *American Journal of Psychiatry, 156*, 1312–1321.

Pfohl, B., Blum, N., & Zimmerman, M. (1997). *The Structured Interview for DSM-IV Personality: SIDP-IV*. Washington, DC: American Psychiatric Publishing.

Piedmont, R. L., Sherman, M. F., Sherman, N. C., & Williams, J. E. G. (2003). A first look at the Structured Clinical Interview for DSM-IV Personality Disorders Screening Questionnaire: More than just a screener? *Measurement and Evaluation in Counseling and Development, 36*, 150–160.

Pilkonis, P. A., Kim, Y., Proietti, J. M., & Barkham, M. (1996). Scales for personality disorders developed from the Inventory of Interpersonal Problems. *Journal of Personality Disorders, 10*, 355–369.

Pinto, A., Grapentine, W. L., Francis, G., & Picariello, C. M. (1996). Borderline personality disorder in adolescents: Affective and cognitive features. *Journal of the American Academy of Child and Adolescent Psychiatry, 35*, 1338–1343.

Raskin, R., & Terry, H. (1988). A principal-components analysis of the Narcissistic Personality Inventory and further evidence of its construct validity. *Journal of Personality and Social Psychology, 54*, 890–902.

Rathus, J. H., & Miller, A. L. (2002). Dialectical behavior therapy adapted for suicidal adolescents. *Suicide and Life-Threatening Behavior, 32*, 146–157.

Ready, R. E., Watson, D., & Clark, L. A. (2002). Psychiatric patient- and informant-reported personality: Predicting concurrent and future behavior. *Assessment, 9*, 361–372.

Reynolds, W. M. (1998). *Adolescent Psychopathology Scale* (APS). Odessa, FL: Psychological Assessment Resources.

Roberts, B. W., & DelVecchio, W. F. (2000). The rank-order consistency of personality traits from childhood to old age: A quantitative review of longitudinal studies. *Psychological Bulletin, 126*, 3–25.

Roberts, B. W., Walton, K. E., & Viechtbauer, W. (2006). Patterns of mean-level change in personality traits across the life course: A meta-analysis of longitudinal studies. *Psychological Bulletin, 132*, 1–25.

Rogers, R. (2001). *Handbook of diagnostic and structured interviewing*. New York: Guilford Press.

Rogers, R. (2003). Standardizing DSM-IV diagnoses: The clinical applications of structured interviews. *Journal of Personality Assessment, 81*, 220–225.

Rothbart, M. K., & Bates, J. E. (2006). Temperament. In W. Damon & R. Lerner (Series Eds.) & N. Eisenberg (Vol. Ed.), *Handbook of child psychology: Vol. 3. Social, emotional, and personality development* (6th ed., pp. 99–166). New York: Wiley.

Rounsaville, B. J., Alarcón, R. D., Andrews, G., Jackson, J. S., Kendell, R. E., & Kendler, K. (2002). Basic nomenclature issues for DSM-V. In D. J. Kupfer, M. B. First, & D. A. Regier (Eds.), *A research agenda for DSM-V* (pp. 1–29). Washington, DC: American Psychiatric Publishing.

Ruscio, A. M., & Holohan, D. R. (2006). Applying empirically supported treatments to complex cases: Ethical, empirical, and practical considerations. *Clinical Psychology: Science and Practice, 13*, 146–162.

Salekin, R. T., & Frick, P. J. (2005). Psychopathy in children and adolescents: The need for a developmental perspective. *Journal of Abnormal Child Psychology,* 33, 403–409.

Schotte, C., K. W., & De Doncker, D. A. M. (1996). *ADP-IV Questionnaire: Manual and norms.* Antwerp, Belgium: University Hospital Antwerp.

Schotte, C. K. W., De Doncker, D. A. M., Dmitruk, D., Van Mulders, I., D'Haenen, H., & Cosyns, P. (2004). The ADP-IV Questionnaire: Differential validity and concordance with the semi-structured interview. *Journal of Personality Disorders,* 18, 405–419.

Shiner, R. L. (2005). A developmental perspective on personality disorders: Lessons from research on normal personality development in childhood and adolescence. *Journal of Personality Disorders,* 19, 202–210.

Shiner, R. L. (2006). Temperament and personality in childhood. In D. K. Mroczek & T. D. Little (Eds.), *Handbook of personality development* (pp. 213–230). Mahwah, NJ: Erlbaum.

Shiner, R. L., & Caspi, A. (2003). Personality differences in childhood and adolescence: Measurement, development, and consequences. *Journal of Child Psychology and Psychiatry and Allied Disciplines,* 44, 2–32.

Singer, J. A. (2005). *Personality and psychotherapy: Treating the whole person.* New York: Guilford Press.

Skodol, A. E. (2005). Manifestations, clinical diagnosis, and comorbidity. In J. M. Oldham, A. E. Skodol, & D. S. Bender (Eds.), *The American Psychiatric Publishing textbook of personality disorders* (pp. 57–87). Washington, DC: American Psychiatric Publishing.

Skodol, A. E., Gunderson, J. G., Shea, M. T., McGlashan, T. H., Morey, L. C., Sanislow, C. A., et al. (2005). The Collaborative Longitudinal Personality Disorders Study (CLPS): Overview and implications. *Journal of Personality Disorders,* 19, 487–504.

Skodol, A. E., Oldham, J. M., Bender, D. S., Dyck, I. R., Stout, R. L., Morey, L. C., et al. (2005). Dimensional representations of DSM-IV personality disorders: Relationships to functional impairment. *American Journal of Psychiatry,* 162, 1919–1925.

Svartberg, M., Stiles, T. C., & Seltzer, M. H. (2004). Randomized, controlled trial of the effectiveness of short-term dynamic psychotherapy and cognitive therapy for cluster C personality disorders. *American Journal of Psychiatry,* 161, 810–817.

Torgersen, S. (2005). Epidemiology. In J. M. Oldham, A. E. Skodol, & D. S. Bender (Eds.), *The American Psychiatric Publishing textbook of personality disorders* (pp. 129–141). Washington, DC: American Psychiatric Publishing.

Trull, T. J., & Durrett, C. A. (2005). Categorical and dimensional models of personality disorder. *Annual Review of Clinical Psychology,* 1, 355–380.

Trull, T. J., & Widiger, T. A. (1997). *Structured Interview for the Five-Factor Model of Personality (SIFFM): Professional manual.* Odessa, FL: Psychological Assessment Resources.

Vaughn, M. G., & Howard, M. O. (2005). Self-report measures of juvenile psychopathic personality traits: A comparative review. *Journal of Emotional and Behavioral Disorders,* 13, 152–162.

Verheul, R., & Widiger, T. A. (2004). A meta-analysis of the prevalence and usage of the personality disorder not otherwise specified (PD-NOS) diagnosis. *Journal of Personality Disorders,* 18, 309–319.

Vinnars, B., Barber, J. P., Noren, K., Gallop, R., & Weinryb, R. M. (2005). Manualized supportive–expressive psychotherapy versus nonmanualized community-delivered psychodynamic therapy for patients with personality disorders: Bridging efficacy and effectiveness. *American Journal of Psychiatry,* 162, 1933–1940.

Vito, E. D., Ladame, F., & Orlandini, A. (1999). Adolescence and personality disorders: Current perspectives on a controversial problem. In J. Derksen, C. Maffei, & H. Groen (Eds.), *Treatment of personality disorders* (pp. 77–95). Boston: Kluwer Academic.

Wachtel, P. L. (1994). Cyclical processes in personality and psychopathology. *Journal of Abnormal Psychology,* 103, 51–66.

Westen, D. (1997). Divergences between clinical and research methods for assessing personality disorders: Implications for research and the evolution of Axis II. *American Journal of Psychiatry,* 154, 895–903.

Westen, D. (2004). *Clinical Diagnostic Interview.* Unpublished manual, Emory University, Atlanta, GA. Available online at *www.psychsystems.net/lab*

Westen, D., & Bradley, R. (2005). Empirically supported complexity: Rethinking evidence-based practice in psychotherapy. *Current Directions in Psychological Science,* 14, 266–271.

Westen, D., & Chang, C. (2000). Personality pathology in adolescence: A review. In A. H. Esman, L. T. Flaherty, & H. A. Horowitz (Eds.), *Adolescent psychiatry: Developmental and clinical studies* (Vol. 25, pp. 61–100). Mahwah, NJ: Analytic Press.

Westen, D., Dutra, L., & Shedler, J. (2005). Assessing adolescent personality pathology. *British Journal of Psychiatry,* 186, 227–238.

Westen, D., & Shedler, J. (1999). Revising and assessing Axis II: Part I. Developing a clinically and empirically valid assessment method. *American Journal of Psychiatry,* 156, 258–272.

Westen, D., Shedler, J., Durrett, C., Glass, S., & Martens, A. (2003). Personality diagnoses in adolescence: DSM-IV Axis II diagnoses and an empirically derived alternative. *American Journal of Psychiatry,* 160, 952–966.

Widiger, T. A. (1999). Millon's dimensional polarities. *Journal of Personality Assessment,* 72, 365–389.

Widiger, T. A. (2002). Personality disorders. In M. M. Antony & D. H. Barlow (Eds.), *Handbook of assessment and treatment planning for psychological disorders* (pp. 453–480). New York: Guilford Press.

Widiger, T. A., & Coker, L. A. (2002). Assessing personality disorders. In J. N. Butcher (Ed.), *Clinical personality assessment: Practical approaches* (2nd ed., pp. 407–434). New York: Oxford University Press.

Widiger, T. A., Costa, P. T., & Samuel, D. B. (2006). Assessment of maladaptive personality traits. In S. Strack (Ed.), *Differentiating normal and abnormal personality* (2nd ed., pp. 311–335). New York: Springer.

Widiger, T. A., Mangine, S., Corbitt, E. M., Ellis, C. G., & Thomas, G. V. (1995). *Personality Disorder Interview—IV: A semistructured interview for the assessment of personality disorders.* Odessa, FL: Psychological Assessment Resources.

Widiger, T. A., & Mullins-Sweatt, S. N. (2005). Categorical and dimensional models of personality disorders. In J. M. Oldham, A. E. Skodol, & D. S. Bender (Eds.), *The American Psychiatric Publishing textbook of personality disorders* (pp. 35–53). Washington, DC: American Psychiatric Publishing.

Widiger, T. A., & Samuel, D. B. (2005). Evidence-based assessment of personality disorders. *Psychological Assessment, 17,* 278–287.

Widiger, T. A., & Simonsen, E. (2005). Alternative dimensional models of personality disorder: Finding a common ground. *Journal of Personality Disorders, 19,* 110–130.

Wiggins, J. S., & Trobst, K. K. (1999). The fields of interpersonal behavior. In L. A. Pervin & O. P. John (Eds.), *Handbook of personality: Theory and research* (2nd ed., pp. 653–670). New York: Guilford Press.

Zanarini, M. C., Frankenburg, F. R., Hennen, J., Reich, B., & Silk, K. R. (2005). The McLean Study of Adult Development (MSAD): Overview and implications of the first six years of prospective follow-up. *Journal of Personality Disorders, 19,* 505–523.

Zanarini, M. C., Frankenburg, F. R., Ridolfi, M. E., Jager-Hyman, S., Hennen, J., & Gunderson, J. G. (2006). Reported childhood onset of self-mutilation among borderline patients. *Journal of Personality Disorders, 20,* 9–15.

Zanarini, M. C., Frankenburg, F. R., Sickel, A. E., & Yong, L. (1996). *Diagnostic Interview for DSM-IV Personality Disorders.* Cambridge, MA: Laboratory for the Study of Adult Development, McLean Hospital, and the Department of Psychiatry, Harvard University.

Zanarini, M. C., Gunderson, J. G., Frankenburg, F. R., & Chauncey, D. L. (1989). The Revised Diagnostic Interview for Borderlines: Discriminating BPD from other Axis II disorders. *Journal of Personality Disorders, 3,* 10–18.

Zanarini, M. C., Skodol, A. E., Bender, D., Dolan, R., Sanislow, C., Schaefer, E., et al. (2000). The Collaborative Longitudinal Personality Disorders Study: Reliability of Axis I and II diagnoses. *Journal of Personality Disorders, 14,* 291–299.

Zimmerman, M. (1994). Diagnosing personality disorders: A review of issues and research models. *Archives of General Psychiatry, 51,* 225–245.

Author Index

817

Subject Index

Page numbers followed by *f* indicate figure, *t* indicate table